Nursing the Critically Ill Adult

Fourth Edition

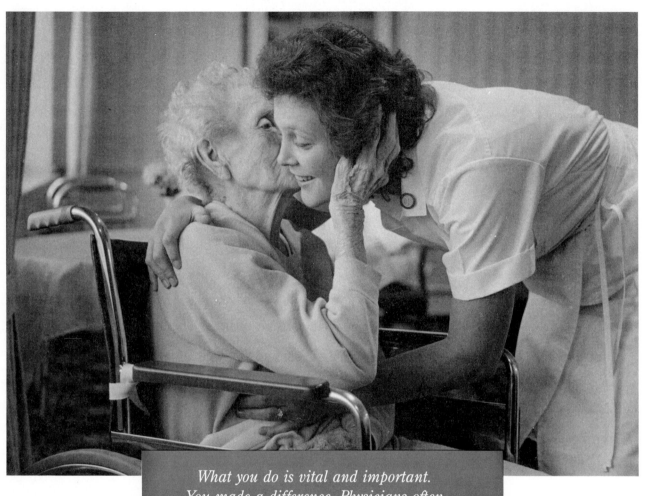

What you do is vital and important.
You made a difference. Physicians often
get all the credit. But the patients know
who performs the miracles. Some
remember the brilliance of the surgeon.
But most of us remember the nurse.

Gerard F. Humphreys

Nursing the Critically Ill Adult

Fourth Edition

Nancy Meyer Holloway, RN, MSN

Critical Care Nursing Educational Consultant
Nancy Holloway & Associates
Orinda, California

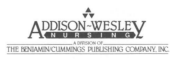

ADDISON-WESLEY
NURSING
A DIVISION OF
THE BENJAMIN/CUMMINGS PUBLISHING COMPANY, INC.

Redwood City, California   Menlo Park, California
Reading, Massachusetts   New York   Don Mills, Ontario
Workingham, U.K.   Amsterdam   Bonn   Sydney   Tokyo   Madrid   San Juan

Sponsoring Editor: Mark McCormick
Production Editors: Gail Carrigan, Cathy Lewis
Art Supervisor: Kay Brown
Text Designer: Rob Hugel
Cover Designer: Yvo Riezebos
Editorial Assistant: Bob Bledsoe
Copyeditor: Tärna Rosendahl
Compositor: Graphic World, Inc.

Care has been taken to confirm the accuracy of information presented in this book. The author, editors, and publisher, however,
cannot accept any responsibility for errors or omissions or for consequences from application of the information in this book and
make no warranty, express or implied, with respect to its contents.

The authors and publisher have exerted every effort to ensure that
drug selections and dosages set forth in this text are in accord with
current recommendations and practice at the time of publication.
However, in view of ongoing research, changes in government regulations, and the constant flow of information relating to drug therapy and drug reactions, the reader is urged to check the package
inserts of all drugs for any change in indications of dosage and for
added warnings and precautions. This is particularly important
when the recommended agent is a new and/or infrequently employed drug. Mention of a particular generic or brand name drug is
not an endorsement, nor an implication that it is preferable to other
named or unnamed agents.

Library of Congress Cataloging-in-Publication Data
Nursing the critically ill adult / [edited by] Nancy Meyer
Holloway.—
    4th ed.
        p.   cm.
    Includes bibliographical references and index.
    ISBN 0-8053-2544-1
    1. Intensive care nursing.   I. Holloway, Nancy Meyer,
    1947-   .
    [DNLM: 1. Critical Care—nurses'
    instruction.   2. Intensive Care
Units—nurses' instruction.   3. Nursing
Assessment.   4. Nursing
Process.   WY 154 N9745]
RT120.I5H64   1993
610.73'61—dc20
DNLM/DLC
for Library of Congress   92-49611
                                            CIP

1 2 3 4 5 6 7 8 9 10 -MU- 97 96 95 94 93

About the Cover
Addison-Wesley Nursing has presented quilts on the covers of our
clinical nursing books for a few years now. This particular quilt by
Sally A. Sellers of Vancouver, Washington, had a particular resonance for us when we found out that the artist was inspired to create the quilt in response to her daughter's illness, a neurological
condition. She writes, "I was struggling with unknowns, the opposite of control. In my quilts, I began playing with ambiguity, uncertain boundaries, and transition . . ." We hope the image inspires you,
as it did us, to consider the human element fundamental to all nursing science. *The Editors.*

Addison-Wesley Nursing
A Division of The Benjamin/Cummings Publishing Company, Inc.
390 Bridge Parkway, Redwood City, CA 94065

Brief Contents

Contents

Chapter 4: Neurologic Assessment   51

Chapter 5: Neurologic Disorders   89

Chapter 6: Neurologic Interventions   130

Chapter 21: Trauma   611

Appendix: Pharmacology   656

Index   682

Preface

This book is for you:

- The nursing student wanting a solid foundation on which to base your clinical experience
- The graduate nurse beginning your career in critical care
- The experienced critical-care nurse wanting to update and strengthen your knowledge base
- The critical-care educator wanting to convey both the science of critical-care nursing and the importance of clinical insight and caring

Clinical insight is that intuitive "knowing" or grasp of a situation that enables you to be intimately involved in a patient's care and yet "there" for the patient on an emotional level. It is an amalgam of perceptual awareness, practical knowledge, expertise, and clinical experience—and its foundation is caring.

But just how important is caring in the high-technology world of the critical-care unit? Given the day-to-day reality of a busy critical-care unit, can you translate caring into practice? And more importantly, does caring actually improve the quality of patient care?

This text is founded on three key beliefs: that clinical insight distinguishes the novice nurse from the expert clinician; that nursing diagnosis is central to the provision of professional nursing care; and that caring is the link between technology and humanism in the critical-care environment.

Continuing Features

The fourth edition continues the tradition of excellence established by earlier editions. This tradition includes the first edition, winner of an *American Journal of Nursing* Book of the Year award; the second edition, the first critical-care text to use nursing diagnosis as an organizing theme; and the third edition, the first critical-care text to illuminate critical-care nursing practice by including critical-care nurses' "clinical insights".

This book retains many popular features, including:

- Anatomy and physiology integrated into all the steps of the nursing process

The emphasis on nursing diagnosis, utilizing diagnoses approved by the North American Nursing Diagnosis Association (NANDA). The text is specially designed to help the reader develop confidence and competence in applying nursing diagnosis in day-to-day critical-care nursing practice. Easy-to-find screened boxes emphasize the most appropriate nursing diagnoses for each disorder discussed. The diagnoses also provide structure for the presentation of related nursing interventions.

An emphasis on practical applications of clinically relevant information

Specific outcome criteria for evaluating the effectiveness of nursing care

Critical-care pharmacology in an easy-to-use format that emphasizes anticipated effects and nursing responsibilities

New Features

Several distinguishing features characterize this new edition. They include:

Nursing Tips pragmatic pointers from expert nurses that convey practice wisdom, such as "red flags" that tell you a patient's in trouble or tricky steps in performing a procedure

Critical Care Gerontology boxes on special nursing concerns related to the elderly critical care patient

Advances in Critical Care Technology boxes on cutting-edge technological developments in critical care

Research Boxes that concisely report research studies on topics of importance to critical-care nurses, including their clinical application and critical thinking about their strengths and limitations

New content, including new chapters on: Caring: The Essence of Critical Care, which includes the spiritual dimension of critical care; Immunologic Disorders, including an extensive discussion of AIDS; Multisystem Disorders, including multiple organ systems failure (MOSF); carotid endarterectomy; pressure support ventilation; cardiomyopathy; aortic dissection; emergency sternotomy; ventricular assist devices; heart transplantation; renal transplantation; thyroid crisis; and other topics.

Expanded content exploring the intricacies of the intensive care unit: technological advances, nursing role changes, stress, ethical dilemmas, legal issues, and organ donation; critical care physiology; immunologic disorders; cerebral aneurysms; pacemakers; intra-aortic balloon pumping; hepatitis and pancreatitis; and critical care pharmacology.

Nursing Care Plans on ruptured cerebral aneurysm, adult respiratory distress syndrome (ARDS), congestive heart failure, acute myocardial infarction, percutaneous transluminal coronary angioplasty (PTCA), acute renal failure, diabetic ketoacidosis, and gastrointestinal bleeding.

Clinical Insights open each chapter. These are powerful first hand stories of nurses caring for patients and each other.

These insights, unique among critical-care texts, are paradigms that illuminate the day-to-day practice of critical-care nursing. (A paradigm case is a clinical experience that forever alters the nurse's way of perceiving and interpreting clinical situations.) Although the paradigms describe the utilization of a skill or care of a person with a disorder described in the chapter, they also are designed to be appreciated on their own. Taken together, the paradigms poignantly present the issues important to critical-care nurses and illuminate with crystalline clarity the individual acts of grace and mercy that form caring nursing practice in critical care.

The paradigms draw on the research of Benner, Diekelmann, Crabtree, Jorgenson, and Tanner.[1] In her groundbreaking work, Benner (1984) provided a description of expert nursing care within the context of everyday practice. Her journey of exploration, intended to uncover the knowledge embedded in clinical nursing practice, asked nurses to describe critical incidents, as well as typical and atypical days at work. Analysis of their responses revealed 31 expert compe-

[1]Benner, Patricia (1984): *From novice to expert: Excellence and power in clinical nursing practice.* Menlo Park: Addison-Wesley Publishing.

Benner, Patricia and Christine Tanner (1987): "Clinical judgment: how expert nurses use intuition." *Am J Nurs* 87:23–31.

Crabtree, Anne and Marcy Jorgenson (1986): "Exploring the practical knowledge in expert critical-care nursing practice." Unpublished master's thesis, University of Wisconsin, Madison.

Diekelmann, Nancy, Anne Crabtree and Marcy Jorgenson (1987): "Preserving personhood in the ICU—a Heideggerian hermeneutical analysis of the paradigm cases of expert critical-care nurses." Unpublished research manuscript, University of Wisconsin, Madison.

tencies derived from actual nursing practice. (Benner defines a competency as an "interpretively defined area of skilled performance identified and described by its intent, function, and meanings, as in a competency statement"). The competencies were grouped into 7 domains, defined as a "cluster of competencies that have similar intents, functions, and meanings". Benner emphasizes that these competencies and domains are not intended to be a complete description of nursing expertise. They can only be understood within the context of a situation; and that is why these insights are brought to you in the nurse's own words.

The Crabtree and Jorgenson study, a part of Diekelmann's research, extended Benner's work by focusing exclusively on critical-care nurses and asking them to compare their practice to Benner's competencies. Their research provided further insight into the values and behaviors of expert nurses. Benner and Tanner honed in on how expert nurses use intuition.

Each paradigm uncovered in these studies is an exemplar—an "example that conveys more than one intent, meaning function, or outcome and can easily be compared or translated to other clinical situations whose objective characteristics might be quite different" (Benner 1984). Together, they represent a wide variety of the 31 competencies, and a stimulus for thoughtful reflection on your own practice.

Overview

Chapter 1 introduces the concepts central to the book, particularly nursing diagnosis, the development of excellence in critical-care nursing, and the competencies of expert nurses. Chapter 2 highlights caring as the essence of critical care nursing. Chapter 3 discusses professional issues in critical care, such as ethical dilemmas and legal issues. Chapters 4–21 present clinical information, grouped into units that progress from patient assessment techniques through diagnostic techniques, clinical disorders, and related interventions. The appendix presents critical-care pharmacology you'll want to have at your fingertips.

Instructor's Guide

The instructor's guide for this text contains learning objectives, teaching strategies, sample questions, and transparency masters.

In conclusion Enjoy yourself, have fun with this book, and never forget that your human caring is the most valuable gift you have to offer the critically ill.

Acknowledgments

An author is only one member of the team necessary to publish a book. Although a book flows from the author's vision, it takes many talented, committed people to produce it. To each, I extend my gratitude and appreciation:

- The contributors (acknowledged by name on a separate page), who gave so generously of their expertise

- Contributors of clinical stories for the chapter on caring: Dawn Redlaczyk, RN, BSN, CCRN; Michael Adams, RN, BS, CCRN, CEN; Barry Tabel, RN, CEN; Debbie Harika, RN, BS, CEN; Robert Auen, RN, BS, CCRN; Nancy Bell, RN, MN, CCRN, CEN; and others who wish anonymity

- Contributors to former editions, including the late Edward Glogowski and the late Gary Sparger, Catherine Gregory, Julie Shinn, Charleen Strebel, Betsy Todd, and Alice Whittaker

- Barbara Scott, my assistant, whose cheerful demeanor and willingness to work within seemingly impossible deadlines eased project management considerably

- Jane Harper, colleague and editorial assistant, whose conceptualizations of new chapters intrigued me and who assisted with preparation of the manuscript

- Patricia Benner, Christine Tanner, Anne Crabtree, Marcy Jorgenson, and Nancy Diekelmann for their generosity in sharing paradigms

- Mark McCormick, editor; Gail Carrigan, production editor; Cathy Lewis, production editor; and Kay Brown, art supervisor at Addison-Wesley Publishing Co.

- A special thank you to our reviewers:

Reviewers

Margaret Barnett, MSN, FMP, CCRN
University of Alaska, Anchorage
Anchorage, Alaska

Sally Baumeier, RN, MA, CCRN
Daytona Beach Community College
Daytona Beach, Florida

Susan Bennett, RN, DNS
Indiana University
Indianapolis, Indiana

Diane M. Billings, EdD, RN, FAAN
Indiana University School of Nursing
Indianapolis, Indiana

Vicki Buchda, RN, MS
Maryvale Samaritan Medical Center
Phoenix, Arizona

Barbara Bunker, RN, MSN
University of North Carolina at Chapel Hill
Chapel Hill, North Carolina

Barbara J. Hogan, RN, MSN
St. Vincent's Medical Center
Toledo, Ohio

Ann Hotter, RN, MSN, CCRN, CF
Mayo Foundation Hospital
Rochester, Minnesota

Linda M. Haggerty, RN, MS, CCTC
Caremark Inc.
Lincolnshire, Illinois

Nancy Johnson, RN, MS, CCRN
Maricopa Medical Center
Phoenix, Arizona

Pamela Kidd, RN, PhD
University of Kentucky
University Hospital
Lexington, Kentucky

Deborah Klein, RN, MSN, CCRN, CS
MetroHealth Medical Center
Cleveland, Ohio

Kathryne M. LaGrange, RN, MS, CCRN
Stanford University Hospital
Stanford, California

Mary L. Morgan, PhD
Fort Hays State University
Hays, Kansas

Jim Rankin, RN, RGN, MSC
University of Calgary
Calgary, Alberta, Canada

Marlene Reimer, RN, MN, CNNC
University of Calgary
Calgary, Alberta, Canada

Carleen J. Ronchetti, MS
St. Luke's Hospital
Duluth, Minnesota

Amy Perrin Ross, RN, MSN, CNRN
Loyola University Medical Center
Maywood, Illinois

Julie A. Shinn, MA, CCRN, FAAN
Stanford University Medical Center
Stanford, California

Karen L. Then, RN, BN, MN
University of Calgary
Calgary, Alberta, Canada

Marla Weston, RN, MS, CCRN
Desert Samaritan Medical Center
Mesa, Arizona

On a personal level, I appreciate the love and support of my family. My husband, Mike, keeps me centered and upbeat even during the "tough times"; and our son, Jason, shares his wonder and excitement in the ever-expanding world around him. They both remind me of the central importance of love in a meaningful life.

Nancy Meyer Holloway

Contributors

Jo Barr, RN, MS
Critical Care Educator
Neurosurgical Nurse Specialist
Santa Clara Valley Medical Center
San Jose, California
Neurologic Disorders; Neurologic Interventions

Nancy Newell Bell
RN, MN, CCRN, CEN
Trauma Clinical Nurse Specialist
Eden Hospital Medical Center
Castro Valley, California;
Assistant Clinical Professor
School of Nursing
University of California
San Francisco, California
Caring: The Essence of Critical Care Nursing; Trauma

Diane Sadler Benson
RN, MS, MEd
Nurse Educator and Consultant
Benson-Sadler Enterprises
Eureka, California;
Clinical Nursing Faculty
Humboldt State University
Aracta, California
Critical Care Pharmacology

Gregory A. DeBourgh
MS, RN, CS, CCRN
Director of Nursing, Critical Care
California Pacific Medical Center
San Francisco, California;
formerly Surgical Clinical Nurse Specialist
(Gastrointestinal System and Wound Care)
Merritt-Peralta Medical Center
Oakland, California
Gastrointestinal System

Claire Dyer
RN
Clinical Manager
Bothin Burn Center
Saint Francis Memorial Hospital
San Francisco, California
Burns

Madeline Dignan Fassler
RN, BSN, CEN
Manager, Nursing and Clinical Education
Kaiser Permanente Medical Center
Hayward, California
Dysrhythmias and Conduction Defects

Anna Gawlinski
RN, MSN, CCRN
Cardiovascular Clinical Nurse Specialist
University of California Medical Center
Los Angeles, California
Cardiovascular Physical Assessment; Cardiovascular Diagnostic Techniques

Teresa Gwin
RN
Staff Nurse
California Pacific Medical Center
San Francisco, California
Chest X-ray Interpretation

Jane Harper
RN, MS, CCRN
Doctoral Student
University of California
San Francisco, California
Immunologic Disorders; Multisystem Disorders

Susan S. Jacobs
RN, MS, CCRN
Clinical Coordinator, Pulmonary Rehabilitation
Seton Medical Center
Daly City, California
Pulmonary Assessment; Pulmonary Disorders; Pulmonary Interventions

Leslie S. Kern
RN, MN
Cardiovascular Clinical Nurse Specialist
University of California Medical Center
Los Angeles, California
Cardiovascular Disorders; Emergency Exploratory Sternotomy

Linda M. Kresge
RN, MPA, CCRN
Neurological Nurse Specialist
San Jose, California
Neurologic Assessment

S. Jill Ley
RN, MS, CCRN
Clinical Nurse Specialist, Cardiovascular Surgery/Transplant
California Pacific Medical Center
San Francisco, California
Cardiovascular Interventions

Mary L. Morgan
BSN, PhD
Professor of Nursing and Biological Sciences and Allied Health
Fort Hays State University
Hays, Kansas
Immunologic Disorders

Susan A. Pfettscher
RN, DNS
Clinical Specialist, Nephrology Nursing
Treatment Options Educator
Satellite Dialysis Centers, Inc.
Redwood City, California
Dimensions in Critical Care; Renal Disorders

Barbara Tueller Steuble
RN, MS
Education Coordinator
Amador Hospital
Jackson, California
Fluid, Electrolyte, and Acid-Base Imbalances; Endocrine/Metabolic Disorders

Tanya Wapensky
RD, MS
Clinical Dietitian
California Pacific Medical Center
San Francisco, California
Nourishment of the Critically Ill

1

Introduction

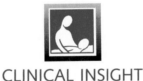

CLINICAL INSIGHT

Domain: The helping role

Competency: Providing comfort measures and preserving personhood in the face of pain and extreme breakdown.

In the emotionally treacherous atmosphere of the intensive care unit, acts of simple human kindness take on special poignancy. In this excerpt, from Crabtree and Jorgenson (1986, pp. 96–99), Kim, a nurse, describes the bond that she developed with Jack, a gravely ill cardiac surgical patient dying after numerous surgeries, and his wife Kate, who has resisted the painful realization that her husband will not survive much longer. Shortly after Jack survives a code, his 40th birthday occurs:

> *It was the night of Jack's 40th birthday, and I was working nights, and another nurse and I went nuts; we decorated his room; we had balloons all over.*

We got him a corsage, and we got Kate a corsage, too. We decorated the whole room. And, when Kate came in the next morning, she just went nuts! She was so touched that somebody would do this. I don't think she knew that we knew that it was his birthday, except for the fact that it's on the admission sheet. And, we had gone to the hilt. We had a birthday party to behold! . . . Kate was so touched that I think it made all the difference in the world. She was a different lady after that; she was even to the point where she was saying things like, I know that this is probably going to be Jack's last birthday. Because, I've seen how he does better, and then how he's gotten worse.

Later, Kim shares her reflections on the bond that developed among them and her gratitude for their gifts of love to each other:

1

That's the kind of situation (where) I think it's so important to become emotionally involved. You can have all the book knowledge in the world, and I think it's important. Maybe it's important not to get too involved, but maybe we need to be slapped in the face sometimes with reality. That's the kind of situation where I knew what the full picture was; I knew the man was dying, and I got so emotionally involved, but it felt so good. It felt so good to feel like I touched that lady and her family . . . and Jack; even if she didn't admit that he was dying, at least she could feel good, you know. She didn't have to say to me, I know my husband has a dying heart, and he's not going to live very long but, for even just one day, to make them feel good. They had a nice day. And, to a certain degree, I think that is very important in nursing. . . . Not only do I think that we need to represent patients and their families, and be their advocates, but who else is going to make them feel good? And, I, maybe for that reason . . . maybe I should thank them for that. We had just had a horrendous stretch, and it was kind of like he and his wife slapped me in the face, you know; like, don't forget about us poor souls here who, even though you might not be able to give him this drug and make him better, or you might not be able to put me on this drip and I'll be all better. . . . You know, don't forget about us and feel good about the fact that you can cry and feel bad, but you're still human, and you haven't lost that. And, you know, after that time it was like yes, I do want to be a nurse, and, yes, I do want to keep doing what I'm doing. I don't want a new job, and I want to stay here and keep doing what I'm doing because I feel good about it. And, they gave that back to me, and I think that's really important. So . . . he's my favorite patient. I'll never forget him as long as I live.

The American Association of Critical Care Nurses (AACN) defines critical-care nursing as follows:

"In *Nursing: A Social Policy Statement* the American Nurses' Association (ANA) defines nursing as 'the diagnosis and treatment of human responses to actual or potential health problems' (ANA 1980). Critical-care nursing is that specialty within nursing which deals specifically with human responses to life-threatening problems." (AACN 1984)

As a critical-care nurse, you offer your patients and their families something very special: direct assistance with life-and-death crises. This assistance can be both an awe-inspiring responsibility and a tremendously exciting challenge. This Clinical Insight is eloquently describes a further special contribution of the critical-care nurse: preserving personhood in the face of such crises.

AACN defines the scope of critical-care nursing as encompassing three components: the critically ill patient, the critical-care nurse, and the critical-care environment (Table 1–1). As implied in the AACN Scope of Practice, the essence of critical-care nursing is anticipation and early intervention in problems besetting the critically ill. Nursing diagnosis of patient problems must be based on a sound understanding of anatomy and physiology and astute patient assessment. For this reason, significant portions of this book are devoted to helping you acquire this knowledge base. Critical-care nursing also requires adeptness at nursing care planning, intervention, and evaluation. These subjects also are discussed in depth in this book.

Three unifying concepts guided the selection and organization of the material in this book:

- The importance of a nursing model in guiding practice.
- The concept of core knowledge and skills.
- The nursing process, incorporating nursing diagnosis.

Nursing Model

Nursing education long has been patterned upon the traditional "body systems" approach. That approach reflects the biomedical model, which is based on the Cartesian view that distinguishes between the body and the mind or soul (Feild and Winslow 1985). Although a biomedical model is appropriate for use in fulfilling the responsibilities that nurses share with physicians (nursing's interdependent role), a nursing model is needed to focus attention on nursing's unique concerns (its independent role). Feild and Winslow point out that a nursing model is used *with*—not in place of—a medical model. This text utilizes both a nursing process model and the biomedical model as an organizing framework. By integrating a nursing model with the biomedical model, this framework promotes a holistic approach to patient care, one that integrates nursing's independent functions with its collaborative ones.

TABLE 1–1

Scope of Critical Care Nursing Practice

Introduction

AACN builds on the ANA definition of nursing[1] and defines critical care nursing as that specialty within nursing which deals with human responses to life-threatening problems.[2] The scope of critical care nursing is defined by the dynamic interaction of the critically ill patient, the critical care nurse, and the critical care environment.

The goal of critical care nursing is to ensure effective interaction of these three requisite elements to effect competent nursing practice and optimal patient outcomes within an environment supportive of both. The framework within which critical care nursing is practiced is based on a scientific body of knowledge, the nursing process, and multidisciplinary collaboration in the care of patients.

Although a distinct specialty, critical care nursing is inseparable from the profession of nursing as a whole. As members of the profession, critical care nurses hold the same commitment to protect, maintain, and restore health as well as to embrace the *Code for Nurses*.[3]

The Critically Ill Patient

Central to the scope of critical-care nursing is the critically ill patient, who is characterized by the presence of, or being at high risk for developing, life-threatening problems. The critically ill patient requires constant intensive, multidisciplinary assessment and intervention in order to restore stability, prevent complications, and achieve and maintain optimal responses.

In recognition of the critically ill patients' primary need for restoration of physiologic stability, the critical care nurse coordinates interventions directed at resolving life-threatening problems. Nursing activities also focus on support of patient adaptation, restoration of health, and preservation of patient rights, including the right to refuse treatment or to die. Inherent in the patients' response to critical illness is the need to maintain psychological, emotional, and social integrity. The familiarity, comfort, and support provided by social relationships can enhance effective coping. Therefore, the concept of the critically ill patient includes the interaction and impact of the patient's family and/or significant other(s).

The Critical Care Nurse

The critical care nurse is a licensed professional who is responsible for ensuring that all critically ill patients receive optimal care. Basic to accomplishment of this goal is individual professional accountability through adherence to standards of nursing care of the critically ill and through a commitment to act in accordance with ethical principles.

Critical care nursing practice encompasses the diagnosis and treatment of patient responses to life-threatening health problems. The critical care nurse is the one constant in the critical care environment. As such, coordination of the care delivered by various health care providers is an intrinsic responsibility of the critical care nurse. With the nursing process as a framework, the critical care nurse uses independent, dependent, and interdependent interventions to restore stability, prevent complications, and achieve and maintain optimal patient responses. Independent nursing interventions are those actions which are in the unique realm of nursing and include manipulation of the environment, teaching, counseling, and initiating referrals. Dependent nursing interventions are those actions prescribed by medicine. Interdependent nursing interventions are actions determined through multidisciplinary collaboration. Underlying the application of these interventions is a holistic approach that expresses human warmth and caring. This art, in conjunction with the science of critical care nursing, is essential to the interaction between the critical care nurse and critically ill patient in attaining optimal outcomes.

The critical care environment is constantly changing. The critical care nurse must respond effectively to the demands created by this environment for the broad application of knowledge. Realization of this goal is accomplished through entry preparation into professional nursing practice at a baccalaureate level and a commitment to maintaining competency in critical care nursing through ongoing education concurrent with an expanding base of experience.

The Critical Care Environment

The critical care environment can be viewed from three perspectives. On one level the critical care environment is defined by those conditions and circumstances surrounding the direct interaction between the critical care nurse and the critically ill patient. The immediate environment must constantly support this interaction in order to effect desired patient outcomes. Adequate resources, in the form of readily available emergency equipment, needed supplies, effective support systems for managing emergent patient situations, and measures for ensuring patient safety are requisites. The framework for nursing practice in this setting is provided by standards of nursing care of the critically ill.

The institution or setting within which critically ill patients receive care represents another perspective of the critical care environment. At this level, the critical care management and administrative structure ensures effective care delivery systems for various populations of critically ill patients through provision of adequate human, material, and financial resources, through required quality systems, and through maintenance of standards of nursing care of the critically ill.

Additional elements contributing to effective care delivery include:

- Participatory decision-making which ensures that the critical care nurse provides input into decisions affecting the nurse-patient interaction.

- A collaborative practice model that facilitates multidisciplinary problem-solving and ethical decision-making.

- Education of critical care nurses consistent with standards for critical care nursing education and practice.

(Continues)

TABLE 1–1

Scope of Critical Care Nursing Practice (Continued)

The broadest perspective of the environment encompasses a global view of those factors that impact the provision of care to the critically ill patient. Monitoring of legal, regulatory, social, economic, and political trends is necessary to promote

early recognition of the potential implications for critical care nursing and to provide a basis for a timely response. (Adopted by AACN Board of Directors, November 1986)

[1]American Nurses' Association: *Nursing: A social policy statement.* Kansas City, MO: ANA, 1980.
[2]American Association of Critical Care Nurses: *Definition of critical care nursing* (AACN Position Statement). Newport Beach, CA: AACN, 1984.
[3]ANA, Code for Nurses, ANA, Kansas City, Missouri, 1985.
Reprinted with permission of the American Association of Critical-Care Nurses, Laguna Niguel, CA.

Core Concepts and Skills

The concept of core knowledge and skills implies that standard principles and techniques guide the nurse in the care of critically ill patients. These core elements provide a fruitful approach to mastering the general principles and skills of critical-care nursing, which can be applied to a wide variety of patients and which form the foundation for individualized care based on professional judgment.

Nursing Process

The critical-care nurse must be assisted in developing a nursing style that both nurtures him or her and enables him or her to provide optimum patient care. The keys to such a nursing style—anticipation, judgment, and creativity—depend on skillful application of the nursing process in critical-care situations. *Nursing the Critically Ill Adult* recognizes five phases of the nursing process: (1) assessment; (2) diagnosis; (3) planning; (4) intervention; and (5) evaluation (Figure 1–1). Although separated in this book for analysis, the phases of the nursing process interact synergistically in practice.

Assessment

Any scientific process starts with data collection and analysis. What distinguishes medical from nursing assessment is the use to which the data will be put; that use determines the goal of each professional's assessment.

The nurse's goal in the assessment phase is the acquisition of a nursing database, that is, information

from which the patient's nursing care needs can be identified. Comprehensive nursing assessment thus necessitates collection of data from many sources: the health record, your own physical assessment of the patient, interviews with the patient and family, monitoring devices, diagnostic studies, and laboratory tests. When gathering data from these sources, remember that your focus is on the patient's current condition and on information with nursing implications. The sections of this book addressing patient assessment present one way to examine these data systematically. By following a logical sequence in assessment, you avoid accidentally overlooking an important source of information about your patient.

In contrast, the physician's goal in the assessment phase is the acquisition of a medical database. To this end, the physician performs a comprehensive history and physical examination to the extent appropriate to the patient's current status. The health history usually consists of the patient's chief complaint, profile, family history, past health history, history of the present problem, and a review of systems. To perform the review, the physician questions the patient about the presence and characteristics of symptoms. A detailed physical examination follows.

There is no one "right" way to assess a patient; many nursing assessment formats have been developed. Those most commonly used are head-to-toe and body systems. Close comparison of these two formats reveals that each includes the same items for assessment; what varies is their organization. Other nursing assessment tools are based on conceptual models you might wish to explore; such models include Roy's adaptation model (1976), Orem's self-care competency model (1980), Rogers' unitary-man model (1969), King's systems model (1971), and Gordon's model of eleven functional health patterns (1987). You may choose to use one of these formats or you may develop one appropriate to your own patients and practice setting.

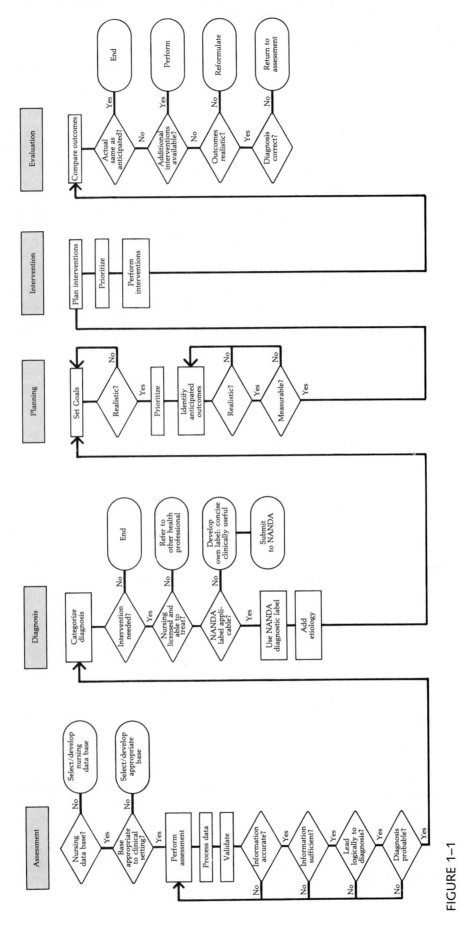

FIGURE 1-1

Nursing process flowchart.

Assessment in critical care differs from that in most other clinical areas because the needs of patients undergoing life-threatening physiologic crises change so rapidly. Obviously, it is neither expedient nor appropriate to collect for every patient all the data presented via any assessment tool. As critical-care nurses, our approach is a *focused* assessment: within the first 5–10 minutes of admission, we obtain a brief nursing history and perform a rapid examination guided by the patient's symptomatology. In this rapid assessment, we seek to identify the patient's major problems, the rapidity with which they are developing, and how well he or she is compensating for them. We then are able to determine priorities and initiate any urgent care. More complete assessment can be undertaken once care for the patient's immediate life threats has been instituted.

By developing knowledge and skill in patient assessment, you can enhance your ability to deliver comprehensive, high-quality patient care. You will be better able to detect significant changes early, institute care, and evaluate the results of your actions. You also will be better able to understand the detailed examinations performed by physicians and appreciate the significance of their findings. Finally, you will be able to demonstrate to patients, visitors, and other staff the increasing responsibility nurses are assuming for anticipation, prevention, and early intervention in the myriad disorders that can plague the critically ill.

Whatever assessment tool you choose, it should be practical, flexible, and systematic, and should lead naturally into the next phase of the nursing process—*nursing diagnosis*.

Diagnosis

A *nursing diagnosis* is defined as "a clinical judgment about an individual, family, or community response to actual or potential health problems/life processes which provides the basis for definitive therapy toward achievement of outcomes for which the nurse is accountable" (North American Nursing Diagnosis Association 1989). Although the term "nursing diagnosis" is relatively recent, the process itself is not. Nurses have been diagnosing for years, but the accepted labels for their decisions have been "patient problems" or "needs." Nurses' diagnostic efforts often have been intuitive, haphazard, not shared explicitly with colleagues or patients, and in some cases poorly differentiated from medical diagnoses.

Nursing diagnosis was formally recognized as a professional nursing function in 1973 when it was included in the ANA *Standards of Nursing Practice*. A major contribution to the profession has been the systematic definition and classification of diagnoses by the National Group for the Classification of Nursing Diagnoses. This pioneering group has met biannually in St. Louis, Missouri, since 1973. At the Fifth National Conference in 1982, the group was formalized as the North American Nursing Diagnosis Association (NANDA).

The goals of NANDA include formal acceptance of diagnostic labels for clinical testing. A list of approved nursing diagnoses is shown in Table 1–2. The list incorporates both actual diagnoses and "high risk" diagnoses (i.e., those that include the term "high risk"). A high risk nursing diagnosis is "a clinical judgment that an individual, family or community is more vulnerable to develop the problem than others in the same or similar situation" (NANDA 1990). A high risk diagnosis was formerly designated by the terminology "potential for . . ." in the diagnosis.

NANDA maintains a national clearinghouse to serve as a central information exchange. Clearinghouse activities include storing materials on nursing diagnosis, providing bibliographies on diagnostic categories, disseminating information about activities of nurses using nursing diagnosis, publishing a journal, and coordinating arrangements for national conferences.

Nursing Diagnosis in Critical Care Critical care poses a unique challenge in the use of nursing diagnosis. There are several reasons for this challenge:

1. The very nature of the problems with which critical-care nurses deal. As noted at the start of the chapter, critical-care nursing involves the care of people undergoing life-threatening physiologic crises. As such, the prominence of physiologic problems is undeniable.

2. The inseparability of physiologic and psychologic factors underlying patient problems, for example, postcardiotomy delirium, which can result from postoperative chemical imbalances as well as anxiety, powerlessness, and so on.

3. The close collaboration between nursing and other disciplines. This collaboration exists both in assessing patients and in making and carrying out therapeutic decisions.

4. The theoretical and practical confusion regarding the dependent, interdependent, and independent roles of the nurse. These roles have been the source of major philosophic disagreements and controversy in nursing. Nowhere is this more apparent than in the field of critical-care nursing. In a classic article, Guzzetta and Dossey (1983) asserted:

TABLE 1–2

Approved Nursing Diagnoses

North American Nursing Diagnosis Association (NANDA)
1992 Approved Nursing Diagnostic Categories

Activity intolerance
Activity intolerance: High risk
Adjustment, Impaired
Airway clearance, Ineffective
Anxiety
Aspiration: High risk
Body image disturbance
Body temperature, Altered: High risk
Bowel incontinence
Breast-feeding, Effective (potential for enhanced)
Breast-feeding, Ineffective
Breathing pattern, Ineffective
Cardiac output, Decreased
Caregiver role strain
Communication, Impaired: Verbal
Constipation
Constipation, Colonic
Constipation, Perceived
Coping, Defensive
Coping, Family: Potential for growth
Coping, Ineffective family: Compromised
Coping, Ineffective family: Disabling
Coping, Ineffective individual
Decisional conflict (specify)
Denial, Ineffective
Diarrhea
Disuse syndrome: High risk
Diversional activity deficit
Dysfunctional ventilatory weaning response
Dysreflexia
Family processes, Altered
Fatigue
Fear
Fluid volume deficit
Fluid volume deficit: High risk
Fluid volume excess
Gas exchange, Impaired
Grieving, Anticipatory
Grieving, Dysfunctional
Growth and development, Altered
Health maintenance, Altered
Health-seeking behaviors (specify)
High risk for caregiver role strain
High risk for peripheral neurovascular dysfunction
High risk for self-mutilation
Home maintenance management, Impaired
Hopelessness
Hyperthermia
Hypothermia
Inability to sustain spontaneous ventilation
Ineffective infant feeding pattern
Infection: High risk
Ineffective management of therapeutic regimen (individual)
Injury: High risk
Interrupted breast-feeding
Knowledge deficit (specify)

Mobility, Impaired physical
Noncompliance (specify)
Nutrition, Altered: Less than body requirements
Nutrition, Altered: More than body requirements
Nutrition, Altered: High risk for more than body requirements
Oral mucous membrane, Altered
Pain (Acute)
Pain, Chronic
Parental role conflict
Parenting, Altered
Parenting, Altered: High risk
Personal identity disturbance
Poisoning: High risk
Post-trauma response
Powerlessness
Protection, Altered
Rape-trauma syndrome
Rape-trauma syndrome: Compound reaction
Rape-trauma syndrome: Silent reaction
Relocation stress syndrome
Role performance, Altered
Self-care deficit: Bathing/hygiene
Self-care deficit: Dressing/grooming
Self-care deficit: Feeding
Self-care deficit: Toileting
Self-esteem disturbance
Self-esteem, Low: Chronic
Self-esteem, Low: Situational
Sensory/perceptual alterations: Visual, auditory, kinesthetic, gustatory, tactile, olfactory (specify)
Sexual dysfunction
Sexuality patterns, Altered
Skin integrity, Impaired
Skin integrity, Impaired: High risk
Sleep pattern disturbance
Social interaction, Impaired
Social isolation
Spiritual distress
Suffocation: High risk
Swallowing, Impaired
Thermoregulation, Impaired
Thought processes, Altered
Tissue integrity, Impaired
Tissue perfusion, Altered: Renal, cerebral, cardiopulmonary, gastrointestinal, peripheral (specify type)
Trauma: High risk
Unilateral neglect
Urinary elimination, Altered
Urinary incontinence, Functional
Urinary incontinence, Reflex
Urinary incontinence, Stress
Urinary incontinence, Total
Urinary incontinence, Urge
Urinary retention
Violence, High risk: Self-directed or directed at others

One of the major problems with using nursing diagnosis in critical care is related to the so-called "dependent" role vs. the interdependent and independent roles of the critical-care nurse.... Although the "dependent" and independent roles of the nurse can be *theoretically* defined, the lines that separate these roles in practice become fuzzy. Perhaps it is time to rethink these concepts and reexamine the premises on which they are based.... Perhaps the reason that the nurse's "dependent" and independent roles cannot be clearly defined in critical care is that *in practice* these roles do not exist. Perhaps we should stop wasting our time trying to delineate these roles and realize that the *critical-care nurse's role is one of interdependence* and coparticipation with the patient, the family, the physician, and other members of the health team.

5.   The nature of the NANDA list of diagnoses. The levels of conceptualization vary from very concrete to very abstract. Some of the diagnoses appear to rename medical problems, for example, *decreased cardiac output* and *altered tissue perfusion.*

To enrich the development and utilization of nursing diagnosis from a critical-care perspective, National Conferences on Nursing Diagnosis in Critical Care, jointly sponsored by AACN and Marquette University, have been held biannually since 1983. The purpose of the conferences is to move beyond conceptual controversy to address the clinical use of nursing diagnosis in critical care.

Other leaders in critical care support the use of nursing diagnosis as well. For example, the nursing diagnosis model now serves as the organizing framework for *Outcome Standards for Nursing Care of the Critically Ill* (Kuhn et al. 1990) and the *Core Curriculum for Critical Care Nursing,* 4th ed. (Alspach 1991). An exciting development occurred as part of the Outcome Standards project in 1988, when AACN sponsored a consensus conference of 25 critical care nurse experts to determine which diagnoses to include in the book (Kuhn 1991). The nurses selected 30 diagnoses judged relevant to critical care and then ranked them using Likert-type scales and magnitude estimation. (Likert-type scales ask people to indicate their degree of agreement with a statement.) The result was a list of 30 nursing diagnoses ranked in order of importance to critical care, in the 1988 judgment of these experts (Table 1–3).

Several points are worth considering about this list. First, when reading this list, one must keep in mind the purpose for which it was generated: to guide develop-

TABLE 1–3

Categories of Nursing Diagnoses

High Frequency, High Priority (Importance)

Fluid Volume/Dynamics, Alterations in
Gas Exchange, Impaired
Tissue Perfusion, Alterations in
Injury, Potential for
Airway Clearance, Ineffective
Infection, Potential for
Nutrition, Alterations in
Skin Integrity, Impaired
Comfort, Alterations in
Activity Intolerance
Sensory-Perceptual Alterations
Mobility, Impaired Physical

Low Frequency, High Priority (Importance)

Thermoregulation, Ineffective
Breathing Pattern, Impaired
Adaptive Capacity, Decreased

High Frequency, Low Priority (Importance)

Anxiety
Communication, Ineffective
Coping, Ineffective
Self-Care Deficit
Fear
Family Process, Alteration in
Role Performance, Alteration in

Borderline

Elimination, Alteration in: Urinary
Elimination, Alteration in: Bowel

Low Frequency, Low Priority (Importance)

Powerlessness
Grieving
Self-Concept, Disturbance in
Spiritual Distress
Growth and Development, Alterations in
Noncompliance

American Association of Critical-Care Nurses, *Outcome standards for nursing care of the critically ill.* Laguna Niguel, CA: AACN, 1990. Reprinted with permission, American Association of Critical-Care Nurses.

ment of a book. As Kuhn (1991) points out, it may or may not be useful for other purposes. Second, all the high-frequency, high-priority diagnoses are physiologic. Third, the psychosocial and spiritual diagnoses ranked lower in priority. This ranking should not be interpreted as meaning these diagnoses are unimportant in critical care, but rather that, in critical illness, basic physiologic needs take precedence over psychologic and spiritual needs.

Nursing diagnosis in critical care is in an evolutionary phase. The issues of the appropriateness of including physiologic diagnoses in patient care plans and the type and degree of nursing autonomy necessary to treat nursing diagnoses will remain an area of stimulating debate. Until these issues are resolved, the following guidelines are appropriate for those of us engaged in clinical practice who want to use nursing diagnosis.

1. *Remember that a physiologic diagnosis is not synonymous with a medical diagnosis.* The finding that critical care experts who participated in the consensus conference indicated that physiologic diagnoses are relevant and important to critical care nursing practice clearly supports the value of including physiologic diagnoses in the NANDA taxonomy.

2. *Include in the plan of patient care all the problems with which the critical-care nurse must deal.* Whether the medical and nursing diagnoses and interventions are listed in separate areas of the care plan, or whether the list of nursing diagnoses includes all problems encountered by the critical-care nurse, is less important than having accessible to the nurse all the data he or she needs to get a clear picture of the patient and his or her problems.

3. *Use the diagnoses that have meaning for you.*

Benefits of Nursing Diagnosis Considerable confusion has surrounded the term "nursing diagnosis" in the minds of nurses, physicians, and the public. By custom, "diagnosis" has been so strongly associated with medicine for so long that many people think the use of this term automatically implies that the nurse is trying to practice medicine. In actuality, diagnosis simply is the generic term for the intellectual process by which a person makes judgments from data gleaned during the assessment phase.

What are the benefits of using nursing diagnosis? Benefits fall into two major areas: the impact on day-to-day nursing practice, and the influence on the nursing profession. Clinical benefits from nursing diagnosis include (1) clear identification of the problem, which directs specific planning, implementation, and evaluation of care; and (2) clear identification of the nurse's accountability. Nursing diagnosis provides a clinical language that facilitates reporting, team conferences, charting, computerization, teaching, research, and publishing. Even more important, nursing diagnosis facilitates accountability, in the nurses' own eyes, their colleagues' eyes, and the public's eyes. As Diers (1981) has written:

Nursing is exceedingly complicated work since it involves technical skill, a great deal of formal knowledge, communication ability, use of self, timing, emotional investment, and any number of other qualities. What it also involves, and what is hidden from the public, is the process of thinking that leads from the knowledge to the skill, from the perception to the action, from the investment to the touch, from the observation to the diagnosis. Yet it is the process of nursing care that is at the center of nursing's work and is so little attended to, so little described, that no wonder people think nurses are just nice people with a minimum of training, dumbly following doctors' orders.

Nursing diagnosis represents an important way for us to document nursing thinking and thus to differentiate ourselves from other professions and to validate ourselves as autonomous professionals.

Nursing vs Medical Diagnosis Many nurses have trouble articulating the distinctions between medical diagnosis and nursing diagnosis. This difficulty is particularly serious in critical care, where nurses may be called upon in emergencies to make medical diagnoses and to treat patients under standing orders or protocols. A delineation of the most distinct differences follows.

1. The physician focuses on the diagnosis of a specific disease process. In contrast, the nurse focuses on the diagnosis of human responses, both those resulting from the disease and those unrelated to it. The nursing diagnosis considers the medical diagnosis and treatment but zeroes in on the patient's physical, emotional, and social responses to disease, treatment, surroundings, other people, and him or herself (Shoemaker 1979). As every experienced nurse knows, two patients with the same disease label may have widely varying problems, depending on their personal differences and on their progress along the health–illness continuum.

2. The intent of medical diagnosis is to prescribe treatment to cure the disease process. Medical treatment typically consists of diet, medication, surgery, and physical therapy. The intent of nursing diagnosis is to prescribe treatment to relieve patient problems falling within nursing's independent area of practice. Nursing treatment typically consists of physiologic interventions, health education, crisis intervention, counseling, therapeutic use of self, and referral to other professionals.

3. Medical diagnoses usually are limited and static during the course of an illness. In contrast, nursing diagnoses are numerous and flexible, reflecting dynamic alterations in the patient's status during illness and recovery.

4. Medical diagnoses are short, commonly accepted phrases. Nursing diagnoses are not—yet. Nursing diagnostic terminology is not yet universally accepted. As a result, nurses may use different phrases to describe the same problem, further contributing to confusion in the development and use of nursing diagnoses. NANDA is working to develop a universally acceptable taxonomy. As it struggles with the balance between conciseness and comprehensiveness in terminology, it sometimes adopts phrases that appear long and somewhat awkward to use. To support this important move toward nursing unity, this text uses the diagnoses approved by NANDA for clinical testing, in spite of any difficulties with length or awkward phrasing. The order of words in accepted diagnoses has been revised to reflect the order used in ordinary conversation, for example, the accepted diagnosis of "coping, ineffective individual" appears in this book as "ineffective individual coping." In situations where NANDA has not yet identified or accepted specific diagnoses for clinical testing, new ones have been created. These are identified clearly as such, by an asterisk (*) following the diagnosis.

Process of Nursing Diagnosis The two essential components of a nursing diagnosis are the problem and the etiology. The *problem* is a statement of an undesirable health response. It reflects a nursing judgment that the problem's outcomes are ones for which nurses are accountable. The *etiology* is a statement of the most probable cause of the problem.

Because many nurses are uncertain about how to identify nursing diagnoses in their day-to-day practice, the following section includes some clear, useful guidelines drawn from the classic works of Shoemaker (1979) and Dossey and Guzzetta (1981).

Step 1. Assess Your Patient Do a baseline physical and emotional assessment as early as possible in your care of the patient. Use a nursing database, as it is difficult to derive nursing diagnoses from a medical database. Many nursing databases are available in the literature, or you can develop your own to assess the nursing data you consider important.

Step 2. Process the Information Shoemaker (1979) suggests you use three general steps: cognitive processing, pattern recognition, and validation. *Cognitive processing* means comparing the data you have assessed against your knowledge base of normal versus abnormal findings. *Pattern recognition* is the clustering of related findings and the identification of possible causes. For instance, the signs of restlessness, tachycardia, sweating, and dilated pupils can be clustered together in a pattern that may be associated with pain, shock, or anxiety. Pattern recognition enables you to form tentative diagnoses and then gather further data to rule out inappropriate diagnoses. Pattern recognition thus is essentially the same step as the identification of the signs and symptoms that define the problem and the identification of a tentative diagnosis. *Validation* involves careful review of each step to be certain that you have sufficient, accurate information, that the information leads logically to the diagnosis, and that the chosen diagnosis is reasonably probable. It is validation that differentiates nursing diagnosis from nursing intuition.

Step 3. Diagnose the Problem For each problem recognized in Step 2, decide whether you are accountable for its outcomes. If not, collaborate with a physician or other appropriate professional about it. If the problem does fall within the nursing realm, try to label it using an accepted diagnosis. The NANDA list is alphabetical, making it somewhat impractical to use for quick location of an appropriate label. It is easier to use a categorized list, which groups related diagnoses together. Such lists include Bockrath's (1982) grouping of diagnoses under 10 common responses to illness, and Gordon's (1982) grouping of diagnoses under 11 functional health patterns. Whatever list you choose, carry a copy of it with you for easy reference when you are on duty.

Step 4. Add the Etiology The etiology should be a concise, clinically useful description of the factor(s) maintaining the problem. Use the words "related to" to join the problem and the etiology, for example: "Ineffective individual coping related to lack of support system."

For most nursing diagnoses, the problem–etiology linkage is an inference based on clinical judgment (Gordon 1987). In this book, the editor and contributors take the position that is unnecessary to limit etiologies only to factors within the area of independent nursing practice. Based on the criterion of clinical usefulness, they believe that acceptable etiologies may be pathophysiologic factors (e.g., anemia) or medical or surgical disorders or interventions (e.g., thoracotomy). Limiting etiologies to factors amenable only to independent nursing interventions, as has been advocated by some nursing diagnosis proponents, can lead to convoluted attempts to "force-fit" phraseology, for example, "high risk of wound infection related to impaired skin integrity secondary to surgical incision resulting from thoracotomy" rather than concise, easily understood "high risk for wound infection related to thoracotomy."

Step 5. Write Your Own Diagnosis If Necessary If there is no accepted diagnosis that fits the problem you have identified, *write your own.* You may wish to consult the nursing literature or simply to state the problem clearly. Remember to use concise, clinically useful terms that describe problems for whose outcomes nurses are accountable. Avoid jargon and terms with legal implications, such as "pain related to fall from bed when siderails left down."

Don't be afraid of physiologic diagnoses. Try them out and see how they work for you. Do they make your practice clearer? easier to explain to others? more satisfying? Keep notes on your experiences—and be sure to share them with NANDA members.*

Planning and Intervention

An analogy can be made between a neophyte cook and a neophyte critical-care nurse. When you are learning to cook, a cookbook guides you into selecting the proper ingredients in the proper proportions and informs you what others have found to be the most effective ways to prepare the dish so that it ends up a delight instead of a disaster. As you develop skill in cooking, you begin to experiment, adapting the ingredients and techniques to fit what you have on hand. Eventually, for familiar dishes you may not need the cookbook at all, consulting it only when you prepare a dish you serve infrequently. You may even become a gourmet cook, inventing your own recipes. Although this book describes concepts and techniques used in critical-care nursing, just as you cannot become a great cook by blind adherence to recipes, you cannot become an excellent critical-care nurse by rote application of concepts; nor can you learn motor skills from written descriptions only. Benner's (1984) ground-breaking study of clinically expert nurses illuminates some of the competencies that contribute to their excellence. These competencies, derived from actual practice, are presented in Table 1–4.

Based on the Dreyfuss model of skill acquisition, Benner discusses five levels of skill acquisition in nursing: novice, advanced beginner, competent, profi-

cient, and expert. Briefly, these stages can be characterized as follows:

- *Novice.* Because the person has no experience in the situation, he or she must use previously taught rules to guide action. Behavior is inflexible and limited.
- *Advanced beginner.* The person has coped with enough situations to begin to recognize recurring meaningful aspects of a situation. Performance is barely acceptable. He or she can't yet sort out priorities.
- *Competent.* The person feels a growing ability to cope with the demands of nursing. Plans are conscious and deliberate, so the person is organized and efficient. Actions are beginning to be based on long-term goals.
- *Proficient.* The person understands the situation as a whole. Having learned from experience what typical events to expect, he or she recognizes when something unusual is happening. He or she is able to quickly zero in on the most important aspects of a situation.
- *Expert.* The person intuitively grasps a situation, no longer relying on rules and guidelines. The meaning of events and actions depend on the context of the situation.

These levels of skill reflect changes in three characteristics of skilled performance:

- Transformation from relying on abstract principles to using prior concrete experience to predict and project events.
- Growing recognition of salience, that is, a change in perception from seeing all parts of a situation as equally important to viewing the situation as a complete whole in which only some parts are important.
- Transformation from a detached observer to an involved participant.

Benner points out that experience is required for developing expertise, and that a sound educational base is necessary for acquiring advanced skills because it forms the best position for developing salience. *Nursing the Critically Ill Adult* is intended to help provide the basis on which you can develop expertise. Accordingly, the experts who have contributed to the book focus on the salient aspects of various types of patient care situations, indicate nursing priorities, and offer guidelines for action.

TABLE 1–4

Competencies of the Expert Nurse

DOMAIN	COMPETENCIES
Helping role	The healing relationship: creating a climate for and establishing a commitment to healing
	Providing comfort measures and preserving personhood in the face of pain and extreme breakdown
	Presencing: being with a patient
	Maximizing the patient's participation and control in his or her own recovery
	Interpreting kinds of pain and selecting appropriate strategies for pain management and control
	Providing comfort and communication by touch
	Providing emotional and informational support to patients' families
	Guiding a patient through emotional and developmental change by providing new options and closing off old ones through channeling, teaching, mediating
	Acting as a psychologic and cultural mediator
	Using goals therapeutically
	Working to build and maintain a therapeutic community
Teaching-coaching function	Timing: capturing a patient's readiness to learn
	Assisting patients to integrate the implications of illness and recovery into their lifestyles
	Eliciting and understanding the patient's interpretation of his or her illness
	Providing an interpretation of the patient's condition and giving a rationale for procedures
	The coaching function: making culturally avoided aspects of an illness approachable and understandable
Diagnostic and monitoring function	Detection and documentation of significant changes in a patient's condition
	Providing an early warning signal: anticipating breakdown and deterioration prior to explicit confirming diagnostic signs
	Anticipating problems: future-think
	Understanding the particular demands and experiences of an illness: anticipating patient care needs
	Assessing the patient's potential for wellness and for responding to various treatment strategies
Effective management of rapidly changing situations	Skilled performance in extreme life-threatening emergencies: rapid grasp of a problem
	Contingency management: rapid matching of demands and resources in emergency situations
	Identifying and managing a patient crisis until physician assistance is available
Administering and monitoring therapeutic interventions and regimens	Starting and maintaining intravenous therapy with minimal risks and complications
	Administering medications accurately and safely: monitoring untoward effects, reactions, therapeutic responses, toxicity, and incompatibilities
	Combating the hazards of immobility: preventing and intervening with skin breakdown, ambulating and exercising patients to maximize mobility and rehabilitation, preventing respiratory complications
	Creating a wound management strategy that fosters healing, comfort, and appropriate drainage
Monitoring and ensuring the quality of health care	Providing a backup system to ensure safe medical and nursing care
	Assessing what can be safely omitted from or added to medical orders
	Getting appropriate and timely responses from physicians
Organizational and work-role competencies	Coordinating, ordering, and meeting multiple patient needs and requests: setting priorities
	Building and maintaining a therapeutic team to provide optimum therapy
	Coping with staff shortages and high turnover: contingency planning
	Anticipating and preventing periods of extreme work overload within a shift
	Using and maintaining team spirit: gaining social support from other nurses
	Maintaining a caring attitude toward patients even in the absence of close and frequent contact
	Maintaining a flexible stance toward patients, technology, and bureaucracy

Adapted from Benner P: *From novice to expert: Excellence and power in clinical nursing practice* (compiled from individual boxed tables in Benner). Menlo Park, CA: Addison-Wesley, 1984.

To become an expert, you must care for patients under the guidance of an experienced practitioner who can help you develop your ability to sort through concepts and facts, select the ones pertinent to your patient and practice setting, and synthesize them into a plan of action. Even in seemingly routine situations, you must be alert to special circumstances and adapt your care accordingly. With practice, you may discover that you no longer need this book's guidelines in familiar situations. Instead, you will return to them from time to time to refresh your memory and to guide your care in unfamiliar circumstances.

Evaluation

Evaluation is a crucial phase of the nursing process because it enables you to judge the accuracy of your decisions and effectiveness of your actions during the earlier phases. To help you evaluate your assessments, plans, and interventions, each chapter of this book contains a list of patient outcome criteria, that is, the desirable outcomes toward which your care is oriented. These are *ideal* outcome criteria, and you must use your judgment about their applicability in a given situation.

Conclusions

In the past, nursing has functioned largely on a perceptual basis; that is, the nurse perceived a problem and then acted upon it. His or her behavior often was prescribed by common sense or ritualistic practice. In recent years, the profession increasingly has emphasized an intellectual approach to patient care. Such an approach is crucial for developing the body of nursing knowledge, but it must be tempered by an awareness of the realities of day-to-day practice in the clinical setting. According to Doona (1976), the dynamic interaction of perceptual and conceptual data is the key to ideal judgment. Tempering your scientific knowledge with imagination will enable you to become a creative critical-care nurse. Add judgment to the mix, and you also will become a wise one.

REFERENCES

Alspach J (ed.): *Core curriculum for critical care nursing,* 4th ed. Philadelphia: Saunders, 1991.

American Nurses' Association: *Standards of nursing practice.* Kansas City, MO: The Association, 1973.

American Nurses' Association, Congress on Nursing Practice: *Nursing: A social policy statement.* Kansas City, MO: The Association, 1980.

American Association of Critical-Care Nurses: *Definition of critical care nursing.* Newport Beach, CA: The Association, 1984.

Benner P: *From novice to expert: Excellence and power in clinical nursing practice.* Menlo Park, CA: Addison-Wesley, 1984.

Bockrath M: Your patient needs two diagnoses—medical and nursing. *Nurs Life* (Mar/Apr) 1982; 29–32.

Crabtree A, Jorgenson M: Exploring the practical knowledge in expert critical-care nursing practice (unpublished Master's thesis, University of Wisconsin, Madison, 1986).

Diers D: Why write? Why publish? *Image* 1981; 13:1–7.

Doona M: The judgment process in nursing. *Image* 1976; 8:27–29.

Dossey B, Guzzetta C: Nursing diagnosis. *Nursing 81* (Jun) 1981; 34–38.

Feild L, Winslow EH: Moving to a nursing model. *Am J Nurs* (Oct) 1985; 1100–1101.

Gordon M: Nursing diagnosis and the diagnostic process. *Am J Nurs* 1976; 76:1298–1300.

Gordon M: Historical perspective: The national conference group for classification of nursing diagnosis. Pages 2–8 in *Classification of nursing diagnosis: Proceedings of the third and fourth national conferences.* Kim M, Moritz D (eds). New York: McGraw-Hill, 1982.

Gordon M: *Nursing diagnosis: Process and application,* 2d ed. New York: McGraw-Hill, 1987.

Guzzetta C, Dossey B: Nursing diagnosis: Framework-process-problems. *Heart Lung* 1983; 12:281–291.

King I: *Toward a theory of nursing.* New York: Wiley, 1971.

Kuhn R: Letter to the editors. *Heart Lung* 1991; 20(4):425–426.

Kuhn R et al. (eds.): *Outcome standards for nursing care of the critically ill.* Laguna Niguel, CA: The Association, 1990.

North American Nursing Diagnosis Association: NANDA news. *Nursing diagnosis* 1990; 1(3):124–128.

Orem D: *Nursing: Concepts of practice,* 2d ed. New York: McGraw-Hill, 1980.

Rogers M: *Introduction to the theoretical basis of nursing.* Philadelphia: Davis, 1969.

Roy C: *Introduction to nursing: An adaptation model.* Englewood Cliffs, NJ: Prentice-Hall, 1976.

Shoemaker J: How nursing diagnosis helps focus your care. *RN* (August) 1979; 57–61.

Caring: The Essence of Critical-Care Nursing Practice

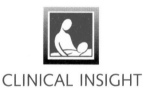

CLINICAL INSIGHT

He (the patient's father) pulled a knife on me. I was devastated. We had been caring for his son for a week, and he wasn't getting better. His (spinal) cord was transected at T_{12}; he had ARDS (Adult Respiratory Distress Syndrome) and acute renal failure. I think we really thought he would die, even hoped that he would. But when his Dad came in with a gun in his pocket and a knife on his belt, I was terrified. Eventually, after talking for a long time, we understood that he loved his son so much he wanted to help him kill himself. His son would have to live as a paraplegic. He didn't want to; he was a race car driver. We didn't share his values and certainly didn't feel comfortable with all that hardware in the unit. I've practiced critical care nursing almost twenty-five years and I've never had such anger, resentment, and fear all at once. I was devastated.

Dawn Redlaczyk RN, BSN, CCRN

This chapter takes a broad approach to examining caring. As it presents several nurses' stories of caring and being cared for, it illuminates three related concepts: (1) caring; (2) emotional growth and development of the critical-care nurse; and (3) spiritual needs of patients, because attention to these needs is part of the nurse's complete approach to human caring within the critical-care setting. It is only through comprehending the interdependence of the patient's body, mind, and spirit and the nurse's mind and spirit that we can hope to understand the effect of caring on outcome.

Caring

What Is Caring?

Caring means that persons, events, projects, and things matter to people (Benner & Wrubel 1989). Human

TABLE 2–1

The Major Components of Five Perspectives on Caring

HUMAN TRAIT	MORAL IMPERATIVE	AFFECT INTERACTION	INTERPERSONAL INTERVENTION	THERAPEUTIC
Essential for being human	Foundational basis: Nurse virtue	Empathy, feeling, and concern for another	An exchange characterized by respect and trust	Nursing actions that meet patient's needs
Universal	Nurse-centered	Nurse-centered	Mutual involvement	Patient-centered
Necessary for survival	Maintain dignity of patients	Nurse must feel compassion to be able to nurse	Develop a type of intimate relationship	Implementation meets patient's goals
Essential way of being	Guides decision-making, provides the "oughts" behind the "shoulds"	Feeling motivates the nurse. Nurse feels better when able to "really nurse."	Process that can enhance growth of both patient and nurse	If actions are appropriate, the patient improves regardless of how nurse feels
Constant, long-lasting	Constant concern for patient	Nursing is defined in relation to affect. However, affect may vary with kind of patient, stage of relationship, and/or situational demands	Is likely to vary with ability or desire of patient to be involved with nurse and situational demands	Varies with situational demands and in relation to knowledge and skill of nurse

From Morse J et al.: Comparative analysis of conceptualizations and theories of caring. *Image* 1991; 23(2): 119-126.

caring is a combination of physical, mental, spiritual, environmental, and interactive forces to be held in the highest respect, honored, cherished, and emulated (Watson 1985). Caring fuses feeling and action, knowing and being. Caring creates a willingness to enter into a relationship. Caring is primary because it creates the opportunity for giving and receiving help (Benner and Wrubel 1989).

The process of caring for individuals, for families, and for groups is a major focus in nursing today. Caring in nursing is a powerful force which involves the nurse, the patient, and the environment. The nurse and patient bring to the caring experience knowledge, prior experience, self-concept, power, values, limitations, needs, and hopes which determine or predict the outcome of the caring relationship.

Caring Theory

Morse et al. (1991) have analyzed articles on nursing that describe caring or use caring as the focus of a research project and identified the authors' underlying or implied assumptions about caring. They identified five conceptualizations of caring: caring as a human trait, caring as a moral imperative, caring as an affect, caring as an interpersonal interaction, and caring as a

therapeutic intervention. Capsule descriptions of the five conceptualizations follow:

- Caring as a human trait: Caring is a part of human nature necessary for survival.

- Caring as a moral imperative: Caring is morally good. It enables the nurse to identify appropriate behavior and preserve the patient's dignity and humanity.

- Caring as an affect: Caring is an emotion, a feeling of compassion which motivates the nurse to provide care.

- Caring as an interpersonal interaction: Caring is a mutual exchange characterized by respect and trust. It can enrich the lives of both patient and nurse.

- Caring as a therapeutic intervention: Caring is action that the nurse uses to meet the patient's unique needs, for example, providing information and reassurance.

The major components of these perspectives on caring are compared in Table 2–1.

Table 2–2 presents Morse and colleagues' grouping of specific caring theorists under one of the five conceptualizations. Direct linkages to other conceptualizations are shown by solid arrows, and implied

TABLE 2–2

Selected Caring Theorists Grouped by Conceptualization of Caring

AUTHOR(S)	DEFINITION	LINKAGES	PURPOSES	OUTCOME/GOAL
Caring as a Human Trait Leininger (1981, 1988)	• "...powerful means to help..." (1988, p. 152) "...actions directed toward assisting, supporting, or enabling..." (1988, p. 156)	◆Therapeutic Intervention ◇Affect ◇Interpersonal Interaction ◆Patient's Subjective Experience ◆Patient's Physical Response	• "...ameliorate or improve a human condition or lifeway" (1988, p. 156)	• "...provide quality care-...that is congruent, satisfying, and beneficial..." (1988, p. 155) • "...care constructs influence the health or well-being..." (1988, p. 158) • "...to improve health care to people" (1981, p. 12).
Caring as a Moral Imperative Gadow (1985)	• "...attending to the 'objectness' of persons without reducing them to the moral status of objects" (p. 33)	◆Therapeutic Intervention ◆Interpersonal Interaction ◆Patient's Subjective Experience	• "...overcomes objectivity by touching the self of the patient..." (p. 41)	• "...protection and enhancement of human dignity" (1985, p. 32).
Watson (1988)	• "...involves values, a will and commitment to care, knowledge, caring actions and consequences" (p. 29)	◆Interpersonal Interaction ◆Therapeutic Intervention ◆Patient's Subjective Experience	• enhance development of "a higher sense of self and harmony with his or her mind, body, and soul" (p. 70)	• "...the protection, enhancement, and preservation of the person's humanity, which helps to restore inner harmony and potential healing" (p. 58)
Caring as an Affect Bevis (1981)	• "...a feeling of dedication to another to the extent that it motivates and energizes action to influence life constructively and positively by increasing intimacy and mutual self actualization" (p. 50)	◆Interpersonal Interaction ◆Patient's Subjective Experience	"facilitate mutual self-actualization" "facilitate an improvement in the cared one's state, condition, experiences, and being" "further the caring relationship" • express feeling about the relationship" (p. 51)	• nurse and client personal growth and selfactualization • reaching full human potential
Caring as an Interpersonal Interaction Benner & Wrubel (1989)	• "...being connected...it fuses thought, feeling and action-knowing and being" (p. 1) • "...basic way of being in the world" (p. 398)	◇Affect ◆Therapeutic Intervention ◆Patient's Subjective Experience	• "...essential requisite for all coping" (p. 2) • enables one to be connected and concerned • "...sets up possibility of giving help and receiving help" (p. 4)	"the one caring is enriched in the process" (p. 398)

Author	Definition	Concept	Outcomes
Horner (1988)	"... a complex interpersonal interaction between a nurse and a client, in which each perceives the other as a unique responsive individual, and which incorporates both feeling and behavioral, or commitment, responses which are directed toward humanistic goals" (p. 169)	" "	•increasing attainability of humanistic goals; "... client identified goals, the support development, and health" (p. 171)
Knowlden (1988)	"... an interpersonal communication between nurses and patients in which the content and the relationship aspect of the communication are integrated in the nurses' action" (p. 321)	◊Therapeutic Intervention	

Caring as Therapeutic Intervention

Author	Definition	Concept	Outcomes
Larson (1984)	"... the acts, conduct and mannerisms enacted by professional nurses that convey to the patient concern, safety and attention" (p. 47)	" "	"feeling cared for, the sensation of well-being and safety that is the result of enacted behaviors of others" (p. 47)
Orem (1985)	"... attention, service, and protection provided by persons in a society who are in a position that requires them to be 'in charge of' or 'take care of others'; "... signifies a state of mind of an individual characterized by concern for, interest in, and solicitude for another" (p. 9)	◊Human Trait ◆Patient's Subjective Experience ◆Patient's Physical Response	•promotion of normalcy •develop self-care capacity •prevent hazards to well-being •maintain a realistic self-concept •human development •integrity of one's human structure and functioning; •achievement of optimal self-care so patient can achieve and maintain optimal health
Swanson-Kauffman (1988)	"... behaviors that were perceived as caring; Knowing, being with, doing for, enabling and maintaining belief" (p. 58)	◊Interpersonal Interaction	•promote recovery •sensitive to ongoing fears •supportive of patient decision.

Abridged from Morse J et al.: Comparative analysis of conceptualizations and theories of caring. *Image* 1991; 23(2):119-126.

linkages are shown by hollow arrows. (A thorough discussion of the conceptualizations is beyond the scope of this chapter, and the interested reader is encouraged to read the source documents.)

The work of the following theorists guides this chapter's examination of several stories told by nurses:

Leininger (1988), whom Morse and colleagues have classified under the conceptualization "Caring as a Human Trait"

Gadow (1985) and Watson (1988), classified as conceptualizing "Caring as a Moral Imperative"

Benner and Wrubel (1989), conceptualizing "Caring as an Interpersonal Interaction"

Larsen (1987), perceiving "Caring as a Therapeutic Intervention"

Descriptions of Caring at the Bedside The following stories told by nurses caring at the bedside provide explorative descriptions of the phenomenon of caring. The stories were told by staff in a community critical-care service in a large tertiary-care referral center and designated trauma center in the San Francisco Bay Area. Twenty-two of the 74 staff members had practiced nursing for less than five years. Some nurses were students in the hospital's critical-care nursing residency program, a 360-hour precepted classroom and clinical program. Nine nurses had practiced for less than 6 months. The remainder of the staff had had between 10 and 22 years of practical experience. Most nurses had practiced nursing from 10 to 15 years. In this chapter, the term "novice" refers to a critical-care nurse with less than 5 years of experience. The term "expert" is used to refer to a critical-care nurse with more than 5 years of experience.

The opportunity to create this chapter occurred at a time when the author noticed a change of behavior in her organization's critical-care staff. She observed that the critical-care staff members were experiencing a period of isolation or social withdrawal from the group. This isolation was perhaps related to their moving into a new stage of growth and development. This phase was characterized by reevaluation of behavior; withdrawal into anger, restlessness, and depression; and a transient inability or unwillingness to see the result of their caring practice. The author believed that with such a large novice group, the novices may have been "depleting" the experienced staff who were caring for (mentoring) them. The author also believed that encouraging a discussion of the efficacy of caring might enhance staff self-esteem and communication. Senior staff would be recognized by the novices; novices would be nourished by the sharing. Communication would be enhanced, a sense of well-being

reestablished, and collaborative practice strengthened as the result of building new relationships and giving and receiving support.

The study participants represented an outstanding staff of nurses who care and whose caring makes a difference, every day, to the patients to whom they deliver care as well as to each other, those with whom they care. The cases included here support the efficacy of the caring practices within this group. The staff was excited about sharing their stories. It was not possible to include everyone, but everyone could have been included, since each was important and significant. All participants consented to have their stories mentioned in this chapter.

On Bonding: Caring as a Moral Imperative

My gut ached, but there was nothing more to do. . . . This was a horrible case and I instantly identified with the patient laying on the trauma re-sus (resuscitation) table. He was a Vietnam vet who had a history of abusing alcohol. He had gone through detoxification and restarted his life. He kept saying, "Don't leave me man, don't leave me." I responded, "I am not going to leave you, I am staying right here with you."

He couldn't stand the city and (had) decided to jump a train. I don't know exactly what happened, but trying to get off, he missed the step and was sucked under the train in an arc. It took both of his legs off and most of his left arm. . . . There was a bit of the elbow joint but the avulsion was so bad I knew that he'd lose it at the shoulder. Reimplantation was not an issue when we looked at what was left.

He was totally lucid—he answered questions. All he wanted was for us to put his legs back on. At one point he tried to sit up and screamed. . . . I'll remember the scream forever. I felt like running away, I wanted to "put him down" (give him narcotics to make him sleep so I wouldn't have to talk to him about what was going on). I could never do that, though. He refused narcotics for relief of his pain. For me, when he refused, to put him to sleep was to end his life. I was pretty sure he wouldn't wake up. Sleep, no matter how peaceful, would in some way diminish his last moments and that seemed wrong. He had the right to stay awake now, he knew it was over for him. He deserved the opportunity to be able to experience and understand what had happened. Well, he had terrible pain from an ischemic contracture of his left elbow. That was his only pain, though, and I would push down on the ulnar stump and that helped; he didn't want narcotics.

There was so much bonding between us. I had such a connection with him; I told him where I'd been in Nam and he told me he'd been there too. He kept turning back to me for support. I felt so helpless, there was really nothing to say. I did all the stuff you do to save his life, I told him the surgeons were terrific, that there was plenty to live for. He told me that if we couldn't fix his legs not to do anything. I knew he meant it but we couldn't stop. Maybe we never considered stopping.

I was there the whole time, he trusted me, he changed from terrified to . . . I don't know . . . calm, his eyes softened, you know the way they do when you are tight with the guy, when they trust you. There was no more look of panic, I can't describe it. It's like running an alpha code (a trauma admission which requires massive resuscitation with intubation); you can talk about it but until you've experienced it there are no words to help to understand the bond that comes when you are doing it together, you've been there.

I went home, I guess a couple of hours after we got him to the units and settled. I just knew that he wasn't going to make it even though we'd done everything we could. We still don't know . . . . Well, he literally exsanguinated during the night . . . . I guess he DIC'd (developed disseminated intravascular coagulation, a bleeding disorder). Nothing was enough. He was dead to start with but we bonded, we'd been there.

> *Michael Adams RN, BS, CCRN, CEN*
> *Trauma Nurse Clinician, EHMC*

This story provides insight about the power and impact of a shared past experience on a patient's comfort and on the intensity of the nurse's pain in caring for a dying patient. We are able to see this nurse's desire to distance himself from caring ("I wanted to put him down") and the patient's invitation to share the last moments of his life ("Don't leave me man, please don't leave me"). The cost to the patient of exposing his or her suffering, woundedness, and grief is high (Pettigrew, 1990). The caring process for this nurse was affected by past experience, both social and professional (Benner 1984). Presence and sharing in the last moments of another's life is an invaluable gift to the nurse and can be of great comfort to the patient. Presence risks vulnerability and requires the capacity for silence.

Four ethical principles are demonstrated here as well. (For a detailed discussion of ethical principles, refer to Chapter 3.) First, the nurse displayed the principle of beneficence, the duty to do good: "I did everything to save his life." Secondly, the nurse also acted from nonmaleficence, or the duty to do no harm. The nurse did not try to distance and thus shield himself (by administering narcotics). Neither did he try to protect the patient from the imminent reality of his death, perhaps depriving this patient of an opportunity to experience his life at its conclusion. The principle of fidelity, the duty to keep one's promise or word, was the most difficult for the nurse in this situation. As nurses, we commit ourselves to "whole person" care; this nurse kept his promise to stay with the patient. Finally, the principle of autonomy respects the invitation to share the suffering. When the nurse enters the suffering, it is always a privilege, never a right; it is always done with respect for the other person's autonomy.

On Perseverance: Caring as an Interpersonal Interaction

I relate the following anecdote not because it's a good "war" story, but because it illustrates my heartfelt conviction that one of the most powerful weapons a nurse can add to the healing process is the ability to connect with patients on a personal level, to really care. When one is able to establish an intimate link with the patient, it is possible to engineer an amazing array of outcomes. You can help relieve pain and anxiety and even save lives. All it takes is acknowledging the common link of humanity and the commitment, but the process may be painful.

I add variety to my work by doing interfacility transfers of critical-care patients for the major ambulance company in my community. Often, the patients are so stable you could let them drive, but every so often you run into someone who's sick enough to scare you. So when the beeper goes off, I always get a little blast of adrenalin; I never know what I'm going to get involved in.

One night I was dispatched to my own hospital to take a gentleman to UCSF where he was followed for his renal problems. Forty-five minute drive; no big deal. When I arrive, my patient is in Trendelenburg with a systolic pressure of 60, white as the sheets, pouring sweat and moaning in pain. The ED doc is struggling to get a triple lumen catheter in without much success. I have a great working relationship with this physician and I tell him, "I can't take this guy in this condition. What's going on here?"

The patient was three weeks status post kidney transplant and had been doing very well. While enjoying an evening walk with his wife, he felt abrupt, excruciating pain in his flank accompanied by a syncopal episode. A CAT scan showed a massive ac-

cumulation of fluid around the kidney that was thought to be either urine or lymph fluid.

The physician gives me this little bit of history and then states, "If you don't take him he's going to die." So I step out to the clerk and ask her to get this man's nephrologist on the phone. I knew him very well, too. I tell him that I don't feel comfortable moving this man in this condition. Very calmly, he asks for an update and after I describe his patient's condition, he says, "I understand your concern, but if he doesn't get there ASAP, he is going to die." "There is no one here who can help him?" Very matter of fact, no histrionics or hoo rah-rah. Just, "He's going to die."

By now, I'm sweating like everybody else and all my internal alarms are going crazy: what if he codes en route, liability, blah, blah, blah. All that stuff is banging around in my head like a horse in a burning barn. I am not happy.

I decide to go to have a chat with my patient, who is conscious despite his profound shock state. I start to tell him very gently what is going on and he interrupts me and asks me, no BEGS me, to take him. As far as I was concerned, that was all that needed to be said. When a man looks you in the eye and begs you to save his life, all bets are off. I was flooded by a sense of purpose and determination, and humility. Still scared silly, but determined to give this dying man his last wish. By now we have an EJ (external jugular intravenous line) in place along with another peripheral line and the saline is running wide open. Somehow I get a systolic of 90 and it's time to go.

I had already briefed my EMT crew and we moved double-speed to get our man into the rig. My practice is to obtain baseline VS in the rig before moving; his were systolic 70 by Doppler, heart rate around 120, respirations 36, and he was pale, clammy and in pain. You can't hear squat in the back of an ambulance so I'm racking my brain for something on which I can hang my evaluation of this man's status for the duration of the transport and finally decide on the carotid pulse. I find it and tell our driver to go fast.

Maybe it is sympathetic release or determination on the patient's part, but he actually improves a little for the first ten minutes of the transport. I'm talking non-stop and making him answer me so I can tell if he's still with me . . . no sleeping. The first clue I have that things are getting out of control is [that] his peripheral oxygen saturation starts dropping. I quietly say to the EMT, "Get the Ambu bag and hit it, we're code 3" (a life-threatening emergency which requires high-speed transport with sirens and lights).

By now we can't hear a thing. The patient's eyes roll back in his head and his hand slides off his chest and hits the deck with a sickening thud. And we are on the long span of the Bay Bridge at three o'clock in the morning. Closest Emergency Department is 10 minutes away. I don't recall looking at the monitor. I lean over, whack him a good crack on the sternum and scream in his face, "Don't die on me! Please don't go now." He's still breathing, but his pulse is up in the 140s and his skin signs are deteriorating. The carotid pulse is thready. So I dig my knuckles into his chest and yell his name. His eyes flutter and open. I get a pulse. He says, YES, when I ask if he's still with me. Keep talking to me. . . . I babble, pray and bag. I remember he had been walking with his wife Barbara. "She needs you, man, don't give up now." I keep him listening and talking.

When we wheel him into the ED at UCSF there is a very cheerful fellow who almost loses his life, waving a requisition for a scan and mumbling something about delay. I am still enjoying the ultra-clarity of the megadose of epinephrine my body has given me. I smile my sweetest smile ever and yell, "Get a DOC STAT." Things begin to happen quickly then. I lean over the gurney still muttering, "Barbara loves you, man, and she needs you. Don't give up now. . . ."

He'd ruptured his renal artery. The fluid around his kidney we had seen earlier was not urine; it was about three liters of blood. He had missed the last transplant opportunity because he was in Tahoe (honeymooning the second time) with Barbara.

Barry Tabel, RN, CEN,
Emergency Department

Barry has entered a caring relationship. In a caring relationship a person or idea is experienced both as an extension of and as something separate from oneself. One experiences the person who is cared for as having dignity and worth (they matter) in their own right, with a potential and ability for growth. Caring cannot occur by sheer habit; nor can it occur in the abstract.

Mayeroff (1971) considers the following eight criteria essential to a caring relationship: knowledge, alternating rhythms (the ability to modify behavior with circumstance or perspective), patience, honesty, trust, humility, hope, and courage. These elements are contained in Barry's story.

On Connecting: Caring as a Human Trait

Caring is not the exclusive domain of nurses or even of health care providers. Caring is a human trait, the manner in which activities are enacted (Corless 1990). The following story illustrates the interplay be-

tween the caregiver and other people in the clinical environment as caring happens within the context of nursing care. The message within this story is that you can care about yourself when you see yourself reflected in the eyes of another.

About ten years ago, I decided to quit nursing. I had worked in the ED of a hospital with extremely limited resources for two years. I was right out of school. Because of my degree and my experience in trauma resuscitation, they put me on the front line immediately. I was tired of seeing the same guys in for drugs and the same PID (pelvic inflammatory disease) and homemade TABs (therapeutic abortions). I wanted to see somebody get well and it seemed that nobody I knew had gotten better. I felt like I didn't have a friend, ya . . . .Well, we all went drinking after work and crabbed about the administration and schedules but I didn't care about nursing any more. I was just burned out until this one night.

We waited, all huddled against the walls of the receiving corridor for the [ambulance] rig to pull into the back . . . . It (the ED) was full and we were tired, bone tired . . . . The tired you feel at 4 A.M. on the first night back.

The back door of the rig opened and blood ran out the back door. All I could think was, I'm too tired to clean this mess up. Why did she have to use a knife? Why can't they use pills or jump off a bridge? Then I saw the tiny body of a maybe thirty-year-old blonde. Her skin color was waxy . . . you know, the color of dead.

I started to work on her and the (Admitting) Clerk came into the room. She came to get basic information; I'd heard the questions a thousand times. With her lips the patient said, "It doesn't matter, no one cares." I looked under the dressing and realized that she had transected her left carotid artery and trachea. She got her left femoral artery and maybe vein, I couldn't tell . . . and her left radial. How could she do this to herself? This was the worst I'd seen in my career . . . but I heard this new clerk say, "Oh, honey, I care. I left my six kids alone today to be here. I care, that's why I do this. Do you think for one minute that I could stand here with your blood running into my shoes if I didn't care whether you lived? I know you . . . you check at the store where I get food and you always make me feel glad when I see you. I care for you, honey, I need ya, and my kids need ya . . . .Don't you give up."

There, in an instant, you know, it seems like hours and it's three seconds, I saw my career flash in front of me. I couldn't quit; I cared desperately. I

was so tired of seeing mangled bodies but I really cared and hoped that she could find the strength to get better, to live through what was a 12-hour surgery, to have enough hope to get better on the other side. I sent her to the OR and began to cry.

"Who cares for me? We're so short and I'm so tired." I sat there for awhile. I couldn't even get mad. One of my old instructors came out of nowhere. "It's the middle of the night; what are you doing here?" I collapsed into her arms. We met several times after that. She helped me. She really cared about me; she helped me care about myself. She helped me understand the pain I always felt with death and dying, and my feelings and philosophy. She helped me set goals and get some playtime into my life. I was taking things too seriously and working too long and too many days. I guess my patient and I had so much in common.

I saw her (the patient) again. She came in one night with a card and I recognized her. Our eyes met, I might never have seen her otherwise, if you know what I mean. All she said was, "You saved my life, thank you." She left in an instant but I'll remember her forever because she saved my life, too.

Anonymous

Growth and Development of Caring by the Critical-Care Nurse

Critical-care nursing activities require specific technical skills applied in patient care situations requiring an advanced level of professional expertise. Caring is an added component within the process.

Caring requires a tremendous body of knowledge, commitment, clear human values and personal, social, and moral engagement of the nurse in time and space (Watson 1985). Caring involves continuous learning and an awareness of the uniqueness of each new situation, regardless of how extensive the nurse's basic education or experience has been.

Caring demands that the nurse surrender some control. It puts the nurse in a position of emotional vulnerability. There is always the choice to escape by becoming detached and creating a psychologic haven through "controlled caring." If, however, the nurse adopts a noncaring or distanced relationship, he or she becomes unable to enact healing through caring practice and may even impede progress toward wellness, thus extending the patient's hospital stay. Noncaring amounts to not being emotionally present with patients. Patients feel dehumanized, devalued, angry, and fearful when nursing care is hurried and distant (Drew 1986, Larson 1987, Mayer 1986, Reiman 1986).

For Barry, the nurse who cared for the renal transplant patient described earlier, abandoning a focus on physical needs is essential to caring. Peplau (1988) suggests that caring is an integration of art and science. There is a point during the critical-care nurse's developmental process at which the technology (science) becomes transparent or automatic, the surveillance behaviors (Harper [in press]) and caring behaviors and attitudes are established, and the caring relationship is readily formed.

The author sees a linear relationship in the development of caring which is based on surveillance transparency as a precursor to caring practice. The nurse must progress past an intense focus on technology before he or she is able to feel the real suffering inherent in critical illness.

On Mentoring: Caring as an Interpersonal Interaction

The next story is about mentoring: a willingness to enter into a relationship, to care, to relate, to develop and persist. When a critical-care nurse is unable to cope with practice demands, one common attempt to escape the pain and suffering is the recreational use of legal and/or illegal drugs. The following story is about caring for your colleagues, caring that nurses find meaning in their lives and support for the difficult, sometimes unrecognized job that we do. It describes an effective mentoring relationship which ultimately brings this nurse back to the practice setting.

You asked me to suggest a controversial topic of personal interest to nurses to present at a national conference in San Francisco. I told you that you needed to talk about the impaired professional: the Impaired Nurse bill was before the legislature in California. I have known you a long time and I sat in the front row through both sections of the presentation. I admired you and watched you express a personal caring for each person in that room. I believed for the first time that my experiences counted, they were valuable and I was important and too special to be hurting myself.

You described the signs and symptoms. I had every one: calling in sick too late to be replaced—or not coming in at all, diverting drugs from my patients, falsifying charting. I was even diluting PCA (patient-controlled analgesia) syringes in the bathroom with tap water. My practice was terrible; I was making all kinds of mistakes and nobody called me on them. My colleagues just kept covering for me because we were so short-staffed.

You got me into recovery, not that day or even the next. I resigned that position because I was afraid someone would call in the "Feds." I called you in January to come and talk to the nurses here, and I listened again, and we went to lunch and then to dinner, and we talked. You loved me and told me I was too special to be this distressed. You told me I was different, not the same friend, frightened, cold, and nervous. I laughed. Then, I called anonymously from Canada to ask for help; you were there again. I fell out of recovery, but you helped me back. I won't need a recovery program again. I live and walk and talk my recovery every day. I want to practice nursing for as long as I live. I love caring again, I love feeling. Thank you, you saved my life and my career.

Anonymous RN

Another story demonstrates the validity of Noddings' (1984) ethic of caring, which depends on the maintenance of conditions that will permit caring to flourish. When these conditions are not present, we are faced with stories like this:

Twelve years ago, I had been in ICU practice for about five years and I knew everything I needed to, I thought. I could do everything, fast, and not be affected by the tremendous morbidity and mortality by which I was surrounded. The staff around me were stoic, they never cried, they never needed each other, never hugged or touched. The supervisor would make sure that we never cried or hugged one another in a tough moment; we were to have no feelings, it was dangerous. I was about six months pregnant with my youngest child. We admitted a 34-year-old male patient earlier in the week. He had been exposed to Agent Orange and had suffered hepatic failure and GI bleeding. We had used a Sengstaken-Blakemore tube, pitressin drip, dopamine, and so much blood I can't even remember. Saturday morning I bathed him. He looked great, although unconscious. When he began to bleed, liters of blood poured out of him. We were unable to keep up and he died. His wife, seven months pregnant, came to the bedside to say goodbye. She told me that she would be all right. But she also said, "How am I going to tell our three-year-old that Daddy is never coming home?"

I cried, I dreamed about this woman for weeks, there was no escape. I needed to talk but I was too afraid to admit I had feelings or fears. But I left critical-care practice. I never went back. I couldn't take it any more. There was just too much contact, too much giving. With three children there was nothing more for me to give.

Debbie Harika RN, BS, CEN
Surgical Staff, EHMC

Caring for oneself is critical to surviving and thriving in nursing. "Letting go" is a term used in some settings to indicate patient death and intrapsychic release by the caregiver (Corless 1990). Not letting go is related to burnout, to leaving nursing, and to personal loss of the will to care. Letting go, the kind that happens about 20 minutes into a code when the futility of the interventions becomes apparent, is an essential part of the caring process. When we fully understand how presence and distancing affect the nurse, both now and in the future, we will be more effective in debriefing these critical situations.

Being Cared For: Caring as an Interpersonal Interaction *This story is about real caring by an expert, about to die, indelibly imprinted on the heart and mind of a novice. The story is told by a novice who is vulnerable and open in his caring. Because of that vulnerability and openness, he is easy to care for. This nurse can tell when he is hurting or depleted, or insecure in his knowledge base or skill performance. Caring about yourself means being able to say, "I don't know," asking for help, and having a mentor (Bell 1991).*

I've only been doing this for two years, but my patients seem to take care of me sometimes. An 82-year-old lady came in with multiple pulmonary emboli. She was stable and didn't have too much impairment, but some weakness was apparent. Her dyspnea was really frustrating for her. She had recently retired as a nursing administrator who was well known in the Bay Area. I admitted her and felt nervousness. You know, I really wanted to take great care of her, but I was afraid I'd make a mistake or she wouldn't like the way I did something. When I asked about her history, she answered my questions, but later when we were through she began to cry and she looked sort of panicky. I didn't know what to do, I hate it when my wife starts to cry. I stayed with her. It seemed like what she wanted and I didn't want to leave her this scared. I got tears too. It was just incredibly sad, because she knew that she was dying, and she was afraid. All I could do was stay with her. Suddenly she stopped crying and a tremendous peace came over her. She smiled and invited me to sit beside her. I did. She told me the following story, which I will never forget. I think she told me because she could see how badly I felt.

"Do you understand?" she started, "I have always looked at the best. Life is like a rose. I'm a gardener. I have studied the roses in my flower beds. Every inch or so there is a thorn and leaves, but the last 6 inches or so are clear sailing until the bud. The bud blossoms and is so beautiful and that's the last work it does. . . . It makes this incredibly beautiful blossom and then it dies. . . . Well, Bob, it occurs to me that I am about to bloom. My whole life I've been working . . . budding, if you will, and today I am going to bloom."

Robert Auen, RN, BS, CCRN
Staff Nurse, Surgical/Trauma Intensive Care Nursing Services

Critical-care nurses know how focusing on "the routine" can be used for protection, that is, for keeping a safe distance and preventing the formation of the kind of caring relationship that can result in pain for the nurse. Both the novice and the expert use this "safe withdrawal" frequently and effectively. In the following story, the nurse discusses how he sometimes hides in the routine and a particular situation in which he chose not to do so.

This just happened and it made me feel so good. You know Doug, the 16-year-old kid in 22. Last week when they revised his stump and debrided that right leg, he stayed a long time in recovery. We sent him over in his bed so he'd feel safer when he woke up. To help establish Doug's level of consciousness after returning to the recovery room, Tina asked him what his monkey's name was. He said he didn't know. Tina insisted that he figure out a name quick because it was not OK for unnamed monkeys to roam the halls of the recovery room. Immediately, even through his anesthesia, he said, "Bob . . . his name is Bob." Confused, Tina said, "Why would you name a monkey Bob?" "For my favorite nurse, Bob."

It was really important to be his "favorite" nurse, because he has been through so much and he deserves the best. I really cared for him, it really matters to me that he does well, and we have worked really hard. You know exactly how it feels don't you, you've been there. I really care about this kid and even though one day I thought he might die, I didn't back off. You know the way you withdraw when you think they aren't going to make it. I sometimes hide in the routine, it's not really that I stop caring but it's a way of protecting myself from feeling too sad.

Robert Auen, RN, BS, CCRN
Staff Nurse, Surgical/Trauma Intensive Care Nursing Services

On Being a Role Model: Caring as a Therapeutic Intervention *The following stories demonstrate the importance of role models in supporting caring and* *healing behaviors in nurses. The mentors are expert clinical nurses and experienced mentors. The novices are learning, and they are persistent, noting every detail of interventions for further use. These stories show how caring skills and behaviors can be taught and modeled from one generation of nurses to the next. Certainly, caring touch can be taught to students who are willing to learn and are confident in applying their skills.*

As an undergraduate student I watched my mentor (now friend and colleague) with an elderly female who was newly diagnosed with type I diabetes. The patient was so anxious about going home that she was diaphoretic and tachypneic. I was sure she was having a reaction, or dying, or something terrible was about to happen. My mentor took my patient's hand, sat on the edge of the bed, and talked with her for a few minutes. After the conversation, the patient stood up, confidently picked up her bag, and directed me to tell her husband that she was ready to go. I was sure my mentor had worked a miracle, right there before me. I remember thinking that this was a special gift; she had it and I didn't. Surely she couldn't teach me to be this significant in my interventions, or had she already done just that in that one moment?

Several years ago, in the days before thrombolytics, I accepted a position as Critical-Care Clinical Specialist in an inner-city hospital. My job was wonderful. I wondered if I was crazy accepting a career-track position like this. There were so many physical demands; the hours were so long; it had 24-hour responsibility; the patient acuity rivaled those I'd seen at the Med Center during graduate school; and I loved every minute in that building.

We'd just finished a 360-hour Critical-Care Residency Program and the students were taking their positions on the night shift. As we came out of report, I heard the cry . . . "Oh my God, he's in bed with her again." A very confused elderly gentleman had tried to find his way to the bathroom and passed through the wrong doorway. I put him back to bed with soft restraints and sedation. One of the novices said to me, "Come and see my patient, she's really bad, she's crashing, she has chest pain, tachypnea, tachycardia, and hypotension." I said, "Start the oxygen; recheck all the data; call the primary attending physician." The novice said, "He's not to be found; there's no one on call." I went to the patient's room with an obviously anxious new nursing resident. I sat on the side of her patient's

bed, put my hand on this frail lady's chest, and began to talk with her. Her eyes became calm, her respirations became regular at 16, and her heart rate dropped down from 100 to 74. Within 15 minutes she began to sleep. No narcotics. By 0630 we were able to reach the physician to tell him of the events of the night . . . .He ordered an ECG, which revealed an inferior infarct. Nothing to do, she was pain-free and had experienced a comfortable night's sleep.

A couple of years ago, that "new nursing resident" called to tell me she had just been admitted to a graduate school of nursing. She reminded me of that night and she shared this story.

You told me there would be one day when there was no longer any doubt that my touch, my skills, and my communication had made an undeniable difference, both to me and to the people involved. This patient was a 45-year-old executive with an oil company. He was so anxious and afraid that he was going to die. I felt that if I couldn't get him settled down he would die. Narcotics hadn't worked; benzodiazapines were just blunting his anxiety. I turned on a relaxation tape with birds, music, water, and surf. I rubbed his feet. He slept for the first time in two weeks.

Nancy N. Bell RN, MN, CCRN, CEN
Critical Care/Trauma Clinical Nurse Specialist

Sharing caring with colleagues at the same developmental level is important. Also, being nurtured by your predecessors is as important as sharing with those who admire your work and are learning from you. Expert nurses often use humor, healing touch, and prayer, but are hesitant to discuss their use or outcome because they are so easily misunderstood or judged. Their methods are so personal and individual, yet, as you can see from the stories in this chapter, they are among the very actions that demonstrate the art of nursing. Sharing these stories with novices can be a way of both validating the expert and empowering the novice.

Spiritual Distress

Human spirituality and the need for autonomous expression is included in many theories of caring (Watson 1985, Benner and Wrubel 1989, Leininger 1977, Gadow 1985, Noddings 1984). Watson (1985) includes spiritual and metaphysical dimensions in the philosophy of action in caring.

Identification of Spiritual Distress: An Ethical Imperative

Many who practice nursing have made a commitment to the moral imperative of spirituality in the caring relationship. Once a nurse supports the principles of autonomy and beneficence, he or she may not ethically choose to ignore a patient's spiritual distress. If the nurse's personal philosophy includes a promise to support the body, mind, and spirit as essential components to human healing, ignoring the patient's spiritual needs violates the principle of fidelity. This is not to say that the nurse should violate a personal spiritual commitment, but to reinforce the nurse's duty to ensure that the patient's needs are met by persons who share a congruent spirituality.

NANDA (1991) identifies spiritual distress as "a disruption in the life principle which pervades a person's entire being and which integrates and transcends biopsychosocial nature." Although NANDA recognized spiritual distress in its initial list of diagnoses, we nurses find it difficult to implement interventions for it—with the exception of calling appropriate clergy. There has been little research to validate interventions related to this diagnosis. Carson (1989) helps identify a nursing process that is effective in spiritual distress. The following guidelines for the caring related to spirituality are offered to help you identify spiritual distress and apply effective interventions.

Assessment of Spiritual Distress

Assessment of the patient may include the following questions:

- What do you usually do during times of great stress? Try to avoid the appearance of cultural or language bias when asking this question. Patients need to feel that they are not being judged by the values or standards of the interviewer.
- What do you do to feel hope or feel stronger? This is one of this author's favorite questions. This author rarely asks about God specifically (Shaffer 1991). If patients pray, irrespective of their specific preference, they usually will express spiritual distress or needs.
- Can I call someone who would want to know that you are in the hospital? Patients need to feel spiritually connected with their significant others.
- When you feel sad, what do you usually do?

- Why do you think you have this problem (be specific to the individual)? Most of the patients this author sees are trauma patients. Trauma is rarely an accident, and you usually can find evidence of extreme distress prior to the event. The answer to this question usually helps to identify the person's health locus of control as being internal or external. This question also may uncover whether the patient feels that he or she is being punished or "cursed."

The number of questions in the assessment of spiritual distress should be very brief initially. Further questions require a level of caring and trust which may not be possible to reach in a short period of time. Generally when nurses "get into trouble" when dealing with patient spirituality, it is due to a perception of intrusive assessment and imposition of the nurse's values or beliefs on an already overly stressed patient. Perhaps the difficulty is a result of dissonance between the type of caring being offered by the nurse and the type needed by the patient at a particular time. Patients may become angry—possibly because of feelings of powerlessness or abandonment or because of a lack of pain relief—and may project this anger on the nurse who makes any spiritual move because the priorities are not in harmony. This type of dissonance rarely occurs between experienced nurses and their patients.

Nursing Diagnosis

The following defining characteristics and etiologies assist in making the diagnosis of spiritual distress. (This particular diagnosis may need to be expanded; each of us may contribute to the research for further elaboration and definition.)

Defining Characteristics The following characteristics are drawn from Carpenito (1991).

Expresses concern with meaning of life, death, and/or belief system.

Expresses anger toward God or representatives of the community.

Questions meaning of suffering.

Refuses to participate in or practice usual rituals.

Seeks support from spiritual leaders or community.

Demonstrates changes in behavior or mood evidenced by anger, crying, withdrawal, preoccupation, anxiety, hostility, or apathy.

Etiologies

Loss (e.g., of wellness, body part or function, fetus, or family member).

Separation from religious or cultural ties.

Challenges to belief and value system (e.g., due to moral or ethical implications of therapy, intense suffering).

Pain.

Planning and Implementation of Care

The effectiveness of intervention in the spiritual distress of patients depends to a large extent on the quality of the relationship between nurse and patient. Multiple factors influence the interaction and apply equally to both participants: age, spiritual growth and development, state of mind, belief system (including atheistic or agnostic belief), recent experience, values, culture, and stress levels, to name just a few. A clear knowledge of the patient's cultural values will be enhanced by ongoing exploration of transcultural caring practices. Remember, however, that each patient will have a different set of values and beliefs.

Human beings need to be able to express their unique needs and ask for spiritual support based upon their unique perspective of the world. As nurses, we are challenged to help patients meet their needs for prayer, meditation, or supportive visitors. We do not need to feel responsible for helping patients pray or read spiritual literature in a way that conflicts with our own values, but we do need to find support for our patients.

General Guidelines The following discussion of spiritual needs and practices is presented to assist with some guidelines for meeting the self-identified spiritual needs of the patient.

- Communicate acceptance of the patient's spiritual needs and acknowledge their importance.

- Express a willingness to assist and cooperate with religious practices not detrimental to anyone's health or to the treatment setting, including the need for privacy. (Experience teaches us to remind patients that no fires or spilling of large quantities of water are allowed in the critical-care areas because of nearby equipment and oxygen.)

- Contact an appropriate spiritual leader or community if the patient wants assistance in conducting his or her usual rituals. Frequently, people assume that members of their spiritual community know that they have been hospitalized. Notifying the community ensures that the person will not be overlooked inadvertently.

- If the patient asks about your personal beliefs or values, first clarify the reason for the question with the patient. Often, patients will ask about your values, when in fact they are looking for an opportunity to explore and verbalize their own situation. If you do share your own beliefs, be brief, because a distressed patient may view this sharing as an intrusion.

- Do not feel that you should or ought to do things in conflict with your own philosophy. Delegate or reassign support for your patients, if appropriate. For example, a Christian nurse who has great difficulty reading from literature with a non-Christian theology or who finds it impossible to pray with non-Christian patients should call someone else to meet his or her patients' needs.

- Occasionally, patients' values and religious beliefs conflict with the policies and practices within the health-care system. When such conflicts occur, encourage assembly of the patient's usual support group; provide a private area when possible. Alert your institution's ethics committee and other appropriate administrators. Some interventions can include specialists in bloodless procedures. Usually, senior members of the patient's community can provide resources; for example, the Hispanic community, Native American Indian Councils, and Asian communities can assist in some cases. It may be helpful to develop institutional guidelines or policies for assisting with patients who refuse treatment. Ethics committees may be quite helpful in drafting guidelines if none are available.

Spiritual Artifacts We need to respect and support the use of artifacts integral to the spiritual comforting of our patients. Some patients will want a book, such as the *Bible, Torah, Koran,* or *Bhagavad-Gita,* or a piece of jewelry, such as a rosary, cross, or pendant. Bradley, the patient described in the story below, needed something more. He taught us how to help him establish his best prayer environment. He believed that the prayer wheels made him strong and fruit fed the spirits of ancestors who were watching over him.

On Empathy: Caring as an Affect

I remember Bradley; he had Duchenne's dystrophy and was severely disabled and contracted, but he was great fun—intelligent, witty, a fabulous chess player, and a worldly scholar with several books to his credit.

When I met him, he was in our ED in respiratory arrest. On a previous admission he had requested that he not be intubated, but the paramedics had no choice when Chris called 911. We were able to clear his pneumonia and extubate him.

Brad's tidal volumes were very low during the day and when he was discharged, he went home to sleep in an iron lung at night. His discharge teaching included use of an iron lung—don't think that wasn't a clinical specialist's challenge in 1985. (The literature was virtually void of nursing experiences with the iron lung; they had been purged to the archives 20 years earlier.) His tidal volumes were insufficient during the day to keep him from developing pneumonia. . . . He did well in his lung with regular home visits to check night-time oxygen saturation and tidal volumes. When he came to the hospital, he came with the lung, three electric prayer wheels, an altar, and "unauthorized flowers and fruit." We all knew the "rules"—we had terrible preexistent iatrogenic Pseudomonas and Serratia contamination problems—but Brad's spiritual needs and the physical artifacts were too important; they all stayed. If we had been required to do a code in his room it might have been different, there just wasn't room. But then we did not need room to code . . . just room to sit, to listen and to shampoo.

Brad couldn't feel anything below his clavicles as a result of a cervical spinal fracture several years earlier. He could not feel touch unless you touched his face or shampooed his hair. We did that every day. We also did the required skin care for the rest of his body. I watched his nurses touch him after identifying his lack of "feeling" in the rest of his body. We knew he had no sensation below the clavicles, but the character of our touch changed when our "hearts knew" that his face felt our touch and that "feeling touched" helped Brad feel cared for and cared about.

Nancy N. Bell RN, MN, CCRN, CEN
Critical Care/Trauma Clinical Nurse Specialist

Prayer Praying, reading, and meditating with the patient should be guided by the patient and your own ethic, theology, spirituality, and development. Prayer is very personal and every nurse needs to assert the right to make choices in this matter. You need to know what you believe and what you will and will not do.

Should you choose not to pray with the patient, tell the person you would prefer to call appropriate clergy or some other person of his or her choice. When or if you choose to accept the interaction, it is imperative that the patient's own words be used for specific personal needs. If the patient usually prays silently, do not interrupt.

The final story helps to set a model for caring practice in meeting the needs of the patient in spiritual distress.

On Praying Together: Caring as a Human Trait

I remember the nurse who cared for our daughter after she was hit by a drunk driver. We were angry. I was so confused; I wanted to take care of her but I knew I couldn't. I couldn't touch her without feeling scared. All my education and experience was useless, she was my daughter. This special nurse came to us to help to get information for Traci's history. We talked, she listened. At the end of our conversation, she asked if there was anyone that she could call to stay with us or to be close in the event we needed anything. She asked if we had a . . . how did she put that? . . . a member of the clergy, a spiritual advisor . . . no . . . she asked if we wanted someone who could help us with hope or prayer or wait with us. I would have died if she had asked us if she could call a priest. Our family never called a priest except for funerals; well, maybe a wedding or baptism. We all believed in prayer, though, and I used to pray all the time, mostly when I wanted something. It gave me hope. I guess I got busy and stopped, but I asked her to pray with us. She said yes, almost as if she did it every day, it was nothing extraordinary. She asked us what that prayer might be like for us. I felt awkward until she asked what would Traci want us to pray for, and I knew instantly. We prayed that she would be free from pain, and that the Lord (we're Christians) would heal her leg. I remember she held my hand and I felt so safe. She asked me again if there was someone I would like to call; again I said no. I went home to call my sister for the first time in five years. We had had a falling out but I needed her now and I missed her. That nurse prayed with us when we asked. We don't know if she was a Christian, Jew, or Moslem; it didn't matter. She helped us reunite our family and begin to see our life with Christ in a new way that has helped me every day of Traci's rehabilitation. Oh, Traci's just fine now. She still can't balance her checkbook, but she couldn't before her accident. Her leg is just fine; she rides her bike about 12 miles a day now and has a 25-mile marathon scheduled for later this year.

Anonymous RN, mother

This is an important story for nurses who want to facilitate and enable autonomy in prayer when their per-

sonal type of prayer may sound quite different. There may be a dissonance with this "generic" approach to bedside prayer; however, each person will take what he or she needs from the interaction and the attitude with which it is offered.

Patients Without Specific Spiritual or Religious Preferences The following discussion concerns techniques that can be used with those patients who do not have or choose not to express a specific spirituality or religious preference. These techniques have been included because they are caring practices or interventions that have to do with spirituality in the most existential way. They may help the patient create a more positive mental attitude in much the same way that prayer may facilitate hope, grace, and peace for those who believe in its use.

- For patients without formal religious preference several interventions may be very helpful in fostering a sense of well-being establishing meaning for their illness, and providing some distraction and comfort. These include humor; relaxation, guided imagery (Dossey 1988, 1991); and touch and massage (Krieger 1979).

- Music may be very helpful for all patients. The patient and/or family members should participate in assessment and planning. Effects often noted include decreased restlessness and/or increased positive imagery in patients who are confused (Dossey 1988). It may be helpful to encourage family members to bring the patient a personal tape player and tapes which have familiar sounds and voices from home.

Outcome Evaluation

Carpenito (1991) suggests these criteria as indicators for the effectiveness of spiritual interventions:

- Cardiac output increases or decreases to optimum level.

- Restlessness, anger, and fear are decreased or eliminated.

- Patient expresses feelings of peace and comfort or connectedness.

- Patient continues spiritual practices not detrimental to health.

- Patient expresses decreasing feelings of anxiety and guilt.

- Patient expresses satisfaction with spiritual condition.

Conclusion

Caring is not unique to nursing. We can see caring in the teachers who educate our children, the physical therapists who assist with rehabilitation, and the physicians with whom we practice. Our challenge, as scientists, is to describe the impact of nurse caring on patient outcome. If caring does not permeate the task performance, the outcome will not be the same. Parceling out aspects of patient care to various team members undoubtedly has contributed to the increasing dissatisfaction and impotence expressed by patients. Just as the child who is warm and nourished often will fail to thrive without touch and caring, the critically ill adult will not survive without hope, touch, and caring provided by critical-care nurses.

REFERENCES

Bell N: Letter to the editor. *Nurseweek* 1991; (Jan) 7:19.

Benner P: *From novice to expert: Excellence and power in clinical nursing practice.* Menlo Park, CA: Addison-Wesley, 1984.

Benner P, Wrubel J: *The primacy of caring: Stress and coping in health and illness.* Menlo Park, CA: Addison-Wesley, 1989.

Bevis, E.: Caring: A life force. In M. Leininger (Ed.), *Caring: An essential human need. Proceedings of Three National Caring Conferences.* Thorofare, NJ: C. Slack, 1981; 49–59.

Carpenito L: *Handbook of nursing diagnosis.* Philadelphia: Lippincott, 1991.

Carson V: *Spiritual dimensions of nursing practice.* Philadelphia: Saunders, 1989.

Dossey B: *Holistic nursing: A handbook for practice.* Rockville, MD Aspen, 1988.

Dossey B: Awakening the inner healer. *Am J Nurs* 1991; 91(8):31–34.

Drew N: Exclusion and confirmation: A phenomenology of patients' experiences with caregivers. *Image* 1986; 18(1):39–43.

Gadow S: Nurse and patient: The caring relationship. In *Caring, curing, coping: Nurse, physician, patient relationships.* Bishop A, Scudder J (eds). Birmingham: University of Alabama Press, 1985:31–43.

Harper J: *Surveillance.* Submitted for publication, unpublished paper, University of California, San Francisco, 1992.

Horner, S: Intersubjective co-presence in a caring model. In *Caring and nursing explorations in the feminist perspective.* Denver, CO: Center for Human Caring, University of Colorado Health Sciences Centre, 1988; 166–180.

Knowlden, V: Nurse caring as constructed knowledge. In *Caring and nursing explorations in the feminist perspective.* Denver, CO: Center for Human Caring, University of Colorado Health Sciences Centre, 1988; 318–339.

Krieger D: *The therapeutic touch: How to use your hands to help or heal.* Englewood Cliffs, NJ: Prentice Hall, 1979.

Larson P: Comparison of cancer patients and professional nurses' perceptions of important nurse caring behaviors. *Heart Lung* 1987; 16(1): 187–192.

Larson, P: Important nurse caring behaviors perceived by patients with cancer. *Oncology Nursing Forum,* 1984; 11(6):46–50.

Leininger M: Caring: The essence and central focus of nursing. In *The phenomenon of caring, Part V.* American Nurses' Foundation, Nursing Research Report 1977; (Feb) 77:2–14.

Leininger, M: Leininger's theory of nursing: Cultural care diversity and universality. *Nursing Science Quarterly,* 1988; 1:152–160.

Leininger, M: The phenomenon of caring: Importance, research questions and theoretical considerations. In M. Leininger (Ed.), *Caring: An essential human need.* Thorofare, NJ: C. Slack, 1981; 3–16.

Mayer D: Cancer patients' and families' perceptions of nurse caring behaviors. *Top Clin Nurs* 1986; 8:63–69.

Morse J et al.: Comparative analysis of conceptualizations and theories of caring. *Image* 1991; 23(2):119–126.

Noddings N: *Caring: A feminine approach to ethics and moral education.* Berkeley: University of California Press, 1984.

North American Nursing Diagnosis Association: *Proceedings of the Ninth Conference. Approved Nursing Diagnostic Categories.* Philadelphia: Lippincott, 1991.

Orem, D: *Nursing: Concepts of practice.* Chevy Chase, MD: McGraw-Hill, 1985.

Pettigrew J: Intensive care nursing: The ministry of presence. *Critical Care Nurs* 1990; 2(3):503–508.

Reiman D: Noncaring and caring in the clinical setting: Patients' descriptions. *Top Clin Nurs* 1986; 8:30–36.

Shaffer J: Spiritual distress and critical illness. *Crit Care Nurse* 1991; 11(1):42–45.

Swanson-Kauffman, K: Caring needs of women who miscarried. In M. Leininger (Ed.), *Care discovery and uses in clinical and community nursing.* Detroit, MI: Wayne State University Press, 1988; 55–70.

Watson J: *Nursing: Human science and human care: A theory of nursing.* Norwalk, CT: Appleton-Century-Crofts, 1985.

Watson, J.: *Nursing: Human science and human care. A theory of nursing.* New York: National League for Nursing, 1988.

3

Dimensions in Critical Care

CLINICAL INSIGHT

Domain: The helping role
Competency: Presencing: being with a patient

Ethical dilemmas, especially those related to impending death, are a poignant part of critical-care nursing. Although ICU nurses are committed to making the culturally avoided subject of death approachable, the ethical dilemmas surrounding death in the ICU can be wrenching. In the following paradigm, from Crabtree and Jorgenson (1986), pp. 110–111), Chris, a nurse, reflects on a situation in which a family is paralyzed over whether to discontinue ventilatory support. The patient, a male, has had respiratory disease for over 30 years and multiple hospitalizations. After being transferred out of the unit, he suffers a cardiac arrest and is returned to the unit brain-dead.

When I finally took him as a primary nurse, because I knew this man needed to be allowed to die,

and there was an impasse between the family and the physician, the family was angry at the physicians and wouldn't speak to them. I didn't know much more about it than that. I looked in the chart, and it was plainly evident why the family was unwilling to speak with the physicians that day he arrested; when the family came back and said, "Why did you move him out? Why did you do this?", the resident told the family, and recorded a note in the chart, that this family was totally unrealistic. They should have understood from the day he was admitted to this hospital that there was very little we could offer him. And that . . . and this was what the resident said . . . that he was unable to help himself in any way; he was too weak to feed himself, too weak to breathe on his own, and this family should have known from the start that he was terminal.

Fighting to honor the patient's previously expressed wish to die naturally, Chris makes concerted efforts to improve communication between the family and the medical staff. One daughter strongly resists discontinuing ventilatory support—and after lengthy discussion with her, Chris discovers why. Chris's attempts to draw out this daughter reveal a powerful reason for the daughter's resistance.

She said, look, the reason why I can't stop this ventilator, why I can't say, go ahead and do this, is because my father's suffered for 30 years with a disease where he couldn't breathe. His father was hanged, and he talked many times with me about how he couldn't bear the thought of dying for lack of air, because that's the way his father died. She said, I am not going to agree to stop a ventilator. So that was the basic issue. That was why this woman was holding out. I had no idea. I had no idea about any of this. And, everybody else just thought she was being unreasonable. Because they had been, at a certain time, unreasonable in the past. But, nobody had any idea that there was some promise between father and daughter.

This insight provokes considerable soul-searching for Chris, following which she is able to use compassion and wisdom to resolve the impasse:

So, then I had to rethink my whole position on this thing, because I was arguing that it's unethical to prolong the death and suffering of a dying person. Which is a reasonable argument. But, on the other hand, there's a very good chance that this man wasn't suffering; this patient wasn't suffering. And, yet, stopping the ventilator would cause an enormous amount of suffering for the daughter. Well, in that case, it seems much less reasonable to stop the ventilator on the patient when we could do all sorts of other things, like stopping all labs and all other kinds of treatment, and put the patient on at least morphine and Valium or some combination like that, so we were certain he wasn't suffering, and let him go.

In the intensive care unit (ICU), advanced technology gives us the power to view death as a symptom—to be treated and reversed when possible—rather than as a life event (Crabtree and Jorgenson, p. 189). But with this power comes terrible knowledge, for we nurses have seen the consequences of defying death. Assisting patients and families to experience death in a way meaningful to them is an act of grace and mercy.

This chapter examines many of the threads that make up the tapestry of life and death in the intensive care unit: the critical-care environment, the patient and family, the changing role of the nurse, and the ethical and legal issues that define the care we administer. All of these threads are integrated and illuminated in the concluding section, which uses the example of organ donation.

The Critical-Care Environment

The explosion of biomedical technology in the second half of the twentieth century has created the environment of the critical-care unit, a specialized unit viewed as the ultimate site for delivery of the "best" in acute life-saving health care. This environment is successful not only because of its technology but also because of the expertise of its nursing staff and other members of the health-care team.

The specific functions of critical-care units are as variable as the hospitals in which they exist. The nursing staffs of these units, which range from the small units in a primary community hospital to the large, multiple units in a major tertiary-care facility, are responsible for care of the critically ill patient who requires both constant surveillance and multiple technically sophisticated interventions.

Hospitals increasingly have designated subspecialty critical-care units (e.g., cardiac, neurologic, general surgical, trauma, medical) with subspecialized nursing staffs. The type of patients admitted to these various critical-care units depends on specific facility criteria, which may consider such variables as patient diagnosis, age, individual physician practice, community standards, bed availability, and nursing staff availability (both within the critical-care unit and elsewhere in the hospital). Thus, patients may be admitted for observation and surveillance of their primary medical condition or its complications, care and treatment of an acute illness or injury, postoperative care (routine or for complications), or delivery of specialized technologic monitoring or treatment.

The physical environment of a critical-care unit is also as variable as the hospital itself. In general, however, the critical-care unit is isolated behind closed doors with multiple cubicles placed around a central nursing station. The cubicles may be separated by either walls or curtains. Even when walls exist between patients' beds, the front of each cubicle either has no door or has a clear glass wall or door that allows the nursing staff easy and immediate visibility of the patient. Critical-care units are often noisy, due to the function and alarms of multiple monitors and ventilators as well as the sounds made during the normal work of multiple staff, including the ringing of the telephone. Lights are constantly left on, both in patient cubicles and in other areas of the unit, to allow for ongoing observation and performance of work. These physical aspects of the environment have been implicated as the cause of "ICU psychosis," a syndrome characterized by the patient's apparent loss of contact with time or place and/or hallucinations. This syndrome, still poorly understood, will be discussed more completely in a later section.

Finally, the critical-care unit has a specific ancillary area which is a vital extension: the family waiting room, with its telephone communication into the unit, as well as a public telephone by which the family can remain in touch with others. This part of the critical-care environment has special impact on both families of patients and the nursing staff. It easily can create feelings of hostility and isolation in the family, as it separates them from their loved one. Nurses may see it as a necessary barrier that allows patients to rest and provides privacy during invasive procedures and personal care. The interactions between the family and staff can be either positive or negative depending on how communication between them is established and maintained.

The Critical-Care Patient

While the patient population admitted to critical-care units may be influenced by the factors previously outlined, nurses can also identify potential clients by understanding the community that the hospital serves. The location of an individual hospital may determine who becomes a patient in the critical-care unit. Is the community that the hospital serves primarily a young adult population or an elderly population? Age of patient population also predicts the nature of illness; younger patients are more likely to suffer from an acute illness or injury, whereas older patients are more likely to be hospitalized with a combination of acute and chronic illness or with complications of a chronic illness.

In addition to the aging of the United States population, other demographic factors in an individual community define the population receiving care in the hospital's critical-care units. Such factors include socioeconomic status, ethnicity, immigration status, primary language spoken, and the cultural beliefs of the patients that the hospital serves.

Critical-care units in specialty hospitals and/or tertiary-care facilities serve a different patient population than do community facilities. Hospitals which carry out clinical research protocols may also serve a different critical-care patient population with unique diseases and different care requirements.

The extension of life of patients suffering from chronic illnesses may also affect the patient population admitted to the critical-care unit. As medical knowledge is employed to maintain the lives of these individuals, disease or illness' acute episodes or complications may bring these patients to the critical-care unit repeatedly. New units are being organized to provide care to this population, which is different from other critical-care patients. A unit for these "chronically critically ill" patients was described as having limited technology and focusing on family involvement and patient rehabilitation (Daly et al. 1991). With some variations in nursing organization, this design appears to be similar to other step-down (intermediate-care) units which receive patients from a critical-care setting.

As noted in the introductory vignette, terminally ill patients often are transferred from the critical-care unit to other hospital units or even to other facilities for continued care, even though they may still require high-technology care and monitoring. Thus, a new definition of patient appropriateness for critical care may be not the need for high-technology care, which may be provided in other settings, but rather the potential for recovery.

Patient Responses to the ICU

The proportion of patients who suffer sensory disturbances in critical-care units is uncertain. Some reports of postcardiotomy patients reveal the occurrence of sensory disturbances, usually classified as "ICU psychosis." Very little research has been performed to measure this phenomenon. A classic experimental study by Downs (1974) provides some information about the ICU environment. She placed 180 normal subjects between the ages of 18 and 35 on bedrest for 2¾ hours in a room that simulated a semi-private hospital room to measure the effects of personality and varied auditory input on cardiovascular function, motor activity, and time perception. A serendipitous finding was that 20% of the subjects experienced sensory distortions including odors, falling objects, body distortion and floating sensations, and changes in the environment in regard to temperature, light, and sound. Finally, they reported being bored, unable to concentrate, and irritated because of aimless thinking.

The environment of the critical-care unit (light, sounds, activity, and strange equipment), as previously described, is even more stressful than the environment described by Downs, which led to disorientation in a short time.

As critical-care nurses, we can maintain our patient's sensory stimuli and orientation in a number of ways:

1. Introduce yourself and your functions; describe what tasks you will be doing, even if you will not be touching the patient.

2. Establish a pattern of activities and a schedule for the patient; describe that pattern and review it with the patient.

3. Orient the patient and family to the unit, its equipment, and its schedule.

4. Keep clocks and calendars in the patient's room or cubicle to maintain a sense of time.

5. Minimize unnecessary stimuli. Decrease monitor sounds in the room if possible, dim lights when activities are not being performed, and decrease other noises such as ringing telephones, paging systems, door buzzers, etc.

6. Decrease conversations with others in the patient's field of hearing. To prevent the patient from overhearing conversations or interpreting them incorrectly, avoid gathering with other staff inside or outside the room or cubicle. Even when caring for the comatose or otherwise noncommunicative patient, do not hold conversations in the patient's presence, whether they relate to the patient's condition or other professional or personal matters.

7. Allow the patient to have personal items. Eyeglasses and hearing aids are critical to processing visual and auditory stimuli for many patients. Restricting their use may lead to sensory distortion and disorientation.

While most reports of patients' critical-care experiences are singular or anecdotal, Compton (1991) interviewed ten patients in depth about their experience in the ICU to determine what critical illness and the ICU experience mean to the patient. While this sample is small, the findings of these unstructured interviews give us some updated information about patient perceptions.

These patients ranged in age from 19 to 68 years and were hospitalized in critical-care units for 2–10 days in three different facilities. All suffered from acute medical problems rather than being placed in the critical-care unit following scheduled surgery or hospitalization. Significantly, most patients remembered very little about their stay in the ICU but did recall feeling very tired and energy-depleted. They described the medical and nursing interventions as being bothersome but not especially anxiety-provoking. In addition,

they reported that they felt very safe and well-protected in the ICU; they felt that they had handed themselves over to the staff for care. They were aware of assessing their own medical status by comparing themselves to other patients and by "reading" the reactions of the staff and their own families. Patients also reported that they did not think about or reflect on their experiences after leaving the critical-care unit; they apparently did not feel the need to interpret it as a significant event. Importantly, none of these patients reported having any sensory changes (deprivation or overload). In fact, all of them reported that they slept through most of their ICU stay.

Compton's research raises some major questions about the patient in the critical-care unit. Do her results reflect the experience of patients today? Have the problems previously observed and reported been resolved? Compton suggests that there may be dissonance between the observations of the health care professionals and the perception of the patients in regard to the various psychologic aspects of the ICU environment. Does a shortened length of stay influence the patient's perception of the critical-care environment? What other specific variables of patient condition or treatment alter his or her perception of the unit and the care being given? Has the public's general education about health care also diminished the patient's anxiety about the ICU environment? It is certainly evident that much more study of patients' perceptions as well as nurses' observations is needed to determine the effect of the critical-care environment and the care patients receive there on their total experience and recovery.

Patient and Family Communication

The clinical insight at the beginning of this chapter is rich in issues confronting the critical-care nurse. One of these issues, which often creates both stress and satisfaction for the critical-care nurse, is that of communication with the patient and the patient's family.

Communication is the dynamic, multisensory interaction in which a person shares thoughts and feelings with other people in his or her psychosocial environment. The interaction between two persons can be simple or complex and performed in many ways. During a critical illness, the patient's communication with health professionals and family is crucial to your planning and implementation of care as well as to the patient's eventual recovery.

Communicating with the Patient   Communication consists of both process and content. The identification of both of these aspects of communication is necessary to the care of the critically ill individual. Initial assessment of the patient admitted to an ICU can identify how well that individual will be able to communicate with his or her caregivers.

The patient's ability to communicate with staff may be intact or affected by an acute or chronic condition. The immediate assessment of communication ability may be undertaken by other staff prior to the patient's admission to the critical-care setting and should be emphasized in nursing reports. In addition, the family may be aware of special problems; this information should be elicited on patient admission. Also, the family can provide special techniques that may enhance effective communication with the patient.

Auditory input is usually necessary for verbal communication between people. If the person fails to respond normally to sound, a conductive or sensorineural hearing loss may be present. Such losses are due to transport of sound to the middle ear or to the inner ear's inability to transmit sound energy to the brain. If the patient has a hearing loss which predates hospitalization, the person may communicate via sign language, reading lips, or by wearing hearing aid(s). The patient with a hearing aid should be allowed to use it in the ICU so that he or she can communicate in the normal fashion.

Visual input is also important to communication. Vision assists in communication by allowing the individual to assess his or her environment, visualize the others involved in the communication process, and visually perceive the emotional aspects of the communication (appearances, expressions, posture, etc.). Loss of vision (blindness) is a most profound change; when it occurs on an acute basis (secondary to accident or injury), the patient may become withdrawn or disoriented. Other visual changes may also interfere with communication. The use of corrective lenses (either eyeglasses or contact lenses) allows the individual to clearly view his or her environment and the persons in it. If visual deficits are severe, the patient may not be able to perform certain activities. The patient also may suffer from varying stages of cataract development, which compromises visual acuity. Brightly lighted or darkened environments may further compromise a patient's visual acuity. The patient admitted to the critical-care unit should be asked about visual acuity. To enhance communication, the patient who is alert to his or her environment and who normally wears glasses should wear them. A patient who is admitted acutely should be assessed for the presence of removable contact lenses either in the Emergency Department or in the ICU. To prevent corneal abrasions or ulcerations, either the patient or staff should remove contact lenses.

Special consideration of visual acuity is necessary for the elderly patient or those with other medical conditions that involve visual acuity (e.g., diabetes mellitus). Changes in blood pressure (increased or decreased) may also cause sudden changes in visual acuity; blurriness or even transient visual loss are not uncommon but may remain unreported by the critically ill patient.

Tactile perception may also play a role in communication. The patient may need to feel objects to understand their meaning or verbal description; he or she also needs to be able to feel the touch of others which may be used to express emotion. Finally, pain as a tactile perception may also be felt and expressed by the patient.

Communication is expressed by speaking, writing, and/or gesturing. Expression can be altered or diminished by a variety of physical problems or diseases. Cerebrovascular accidents resulting in expressive aphasia (inability to speak clearly), brain tumors, paralysis, or other neurologic diseases or events may interfere with or prevent the patient from verbally communicating. Laryngeal tumors and/or their resection may prevent speech. Speech complications may have occurred prior to the patient's admission to the critical-care unit or may be a part of the reason for the patient's admission.

In the critical-care setting, there are two other major reasons why a patient is unable to verbally communicate with his or her nurses and physicians: the patient may be in a comatose state, or he/she may be intubated for respiratory support. The intubated, alert patient in the critical-care unit is processing all the inputs for communication (seeing, hearing, feeling) but is unable to express his or her thoughts, feelings, or fears. One ventilator patient, a physician, later described his communication difficulties vividly (Chaney 1975):

> I was lying there on my back with the respirator humming away, when I suddenly felt a wave of nausea. I immediately knew I'd developed gastric distention and that I was vomiting and aspirating a lot of gastric fluid. Since I couldn't talk with the endotracheal tube, I frantically signaled the nurse and tried to communicate I was aspirating. She tried to reassure me that I wasn't but there was no doubt. It felt like it was at least a gallon, and I felt like I was drowning.... I still feel that had I been successful in my desperate attempts to pull the bite block and the tube out so I could vomit over the side of the bed, I would have been able to prevent much of the damage.... I just lay there waiting for my aspiration pneumonia to develop—which is exactly what happened.

An intubated patient who is paralyzed with pancuronium bromide or curare is even more limited in his or her ability to communicate. In addition to the terror of being unable to speak, this patient is also unable to move, gesture, or otherwise physically express their discomfort, pain, or fear. Without special awareness, staff may treat this patient as if he/she was comatose. This patient needs exceptional emotional support from a caring, sensitive staff and family. He/she also may benefit from sedation to blunt his or her perceptions and fears of paralysis. In addition, continued attention to pain control should remain a priority.

Finally, the stimuli given to the comatose patient deserve attention. Humanistic care mandates that we provide gentle physical care, creating minimal pain to patients. In addition, many nurses and families believe that even patients who do not appear cognitively alert may continue to integrate auditory stimuli and choose to speak to them, explaining what tasks are being performed or providing other types of auditory stimulation (e.g., music, television, recorded family messages). While some preliminary research has been done regarding auditory and tactile sensations experienced by the sedated or comatose patient, we know very little about these physiologic phenomena.

Other considerations for communication with patients suffering from input deficits (vision or hearing) include the following:

1. For the patient with visual field defects (hemianopsia), perform tasks from the patient's sighted side and teach the patient to turn his or her head to compensate for the defect.

2. Determine how the blind patient has compensated in the past and his / her preferences in interacting with the environment. Always identify yourself verbally to the visually impaired patient and describe the activities you will be performing.

3. For the hearing-impaired patient, speak slowly and directly facing the patient (particularly if he / she reads lips). Gesture to describe activities and show him or her items or equipment to enhance his / her visual understanding of procedures to be performed.

4. Assess the patient's wish for tactile comfort or stimulation; a patient may or may not wish to be touched or comforted in this manner. Confirm with family and friends what the patient's preferences are in regard to tactile stimulation.

If a patient is unable to express his or her thoughts through speech, interventions may include:

1. Paper and pencil or a magic slate for writing responses if the patient can perform such activity. Keep responses simple to minimize the patient's physical fatigue.

2. Large cards or flip-charts to identify frequently used phrases, requests, or questions.

3. Eye motion or blinking for simple yes-no

communication when the patient has no other method of expression available because of his or her physical status.

For all communication difficulties, patience and a sense of calm during our "conversations" with the patient is essential. Acknowledging the difficulties of communication may also relieve the patient. If these problems will be short-term (i.e., intubation), assure the patient of that; if they may be longer-term, we can encourage the patient by reminding him or her that this communication process may become easier with time and technologic support or education. Constant presence or availability of a nurse is also very comforting to the patient who has difficulty or is unable to communicate verbally; it promotes a feeling of safety and security. Call systems that can be triggered with minimal movement of the head, shoulder, or mouth are also becoming increasingly available.

In United States acute care facilities, language differences may also create serious communication difficulties. If we cannot speak in the same language as our patients, special assignment of staff who are fluent in the patient's language or the use of cards with relevant foreign language and English terms (assuming that the patient can read), may resolve some communication problems. Family members may also be able to assist in adequate communication between patient and staff.

Communicating with the Family A review of the critical-care nursing literature suggests that family communication and family needs are "hot" issues. The early findings of Breu and Dracup (1978) documented the losses and needs of spouses of critical-care patients. They found that these spouses were concerned about the following issues:

1. Threat of their mate's death.
2. Deprivation of their primary source of social contact, gratification, and self-esteem.
3. Interruption of all daily routines, including eating and sleeping.
4. Sudden role reversal.
5. Involuntary independence.
6. Disruption of social contacts.
7. Financial instability.
8. Disturbed system of interpersonal rewards.
9. Relocation to a strange environment for most of the day.

Bedsworth and Molen (1982) identified similar types of threats faced by spouses of myocardial infarction patients. While these findings have been widely cited and used as a theoretical basis for interventions, one should also recognize that findings are fairly sex-specific (female spouses) and reflect a very different era of treatment and outcome of myocardial infarction.

More general studies of family needs done by Molter (1979), Daley (1984), and Leske (1986) have validated the ranking of 30 of these needs (Table 3–1). Such needs, expressed on multiple occasions by family of critical-care patients, are neither unique nor difficult to satisfy. Indeed, medical, philosophic, and nursing literature identify these needs as basic human rights. If we nurses were to experience being a family member of a critical-care patient, we would wish for the same needs to be met.

Communicating with families and meeting their needs are important aspects of critical-care nursing. As

such, they can become stressors that create ethical dilemmas for critical-care nurses as well as challenge their expertise. Three issues in particular confront critical-care nurses as they try to meet family needs: determining family membership, explaining visiting policies, and providing information.

While a discussion of the definition of the family in United States society is beyond the scope of this chapter, it is clear that family membership continues to be characterized by changing relationships. Thus, the question of what the term "immediate family" means to the individual patient becomes important. Generally, it is defined as including only blood relationships (parents, sisters and brothers, or offspring) or legal marital relationships (married spouses). The critical-care nurse, often asked to serve as a "gatekeeper" to visitor access, may well wonder what identification is required. As emotional, non-legal relationships between adults have become increasingly recognized as being important to one's well-being, the extension of visiting privileges to individuals seems only appropriate. However, doing so would violate the strictest definition of family which exists in some hospitals.

After withstanding the stress of determining who might be allowed to visit the patient, the critical-care nurse is confronted with deciding when and for how long. If the purpose of visiting the critical-care patient is to be updated on his or her current medical condition, a brief visit, rather like an inspection, is probably sufficient. If the family's purpose for visiting is to provide emotional support and comfort during the period of critical illness, more extended visits are essential. Multiple studies have reached conflicting conclusions about the stress of visitation on critically ill patients. Does it cause them greater or lesser stress? Is a visit of limited duration more stressful than a longer one would be? In Compton's (1991) sample, patients reported that they were more concerned about the well-being of their families than they were about their own condition. What role does this worry play in the patient's outcome, and what kind of visitation arrangements would minimize it? If nurses believe that knowing the patient's history is important to planning and implementing their care, should this history be obtained from the patient and family during more extended visiting times? Should families be allowed to observe the nursing care administered to patients during their visits or should they always be asked to leave? Consider that some of the most important family needs in the sample concerned the quality of patient's care, especially the need to be assured that the patient was cared for. Perhaps the direct observation of nursing care would satisfy this need well. Would families be better able to make decisions about

---

TABLE 3–1

Needs of Family Members

1. To feel there is hope.
2. To have questions answered honestly.
3. To know the prognosis.
4. To know specific facts concerning the patient's progress.
5. To have explanations given in terms that are understandable.
6. To receive information about the patient once a day.
7. To be called at home about changes in the patient's condition.
8. To feel that the hospital personnel care about the patient.
9. To see the patient frequently.
10. To know why things were done for the patient.
11. To have the waiting room near the patient.
12. To be assured that the best care possible is being given to the patient.
13. To know exactly what is being done for the patient.
14. To know how the patient is being treated medically.
15. To visit at any time.
16. To have visiting hours changed for special conditions.
17. To have a place to be alone in the hospital.
18. To feel accepted by the hospital staff.
19. To have explanations of the environment before going into the critical-care unit for the first time.
20. To talk about negative feelings, such as guilt and anger.
21. To have directions regarding what to do at the bedside.
22. To have visiting hours start on time.
23. To be told about transfer plans while they are being made.
24. To be assured it is all right to leave the hospital for a while.
25. To talk to the doctors every day.
26. To be alone at any time.
27. To have friends nearby for support.
28. To be encouraged to cry.
29. To talk about the possibility of the patient's death.
30. To have a telephone near the waiting room.

From Molter N: Needs of relatives of critically ill patients: a descriptive study. *Heart Lung* 1979; 8:332–339.

continuation or discontinuation of treatment if they had directly observed that treatment for more extended periods of time? Finally, should visiting times be different for patients with different acuity levels? Should families of terminally ill patients be allowed to spend more time with them and to remain at the bedside until death occurs?

Information about the patient's status is a major concern for families. How do critical-care nurses perceive their role in providing such information? Several reports indicate that staff nurses in critical-care feel that the physician staff or the clinical nurse specialist in the facility should inform family of the patient's status. Nurses have reported that they feel uncomfortable about their ability to interpret and provide such information. Younger, less experienced critical-care nurses especially may be unable to perform this task. However, the necessary skills can be obtained through preceptorship and additional staff education.

The role of critical-care nurses in meeting the needs of the family group is an increasingly important challenge. The integration of this aspect of nursing into nursing practice results in a more holistic approach to patient care.

The Nurse in Critical Care

Critical-care nurses work on the cutting edge of technologic developments in acute medical care. The development and implementation of life-saving equipment and procedures occur routinely in the critical-care setting. These technologic advances and changes require that critical-care nurses be flexible in their practice and able to quickly integrate such advances into their knowledge base and skills. Because our technologies are so diverse, we have witnessed the subspecialization of critical-care nurses, who have become expert practitioners in areas such as coronary care, open heart surgery, burn care, and trauma.

Satisfactions of Critical-Care Nursing

Critical-care nursing is intellectually and emotionally demanding. To provide care to desperately ill, unstable patients successfully, the nurse must have a more extensive base of scientific knowledge and be more technologically astute than at any previous time. The opportunity to exercise intellectual skills and receive recognition for them is satisfying. In addition, many nurses thrive in the fast-paced atmosphere of the critical-care unit. The very intensity of the experience is thrilling, and the opportunity to help save someone's life can be profoundly satisfying.

In a 1988 readership survey conducted by *Critical Care Nurse* (Alspach 1988), 39% of the nurses responding indicated that they "enjoyed the challenge" of working in the ICU, especially the challenge of caring for complex and seriously ill patients and having frequent learning experiences. In addition, they reported that the lower nurse-patient ratios and the chance to perform bedside nursing in a holistic manner were also reasons that they remained in critical care.

Stresses of Critical-Care Nursing

The practice of critical-care nursing may exact a price, however. The sources and impact of stress on the critical-care nurse have been the subjects of study for over a decade. In spite of much study and recommendations for resolution, nurses report that they continue to feel stress and suffer from "burnout" leading to multiple job changes and even to leaving the field of nursing.

When Gentry and Parkes (1982) published a classic perspective on stress recognition and management in critical-care nursing, they determined that although study of this problem had become more empirical than anecdotal, it had provided few, if any, answers about the real causes of stress and how to resolve it. Bailey et al. (1980) performed one of the early studies of stress in critical-care nurses. Their study of 1,800 ICU nurses determined that the greatest stressors were management of the unit, interpersonal relationships, and patient care. Using these findings in a smaller study and additionally addressing the question of whether stress is greater for ICU nurses than for non-ICU nurses, Vincent and Coleman (1986) studied the nursing staff at a single institution. Their data indicated that management of the unit and interpersonal relations (conflicts) are the leading problems for both ICU and non-ICU nurses.

Such interpersonal conflicts are generic to the nursing profession and emanate from the historical structure and function of nursing in the hospital setting (Ashley 1976; Jervik and Martinson 1979). In the critical-care setting, interpersonal conflicts may be intensified by the relatively closed environment and the smaller number of staff working together. According to Mendenhall (1982), lack of control or effectiveness contributes to the stresses of interpersonal conflicts. Issues of decision-making, autonomy, responsibility, feeling needed and helpful, and recognition and respect from others all relate to the nurse's self-esteem and self-actualization. Christopherson (1986) discussed these stressors within the context of control and power in the critical-care setting. She encouraged the nurse to be self-reflective in identifying the extent of control that he or she needs to reduce stresses or resolve conflicts in the critical-care setting.

Robinson and Lewis (1990) have also quantified some of the stressors which may be affecting critical-care nurses. Their study of 577 ICU nurses working in Veterans' Administration hospitals found that the stressors which these nurses identified as occurring frequently or being the most severe included a lack of reward, the crisis atmosphere, and the experience level of medical residents. In addition, shift rotation, clinical nurse–nursing administration relationships, crowded work space, frequent negative feedback, and too much responsibility also ranked highly as stressors.

To completely understand and resolve the stress of unit management and interpersonal relations, we may have to change the structure and function of nursing and even that of women in the workplace. Burnout is not an exclusive problem of ICU nurses; it is shared by many in the workplace. Freudenberger and North's (1985) research on burnout in women provided significant information to all nurses at risk for job-related stress or burnout. They identified several general risk factors, such as being taken for granted as the "resident" nurturer, feeling alone and lonely, having a sense of powerlessness about one's professional and personal life, and being frustrated by notions of autonomy and dependency.

Stress and Staff Shortages

Our discussion of stress and stressors would be incomplete without a discussion of staff shortages, staff turnover, and job dissatisfaction. The real or perceived shortage of nursing staff in acute care facilities extends into critical-care units. While the problem of staffing shortages varies from facility to facility and in specific areas of the United States, it is an obvious cause of stress when it occurs. The *Critical Care Nurse* survey (Alspach 1988) identified understaffing as the second most important reason for nurses leaving critical-care setting. Benner (1984) has noted that the need to work with temporary or inexperienced staff alters the quality of care that nurses give to their patients, limits their coping strategies, and decreases the work satisfaction they are able to enjoy. The nurses interviewed by Benner said that they felt they had little time for reflection and were performing only "emergency nursing"—that their own learning and growth had stopped. These observations are shared and analyzed by Prescott (1989), who noted that shortage problems are not solved simply by substituting nurses, and that "inexperienced staff members sent to help may place a greater burden on the regular staff than would be felt without any assistance." Numerous methods and interventions have been suggested and implemented to decrease staff turnover in critical-care units. Improved salaries, changes in the organization of nursing practice to resolve administrative conflicts, and innovative scheduling of staff all have been used to assist in retention of nursing staff.

Another important source of stress for the critical-care nurse relates to expertise and excellence in practice, for example, the stress and anxiety experienced by the critical-care novice. Mastering skills and developing expert knowledge and practice greatly reduce stress in the critical-care setting. Benner's (1984) work has provided us with much information about the development of expert practice. In particular, the continuing mastery of the ever-changing technology of the critical-care unit does much to reduce the stress experienced by the practicing nurse.

Finally, the role that patient death plays in creating stress for the critical-care nurse is poorly understood. Gardner et al. (1980) suggested that high mortality rates in critical-care units presented staff with repetitive losses without giving the staff time to "mourn the loss of a former patient to whom they have become attached emotionally." Based on that observation, staff members at the Washington Hospital Center in Washington, D.C. organized sessions called "Timeout," which gave staff a special time to deal with patient death (Richmond and Craig 1985). Similar approaches have been employed in critical-care units throughout the United States. The *Critical Care Nurse* survey (Alspach 1988) did not identify high mortality rates or patient deaths in the critical-care unit as influencing nurses' level of satisfaction with their work. Robinson and Lewis (1990) also found that only 8.1% of their subjects reported that they felt exposure to death and dying was a frequent or severe cause of work-related stress.

Stress-Reduction Mechanisms

Individually identifying the stressors in one's own professional practice and ways to resolve them are essential to success as a person and a nurse. For example, nurses who work to prevent or resolve staff shortage problems may alleviate a major source of stress. According to Gentry and Parkes (1982), "if adequate staffing is maintained, nurses are able to take all other frustrations in their stride."

As with everyone else, critical-care nurses benefit from identifying the source of stresses in their lives. If they arise from your personal life, individual methods of resolution may be needed; the work setting cannot be considered responsible for creating such stresses. However, the intimate relationship of your work and personal life may make it difficult to determine which stress leads to another—a personal problem may lead to work stress, or a work-related problem may lead to stress in personal life. If you find that your stress is due to the work environment and activities, professional support and collegiality can be used as a buffer and may provide a supportive environment in which to discuss and resolve shared problems. According to Robinson and Lewis' (1990) study, over half of their respondents reported that they discussed problems with their coworkers; another 38% reported that they used problem-solving techniques as their coping mechanism. The other coping mechanisms were personal ones which the authors classified as either adaptive (e.g., hobbies) or maladaptive (e.g., overeating).

Institutional interventions and changes may be required to reduce stress for staff in the critical-care unit. Professionals must be able to work together to implement changes such as altering work schedules (for example, 10–12-hour days), not splitting days off (to allow for adequate recovery from work-related stress), utilizing effective methods of nurse staffing (either rotating assignments or primary-care assignments depending on which will better reduce stress), and setting up special staff conferences and programs to deal with both the stress experienced and the causes for the stress.

Critical-care nurses suffering from work-related stress are not solely responsible for resolving these problems. Managers and administrators must be aware of the stressors affecting nursing practice; different management techniques such as primary nursing, decentralized administration, and collaborative practice methods have been employed successfully to decrease stress and enhance professional nursing practice.

Ethics: Principles and Dilemmas

The delivery of health care traditionally has been directed by ethical principles. From the time of Hippocrates, certain ethical principles have influenced both medical care and nursing care. During the latter half of the twentieth century, however, increasing attention has been paid to ethics in health care. A new term, *bioethics,* has been coined to describe this new area of ethics. The explosion of interest and concern can be attributed to a number of factors, including the extension of life by the development and application of high technology, the rapidly increasing cost of medical care, and growing emphasis on one's quality of life. In addition, the delivery of medical care and the actions of practitioners are no longer private or mystical situations. The dissemination of knowledge and information in our modern world is supported by our individual and collective belief in a right to know and understand everything that affects our physical and emotional well-being; our abilities to communicate via modern communication media make information about medical advances and their utilization accessible to most people in the United States and other Westernized countries. As the public has gained this information about the state of health care, it also has been introduced to and become a part of the ethical decision-making and dilemmas that health care practitioners and our system are confronting.

The following section reviews selected ethical principles that are particularly cogent to the functions of the intensive care unit, the dilemmas that may arise from ethical conflicts, and methods by which such dilemmas may be resolved. Nurses in critical-care units have a vital role in these situations, ranging from their identification to assuring and participating in their resolution.

Ethical Principles

The principle of *beneficence* is a foundation stone of nursing practice in all settings, including the critical-care unit. *Beneficence* means that our care and actions are directed toward "doing good" (Table 3–2). Our actions are dominated by our belief that our care and interventions should be directed toward ensuring a positive outcome—saving the patient's life, relieving suffering, preventing complications. Care guided by the principle of beneficence is usually active—employing major and minor procedures that lead to a positive benefit to the patient.

The principle of *nonmaleficence* is a corollary to beneficence. *Nonmaleficence,* most simply described as "doing no harm," is the principle most commonly associated with the Hippocratic Oath. Because of that association, it traditionally has been considered the dominant principle of medical and nursing practice. This principle is defined as one of restraint or constraint; when applied to a patient situation, it may prevent the practitioner from carrying out procedures

RESEARCH NOTE

Knaus W et al.:
An evaluation of outcome from intensive care in major medical centers.
Ann Intern Med 1986; 104:410–418. (with update by Elizabeth Draper, 1992)

CLINICAL APPLICATION

Does close collaboration between physicians and nurses really improve ICU patient survival? For years, nurses believed so; this classic study actually documented the crucial impact of quality nursing care on patient outcome. The study was designed to test the validity of a simplified Acute Physiology and Chronic Health Evaluation (APACHE) in predicting risk of death; its findings about the importance of nurse–physician collaboration were serendipitous.

The researchers prospectively studied treatment and outcome in 5,030 patients in 13 tertiary-care hospitals' intensive care units. Utilizing diagnosis, treatment indication, and APACHE score, they stratified each hospital's patients by individual risk of death; then, using group results as the standard, they compared actual and predicted death rates. (Research methodology in the first step utilized a multiple logistic regression analysis; the second step utilized a multivariate logistic regression analysis, a t-test, and partial chi-square tests. The reader interested in the details of the research methodology should consult the original source.)

One hospital had a significantly lower death rate and one a signifi-

cantly higher death rate than the others ($p < 0.0001$). Further investigation revealed profound differences in the intensive care in these two hospitals. The hospital with the significantly lower death rate utilized carefully planned clinical protocols, implemented by senior physicians in the unit. Within these protocols, nurses had independent responsibilities; for example, they could cancel surgery if adequate nursing staff were not available. Primary nursing was used, and communications between nurses and physicians were ongoing and respectful. An extensive support system included comprehensive educational programs and clinical specialists with Master's degrees and extensive ICU experience.

In contrast, the hospital with the significantly higher death rate had no dedicated unit physician, centralized nursing authority, formal educational program, primary nursing, or other provision for continuity of care. Physician and nurse communication was marked by frequent disagreement and an air of distrust. Staff shortages sometimes meant that non–ICU-prepared nurses cared for patients.

The researchers considered a number of possible measurement biases but found none that would have systematically favored one hospital over another. They there-

fore concluded that the quality of nurse–physician interaction in this sample has a profound influence on patient survival in the ICUs used for the study.

CRITICAL THINKING

Limitations: This finding needed further investigation. At the completion of this original study, Elizabeth Draper, RN, a senior research scientist in the study, indicated that the researchers would carry out a major national survey to further evaluate the effect of nurse–physician interaction on patient survival. [*Am J Nurs* (March) 1987; 87:283–284.] According to Ms. Draper (personal communication, February 1992), Apache III, a study of 40 hospitals and 15,000 patients, is now complete and the results are being analyzed. This variable is included as part of the data to be analyzed from all of the participating 40 hospitals. Reports should be forthcoming soon from this study.

Strengths: This large, well-designed study has important implications for practice. If, as nurses long have "known," the quality of nurse-patient interaction profoundly influences patient survival, this study provides credibility to nurses' efforts to establish more respectful relationships between nurses and physicians to enhance collaborative practice.

that could cause harm to the patient. The way one defines *harm* becomes significant to the interpretation and application of this principle. The harm that would occur generally is interpreted as irreversible. It is associated either with a procedure where harm outweighs the benefit or negligence or malpractice on the part of the practitioner. While we often assume that doing no harm automatically means we will be benef-

icent, these two principles are not opposites. Practicing nonmaleficence only prevents harm; it does not automatically include an active beneficial process. In the critical-care setting, both principles are employed simultaneously to guide patient care.

Veracity as an ethical principle usually is known as "telling the truth." As public awareness and knowledge about health and disease have increased, our patients

TABLE 3–2

Ethical Principles

Beneficence: doing good acts.

Nonmaleficence: doing no harm.

Autonomy: an individual's right to make choices and decisions for self.

Parentalism (paternalism): actions or decisions by one individual for and in the best interests of another.

Veracity: telling the truth.

Fidelity: faithfulness to one's agreements or contracts.

Justice as Fairness: the allocation of resources to achieve equal shares or benefits to all.

---

have come to expect that they will be told the truth about illness, treatments, and the outcome of their disease or condition. The emphasis on consumerism and health care as a commodity assumes that patients are capable of making and will make choices and decisions about their care. To help them do so, the professional caregiver should provide patients with truthful information as completely as possible to the greatest extent possible.

Closely associated with the principle of veracity is the principle of *autonomy.* This modern ethical principle is defined as the individual's right and responsibility to make decisions about all aspects of his or her life to the degree that they do not violate the well-being of another. When applied to the medical setting, this principle requires that every patient has the right to make decisions about the care he or she wishes to receive. It further assumes that the patient has the right to accept or refuse care and that the patient's decision is honored (not overruled by another).

Paternalism is the principle which holds that certain individuals are better able to, and have the right to, make decisions for another. In the health care setting, this principle usually is applied to physicians but may easily include nurses as well. Paternalism (parentalism) is practiced in circumstances when we make decisions for patients in non–life-threatening situations or when we attempt to coerce or influence the patient's decision-making to meet the practitioner's objectives. Thus, the principle of paternalism is traditionally seen as conflicting with the principle of autonomy.

The principle of *fidelity* also is important in our patient relationships and care. Fidelity in health care is interpreted as meaning faithfulness to our contract for care or to achievement of outcome as it has been presented to the patient. It also means that we will meet our duties and obligations to our patients as they are agreed upon; the promises we make to patients will be kept.

The principle of *justice as fairness* is a modern ethical principle often applied to our modern health care system. The usual definition of justice as fairness means providing resources so that all will receive essentially the same level of benefit. The use of triage is the common application of this principle to individual patient situations. This principle also guides and often dominates discussions and decisions about the allocation of health care resources, equity in access to care, and delivery of care to certain groups or to all.

The existence and employment of these ethical principles in the critical-care unit does not necessarily constitute an ethical dilemma. Dilemmas are created when human beings apply differing or conflicting ethical principles in the same situation. These people can be any health care professional, the patient, any person significant to the patient, or outside agents or agencies. Determination of whether an ethical dilemma exists requires first that each person involved be clear about what is creating the conflict. This clarity requires that everyone understand his or her own set of values, which are personal and individual and arise from life experience. A majority of individuals commonly shares ethical principles; in fact, many people believe that people share ethical principles and beliefs universally. In resolving an ethical dilemma, everyone involved must understand the nature and meaning of the relevant ethical principles, regardless of whether or not these principles reflect the individual's values. Such understanding is necessary before the dominant principle to be employed in resolving the dilemma can be determined.

The actual process of ethical decision-making can be undertaken when everyone is familiar with the meaning of the ethical principles and agrees that a dilemma exists. Finally, the group involved in the decision-making should be familiar with the various theoretical methods by which to arrive at a decision.

When it is clear that a dilemma exists, there are two theoretical methods for resolution or decision-making (Figure 3–1). The *deontological method* dictates that, in any dilemma, there is only one right action that is consistent with ethical principles or rules. If conflict between ethical rules occurs, the higher-level principle dominates and determines the right action to be taken. The second ethical method is the *utilitarian approach,* which defines the problem, alternative solutions, and each alternative's consequences and happiness value (best outcome for all). The alternative with the highest value then becomes the ethically right choice. This

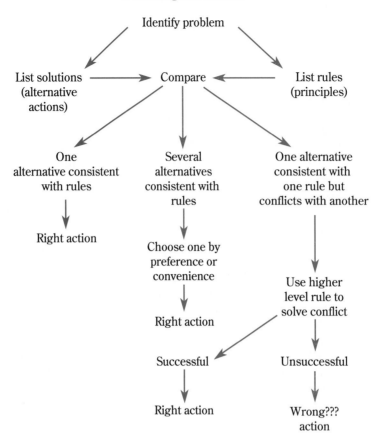

Deontological Method

Identify problem

List solutions (alternative actions) → Compare ← List rules (principles)

One alternative consistent with rules

Several alternatives consistent with rules

One alternative consistent with one rule but conflicts with another

Right action

Choose one by preference or convenience

Right action

Use higher level rule to solve conflict

Successful

Unsuccessful

Right action

Wrong??? action

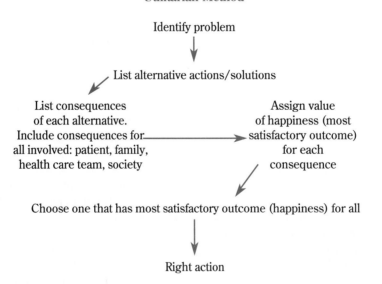

Utilitarian Method

Identify problem

List alternative actions/solutions

List consequences of each alternative. Include consequences for all involved: patient, family, health care team, society

Assign value of happiness (most satisfactory outcome) for each consequence

Choose one that has most satisfactory outcome (happiness) for all

Right action

FIGURE 3-1

Two methods of resolving ethical dilemmas. Courtesy of Susan Pfettscher, DNS, RN.

method also has been identified as "consequential" ethical theory and decision-making. (For a more complete discussion of these two methods and their variations, refer to Davis and Krueger 1980). Jonsen et al. (1982) have developed a model of ethical decision-making that is specific to the medical setting; it takes into account the medical situation (indications for care and treatment), patient preferences, quality of life, and external factors which may influence or be influenced by the decision to be made.

Although theoretically any group can undertake the decision-making process, an experienced group of people from within the unit or hospital usually resolves ethical dilemmas in the critical-care setting. Because of a growing emphasis on ethical dilemmas in hospitals, an increasing number of hospitals have organized bioethics committees and called on experts to assist in resolving ethical dilemmas. There is an increasing amount of literature in nursing, medical, and ethics journals regarding the functions of these committees, but there is currently no single approach to the organization and function of such committees in the individual hospital. The concerns and interests of nurses should be represented on such committees; in particular, critical-care nurses should be familiar with the existence and function of bioethics committees in their hospitals and should be able to refer patient cases for review.

Critical-care nurses must be familiar with the increasingly important area of bioethics—understanding the principles, recognizing dilemmas, and being actively involved in their resolution. Because ethical dilemmas add to the stress of working in the critical-care unit, it is especially important to critical-care nurses that these dilemmas be resolved appropriately. To assure the quality of patient care in their unit, nurses should insist on being a part of this special process.

Types of Ethical Dilemmas

Critical-care nurses often question the benefit that arises from use of the critical-care environment for certain patients, such as the terminally ill patient (very often also elderly) or the patient admitted to the ICU whom nurses do not view as being critically ill. For the terminally ill patient, the ICU interventions often necessary (beginning with simple procedures such as drawing blood and IV placement) may appear to "harm" the patient more than they benefit. If one works in a unit that carries out research protocols, similar questions may be raised about the perceived conflict between benefit and harm of such research.

The conflicts between paternalism and autonomy still exist in many ICUs. Many practitioners still believe *they* know what is "best" for their patients, although they may perhaps express such beliefs more subtly than in the past. Recommending procedures and treatments, as well as minimizing discussion about alternatives, is still a typical approach of some physicians. Nurses often witness such practices with patients or families during the stay in critical-care units. Before we identify paternalism as a dilemma, however, we need to be sure that the patient or family identifies it as a dilemma. Not all patients and their families feel capable of making decisions about their medical care and some choose instead to rely on the expertise of physicians and nurses during an acute illness. Requiring them to make new and difficult decisions may be inappropriate during the critical-care experience. Similarly, nurses may often attempt to influence patients' decision-making about a treatment or care or to be the professional from whom the patient or family seeks advice and guidance about treatment.

Critical-care nurses must listen closely to patients and their families to determine whether the patient's autonomy is being acknowledged or violated. We also should be familiar with ways in which patients have expressed their wishes regarding care. The most common expression of the patient's wishes regarding immediate treatment is via informed consent documentation. *Living wills* have been implemented by many individuals; from state to state, the legality and form of such documents differs, so we must all be familiar with what laws and regulations exist in our particular state. More recently, another form of document has been implemented to ensure a person's autonomy in the medical setting. The *durable power of attorney* allows an individual to assign legal power of attorney to another person (not necessarily the legal next-of-kin) to make decisions about medical care when the individual is rendered incapable of doing so. Public awareness and utilization of this document has been enhanced by a recent United States Supreme Court decision *(Cruzan v. Director of Missouri Department of Health)* regarding an individual's expressed wishes about medical intervention. In upholding the state of Missouri's position to maintain nutrition for this patient who was in a persistent vegetative state, the Court indicated that the person must express his or her wishes in a "clear and convincing" manner (Guarino 1991). The court did not accept that the verbal communications Ms. Cruzan had with friends regarding her wishes about medical treatment met the "clear and convincing" criteria. This ruling strengthens the need for patients' expressions of their wishes through written documentation (such as living wills, durable power of attorney documents, or both). Through education about and implementation of such documents, our current patients and future patients will be able to exercise more autonomy in regard to their medical care.

A typical example of potential conflict between paternalism and autonomy is that related to the order "Do not resuscitate." Patients and families who request such an approach to terminating care must resolve any potential conflict with the physicians and nurses providing care. Discontinuation of life-extending or life-saving treatment also requires resolving any conflict between the principles of paternalism and autonomy.

The principle of justice as fairness is applied more often to situations involving the entire critical-care unit and general delivery of care (rather than an individual patient situation). This ethical principle is usually cited during discussions of the use and allocation of resources—human, financial, and technologic. The cost of critical care remains a major problem for both patients and third-party payers. In addition, there are continuing discussions regarding the use of critical-care beds for certain patients and the decisions made regarding which patients will receive care in the ICU. Engelhardt and Rie (1986) have described the problems of allocating ICU beds as a distribution issue (under the principle of justice as fairness) by identifying three areas of conflict:

(1) when further admissions to an ICU will jeopardize the standard of health care for all those in the ICU, (2) when those eligible for admission to an ICU (newcomers) appear to show greater promise of benefiting from treatment than those already allocated ICU beds (early arrivers), or (3) when the investment of resources appears disproportionate given the marginal benefits likely to be obtained.

A study by Strauss et al. (1986) reviewed the issue of decision-making about patient admission and discharge from the ICU. They found that, during episodes of bed shortage, patients were generally more severely ill at the times of admission and discharge from the unit and had shorter stays in the unit. When beds were available, patients were less severely ill at the time of admission and stays were longer. Of interest is that bed availability had no effect on rates of death in the ICU, after discharge from the ICU, or upon readmission to the ICU.

Most of the ethical dilemmas that receive attention in the popular media or in professional reports (journals or texts) relate to conflicts between health care providers and patients, their families, or both. However, there are other general ethical dilemmas that may affect nurses. For example, the stressors and issues regarding family communication have ethical dimensions. Patient–staff ratios, other administrative conflicts, use of sedation or pain medication, or rules and issues regarding visitation may all create ethical dilemmas for nurses, which may lead to conflict with each other and other health care staff or administrators or even within ourselves. Discussions with colleagues on a more informal basis can assist in resolving these issues. Nursing ethics committees also have been formed to deal with issues particularly or uniquely relevant to nursing practice and care (Fowler 1988).

Nurses must be familiar with the ethical principles that dictate the allocation of ICU resources and must protect the established ICU policies and procedures from frivolous or inappropriate use. Even nurses who are not directly involved with families and decision-making regarding admission to the ICU may be involved in explaining the transfer of patients from the ICU. Such interaction requires that the critical-care nurse fully explain to the family the reasons for discharge and the way in which it was determined that the patient could be discharged. Assurance that care will be adequately and appropriately given by other nursing staff following discharge from the ICU also needs to be provided to the family.

Another issue with which critical-care nurses often must deal is that of terminal care being delivered in the critical-care unit, when it seems clear that the resources being used will not be able to save the patient's life. This dilemma is exacerbated by conflicts and decisions about resuscitation for these terminal patients. Should such patients be automatically transferred from the ICU? Is transfer seen as abandonment by family members? Can nurses explain this decision so that families understand its medical intent? The case example at the beginning of this chapter identifies this dilemma.

An issue in allocation of ICU resources that has a direct impact on the critical-care nurse is that of professional staff. While Engelhardt, Rie, and Strauss focused on bed availability, the availability of critical-care nurses also may limit admission of patients to the unit. Establishment and maintenance of appropriate patient–nurse ratios is critical to the continued provision of ICU services to the patient population. Adverse effects of shortages will be felt in a variety of ways by the institution and the patient—lowered quality of care, decreased patient admissions, changes in physicians' use of the hospital if they are not guaranteed quality critical care for their patients, and increased stress on critical-care nurses leading to staff shortages (see previous discussion). Appropriate staffing patterns have been addressed by a number of groups including hospital-based nursing committees, professional nursing organizations via contractual agreements, and most recently, the Joint Commission on Accreditation of

Healthcare Organizations (JCAHO). Nurses need to remain very aware of and alert to potential problems in critical-care staffing. In addition to the ethical issues involved, there are legal implications in the allocation of resources in the critical-care unit (see next section).

In summary, ethical principles, ethical dilemmas, and ethical decision-making are frequent concerns for critical-care nurses. Unresolved issues or dilemmas can create stress for critical-care nurses and may have adverse effects on the nurse's patient care and interactions with patients' families. Assurance of ethical practice and care in the critical-care unit can only help to maintain high-quality nursing practice, professional satisfaction, and patient care.

Legal Issues

Critical-care nursing is a high-risk occupation from a legal standpoint. According to Kimberly et al. (1982), nurses are often abysmally ignorant of the situations that place them at legal risk. Nurses face an increasing likelihood of becoming involved in a lawsuit in this era of increasing health care litigation. A general legal principle that critical-care nurses need to know is that civil law, specifically tort law, is the area with which they are most likely to be involved.

Tort law applies to situations in which a person is injured or damaged by another person. In contrast, *criminal law* applies to injury or damage committed against the state or society by violation of statutes (laws). Typical torts cited in cases involving medical care are:

- *Negligence*—when harm comes to someone because the professional has failed to conform to an identified standard of care or practice.
- *Malpractice*—when a negligent act or omission in care or practice causes harm or injury.

The principle of *respondeat superior* is of special interest to nurses; it holds that the employer may be held vicariously liable for the acts of nurses. Traditionally, a hospital has provided full-time nurses with professional insurance as an employment benefit and thus would seem to protect and represent them should a legal matter arise. Depending on your actions (or inactions) in certain situations, however, the hospital may or may not be obligated to provide legal counsel and support. You should be aware that the protection provided by the hospital has its limitations. It is your responsibility to know what coverage and services the hospital will provide; any gaps in coverage should be assumed privately by you. The hospital's policy will cover nurses only when they are functioning within the scope of their job description. Moreover, your memory or viewpoint may differ from that of other staff; if such a conflict occurs, the hospital's attorney may not provide adequate representation. In addition, if the hospital pays a claim because of a nurse's negligence, it does have the legal right to sue you for reimbursement of its payment (George 1982).

Additional insurance coverage is available and usually provided through groups such as a specialty organization (AACN), the American Nurses Association (ANA), or the state nurses' association. Nurses who are employed part-time, in a "casual" category, or on per-diem status may not have the insurance coverage afforded the full-time nurse; nurses working in these capacities should determine what insurance coverage they do or do not have and what they need. Nurses working via registries also must be cognizant of what coverage, if any, is provided by their agency.

Whether your behavior and practice in any situation is negligent is determined by comparing it to the acceptable standard of care, defined as that which a reasonably prudent nurse would have applied in the same situation. Scope and standards of practice as defined by state Nurse Practice Acts are the primary legal standards used to judge the nurse's practice. In addition, standards of practice promulgated by professional organizations (e.g., AACN, ANA) also serve as definitions of standards of care.

Reasons for Lawsuits

Experience indicates reasons why lawsuits are filed against nurses (or physicians and nurses). The most important cause is usually that one has not established rapport or has lost rapport with the family or the patient, who feel they have been treated badly. The actual incident is often secondary and relates to breaks in established techniques or procedures, a sudden, unexpected negative change in the patient's condition, or an unexpected poor outcome of care leading the family or patient to charge that the nurse failed to observe the patient adequately or communicate to the physician significant changes in the patient's condition (Grane 1983).

Protection Against Lawsuits

Nurses often dismiss the possibility of a lawsuit by saying, "It can't happen to me. I am a professional." However, assumptions about one's expertise and denial of the possibility simply are not enough.

Stabler-Hass and McHugh (1989) believe that many nurses have lost their compassion while focusing on and developing their technical skills. They exhort us to regain this aspect of our practice and care, suggesting that compassion is an appropriate strategy for avoiding a lawsuit; they enumerate 15 examples of compassionate care which would prevent legal action by patients and/or their families. If that is actually the case, one would hope that the nurse would give compassionate care not primarily to prevent lawsuits, but because compassion is an intrinsic and valuable aspect of nursing, perhaps the most valuable. However, there are a number of specific measures that one can take to avoid lawsuits; Table 3–3 presents some of them.

Special Legal Problems

There are a number of particular areas of critical care that may pose potential legal problems for the nursing staff. Legal experts have made some recommendations for preventing problems in these areas.

The *medically questionable order* is one of the most common dilemmas faced by the critical-care nurse and has been the subject of several legal decisions. To protect yourself, there are several kinds of orders you should question. These include ambiguous orders, any order the patient questions, any order that will compromise a preexisting patient condition, and standing or PRN orders if you cannot judge whether they are appropriate for the situation.

The courts have clearly indicated that when there is a question about a written medical order, you are responsible for contacting the physician who wrote it (Roach 1980). If you disagree with the order and the physician still directs you to carry it out, you have a duty to refuse. When the situation is less clear and you are unclear about the order or its rationale, you can discuss the order with other physicians involved in the case or consult with the medical director of the critical-care unit. Finally, always read back verbal orders and ask the physician any questions about them to be sure you have understood and noted them correctly. Some units require a second nurse to listen to verbal orders. The safest form of documentation would, of course, be to tape record all such telephone orders (Bennett 1981).

The use of *"standing orders"* has become increasingly popular but remains variable from facility to facility. Standing orders that have been appropriately drafted and reviewed can prevent errors in orders being given emergently but may also require the nurse to think and act more independently than he or she would under more traditional, patient-specific orders.

"Do not resuscitate" (DNR or no code) orders have already been mentioned as a potential ethical dilemma. Without written information provided by the patient, such orders are more difficult to carry out within the ICU. Individual states have made different rulings on such orders, so it is necessary to be aware of established case law. The issuance of verbal orders regarding DNR and "slow codes" (which may be both unethical and illegal) creates even greater dilemmas and should be avoided through procedural mechanisms in the ICU setting.

As reviewed above, *withdrawal of life support* for the terminal, comatose patient is a more current dilemma which is being resolved in case law. Often life-support withdrawal occurs after transfer from the ICU and thus does not impact as directly on the critical-care nurse.

TABLE 3–3

How to Protect Yourself from Legal Action by Patients and Families

Know your job. Know exactly what job you are supposed to be doing—its scope and its limitations. Know what the job description says that you are to be doing; know that it reflects the current responsibilities and practices of you and your colleagues.

Document promptly, completely, clearly, and accurately. Carefully record the time that events occurred as well as the time of documentation (especially if there has been a time lapse). Note corrections in your charting with a single line through the entry and the word "error" and reason for error noted. Never totally obliterate an entry by crossing over or with use of "white-out." Because lawsuits often are filed several years after the event, develop a charting style that you will recognize and perhaps will allow a greater sense of recall about the events. Review physician notes and charting about especially important or problematic incidents and resolve discrepancies with the physician at the time of the event; it is often too late at the time of deposition and trial.

Never be too busy to talk to the patient or family (or significant others). At the end of the crisis or the resuscitation procedure, take a moment to talk to the family; make this the first priority (when you would surely prefer a moment of rest and quiet for yourself). Be as honest as possible about what is happening; do not try to minimize crises or simply dismiss the apparent gravity of the situation (these actions adhere to the ethical principles of veracity and fidelity). Remember that events that we consider usual or expected in the critical-care setting remain frightening and unexpected for families and loved ones.

However, it has the potential for creating both ethical and legal dilemmas for the nursing staff.

Remaining aware of ways in which legal action can be prevented and ensuring that our nursing practice is professional at all times are the best defenses against lawsuits. In our increasingly litigious society, however, nurses should no longer believe that they will not be sued. Nurses individually and collectively are increasingly at great risk. For example, Engelhardt and Rie (1986) reviewed the case of a lawsuit against critical-care nurses and a hospital because of inadequate staffing in the ICU that caused patient complications. Nursing liability increases as we assume more and more responsibility in an increasingly technical environment.

Example: The Case of Organ Donation

The following discussion of organ donation is used as an example to integrate all of the various threads of critical-care nursing practice illuminated in this chapter—stress and emotional aspects of critical-care nursing, patient and family communication, ethical dilemmas and decision-making, and legal considerations of practice—all occurring in a highly technologic environment. While a number of issues could be discussed, organ donation has been chosen because it has a fairly long history of development, many (although not all) of the issues have been resolved, and, most importantly, it is a universal process—one that can be accomplished in every ICU in the United States. (This section is not intended to serve as a guideline for organ donation activities, however.)

For purposes of this discussion, organ donation includes the donation of all cadaver organs and tissues currently being used for both research and clinical transplants. The history of organ donation is a long one, with the first solid organs (kidneys) being removed in the 1950s and 1960s (Moore 1964). The development of the ICU made the concept of organ donation a possibility by providing complete artificial respiratory function; without such treatment, brain death would never have become an identified phenomenon (Hopper 1983).

Organ donation is achieved when a number of factors are met through the efforts of a number of people. At the center of the process is an individual (usually young and healthy) who has suffered brain death secondary to an unexpected accident, injury, or disease. The patient's next-of-kin and other loved ones are intimately involved in the donation. Physicians representing a number of specialties are providing medical care to the patient, initially directed toward life-saving treatments and procedures. Critical-care nurses are providing direct care to the patient and share the goal of patient recovery; in addition, they closely interact with the family and other loved ones. Law enforcement officials and medical examiners or coroners also are involved frequently (although not universally).

Stress of Organ Donation

The stress of caring for the organ donor has been poorly measured and documented. Sophie et al. (1983) measured the responses of critical-care nurses to organ donation. They found that many nurses report organ donation is often a frustrating experience that conflicts with their goals. The distress and concern that nurses have regarding the organ donor process has not lessened over the years; a later study by Bidigare and Oermann (1991) identified responses similar to Sophie's earlier study. Physicians as well feel these conflicts when their attempts to save a life are negated by brain death. It is not uncommon for physicians to seem to withdraw in such situations, providing necessary supportive care but referring the patient to appropriate transplant agencies and physicians for continued care.

Stress is intensified as nurses continue to provide direct care to the organ donor and struggle with the issue of caring for someone who is dead. An additional stressor is present in this nursing care: the nurse is the direct protector of the critically important vital organs that will be removed and used for transplantation. The need to provide expert care, to monitor and maintain excellent cardiac, respiratory, liver, and kidney function in a hemodynamically fragile or unstable patient, is a challenge to the critical-care nurse. Goldsmith and Montefusco (1985) outlined in detail these nursing care responsibilities and interventions. The stress of caring for an organ donor may be intensified by the responsibility nurses may have in contacting the appropriate organ procurement agency in their community. As organ procurement agencies have become more numerous and prominent in the past several years, some hospitals have identified their own staff person who will interact with the appropriate organ procurement agency and coordinate this activity in a specialized capacity. Lastly, the critical-care nurse provides emotional support and information to the family of the organ donor in a way that assures donation will be a positive experience for them. A major finding of the Bidigare and Oermann study (1991) is that nurses' knowledge about organ donation was significantly and inversely related to the comfort they felt about participating in the organ donation process.

Communication and Organ Donation

Patient and family communication is a critical aspect of organ donation. Obviously, the patient cannot communicate his or her wishes about organ donation at this time. Thus, the nurse is responsible for determining whether prior instructions have been given via signed organ donor cards, living wills, or durable power of attorney documentation.

The concept of *required request* ensures that all hospitals and their staffs (including physicians and nurses) approach families about organ and tissue donation at the time of death of every patient. Required request, a federal regulation associated with Medicare and Medicaid hospital reimbursement, is supported by Joint Commission for the Accreditation of Healthcare Organizations (JCAHO) regulations. (Required request is not statutory in all states, so it only applies to Medicare and/or Medicaid patients at present.) Appropriate documentation of this request is required in the patient's chart.

These regulations affect nurse and family communication. It is clear that a nurse's discomfort with the process, lack of knowledge or understanding about it, or both, will diminish therapeutic communication with families about organ and tissue donation. Norris (1990) noted that education and training about how to talk with families about donation has been insufficient. She believed that poorly presented requests give families inaccurate perceptions and uncomfortable feelings. Thus, the organ donation situation exemplifies the challenges in regard to family communication that are faced—and can be met—by critical-care nurses.

Ethical Aspects of Organ Donation

The developing awareness of ethical considerations of organ donation and the related transplant seem to parallel the development of bioethics. In conjunction with the problems of those awaiting organ transplants (such as selection for and treatment with dialysis or death of children and young adults from cardiac or liver disease), organ donation raised issues of beneficence, autonomy, and allocation of resources. These ethical issues and attendant dilemmas continue to exist, although their form has changed. Health professionals and the public have had to clarify their values about the very definitions of life and death (brain death vs cardiorespiratory death). With the first heart transplant in 1967, everyone had to confront the fact that biologic life depended on brain function, not cardiac function as tradition had taught. The survival and function of a transplanted heart created conflicts of biology and spirit (soul); individuals had to rethink the meaning of life and death. This dilemma of redefinition has continued through more recent discussions of the use of anencephalic newborns as organ donors at the time of birth (Harrison 1986).

The ethical principle of beneficence may be achieved through organ donation, albeit indirectly. While the organ donor receives no direct benefit, it is held ethically good that the organs and tissues donated provide life, improve quality of life, and relieve suffering for those who receive the transplants. Beneficence also is provided to families who are comforted by the knowledge of benefit to the transplant recipients.

The principle of autonomy in organ donation was defined in 1964 with the Uniform Anatomic Gift Act, which provided adults with the right to make decisions regarding organ and tissue donation following their death. The right to sign a donor card as a legal document expressing one's wish about organ donation has stood the test of time without controversy. This autonomous decision rarely is overridden by family members; when this occurs, professionals deem it necessary for the psychologic well-being of the family not to carry out the wishes of the deceased individual. Changes affecting the autonomy of patients in regard to organ donation have been made; some states allow for the removal of corneas without the donor's express consent (via a donor card) or without consent of the next-of-kin. Caplan (1983) advocated the principle of *presumed consent* for organ donation, which would allow anyone to serve as an organ or tissue donor unless the person had, in writing, expressly opposed donation. However, this method (which would minimize or overrule the principle of autonomy) still has not been adopted.

The principle of justice as fairness usually is applied to organ donation in regard to the maintenance of donors in the critical-care unit; also, the benefit of fairness often is discussed in regard to transplant recipients. When resources are scarce or unavailable, is it appropriate to continue the life-support maintenance of the potential organ donor while consent is being obtained, arrangements made, and transplant teams travel to the donor hospital? Does the benefit outweigh the risks to other patients that may come from the additional activity of organ donation, that may tax the nursing resources in the ICU? Is the brain-dead patient to be admitted to the busy critical-care unit to receive supportive care until organs can be recovered?

These questions are not easily resolved by policy or regulation and create continuing ethical dilemmas for the nurse involved with organ donation.

Legal Aspects of Organ Donation

Consent for organ donation was established by statute, as previously described. That same legislation describes the legal order of consent by next-of-kin. Critical-care nurses must be familiar with the legal aspects of consent for organ donation; they often are responsible for ensuring that the legal next-of-kin is identified for purposes of consent. In some circumstances this is not as simple as it may seem. Careful attention to the legal aspects (as well as donor care) can prevent potential litigation. If questions arise regarding consent for organ donation, you should consult a member of the transplant team, the organ procurement agency, or the hospital's attorney for expert advice.

The definition of brain death moved from being a medical diagnosis in the 1960s (Ad Hoc Committee 1968) to becoming a recognized legal definition. Medical criteria and assessment determine the total and irreversible cessation of brain function, including that of the brain stem. Brain death is recognized legally in all 50 states and the District of Columbia through statutory legislation or court decisions. Though the President's Commission for the Study of Ethical Problems in Medicine and Biomedical and Behavioral Research (1981) recommended uniform legislation for the determination of death (including brain death), such legislation has not been forthcoming. You must therefore be very familiar with the legal determination of brain death in your state to ensure that this process is carried out properly.

Other legal parameters of organ donation may involve traditional state laws about reporting deaths in the hospital to law enforcement personnel or medical examiners or coroners. States have lenient to rigid laws regarding the reporting of unexpected or sudden deaths (even from "natural" causes) as well as those associated with accidents or at the hand of others. Medical examiners or coroners are considered to be the recipients of the patient's body in cases where an autopsy must be performed to determine the legal cause of death. Thus, organ donation often must be approved by the coroner to ensure that the removal of organs will not interfere with or compromise the ability to determine the legal cause of death. Medical examiners or coroners interpret their role in organ donation in very different ways and have established local (county) policies and procedures regarding organ donation. You also must be familiar with these policies.

In summary, organ donation is a complex procedure carried out in the critical-care unit. Nurses should have available written policies and procedures for organ donation specific to their institution, county, and state. Personnel also are available from the various transplant or organ procurement programs to advise and assist the critical-care nursing staff.

Organ donation is simply one of many of the issues (ethical, legal, and professional) that impact on the practice of critical-care nurses. Nurses who work in critical-care settings must be expert practitioners in a variety of specialty and subspecialty areas. A nurse's expertise and care are the keys to assuring the successful completion of this process and all others that are currently a part of critical care.

REFERENCES

Ad Hoc Committee: A definition of irreversible coma: Report of the ad hoc committee of the Harvard Medical School to examine the definition of brain death. *JAMA* 1968; 205(6):337–341.

Alspach J: The shortage of critical care nurses: Readership survey results. *Crit Care Nurse* 1988; 8(3):14–21.

Ashley J: *Hospitals, paternalism, and the role of the nurse.* New York: Teachers College Press, 1976.

Bailey J et al.: The stress audit: Identifying the stressors of the ICU nurse. *J Nurs Ed* 1980; 19:15–25.

Bedsworth J, Molen M: Psychological stress in spouses of patients with myocardial infarction. *Heart Lung* 1982; 11:450–456.

Benner P: *From novice to expert: Excellence and power in clinical nursing practice.* Menlo Park, CA: Addison-Wesley, 1984.

Bennett H: The legalities of critical care. *Crit Care Nurse* (March/April) 1981; 54–55.

Bidigare S, Oermann M: Attitudes and knowledge of nurses regarding organ procurement. *Heart Lung* 1991; 20(1):20–24.

Breu C, Dracup K: Helping the spouses of critically ill patients. *Am J Nurs* 1978; 78:51–53.

Caplan A: Organ transplants: The costs of success. *The Hastings Center Report* Dec. 1983; 23–25.

Chaney P: Ordeal. *Nurs 75* 1975; 5:27–40.

Christopherson D: Control and power in critical care. *Dimen Crit Care Nurs* 1986; 5(5).

Compton P: Critical illness and intensive care: What it means to the client. *Crit Care Nurse* 1991; 11(1):50–56.

Daley L: The perceived immediate needs of families with relatives in the intensive care setting. *Heart Lung* 1984; 13:231–237.

Daly B, Rudy E, Thompson K, Happ M: Development of a special care unit for chronically critically ill patients. *Heart Lung* 1991; 20(1):45–51.

Davis J, Krueger C: *Patients, nurses, ethics.* New York: American Journal of Nursing Co., 1980.

Downs F: Bed rest and sensory disturbances. *Am J Nurs* 1974; 74:434–436.

Engelhardt H, Rie A: Intensive care units, scarce resources, and conflicting principles of justice. *JAMA* 1986; 255(9):1159–1164.

Fowler M: Nursing ethics committees. *Heart Lung* 1988; 17(6):718–719.

Freudenberger H, North G: *Women's burnout.* Garden City, NY: Doubleday, 1985.

Gardner D et al.: The nurse's dilemma: Mediating stress in critical care units. *Heart Lung* 1980; 9:103–106.

Gentry W, Parkes K: Psychologic stress in intensive care unit and non-intensive care unit nursing. A review of the past decade. *Heart Lung* 1982; 11:43–47.

George J: Malpractice insurance. *J Emerg Nurs* 1982; 6:319–320.

Goldsmith J, Montefusco CM: Nursing care of the potential organ donor. *Crit Care Nurse* 1985; 5(6):22–29.

Grane N: How to reduce your risk of a lawsuit. *Nurs Life* (January-February) 1983; 17–20.

Guarino K, Antoine M: The case of Nancy Cruzan: The Supreme Court's decision. *Crit Care Nurse* 1991; 11(1):32–40.

Harrison M: Anencephalic newborns as organ donors. *The Hastings Center Report* (April) 1986; 16(2):21–23.

Hopper S: Science, technology, and organ recovery (Unpublished Paper). 1983.

Jervik D, Martinson I: *Women in stress: A nursing perspective.* New York: Appleton-Century-Crofts, 1979.

Jonsen A et al.: *Clinical ethics.* New York: Macmillan, 1982.

Kimberly R et al.: What do the courts expect from nurses? *Nurs Life* (September/October) 1982; 34–37.

Leske J: Needs of relatives of critically ill patients: A follow-up. *Heart Lung* 1986; 15:189–193.

Mendenhall J: Factors affecting job satisfaction/dissatisfaction among critical care nurses. *Focus* (October/November) 1982; 14–18.

Molter N: Needs of relatives of critically ill patients: A descriptive study. *Heart Lung* 1979; 8:332–339.

Moore F: *Transplant: The give and take of tissue transplantation.* New York: Saunders, 1964.

Norris M: Required request: Why it has not significantly improved the donor shortage. *Heart Lung* 1990; 19(6):685–686.

Prescott P: Shortage of professional nursing practice: a reframing of the shortage problem. *Heart Lung* 1989; 18(5):436–443.

President's Commission: *Defining death: Medical, legal and ethical issues in the determination of death.* President's Commission for the Study of Ethical Problems in Medicine and Biomedical and Behavioral Research. Washington, D.C.: U.S. Government Printing Office, 1981.

Richmond T, Craig M: Timeout: Facing death in the ICU. *Dimen Crit Care Nurs* 1985; 4(1):41–45.

Roach W: Responsible intervention: A legal duty to act. *J Nurs Admin* (July) 1980; 18–24.

Robinson J, Lewis D: Coping with ICU work-related stressors: A study. *Crit Care Nurse* 1990; 10(5):80–88.

Sophie L et al.: Intensive care nurses' perceptions of cadaver organ procurement. *Heart Lung* 1983; 12:261–267.

Stabler-Haas S, McHugh M: Compassion: A strategy for avoiding a lawsuit. *Crit Care Nurse* 1989; 9(2):12–13.

Strauss M et al.: Rationing of intensive care unit services. *JAMA* 1986; 255(9):1143–1146.

Vincent P, Coleman W: Comparison of major stressors perceived by ICU and non-ICU nurses. *Crit Care Nurse* 1986; 6(1):64–69.

4

Neurologic Assessment

CLINICAL INSIGHT

Domain: The diagnostic and monitoring function

Competency: Anticipating problems: future think

Diagnostic and monitoring skills are vital components of critical-care nursing that permeate all phases of the nursing process. Nurses routinely identify minor physical and emotional changes and search among multiple possibilities for their cause. As such, they become masters at interpreting subtle shifts. They must react promptly to seemingly minor, yet significant changes—but not overreact to insignificant ones. Learning to differentiate the two requires continual awareness of what could be happening with a particular patient—not just what happens with nine of ten other patients. Caring for unstable patients requires an ability to titrate interventions so that precursors of catastrophe remain detectable. In the following exemplar, from Benner and Tanner (1986, pp. 26–27), an
expert nurse elegantly describes the tightrope walk involved in anticipating critical-care problems.

Vasospasm can be devastating. It is like a stroke. Everybody is so individual. If they have severe subarachnoid hemorrhages and are agitated, restless, and combative, their blood pressures go up, and then they get very quiet and their blood pressures drop down. You are worried about bleeding, and then you are worried about their stroking. You just play a game. And you play with these drugs and you try to keep it within the limits as well as you can.

Some of the time, if the bleed is bad enough, the people are pretty confused and agitated. So they are combative, and there is not anything you can really do for that. You don't want to snow them because you don't want to put them out, even enough to keep them quiet, because you won't know if the quietness is neurological, an indication of a rebleed, or whatever. It's very difficult.

The ability to anticipate problems rests on a solid foundation of theoretical knowledge, assessment skills, and rich background experience. This chapter presents the theoretical framework a nurse should have at his or her command to assess a person's ability to receive, interpret, and integrate impulses into a unified response. This ability is mediated by the nervous system, a wondrously complex constellation of structures. These structures can be divided anatomically into those inside the skull and vertebral column—that is, the central nervous system (CNS), consisting of the brain and spinal cord—and those outside the bony structures—that is, the peripheral nervous system, consisting of the cranial and spinal nerves (Figure 4–1). The peripheral nervous system can be subdivided further into a sensory (afferent) division and a motor (efferent) division. Although these distinctions are helpful in developing a cognitive framework for understanding the nervous system, they blur in practical application to patient assessment. The discussion that follows offers an overview of the nervous system's structure and function.

Central Nervous System

The central nervous system (CNS) includes the brain and spinal cord and carries out its function through sensory and motor pathways and association centers.

Brain

For easy reference, the functions of brain structures are listed in Table 4–1.

Cerebrum The major divisions of the brain are the bilateral cerebral hemispheres, the diencephalon, the brainstem, and the cerebellum. Divisions within the brain are identifiable by various folds on the surface referred to as gyri, sulci, and fissures (Figure 4–2). The *cerebrum* consists of two hemispheres connected by the corpus callosum (Figure 4–3). The corpus callosum allows fibers to pass from one hemisphere to the other. The basal ganglia are islands of nuclei deep in the cerebral hemispheres that control fine body movements (Figure 4–4). The cerebral cortex is subdivided

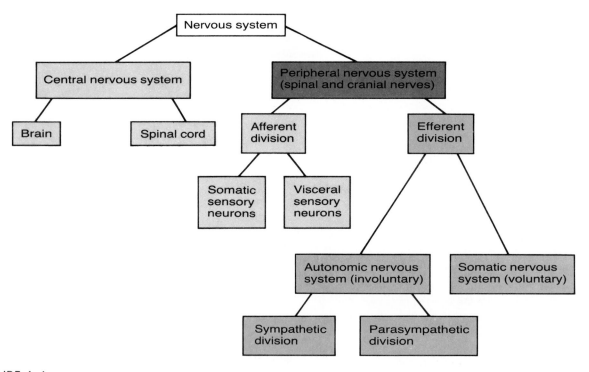

FIGURE 4–1

Organization of the nervous system. (From: Spence A: *Basic human anatomy,* 3d ed. Redwood City, CA: Benjamin/Cummings, 1989, p. 352.)

into four lobes: the frontal, parietal, temporal, and occipital (Figure 4–5).

The frontal lobe is the largest lobe of the brain. In addition to its control of voluntary movement, it also functions to control one's affect or personality. Most voluntary activity originates in the primary motor cortex (precentral gyrus), which is a narrow strip in each frontal lobe, anterior to the central sulcus. Broca's area, within the inferior gyrus of the frontal lobe, mediates the formation of words. Damage to Broca's area produces expressive aphasia.

The parietal lobe gives one the ability to distinguish the sensations of touch. In addition, awareness of body parts and orientation in space are interpreted in this lobe. A stroke that interrupts blood supply to the parietal lobe can produce perceptual impairments.

The temporal lobe receives and interprets auditory information. Wernicke's area, within the temporal lobe, houses the primary reception station for speech; damage to this area produces receptive aphasia. The superior portion of the temporal lobe integrates complex thought and memory. Seizures in this area result in auditory, visual, or sensory hallucinations. The medial portion of the temporal lobe, the hippocampus, functions to transfer short-term memory to long-term memory. This function is disturbed in

TABLE 4–1

Brain Structures and Functions

STRUCTURE	FUNCTIONS
Cerebrum	Gray and white matter with sensory, motor, and integrative functions
A. Cerebral cortex	Outer layer consisting of gray matter
1. Frontal lobe	Complex intellectual functions such as memory, judgment, and problem solving; personality
Precentral gyrus	Primary motor area
2. Parietal lobe (specifically, postcentral gyrus)	Primary somatic sensory area
3. Temporal lobe	Primary auditory area: taste, smell; comprehension of speech
4. Occipital lobe	Primary visual area
B. Basal ganglia	Gray matter deep in each hemisphere; coordination of muscular activity; automatic movements of expression
Diencephalon	Gray matter between cerebrum and midbrain; structures around third ventricle, particularly thalamus and hypothalamus
A. Thalamus	Gray matter located against lateral walls of third ventricle; reception of sensory impulses; participation in arousal mechanism: conscious awareness of crude sensations; relay of sensations to cortex for fine discrimination
B. Hypothalamus	Regulation of activity of autonomic nervous system; secretion of hormonal releasing factors, antidiuretic hormone and oxytocin; participation in arousal mechanism; control of appetite and body temperature
C. Internal capsule	White matter; sensory and motor tracts located between thalamus and basal ganglia
Brainstem	
A. Midbrain	White and gray matter connecting cerebrum and pons; contains nuclei of third cranial nerve (including the pupillary reflex center) and nuclei of fourth and part of fifth cranial nerves
B. Pons	White matter and nuclei of fifth to eighth cranial nerves; participation in regulation of respiration; projection tracts between brain and spinal cord
C. Medulla oblongata	Mostly white matter and nuclei of ninth to twelfth cranial nerves; cardiac, vasomotor, and respiratory reflex centers; also reflex centers for sneezing, coughing, vomiting, swallowing; projection tracts between brain and cord
D. Reticular activating system	Diffuse gray and white matter in brainstem core; relays impulses from cord and specialized sensory tracts to thalamus and then to cortex; portion rostral to midpons functions to arouse cerebral cortex and to maintain consciousness
Cerebellum	Coordination of muscular activity; maintenance of muscle tone, equilibrium, and posture

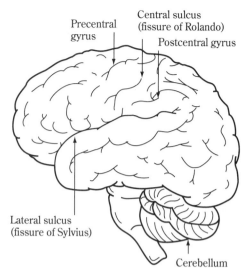

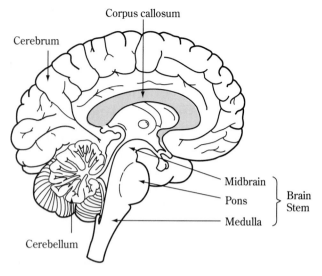

FIGURE 4–2

Folds on brain surface. (From Ahrens T: *Critical care certification preparation and review,* 2d ed. East Norwalk, CT: Appleton & Lange, 1991, p. 152.)

FIGURE 4–3

Midsagittal section showing the corpus callosum. (From Ahrens T: *Critical care certification preparation and review,* 2d ed. East Norwalk, CT: Appleton & Lange, 1991, p. 151.)

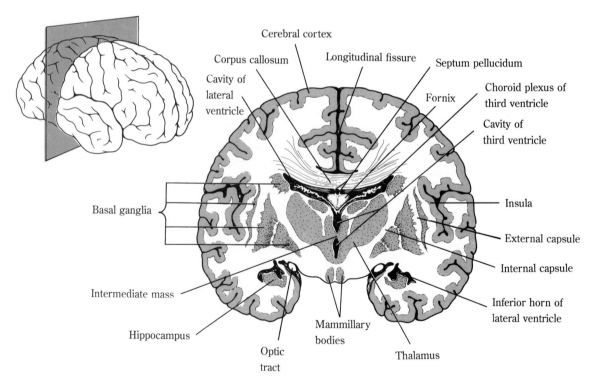

FIGURE 4–4

Frontal section of the cerebrum and the diencephalon *(shaded)* showing the cerebral cortex (gray matter) surrounding the white matter and, deep within the white matter, the basal ganglia. (From Spence A: *Basic human anatomy,* 3d ed. Redwood City, CA: Benjamin/Cummings, 1989, p. 380.)

(a)

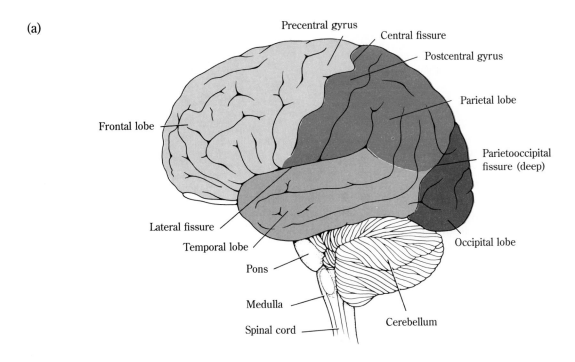

(b)

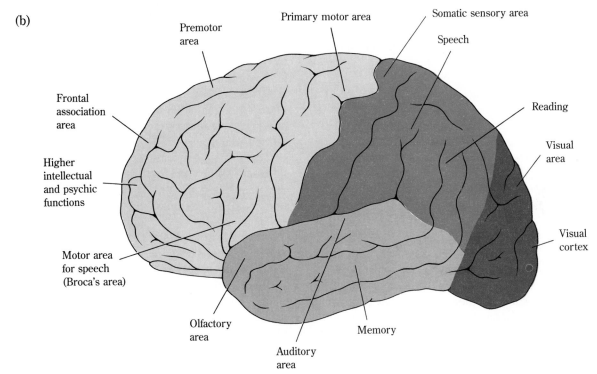

FIGURE 4–5

Left lateral view of the brain. Major **(a)** structural and **(b)** functional areas of the cerebral hemispheres. (From Marieb E: *Essentials of human anatomy and physiology,* 3d ed. Redwood City, CA: Benjamin/Cummings, 1991, p. 184. Reprinted by permission.)

head injury, hypoxia, or ischemic insults (Marshall et al. 1990).

The temporal lobe has connections to the hypothalamus and cingulate gyrus, parts of the limbic system. The limbic system influences the expression of instinctive behaviors, emotion, and control of autonomic functions. Areas of the temporal lobe are also important in memory and the sense of smell. A certain song may evoke emotion in you each time you hear it, or the smell of a favorite food may remind you of a certain event. This association demonstrates the integration of the limbic system.

The occipital lobe receives and interprets visual information. It is separated from the cerebellum by the tentorium, a tent-like structure with an opening that allows passage of nerves and blood vessels. Herniation develops when edema or a mass causes the brain to shift. If the shift occurs above the tentorium, it is described as supratentorial herniation. Shifts that occur below the tentorium result in infratentorial herniation. The pressure that is placed on the cerebral vessels and vital functional centers of the brain can lead to death. Neurologic assessment is key to initiating treatment to prevent herniation. See Chapter 5 for a detailed description of appropriate preventive actions.

Diencephalon The *diencephalon* is the part of the brain located between the cerebrum and midbrain. It contains several structures around the third ventricle, the most important ones being the thalamus and the hypothalamus. The *thalamus* integrates sensory signals and relays them to higher brain structures. The *hypothalamus* regulates the internal environment, including body temperature. The *internal capsule* refers to the bundle of motor and sensory nerve fibers that meet in the diencephalon within the thalamic region (Figure 4–4). These nerve fibers connect areas of the brain and spinal cord. Damage to the internal capsule can cause selective loss of motor and sensory function. An example of such damage is a lacunar stroke, in which occlusion of a small vessel results in paresis in the contralateral hand without affecting the leg or face (Marshall et al. 1990).

Brainstem The next major part of the brain is the *brainstem,* the most primitive part of the brain, which consists of the midbrain, pons, and medulla oblongata. Consciousness is mediated by the reticular activating system (RAS), which originates in the brainstem and terminates in almost all areas of the diencephalon and the cerebrum.

The RAS receives input from sensory stimuli via ascending tracts from the spinal cord and brainstem,

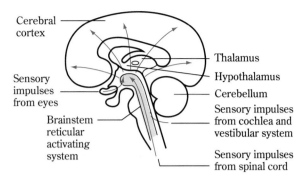

FIGURE 4–6

Reticular activating system.

as depicted in Figure 4–6. Retrograde stimulation of the RAS by the cerebrum is mediated through direct fiber pathways into the reticular formation from (1) the somatic sensory cortex, (2) the motor cortex, (3) the frontal cortex, (4) the basal ganglia, (5) the hypothalamus, and (6) the limbic structures. The brainstem reticular formation integrates these stimuli and transmits them over discrete pathways to the diencephalon and the cerebrum. The RAS is believed to be responsible for arousal and wakefulness; when it is stimulated, it causes diffuse activation of the entire brain. For full consciousness, the person must have both a functioning reticular activating system and relatively intact cerebral hemispheres (Plum and Posner 1980).

The primary involuntary respiratory centers are housed in the brain stem. The basic rhythm of respiration is generated in the dorsal neurons of the medulla. The pneumotaxic center in the pons functions to limit the duration of inspiration and to increase the respiratory rate. An apneustic center in the lower pons also may provide extra inspiratory drive. It does not influence normal respiration because it is overridden by the pneumotaxic center. Influences from stretch receptors in the lung, peripheral and central chemoreceptors, the spinal cord, midbrain, and cerebral cortex also modify respiratory rate, depth, and pattern.

Cerebellum The *cerebellum* sits below the occipital lobes and posterior to the brainstem. It has two hemispheres, which are connected to each other and the brainstem by tracts called cerebellar peduncles. The cerebellum receives input from the motor cortex, brain stem, and peripheral areas. It modifies motor activity in numerous ways, which can be grouped into regulation of muscle tone, coordination of muscle movements, and maintenance of equilibrium.

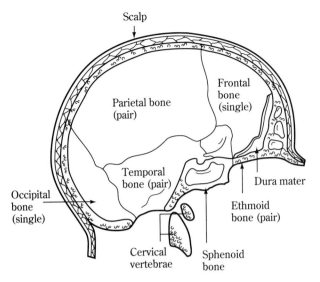

FIGURE 4–7

The cranium. (From Ahrens T: *Critical care certification preparation and review,* 2d ed. East Norwalk, CT: Appleton & Lange, 1991, p. 150.)

Skull

Bones   Many bones form the skull; the major ones are the frontal, parietal, temporal, occipital, and sphenoid bones and the paired ethmoid bones, also referred to as the cribriform plate (Figure 4–7). Disruption of these bones implies potential damage to the underlying structures.

The interior floor of the skull is a relatively thin shell of bone divided into three areas (Figure 4–8). The *anterior fossa* contains the frontal lobes of the brain. The *middle fossa* contains the temporal lobes, the upper brainstem, and the pituitary gland. The *posterior fossa* contains the brainstem and cerebellum. At the base of the skull is an opening, called the foramen magnum, through which the spinal cord emerges. Other openings in the skull provide passageways for the cranial nerves.

Meninges   Between the skull and the brain, and between the vertebral column and spinal cord, are

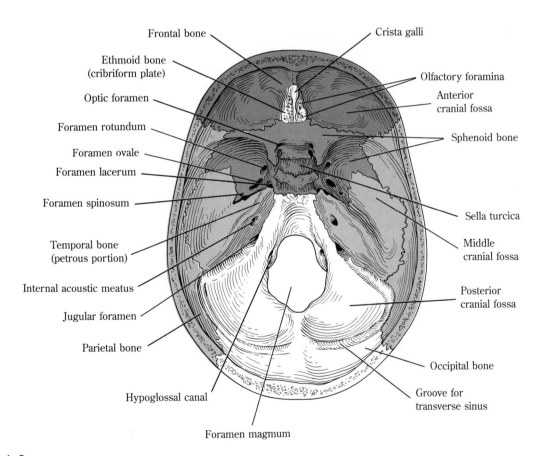

FIGURE 4–8

Internal view of skull floor. (From Spence A: *Basic human anatomy,* 3d ed. Redwood City, CA: Benjamin/Cummings, 1989, p. 110.)

membranes called *meninges* (Figure 4–9). The outermost layer, the dura mater, is a tough membrane that adheres to the skull though not to the vertebral column. The middle layer is the arachnoid. The innermost membrane, the pia mater, adheres to the brain and cord.

Folds of the dura support the brain (Figure 4–10). The midsagittal fold that divides the cerebral hemispheres is known as the *falx cerebri.* Its posterior portion swoops out laterally and anteriorly to form the *tentorium cerebelli,* which separates the middle and the posterior fossae, that is, the temporal and occipital lobes from the cerebellum and most of the brainstem. Structures contained in the anterior and middle cranial fossae thus are described as supratentorial, while those in the posterior fossa are infratentorial.

The spaces outside and between the meninges are named for their locations: between the skull and dura is the epidural space; between the dura and arachnoid is the subdural space; and between the arachnoid and the pia is the subarachnoid space. The larger subarachnoid spaces are called cisterns, with the largest, the cisterna magna, being located between the foramen magnum and the first cervical vertebra. The meninges provide potential spaces for accumulation of blood and cerebrospinal fluid. The dura and large arterial vessels are the only pain-sensitive structures within the skull (Marshall et al. 1990).

Blood Supply

The arterial blood supply to the brain arises from the two internal carotid arteries anteriorly and the two vertebral arteries posteriorly (Figure 4–11). You may recall that the first three branches of the aorta are the brachiocephalic (which subdivides into the right common carotid and right subclavian arteries), the left common carotid, and the left subclavian arteries. The common carotid arteries give rise to the *internal carotid arteries,* which enter the skull through the cranial floor. The subclavian arteries give rise to the vertebral arteries, which travel up through the transverse processes of cervical vertebrae and through the foramen magnum to unite into the *basilar artery* (Figure 4–12). The internal carotid arteries give rise to the anterior and middle cerebral arteries. The basilar artery gives rise to the posterior cerebral arteries.

At the base of the brain, the anterior and posterior cerebral arteries and their communicating (interconnecting) arteries form the cerebral arterial circle (circle of Willis).

The anterior cerebral artery supplies the medial part of the frontal and parietal lobes and the corpus callosum. The middle cerebral artery nourishes the lateral part of the hemisphere, including portions of the frontal, parietal, and temporal lobes, and supplies

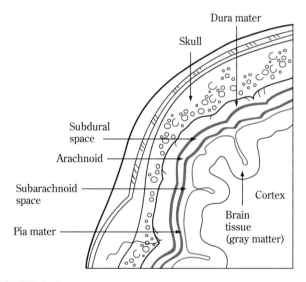

FIGURE 4–9

The meninges. (From Ahrens T: *Critical care certification preparation and review,* 2d ed. East Norwalk, CT: Appleton & Lange. 1991, p. 150.)

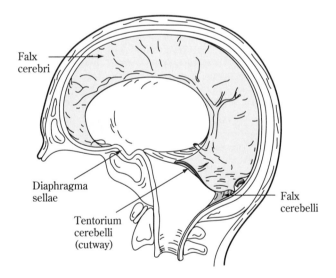

FIGURE 4–10

Folds of the dura. (From Ahrens T: *Critical care certification preparation and review,* 2d ed. East Norwalk, CT: Appleton & Lange, 1991, p. 151.)

branches to nourish the deep structures such as the basal ganglia. The posterior cerebral artery serves the posterior surface of the hemisphere, including part of the temporal lobes and all of the occipital lobes. Branches of the vertebral and basilar arteries nourish the cerebellum and brainstem.

Branches of the external carotid arteries give rise to the meningeal arteries, which course between the skull and dura and nourish the dura. The pia and arachnoid are nourished from branches of the internal carotid and vertebral arteries.

Venous sinuses are located throughout the cranium. They drain blood into the internal jugular vein, which empties into the right atrium via the superior vena cava.

NURSING TIP

Internal Jugular Veins

To promote normal venous drainage and intracranial pressure, take care to prevent compression of the internal jugular veins. Avoid securing endotracheal tubes by taping over the internal jugular veins, as this will impede venous outflow.

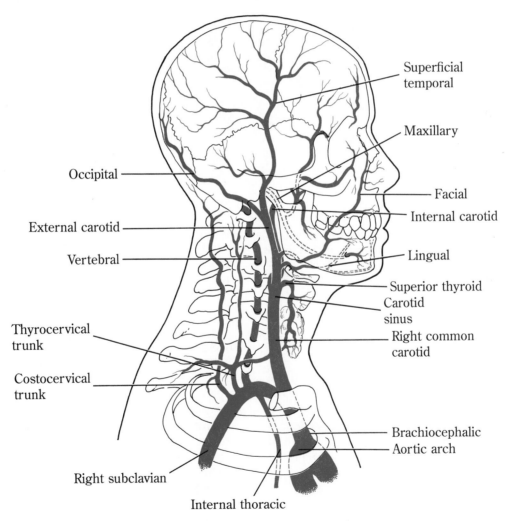

FIGURE 4–11

Arteries of the right side of the head and neck. (From Spence A: *Basic human anatomy,* 3d ed. Redwood City, CA: Benjamin/Cummings, 1989, p. 313.)

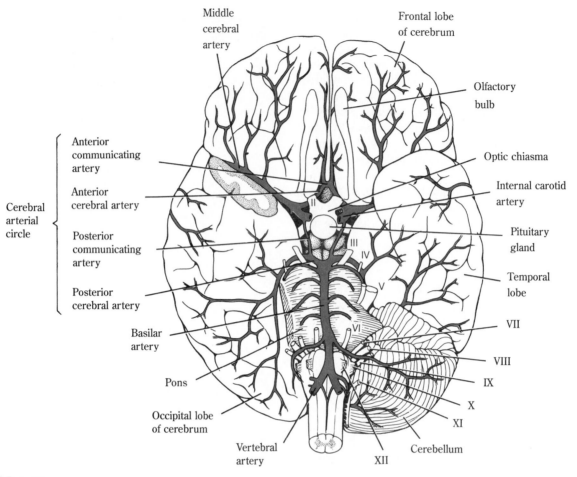

FIGURE 4–12

Arteries of the base of the brain, forming the cerebral arterial circle around the pituitary gland. To provide an unobstructed view, part of the right temporal lobe and the right cerebellar hemisphere have been removed. Roman numerals indicate cranial nerves. (From Spence A: *Basic human anatomy,* 3d. ed. Redwood City, CA: Benjamin/Cummings, 1989, p. 314.)

Cerebrospinal Fluid

Cerebrospinal fluid (CSF) is formed primarily in the choroid plexus of the lateral ventricles. The plexus consists of tufts of capillaries and epithelium lining the brain's ventricular system. The ventricular system is composed of two lateral ventricles, a central third ventricle, a fourth ventricle located between the brainstem and cerebellum, and interconnecting canals (Figure 4–13).

One lateral ventricle sits in each cerebral hemisphere and consists of an anterior horn in the frontal lobe, a body in the parietal lobe, a posterior horn in the occipital lobe, and an inferior horn in the temporal lobe. From each lateral ventricle, CSF passes through a foramen of Monroe into the third ventricle and then through the aqueduct of Sylvius into the fourth ventricle. It then passes through openings in the fourth ventricle (foramens of Luschka and Magendie) into the subarachnoid space. After flowing over the brain and down around the spinal cord, it is drained from the subarachnoid space through the arachnoid villi, which project into the superior sagittal sinus, the large superficial midline sinus of the dura mater.

CSF functions to cushion and nourish the brain. It is formed and absorbed constantly, at the rate of 400–500 ml in 24 hours; at a given moment, about 140 ml is circulating. It is clear, colorless, and odorless and normally contains no red cells and a few white cells. Glucose content varies with the serum glucose level, averaging about 60% of the serum glucose. The normal value is approximately 50–75 mg/100 ml. Protein

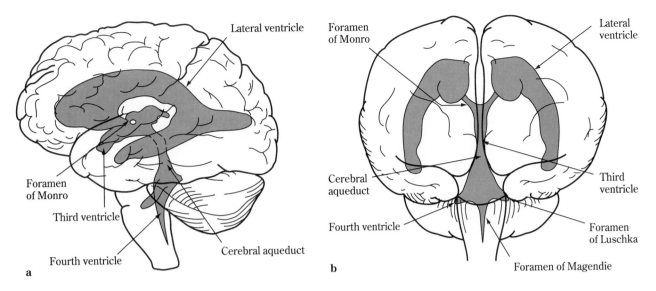

FIGURE 4–13

a, Lateral view of the ventricular system of the brain; **b,** anterior view of the ventricular system of the brain. (From Ahrens T: *Critical care certification preparation and review,* 2d ed. Appleton & Lange, 1991, p. 155.)

concentration varies with the sampling site, normally measuring 5–15 mg/100 ml in the ventricles, 15–25 mg/100 ml in the cisterna magna, and 15–45 mg/100 ml in the spinal canal. Normal specific gravity is 1.007. Opening pressure is up to 180 mm H_2O recumbent.

Disturbances in CSF circulation cause hydrocephalus (excessive fluid accumulation causing ventricular dilatation). For example, the aqueduct of Sylvius may be obstructed by congenital abnormalities or a tumor. The arachnoid villi may become obstructed by clotted blood as the result of a subarachnoid hemorrhage. A nonobstructive hydrocephalus may result from a choroid plexus tumor resulting in over-production of CSF (Marshall et al. 1990). Hydrocephalus is discussed further in Chapter 6.

Spinal Cord

Cord The vertebral column is made up of seven cervical, twelve thoracic, and five lumbar vertebrae plus the sacrum and coccyx. Central openings in the vertebrae form the spinal canal, which contains the spinal cord. The cord proper extends from the base of the brainstem through the foramen magnum to the second lumbar vertebra, from which a fibrous band attaches to the coccyx.

Between the vertebrae and the spinal cord are the spinal meninges (dura, arachnoid, and pia). The cord is supplied by the anterior and posterior spinal arteries, which arise from the vertebral arteries at the foramen

magnum, and by the lateral spinal arteries. Cerebrospinal fluid circulates in the subarachnoid space. In addition, the spinal cord has a central canal which is a small opening in the center. The central canal houses CSF and is an extension of the fourth ventricle.

Tracts Synapses within the spinal cord enable sensory impulses to: (1) enter a spinal reflex arc back to the motor root (Figure 4–14); and/or (2) ascend the spinal cord to the cerebellum via the spinocerebellar tract; and/or (3) ascend the spinal cord to the cortex. To reach the cortex, impulses travel up spinal tracts to the thalamus and pass through the internal capsule to the sensory cortex, which is located behind the Sylvian fissure in the parietal lobe.

Different types of sensory information ascend different tracts. Almost all of the sensory information from the body's somatic segments enter the cord through the posterior roots. After entering the cord, the sensory signals are carried through one of two pathways: the dorsal-column–lemniscal-system (made up of the dorsal column and the spinocervical pathways in the dorsolateral columns) and the anterolateral spinothalamic tracts (Guyton 1991).

The dorsal columns transmit only mechanoreceptive stimuli (Guyton 1991). Fibers carrying fine touch and pressure impulses from the skin, and position and vibration impulses from muscles, tendons, and joints enter the cord and ascend uncrossed in the dorsal columns (posterior tract) to the medulla. (Impulses from the arm and upper body ascend in the column

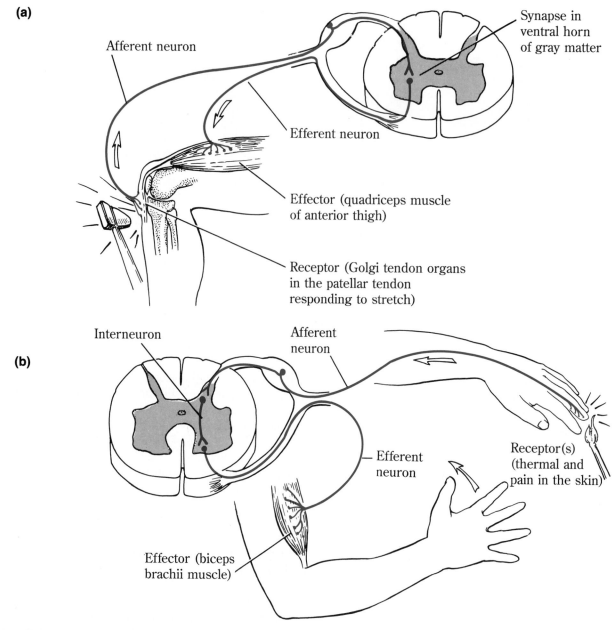

(a)

Afferent neuron

Synapse in
ventral horn
of gray matter

Efferent neuron

Effector (quadriceps muscle
of anterior thigh)

Receptor (Golgi tendon organs
in the patellar tendon
responding to stretch)

(b)

Interneuron

Afferent
neuron

Efferent
neuron

Receptor(s)
(thermal and
pain in the skin)

Effector (biceps
brachii muscle)

FIGURE 4–14

Simple reflex arcs. (a) Two-neuron reflex arc. (b) Three-neuron reflex arc. (From
Marieb E: *Essentials of human anatomy and physiology,* 3d ed. Redwood City, CA:
Benjamin/Cummings, 1991, p. 182.)

called the fasciculus cuneatus, those from the leg and
lower body in the fasciculus gracilis, as shown in
Figure 4–15.) In the medulla, they synapse with another
neuron. This neuron crosses within the medulla and
ascends to the thalamus, which perceives the general
sensation. From the thalamus, a third neuron passes
through the internal capsule to the sensory area in the
parietal lobe.

The anterolateral spinothalamic tracts carry information about pain, temperature, crude touch, and
pressure. Pain and temperature impulses ascend the
lateral spinothalamic tract (Figure 4–16); crude touch
and pressure impulses ascend the ventral (anterior)
spinothalamic tract. In each case, the fibers carrying
the impulses enter the dorsal root and synapse with
another neuron. This neuron crosses to the opposite
side of the cord and ascends the appropriate tract to the
thalamus. In the thalamus, the crude sensation is
perceived and the neuron synapses with a third neuron.
This third neuron travels through the internal capsule

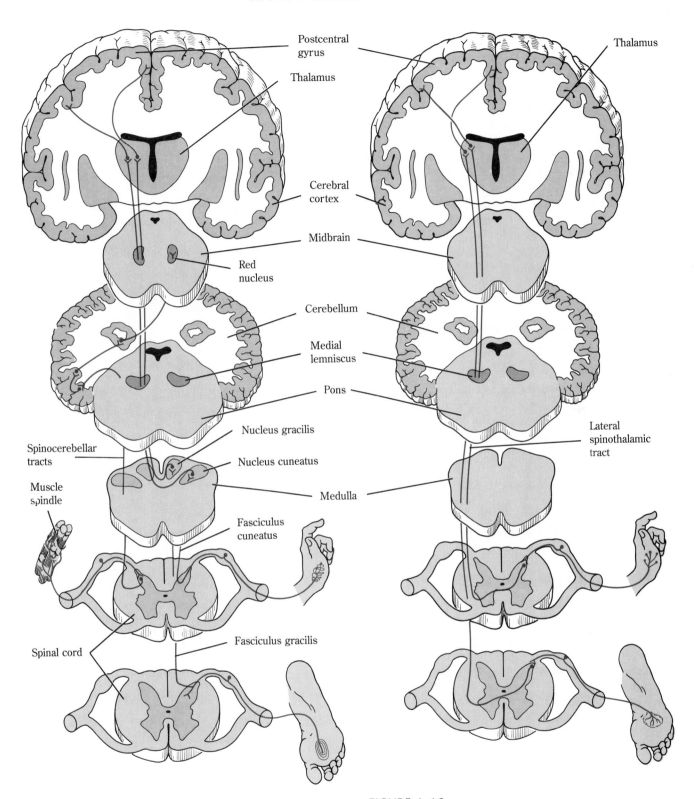

FIGURE 4–15

Sensory pathways for touch, pressure, and proprioception (conscious and unconscious) within the fasciculi gracilis, the fasciculi cuneatus, and the spinocerebellar tracts (posterior tracts). (From Spence A: *Basic human anatomy,* 3d. ed. Redwood City, CA: Benjamin/Cummings, 1989, p. 400.)

FIGURE 4–16

Sensory pathways for pain and temperature within the lateral spinothalamic tracts. (From Spence A: *Basic human anatomy,* 3d ed. Redwood City, CA: Benjamin/Cummings, 1989, p. 400.)

to the sensory cortex, where the stimulus is discriminated and localized.

The spinal cord also contains motor tracts. From each motor cortex, fibers pass through the internal capsule on the same side. The fibers continue to the medulla, where they are grouped to form the corticospinal (pyramidal) tracts (Figure 4–17). In the medulla, most pyramidal fibers cross to the opposite side and continue down the cord as the crossed pyramidal (lateral corticospinal) tract. Motor impulses leave the cord via the anterior (ventral) horn and traverse spinal nerves, peripheral nerves, and neuromuscular junctions before they reach the muscle itself. Because the fibers cross in the medulla, voluntary movement initiated by the motor cortex is manifested on the opposite side of the body.

Peripheral Nervous System

The cranial nerves, spinal nerves, and autonomic nervous system form the peripheral nervous system (PNS). The PNS includes afferent sensory receptors (organs) that detect changes in the internal or external environment and communicate these signals to the CNS via afferent sensory nerves. Efferent motor nerves, which are responsible for body movements, visceral organ motility and secretions, are also part of the PNS. There are 43 sets of peripheral nerves, 12 pairs associated with the brain (cranial nerves) and 31 pairs associated with the spinal cord (spinal nerves).

Cranial Nerves

Twelve pairs of cranial nerves emanate from the brain (Figure 4–18). The critical-care nurse may perform a screening evaluation of cranial nerves, particularly focusing on those whose dysfunction may indicate life threats or seriously interfere with activities of daily living (Table 4–2).

Spinal Nerves

Sensory information reaches the spinal cord and brain from a variety of sources. Impulses pass from a sensory receptor to a peripheral nerve, which carries sensory, motor, and autonomic fibers from a fairly wide area of the body. The peripheral nerves are regrouped closer to the spinal cord into nerve plexes (Figure 4–19) and

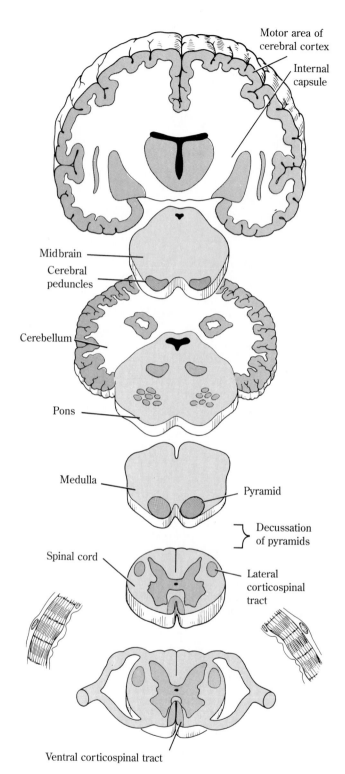

FIGURE 4–17

Pathways of the pyramidal tracts (lateral and ventral corticospinal tracts) carrying motor impulses to skeletal muscles. (From Spence A: *Basic human anatomy,* 3d. ed. Redwood City, CA: Benjamin/Cummings, 1989, p. 402.)

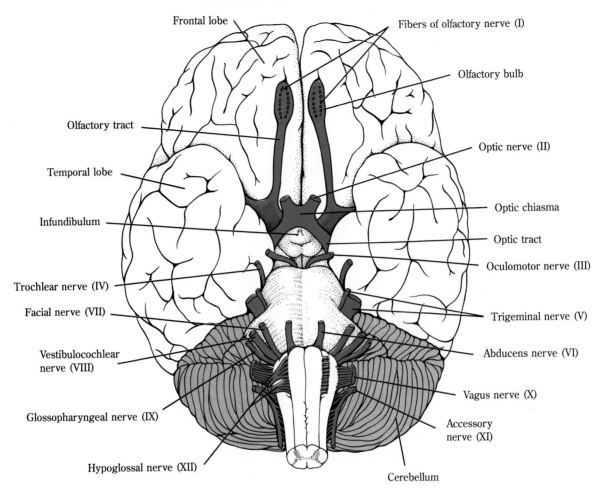

FIGURE 4–18

Cranial nerves. (From Spence A: *Basic human anatomy,* 3d ed. Redwood City, CA: Benjamin/Cummings, 1989, p. 416.)

NURSING TIP

Nursing Assessment After Carotid Endarterectomy

The most important aspects of postoperative neurochecks are level of consciousness, extremity movement, and facial symmetry. To evaluate cranial nerve function quickly, ask the patient to puff his cheeks, stick his tongue out to the right and the left, and open his eyes widely and then close them tightly. Temporal pulses no longer are checked routinely.

TABLE 4–2

A Practical ICU Screening Test for Cranial Nerve Function

NERVE		TEST PROCEDURE
II	Optic	Shine a light into each eye and note whether the pupil on that side constricts (*direct light reflex*). Then shine a light into each eye and note whether the opposite pupil constricts (*consensual light reflex*).
III	Oculomotor	
V	Trigeminal	Touch the cornea with a cotton wisp. (Approach the eye from the side, and avoid the eyelashes.) Note whether a blink reflex is present.
VII	Facial	
IX	Glossopharyngeal	Touch the back of the throat with a tongue blade and note whether a gag reflex is present.
X	Vagus	

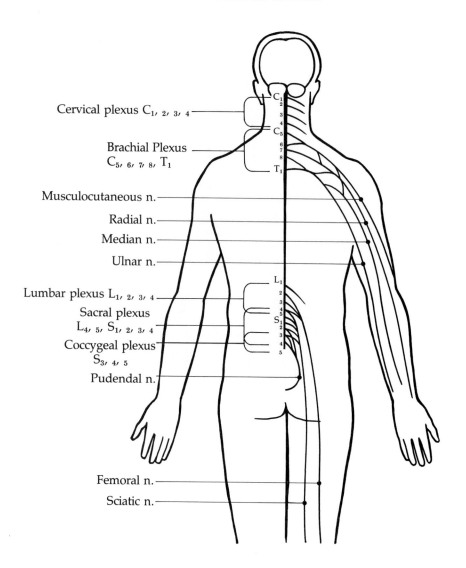

Cervical plexus $C_{1, 2, 3, 4}$

Brachial Plexus
$C_{5, 6, 7, 8}, T_1$

Musculocutaneous n.

Radial n.

Median n.

Ulnar n.

Lumbar plexus $L_{1, 2, 3, 4}$

Sacral plexus
$L_{4, 5}, S_{1, 2, 3, 4}$

Coccygeal plexus
$S_{3, 4, 5}$

Pudendal n.

Femoral n.

Sciatic n.

FIGURE 4–19

Spinal nerve plexes and major peripheral nerves arising from them.

then into 31 pairs of spinal nerves. The pairs of spinal nerves correspond to the 31 spinal segments (eight cervical, twelve thoracic, five lumbar, five sacral, and one coccygeal). Near the cord, the spinal nerves split into posterior and anterior roots (Figure 4–20). The roots connect with gray matter shaped like two pairs of horns within the spinal cord. The posterior (dorsal) root carries sensory fibers into the cord. The anterior (ventral) root carries motor fibers out from the cord. Specific skin segments innervated by the sensory roots are called dermatomes. Dermatomes overlap each other considerably; a simplified diagram appears in Figure 4–21. Knowledge of dermatome innervation aids the physician or nurse in localizing a lesion causing a sensory abnormality.

Autonomic Nervous System

Vital signs are controlled primarily by the involuntary or autonomic nervous system (ANS). This complex system is responsible for unconscious control of involuntary muscles and most glands. It therefore regulates vital signs, fluid intake and output, appetite, gastrointestinal activity, carbohydrate and fat metabolism, sleep, and sexual functioning. Its effects are widespread because they are exerted both by nerves and by chemical mediators.

Overall control of the ANS resides in the hypothalamus. From the hypothalamus, neurons descend through the brainstem and spinal cord and end in three groups. One group of neurons is clustered in the

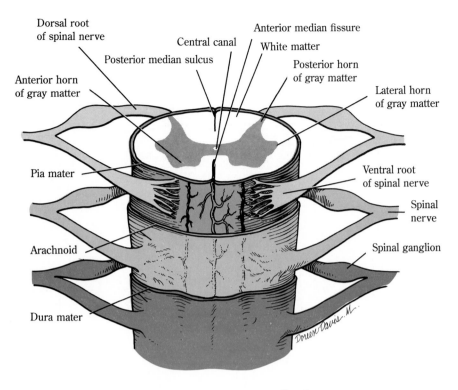

FIGURE 4–20

General internal structure of the spinal cord and the meninges surrounding it.
(From Spence A: *Basic human anatomy,* 3d ed. Redwood City, CA: Benjamin/
Cummings, 1989, p. 396.)

brainstem (around the nuclei of the third cranial nerve in the midbrain and the seventh, ninth, and tenth cranial nerves in the medulla). Another group of neurons is located in the cord around the thoracic and upper lumbar vertebrae, and the last group is centered around the sacral portion of the cord (Figure 4–22). The thoracolumbar outflow powers the *sympathetic* division of the ANS, and the craniosacral outflow powers the *parasympathetic* division.

Sympathetic System Neurons from the thoracic and lumbar area leave the cord through its anterior roots and form an interconnected chain of ganglia near the cord, on either side of the vertebral column and along its complete length. From these ganglia, long postganglionic fibers carry impulses to visceral structures. The primary chemical mediator secreted by sympathetic postganglionic endings is norepinephrine (noradrenalin); drugs that mimic its effects are called *adrenergic* or *sympathomimetic* agents.

Parasympathetic System In contrast to the sympathetic system, neurons from the cranial and sacral parts of the ANS form parasympathetic ganglia near

the effector organs. From these ganglia, short postganglionic fibers carry impulses to visceral structures. The parasympathetic postganglionic endings primarily secrete acetylcholine, and drugs mimicking its effects are known as *cholinergic* agents.

The distribution of fibers to effector organs does not necessarily follow the distribution of spinal nerves and is determined partially by the embryonic origin of the organ. Most muscles and glands are innervated by both sympathetic and parasympathetic fibers; their effects are antagonistic but balanced.

Primary Neurologic Assessment (Neuro-checks)

The nursing process begins with the initial clinical assessment of the patient who presents to the critical-care unit. Noting subtle changes and reporting them promptly is an important aspect of critical-care nursing that requires a baseline assessment from which to measure patient progress, stabilization, or deterioration. All critically ill patients require *neuro-checks*. This

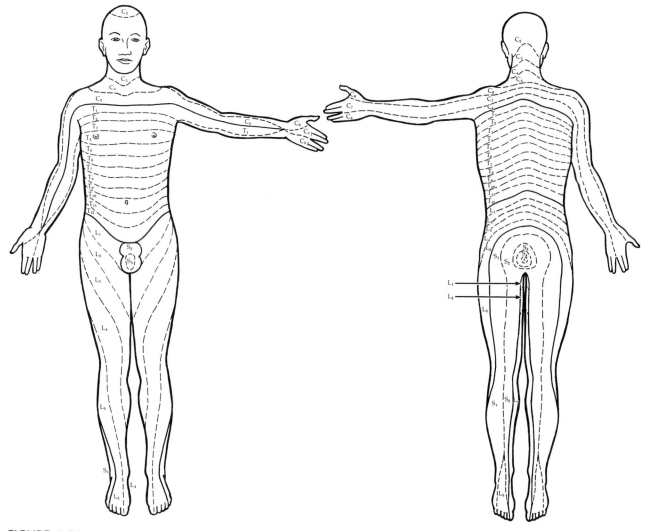

FIGURE 4–21

Dermatomes.

term refers to a brief, systematic approach to assessing key neurologic functions. Patients with identified neurologic deficits may require a more in-depth examination, which will be discussed after the presentation of neuro-checks.

Information obtained on neurologic assessment will shape the medical and nursing care plans; therefore, the neurologic examination must be accurate and reproducible. Charting must be succinct and should identify the mode of stimulation that evoked a patient response. To simplify documentation and evaluation, a flow sheet may be used. A sample is shown in Table 4–3.

An initial, rapid neurologic assessment focuses on the following indicators:

- Level of consciousness.
- Pupil responses.
- Motor function.
- Vital signs.

Level of Consciousness

Level of consciousness (LOC) is the most sensitive indicator of neurologic dysfunction because it reflects the functional integrity of the brain as a whole. Describe the LOC in general terms only if those terms are known and agreed upon by all staff with whom you communicate (Table 4–4).

It is important to arouse the patient maximally before evaluating and noting the LOC. Start with the least noxious stimulus, such as calling the patient's name. If there is no response, gentle tactile stimulation,

Sympathetic
nervous system

Parasympathetic
nervous system

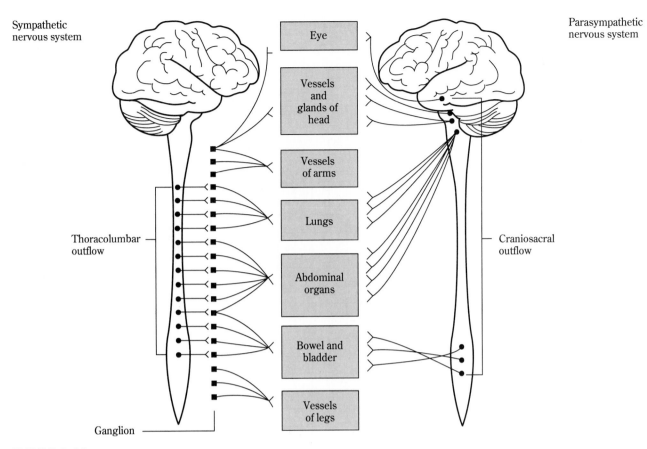

Thoracolumbar
outflow

Craniosacral
outflow

Ganglion

Eye

Vessels
and
glands of
head

Vessels
of arms

Lungs

Abdominal
organs

Bowel and
bladder

Vessels
of legs

FIGURE 4–22

Autonomic nervous system. (From Peck V: *Nurse review: neurological problems.*
Springhouse, VA: Springhouse Corp., 1987, p. 44.)

such as a shoulder shake, may be necessary. Systematically intensify the stimulus to evoke a response. Remember, any stimulus used to evaluate LOC should not scratch, bruise, or otherwise injure the patient. If noxious stimuli are required to evoke a response, one might lay a pen or pencil across the patient's fingernail bed and press firmly. If this does not elicit a response, a sternal massage may be attempted. Rub your open hand firmly over the middle of the sternum, taking care to avoid pressing the xiphoid process at the lower end of the sternum. Another painful stimulus involves applying firm pressure to the Achilles tendon.

Glasgow Coma Scale

The Glasgow Coma Scale (GCS) was designed to measure the functional state of the brain as a whole, since the unconscious state may be brought on by focal or diffuse pathology. It is objective enough to give it high interrater reliability. The scale relates consciousness to three parameters: *eye opening, verbal response,* and *motor response.* Points are assigned to the best level

of response in each category and the total score computed. The fully alert, responsive patient will score 15; the comatose patient will score 7 or less. When assessing a patient, always observe for spontaneous activity before stimulating the patient. If spontaneous activity is not present, then proceed to verbal stimulation and ultimately to tactile (painful) stimulation, if necessary. The Glasgow Coma Scale may be incorporated in ICU and ED flow sheets to detect early changes in neurologic function.

Drawbacks of the Glasgow Coma Scale include the difficulty of use with very young or very old patients and the possibility of a falsely low score with patients who are deaf, intoxicated, uncooperative, or unable to speak English. In addition, patients suffering from "locked-in syndrome" may be fully conscious with extremity and lower cranial nerve paralysis. Movement of extremities and speech will not be possible; therefore, assessment must focus on vertical eye movement and blinking. The scale, therefore, should be viewed as a rapid method for assessing consciousness to be followed by history-taking, a more thorough neurologic examination, and diagnostic testing.

TABLE 4–3

Neurologic Flow Sheet

ST. FRANCIS MEDICAL CENTER
La Crosse, Wisconsin
Neurologic Flow Sheet

92-626   Nurse's Signature and Initials

Pt. Name Plate

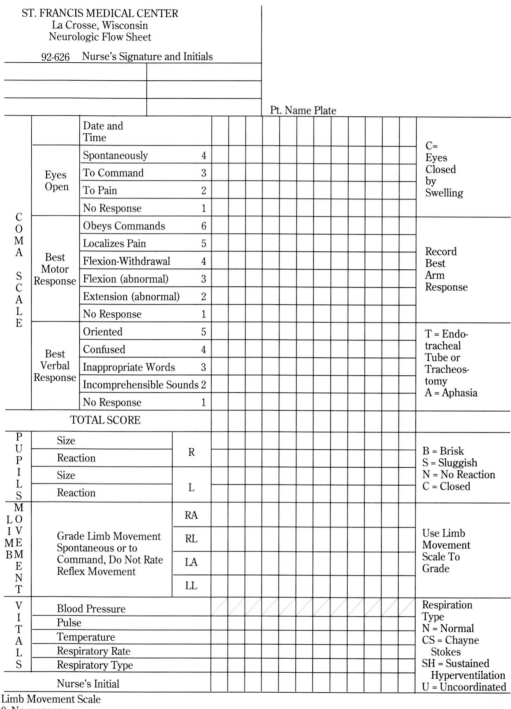

COMA SCALE		Date and Time												C= Eyes Closed by Swelling
	Eyes Open	Spontaneously	4											
		To Command	3											
		To Pain	2											
		No Response	1											
	Best Motor Response	Obeys Commands	6											Record Best Arm Response
		Localizes Pain	5											
		Flexion-Withdrawal	4											
		Flexion (abnormal)	3											
		Extension (abnormal)	2											
		No Response	1											
	Best Verbal Response	Oriented	5											T = Endotracheal Tube or Tracheostomy A = Aphasia
		Confused	4											
		Inappropriate Words	3											
		Incomprehensible Sounds	2											
		No Response	1											
	TOTAL SCORE													
PUPILS	Size	R												B = Brisk S = Sluggish N = No Reaction C = Closed
	Reaction													
	Size	L												
	Reaction													
LIMB MOVEMENT	Grade Limb Movement Spontaneous or to Command, Do Not Rate Reflex Movement	RA												Use Limb Movement Scale To Grade
		RL												
		LA												
		LL												
VITALS	Blood Pressure													Respiration Type N = Normal CS = Chayne Stokes SH = Sustained Hyperventilation U = Uncoordinated
	Pulse													
	Temperature													
	Respiratory Rate													
	Respiratory Type													
	Nurse's Initial													

Limb Movement Scale
0–No response
1–Flicker or Trace of Contraction
2–Active Movement with Gravity Eliminated
3–Active Movement Against Gravity
4–Active Movement Against Gravity and Resistance
5–Normal Power

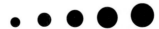

1MM 2MM 3MM 4MM 5MM 6MM 7MM 8MM 9MM

Source: Davenport-Fortune P, Dunnum L: Professional nursing care of the patient with increased intracranial pressure: planned or "hit and miss"? *J Neurosurg Nurs* 1985; 17:367-370.

TABLE 4–4

General Terms Describing Level of Consciousness

Conscious	Awake, alert, aware of environment, able to provide appropriate responses.
Demented	Awake, may be aware of environment, forgetful (mild dementia) to severe mental deterioration, irreversible.
Delirious	Awake or drowsy (hyper- or hypoactive), disoriented, easily distracted, unable to cooperate, inappropriate behavior, disrupted sleep-wake cycle, reversible.
Lethargic	Very drowsy, arousable with stimulation, aware of environment with slow responses that may be appropriate.
Stuporous	Very drowsy, arousable only by noxious and repeated stimulation.
Comatose	Presumably unarousable and unaware with no purposeful response to noxious stimulation.

Adapted from: Stewart-Amidei C: Assessing the comatose patient in the intensive care unit. *AACN Clin Issues Crit Care Nurs* 1991; 2(4):613–622.

Pupil Response

Size and Shape Pupils should be equal in size, unless a congenital disparity exists or constricting or dilating eyedrops have been used in one eye. Anisocoria (unequal pupils) is probably unimportant unless other evidence of a third cranial nerve lesion exists, such as sluggish pupil constriction or diminished medial rectus function (inability to move the eye toward the nose).

NURSING TIP

Constricted and Dilated Pupils

Cranial nerve damage is not the only cause of pupil abnormalities. An awareness of other causes will enhance your assessment skills. Causes of mitotic (constricted) pupils include opiates (morphine), ophthalmic drugs, and intraocular inflammation. Causes of mydriatic (dilated) pupils include ophthalmic dilating medications (used to enhance eye examinations), amphetamines, atropine, scopolamine, and orbit injuries.

To enhance accuracy in communication, specify pupil size in millimeters. Also specify the degree of light in which you observed the eyes; for example, "dilated pupils" is less informative than "pupils 8 mm in brightly lit room." Normal pupils are 2–6 mm in diameter, are round, and have smooth edges.

Response to Light Testing pupillary response to light involves testing both the optic and oculomotor nerves. The following procedure is recommended. Darken the room if possible. If the patient is conscious, ask him or her to focus on a distant point. This will minimize the reflex constriction that occurs when focusing on a nearby point.

Place the edge of your hand along the patient's nose (to avoid the consensual response, explained later). Shine a bright light into one eye and observe the speed with which it constricts (*direct light reflex*). Repeat the procedure with the other eye. Each eye should constrict briskly. Next, shine the light in one eye and observe whether the other eye constricts; then test the other eye. When one eye is stimulated, both pupils should constrict (*consensual light reflex*). The reason this occurs is that one eye perceives the light and transmits impulses to the brain via the optic system; the brain, however, stimulates both oculomotor nerves.

Accommodation To test accommodation, hold your finger 8–12 inches from the bridge of the patient's nose. Have the patient focus on your finger as you move it toward the patient's nose. As you approach the nose, the pupils should constrict and the eyes converge bilaterally and equally to maintain a clear visual image.

The normal pupil response is recorded as **PERRLA**—Pupils Equal, Round, and Reactive to Light and Accommodation.

Abnormal Pupils Some important pupillary abnormalities are shown in Figure 4–23 (Plum and Posner 1980). *Small reactive pupils* often are seen in (1) bilateral diencephalic damage during rostral-caudal deterioration in supratentorial lesions, and (2) metabolic encephalopathies.

Large fixed pupils (5–6 mm) that spontaneously fluctuate in size and may show spasmodic contractions (hippus) result from lesions in the tectal area (roof) of the midbrain.

Midposition fixed pupils (4–5 mm) that are often slightly irregular and unequal are caused by midbrain lesions that interrupt both sympathetic and parasympathetic innervation of the eye. They usually are caused by midbrain damage from transtentorial herniation but also are seen with midbrain tumors, hemorrhages, or infarcts.

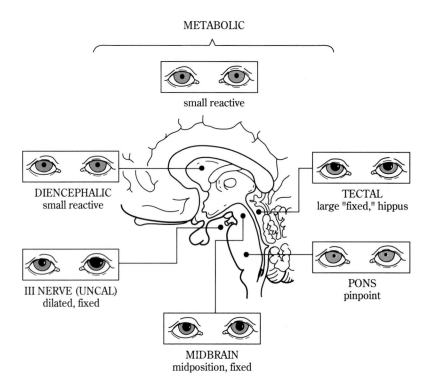

METABOLIC

small reactive

DIENCEPHALIC
small reactive

TECTAL
large "fixed," hippus

III NERVE (UNCAL)
dilated, fixed

PONS
pinpoint

MIDBRAIN
midposition, fixed

FIGURE 4–23

Pupils in comatose patients. (From Plum F, Posner J: *The diagnosis of stupor and coma,*
3d ed. Philadelphia: Davis, 1980.)

Pinpoint pupils are seen with pontine hemorrhage, which interrupts sympathetic pathways to the eye and produces bilaterally small pupils, and with opiate overdose.

A *dilated, fixed ("blown") pupil* is seen with third cranial nerve damage when uncal herniation compresses the oculomotor nerve against the tentorial edge. Recall that a fold of dura, the tentorium, separates the cerebral hemispheres from the cerebellum. An opening in it, called the *incisura* or *tentorial notch,* allows the upper brainstem and its nerves and blood vessels to pass through. When supratentorial pressure increases, the structures near the notch become compressed. One of these structures is the third cranial (oculomotor) nerve. This nerve contains motor fibers (for eye movement) in the center and parasympathetic fibers (for pupillary constriction and eyelid elevation) on the outside. Compression of one oculomotor nerve causes loss of parasympathetic stimulation to the eye on the same side. Sympathetic stimulation continues unopposed, because the sympathetic fibers are not compressed. (The sympathetic pathway originates in the hypothalamus and courses through the brainstem to the upper three segments of the thoracic spinal cord, where the sympathetic nerves to the eye originate.) The result is pupillary dilation and loss of the reflex response to light on the same side as the compression. Associated symptoms may include lateral, downward deviation of the eye and ptosis.

Bilaterally *wide, fixed pupils* are seen in profound hypoxia, such as cardiac arrest, and in anticholinergic poisoning.

Motor Function

When assessing the patient's motor function, note muscle tone, asymmetry, atrophy, fasciculations (signs of a lower motor neuron lesion), or increased tone and spasticity (signs of an upper motor neuron lesion). Motor function can be classed conveniently into voluntary and involuntary (reflex) activity.

Voluntary Activity   Assess voluntary motor activity in the upper extremities with hand grips, by asking the patient to grip the second and third fingers of your hands. Note whether she or he is able to do so, and compare the strength of the grip bilaterally. In addition, ask the patient to close the eyes and extend the arms upright, with the hands supine, for a few seconds. A drifting arm is an early sign of weakness. Assess voluntary motor activity in the legs by asking the

Evaluating Response to Command

Differentiating a grasp-to-command (hand grip) from a grasp reflex may be difficult in the critical-care patient who is weak or slow to respond. Command the patient to grip the second and third fingers of your hands. Note the response. Then direct the patient to release only his or her second and third fingers from yours. Observing the response will help you distinguish a response to command from a coincidental release of grasp.

patient to push her or his feet against your hands. Note spontaneous movement in those patients unable to obey commands.

Reflex Activity If the person does not display voluntary motor activity, a loud voice, vigorous shaking, pressure, or pain should be used to elicit reflex activity. Avoid pinching the patient, as repeated pinching will bruise the patient. Instead, try light pressure by stroking the extremity; if no response, try deep pressure by pressing intensely on the fingernail bed, the Achilles tendon, or the sternum. Note any specific response and evaluate it as appropriate, inappropriate, or absent. Appropriate responses include pushing your hand away or withdrawing from the stimulus. They indicate that sensory function is intact and motor function from the cortex to the muscle is present to some degree. Inappropriate responses include unilateral or

Neurochecks Postanesthesia

To evaluate the neurologic function of the postoperative patient, check hand grips, lower extremity strength (feet pushing against your hands) and ability to raise the head off the pillow. Normal findings are indicators that the patient has adequate muscle strength postanesthesia.

bilateral abnormal flexion (decorticate) or abnormal extension (decerebrate) postures (Figure 4–24).

The following information on abnormal postures is from Plum and Posner's (1980) classic descriptions. If the patient's response is to bring the arm next to the body; flex the fingers, wrist, and arm; and extend the leg, rotate it internally, and plantar flex the foot, then the patient is showing *abnormal flexion* posturing (Figure 4–24 *a, b*). This response is typical of the interruption of corticospinal pathways produced by a lesion in the motor cortex or internal capsule. If the patient's response is to rigidly extend the arms and legs, bring the arms close to the body and hyperpronate them, plantar flex the feet, and sometimes to arch the back (opisthotonos), then the patient is displaying *abnormal extension* posturing (Figure 4–24*c*). This sign indicates a more life-threatening situation than abnormal flexion posturing. It indicates a cerebral lesion that is compressing or destroying the lower thalamus and midbrain, or all the brainstem above the middle of the pons. Abnormal extension in the arms with flaccidity or weak flexor responses in the legs are primitive reactions seen in patients with extensive brainstem damage (Figure 4–24*d*).

There are some important points to remember about abnormal flexion and extension postures. The above descriptions are of full-blown responses; often, you will see only fragments of a posture, such as flexion of one arm. These fragments are important to note and report to the physician, as they are early indicators of abnormal responses. The postures may occur with or without your stimulation, and they may be intermittent or continuous.

Vital Signs

Vital signs can provide valuable clues to nervous system function but must be interpreted with caution due to the multiplicity of factors that influence them. It is also important to remember that changes in level of consciousness are earlier, more sensitive indicators of central nervous system dysfunction than are vital sign changes.

Temperature Changes Although temperature is regulated by the hypothalamus, changes in temperature more often reflect infection in other body sites than hypothalamic dysfunction. Metabolic coma, exposure to extreme cold, and hypothalamic disorders may produce a temperature drop (Plum and Posner 1980), whereas a rise may occur with cerebrospinal fluid infection, blood in the CSF, dehydration, or exposure to extreme heat.

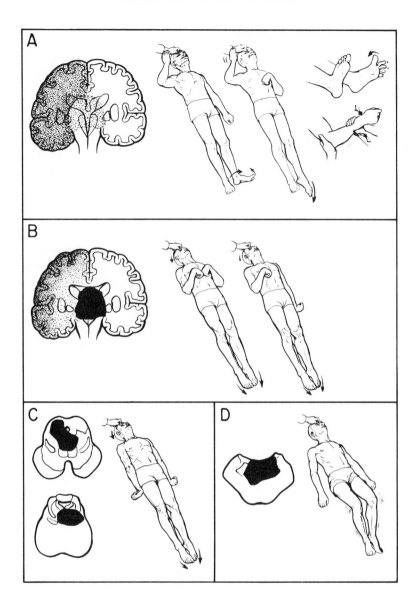

FIGURE 4–24

Motor responses to noxious stimulation in patients with acute cerebral dysfunction.
Noxious stimuli can be delivered with minimal trauma to the supraorbital ridge,
the nail bed, or the sternum. Levels of associated brain dysfunction are roughly indicated at left. The text provides details. (From Plum F, Posner J: *The diagnosis of
stupor and coma,* 3d ed. Philadelphia: Davis, 1980.)

Blood Pressure Changes Blood pressure is influenced by the vasomotor center in the lower pons
and upper medulla. The lateral portions send excitatory impulses via the sympathetic nerves to the
heart, thus increasing pulse rate and myocardial
contractility. The medial portion sends inhibitory
impulses to the heart via the vagus nerves (part
of the parasympathetic system), thus slowing the
heart rate. Dysrhythmias may occur due to pres-

sure on the vasomotor center, or more commonly,
due to blood gas alterations that accompany brain
disorders.

Cushing's triad refers to an increased systolic blood
pressure, bradycardia, and decreased respiratory rate.
These signs result from pressure on the medulla due
to increased intracranial pressure or herniation. Cushing's triad is a late sign of neurologic deterioration. See
Chapter 5 for further details.

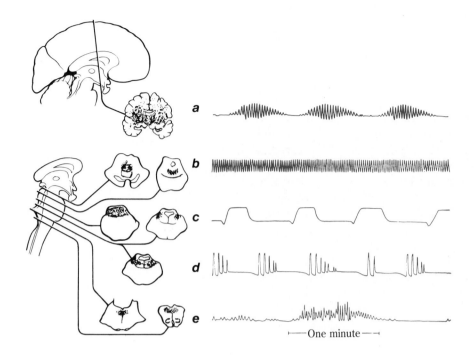

——One minute——

FIGURE 4–25

Abnormal respiratory patterns associated with pathologic lesions (shaded areas) at various levels of the brain. Tracings by chest-abdomen pneumograph, inspiration reads up. **a,** Cheyne-Stokes respiration; **b,** central neurogenic hyperventilation; **c,** apneusis; **d,** cluster breathing; **e,** ataxic breathing. (From Plum F, Posner J: *The diagnosis of stupor and coma,* 3d ed. Philadelphia: Davis, 1980.)

Respiratory Changes Respiration is influenced by many levels of the brain and depends on central nervous system regulation of skeletal muscles. Since metabolic factors also influence respiration, they must be ruled out before one assumes a neurologic basis for abnormal respiration.

As explained in Chapter 7, the most potent stimulus to respiration is the CO_2 concentration or pH of cerebrospinal fluid bathing the respiratory center. The CSF in turn is influenced by changes in CO_2 concentration or pH in arterial blood. Increased CO_2 concentration (decreased pH) causes the rate and depth of respirations to increase (hyperventilation); decreased CO_2 concentration (increased pH) causes the respiratory rate and depth to decrease. Plum and Posner (1980) state that when hyperventilation reduces arterial CO_2 tension below its normal resting level, the stimulus that causes rhythmic breathing appears to arise from the forebrain. In other words, rhythmic breathing due to normal variation in CO_2 appears to originate in the respiratory center in the medulla, whereas that following hyperventilation appears to originate in the forebrain.

Respiratory patterns thus can be used as a reliable guide to the level of neurologic involvement once

metabolic causes (such as diabetic ketoacidosis) have been ruled out. Following are the most common respiratory changes in neurologic patients, based on Plum and Posner's descriptions (Figure 4–25).

After taking five or six deep breaths, the normal person experiences either no apnea or apnea of less than 10 seconds; presumably, the lowered arterial CO_2 tension produced by this hyperventilation has been followed by a forebrain respiratory stimulus. If breathing ceases for more than 12 seconds after this maneuver (posthyperventilation apnea), forebrain response is lacking and the person will resume breathing only when the CO_2 accumulating in the blood again stimulates the respiratory center. Posthyperventilation apnea indicates a diffuse process affecting both cerebral hemispheres, such as metabolic disease.

Smoothly alternating crescendo/decrescendo breathing followed by apneic periods is known as *Cheyne-Stokes respiration*. It results from the combination of an increased respiratory center response to CO_2 stimulation (which produces the hyperpnea) and a decreased cortical response to lowered CO_2 (which produces the apnea). The neurologic cause usually is bilateral lesions deep in the cerebral hemispheres or diencephalon. (Cheyne-Stokes respiration may occur in other disorders, most often in profound cardiac failure, where it probably results from prolonged circulation time between the lungs and brain. This delay allows large changes in blood gas concentration to occur before the respiratory center detects and reacts to them.)

A pattern of prolonged, rapid hyperpnea occurs in some patients with lesions in the low midbrain and upper pons, and in many patients in whom cerebral hemorrhage has caused herniation through the tentorial notch and resulting midbrain compression. Evidence indicates that true central *neurogenic hyperventilation* is rare (Marshall et al. 1990). Instead, the hyperventilation so often seen in unconscious patients probably results from pulmonary congestion due to aspiration, dependent congestion, and infection.

Brief (2–3-second) pauses at the end of inspiration characterize *apneustic breathing*. Expiratory pauses and other irregularities may be present as well. This pattern indicates extensive pontine lesions. Varying groups of breaths with irregular in-between pauses *(cluster breathing)* typify lesions in the lower pons or upper medulla.

Totally irregular respiration indicates damage to the respiratory center in the medulla, such as that produced by downward herniation of supratentorial contents, upward herniation from rapidly expanding posterior fossa lesions, or pontine or medullary hemorrhage. Called *ataxic breathing* (Biot's respirations), this type consists of random shallow and deep breaths with irregular apneic pauses. It indicates disrupted coordination between inspiratory and expiratory neurons in the medulla. This type of breathing necessitates mechanical ventilation if the patient is to survive.

Supplemental Neurologic Assessment

The initial neurologic examination serves as the baseline for subsequent assessment. As patient condition warrants, assessment beyond the neuro-checks will be required. Supplemental neurologic assessment strategies include:

- Patient history.
- Assessment of mentation.
- Examination of the head and neck.
- Eye signs, including corneal reflex and eye position and movement.
- Reflex testing, including oculocephalic reflex, oculovestibular reflex, and spinal reflexes.
- Sensory evaluation.

Patient History

Although a very detailed history can provide valuable insight into a patient's condition, history-taking in the patient with neurologic dysfunction may be difficult due to an altered level of consciousness, communication problems, or memory impairment. Patient interviewing should be done to the extent possible. Questioning should elicit presenting symptoms and their interference with activities of daily living. Particularly note any history of loss of consciousness (onset, duration, behavior after regaining consciousness), seizure activity, behavioral changes, headache, pain, visual abnormalities, dizziness, weakness, decreased level of consciousness, memory loss, and impaired speech. Family members should always be interviewed, because most neurologic patients do not have good insight into the extent of their symptoms.

Assessment of Mentation

Mentation can be defined as the content of consciousness. It reflects general cerebral function and is evaluated with a mental status examination. The components of this examination are: (a) general appearance and behavior; (b) mood and affect; and (c) cognitive functions. To assess general appearance, note the person's dress and grooming. In evaluating behavior, note speech patterns, body language, and the appropriateness of behavior. Next, note mood and affect, that is, the appropriateness, diversity, and speed of change of the person's emotions. Finally, evaluate cognitive functions. These include orientation, attention and concentration, memory, ability to reason, insight, judgment, and thought content.

To evaluate *orientation,* ask the person questions to test awareness of person, place, and time. Test *attention* and *concentration* by asking the person to count backward from twenty by threes or name the months of the year backward, starting with December. Most people can respond to this request within 20 seconds.

Memory consists of short-term, recent, and remote memory. Evaluate *short-term memory* by asking the patient to repeat a phrase given a few minutes earlier. Evaluate *recent memory* by asking what brought the patient to the hospital. Ask about events that occurred several years ago to test *remote memory.* When caring for patients in the same room, it is wise to avoid asking the same questions. Minimizing distractions, such as the television, also will enhance the assessment process.

CRITICAL-CARE GERONTOLOGY

Neurologic Assessment of the Elderly

Neurologic assessment of the geriatric patient may prove difficult due to preexisting illnesses, sensory deficits, and the normal effects of the aging process. Enlist the assistance of family members and friends to obtain valuable baseline information. Remember that normal aging may increase a patient's response time and cause gradual memory impairment. However, deterioration of cognitive functions is not a part of the normal aging process. To maximize a patient's cognitive function, it is important to correct biochemical imbalances and prevent sensory overload or deprivation (Kroeger 1991).

The elderly patient's cooperation may be limited by uncompensated sensory impairments, such as impaired vision or hearing. The patient should be assisted in wearing eyeglasses or hearing aids. These should be clean and in working order. Familiar objects, such as clocks, calendars, and newspapers, and television are helpful in reality orientation. It is important to reassure patients and family that disorientation often occurs in an intensive care unit and does not indicate senility (Stewart-Amidei 1991).

Test *abstract thinking* by asking the person to identify similarities in two objects and to interpret a proverb or solve a problem appropriate to her or his education level. Evaluate *insight* and *judgment* by asking about the cause of the patient's illness and what she or he would do in a given situation, such as discovering a fire. To assess *thought,* note the clarity, content, and flow of thought. Especially note hallucinations and delusions, as they likely will be present in the patient with delirium.

The assessment of mentation should not take more than 5 minutes. Baseline data coupled with well-documented follow-up assessment can assist you to detect delirium early. Report findings objectively. Documentation that a patient made errors in response because of fatigue would be an interpretation, not an observation.

Delirium and Dementia Baseline data are necessary to establish the possibility of pre-existing dementia or developing delirium, both of which may alter the prognosis (Guin 1992). Delirium is a transient disorder of global cognition, while dementia is a chronic brain disorder that produces permanent cognitive dysfunction. In delirium, disorientation may be complete or only partial. Impairment may be more prevalent at night (Inaba-Roland and Maricle 1992). In delirium, you may note slowed speech responses or an inability to comply with the request to count backward or name months backward (Inaba-Roland and Maricle 1992). It is important to note that patients with dementia are at increased risk of developing delirium. (Delusions and hallucinations differentiate delirium from dementia.)

Delirium in the critically ill patient can drastically impact mortality. The delirious patient may pull out lines and tubes, disrupt sutures, or fight mechanical ventilation. In addition, ventilator weaning is delayed when the patient is unable to cooperate. Restraints and sedation may be required to protect the delirious patient. As a result of this immobilization, the patient is at risk of developing deep vein thrombosis, pulmonary embolus, and atelectasis.

An awareness of the common causes of delirium will assist in identifying patients at risk (Table 4–5). The diagnostic criteria for delirium are described in Table

NURSING TIP

Initiating the Mental Status Examination

It is interesting to note that some examiners find the mental status examination more intrusive than starting an intravenous line. Tactful, professional approaches can alleviate the fear of insulting patients. To introduce your exam, you might say, "Some of the questions I will ask you may seem unusual. We ask all our patients these questions. This information helps us to take better care of you" (Inaba-Roland 1992).

TABLE 4–5

Common Causes of Delirium

Organ failure

Renal (uremia)

Hepatic (e.g., hyperammonemia)

Pulmonary (e.g., hypoxia, hypercarbia)

Cardiac (e.g., hypotension, low perfusion states)

Nutritional (e.g., hypoglycemia; hypovitaminosis; B_{12}, folate, thiamine)

Endocrine

Hypothyroidism, hypercorticism

Hyperparathyroidism, hypopituitarism

Structural-vascular-epileptic

Trauma (postconcussive syndrome, subdural hematoma)

Cerebrovascular events (thrombotic, embolic, hemorrhagic)

Neoplastic (primary and secondary)

Infectious (encephalitis)

Epilepsy (postictal, temporal lobe)

Infectious

Septic shock

Central nervous system, non-central nervous system, and systemic (e.g., bacterial, fungal, viral)

Toxic

Intoxication and withdrawal

Alcohol

Anticholinergics

Sedative-hypnotics

Barbiturates

Benzodiazepines

Hallucinogens

Stimulants (cocaine, amphetamines)

Psychotropics (therapeutic and illicit use) (e.g., antidepressants, sedative-hypnotics, lithium)

Anticonvulsants

Corticosteroids

Opiates

Histamine 2 blockers

Digitalis, antiarrhythmics, and other cardiac drugs

Antihypertensives

Electrolyte and acid-base disorders

Sodium, potassium, magnesium

Calcium, acidosis, alkalosis

Source: Inaba-Roland K, Maricle R: Assessing delirium in the acute care setting. *Heart Lung* 1992; 21(1):48–55.

4–6. Evaluation of the delirious patient should focus on identifying treatable physiologic abnormalities that cause cerebral dysfunction.

Medications are implicated in the development of delirium. Lidocaine, digoxin, and aminophylline, which are frequently administered in the critical-care unit, can cause mental status changes. In addition, withdrawal from sedatives or alcohol can cause delirium; onset is usually 24–72 hours.

Treatment of delirium focuses on correcting physiologic abnormalities. Unnecessary drugs should be discontinued and dosages reduced when possible. Uninterrupted sleep should be encouraged as patient condition permits. Clarifying misconceptions, explaining procedures, and reorienting patients may be necessary, as the unfamiliar, technology-filled critical-care environment significantly contributes to cases of delirium (Inaba-Roland and Maricle 1992).

When the strategies discussed are ineffective, pharmacologic approaches are indicated. For mild symptoms, medications that normalize the sleep pattern may suffice. Antipsychotic drugs, such as haloperidol (Haldol) may be required to calm the patient with severe delirium. Haloperidol is the drug of choice for many critically ill patients due to its relative lack of hemodynamic effects (Lyerly 1989).

In the treatment of *delirium tremens* associated with alcohol or sedative withdrawal, antipsychotics are not used because they lower the seizure threshold. Benzodiazepines raise the seizure threshold to help prevent this complication and substitute for alcohol in the brain to allow for a gradual withdrawal (Lyerly 1989).

Examination of the Head and Neck

While inspecting and palpating the cranial bones, look for cerebrospinal fluid leaks, which usually appear as clear, colorless fluid oozing or dripping from the ear *(otorrhea)* or nose *(rhinorrhea)* or down the posterior pharynx. To differentiate this fluid from mucus, test it for glucose—CSF contains glucose, but mucus does not. The presence of blood in the fluid will invalidate this assessment tool, because blood, too, contains glucose. However, the drainage may separate, leaving a "halo effect" of pale yellow CSF around the denser sanguinous drainage. Initiate body substance isolation procedures when handling CSF.

While examining the skull, note also whether the person can touch chin to chest or whether *nuchal rigidity* (a sign of meningeal irritation) is present. (Do not flex the neck if trauma to the cervical spine is suspected.)

TABLE 4–6

Diagnostic Criteria for Delirium*

A. Reduced ability to maintain attention to external stimuli (e.g., questions must be repeated because attention wanders) and to appropriately shift attention to new external stimuli (e.g., perseverates answer to a previous question)

B. Disorganized thinking, as indicated by rambling, irrelevant, or incoherent speech

C. At least two of the following:

    1. Reduced level of consciousness, e.g., difficulty keeping awake during examination

    2. Perceptual disturbances: misinterpretations, illusions, or hallucinations

    3. Disturbance of sleep-wake cycle with insomnia or daytime sleepiness

    4. Increased or decreased psychomotor activity

    5. Disorientation to time, place, or person

    6. Memory impairment, e.g., inability to learn new material, such as the names of several unrelated objects after 5 minutes, or to remember past events, such as history of current episode of illness

D. Clinical features develop over a short period of time (usually hours to days) and tend to fluctuate over the course of a day

E. Either 1 or 2:

    1. Evidence from the history, physical examination, or laboratory tests of a specific organic factor (or factors) judged to be etiologically related to the disturbance

    2. In the absence of such evidence, an etiologic organic factor can be presumed if the disturbance cannot be accounted for by any non-organic mental disorder, e.g., manic episode accounting for agitation and sleep disturbance

Source: American Psychiatric Association: *Diagnostic and statistical manual of mental disorders.* 3d ed., revised. Washington, D.C.: American Psychiatric Association, 1987.
*Each of the main criteria A through E must be satisfied for diagnosis of delirium.

Corneal Reflex

Eye examinations are particularly important in critical care. When examining a patient's eyes, note whether a corneal reflex is present. If the person does not blink spontaneously, test the reflex. With a fine wisp of cotton, approach the eye from the side. Avoid the eyelashes and touch the cornea lightly. Normally, this sensation is perceived by the trigeminal nerve and provokes intense blinking. If this reflex is absent, the cornea may become inflamed or ulcerated due to dryness, scratches, or the presence of a foreign particle. These conditions can deteriorate into inflammation of the iris and blindness. To prevent damage, lubricate the eye with artificial tears and cover with an eye patch. Periodically remove the patch, clean the eye area, and check for inflammation.

Eye Movement

In the resting state, the eyes normally are in midposition. Extraocular movement can be tested in the conscious patient by having him or her follow the movement of your finger. If the eyes move as a pair, conjugate eye movement is present. The presence of conjugate eye movement upward, downward, and diagonally indicates an intact brainstem (Steward-Amider 1991). If the eyes move in different directions, dysconjugate eye movement is present, indicating abnormal function of the third, fourth, or sixth cranial nerve. It is important to document which eye fails to move and what direction causes the problem, for example, "on right lateral gaze, the right eye does not move past midline."

Oculocephalic Reflex   Testing for the oculocephalic reflex *(doll's eyes phenomenon)* is done to evaluate the intactness of the brainstem in the patient in a coma. It is not performed on a conscious patient or one with cervical injuries. The examiner holds the patient's eyelids open and rotates the head to one side and holds it there. If the brainstem reflex is intact, the eyes will move in the opposite direction to the head rotation (Figure 4–26). The doll's eyes reflex can be tested by moving the patient's head to the left, right, up and down. When the head is turned to the left, the eyes should move to the right. Similarly, when the neck is flexed, the eyes should move up. This result is referred to as a positive doll's eyes response and confirms that the brainstem reflex is intact.

Head in neutral position   Head rotated to patient's left

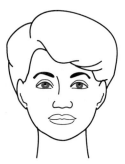   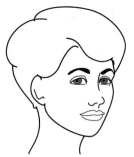   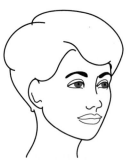

Eyes midline   Positive response   Negative response
                                eyes move in   eyes do not move
                                relation to head   in relation to head

FIGURE 4–26

Doll's eyes phenomenon.

To understand the significance of this response, recall that the vestibular apparatus transmits information about head position along the acoustic nerve to the pons. The nerves controlling lateral gaze are the sixth cranial nerve from the pons and the third cranial nerve from the midbrain. A positive doll's eyes response indicates that information enters the lower pons, ascends to the upper pons and midbrain, and exits the appropriate cranial nerves, in other words, the brainstem is intact. A positive doll's eyes response thus means the coma-producing lesion is either supratentorial or metabolic.

An absent (negative) doll's eyes reflex in a comatose patient usually indicates that the lesion is in the brainstem itself; when the brainstem is damaged, the eyes do not move. An exception is the negative doll's eyes response seen in sedative drug intoxication (the only metabolic encephalopathy in which negative doll's eyes is seen). This exception is important to remember, since drug-induced coma is common.

Oculovestibular Reflex In addition to testing the pupillary and corneal reflexes and the doll's eye phenomenon, the examiner may use the oculocephalic reflex (ice water stimulation; cold calorics) to evaluate the intactness of the brainstem. This maneuver is physiologically identical to the doll's eyes maneuver but is more powerful in inducing eye movements. The following descriptions are based on Plum and Posner (1980). After examining the ear for intactness of the tympanic membrane, the examiner places the patient with the head elevated 30 degrees to provide maximal stimulation of the semicircular canal. The examiner then uses a large syringe,

filled with ice water, and a small catheter to slowly irrigate the canal until nystagmus or ocular deviation occurs. Approximately 120 ml of water may be used in an attempt to elicit a response. The response in the normal awake patient is nystagmus after 20–30 seconds, with slow movement toward the irrigated ear and rapid movement away. In the comatose patient, you may see the eyes move slowly toward the irrigated ear and remain there for 2–3 minutes; the fast return to midline (quick phase) has disappeared. This response indicates that the lesion is supratentorial or metabolic. If you see an extremely abnormal response, such as downward deviation and rotary jerking of one eye, the lesion is in the brainstem. An absent cold caloric response indicates severe brainstem damage or depression.

Motor Responses

Spinal Reflexes Spinal reflexes include superficial (or cutaneous), pathologic (seen only in neurologic diseases) and deep tendon (or stretch) reflexes. Superficial reflexes are tested by stroking the skin. One superficial reflex you may have observed in males is the cremasteric reflex: stimulating inner thigh skin (such as when you manipulate a urinary catheter) causes testicular elevation on the same side. The abdominal reflex is tested by stroking the abdomen toward the midline with the handle of a reflex hammer. The umbilicus should move toward the stimulus. This response may be difficult to detect in the obese patient.

Critical-care nurses evaluate pathologic reflexes when they check the plantar reflex for the Babinski sign. To evaluate the plantar reflex, use a semisharp

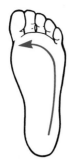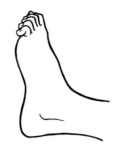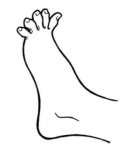

Stroke up sole of foot and across ball

Normal response—plantar flexion of all toes

Abnormal response—dorsiflexion of big toe with or without fanning of other toes

FIGURE 4–27

Babinski sign.

object such as the handle of a reflex hammer. Start at the outer edge of the heel. Stroke up the outer side of the sole and across the ball of the foot (Figure 4–27). Watch the big toe. Normally, the person will plantar flex the big toe. The abnormal response of dorsiflexing the big toe (and sometimes flaring the other toes) is called a positive Babinski sign and indicates damage to the pyramidal tract.

The critical-care nurse usually does not test deep tendon reflexes. An examiner can test them by briskly striking a partially stretched tendon or bony prominence with a reflex hammer and evaluating the resulting muscular contraction. Examples are the biceps and patellar reflexes.

Motor Neuron Lesions Disorders causing loss of voluntary or reflex movement commonly are described as upper motor neuron or lower motor neuron lesions (Table 4–7). As mentioned earlier, peripheral nerves can carry motor and sensory fibers. The motor fibers eventually subdivide so that one motor fiber serves one muscle fiber. This last motor neuron innervating a muscle fiber is called the final common pathway because all motor impulses must pass through it to the muscle fiber.

Motor neurons serving the final common pathway are of two types. Those between the cerebral cortex and the motor nuclei of the brainstem or spinal cord are called *upper motor neurons.* Those between the motor nuclei of the brainstem (for cranial nerves) or the anterior horn cell in the spinal cord (for spinal nerves) and the muscle are called *lower motor neurons.*

Upper motor neuron lesions produce hyperactive reflex activity: while the reflex arc remains intact, cortical inhibition is lost. Although reflex activity is retained, voluntary motor function is lost (spastic paralysis). An example of an upper motor neuron lesion is hemiparesis following a cerebrovascular accident. Lower motor neuron lesions produce hypoactive reflexes, loss of voluntary movement, and muscle atrophy (flaccid paralysis). Examples are poliomyelitis and Guillain-Barré syndrome.

Impulses from the cerebellum and basal ganglia are transmitted to the muscles via extrapyramidal pathways in the spinal cord. During your assessment of motor activity, note whether movements are smooth and coordinated. Specific tests of cerebellar function (such as finger-to-nose, heel-to-shin, and rapid alternating movements, to test coordination; heel-to-toe walking to evaluate gait; and the Romberg test to assess balance) are part of the comprehensive neurologic

TABLE 4–7

Comparison of Motor Neuron* Lesions

UPPER MOTOR NEURON	LOWER MOTOR NEURON
Involves cortex, internal capsule, corticospinal or corticobulbar tracts	Involves anterior horn, anterior nerve root, and peripheral nerve to motor end plate
Muscle spasticity and slight atrophy	Muscle flaccidity and extensive atrophy
Hyperreflexic	Hyporeflexic
+Babinski sign	–Babinski sign
–Fasciculations	+Fasciculations

*Motor neurons are functional units that convey motor impulses.

examination of the ambulatory patient but not the patient with a critical neurologic problem. Loss of smoothness and coordination can result from damage to the cerebellum, basal ganglia, and/or extrapyramidal pathways in the cord.

Sensory Evaluation

The sensory examination is designed to test both of the primary afferent pathways: the spinothalamic tract and the posterior columns.

Spinothalamic Tracts The spinothalamic tracts convey pain and temperature sensations. Pain perception is tested by asking the patient to close his or her eyes. The examiner uses the sharp end of a reflex hammer and rubs against the skin. The blunt end of the hammer will provide a contrast between sharp and dull stimulation. Responses are recorded as sensation is felt in relation to anatomic landmarks such as the nipples, umbilicus, iliac crest, or knees. Temperature sensation may be tested by rubbing an alcohol wipe across the skin. Testing of pain *or* temperature sensation is appropriate because both functions are carried in the same tract. Remember to evaluate both sides and the upper and lower extremities.

Posterior Columns Posterior columns convey fine touch, vibration, and proprioception. Fine touch perception is evaluated by rubbing a wisp of cotton, or the corner of a gauze pad, across the patient's skin while his or her eyes are closed. Vibratory sensation is evaluated bilaterally by placing a tuning fork on the bony prominences or soft tissue. Proprioception is tested by asking the patient, whose eyes are closed, to identify if you are moving the patient's finger toward or away from his or her head.

Lesions above the thalamus may not cause demonstrable deficits in the primary sensory modalities as described above (Lyerly 1989).

Patterns of Pathology

So far, correlation of signs and symptoms and sites of dysfunction has been presented beginning with the sign and then identifying possible sites. As you have seen, most signs can be due to lesions in a variety of sites. The differential diagnosis of pathology requires extensive education and experience in neurology and is based upon the level and extent of symptomatology and a knowledge of the patterns of findings produced by lesions in different sites. Some patterns of pathology you may observe are presented in Table 4–8. It is useful to acquaint yourself with them, both to understand how one identifies the site of a lesion and to predict a patient's deficits from a medical diagnosis so you can better plan nursing care.

Diagnostic Procedures

Numerous diagnostic procedures are available to aid the clinician in assessing the location and extent of neurologic damage and the prognosis for recovery. The ones reviewed here are: cerebrospinal fluid sampling, electroencephalography, computerized tomography, magnetic resonance imaging, cerebral arteriography, and evoked potential tests. Intracranial pressure monitoring is discussed in the next chapter.

Cerebrospinal Fluid Sampling

Samples of CSF can be obtained from the lumbar subarachnoid space of the spinal canal or the lateral ventricles. For sampling at any site, the patient and/or family should be prepared psychologically with a description of the benefits and risks, steps in the procedure, and normal sensations. An informed consent should be signed and the patient sedated if necessary. Lumbar and ventricular punctures may be done in the critical-care unit.

Lumbar Puncture A *lumbar puncture,* the most common, is done to measure CSF pressure, sample CSF, remove CSF to lower intracranial pressure, or inject contrast media or medications. Contraindications to a lumbar puncture are inflammation at the proposed injection site and greatly increased intracranial

TABLE 4–8

Patterns of Pathology

TYPE OF LOSS	LOCATION OF LESION
Sensory	
1. Decrease or loss of all sensation in area served by peripheral nerve	Peripheral nerve
2. Decrease or loss of all sensation in dermatome	Sensory (dorsal) root
3. Decrease or loss of pain and temperature sensation on one side of body	Lateral spinothalamic tract on opposite side of body
4. Decrease or loss of fine touch discrimination, vibration awareness, awareness of limb position	Dorsal column (fasciculus gracilis or cuneatus) on same side of body
5. Decrease or absence of all sensation on one whole side of body	Thalamus on opposite side of body
6. Retention of crude sensation with loss of fine discrimination on one whole side of body	Sensory cortex on opposite side of body
Motor	
1. Loss of voluntary activity below level of lesion with retention of reflex activity (spastic paralysis)	Corticospinal (pyramidal) tract (upper motor neuron); side of body depends on level of lesion
2. Loss of voluntary and reflex activity below level of lesion (flaccid paralysis)	Lower motor neuron on same side of body
3. Decrease or loss of fine sensation and voluntary movement on entire side of body, with retention of crude sensation and reflex activity	Internal capsule
4. Decrease of muscle tone; inability to synchronize movements, gauge distance and speed, alternate movements quickly; intention tremor; poor equilibrium; voluntary and reflex motor activity present	Cerebellum
5. Rigidity, resting tremor, involuntary movements such as in Huntington's chorea; voluntary and reflex motor activity present	Extrapyramidal system

pressure; in the latter case, removal of CSF from the spinal canal could precipitate brain herniation.

To assist with a lumbar puncture, explain to the patient that the procedure will last only a few minutes and usually is not painful; that the doctor will give a local anesthetic to reduce the feeling of pressure from the needle insertion; that the patient will lie on his or her side and should stay very still; and that brief pains in the legs or pelvis may be experienced if the needle brushes nerves to those areas. Bring to the bedside a lumbar puncture tray, local anesthetic, sterile gloves, and a small bandage. Place the patient on his or her side with the back at the edge of the bed and the spine curved; or have the patient sit up and bend over a bedside table. You may need to hold a restless patient. The physician will clean the skin and infiltrate it with a local anesthetic. She or he then will insert the needle and stylet at the level of the iliac crests. Insertion of the needle at this level places its tip in the spinal canal below the termination of the cord. After removing the stylet, the physician will connect the manometer, measure opening pressure, drain off fluid into labora-

tory tubes, measure closing pressure, remove the needle, and cover the puncture site with a small bandage.

During the procedure, reassure the patient, remind him or her not to move, and observe for a change in the level of consciousness, which may signify herniation. After the procedure, observe for changes in the level of consciousness or vital signs, meningeal irritation, edema or hematoma at the puncture site, and motor power in the lower limbs. Headache may be eased by (1) having the patient remain lying flat for 1–6 hours, (2) increasing fluid intake (by mouth or intravenously), and (3) giving analgesics. Transient back and leg pain may result from nerve root irritation.

Ventricular Puncture   A *ventricular puncture* is done if lumbar puncture is contraindicated or if ventricular drainage is necessary for increased intracranial pressure. In the critical-care unit, ventricular puncture most likely will be done to monitor intracranial pressure. For details, see the section in Chapter 5 on measuring intracranial pressure. Nursing care following a ventricular puncture consists of 10–15 degree elevation of the head; bedrest for 24 hours; neurologic checks every 30–60 minutes until stable; and maintenance of a dry, sterile dressing over the sutured skin incision. The patient should be watched closely, as she or he may develop a headache, respiratory distress, convulsions, or increasing intracranial pressure.

Electroencephalography

In this procedure, the electrical activity of the brain is recorded from scalp electrodes. The electroencephalogram (EEG) is used to diagnose disorders that cause changes in electrical patterns, such as epilepsy, tumors, and brain death.

Other than an explanation to the patient, no particular preparation is necessary. Either the patient will be taken to a soundproofed, electrically shielded room or, if he or she is too sick to be moved, the EEG will be recorded at the bedside. Electrodes are applied with paste or needles to the scalp over the various lobes, and the tracing is recorded while the patient remains relaxed and still to avoid creating electrical artifacts. The EEG may take up to 2 hours and will be interrupted periodically so the patient can change position. Alert the patient in advance that he or she will be asked to hyperventilate for a short time to provoke any abnormal discharge and can anticipate transient lightheadedness or dizziness during this hyperventilation. An EEG is not painful and does not produce any postprocedure complications.

Computerized Tomography (CT)

Computerized tomography (CT) scanning is a neurodiagnostic procedure that utilizes a computer to analyze x-ray data. Although a beam of x-ray photons is used, the data are recorded numerically rather than in a conventional x-ray. CT scanning shows horizontal cross-sections of the brain. CT scans are much more sensitive than conventional x-ray studies.

Patient Preparation Patient preparation for a CT scan should include a brief description of the equipment and the procedure. The patient must hold very still, as even small movements induce artifact. If the patient is unable to hold still, sedation may be necessary. The scan is safe and painless; the only unpleasant sensation the person might experience is a brief burning sensation if contrast medium is used. It is imperative that information about patient allergies and renal function be ascertained before the injection of iodine-based contrast media.

Procedure The patient lies on a table with his or her head positioned within the section of the scanner containing the x-ray tube. The x-ray tube rotates 360° around the head, transmitting an x-ray beam (a scan) through the head. Clicking sounds normally are heard from the scanner.

The duration of the scan is about 10 minutes without contrast medium and 25 minutes with contrast medium. After each scan, the table moves so the patient's head is progressively withdrawn from the apparatus. On the opposite side of the head from the beam is a crystal detector that reads the transmission. The readings form the basis of complex equations that the computer solves and transforms into absorption coefficients indicating the density of predetermined volumes of brain tissue. The data from the scan are available in three forms: a computer printout, television monitor display, and hard-copy print on standard x-ray film or Polaroid film.

Abnormalities Detected Abnormalities are detected by deviations from normal density and sometimes also by displacement of normal structures. Lesions that can be located by CT scanning are tumors, cysts, abscesses, hematomas, infarctions, aneurysms, and arteriovenous malformations. Although CT scans have reduced the use of cerebral arteriography for tumor screening, the cerebral arteriogram is more precise than the scan for visualizing vascular anatomy and abnormalities such as aneurysms and occlusions. Since the amount of radiation exposure is relatively low, serial CT scans can be taken to follow the resolution of cerebral disorders.

No special physiologic care is necessary after a scan without contrast medium. If contrast medium is used, observe for a possible allergic reaction.

Magnetic Resonance Imaging (MRI)

Magnetic resonance imaging (MRI) is a procedure that has proven especially effective for imaging the nervous system. The availability of magnetic resonance contrast-enhancing medium (gadopentetate dimeglumine) allows for an even more sophisticated resolution of the brain. This medium is injected intravenously and, although not required for MRI, produces enhanced resolutions. MRI utilizes a magnetic field and radio frequency to generate body organ images of such quality and precision that you feel you are looking at the anatomic specimen. The high reliability and minimal patient risk associated with the use of CT and/or MRI have almost eliminated the need to perform pneumoencephalograms or ventriculograms.

Use of magnetic resonance imaging is indicated when lesions are poorly demonstrated on CT scan or patients are allergic to iodinated contrast media. Sequential exams may be carried out with minimal patient risk, since MRI does not employ ionizing radiation. MRI appears to be more sensitive than CT in detecting: (1) demyelinization associated with multiple sclerosis, (2) lesions located in the brainstem, craniocervical junction, or spinal cord, (3) small hemorrhages deep within the brain, and (4) tumors.

The major disadvantage of MRI results from the use of a strong, static magnetic field. Since the magnetic field attracts ferromagnetic devices, sheet metal workers (who may have metal slivers imbedded in their tissues) and patients with prosthetic devices such as cardiac valves, aneurysm clips, and orthopedic pins may be excluded from MRI screening. Recent changes in the type of metals used for procedures has made MRI accessible to more patients with the prosthetic devices described.

Patient Preparation Patient education focuses on the potential problems related to the MRI housing unit and the magnetic environment. The table the patient lies on and the opening (bore) in the housing unit are narrow. When the table moves inside the unit, the patient may experience claustrophobia. To minimize this feeling, most units have mirrors so the patient can see out into the room and not feel so enclosed. Also, the technicians move the table slowly into the unit so the patient can adjust to the space. Sedation may be necessary for claustrophobic patients. Although the technicians must be out of the room while the test is in progress, the patient can still communicate with them. Assure the patient that it is normal to hear a continuous knocking sound during the test.

Prior to entering the magnetic area, the patient must remove any items that might be ferromagnetic, including nondigital watches, rings, bobby pins, hair clips, eyeglasses, and any articles of clothing with metal snaps, zippers, or buckles.

The magnet used is in a housing similar to that for CT scanning (Figure 4–28). When the patient is placed inside the unit and the magnet is turned on, the magnet aligns, or polarizes, the hydrogen protons. Radio frequency (RF) waves are then transmitted into the magnetic field, causing the protons to change alignment, or depolarize. Termination of the RF waves allows the protons to return to their original state. The energy emitted and the speed with which the protons return to their polarized state differentiate healthy tissue from diseased tissue.

Based on this information, the computer constructs an image of the tissue in one of three projections—

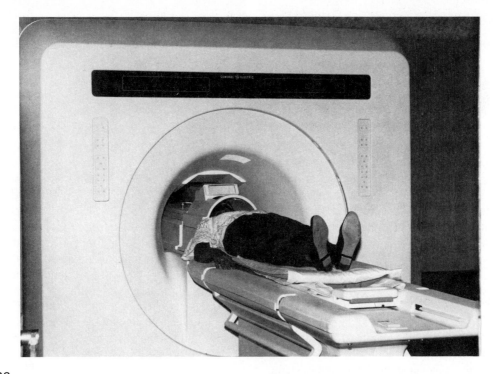

FIGURE 4–28

MRI housing unit, showing a patient lying on a table with head inside the bore.
(Photo courtesy of Santa Barbara Cottage Hospital, Glenn Dubock photographer.)

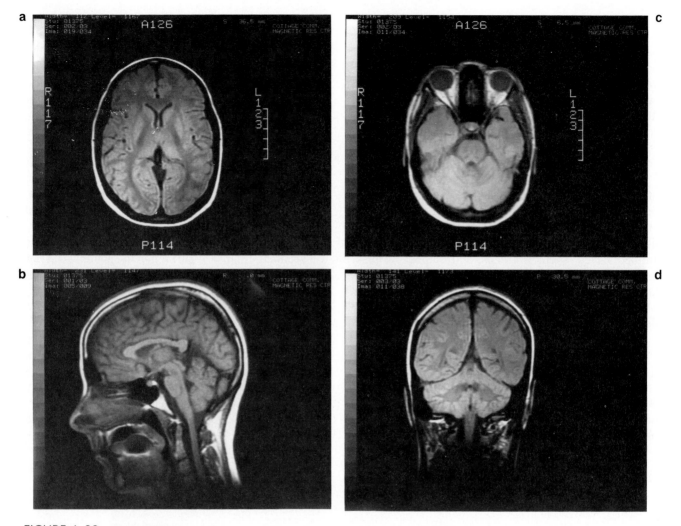

FIGURE 4–29

Magnetic resonance images. **a,** Axial view at midthalamic level; **b,** midline sagittal image; **c,** axial image at level of upper pons; **d,** coronal image through occipital lobe and cerebellum. (Photos courtesy of Cottage Community Magnetic Resonance Center.)

axial, coronal, or sagittal—depending on the program (Figure 4–29). All planes can be obtained in approximately 35 minutes, with each plane consisting of 20 slices. Still images are permanently recorded on x-ray–type film.

Cerebral Arteriography

In this diagnostic maneuver, contrast medium is injected into the cerebral circulation to visualize the arteries and veins. It is used to detect aneurysms, occlusions, hematomas, tumors, and other lesions sizable enough to destroy cerebral vessels.

Patient Preparation Before the procedure, assist the physician to explain its benefits and risks and secure informed consent. Particularly prepare the patient for the sequence of steps and the intense burning sensation that may be experienced when dye is injected. This sensation is normal and lasts 20–30 seconds.

Preprocedure preparation usually includes a sedative the night before, nothing by mouth for 8 hours before the procedure, and shaving of the proposed injection site. Just before the patient leaves the unit, you should record a current neurologic assessment and then premedicate.

Procedure The patient will be taken to the neuroradiology department and placed on a movable x-ray

ADVANCES IN CRITICAL-CARE TECHNOLOGY

POSITRON EMISSION TOMOGRAPHY (PET)

The Technology PET is a process by which pathways of brain activity are studied. A glucose compound containing a radioactive isotope is delivered to a patient by inhalation or injection. This radioactive isotope is then observed as a means of studying the brain's metabolism by monitoring cerebral blood flow and biochemical reactions. Detectors outside the head measure the activity of the isotopes in the patient's head.

Patient Care Considerations PET scanning can be used to differentiate areas of brain tumor recurrence from areas of radiation necrosis. Seizure activity in the brain can also be localized by PET. PET scanning is costly and is used primarily as a diagnostic tool in research. With progress in research and technology, PET may prove to be a valued neurodiagnostic tool (Jamieson 1988).

SINGLE PHOTON EMISSION COMPUTED TOMOGRAPHY (SPECT)

The Technology SPECT is a process by which the regional differences in the brain's blood flow are studied (cerebral blood flow and metabolic activity are studied with PET). SPECT was developed as an alternative to the complex and costly PET. SPECT can be performed with conventional nuclear medicine cameras that are modified to rotate around the patient's head. Radioactive isotopes are administered so that cerebral blood flow may be measured.

Patient Care Considerations SPECT identifies areas of perfusion defects before CT scans show evidence of infarction. SPECT shows promise in replicating the more expensive PET studies (Marshall et al. 1990).

---

table. Depending upon the anticipated site of pathology, the physician will plan to inject either the carotid artery (to visualize the anterior, middle, and posterior cerebral arteries) or the vertebral artery (to visualize it and the basilar artery). The carotid and vertebral arteries can be either punctured directly or, as is more commonly done, reached by a catheter advanced from other arteries, such as the femoral or brachial artery.

The physician will prepare the skin, inject local anesthesia, make a percutaneous entry into the vessel, introduce and advance a catheter under fluoroscopic examination, and inject radiopaque contrast medium while repeated x-rays are taken. During this time, the patient will be monitored closely for an anaphylactic reaction and signs of increased intracranial pressure.

After the procedure is completed, the patient will be returned to his or her room. Perform neuro-checks, peripheral pulse checks, and site inspection every 30 minutes to 4 hours, depending upon the patient's stability. Also follow the measures outlined in the section on cardiac catheterization (Chapter 11) for potential complications after catheterization. Patients usually recover from this procedure in a few hours and without severe reactions.

To understand better the experience of cerebral arteriography, talk with patients who have undergone the procedure. Seeking this information will sensitize you to the concerns of patients and help increase your ability to alleviate their worries.

Evoked Potentials (EP)

Evoked potentials (EP) are electrical manifestations of the brain's response to an external stimulus. The monitoring of EP has become a useful diagnostic tool in clinical neurophysiology. The EP test provides an objective measurement of the functional status of certain sensory pathways.

Visual EPs are tested by flashing bright lights through special goggles placed over the patient's eyes. Somatic EPs rely on tactile stimuli to evoke a response. Auditory EPs involve the use of sound delivered via headphones. Electrodes are placed on the patient's scalp, and the brain's response to the stimulation is captured by the electrodes and recorded on an oscilloscope as a waveform.

The ability of the EP tests to aid in the evaluation of whether sensory pathways are functioning properly makes them useful in monitoring central nervous system surgical procedures. Muscle relaxants do not alter test results. EP tests have also proven useful for patients who are in barbiturate coma with a flat EEG (Marshall 1990).

REFERENCES

Ahrens T: *Critical care certification preparation and review,* 2d ed. Norwalk, CT: Appleton & Lange, 1991.

Guyton A: *Textbook of medical physiology,* 8th ed. Philadelphia: Saunders, 1991.

Inaba-Roland K, Maricle R: Assessing delirium in the acute care setting. *Heart Lung* 1992; 21(1):48–55.

Jamieson D et al.: Positron Emission Tomography in the investigation of central nervous system disorders. *Radiol Clin North Am* 1988; 26(5):1075–1088.

Kroeger L: Critical care nurses' perception of the confused elderly patient. *Focus Crit Care* 1991; (Oct) 18(5):395–400.

Lyerly H: *The handbook of surgical intensive care,* 2d ed. Chicago: Yearbook Medical, 1989.

Marshall S et al.: *Neuroscience critical care.* Philadelphia: Saunders, 1990.

Plum F, Posner J: *The diagnosis of stupor and coma,* 3d ed. Philadelphia: Davis, 1980.

Stewart-Amidei C: Assessing the comatose patient in the intensive care unit. *AACN Clin Issues Crit Care Nurs* 1991; 2(4):613–622.

Neurologic Disorders

CLINICAL INSIGHT

Domain: Administering and monitoring therapeutic interventions and regimens

Competency: Combating the hazards of immobility: preventing and intervening with skin breakdown, ambulating and exercising patients to assure maximum mobility and rehabilitation, preventing respiratory complications

Combating hazards of immobility requires not just deciding what activity a patient needs but also inspiring the patient to exercise despite pain and fatigue, controlling any pain provoked by the activity, and, when necessary, setting and enforcing limits. In the following exemplar, from Crabtree and Jorgenson (1986, pp. 112–114), a nurse reflects on the challenge presented to her and a second nurse by Liz, a 16-year-old Guillain-Barré patient whose natural adolescent limit-testing was exacerbated by her months-long hospitalization in the critical-care unit. After being com-

pletely dependent—mechanically ventilated and unable even to open her eyes—Liz gradually regains muscle function. Unfortunately, Liz has become both manipulative in response to her forced dependency and addicted to narcotics. Recognizing that Liz desperately needs some control restored to her life, the two nurses become instrumental in using behavior modification to manage her acting out—and try to enlist her parents' support.

We had care conferences on Liz. Her mother came to the first one we had, although we talked to both of her parents, but she was there during the day more. They always stated they were aware of it (referring to giving in to Liz), but they just couldn't stop themselves. You know, they always said that they would try, and then her father would take that role and be stern and say, this is what you do; the nurses are telling you to do this, but then Liz would cry. And, her dad would fall apart. And, so, it was like being that intimate with her father; he couldn't do it. He could do it until Liz cried, he fell apart, and then he turned around and took back everything he'd said and said, okay, I'll go get the nurses to put you back to bed. And, Liz knew it! She knew that, if she didn't like her parents' behavior, all she had to do was cry and that would change everything.

Recognizing that soliciting the parents' support in setting limits was unsuccessful, the two nurses assume a more parental role. Liz's crying has been effective in interrupting badly needed physical activity, until . . .

. . . she hit up with Chris and I, and then it didn't work any more—and we did not back down; that was the biggest thing. We did not back down. If you want to cry, you cry then. But, you're still going to sit in the chair, and I'll draw the curtain so that you can sit in here and cry, and you don't have to feel like everybody walking by is watching you cry, but you're going to stay in the chair. You know? And, yes, I do feel sorry for you, but crying doesn't put you back in bed.

As the months pass, the nurses use the reward of walking outside, which Liz loves, for sitting in the chair, which she dislikes.

Basically, we only went out the door. But, that worked then. She loved to be outside. It worked remarkably. We had a changed young lady by April, by the time we transferred her out to the floor. She was very motivated when she went to rehabilitation in April. She was motivated to work; she was up walking in days after she started her rigorous physical therapy. She was up in the wheelchair independently by herself very quickly once she transferred down there. And Chris and I, the other nurse who co-primaried her, we transferred that information to rehabilitation, and they continued it.

Though Liz struggled against the limits, it was the nurses' very act of setting them that allowed her to grow beyond adolescent limit-testing in dealing with her devastating illness.

She's come back to visit several times, and she said, you know, I hated you with a passion. But, she said, if I ever really wanted anything or needed anything, I knew you two would do it. You know, you wouldn't put up with the bullcrap, but if I really needed something, you'd be there. And, it got to a point when she's come back to visit and said, it was the two of you who sorted through that constantly for me, what was real and what was not real.

Neurologic disorders present challenging problems to nurses, particularly disorders that are chronic or marked by prolonged recovery. This chapter reviews not only acute disorders involving the neurologic system—increased intracranial pressure, herniation syndromes, and status epilepticus—but more chronic ones as well—stroke, Guillain-Barré syndrome, and myasthenia gravis. As the Clinical Insight demonstrates, nurses can be instrumental in helping a patient adjust to the pervasive life changes necessitated by these disorders. (Head and spinal cord trauma are discussed in Chapter 21.)

Increased Intracranial Pressure

The intracranial contents (or volume, ICV) consist of brain tissue (BT), blood volume (BV), and cerebrospinal fluid (CSF).

$$ICV = BT + BV + CSF$$

Brain tissue accounts for 80% of intracranial contents, blood volume 10%, and CSF 10%. Intracranial pressure (ICP) is a reflection of volume or pressure within the intracranial space. The normal value for ICP ranges from 1–15 mm Hg (Marshall S. et al. 1990). Intracranial hypertension is present when ICP exceeds 15 mm Hg.

Assessment

Risk Conditions Be alert for patients with actual or potential increases in ICP. Using the above formula, it is convenient to group risk conditions for increased ICP according to the three categories of intracranial contents. Conditions increasing the patient's risk include: mass lesions such as cranial tumors, hematomas, and brain swelling; cerebral vascular congestion due to vasodilation, loss of autoregulation, or increased systemic venous pressure; and diminished CSF absorption, such as when the meninges are covered with breakdown products *(subarachnoid hemorrhage)* or exudates *(meningitis)* or when there is a blockage of CSF pathways *(obstructive hydrocephalus)*.

A common misconception is that ICP is a static phenomenon and normally never elevated. As Mitchell (1982) points out, many everyday activities such as sneezing, coughing, and straining at bowel movements cause spikes of pressure far above normal levels. Moreover, patients with benign intracranial hypertension (caused by jugular venous or vena caval obstruction) can have extremely high intracranial pressures that nevertheless are well tolerated.

Although these exceptions are important, it is imperative to realize that acute increases of intracranial pressure can be lethal for patients in critical-care units. In fact, ICP can be dangerously elevated long before signs and symptoms of intracranial hypertension are manifested clinically. This section focuses on methods you can use to anticipate, prevent, and ameliorate detrimental increases in intracranial pressure.

Intracranial Dynamics   The brain is surrounded by nondistensible bone and a series of coverings called meninges. The addition of relatively small amounts of volume to the intracranial space will result in increased pressure, unless compensatory mechanisms are triggered. This compensatory or spatial accommodation, allowing intracranial contents to change or be rearranged, is explained best by the Monro-Kellie hypothesis. According to this hypothesis, when the volume of one of the intracranial contents increases, the total pressure will increase also, unless there is a reciprocal decrease in another of the intracranial contents.

Although the skull is a rigid structure, it has openings for the spinal cord, cranial nerves, and blood vessels. Cranial contents can be displaced through these openings. Accommodation is achieved by decreasing cerebral blood volume, displacing brain tissue, and decreasing CSF volume. The major pressure buffer is CSF, for two reasons: (1) the dura covering the spinal cord is loosely attached and can expand readily to accommodate CSF leaving the cranial subarachnoid space; (2) CSF absorption by the arachnoid villi partially depends on CSF pressure. The ability of CSF to buffer pressure changes is compromised when an expanding mass blocks subarachnoid pathways or when CSF absorption is diminished. In many pathologic states, such as tumor, edema, and aneurysmal rupture, these mechanisms are exhausted and any additional increase in intracranial volume will result in a dramatic and often fatal increase in ICP.

The relationship between volume and pressure is described best by using the volume-pressure curve shown in Figure 5–1. Compliance is the ability to compensate for a volume change without a large pressure increase (Germon 1988).

A direct invasive method of assessing cerebral compliance is possible using the intraventricular catheter. The volume pressure response (VPR) test and the pressure volume index (PVI) test can be performed by injecting a known amount of fluid (1 ml of preservative-free normal saline) into the ventricles. A person with adequate compliance has an intact compensatory

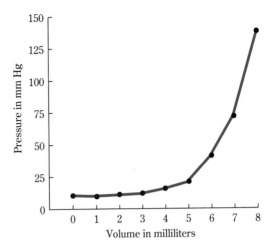

FIGURE 5–1

The relationship between volume and pressure within the intracranial space. As the volume reaches the point where pressure begins to rise, small increases in volume cause large rises in the ICP. (From: Marshall S et al.: *Neuroscience critical care: Pathophysiology and patient management.* Philadelphia: Saunders, 1990, p. 149)

mechanism, that is, reserves for adapting to an increasing volume. If the patient's ICP is relatively normal and compensatory mechanisms are working, instilling a small amount of fluid causes only slight increases in ICP and waveform amplitude. A normal response is a rise in ICP of less than 2 mm Hg (Germon 1988). Increases greater than 2 mm Hg suggest decreased compliance or a "tight brain." If the ICP is increased significantly (greater than 5 mm Hg), compensatory mechanisms are ineffective and the fluid should be immediately withdrawn (Mitchell 1986). These tests are highly invasive and carry serious potential side effects, such as infection, increased ICP, and tissue herniation (Germon 1988). Because this procedure can cause decompensation and rapid neurologic deterioration that is often irreversible, in most institutions this procedure is performed only by a physician.

The ICP value alone is not a reliable measure of the brain's response to injury and its ability to survive. A better measure is the cerebral perfusion pressure (CPP), the pressure at which blood perfuses brain cells.

To calculate CPP, first note the mean arterial pressure (MAP) from an arterial monitoring line. From the mean arterial pressure, subtract the intracranial pressure (ICP) to get the approximate cerebral perfusion pressure (CPP):

$$CPP = MAP - ICP$$

Normal CPP is 60–100 mm Hg (Cammermeyer and Appeldorn 1990). CPP can be reduced by either a drop in MAP or a rise in ICP. As ICP increases, compensatory cerebral vasodilation *(autoregulation)* maintains cerebral blood flow. Autoregulation is an additional compensatory mechanism by which the brain automatically alters the size or diameter of the cerebral arteries to maintain constant cerebral blood flow (CBF). This type of automatic regulation, known as pressure autoregulation, is essential in avoiding drastic changes in CBF.

Autoregulation is maintained when MAP is between 50–150 mm Hg. MAPs below 50 mm Hg will reduce CPP and may result in hypoxia, vascular collapse, and cell death. MAPs greater than 170 mm Hg may disrupt the blood–brain barrier, increasing CBF and causing cerebral edema and hemorrhage. Most authorities recommend maintaining a minimum CPP of at least 50–60 mm Hg in critically ill patients with injured brains (Miller and Williams 1987; Marshall et al. 1990).

Another type of autoregulation is chemical autoregulation. Chemical autoregulation is the ability of the cerebral vasculature to respond and adjust to changes in both arterial carbon dioxide pressure (P_aCO_2) and arterial oxygen pressure (P_aO_2). Within the normal range of P_aCO_2 (35–45 mm Hg), changes in P_aCO_2 level exert more effect on CBF than do changes in P_aO_2 level. As P_aCO_2 increases, cerebral vessels dilate, and as P_aCO_2 decreases, they constrict. Doubling the P_aCO_2 from 40 to 80 mm Hg will result in an almost 100% increase in CBF (Marshall et al. 1990).

The cerebral circulation is less sensitive to changes in P_aO_2. Modest changes in P_aO_2 have little, if any, effect on CBF under normal circumstances. CBF is not affected until P_aO_2 is 50 mm Hg or less. In the presence of hypoxia, cerebral vessels dilate and CBF increases. Lactic acid accumulation also causes vasodilatation. To summarize, hypercapnia, hypoxemia, and lactic acidemia all cause cerebral blood vessels to dilate. Chemical autoregulation is extremely hardy and will not be affected unless severe brain injury has occurred (Marshall et al. 1990).

Autoregulation fails when ICP exceeds approximately 30 mm Hg (Mitchell et al. 1981), MAP falls below 50 mm Hg, or CPP drops below 50 mm Hg (McGillicuddy 1985). When autoregulation fails, CBF no longer alters appropriately with pressure or metabolic needs; instead, CBF fluctuates directly with systemic BP. Increases in MAP pound more blood into cerebral vessels, further elevating ICP and increasing cerebral edema. Conversely, decreases in MAP cause cerebral ischemia. In this situation, even the brain's desperate needs for O_2 and removal of CO_2 and lactic acid cannot provoke improved CBF.

Signs and Symptoms Maintain a high index of suspicion for signs and symptoms of increased ICP. Early findings include: change in level of consciousness, pupillary dysfunction, paresis/paralysis, and headache. Later findings include: continued decrease in level of consciousness, changes in respiratory pattern, abnormal posturing, vomiting, alterations in vital signs, and impaired brainstem reflexes. See Chapter 4 for a discussion of various respiratory patterns and pupillary changes that may be seen.

It has been established that clinical signs do not always correlate with the ICP, since it is dynamic and affected by many variables. Therefore, patients likely to suffer acutely increased ICP ideally should have the benefit of direct ICP monitoring. Such monitoring does not, however, eliminate the need for astute bedside physical assessment.

Measuring Intracranial Pressure The following sections describe techniques of intracranial pressure monitoring.

Types of Pressure Monitoring Although CSF pressure can be evaluated by lumbar punctures, such readings are isolated and inaccurate in the presence of subarachnoid block. More importantly, lumbar punctures present a danger of herniation in those patients who most need pressure evaluation. In contrast, an intracranial transducer, ventricular catheter, subarachnoid screw, or epidural device can monitor ICP accurately and continuously, without danger of herniation through the foramen magnum. The three cranial areas monitored most frequently are the epidural space, the subarachnoid space, and the lateral ventricle (Figure 5–2).

Epidural monitoring is done with an intracranial transducer or with an intracranial balloon connected to an external transducer. The dura is not opened, so there is less danger of cranial infection than with other methods. The internal transducer reduces the danger further, but it is affected by heat and cannot be recalibrated. Epidural monitoring does not allow for CSF drainage or testing of intracranial compliance. In addition, a separate, expensive monitoring system is required.

The *intraventricular catheter* (IVC) is inserted into the nondominant frontal horn of the lateral ventricle via a twist drill. (To review ventricular anatomy, refer to Chapter 4.) The catheter is connected via a stopcock to pressure tubing and a drainage system. A transducer can be attached for the purpose of monitoring ICP. The IVC is considered to be the most accurate method of measuring ICP. The catheter can be used to evaluate the pressure-volume response and is the only device

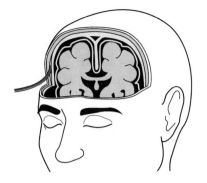

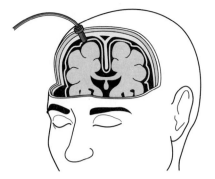

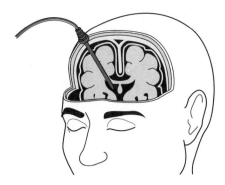

a Epidural sensor. **b** Subarachnoid screw. **c** Intraventricular catheter.

FIGURE 5–2

Three methods of monitoring intracranial pressure. **a,** epidural sensor; **b,** subarachnoid screw; **c,** intraventricular catheter. (From: McQuillan K: Intracranial pressure monitoring: Technical imperatives. *Clin Issues Crit Care Nurs* 1991; 2(4):624–628.

that can provide for CSF drainage. Other advantages include access for CSF sampling and access for administration of medications and contrast material when visualizing the size and patency of the ventricular system. Disadvantages include the technical difficulty of insertion in the presence of marked cerebral edema or ventricular collapse, compression, or displacement. Incorrect positioning of the drainage system can result in inadvertent CSF drainage from the ventricle, which can rapidly decrease ICP and cause a subdural hemorrhage or herniation (Cammelmeyer and Appeldorn 1990). Additional risks are infection, bleeding, edema, and blockage of the catheter by blood clots or debris.

The *subarachnoid screw* is a small, hollow screw whose tip sits in the cranial subarachnoid space. Advantages include ease of insertion (it is not necessary to locate the ventricles or penetrate the brain) and the ability to recalibrate the transducer as necessary. Disadvantages are possible infection, inability to instill contrast media, limited access to CSF, unreliable ICP recording in the presence of high ICP, risk of hematoma during insertion, and possible blockage of the screw by brain tissue.

The newest monitoring device is the *fiberoptic catheter* (Hollingsworth-Fridland et al. 1988; McQuillan 1991). The Camino system provides for intraventricular, subarachnoid or intraparenchymal monitoring. Advantages include ease of insertion, excellent waveforms even in the presence of edema, no risk of tissue herniation, and, since the transducer is in the brain, no effect of head position on pressure readings. It is lightweight and portable. The primary disadvantages are cost and the fact that if the catheter is twisted or

bent, the fiberoptic system will break and a new catheter will need to be inserted. The other potential disadvantage is that recalibration can only be performed if the physician removes the device and rezeros or inserts a new zero-balanced catheter.

Insertion of the ICP Monitoring Device   To prepare the patient and family before insertion, explain that monitoring is a temporary measure to enable the nurses and doctors to detect the onset of increased intracranial pressure and intervene early to prevent or ameliorate its detrimental effects. Explain that the scalp will be numbed with local anesthesia and that the insertion itself will be painless. Briefly explain the setup and monitor so that the family will not be horrified by the tubes and wires connected to their loved one's brain. Ideally, the ICP monitoring device is inserted under sterile conditions in the operating room. If transport to the OR is not feasible, then the following protocol may be followed.

Gather the equipment necessary for the monitoring: the catheter or screw; an insertion tray containing a syringe and needle for anesthesia, scalpel, drill, sutures, and dressing supplies; skin preparation solution; local anesthetic; sterile gloves; monitor; and monitoring system. The type of equipment can vary; therefore, many institutions have assembled an "ICP tray" according to their particular needs and their type of monitoring equipment. Preassembled, presterilized, disposable insertion kits are also available.

The neurosurgeon will explain the procedure to patient and/or family and obtain consent. Using sterile procedure, assist the physician in inserting the catheter or screw. The physician will shave, clean, and infiltrate the insertion site with a local anesthetic. He or she will then incise the scalp, drill a hole, puncture the dura (except when using the epidural system), and insert the catheter or screw. Attach the catheter or screw to the monitoring or drainage system. *Never* attach it to a preassembled transducer (arterial or pulmonary arterial) system which contains a flush device. The physician will suture the incision and apply a sterile dressing.

Nursing Care Responsibilities   The following sections describe nursing responsibilities related to intracranial pressure monitoring.

Obtain Accurate Pressure Measurements   Follow these steps each time you measure the pressure.

1. Place the patient in the baseline position, which is usually 30 to 45 degrees of head elevation. False pressure changes will occur if the level of the head has changed in relation to the transducer, unless the epidural or Camino system is in use.

2. Observe the oscilloscope waveform to verify patency of the line. A flattened (dampened) waveform can result from kinked tubing, an air bubble or other blockage in the system, collapse of the ventricle or dura against the tip of the monitoring device, or herniation of brain tissue into the catheter or screw. First check for kinks, and remove any that are present. Inspect the system for air bubbles, if applicable. If

---

NURSING TIP

Reference Point for ICP Monitoring

The internal reference point for ICP monitoring is the foramen of Monro. The traditional external reference points that have been used are the outer canthus of the eye (Smith 1983), the top of the ear (Horner 1985), and the external auditory meatus. It is most important to always verify that the transducer is level with the external reference point used. Pole-mounted transducers require the use of a carpenter's level to ensure proper alignment. Large transducers may also be secured on a towel roll and kept at the reference level. Miniature transducers can be taped directly to the head to preclude measurement error.

---

bubbles are present, turn off the stopcock closest to the patient and open it to air, maintaining sterile technique. Then, using meticulous aseptic procedures, fill a 10-cc syringe with sterile normal saline (preservative-free solution); open the line or stopcock above the air bubbles, attach the syringe, and flush the line. **DO NOT flush the intraventricular cannula itself.** Upon completion of the procedure, close the stopcock port to the syringe and the distal port (where the air bubbles were flushed out of the system). Then remove the syringe and recap the stopcock ports. Your ICP line should now be a closed system open only to the ICP measuring device. Observe the monitor and waveform. If it still appears dampened, consult the physician immediately.

Follow your institution's protocols and procedures for irrigating ICP devices. Many institutions do not allow the nurse to flush the subarachnoid bolt should dampening occur due to herniation of swollen brain tissue, blood, or debris into the hollow bolt and up into the high-pressure tubing. Flushing the ICP device can introduce contamination and infection into the ICP system as well as the brain. Furthermore, adding even small amounts of volume into the brain may adversely affect the patient by dramatically increasing ICP.

If you are allowed to flush the bolt, the following paragraph describes one method.

Fill a syringe only with the amount of flush solution specified by the physician (usually 0.1 ml of preservative-free saline). Connect it to the 3-way stopcock attached to the catheter or screw. Turn the stopcock so it is off to the transducer, that is, so the syringe and catheter or screw are connected. *Slowly* flush the catheter or screw. (Do not aspirate first, as you would with a line for monitoring vascular pressure. Aspiration may suck brain tissue into the screw.) Turn the stopcock so the catheter or screw and transducer are reconnected. Again observe the waveform. If it remains dampened, notify the physician.

3. Do not measure the pressure when the patient is moving, coughing, sneezing, using abdominal muscles to inspire, or has his or her head turned, since these actions will cause temporary increases in intracranial pressure.

4. Follow your hospital's procedure for balancing and calibrating the transducer. To assure accurate readings, the transducer must be leveled

and rezeroed to the external reference point whenever the head position is changed.

Analyze the Pressures Critically Following are guidelines for pressure analysis.

1. Evaluate the recorded ICP value. Remember that the trend is more significant than any isolated reading. Compare the readings to the patient's norm rather than to an arbitrary standard; the patient with chronically increased intracranial pressure will have a higher "normal" value than the patient being monitored to detect the onset of increased pressure. Reported normal ranges are 1–15 mm Hg or 15–200 mm H_2O (Cammermeyer and Appeldorn 1990). Pressures normally fluctuate with cardiac pulsations (transmitted to the CSF through the choroid plexus) and changes in the thoracic and abdominal pressures (transmitted to the CSF through the vena cava and the jugular veins).

2. Monitor CPP by subtracting ICP from MAP. Again, the trend is more significant than individual values. Obtain specific guidelines for the desired CPP range from the physician, when possible.

3. In addition to evaluating absolute pressure values, note the morphology and amplitude of the waveform. As mentioned above, changes in cardiac pulsations are transmitted to the CSF through the choroid plexus. Normally, as cranial blood pressure rises and falls, blood and CSF escape and return through patent outflow channels in the foramina at the base of the skull. These compensatory mechanisms, along with intact autoregulation, keep the amplitude of each pulsation transmitted from the arterioles throughout the brain and CSF small. Although of low amplitude, the pulse wave has a sharp initial inflection that slopes back to baseline (Figure 5–3). Loss of compensatory mechanisms or autoregulation results in an increased pulse pressure leading to an increased ICP pulse. Progressively larger, more-rounded waves may be an early indicator of changing intracranial dynamics.

4. Look also for spontaneous abnormal variations in pressure called *pressure waves* (Figure 5–4). In a classic article, Lundberg (1960) described three types of pressure waves: A, B, and C. Most important are A waves, commonly called *plateau waves*. These waves raise intracranial pressure 50–100 mm Hg and last for 5–20 minutes. These sustained pressure elevations occur on an already-elevated mean intracranial pressure baseline exceeding 20 mm Hg, that is, with intracranial hypertension. Plateau waves are believed to be clinically significant because the elevated pressure reduces cerebral perfusion pressure and contributes to cerebral ischemia. Supporting this assumption is

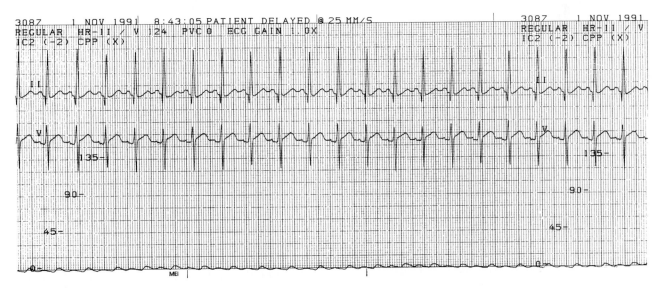

FIGURE 5–3

Normal ICP waveform. (at bottom of tracing.)

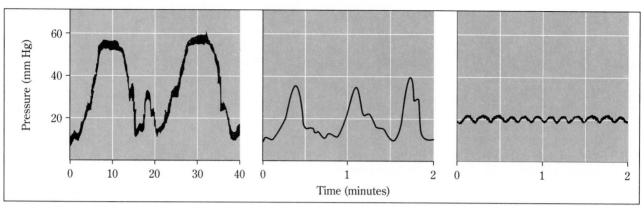

FIGURE 5–4

Intracranial pressure waves. Composite diagram of A (plateau) waves, B waves, and C waves. See text for discussion.

Lundberg's observation that transient displays of the classic signs of increased pressure most often occurred at the peak of plateau waves. B waves are sharp, rhythmic waves with a saw-tooth appearance that occur on a normal baseline ICP. Associated with respiration, they occur every 30 seconds to 2 minutes and last only a few seconds. They are clinically significant, indicating the brain's decreased compensatory capacity, and raise ICP as high as 50 mm Hg. C waves are smaller rhythmic waves that occur every 4–8 minutes and raise intracranial pressure as much as 20 mm Hg. C waves coincide with rhythmic variations in BP, but they are probably not clinically significant.

Anticipate and Prevent Complications of Monitoring Implement the following measures for patients on ICP monitoring.

1. *Prevent infection* by practicing scrupulous aseptic technique. Breaks in technique are particularly likely when you are setting up the system and when you are preparing to flush the system. Good handwashing and cleaning around ports with Betadine prior to changing syringes will decrease the chance of infection. When zeroing the system, a hydrophobic millipore filter should be used. It allows air to communicate with the transducer dome but not bacteria. If the dressing becomes soiled or wet, notify the physician to change it. Otherwise, follow institutional policy or individual physician preference regarding changing a clean, dry dressing.

2. *Observe the system for CSF leaks,* which are dangerous because they allow a pathway for infection and because they lower the pressure

in the system and allow brain tissue to be sucked into the catheter or screw. If you see fluid on the stopcocks or tubing, tighten or replace them. If you are unable to stop the leak, turn the stopcock attached to the catheter or screw off to the direction of the leak, cover the leak with a sterile towel, and notify the physician.

Planning and Implementation of Care

Many maneuvers that nurses commonly use in caring for critically ill patients may have deleterious effects on patients already suffering from increased ICP. To understand why, it is helpful to briefly review intracranial dynamics.

Oxygenation and Ventilation When intracranial pressure rises, venous outflow and therefore cerebral blood flow decrease. As a result, more CO_2 accumulates in cerebral vessels, and less oxygen than normal is available to the cells. The CO_2 excess and oxygen deficit both cause vasodilatation, which reduces resistance and increases cerebral blood flow toward normal (metabolic autoregulation). Unfortunately, the increased blood flow tends to increase intracranial pressure even more. The following sections describe ways of maintaining oxygenation and ventilation to lessen this vicious cycle.

Airway Patency Establish and maintain a patent airway. This may be accomplished simply with oral or nasal airways, or it may necessitate endotracheal intubation. Maintain a P_aO_2 greater than 70 mm Hg.

Hypoxemia and/or Hypercapnia Prevent hypoxemia and/or hypercapnia, either of which can cause vasodilatation and further increase ICP. Particularly important measures are close monitoring of arterial blood gases, preoxygenating and hyperventilating before suctioning, and limiting suction to 10–15 seconds in the apneic patient to minimize CO_2 accumulation. The administration of xylocaine 50 mg IVP, 5 minutes prior to suctioning, is effective in preventing coughing and so limiting elevations of ICP. For other measures to maintain oxygenation and ventilation, see Chapter 9.

Controlled Hyperventilation Controlled hyperventilation is the cornerstone of neurosurgical management for patients with increased ICP. Because of the relationship between P_aCO_2 and cerebral blood flow (refer to previous discussion on autoregulation), hypocapnia effectively reduces ICP. Lowering the P_aCO_2 to 25–30 mm Hg decreases cerebral blood flow and reduces blood volume by vasoconstriction. Hypocapnia also corrects brain tissue acidosis, improves autoregulation, and facilitates the treatment of a ventilated patient (Walleck 1992). Although the benefits of controlled hyperventilation have been documented in the normal brain, they may not apply uniformly to the head injury patient. (See Chapter 21 for further discussion of head trauma.)

When hyperventilation is utilized, monitor P_aCO_2 closely, because decreasing levels below 20 mm Hg can cause severe vasoconstriction, thus producing hypoxemia and worsening the patient's prognosis (Walleck 1989). Many neurosurgeons believe that titrating hyperventilation to assure an adequate cerebral metabolic rate for oxygen (CMR_{O_2}) is more advantageous than seeking the lowest P_aCO_2 (Marshall et al. 1990; Muizelaar et al. 1991). Blood samples from a pulmonary artery catheter or the jugular vein allow for calculation of the arterial-venous oxygen difference (avD_{O_2}), a means to titrate hyperventilation to assure adequate CMR_{O_2} and use of the best-tolerated P_aCO_2.

Other concerns regarding hyperventilation include the length of time hyperventilation can be maintained before beneficial effects are lost, and the effect on outcome of the patients who are hyperventilated. Some authors suggest that the effect of hyperventilation in reducing CBF and controlling ICP is short-lived, lasting only 3–24 hours (Muizelaar et al. 1988; Marshall et al. 1990; Walleck 1989).

Prevention of Obstructions to Venous Outflow
Minimize obstructions to venous outflow from the brain. Such obstructions not only increase pressure in the capillary bed (predisposing toward cerebral swelling) but also diminish absorption of CSF. Because CSF is absorbed by the arachnoid villi into the sagittal sinus and then into the jugular veins, compression of the jugular veins will transmit pressure back into the brain. A continuing rise in pressure may precipitate reduction in one of the other volumes. Blood volume may decrease, causing ischemia, or brain tissue may herniate.

Unless specifically ordered by the physician, do not place the patient with increased ICP flat or in Trendelenburg's position. Instead, keep the head of the bed elevated to increase the pressure gradient between the brain and heart. Although 30° is a common elevation, the degree of elevation often must be individualized. Some researchers have found that ICP can be reduced significantly by placing the patient in a semisitting or sitting (>35°) position (Parsons and Wilson 1984). However, a study by March et al. (1990) suggests that changes in ICP and CPP resulting from changes in backrest position are highly individualized and may not be consistent in all head injury patients or even within a single patient.

Position the head and neck midline to avoid jugular venous compression. Also, maintain a neutral position, avoiding both extreme neck flexion and extension. Research indicates that extreme hip flexion also elevates ICP and should be avoided. For example, if you must catheterize a female with increased ICP, flex the legs as little as possible.

Prevention of Increases in Intrathoracic Pressure
Prevent avoidable increases in intrathoracic pressure. If the physician plans to insert a jugular venous catheter, modify your usual preparation of the patient. Avoid placing the patient in Trendelenburg's position and having him or her execute a Valsalva maneuver, as you do with other patients to minimize the danger of air embolism due to negative intrathoracic pressure. Instead, the physician should prevent air being sucked into the catheter during insertion by maintaining suction on the catheter with a syringe.

Take actions to avoid other Valsalva maneuvers. For example, teach the patient to exhale when moving his or her bowels; assist him or her to turn; and keep fecal contents soft through diet, fluid intake, and/or stool softeners. Though a Valsalva maneuver alone may not be sufficient to cause a plateau wave, in combination with other pressure-increasing actions it can cause a sustained increase in intracranial pressure.

The frequent occurrence of pulmonary complications in patients with increased ICP has encouraged further examination of vigorous pulmonary hygiene therapy. Drainage of pulmonary secretions from the pathology-prone lower lobes may not be achieved by conservative flat chest physiotherapy (CPT). During suctioning and CPT, it is imperative that the nurse and the respiratory therapist pay close attention to the ICP display. If any position causes the patient to experience a rise in ICP or a decrease in CPP, maintain that position as short a time as possible and only if absolutely indicated for pulmonary or skin care.

Positive end-expiratory pressure (PEEP) can increase intrathoracic and intracranial pressure. Monitor patients on PEEP particularly closely and try to avoid doing more than one activity that increases ICP at a time. For example, avoid turning a patient if you have just finished suctioning him or her.

The effects on ICP of nursing care itself have been the subject of several studies. A classic study reported by Mitchell et al. (1981) compared the effects of eight nursing care activities on increased intracranial pressure in 18 neurologic and neurosurgical patients with ventricular drainage. Their findings supported empirical observations that nursing activities do in fact influence ICP and that these effects are potentially dangerous in some patients. The measures evaluated were: (a) two passive range of motion exercises (arm extension and hip flexion); (b) two head rotations (right and left), and (c) turning the body to four positions (supine to right, right to supine, supine to left, left to supine). The passive exercises did not provoke clinically significant changes in ventricular pressure in most patients. Large increases in ICP occurred in the five patients who had head rotations. Turning in any direction caused more variability in ventricular pressure than the head rotations or passive exercises. Activities spaced 15 minutes apart, regardless of their nature, caused a cumulative increase in ICP; those spaced an hour apart did not. This research was supported further by the Tsementzis et al. (1982) study, which documented that small reversible rises in ICP did occur during suctioning, intramuscular injections and nasogastric tube insertion. Boortz-Marx (1985) examined health care activities such as rotation of the head and neck, suctioning, physical assessment, and nursing care (shaving the skin, starting intravenous lines, and cleansing the wound or incision). This research supported previous findings that these activities do influence ICP. However, other activities such as elevating the head of the bed and turning the head and neck to a 90-degree angle reduced ICP. In 1985, Parsons analyzed the effects of hygiene intervention such as oral care, body hygiene, and indwelling catheter care. Variables of arterial blood pressure, ICP, CPP, and heart rate were used to reflect the cerebrovascular status of the patient. Although statistically significant changes in physiologic variables were noted, the findings were not considered clinically significant because at no point in time during an intervention was CPP less than 50 mm Hg, nor did ICP approach dangerous levels.

Nursing research continues to evolve, and further studies to evaluate the effect of current nursing practices are necessary. All evidence suggests that nursing interventions and accumulation of nursing care activities such as bathing, positioning, turning, and painful manipulations can contribute to elevations in ICP. Other nursing care activities such as raising the head of the bed and maintaining neutral head alignment can be effective in reducing intracranial pressure. The controversies presented in this section represent a challenge to the nurse who is caring for these critically ill patients. Hygiene and nursing care activities are important to the care and well-being of the immobile comatose patient. It is imperative that the nurse evaluate the individual's response to such therapy. Although nurses usually are encouraged to group care activities together, doing so may worsen increased ICP. In particular, performing closely spaced activities with the patient supine may be most apt to increase ICP. Mitchell et al. (1981) recommend spacing procedures known to increase ICP, such as suctioning, after the patient has been resting for some time and perhaps with the person in the lateral position. All persons caring for patients undergoing ICP monitoring should continuously assess the patient's response to activities and immediately stop or modify these procedures if elevation of ICP and/or reduction of CPP is documented.

Minimizing Arterial Hypo- or Hypertension Many nursing care activities cause an arousal response accompanied by increased systemic blood pressure. Among the stimuli that can provoke this arousal response are an endotracheal tube, suctioning, chest physiotherapy, and pain. Use BP and intracranial pressure monitors to evaluate your patient's response to these circumstances and adapt your care accordingly. For instance, try timing suctioning or chest PT for intervals of peak sedation; check with the physician about using topical anesthesia if suctioning provokes hypertensive episodes; use muscle relaxants, as ordered by the physician, if repeated explanations are ineffective in calming the patient fighting an endotracheal tube and if your evaluation reveals he or she is not hypoxic. Decrease the occurrence of painful stimuli or any other nonspecific stimuli that provoke the hypertensive response in your particular patient.

Also try to reduce the risk of small pressure increases summating into plateau waves. If you must do two activities each of which causes a pressure increase, time your care judiciously so that pressure can diminish after the first activity before you institute the second.

Prevention of Infection Infection can be catastrophic in patients undergoing ICP monitoring. Meticulous sterile technique and prompt antibiotic therapy if signs of infection appear may protect the patient against meningitis or full-blown sepsis. Because sepsis can lead to increased cardiac output and vasodilatation, it can contribute to a dangerous rise in intracranial pressure.

Implementing Medical Therapy An important aspect of nursing the patient with increased ICP is implementing the plan of medical therapy. Definitive therapy, of course, varies with the cause. General therapeutic measures include hypertonic agents, assisted ventilation with hyperventilation, corticosteroids, CSF drainage, sedation, surgical decompression, and barbiturate coma.

Hypertonic Agents Hypertonic agents are used to reduce cerebral edema by drawing fluid out of brain cells into the hypertonic blood. Hypertonic agents are only temporary measures that buy time for more definitive treatment. Commonly used agents include mannitol (Osmitrol), urea, and glucose. In recent years, mannitol has been by far the most frequently used agent and has been found to be superior to glycerol or pentobarbital in reducing ICP (Levin et al. 1979; Marshall et al. 1990). A 20% mannitol solution (IV bolus of 0.5–1.5 gm/kg) is the first-line drug for reducing ICP (Cammermeyer and Appeldorn 1990). Increased serum osmolality causes water to move from tissue (both brain and systemic) into the vascular system, thus dramatically increasing preload. Therefore, when hypertonic agents are used, be alert for the development of congestive heart failure. Also watch for increasing cerebral edema, which may occur when these drugs pass through the disrupted blood–brain barrier and raise brain osmolality. To reduce the risk of ICP rebound, only a portion of the volume lost during diuresis should be replaced. Mannitol is always administered intravenously through a filter because it

crystallizes; failure to use a filter can cause microemboli to be introduced into the patient's bloodstream. Potential complications of mannitol administration are hyperosmolality and hyperkalemia.

Several studies have indicated that the nonosmotic diuretics such as furosemide (Lasix) may be as effective as mannitol in reducing ICP (Roberts et al. 1987; Walleck 1989). Furosemide, a potent renal loop diuretic, reduces ICP in three ways: it reduces sodium transport into the brain, reduces total body fluid volume, and inhibits cerebrospinal fluid production up to 70%. The major advantage of this drug is that, unlike mannitol, it causes minimal electrolyte and osmolality disturbances and no adverse effects on cardiac dynamics. Some neurosurgeons recommend that furosemide be administered routinely with each mannitol dose, in order to cause a brisk diuresis (Marshall et al. 1990). However, it is important to avoid diuresing patients so briskly that they develop serum osmolarities in excess of 315 mOsm.

Corticosteroids The corticosteroids most often used are *dexamethasone* (Decadron) and *methylprednisolone* (Solu-medrol). It is believed that steroids are effective in reducing vasogenic edema because they stabilize the cell membrane and improve neuronal function by restoring autoregulation and cerebral blood flow. Although they remain in widespread use, their value in treating cerebral edema resulting from trauma is controversial.

Studies have failed to produce conclusive evidence of the efficacy of steroids following head injury. Some investigators have reported no effect on ICP (Gudeman et al. 1979; Marshall and Bowers 1982), while others have demonstrated a positive effect (Faupel et al. 1976; Gobiet et al. 1976). Investigation is underway to determine the therapeutic efficacy of 21-aminosteroid (U74006F), a potent nonglucocorticoid steroid, in the acute treatment of CNS trauma (Hall et al. 1988).

CSF Drainage CSF drainage is particularly helpful when decreased CSF absorption causes increased intracranial pressure. Drainage is safest when done against positive pressure to decrease the risk of ventricular collapse. To provide positive pressure, the drainage reservoir is set at a specified level above the ICP reference point. CSF then drains only when the pressure exceeds the specified level. It is imperative that the level of the head of the bed *not* be altered while a CSF drain is open.

Control of Posturing, Restlessness, and Shivering The use of muscle relaxants such as pancuronium bromide (Pavulon) or vecuronium (Norcuron) to facilitate respiratory management and control posturing, restlessness, and shivering is well documented (Marshall et al. 1990; Walleck 1989). Increased muscle activity, posturing, and shivering may adversely affect ICP by increasing systolic blood pressure, decreasing O_2, and increasing metabolic demands. It is important, however, to remember that these agents do not have analgesic effects and do not protect patients from the delirious effects of noxious stimuli. In many institutions, narcotic sedation has been introduced as an alternative to barbiturates to control agitation, cerebral metabolic rate, and ICP. In the past, the use of narcotics had been regarded as unsuitable for neurologic patients due to the effect of these drugs on mentation, pupils, and respirations. Recently, the use of morphine sulfate in small IV boluses or by continuous infusion and other narcotics has been advocated in the patient with head-injury or aneurysm to blunt the effects of noxious stimuli present in the ICU environment (Marshall et al. 1990; Walleck 1989). Despite the controversial reports on the beneficial effects of narcotic use on cerebral hemodynamics, the major advantage of using narcotic sedation is that it can be reversed with Narcan (naloxone) so that neurologic assessment can be performed. Many clinicians believe that properly monitored use of narcotics can be effective in controlling ICP. Certainly, more research is needed in this area of cerebral management.

Barbiturate Coma   Barbiturate coma is the induction and maintenance of coma by continuous administration of pentobarbital or thiopental. It is used with severe, persistent intracranial hypertension that is refractory to other therapies. The exact mechanism of action is unclear; possible explanations include cerebral vasoconstriction, reduced responsiveness to stimuli, and reduced cerebral metabolic demand. Barbiturate coma necessitates extremely close nursing supervision. The patient must be intubated and on a ventilator. Monitoring devices must include an ICP monitor, cardiac monitor, arterial line, pulmonary artery pressure line, nasogastric tube, and urinary catheter. The blood barbiturate level must be monitored routinely. Because barbiturates may lower blood pressure by reducing cardiac contractility, vasopressors and/or colloid administration may be necessary.

Outcome Evaluation

Evaluate the patient's progress according to these outcome criteria:

- Return to premorbid level of consciousness.

- Pupils of normal and equal size that accommodate briskly to light.
- BP, pulse, respirations, and temperature within normal limits (WNL) for the patient.
- Appropriate responses to stimuli.
- Arterial blood gases WNL for the patient.
- If ICP monitored, ICP <15 mm Hg, CPP >60 mm Hg, and plateau waves absent.

Herniation Syndromes

Herniation may be defined as the protrusion of brain tissue from its normal compartment. Several syndromes exist (Figure 5–5). Tissue may protrude through an opening in the skull from head trauma or craniotomy. If an expanding unilateral cerebral lesion shifts brain tissue (the cingulate gyrus) laterally under the midline dural fold known as the *falx cerebri, subfalcine* herniation occurs. When midline or bilateral cerebral lesions displace the diencephalon downward through the tentorial notch, *central (transtentorial)* herniation occurs. When a laterally located expanding lesion pushes the tip of the temporal lobe (the uncus) through the tentorial notch, *uncal herniation* occurs. An expanding posterior fossa lesion can displace a

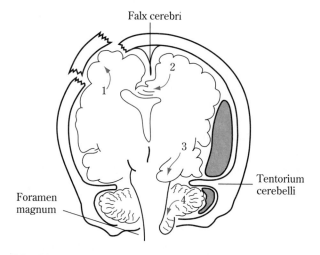

FIGURE 5–5

Brain herniation syndromes. (1) Herniation of brain tissue out through a bony defect in the skull, (2) herniation of the cingulate gyrus under the falx, (3) herniation of the uncus through the tentorial notch, and (4) herniation of a cerebellar tonsil through the foramen magnum. (Reprinted from *Neurological Emergencies: Effective Nursing Care* by J. Raimond and J. Waterman-Taylor, p. 131, with permission of Aspen Publishers, Inc., copyright 1986.)

cerebellar tonsil through the foramen magnum, compressing the brainstem and leading to cardiopulmonary arrest.

Assessment

Risk Conditions   Risk conditions for herniation include tumors, intracranial hematomas, abscesses and cerebral edema. The rapidity of the elevation in pressure and the degree of distortion of the brain and brainstem are important in determining the effect that a given ICP will have. If a lesion expands insidiously over a relatively long period of time, as some tumors do, the brain does not shift and the increase in ICP can have a relatively benign effect on the brain (Marshall et al. 1990). However, if a lesion expands rapidly, as in epidural hematoma, the brain shift obstructs cerebral blood flow or CSF and can lead rapidly to decompensation, herniation, and death.

Signs and Symptoms   Assessment of the patient at risk for herniation includes evaluating level of consciousness, sensorimotor function, respiratory patterns, eye function, and vital signs. Because supratentorial herniation generally progresses in a head-to-toe *(rostral-caudal)* fashion, upper-brain functions are affected first and brainstem functions last. Thus, level of consciousness is the earliest category of brain function to deteriorate, whereas vital signs are the last.

Central and uncal herniation produce distinctly different clinical pictures early in their courses. Nurses should learn to recognize these changes so medical intervention can be instituted rapidly. Once the midbrain and lower levels are involved, the clinical picture is the same for both, and the patient's chance for complete recovery diminishes. The following classic descriptions are taken from Plum and Posner (1980). (Subfalcine herniation will be considered with central herniation because a disorder causing the former also is likely to produce the latter.)

Central Herniation   In central (transtentorial) herniation, an expanding lesion forces the hemispheres and basal nuclei downward. The progressive compression displaces the diencephalon and midbrain downward through the tentorial notch. Displacement of branches of the basilar artery causes ischemia and severe brainstem deterioration. Central herniation also can block the aqueduct of Sylvius, between the third and fourth ventricles. This blockage, which cannot be diagnosed clinically, robs the brain of its ability to displace fluid from the ventricular system to compensate for increased brain volume and causes a severe rise in supratentorial pressure. However, impaired CSF circulation probably is less instrumental in causing herniation than the factor initially causing the increase in intracranial pressure.

Central herniation generally causes ischemia to advance in a rostral-caudal direction. Plum and Posner (1980) describe manifestations typical of four stages of progression: early diencephalic, late diencephalic, midbrain–upper pontine, and lower pontine–upper medullary. These changes are shown in Figure 5–6.

The earliest sign in the *diencephalic stage* is diminished alertness characterized by difficulty in concentration, memory lapses, lethargy, and stupor. Respirations may be a relatively normal pattern interspersed with yawns, sighs, and pauses, or Cheyne–Stokes breathing. Pupils are small (1–3 mm). Although on superficial examination they may appear not to react to light, a closer look reveals that they react rapidly but only within a small range of contraction. The doll's eyes reflex is present. The ice water caloric test provokes normal slow movement but diminished or absent fast movement. There often is a pre-existing hemiparesis or hemiplegia on the opposite side of the body (*contralateral* to the lesion), which may become more severe as this stage develops. In addition, the extremities on the same side of the body (*ipsilateral* to the lesion) develop paratonic resistance, although they continue responding appropriately to noxious stimuli. Bilateral positive Babinski signs are present, although they are weaker on the ipsilateral side. Later, resistance to passive stretch increases and grasp reflexes emerge. Finally, abnormal flexion (decorticate posturing) appears, first on the contralateral side and then bilaterally.

In the *midbrain–upper-pontine stage,* respirations may change from Cheyne–Stokes to sustained hyperventilation. Pupils become somewhat dilated (3–5 mm), fixed in midposition, and unresponsive to light. Their shape often is irregular. The doll's eyes response becomes impaired, and the ice water caloric response becomes harder to provoke. Abnormal extension (decerebrate posturing) occurs in response to painful stimuli or spontaneously. Wide swings of body temperature are common.

In the *lower-pontine–upper-medullary stage,* respirations become more or less regular but rapid and shallow. The pupils remain fixed in midposition and unresponsive to light. Both the doll's eyes and ice water caloric responses are absent. The patient remains flaccid with bilateral Babinski signs and occasional nonpurposeful flickers of movement in response to painful stimuli. In the terminal medullary stage, medullary ischemia causes ataxic respirations, varying pulse rates, hypotension, dilated pupils, and respiratory arrest.

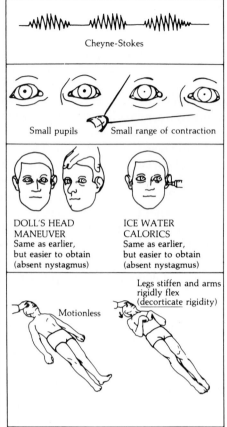

FIGURE 5–6

Signs of central transtentorial herniation. (Adapted from McNealy D, Plum F: "Brainstem Dysfunction with Supratentorial Mass Lesions" from *Archives of Neurology,* July, Volume 7:10–32. Copyright 1962, American Medical Association.)

The authors point out *two exceptions to the generalization of rostral-caudal progression in untreated supratentorial lesions: (1) acute cerebral hemorrhage, and (2) lumbar punctures in patients with impending herniation. In both cases, sudden medullary failure may occur.* In the first case, hemorrhage into the ventricular system compresses structures around the fourth ventricle. In the second case, the extraction of spinal fluid apparently removes support from the brain, allowing it to herniate through the foramen magnum.

Uncal Herniation The uncus, the medial portion of the temporal lobe, overhangs the edge of the tentorial notch. Expanding lesions in the temporal lobe or lateral middle fossa can force the uncus over the edge of the incisura. This uncal herniation compresses the midbrain (which passes through the notch) and opposite cerebral peduncle up against the opposite edge of the

tentorial opening. It compresses the oculomotor nerve and pushes the posterior cerebral artery down, trapping it against the incisural edge. Compression of the oculomotor nerve is discussed below. Posterior cerebral artery compromise can provoke occipital ischemia, edema and infarction. Uncal herniation also can compromise CSF circulation by compressing the aqueduct of Sylvius, with the results indicated above under central herniation.

Because of the anatomic location of the uncus, uncal herniation produces early stages that are different from central herniation: the *third nerve stage* and the *midbrain–upper-pontine stage* (Figure 5–7). The earliest consistent sign is not the level of consciousness (which may vary from diminished alertness to coma) but rather a unilaterally dilating pupil.

In the early third nerve stage, compression of the third cranial nerve first affects the parasympathetic

Mid-brain-upper pons stage   Lower pons-upper medulla stage

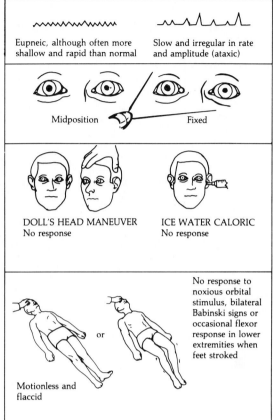

Sustained regular hyperventilation   Rarely, Cheyne-Stokes

Eupneic, although often more shallow and rapid than normal   Slow and irregular in rate and amplitude (ataxic)

Midposition irregular in shape   Fixed

Midposition   Fixed

DOLL'S HEAD MANEUVER
Impaired, may be dysconjugate

ICE WATER CALORICS
Impaired, may be dysconjugate

DOLL'S HEAD MANEUVER
No response

ICE WATER CALORIC
No response

Usually motionless

or

Arms and legs extended and pronate (_decerebrate_ rigidity,) particularly on side opposite primary lesion

Motionless and flaccid

or

No response to noxious orbital stimulus, bilateral Babinski signs or occasional flexor response in lower extremities when feet stroked

5–6 (Continued)

neurons that control reflex pupillary adjustments to light. The result is a moderately dilated pupil on the affected side. When a light is flashed in that eye, the pupil will react sluggishly, although the other eye will respond consensually. Similarly, a light flashed in the nonaffected eye will provoke a normal direct reflex in it but a sluggish consensual response in the affected eye. This unilateral pupillary abnormality may be the _only_ sign of early uncal herniation. Early motor signs may consist of contralateral paratonic resistance and extensor plantar reflex due to compression of the ipsilateral cerebral peduncle.

In the late third nerve stage, the pupil dilates widely and does not respond to light. In addition, the increasing pressure affects the motor neurons that control eyelid muscles and oculomotor-mediated eye movement. As a result, diplopia and ptosis appear, and the eye (when resting) looks downward and outward due to the unopposed action of the sixth cranial nerve. The patient becomes deeply stuporous

and then comatose. Oculocephalic reflexes show absent or dysconjugate doll's eyes. Oculovestibular responses rapidly become sluggish and disappear. Because the opposite cerebral peduncle also becomes compressed against the tentorial edge, bilateral hemiplegia develops. Bilateral motor signs develop, and noxious stimuli elicit abnormal extension of the extremities.

Uncal herniation is particularly dangerous because it tends to progress rapidly to produce irreversible midbrain–upper-pontine damage. In this stage, pressure on midbrain corticospinal and other tracts results in rigid bilateral abnormal extension (decerebrate posturing). The opposite pupil may dilate widely and be fixed to light; eventually both pupils fix in midposition (5–6 mm). Doll's eyes and ice water responses are abnormal, and the respiratory pattern shows sustained hyperventilation. After this stage, the uncal syndrome progresses in the same fashion as the lower-pontine–upper-medullary stage of central herniation.

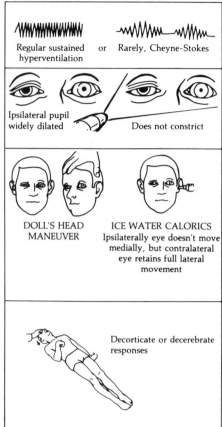

		Early third nerve stage	Late third nerve stage
a.	Respiratory pattern	Eupneic	Regular sustained hyperventilation or Rarely, Cheyne-Stokes
b.	Pupillary size and reactions	Moderately dilated pupil, usually ipsilateral to primary lesion — Constricts sluggishly	Ipsilateral pupil widely dilated — Does not constrict
c.	Oculocephalic and oculovestibular responses	DOLL'S HEAD MANEUVER Present or dysconjugate — ICE WATER CALORICS Full conjugate slow ipsilateral eye movement (impaired nystagmus) or Dysconjugate, because contralateral eye does not move medially	DOLL'S HEAD MANEUVER — ICE WATER CALORICS Ipsilaterally eye doesn't move medially, but contralateral eye retains full lateral movement
d.	Motor responses at rest and to stimulation	Appropriate motor responses to noxious orbital roof pressure Contralateral paratonic resistance — Contralateral extensor plantar reflex	Decorticate or decerebrate responses

FIGURE 5–7

Signs of uncal herniation. (Adapted from McNealy D, Plum F: "Brainstem Dysfunction with Supratentorial Mass Lesions" from *Archives of Neurology,* July, Volume 7:10–32. Copyright 1962, American Medical Association.)

NURSING DIAGNOSIS

One nursing diagnosis for this disorder is: "Altered tissue perfusion (cerebral) related to impending (or actual) herniation."

Planning and Implementation of Care

The above descriptions of downward brain herniation accentuate the importance of conscientious physical examinations by nurses and prompt reactions at the *first* signs of possible impending herniation. Alert the physician if you observe *any* signs of possible incipient herniation, even if they are transient or equivocal. For the patient on continuous intracranial pressure monitoring, notify the physician promptly if there is a consistent rise in ICP, plateau waves, or widening of the pulse pressure, so that CSF drainage, mannitol administration, or other therapy can be instituted.

Outcome Evaluation

The following outcome criteria are ideal:

- Return to premorbid level of consciousness.
- Pupils of normal size, bilaterally equal and briskly responsive to light.
- Vital signs WNL.

- Normal motor response (no posturing, absent Babinski reflex).

Status Epilepticus

Status epilepticus is one of the most common neurologic emergencies encountered by the critical-care nurse. *Status epilepticus* is defined as seizure activity of 30 minutes' or more duration caused by a single seizure or a series of seizures with no return of consciousness between seizures (Niedermeyer 1990). Status epilepticus can occur with any type of seizure activity (Table 5–1). It occurs in up to 10% of all epileptics but can occur in people without a history of epilepsy. The most common and most dangerous form of status epilepticus is generalized tonic-clonic, caused by paroxysmal, uncontrolled electrical activity that spreads across the brain (Niedermeyer 1990).

Assessment

Risk Conditions There are numerous causes for status epilepticus. The most common cause is insufficient serum levels of anticonvulsant drugs caused by the individual's deliberate or inadvertent stopping the drug or by inadequate therapy. Other causes include changing anticonvulsant agents, metabolic imbalances, drug withdrawals, trauma, neoplasm, and acute cerebral edema (Table 5–2).

If not treated promptly, permanent neurologic sequelae may develop or death from cardiovascular

---

NURSING TIP

Emergency Intervention for Suspected Imminent Herniation

Should you suspect imminent herniation, immediately summon medical assistance. Meanwhile, hyperventilate the patient to reduce the P_{aCO_2} and oxygenate with 100% oxygen. This action will constrict the cerebral vessels and temporarily decrease intracranial pressure. It may also avert herniation long enough for more definitive medical therapy to be instituted.

---

failure, respiratory depression, or cerebral edema may intervene. The patient is twice as likely to develop neurologic deficits as to die (Wittman 1985). Neurologic sequelae can range from focal neurologic deficits, behavior disorders, and chronic epilepsy to mental retardation and brain atrophy. Prognosis depends on the cause of the seizures and the period of time between onset and cessation.

Signs and Symptoms There are four distinct phases during tonic-clonic seizures. The *preictal phase,* or *aura,* may or may not be apparent to the patient. The aura may consist of subtle, unusual sensory illusions (smells or patterns of light), mood changes, or focal motor activity. Origin of the seizure may be pinpointed by the characteristics of the aura.

Nursing staff may not be aware of the aura but will note the sudden shrill cry or moan at the beginning of

---

TABLE 5–1

International Classification of Seizure Type

Seizure Classification

I. Partial seizures (focal, local)

  A. Simple partial seizure (SPS)

    1. Motor symptoms

    2. Somatosensory or special sensory symptoms

    3. Autonomic symptoms

    4. Psychic symptoms

  B. Complex partial seizures (CPS)

    1. Simple partial onset followed by impairment of consciousness

    2. Simple partial seizures with impairment of consciousness at onset

  C. Partial seizures progressing to secondary generalized seizures (SGS)

    1. SPS → SGS

    2. CPS → SGS

    3. SPS → CPS → SGS

II. Generalized onset seizures

  A. Absence

  B. Myoclonic

  C. Clonic

  D. Tonic

  E. Tonic-clonic

  F. Atonic

Source: Dupuis R, Miranda-Massari J: Anticonvulsants: Pharmacotherapeutic issues in the critically ill patient. *Clin Issues Crit Care Nurs* 1991; 2(4):639–656.

TABLE 5–2

Common Causes of Status Epilepticus

Insufficient serum levels of anticonvulsant agents
- Noncompliance: deliberate or inadvertent
- Inadequate prescribed therapy

Metabolic disturbances
- Hyperglycemia vs hypoglycemia
- Hypoxia
- Drug or alcohol withdrawal
- Electrolyte imbalances
- Low magnesium, calcium, or phosphorus serum levels
- High P_{CO_2} serum levels
- Hyperpyrexia

Infections

Structural CNS lesions
- Concussion
- Infarctions
- Cerebral or subdural hematoma
- Subarachnoid hemorrhage
- Undetectable structural lesion

Familial predisposition

Idiopathic

Life-threatening dysrhythmias

Focal brain trauma

Environmental stimuli (lights, sounds)

Cerebral neoplasm

Stress

Acute cerebral edema

the *tonic phase*. This cry or moan is caused by air being forced past the closed glottis and larynx by the contraction of thoracic and abdominal muscles. Carefully observe seizure characteristics, particularly noting onset, progression and length, any pupil changes, and any lateralizing signs. Some muscle groups contract; others become flaccid. The person loses consciousness and instantly collapses, increasing the potential for injury. Rigid, intense muscle contractions are exhibited by extended extremities, arched spine, and clamped jaw. Apnea ensues for 10–15 seconds usually but can last up to 1 minute. A concurrent increase in saliva production with sequestering in the mouth and throat increases the risk of aspiration. The saliva may turn bloody if the tongue was bitten as the jaw snapped shut. Pupils become dilated and nonreactive to light and deviate conjugately or rove due to

severe hypoxia; this deviation is not considered as pointing to the seizure focus. Heart rate slows secondary to parasympathetic (vagal) stimulation. There is an abrupt end to the tonic phase as the clonic phase begins.

The muscles begin violent jerking at the onset of the *clonic phase*. This bilateral, global jerking gradually decelerates until it fades when the nutrition and potassium of the brain cells are depleted. There is violent facial grimacing, profuse diaphoresis, and usually incontinence. Respirations become irregular and noisy, with frothing at the mouth from accumulated saliva. Pupil size and reactivity may or may not change. Bradycardia or tachycardia may be present. Clonus usually lasts 2–5 minutes and ends with a deep breath followed by irregular, shallow respirations.

In a generalized seizure, clonus then is replaced by the *postictal phase* of muscle flaccidity and deep sleep that can last from 5 minutes up to several hours. This deep sleep is due to brain and muscle exhaustion from severely depleted cellular glucose and oxygen supplies. Respirations gradually become deep and regular. Pupils react to light. The patient awakens confused and amnesic and may complain of headache, muscle aches, and fatigue.

The status epilepticus patient has continuous seizure activity, without the interictal period of recovery that is typical following a generalized seizure (Marshall et al. 1990). Sometimes, tonic-clonic activity stops briefly between attacks, but the patient remains unconscious. Failure to control seizures can result in systemic exhaustion and can cause severe neurologic deficits or death.

Significant reductions in cerebral cortical oxygenation and insufficient regional oxygenation occur within 20 minutes of seizure onset (Niedermeyer 1990). The intense electrical activity causes a marked increase in cerebral metabolic rate, oxygen and glucose utilization, glycolysis, rapid depletion of adenosine triphosphate bonds (the energy source for cells), and consumption of neurotransmitter substances (Lovely and Ozuna 1982). Cerebral blood flow may increase as much as five times normal (Cammermeyer and Appeldorn 1990) due to increased arterial pressure and vasodilation resulting from CO_2 and lactic acid accumulation. As status epilepticus continues, autoregulation is lost, cerebral vessels dilate, arterial pressure falls, and adequate cerebral perfusion pressure is jeopardized (Lothman 1990; Engel 1989).

During the first 30 minutes of status epilepticus, arterial BP rises, probably due to vasoconstriction resulting from vasomotor center stimulation, mediated by hypoxic or hypercarbic stimulation of aortic arch and carotid body chemoreceptors (Lovely and Ozuna

NURSING DIAGNOSES

The life-threatening nature of status epilepticus makes prompt nursing diagnosis and intervention crucial. The nursing diagnoses for a patient in status epilepticus include:

- Ineffective airway clearance
- Ineffective breathing pattern
- Impaired gas exchange
- High risk for altered tissue perfusion
- High risk for injury
- Sensory-perceptual alteration
- High risk for ineffective individual coping

NURSING TIP

Airway Maintenance During a Seizure

Do not try to place an oral airway when the jaw relaxes, unless there is airway obstruction. The patient may start to seize again and injure him or herself or the nurse. Also, airway placement could stimulate vomiting and increase the chance of aspiration. Side positioning or chin-lift–jaw-thrust maneuver will usually maintain a patent airway.

1982). After the first 30 minutes, mean arterial BP usually falls below normal and may stay depressed in the postictal period (Meldrum and Brierly 1973; Engel 1989).

Permanent cellular damage can occur in the medullary, cerebral, thalamic, hippocampal, and middle cortical layers by 60–90 minutes (Wittman 1985; Gress 1990; Lothman 1990). Severe metabolic imbalances (including hypoxia, hypotension, hypoglycemia, hyperkalemia, and hyperpyrexia) and increased intracranial pressure create an imbalance between supply and demand for glucose and oxygen for which the body may be unable to compensate (Wittman 1985; Engel 1989).

Planning and Implementation of Care

Ineffective Airway Clearance Related to Airway Occlusion by Tongue, Bronchoconstriction, or Increased Secretions Maintenance of a patent airway and adequate ventilation are the first priorities in status epilepticus. Turn the patient on the side to facilitate drainage of secretions. Use low, gentle oropharyngeal suction as needed to aspirate secretions.

Ineffective Breathing Pattern Related to Apnea, Brainstem Depression, or Overmedication Carefully monitor and evaluate the respiratory pattern, rate, and depth for signs of insufficiency. Loosen tight clothing on the chest if necessary. Anticipate intubation when respiratory distress is present and place an intubation tray at bedside. There are no clear-cut guidelines regarding mechanical ventilation; an individual decision must be made by the physician on the basis of ventilatory pattern and arterial blood gas values.

Impaired Gas Exchange Related to Excessive Oxygen Demand or Aspiration If the patient is not intubated, administer supplemental oxygen by nasal prongs, as a mask may impede clearance of emesis. If the patient is intubated, increase the oxygen concentration to 100%. Monitor oxygenation and acid–base status via arterial blood gas sampling. If the status epilepticus does not respond readily to therapy, insert a nasogastric tube, per physician's order, to prevent chemical pneumonitis caused by aspiration of gastric contents or vomitus.

High Risk for Altered Tissue Perfusion Related to Decreased Blood Pressure or Cardiac Output Monitor vital signs closely. Place the patient on continuous ECG monitoring. Establish an intravenous line at a TKO ("to keep open") rate. To avoid cerebral edema, isotonic solutions such as lactated Ringer's or normal saline are preferred; glucose-containing solutions, such as 5% dextrose in lactated Ringer's, frequently are used to provide glucose to the brain (Rich 1986).

High Risk for Injury Related to Tonic-Clonic Movements and Repeated Seizures Never leave the patient unattended during a seizure. Protect the patient from injury by removing any nearby objects. Moving the patient is not advised unless a potentially damaging nearby object cannot be removed. Never try to force anything into the mouth or try to restrain the extremities, because this could tear or stretch the muscles. Gentle guiding of the extremities is acceptable.

If the patient is in a chair, gently lower him or her to the floor. Once the patient is on the floor, place a pad, rolled cloth, or pillow under the head to prevent trauma. When the patient is in bed, lower the head and raise the side rails. Pad the side rails and head and foot boards with special pads or pillows.

Draw blood samples for laboratory studies, including arterial blood gases, serum electrolytes, blood glucose, and toxicology screen. If the patient has been on anticonvulsant therapy, a serum sample should be drawn for determination of baseline blood level of the particular drug(s).

Implement drug therapy as ordered by the physician. Selection of pharmacologic agents may vary with the individual physician as well as the patient's condition. The drugs used most often are a benzodiazepine, phenytoin, and phenobarbital.

A benzodiazepine, such as lorazepam (Ativan) or diazepam (Valium), is regarded as the initial drug of choice by most physicians. An intravenous benzodiazepine is a rapid-acting (2 to 3 minutes), short-lived drug; thus, the dose can easily be titrated according to the patient's response (Dupuis and Miranda-Massari 1991). Seizure activity usually stops during or immediately after the injection. Monitor the patient closely, as respiratory depression, hypotension, and further decreases in level of consciousness may occur. If the patient does not have an artificial airway in place, observe for possible airway obstruction by the tongue due to marked muscle relaxation. Because a benzodiazepine provides only short-term cessation of seizure activity, a prophylactic anticonvulsant also should be administered.

Phenytoin (Dilantin) is used for acute and long-term control of seizure activity. Disadvantages include a slow (15-minute) onset of activity, potential cardiotoxicity, and tendency to crystallize in glucose. Phenytoin often is given in conjunction with a benzodiazepine to provide both immediate and long-term control of seizures. In order to achieve a rapid therapeutic concentration, doses of 15 to 18 mg/kg are administered intravenously in normal saline (to avoid precipitation) at a rate no faster than 50 mg/min (Dupuis and Miranda-Massari 1991). Administration of 1 gram of Dilantin will take 20 minutes or more. In elderly patients with cardiac disease or patients with sepsis, infusion rates as low as 5 mg/min may be necessary (Dupuis and Miranda-Massari 1991). Prior to administration of Dilantin, assess the patency of the IV line. Dilantin is very caustic to tissue, so avoid extravasation. A patient receiving intravenous phenytoin should be under constant ECG surveillance. Very high doses of phenytoin have been associated with CNS toxicity and neurologic manifestations such as severe drowsiness, blurred vision, mental confusion, insomnia, ataxia, tremors, coma, and seizures (Osorio et al. 1989). Side effects, usually due to excessively rapid adminis-

tration, include hypotension, conduction disturbances (QRS widening, AV blocks, and ventricular fibrillation) and cardiorespiratory arrest. Phenytoin should be avoided or used only with extreme caution in patients with sinus bradycardia, SA or AV block, hypotension, or severe myocardial failure.

Barbiturates increase the neuronal threshold for electrical and chemical stimuli, depress physiologic excitation, and enhance inhibition. Phenobarbital is a barbiturate long used to control status epilepticus. Intravenous administration provides long-range (24-hour) control, similar to phenytoin. It is the preferred drug in status epilepticus due to barbiturate withdrawal. Side effects include marked sedation, respiratory depression, and hypotension. Be particularly alert when a patient is given both diazepam and phenobarbital; their interaction may cause severe cardiorespiratory depression.

Phenobarbital and diazepam are not the only anticonvulsant drugs that interact, however. Most of the anticonvulsant drugs interact with each other in some manner as well as with many other drugs given to critically ill patients.

Refractory status epilepticus is present when the patient does not respond to the usual therapy. It may be treated with paraldehyde, neuromuscular blocking drugs, or general anesthesia. Neuromuscular blockade stops motor manifestations of the seizure but not the cerebral seizure activity itself. It requires intubation and mechanical ventilation because of respiratory muscle paralysis. General anesthetics suppress cerebral seizure activity but also require extensive ventilatory support. Other problems with neuromuscular blockade and general anesthesia therapies are the difficulty of determining how long to continue therapy, no guarantee for complete suppression of the seizure activity, and the fact that anesthesia requires full operating room support (Wittman 1985).

Sensory-Perceptual Alteration Related to Postictal Phase
The patient may awaken confused, disoriented, or amnesic. Attempts at reorientation will probably not be effective until the patient is fully alert. Be careful not to speak loudly or make sudden, jerking movements with the patient as this may stimulate another seizure. When clearing the airway, gentle suctioning of the mouth and oropharynx should reduce the risk of this hazard. The patient may be safely left with the family in attendance once recurrence of seizure activity is abated. Monitor general neurologic status between seizures. Neuro-checks should include level of consciousness, pupil size and reaction, and sensorimotor function.

High Risk for Ineffective Individual Coping Related to Loss of Privacy The patient's privacy should be maintained at all times. When a seizure starts, shield the patient from any nearby onlookers. If no other staff are nearby, discreetly notify coworkers of your need for assistance and have them call the physician. Since the patient's hearing may be unaffected by the seizure, use a soft, calm, normal voice to explain what is happening to the patient. When the seizure is over, cover the patient with a blanket. Gently remove the patient to a private place when necessary. Efficient cleansing of the patient for incontinence is important and must be done in complete privacy. The nurse's unbiased attitude toward seizure care and protection of privacy will help the patient, as well as the family, accept the illness and learn to deal positively with it.

Outcome Evaluation

Desirable outcome criteria for a patient with status epilepticus are:

- Prevention of injury.
- Control of abnormal seizure activity.
- Minimal or no loss of privacy during seizure.
- Vital signs WNL.
- Arterial blood gas values WNL.
- Return to a normal level of consciousness.

Cerebral Vascular Disorders

Cerebral vascular disorders include two general categories: ischemic vascular disease and hemorrhagic vascular disease. *Stroke* (cerebrovascular accident) is a sudden, rapid onset of neurologic deficits related directly or indirectly to an interruption of the cerebral blood supply. Approximately 500,000 people in the United States suffer from stroke each year (Marshall et al. 1990). Stroke occurs more frequently in men than in women and in blacks than in whites (Kneisl and Ames 1986). The elderly, ages 75 to 85 years, have the highest incidence of stroke; for people under the age of 65, stroke occurs in one out of seven individuals. The morbidity associated with stroke leads to chronic disability. The continuing decline of stroke mortality has been attributed to several factors, including better control of systemic arterial hypertension, reduction in cigarette smoking, and increased diet consciousness.

Arterial Syndromes

Two arterial systems form the cerebral circulation, the carotid and the vertebrobasilar. The reader is referred to Chapter 4 to review the cerebral circulation. Interruption of blood supply for whatever reason will produce symptoms related to the location of the lesion in the arterial tree and the portion of brain supplied (Table 5–3). The most common presentation is the middle cerebral artery syndrome.

Stroke Classification

Occlusive stroke and hemorrhagic stroke are the two major kinds of stroke. Based on mechanism, occlusive stroke is subdivided into thrombotic and embolic. Cerebral thrombosis, the most common cause of stroke, accounts for 50%–70% of all stroke cases (Marshall et al. 1990).

Occlusive Stroke

Thrombotic Stroke Thrombotic stroke results from thrombosis of the vessel, which leads to ischemia and infarction. Atherosclerosis is the most common cause of ischemic stroke. It affects the carotid vessels five times more often than the vertebrobasilar arteries (Toole 1990). Atherosclerotic plaques form at the branching of the blood vessels and narrow the vessel lumen. Thrombotic stroke is progressive in nature, from partial to total obstruction of the vessel. The resulting clinical picture is evolutionary—from initial warning signs to completed stroke. The common progression is from transient ischemic attack and reversible ischemic neurologic deficit to stroke-in-evolution and completed stroke.

A *transient ischemic attack (TIA)* is an abrupt onset of neurologic dysfunction lasting less than 24 hours and with complete resolution of symptoms. TIAs more commonly present with anterior circulation symptoms that may be traced to internal carotid artery obstruction. Focal ischemic symptoms that persist for more than 24 hours but then clear completely are called *reversible ischemic neurologic deficits, or RINDs.* TIAs are a warning event in 80% of thrombotic ischemic strokes (Toole 1990). The thrombotic *stroke-in-evolution* causes symptoms that progress over hours to days. The *completed stroke* is the residual neurologic deficit.

High blood pressure and diabetes are the most common risk factors for thrombotic stroke. The critical-care nurse should be especially cognizant of

CRITICAL CARE GERONTOLOGY

Neurologic Function in the Elderly

Recently, the United States Congress declared this decade to be the decade of the brain. It has become increasingly apparent that our knowledge of cerebral function is incomplete. We know exceedingly little of the creative process of learning and memory, how the brain recovers from brain trauma or damage, or even the effects of aging. At birth, the human brain contains perhaps as many as one hundred billion nerve cells. From then on, there is a steady but gradual decrease in functional neurons. It has been estimated that over a life span, brain weight decreases about 10%. However, not every part of the brain loses neurons at the same rate. Some areas, such as the brainstem, lose little if any cells with advancing age. On the other hand, the cerebral cortex (the newer, thinking portion of the brain) loses neurons at a maximum rate of 50,000 neurons a day, according to Dr. Stanley Rapoport of the National Institute on Aging (Restak 1988).

Perhaps even more important than cellular death is the loss of interconnections among neurons. Fewer synapses are seen, and dendritic branching is decreased. Like branches in a tree, dendrites thin out and lose their farthest twigs. The neurons are smaller and the quantity of neurotransmitters is decreased as well. Thus, there are fewer messages to be sent, fewer neurotransmitters to dispatch messages, and fewer neurons to receive them.

It is estimated that only 50% of neurons truly are required to carry out a specific task. In theory, one could lose half of the cells in a specific group and still have sufficient numbers to function. Those few remaining neurons become more active and are stimulated to search out new connections and establish alternative communication pathways. The elderly brain is doing the best it can under seemingly adverse conditions to overcome degeneration and cellular death; however, time and disease take their toll.

Death increases exponentially during aging, and stroke is the most common cause of death over the age of 65. A stroke or cerebral vascular accident can result in sudden blockage of a blood vessel and have devastating effects. The end result of a stroke depends on the brain's ability to reorganize itself and reestablish connections. Why do some stroke victims recover and others not? The degree of impairment depends on the site of occlusion, the extent of the damage, as well as the survivability of the existing neurons and their ability to communicate with each other. Some blood vessels serve crucial brain areas responsible for movement, sight, and language. Destruction of these areas leads to serious, often permanent disabilities. Other areas are less critical and the damage is less disabling. The effects of the aging process, neuronal degeneration, and ischemic and anoxic changes all dramatically affect the brain's ability to survive the aftermath of stroke damage. Memory, intelligence, reasoning, decision making, and problem solving skills all may be affected.

As life expectancy increases, the possibility of stroke or dementia increases as well. By the year 2010, one out of every six persons in the United States will be 65 or older. The magnitude of the problems of stroke, dementia, and cognitive decline makes it clear that if we do not find cures for these conditions and diseases that affect the elderly, we may see our nation turned into a huge extended-care facility. Every one of us is growing older, and many of us will some day experience what it is like to be 70 or 80 years of age. In order to locate the keys to unlock the mysteries of the mind, we need extensive research in the field of aging and neuroscience.

---

conditions leading to inadequate cerebral perfusion, such as hypotension and dehydration, since these factors may increase the risk of thrombosis.

Embolic Stroke In an embolic stroke, an embolus travels via the bloodstream and lodges in a cerebral vessel, producing ischemia and infarction. Symptoms develop rapidly without any warning signs. The neurologic deficit relates to the area of brain lacking blood supply. Embolic stroke tends to occur during activity, whereas thrombotic stroke often develops at rest, during sleep, or shortly after arising.

Sources of cerebral emboli include the heart, aorta, neck vessels, foreign substances, and increased blood coagulation. Calcified plaques in the aorta, carotid arteries, or vertebral arteries may break loose and embolize. Cardiac conditions such as myocardial infarction, endocarditis, rheumatic heart disease, and

TABLE 5–3

General Symptoms and Signs of Occlusive CVA

I. CVA involving the anterior cerebral artery:

Mental status impairments

- Confusion
- Amnesia
- Perseveration
- Personality changes: flat affect, apathy
- Cognitive changes: short attention span, slowness
- Deterioration of intellectual function

Urinary incontinence (long duration)

Contralateral hemiparesis or hemiplegia; sensory impairments; foot and leg deficits greater than arm deficits

Footdrop

Apraxia on affected side

Expressive aphasia (for dominant hemisphere involvement)

Deviation of eyes and head toward affected side

Albulia (inability to make decisions or perform voluntary acts)

Gait dysfunction

II. CVA involving the middle cerebral artery:

Dysphasia (dominant hemisphere involvement), dyslexia, dysgraphia

Contralateral hemiparesis or hemiplegia

Contralateral hemisensory disturbances

Rapid deterioration in consciousness from confusion to coma

Vomiting

Homonymous hemianopia

Denial or lack of recognition of a paralyzed extremity

Inability to turn eyes toward affected side

III. CVA involving the posterior cerebral artery:

Peripheral signs

- Visual disturbances:
  - Homonymous hemianopia
  - Cortical blindness
  - Lack of depth perception
  - Failure to see objects not centered in field of vision
  - Visual hallucinations
- Memory deficits
- Perseveration
- Dyslexia

Central signs

- Thalamic or subthalamic nuclei involvement: diffuse sensory loss, mild hemiparesis, intentional tremor
- Cerebral peduncle involvement: contralateral hemiplegia, oculomotor nerve deficits
- Brainstem involvement: pupillary dysfunction, nystagmus, loss of conjugate gaze

IV. CVA involving the internal carotid artery:

Contralateral hemiparesis with facial asymmetry

Contralateral sensory deficits, especially paresthesia

Hemianopia

Ipsilateral episodes of visual blurring or amaurosis fugax (temporary blindness)

Dysphasia (dominant hemisphere involvement)

Carotid bifurcation bruit

Mild Horner's syndrome

V. CVA involving the vertebral-basilar system:

Dysarthria, dysphagia

Vertigo, nausea, and syncope

Memory loss, disorientation

Ataxic gait

Dysmetria

Visual symptoms: double vision, homonymous hemianopia

Tinnitus, hearing loss

Ocular signs: nystagmus, conjugate gaze paralysis, ophthalmoplegia

Akinetic mutism (locked-in syndrome when basilar artery occlusion occurs)

Numbness of tongue

Facial weakness, alternating motor paresis

Drop attacks

VI. CVA involving the anterior-inferior cerebellar artery (inferior lateral pontine syndrome):

Contralateral signs

- Horizontal nystagmus
- Sensory impairments, mainly of trunk and limbs

Ipsilateral signs

- Horner's syndrome
- Tinnitus and deafness
- Ataxia and nystagmus
- Facial paralysis and loss of tactile sensation

VII. CVA involving the posterior-inferior cerebellar artery:

Dysarthria, dysphagia, dysphonia

Vertigo, nystagmus, unsteady gait

Ipsilateral Horner's syndrome

Sensory changes—ipsilateral face and contralateral body

Hiccoughs, vomiting

Paralysis of larynx and soft palate

Wallenberg syndrome: sudden onset of:

- Vertigo, horizontal nystagmus, ataxia
- Nausea and vomiting
- Dysphagia
- Horner's syndrome (ipsilateral)
- Pain and temperature loss on trunk and limbs (contralateral)
- Balance loss on affected side
- Pain and temperature loss on face (ipsilateral)

Source: Kneisl CR, Ames SW. *Adult health nursing: A biopsychosocial approach.* Reading, MA: Addison-Wesley, 1986, p. 1169.

postcardiac surgical procedures all bear the potential to produce an embolus. The risk of embolic stroke for patients with atrial dysrhythmias is five times greater than for those without (Kneisl and Ames 1986). Air embolus may be associated with a disconnected central line or a complication of posterior fossa surgery in the sitting position. Fat emboli may occur after traumatic injury with multiple fractures. Conditions such as polycythemia, sickle cell disease, sepsis, use of oral contraceptives, or hypercoagulable states all carry a risk for embolization.

Hemorrhagic Stroke Hemorrhagic stroke results from the rupture of blood vessels, with blood extravasation into brain tissue. Common causes of hemorrhagic stroke are ruptured cerebral aneurysm, hypertensive intracerebral hemorrhage, and ruptured arteriovenous malformation. Hypertension and abnormalities of the cerebral vessels are major risk factors.

Cerebral Aneurysm A cerebral aneurysm is a localized dilatation of a blood vessel. Congenital weakness in the media of the cerebral vessel allows for a saccular or fusiform aneurysm to develop. Because saccular aneurysms resemble a berry with a stem, they are referred to as *berry aneurysms.* The majority of aneurysms are located on the anterior portion of the circle of Willis.

The incidence of SAH from rupture of an aneurysm is approximately 12 per 100,000 population (Heros and Kistler 1983). Roughly 50% of these patients die or become permanently disabled due to the initial bleed. The majority of patients are asymptomatic until the aneurysm ruptures into the subarachnoid space, pro-ducing a subarachnoid hemorrhage (SAH). Warning symptoms, which precede major aneurysmal rupture 40% of the time, are attributed to an expansion of the aneurysm or a warning leak. Enlargement of the aneurysm may produce symptoms of localized headache (commonly described by the patient as "the worst headache I ever had"), cranial nerve palsies (especially third nerve), and visual deficits. A warning leak can cause a generalized headache, malaise, neck pain, and photophobia. Careful history-taking will assist in identifying the patient at risk for a major bleed.

An acute subarachnoid bleed is followed by an excruciating headache, visual disturbances, nausea and vomiting, motor deficits, or loss of consciousness. Meningeal irritation from the blood in the subarachnoid space causes nuchal rigidity, photophobia, irritability, and low-grade fever. Acute aneurysmal rupture and sudden injection of arterial blood under enormous pressure dramatically elevates ICP and distorts cranial structures. Death almost always is due to severe intracerebral hemorrhage, sudden intracranial hypertension because of the large volume of blood (up to 150 ml), and herniation (Marshall et al. 1990). A grading system based on clinical findings is used as a prognostic indicator and as a guide for surgical intervention. See Table 5–4 for the Botterel scale.

Three major complications of ruptured cerebral aneurysms are rebleeding, cerebral vasospasm, and communicating hydrocephalus. The risk of *rebleed* is highest four to eight days after rupture (Fode 1988). Rebleed carries significant mortality and morbidity. To prevent rebleed, patients are placed on bedrest in a quiet environment. Blood pressure is controlled with hydralazine hydrochloride (Apresoline), methyldopa

TABLE 5–4

The Botterel Scale for Grading Ruptured Cerebral Aneurysms

CATEGORY	CRITERIA	SURVIVAL RATE
Grade I (minimal hemorrhage)	Client alert, neurologically intact, with a minimal headache and slight nuchal rigidity	65%
Grade II (mild hemorrhage)	Client alert, with minimal neurologic deficits, such as CN III palsy (eg, ptosis, diplopia), with a mild to severe headache and nuchal rigidity	55%
Grade III (moderate hemorrhage)	Client has definite change in level of consciousness, is drowsy or confused; nuchal rigidity is present, with mild focal deficits	45%
Grade IV (moderate to severe hemorrhage)	Client stuporous or semicomatose, with mild to severe hemiparesis, nuchal rigidity, and possible early decerebration	30%
Grade V (severe hemorrhage)	Client decerebrate, comatose, with a moribund appearance	5%

Source: Kneisl CR, Ames SW: *Adult health nursing: A biopsychosocial approach.* Reading, MA: Addison-Wesley, 1986, p. 1156.

(Aldomet), reserpine, or a beta-blocker. Aminocaproic acid (Amicar) is an antifibrinolytic agent used to prevent clot lysis. Although Amicar has been shown to reduce rebleeding in patients with SAH, deaths from thromboembolic events and complications such as dysrhythmias have neutralized its beneficial effects (Kassell et al. 1984; Vermeulen et al. 1984; Marshall et al. 1990). In some centers, Amicar is still used if surgical intervention is to occur within a few days (Marshall et al. 1990, MacDonald 1989).

Cerebral vasospasm, the narrowing of portions of the arteries comprising the circle of Willis and its major branches, is a major cause of death and disability in SAH. Vasospasm decreases cerebral blood flow and can result in cerebral ischemia and infarction. The exact cause of vasospasm remains unknown, but there is a high correlation between the existence of blood clots around the vessels at the base of the brain and the development of spasm. SAH patients with no blood seen on CT scan have a very low incidence of vasospasm, while those with a large amount of blood in the cisterns and in the subarachnoid space have an extremely high incidence of cerebral vasospasm (Fisher et al. 1980). Clinical deterioration from vasospasm usually occurs between the fourth and twelfth day after initial bleed (MacDonald 1989; Hummel 1989). Its onset is gradual, with increasing symptomatology depending on the arterial territory. Confusion, disorientation, hemiparesis, or aphasia may be exhibited. Many neurosurgeons are hesitant to operate on patients in vasospasm due to increased morbidity and mortality rates (Adams et al. 1988; Marshall et al. 1990).

A primary objective in the management of cerebral vasospasm is preventing cerebral ischemia by elevating the cerebral perfusion pressure. Hypervolemic hemodilution/hypertension ("Triple H") therapy elevates CPP by expanding intravascular volume and/or using vasopressors to keep the patient hypertensive. These therapies present a challenge in the patient whose aneurysm has not been surgically repaired; maintaining the hypervolemic/hypertensive state significantly increases the risk of rebleed. A variety of techniques may be utilized for volume expansion in the treatment of vasospasm. Both colloid (albumin) and crystalloid (salt) solutions have been used to reduce the hematocrit by 15–20%, increase pulmonary wedge pressure to 16–18 mm Hg, and increase cardiac output to 6–8 L/min. (Marshall et al. 1990; Hummel 1989). Another treatment modality is the use of calcium channel blockers. Nimodipine (Nimotop), a compound similar in structure to nifedipine, has been found more cerebroselective, more potent, and more lipid-soluble than nifedipine. Studies suggest it may benefit patients

who manifest symptomatic cerebral ischemia due to subarachnoid hemorrhage (Ohman et al. 1991). Furthermore, in randomized trials, the incidence of cerebral vasospasm was reduced substantially in patients receiving nimodipine when compared to placebo (Pickard et al. 1989). The recommended dose is 60 mg (two 30-mg capsules) every 4 hours for 21 days. Therapy should commence within 96 hours of the SAH (Petruk et al. 1988). Calcium channel antagonists are administered prophylactically to prevent vasospasm. These drugs prevent calcium from participating in the contraction of smooth muscles, therefore promoting vasodilation. Nimodipine and nicardipine selectively affect cerebral blood vessels by interfering with erythrocyte lysis, preventing platelet aggregation and decreasing endothelial degeneration caused by catecholamines (Oertel 1985; MacDonald 1989). As of 1991, nimodipine is available only in soft gelatin capsules. If the capsule cannot be swallowed, use an 18-gauge needle, extract the contents from the capsule, and administer by nasogastric tube.

Transluminal cerebral angioplasty for treatment of vasospasm was first reported by Zubkov et al. in 1984. Its use appears promising. Investigational studies have demonstrated sustained permanent dilation of vasospastic arteries and improved neurologic function (Higashida et al. 1989; Newell et al. 1989).

Communicating hydrocephalus as a complication of subarachnoid hemorrhage can occur with the initial bleed or weeks later. The products of blood breakdown plug the arachnoid villi, preventing the absorption of CSF into the venous sinuses. Hydrocephalus produces a generalized increase in intracranial pressure. Presenting symptoms in the acute stage include changes in level of consciousness and mental status and may progress to respiratory, pupillary, and motor involvement if not recognized. CT scan confirms hydrocephalus. Temporary relief may be obtained by insertion of an ICP monitoring catheter into a ventricle and draining off some CSF. If the situation does not resolve on its own, long-term management requires ventriculoperitoneal shunt, discussed in Chapter 6.

Diagnosis of Stroke

Patient history is extremely valuable in identifying the onset of symptoms and risk factors. Physical examination may reveal localizing signs, indicating the involved area of the brain.

CT scan may demonstrate occlusive stroke or hemorrhagic stroke. Necrotic areas indicate occlusive stroke, while intracerebral bleeding or blood in the subarachnoid space at the base of the brain indicates hemorrhagic stroke. Due to the rapidity and convenience of CT for critically ill patients, trauma patients, or those suspected of having hemorrhagic strokes, CT remains the neurodiagnostic modality of choice. Magnetic resonance imaging (MRI) is an imaging procedure that does not employ x-rays. MRI is extremely sensitive and is superior to CT scanning in providing contrast between gray and white matter of the brain, visualizing abnormalities in posterior fossa or spinal cord, and detecting subtle changes due to small lucunar strokes or multiple sclerosis. MRI has better resolution and is able to detect more subtle changes in water content and demonstrate intraluminal clots and flowing blood in arteriovenous malformations and aneurysms (Marshall et al. 1990). The time needed to perform an MRI is much longer than that needed for most CT scans and is a distinct disadvantage in emergency situations.

Cerebral angiography is the definitive diagnostic tool. Visualization of the cerebral vessels, including carotid and vertebrobasilar, will locate an aneurysm, arteriovenous malformation, thrombosis, ulcerated plaques, vascular narrowing, or vasospasm. Angiography is not without risk to the patient. When or when not to do it is a critical decision made by the physician.

With the advent of CT, MRI, and digital subtraction angiography, lumbar punctures (LPs) are performed rarely as part of a stroke diagnostic workup. If an LP is to be performed, a CT scan should precede it in order to identify the patient with a mass lesion and increased ICP, because withdrawal of small amounts of CSF and sudden release of ICP may result in herniation. The other major contraindication to LP is documented or suspected coagulopathy, which increases the risk of epidural or subdural hemorrhage with cord compression and paralysis (Marshall et al. 1990).

Noninvasive blood flow studies such as carotid Doppler imaging, carotid phonoangiography, and oculoplethysmography are also used to diagnose disease in the extracranial vessels. Early recognition of lesions in the carotids can guide therapy and may prevent a stroke from occurring.

Management of Stroke

Medical Management The main goal in the acute phase of stroke is to preserve viable brain tissue. Attention to the airway, breathing, and circulation is imperative. Measures to prevent hypoxemia and hypercarbia are crucial. Antihypertensive medications to control the blood pressure may be indicated. Since hypotension may lead to inadequate cerebral perfusion and cause ischemia, the blood pressure should be optimized for the individual. Hyperosmolar drugs and steroids are administered to combat edema and the resultant increased intracranial pressure. Maintenance of hemodynamic stability, adequate circulating volume, and normal fluid balance may be accomplished by administering lactated Ringer's, normal saline or other isotonic solutions. The use of hypotonic solutions, such as 5% dextrose in water, is contraindicated because they will cause water to move passively into the brain (Marshall et al. 1990).

Anticoagulant and antiplatelet aggregation therapy is controversial. It is beneficial in treating patients with TIAs to reduce the risk of further TIAs and subsequent stroke. Obviously, anticoagulant therapy is contraindicated in hemorrhagic stroke. Therefore, the challenge faced by the physician is to accurately diagnose the type of stroke. The treatment of stroke caused by emboli should also be directed at the causative factor. Patients who have mitral stenosis and atrial fibrillation or a prosthetic mechanical heart valve should be placed on anticoagulant therapy.

Research is currently being conducted to determine if cerebral infarction size following a thromboembolic stroke may be reduced by administration of tissue plasminogen activator (t-PA), a fibrinolytic agent. Rabbit model research suggests that t-PA may be efficacious in restoring cerebral blood flow and thus limiting infarction size in acute thromboembolic strokes (Bednar et al. 1990). The National Institute for Neurological Disorders and Stroke is evaluating the use of t-PA in human stroke patients (Dyken 1990). Additional research needs to be conducted to determine the efficacy of t-PA in humans following embolic stroke.

Another experimental drug being investigated for stroke intervention is Arvin (Ancrod), a purified protein factor in the venom of the Malayan pit viper (Jahnke 1991). Currently, a multicenter study to evaluate Arvin is being conducted in 20 major medical centers in the United States. Arvin appears to effectively reduce circulating fibrogen and blood viscosity, and thereby promote a hemodilutional state. If the results of this clinical trial prove favorable, the morbidity and mortality rates of acute ischemic strokes may be significantly reduced. In the meantime, preventive measures, such as control of blood pressure and reduction of cholesterol and lipoprotein levels, and early intervention appear to be the keys in reducing the incidence of stroke.

Seizures frequently occur with thrombotic occlusive stroke. Anticonvulsive drugs may be employed prophylactically or when a seizure occurs.

Surgical Management

Carotid Endarterectomy Carotid endarterectomy is the surgical removal of atheromatous plaque obstructing the carotid artery. It is done to prevent embolization and distal occlusion of a cerebral artery. It is best viewed as preventive surgery for impending thrombotic stroke, done before significant neurologic loss. Carotid endarterectomy is indicated if the patient is symptomatic, has significant obstruction of the carotid artery, or has ulcerated plaque. Nursing care of the carotid endarterectomy patient is presented in Chapter 6.

Craniotomy Surgical clipping of an aneurysm, if approachable, is the definitive treatment modality for impending hemorrhagic stroke from an intracranial aneurysm. The operating microscope and improved anesthetic techniques have greatly assisted the surgeon in reducing operative mortality. The operative procedure involves exposing the aneurysm. Then, while using controlled hypotension, the surgeon applies a self-closing spring clip to the neck of the aneurysm. Aneurysms that cannot be clipped may be wrapped with a gauze material and coated with an acrylic substance.

Postoperative nursing care is similar to that for any patient after craniotomy. For specifics, the reader is referred to the section on craniotomy in Chapter 6. Of major concern is neurologic deterioration due to vasospasm. Early recognition and reporting of decreasing LOC or focal deficits optimizes time for discovering the cause and instituting treatment.

The timing of surgery is controversial. Proponents of early surgery, that is, within 48–72 hours of rupture, argue that it: (1) prevents rebleed; (2) allows for removal of extravasated blood from the subarachnoid space, thereby minimizing vasospasm; (3) allows for hypertensive/hypervolemic treatment of vasospasm if it occurs; and (4) reduces the risk of medical complications that occur while waiting for surgery (Manifold 1990).

Planning and Implementation of Care

Stroke patients may present with minimal to severe neurologic dysfunction. Their actual or high-risk problems range from impaired airway and blood pressure control to sensory-perceptual alterations. Many of the nursing diagnoses discussed in the section on increased intracranial pressure relate to the stroke patient, so they will not be repeated here. Instead we will focus on some of the deficits that interfere with the patient's ability to perceive sensory information, communicate, or be physically active.

A sample nursing care plan addressing the specific needs of the patient with ruptured cerebral aneurysm is found on p. 116.

Sensory-Perceptual Alteration Related to Cerebral Insult Although sensory-perceptual deficits may occur when either hemisphere is involved, they are more pronounced in the patient with a right hemisphere stroke. The right cerebral hemisphere is developed for visual/spatial perception, appreciation of nonverbal information, and music appreciation. Assess the patient's ability to: recognize objects in both visual fields; orient self in space; identify objects by sight, sound, or touch; identify sensations of pain, touch, and temperature; recognize own body parts; and distinguish right from left.

Visual field deficits may occur with right or left hemispheric stroke. Stroke involving the right or left middle cerebral artery may result in *homonymous hemianopia,* the loss of vision in one half of the visual field in each eye, contralateral (opposite) to the lesion. Patients with visual field deficits should be reminded to scan their environment. Place commonly used items on the unaffected side. Approach the patient from the unaffected side and remind them to turn their head to compensate for visual deficits. Impaired sensory interpretation may be handled by presenting the patient with various items to touch while you name them.

Right hemisphere damage may result in left hemiplegia, left hemianopsia, ataxia, and poor judgment. Sensory-perceptual deficits specific to right hemispheric damage include poor abstract thinking, spatial-perceptual deficits, difficulty with bodily perception

---

NURSING DIAGNOSES

The following nursing diagnoses may be utilized to guide patient care for strokes.

- Ineffective airway clearance
- Fluid volume deficit
- Ineffective breathing pattern
- Impaired gas exchange
- Altered cerebral perfusion
- Pain
- Sensory-perceptual alteration
- Impaired verbal communication
- Impaired physical mobility

SAMPLE NURSING CARE PLAN

Ruptured Cerebral Aneurysm, Acute Phase

NURSING DIAGNOSIS	SIGNS AND SYMPTOMS	NURSING ACTIONS	DESIRED OUTCOMES

Altered cerebral perfusion related to:
• Ruptured aneurysm
• Increased intracranial pressure
• Cerebral edema
• Vasospasm
• Hydrocephalus
	• Abnormal respiratory pattern:
	  - Cheyne-Stokes
	  - Central hyperventilation
	  - Apneustic
	  - Cluster
	  - Ataxic
	• Elevated P_{CO_2}
	• Decreased P_{O_2}
	• Increased blood pressure
	• Neurologic deficits
	  - Decreased LOC
	  - Confusion
	  - Agitation
	  - Cranial nerve palsies
	  - Pupil changes
	  - Paresis or paralysis
	  - Abnormal flexion or extension of extremities
	  - Seizure
	• Rhythm and ECG changes
	• Hyperthermia
		1. Establish airway and assess respiratory pattern.
		2. Administer oxygen.
		3. Obtain ABGs.
		4. Monitor vital signs and perform neurologic checks.
		5. Provide for complete bedrest in quiet, nonstimulating environment.
		6. Administer drugs as ordered:
		  • Antihypertensives
		  • Hyperosmolar agents
		  • Steroids
		  • Diuretics (usually Lasix)
		  • Aminocaproic acid
		  • Analgesics
		  • Sedatives
		  • Stool softeners
		  • Laxatives
		7. Notify physician immediately of new or worsening neurologic deficits.
		8. Implement continuous ECG monitoring.
		9. Administer antidysrhythmics as ordered.
		10. Monitor temperature.
		11. Control temperature with antipyretics and/or hypothermia blanket.
		12. Institute seizure precautions.
		13. Administer anticonvulsants as ordered.
			• Normal respiratory pattern
			• ABGs WNL for patient
			• Systolic blood pressure WNL for patient
			• Absence of neurological deterioration
			• Compliance with restricted activities
			• Normal cardiac rhythm
			• Afebrile
			• Absence of seizure activity

Pain: headache related to cerebral hemorrhage; stiff neck and pain in neck related to meningeal irritation	• C/o headache and neck pain • Limited movement, and pain on neck flexion	1. Assess headache for severity and location. 2. Administer analgesics as ordered. 3. Evaluate response to analgesics. 4. Avoid undue neck and head movement. 5. Support head when turning.	Verbalizes relief of headache and minimal neck discomfort.
Pain: photophobia related to meningeal irritation	• C/o discomfort with bright light • Keeps eyes closed	1. Minimize direct lighting; pull curtains or shades. 2. Limit time taken assessing pupils so as not to prolong direct light in the eye. 3. Provide nightshades if patient desires.	Verbalizes less discomfort.

and orientation in space, emotional lability, and short attention span. As a result, these patients tend to be quick and impulsive, exhibit poor judgment, become lost easily, and forget the sequence of steps in a task. Often they are unaware of these deficits and deny they exist.

Left hemispheric strokes may result in right hemiplegia, right hemianopsia, and aphasias (expressive, receptive or global). These patients tend to be slow, cautious, and disorganized. Furthermore, depression, which may significantly affect these patients' health status as well as their rehabilitation, has been found in almost half of this population (Bronstein 1991).

Strategies for coping with sensory-perceptual alterations in the stroke patient include speaking clearly in simple, short sentences and using verbal clues to enhance the patient's understanding. Divide tasks into simple steps, elicit return demonstration of skills, arrange for rest periods, and provide emotional support to the patient and family. For the patient with right hemispheric damage, remind the patient about neglected body parts, help him or her to recognize body position, and distinguish right from left.

Impaired Verbal Communication Related to Cerebral Injury Language is a highly integrated function that involves multiple areas of the brain. The primary centers that control speech are located in the left cerebral hemisphere. *Fluent or receptive aphasia,* a disturbance in Wernicke's area, is a condition in which the patient lacks comprehension of the spoken word and may paraphrase, invent new words, or repeat words over and over. The patient's speech is "fluent" but not related to the conversation. *Nonfluent or expressive aphasia* results from an insult to Broca's area. Comprehension of the spoken word is usually intact, but there is an inability to verbalize. *Dysarthria* is the inability to articulate and phonate due to the primary loss of neuromuscular control of speech. Speech may be slurred and thick or jerky and irregular.

To evaluate the extent of language dysfunction, assess the patient's ability to understand yes/no questions, follow simple verbal directions, follow visual cues, name objects, repeat words, and understand the written word. Most important, take time to listen to the patient and allow aphasic patients sufficient time to process what is being asked and attempt to respond. The speech pathologist is a key person to assist you in communicating effectively with the patient.

Slowed thinking, disorganization, and aphasias characterize the verbal communication of patients with *left hemisphere damage.* Remember to speak slowly, avoid shouting, keep verbal instructions simple and concise,

and use gestures, nonverbal cues, and pantomime. Promote language stimulation by naming objects in the environment and encouraging the patient to repeat the names. Provide ample time for the completion of tasks such as daily hygiene, feeding oneself, and assisted ambulation (Doolittle 1991).

Verbal rambling and use of excessive detail characterize the speech of a patient with *right hemisphere damage.* In addition, such patients may have difficulty interpreting non-verbal communication, such as facial expressions and gestures. Speak slowly and clearly and minimize the use of facial expressions, gestures, and other non-verbal clues.

Impaired Physical Mobility Related to Damage to Motor Pathways Strokes involving the motor cortex or internal capsule will produce contralateral hemiparesis or hemiplegia. Arm involvement is usually greater than leg involvement. Flaccid paralysis may be evident at first. Since the stroke causes an upper motor neuron lesion, reflexes will reappear. Spasticity then becomes a problem. Prevention of contractures and loss of muscle tone is key in rehabilitating the patient to an independent lifestyle.

The affected extremities should be passively exercised and put through their full range of motion. This activity is the responsibility of not only the physical therapist but the nurse as well. The patient and family should be taught early, since exercising will need to be continued in the home setting. Patients should be taught how to use the stronger extremity to move the weaker. Remind patients to look at their weak extremities and get them in position before moving. Also, instruct patients to maintain their weight on the stronger side while pivoting. Caring for the stroke patient is a challenge, and rehabilitation starts on admission. Multifaceted nursing care can improve the emotional, social, and physiological well-being of this unique patient.

Outcome Evaluation

Evaluate the patient's progress according to these outcome criteria:

- Expresses needs/feelings.
- Understands and follows direction.
- Recognizes body parts.
- Knows left from right.
- Assists with acts of daily living (ADLs).
- Has motor function that is the same or improved.
- Assists with exercising of extremities.

- Utilizes adaptive equipment for ADLs and mobility.
- Regains sense of control.

AUTOIMMUNE DISORDERS

Autoimmune diseases currently are in the forefront of medical research. Several neurologic diseases have autoimmune components, but Guillain-Barré syndrome and myasthenia gravis are the ones most often encountered in the critical-care unit.

Guillain-Barré Syndrome

Guillain-Barré syndrome is a disease of the peripheral nervous system typically characterized by an acute, rapidly progressing, ascending, symmetric motor weakness with associated sensory disturbances. The disease is 90–100% reversible (Alter 1990). Spontaneous recovery may occur within one to several months or can take up to a year or more depending on the extent of nerve involvement. Severity varies widely. If the diaphragm becomes involved, the disease can be life-threatening.

Assessment

Risk Conditions   Guillain-Barré syndrome can occur at any age and is nonspecific to gender, race, season, or environment. It is the most common cause of acute weakness in people under age 40 and occurs at the rate of 1.5 per 100,000 population (Morgan 1991). The syndrome is more severe in pregnancy and in the young and the elderly (Kneisl and Ames 1986). In most cases, viral illness commonly associated with the respiratory or gastrointestinal tract precedes the syndrome by 2–3 weeks (Nikas 1991). Less common preceding problems are immunization (swine flu vaccine in 1977), animal bites, and surgery. Guillain-Barré also may occur during the course of lymphoma or systemic lupus erythematosus (Jones 1985). Prompt recognition and intervention has kept the mortality rate at 1.5% (Alter 1990). Mortality is usually due to complications from pulmonary or urinary infections and sepsis.

In order to comprehend the progression of Guillain-Barré, one needs to understand normal nerve conduc-

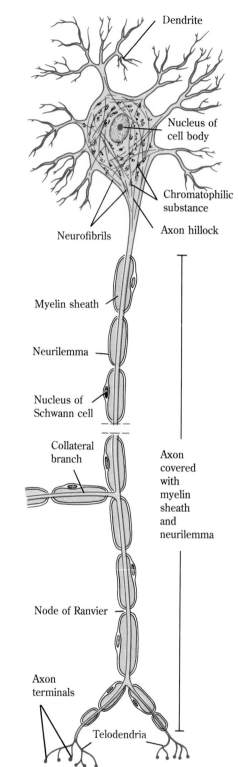

FIGURE 5–8

Structure of a typical motor neuron. (From Spence A: *Basic human anatomy,* 2d ed. Redwood City, CA: Benjamin/Cummings, 1990, p. 356.)

tion. The peripheral nerve has an axon enveloped by a myelin sheath produced by the Schwann cell (Figure 5–8). Motor and proprioceptive sensory nerves are the most heavily myelinated, with the myelin sheath proportional to the nerve diameter (Griswold and Ropper 1984). The sheath insulates the nerve fiber and limits ion exchanges or impulse conduction along the axon (Guyton 1991). A break in the sheath occurs approximately every millimeter. These nonmyelinated areas, called *nodes of Ranvier,* allow impulses to "jump" along the sheath, resulting in faster impulse conduction than nerve fiber or myelin sheath conduction. This saltatory (leaping) conduction, jumping along the gaps, also conserves energy by making impulse conduction possible with less ion shifts at the cell membrane (Guyton 1991).

Diffuse, intense inflammation and demyelination of the peripheral nerves at any level between the nerve's root and distal end is the reason for the progressive muscle weakness. Segmental destruction of myelin between the nodes of Ranvier without axonal destruction is the typical pattern, but secondary axonal damage does occur in severe cases (Pfister and Bullas 1990). The exact mechanism causing the demyelination is unknown, although an autoimmune attack on the myelin sheath is most likely. A cellular immune response may stimulate macrophages and lymphocytes to destroy the myelin or a humoral immune response may produce demyelinating antibodies that destroy it (Ropper and Kennedy 1988). Termination of the inflammatory reaction allows remyelination and reinsulation of the peripheral nerve to occur. When peripheral remyelination is complete, normal neurologic function should return. However, if the inflammatory process damages the axon, remyelination does not take place, the nerve dies, and neurologic dysfunction persists.

Signs and Symptoms   Signs and symptoms reflect the extent of demyelination of peripheral nerves. Motor, sensory, and autonomic nerves are involved. Typically, symmetric weakness, numbness, and tingling begin in the legs and quickly ascend to the trunk and arms, resulting in a generalized limb weakness usually accompanied by areflexia. It is important to note that symptoms can vary and life-threatening symptomatology, especially if the phrenic or intercostal nerves innervating the muscles of respiration are involved, may occur. Many patients complain of deep muscle pain, maddening paresthesias, and skin hypersensitivity. Two-thirds of the patients experience distal paresthesia in a "glove and stocking" pattern (Jones 1985). Since the cranial nerves are part of the peripheral nervous system, facial weakness, dysphagia, dysarthria, and diplopia may occur. Autonomic nerve involvement produces fluctuating pulse rates, labile blood pressures, and diaphoresis (Morgan 1991).

Although all of these symptoms are distressing to the patient, Guillain-Barré is not life-threatening unless dysphagia is present or until the respiratory musculature becomes involved. Serial pulmonary function tests (PFTs) show a gradual or sometimes sudden drop in values for spontaneous and forced vital capacity, inspiratory force, and spontaneous tidal volume. The risks of a precipitous drop in ventilation and labile autonomic function necessitate close monitoring.

Recovery from Guillain-Barré syndrome is spontaneous, and the typical pattern is descending or opposite the pattern of function loss. The extent of underlying axonal damage determines the extent and length of the recovery phase. Typically, deterioration stops within 3 weeks after symptoms onset and then plateaus for several days to weeks before improvements are noted. Full recovery, which correlates with remyelination and axonal regeneration, usually takes a few months but, if damage is extensive, can take up to 18 months (Wechsler and Ropper 1989).

Diagnostic Procedures   Since there is no one cause for Guillain-Barré syndrome, there is no specific test to identify it. Clinical signs and health history are the most important factors. An elevated cerebrospinal fluid protein level with normal cell counts and pressure is common in the first 10 days (Ropper and Kennedy 1988).

Nerve conduction studies permit disorders of peripheral nerves to be distinguished from myopathic and other neuropathic processes. Electrophysiologic studies may reveal marked slowing of motor and sensory conduction velocity (Simon et al. 1989). However, this testing does not correlate well with the severity of clinical symptoms and does not reflect the degree of underlying neuronal damage (Simon et al. 1989). If EMG findings are close to normal, the recovery tends to be quick.

Planning and Implementation of Care

Ineffective Airway Clearance Related to Respiratory Muscle Weakness or Cranial Nerve Involvement   The patient will be unable to clear the respiratory tract effectively if ascending muscle weakness affects the respiratory muscles or cranial nerves 9 and 10 are involved. Inadequate mucociliary clearance, pooling of oral secretions, and retention of secretions in the lung result from an ineffective cough or gag mechanism. Close monitoring for signs of mucus accumulation is necessary to prevent hypoxia, atelectasis, and pneu-

NURSING DIAGNOSES

Because Guillain-Barré syndrome can be life-threatening when respiratory muscles are involved, sophisticated nursing management with prompt effective nursing interventions can be life-saving. Pertinent nursing diagnoses for Guillain-Barré syndrome patients include:

- Ineffective airway clearance
- Ineffective breathing pattern
- Altered nutrition: less than body requirements
- Impaired verbal communication
- Impaired physical mobility
- Impaired skin integrity
- High risk for infection
- High risk for injury to peripheral muscles and nerves
- Pain
- Bowel and bladder dysfunction (altered bowel elimination: incontinence; altered bowel elimination: constipation; total (urinary) incontinence; urinary retention)
- Anxiety, fear, powerlessness
- Ineffective family coping

monia. Listen frequently to breath sounds (anteriorly, laterally, and posteriorly) for signs of compromised air exchange. Suction with aseptic technique to remove secretions when necessary. Encourage deep breathing, holding inspiration, and coughing to prevent atelectasis (George 1988). Keep the physician informed of airway patency, and anticipate intubation if the patient is unable to clear secretions.

Ineffective Breathing Pattern Related to Respiratory Muscle Weakness As mentioned above, vital capacity can drop precipitously. Hypotonia, shallow respirations, mucous plugs, atelectasis, and local consolidation may contribute to neuromuscular respiratory failure (George 1988). Monitor lung sounds, chest excursion, respiratory muscle activity, and ease of breathing at least every 2 hours (more frequently if changes occur). Perform serial PFTs every 2 hours, and as needed for any change. Be alert to the signs of respiratory failure for example, confusion, disorientation, tachycardia, dyspnea; see Chapter 8 for further details. Position the patient for maximal lung expansion: upright, semi-Fowler's, or side positioned with the upper arm off the chest.

Remember, respiratory dysfunction can be either gradual or sudden in these patients. Anticipate intubation when pulmonary function values begin dropping, especially in pregnancy. Also remember that early controlled intubation is less traumatic to the patient than late emergent intubation. Alert the physician to any change in respiratory status.

Altered Nutrition: Less than Body Requirements Related to Impaired Swallowing Adequate intake of essential amino acids, fats, and carbohydrates is mandatory for recovery but can be difficult if the patient suffers from dysphagia. Be aware of the patient's fluid and nutritional status, and notify the physician early of potential needs. This is especially important with severe Guillain-Barré syndrome, which produces neuromuscular dysfunction for several months.

Monitor the swallowing function. Position the patient on his or her side when resting and upright during eating to prevent aspiration. To minimize choking, encourage soft foods and thick liquids. Monitor the fluid status of patients with low oral intake. Assess gastrointestinal function daily. If the patient is unable to eat without choking, anticipate enteral feeding to maintain adequate nutrition and gastrointestinal function. Remember, large feeding tubes are associated with a higher incidence of aspiration. Anticipate total parenteral nutrition therapy when gastrointestinal dysfunction is present.

Impaired Verbal Communication Related to Poor Neuromuscular Transmission When the cranial nerves are involved, the patient may lose the ability to speak, blink the eyes, or move the head to communicate with staff. Effective communication concerning likes, dislikes, comfort positions, effective interventions for pain, and so on *before* the patient becomes uncommunicative will promote consistent, individualized care. If the patient is unable to communicate when admitted to critical care, talk to the family and/or friends to obtain this information. Patients will still be frustrated but may be comforted by the nurses' attempts to make them comfortable.

Set aside time for communication. As the patient recovers partial motor ability, different levels of communication can be established, such as blinking the eyes, squeezing the hands, moving the toes, or using an alphabet board or word list. Use gestures, verbal clues, facial expressions, and posturing to supplement verbal communication. The patient may develop a unique communication style using whatever gross motor movements he or she possesses. Place a soft-pressure-activated nurse call bell within the patient's limited reach for easy notification.

Explain all procedures to the patient before starting. Repeatedly orient the patient to the time of day, the week, the month, and so on. Use television or radio to keep the patient updated on current events. Encourage the family to talk with the patient about everyday family happenings to promote a sense of belonging.

Impaired Physical Mobility Related to Generalized Muscle Weakness Assess motor functions on admission and every shift change thereafter to evaluate the progression of the syndrome. When motor abilities are deteriorating, check motor strength more frequently as needed. Do passive range of motion exercises to maintain joint function and prevent contractures. Reposition every 2 hours or more frequently to prevent pneumonia, skin breakdown, and pressure to peripheral nerves. Monitor extraocular muscle function and suggest eye care to the physician when needed. Rotate an eye patch if such is used to treat diplopia. Explore the use of prism glasses to see if vision can be improved.

Impaired Skin Integrity Related to Multiple Factors Loss of mobility, poor nutrition, and inability to communicate physical needs all can lead to skin problems. Timely, proficient cleansing during daily bathing and after incontinence is necessary to prevent skin breakdown. Oral hygiene, skin massage, use of specialized mattresses to decrease pressure areas, and joint protectors are only a few of the interventions available. Hair washing will not only maintain skin integrity but also promote psychologic well-being in the patient. If antiembolic stockings are ordered, remove them every 8 hours for at least 30 minutes.

High Risk for Infection Related to Multiple Factors Immobility, inadequate nutrition, sequestering of pulmonary secretions, dysphagia with aspiration, steroid therapy, skin breakdown, bowel and bladder dysfunction, and numerous invasive lines are some of the potential causes of infection in Guillain-Barré patients. Monitor closely for signs of local infection from any invasive line. Change invasive lines according to unit protocol. Maintain circulation to the skin and extremities to prevent local hypoxia, tissue destruction, and subsequent opportunistic infection. Observe all drainage from the skin, orifices, and tubes for color or odor changes that suggest infection. Obtain specimens for culture per unit protocol or physician's orders. Evaluate vital signs and general progress for subtle signs of systemic infection. Investigate any areas of tenderness. Notify the physician of any suspicion of infection.

High Risk for Injury to Peripheral Muscles and Nerves Related to Immobility and Communication Deficits Range of motion exercises are performed to maintain joint mobility, and frequent repositioning is done to prevent numerous problems. If either of these procedures is done incorrectly, the peripheral muscles and nerves may be damaged. During the acute phase of Guillain-Barré syndrome, avoid active range of motion exercises and overzealously done passive exercises, because they can stretch the muscles and tendons, causing damage and prolonging recovery. Damage may also occur while turning the patient with inadequate support to the extremities. Also, active range of motion exercises overzealously done by the recovering patient may tire his or her muscles, prolong recovery, and lead to frustration and depression from perceived "poor progress."

Peripheral nerve damage can prolong recovery periods or cause the permanent loss of function in the affected extremity. Throughout hospitalization, care must be taken to avoid excessive pressure on extremities and joints. This is especially important when the patient is unable to communicate. Using pillows or foam pads to decrease pressure and splints to maintain proper alignment is common.

As activity increases, exercise care when first sitting the patient upright. Postural hypotension may be a problem, especially in patients with autonomic dysfunction. Avoid back-muscle injury from premature chair-sitting with weakened muscles.

Pain Related to Sensory Nerve Dysfunction Hypersensitivity of the skin and deep muscle aches are common in the arms, legs, back, and buttocks. Bathing and repositioning become a real challenge because even gentle touch can cause pain. Remember, the paralyzed patient may be unable to communicate the extent of that pain. Mild analgesic agents are usually adequate for pain control.

Altered Bowel Elimination and Altered Urinary Elimination Related to Autonomic Nervous System Dysfunction Autonomic nervous system dysfunction increases the risks of bowel or bladder incontinence in the acute stage, and bladder distention or bowel impaction during the recovery phase. Monitor bowel and bladder function closely. Assess frequently for incontinence, and cleanse the skin thoroughly after incontinence. Insert an indwelling catheter per physician's orders in the acute phase. Anticipate bowel and bladder training once the acute phase is over.

Anxiety, Fear, Powerlessness Related to Sudden Onset of Debilitating Disease The very nature of a sudden, progressive loss of motor function, inadequate breathing, and communication disability leads to feelings of fear, anxiety, and powerlessness. The fact that no health care provider can quantify the extent of disease or length of recovery only magnifies these feelings. Closely monitor the patient during the acute stage not only for signs of disease progress but also to decrease the patient's anxiety and fear of abandonment. Communicating about normal living activities and keeping the patient advised of current events will promote interest outside the self, thereby helping to distract the patient from anxiety and fear.

As paralysis spreads, the patient's feelings of powerlessness increase. Allowing the patient as much control over daily activities as possible will counteract such feelings. Listen to the patient, encourage verbalization of feelings, and offer moral support. Acknowledge improvements and emphasize that function will return with time and physical therapy.

Ineffective Family Coping Related to Sudden Debilitating Disease   The patient's family usually is shocked by the sudden, progressive loss of function in their loved one. Active listening, close monitoring, and emphasizing the expected regain of function should help. If the patient is the main source of income for the family, financial worries may produce feelings of frustration, possibly manifested as anger toward the health care providers for not making the patient better faster. The family life of patients undergoing prolonged recovery is significantly disrupted. Active listening to the family will alert the nurse to problems that may need intervention. Collaboration with the physician and social worker about immediate and long-term needs early in the patient's hospitalization will promote open communication and trust.

Most of the treatment for Guillain-Barré syndrome is supportive and symptomatic. Thus, the nurse and physician plan the patient's care with the goals of recognizing problems early, preventing potential problems, and minimizing the impact of the symptoms.

Some therapies are controversial. Steroids have been used, but studies have shown that these agents may affect the outcome adversely and even increase the time necessary for recovery (Simon et al. 1989; Jones 1985; Miller 1985). Plasmapheresis has been used during the acute phase, with some dramatic

---

NURSING TIP

Assessing the Guillain-Barré Patient

To diminish anxiety in the patient undergoing prolonged recovery, perform daily neurologic checks with the physician, thereby decreasing the number of times per day that the patient is reminded of motor deficits.

---

improvements noted, especially in those with rapidly advancing deficits or respiratory difficulty (Simon et al. 1989).

Outcome Evaluation

Desirable outcome criteria for Guillain-Barré syndrome patients are:

- Return to previous level of sensorimotor function.
- Vital signs within normal limits for the patient.
- Verbalization of fears and anxiety.
- Prevention of complications during disease process.

Myasthenia Gravis

Myasthenia gravis is a progressive, debilitating autoimmune disease involving the postsynaptic membrane of the myoneural junction. The disease is characterized by intermittent, abnormal skeletal muscle fatigue that increases with activity and partially reverses with rest. The occurrence of a crisis is the usual reason for admission to critical care. During crisis, the patient is unable to breathe due to either inadequate neuromuscular transmissions (myasthenic crisis) or to overstimulation by neuromuscular transmitters and resultant muscle fatigue (cholinergic crisis). Without immediate intervention, the patient will die of respiratory failure.

Assessment

Risk Conditions   Myasthenia gravis can strike a person of any age or gender, although two-thirds of stricken women are under 40 and two-thirds of stricken men are over 40 (Herrmann 1985). No specific genetic link has been found, but familial frequency has been noted (Herrmann 1985). No racial or geographic determinants have been discovered (Seybold 1986). Myasthenia is limited to ocular muscles only in approximately 20% of patients, but in the majority, bulbar and extremity muscles become involved either initially or as the disease progresses (Wechsler and Ropper 1989). (Bulbar muscles are those of the face, neck, mastication, and articulation.) Approximately 50% of patients will develop moderate or severe generalized disease and at some time will need ICU care (Wechsler and Ropper 1989). Factors precipitating the onset or exacerbation of the disease include heat, emotional stress, initiation of corticosteroid therapy, infection, surgery, menses, pregnancy, thyrotoxicosis, inadequate medication, and overmedication.

Signs and Symptoms Normally the myelinated nerve branches stimulate muscle fibers by releasing neurotransmittors across the neuromuscular junction (Figure 5–9). The terminal end of the nerve on a skeletal muscle is called the *end-plate*. This end-plate burrows into the muscle fiber, creating a synaptic trough and cleft, the space between the nerve and muscle. The excitatory neurotransmitter acetylcholine is released from the nerve's terminal vesicles into the synaptic cleft and stimulates the muscle fiber membrane at specific receptor sites (Guyton 1991). These receptor sites surround ion-specific channels that open and allow the influx of sodium and calcium ions to enter the muscle and cause depolarization. Acetylcholine is then rapidly destroyed by acetylcholinesterase to prevent further muscle depolarization (Guyton 1991). The acetylcholine receptor sites are regularly removed by endocytosis every 6–13 days and replaced with new receptor sites (Seybold 1986).

Antibodies to acetylcholine receptors have been found in 60–90% of myasthenics, indicating an autoimmune mechanism. These antibodies destroy acetylcholine receptor sites more rapidly than they are replaced. Binding of antibodies to receptor sites on the muscle end-plate results in a blockage and increased degradation of acetylcholine receptor sites and prevents complete depolarization of the muscle. Prevention of normal binding or opening of the ion channel results in depletion of acetylcholine, and neurotransmission is unsuccessful. Repetitive muscle stimulation produces depletion of acetylcholine, progressive decline of muscle action potentials, and neuromuscular fatigue and weakness (Engle 1981; Noroian 1986). Weakness appears to be proportional to the amount of receptor site loss (Seybold 1986).

Onset of symptoms may be sudden or gradual, and their severity varies during the day and from day to day. There are several classifications (Table 5–5), since the course of the disease is unpredictable and spontaneous remissions do occur. It may begin with ocular symptoms and may or may not progress to generalized weakness; or the disease may manifest itself with generalized weakness of mild to moderate severity. Neurologic deficits such as sensory loss, coordination problems, and abnormal reflexes

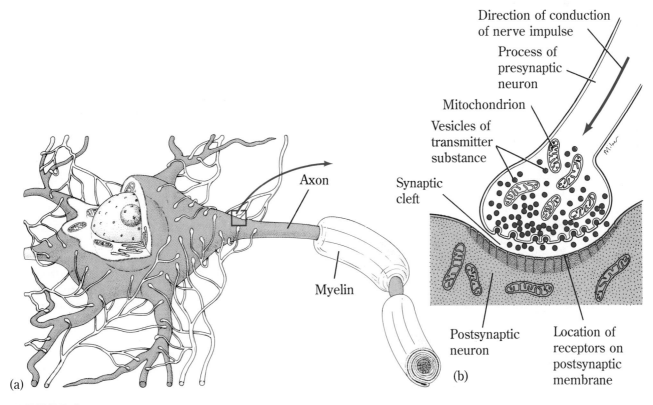

FIGURE 5–9

Synapses between neurons. **a,** Axons of several neurons synapsing with the dendrites and cell body of a neuron; **b,** a single synapse at higher magnification. (From Spence A: *Basic human anatomy,* 3d ed. Redwood City, CA: Benjamin/Cummings, 1990, p. 360.)

TABLE 5–5

Classifications of Myasthenia Gravis

TYPE	CHARACTERISTICS
Ocular	• Cranial nerves III, IV, VI involvement • Only extraocular movements affected • Visual disturbances
Generalized	
Mild	• General muscle involvement • No respiratory involvement • Slow onset
Moderate	• General muscle involvement • Bulbar* and respiratory involvement • Gradual onset
Acute fulminating	• Severe bulbar involvement • Early respiratory involvement • General muscle involvement • Rapid onset

*Bulbar = swallowing and respiratory muscle involvement.

NURSING TIP

Nursing Priorities in the Myasthenic Patient in Crisis

Crisis is characterized by severe muscle weakness that interferes with the patient's ability to maintain a patent airway. This inability may be due to difficulty in clearing secretions, inadequate air exchange, or both. Whether the cause is myasthenic or cholinergic crisis, the initial treatment is the same: maintain a patent airway and support ventilation.

are not associated with myasthenia gravis (Seybold 1986).

The initial symptoms are usually ocular: diplopia and ptosis. Pupillary reaction remains normal (Leahy 1990). Progression is manifested by facial weakness, loss of expression, and a nasal twang to speech. One characteristic may be a snarl when attempting to smile. There is weak chewing and swallowing with nasal regurgitation, which can lead to weight loss or aspiration. Intermittent dyspnea or increases in dyspnea herald respiratory muscle involvement. Involvement of extremity muscles is mostly proximal, but distal involvement is present (George 1988; Noroian 1986). Shoulder girdle weakness is manifested by difficulty in combing hair or shaving. Lower-limb muscle weakness is seen in difficulty in climbing stairs or in rising from a seated position or as sudden falls. There is no associated muscle atrophy or muscular pain. Since stress is the precipitating factor in many cases, a psychiatric diagnosis such as depression, hypochondriasis, or hysteria is not uncommon.

Older patients in a more fragile state of health are more likely to experience crisis than the younger myasthenic patient (Getting 1986). Crisis is also common in summer heat. Other precipitating factors include infections, emotional stress, cardiovascular or pulmonary problems, recent initiation or withdrawal of corticosteroids, drug interactions, alcohol intake, and pregnancy (Jones 1985; Getting 1986).

Myasthenic crisis is caused by insufficient acetylcholine. It occurs in the severe myasthenia patient who is not under treatment, receiving inadequate medica-

tions, or drug resistant, or due to a medication change, infection, or stress. Signs and symptoms may be subtle at first, with no obvious respiratory distress and normal arterial blood gases. Usual signs of respiratory distress such as nasal flaring and accessory muscle use may not be present. Apprehension and insomnia may be the first signs of problems. Eventually chest excursion and air movement will diminish. Dysphagia, dysarthria, dysphonia, and pooled secretions increase the risk of aspiration. Respiratory insufficiency becomes obvious very late, and apnea may be sudden (Kess 1984).

Cholinergic crisis is caused by excessive acetylcholine. This usually results from an overdose of anticholinergic medication or secondary to occasional remissions. Signs of cholinergic overmedication can be muscarinic or nicotinic (Chipps 1991). Muscarinic signs result from smooth muscle stimulation and include excessive pulmonary secretions, diaphoresis and abdominal cramping and diarrhea. Nicotinic signs result from skeletal muscle stimulation and are demonstrated by muscle fasciculations, twitching, and cramps. Thus, except for excessive secretions, abdominal cramps and diarrhea, the weak, dyspneic patient in cholinergic crisis does not look different from the weak, dyspneic patient in myasthenic crisis. It is the physiologic cause that is different and demands different treatment for successful resolution.

Diagnostic Procedures Injection of 2–10 mg edrophonium chloride (Tensilon) is the classic test for myasthenia gravis. It is a short-acting anticholinesterase that blocks the breakdown of acetylcholine. With more acetylcholine to stimulate receptor sites, a transient increase in muscle strength is noted within 1–2 minutes. The test also may be used to differentiate myasthenic from cholinergic crisis. If the patient

NURSING DIAGNOSES

Some of the nursing diagnoses appropriate to myasthenia gravis and the life-threatening nature of crisis include:

- Ineffective airway clearance
- Ineffective breathing pattern
- Impaired verbal communication
- Impaired swallowing
- High risk for infection
- Activity intolerance
- Impaired physical mobility
- Sensory-perceptual alteration: vision
- High risk for injury
- Urinary incontinence
- Bowel incontinence
- Ineffective individual coping
- Knowledge deficit

improves after a cautious injection of Tensilon, a myasthenic crisis is present; if the patient shows no improvement or symptoms worsen, a cholinergic crisis is present (Leahy 1990).

During electromyography, repetitive electrical stimulation of a nerve shows an initial decrease in muscle response by the second stimulation. By the fifth electrical stimulation, this response has fully developed to a drop of 8–10% from the initial muscle response (Jones 1985). Single-fiber electromyography (EMG) measures the time-interval difference between the action potentials of two single, adjacent muscle fibers when their common nerve is stimulated. This difference normally is constant. Variability in the time intervals produces "jitters" on the EMG. The jitters are significantly increased in myoneural junction disorders (Herrmann 1985).

Serum studies show an elevated number of acetylcholine receptor antibodies in myasthenia gravis. They do not correlate with the clinical course and may be normal in some patients (Herrmann 1985; Osterman et al. 1988). Other abnormal serum tests may include sedimentation rates, antinuclear antibodies, thyroid function studies, and creatine phosphokinase.

Planning and Implementation of Care

Treatment of Myasthenia Gravis The treatment of myasthenia is control of symptoms. The patient must understand that no drug will completely restore muscle strength (Kess 1984). Traditionally, control has been accomplished with anticholinesterase medications. Pyridostigmine bromide (Mestinon), neostigmine bromide (Prostigmine), and ambenonium chloride (Mytelase) are those most frequently used (Chipps 1991). Medications must be tailored to the individual patient to control symptoms and prevent cholinergic side effects. When patients are unable to tolerate the cholinergic side effects, atropine is sometimes included. The nurse should be alert to the fact that atropine will mask the symptoms of cholinergic toxicity.

Thymectomy may be performed when conservative drug therapy does not improve the patient's status. Although promoted as a therapeutic measure, thymectomy in patients without thymomas is highly controversial. The rationale is that there is an assumed thymus gland role in antibody formation, and removal of the thymus gland leads to improvement in some patients. In one center a 51% remission rate and a 36% improvement in status was achieved (Mulder et al. 1986; Hatton et al. 1989).

Plasmapheresis, removal of abnormal substances from plasma, has been used for ventilator-dependent patients, for patients in myasthenic crisis and before and after thymectomy to improve the patient's status (Seybold 1986, Chipps 1991). Plasmapheresis may improve symptoms by removing the acetylcholine receptor antibodies that are protein-bound (Leahy 1990). These circulating antibodies are washed from the patient's plasma during the pheresis and temporary improvement can be dramatic (Gracey et al. 1984; Leahy 1990). Frequently, immunosuppressive agents are used adjunctively to prolong the short-term improvement produced by the exchange.

Corticosteroids are used as an adjunct to anticholinesterase medications when the latter have been unsuccessful alone (Seybold 1986; Leahy 1990). In myasthenic patients, steroids have the unique effect of transiently increasing weakness whenever started, increased, or withdrawn (Herrmann 1985). Intensive high-dose therapy versus gradually increased low-dose therapy are currently being debated as the best initial approach. Most authorities agree that maintenance with a moderate dosage every other day for several months followed by a tapered decrease in dosage to a lower level is applicable for all but the most severely ill patients. Due to the risks associated with long-term steroid therapy, patients are gradually tapered off prednisone.

Azathioprine (Imuran), another immunosuppressive agent, has been used in patients unable to take steroids, or in patients with severe or progressive disease despite thymectomy and treatment with anticholinesterases, or as an adjunct to medications (Seybold 1986; Simon et al. 1989). The usual dose is 2–3 mg/kg daily, increased from a lower initial dose (Simon et al. 1989). As with all immunosuppressive therapy, the risk of infection is increased. Other side effects include alopecia and liver toxicity (Seybold 1986). Other therapies utilized less frequently include cyclophosphamide, gamma globulin, antilymphocyte antiserum, and splenic or whole-body radiation (Seybold 1986).

Ineffective Airway Clearance and Breathing Pattern Related to Respiratory Muscle Dysfunction These problems are the reason most myasthenia patients are admitted to critical-care units. Listen to the patient, who is the expert and can warn you of impending crisis. Closely monitor for respiratory insufficiency. Assess lung expansion, pulmonary function, and breath sounds every 2 hours—or more frequently with changing values. Pulmonary secretions are a problem for two reasons. Anticholinesterase drugs increase secretions. Cholinergic crisis further increases secretions, which the patient is unable to clear, since the patient cannot cough and deep breathe. Perform chest physiotherapy and suction audible secretions as needed. Monitor respiratory rate and depth and pulmonary function tests: vital capacity, tidal volume, and inspiratory force. Check vital capacity by having the patient take a deep breath and count for as long as possible before taking another breath. Normally, counting reaches 40 to 50. Assess for subtle signs of muscle weakness, since early signs of respiratory insufficiency may not be present (Noroian 1986). Anticipate a decrease in pulmonary function with the initiation of or withdrawal from steroid therapy. Give anticholinesterase medications on time. Being even 5 minutes late may decrease the blood level, increase muscle weakness, and exacerbate existing pulmonary problems because of rapid drug metabolism (Noroian 1986). Anticipate respiratory arrest, intubation, and mechanical ventilatory support as pulmonary status deteriorates.

Impaired Verbal Communication Related to Poor Neuromuscular Transmission Dysphonia may be an early, subtle sign of impending crisis. Be alert to changes in the patient's speech pattern, which can vary from nasal quality to an imperceptible whisper. Request other staff familiar with the patient to corroborate any suspected changes. Encourage the patient to develop and use an individual means of communication with staff. Detail the communication system in the Kardex for other staff members to use. Allow the patient plenty of time to speak. Talk to the patient, and keep him or her informed of all procedures, plans of action, and current

events. Have the patient use a radio for orientation to current events, since diplopia interferes with reading and with watching television.

Impaired Swallowing Related to Poor Neuromuscular Transmission Dysphagia should alert the nurse to a high risk for aspiration and impending respiratory arrest. Encourage the largest food intake in the morning, to coincide with the normal time of maximal muscle strength. Administer medications 1 hour before meals for best muscle strength. Assist eating by providing mechanically soft foods that require less work to consume. Suggest small amounts of food with frequent rest periods. Be ready to reheat food so it remains appetizing. Encourage liquids to maintain fluid balance. To improve swallowing ability, trigger the swallow reflex with liquids or hot food (Noroian 1986). Keep the patient in a high Fowler's position during meals to reduce the chance of aspiration. If the patient is unable to swallow, suction as needed and/or catch pooled secretions with a towel (change it frequently).

Anticipate use of enteral feeding tubes to maintain nutritional status when oral intake is inadequate. If the patient enters critical care debilitated from previous nutritional deficits, anticipate total parenteral nutrition to prevent muscle wasting and increased potential for infection. Follow standard precautions and unit protocols when using enteral or parenteral feedings.

High Risk for Infection Related to Poor Nutrition, Communication Impairment, Muscle Weakness, Medications, and Invasive Maneuvers Myasthenia gravis patients are bombarded by a multitude of factors that increase their risk of infection. Immunosuppressive agents and steroids are frequently used in the treatment of myasthenia and more recently in the treatment of crisis (Seybold 1986). Recent thymectomy or current plasma exchange also heighten the chance of infection (Noroian 1986). Poor respiratory function and pooled secretions increase the risk of pneumonia. Poor nutrition diminishes the body's normal mechanisms of defense.

Assess the patient, including sites of all invasive lines and any drainage, for signs of infection every 4 hours or more frequently as needed. Alert the physician to any suspicion of infection. Replace all suspicious lines per physician's orders or unit protocol. Use recommended infection control techniques. Use meticulous sterile technique when needed. Reposition the patient every 1–2 hours to prevent skin breakdown and pneumonia.

Activity Intolerance Related to Neuromuscular Dysfunction Schedule the patient's activities to coincide with maximal muscle strength. Plan the heaviest activity in the morning, and allow periodic rest periods. Suggest rest periods for after medication administration. The patient then benefits from the effects of both rest and peak drug effect before engaging in activity. Encourage self-care as much as possible. Assist the fatigued patient. Convey signs of improvement.

Impaired Physical Mobility Related to Neuromuscular Dysfunction During crisis, patients may be either partially or fully paralyzed until their medications are adjusted to their individual needs. Assess motor functions on admission and every shift change thereafter to evaluate progress. When motor abilities are deteriorating, check motor strength more frequently. Do passive range of motion exercises to maintain joint function and prevent contractures. Reposition every 2 hours or more frequently to prevent pneumonia and skin breakdown.

Sensory-Perceptual Alteration (Vision) Related to Neuromuscular and Cranial Nerve Dysfunctions Ocular symptoms are frequently the initial signs of myasthenia gravis. During crisis, patients have ptosis, diminished eye movements, eye deviation, or inability to open the eyes. Assess visual acuity and EOMs. Keep the patient informed of what you are doing. Try experimenting with various methods aimed at restoring the patient's sight. If a patient is unable to open the eyes, tape one eye open while you are present. (Taping both eyes open would result in diplopia.) For the patient who can open the eyes, manage the problem of diplopia with eye patches. Alternate the patch to prevent eye strain. Anticipate use of artificial tears with incomplete lid closure to prevent corneal damage. Use eyeglasses with an eyelid crutch, when available, for patients unable to open their eyes (Noroian 1986).

High Risk for Injury Related to Trauma Assess the patient for skin breakdown or hidden fractures secondary to sudden falls. Anticipate the possible need for support during walking, when increasing activity, or when medications or dosages are changed. Encourage the patient to continue activity. Remind the patient of progress when exhibited.

Urinary Incontinence and Bowel Incontinence Related to Overmedication or Neuromuscular Dysfunction Remember, bowel and bladder incontinence can be signs of cholinergic crisis. Anticipate reduction or discontinuance of anticholinesterase medications. Investigate other causes. Maintain hygiene with immediate, thorough skin cleansing.

Ineffective Individual Coping Related to Acute and/or Chronic Disease Deteriorating pulmonary function is the primary reason for anxiety in crisis patients. Diplopia, dysphonia and dysarthria, misdiagnosis prior to hospitalization, and fear of the unknown could also be causes. Due to facial muscle weakness, the patient does not look anxious. This calm appearance can lead the health care professional to disbelieve the anxious patient. Sensing this disbelief, the patient becomes more anxious. Explain everything you do and plan to do for the patient in a calm, confident manner. Repeated hospitalizations and lifestyle changes also can cause anxiety and feelings of vulnerability. Active listening may clue the nurse into possible interventions.

Myasthenia gravis disrupts a person's normal lifestyle. In crisis, it places the formerly independent person in a position of complete dependence on health care professionals. Assess the patient's psychologic adjustment to the disease. Evaluate whether the patient is in the shock, denial, anger, depression, or acceptance stage. Look for clues such as forgetting to take medication, delaying physician referral until symptoms are severe, or refusing to curtail activity. Having the newly diagnosed myasthenia patient talk with a longer-diagnosed, independent patient could decrease uncertainty and facilitate coping. Adjusting to a new self-image (e.g., expressionless face, scars from surgery, and steroid-induced changes) may take months or years. The nurse can help by directing the patient to supportive outpatient services.

Knowledge Deficit: Disease Process How long the patient has had myasthenia and how well he or she has accepted the diagnosis will determine how much teaching the nurse needs to do. Remember, the patient must at least partially accept the reality of lifestyle changes before teaching can be effective. Including the family or close friends in such teaching is important, because it promotes the family unit, keeps the patient from feeling alone, and is a more efficient use of teaching time. Discuss the signs and symptoms of myasthenic and cholinergic crisis, medication side effects and potential interactions, precipitating factors, and emergency procedures. Practical information on coughing and deep breathing exercises, sighing, chest physiotherapy, suctioning, circumventing swallowing problems, and the care of feeding tubes or tracheostomy will help the patient and family cope with the problems of chronic illness.

Supply written material for future reference. In fact, reading about the disease may be the patient's first step toward acceptance. Stress the need to wear a medic-alert tag to speed emergency care. Encourage the patient and family to contact the Myasthenia Gravis Foundation.

Outcome Evaluation

Outcome criteria appropriate for the patient with myasthenia gravis include:

- Ability to clear airway and maintain normal breathing.
- Normal communication abilities.
- Adequate nutritional status.
- Lack of infection.
- Established schedule to maintain self-care with minimal muscle fatigue.
- Near-normal mobility.
- Regain of visual acuity with or without supportive devices.
- Return of normal bowel and bladder function.
- Diminished anxiety and improved coping mechanisms.
- Knowledge of disease, medications, and available support.

REFERENCES

Adams J et al.: Intracranial operation within several days of aneurysmal subarachnoid hemorrhage: Results in 150 patients. *Arch Neurol* 1988; 45:1065–1069.

Alter M: The epidemiology of Guillain-Barré syndrome. *Ann Neurol* 1990; 27 (supp):S7–12.

Bednar M et al.: Tissue plasma activator reduces brain injury in a rabbit model of thromboembolic stroke. *Stroke* 1990; 21(12):1705–1709.

Boortz-Marx R: Factors affecting intracranial pressure: A descriptive study. *Neurosurg Nurs* 1985; 17(2):89–94.

Cammermeyer M, Appeldorn C (eds): *American Association of Neuroscience Nurses core curriculum for neuroscience nursing,* 3d ed. Chicago: Chicago Press, 1990.

Chipps E: Myasthenia gravis: The patient in crisis. *Crit Care Nurse* 1991; 11(7):18–26.

Doolittle N: Clinical ethnography of lacunar stroke: Implications for acute care. *J Neurosci Nurs* 1991; 23(4):235–240.

Dupuis R, Miranda-Massari J: Anticonvulsants: Pharmacotherapeutic issues in the critically ill patient. *Clin Issues Crit Care Nurs* 1991; 2(4): 639–656.

Dyken M: Safety of tissue plasminogen activator. *Stroke* 1990; 21 (Supp III):III-10-11.

Engel J: Causes of epilepsy. In *Seizures and epilepsy,* Engel J (ed). Philadelphia: Davis, 1989.

Engle A et al.: The immunopathology of acquired myasthenia gravis. In *Myasthenia gravis: Pathophysiology and management.* Grob D (ed). New York: New York Academy of Science, 1981.

Faupel G, Reulen H, Muller D: Double blind study on the effects of steroids on severe closed head injury. In *Dynamics of brain edema,* Pappuis H, Feindel W (eds). New York: Springer-Verlag, 1976.

Fisher C, Kistler J, Davis J: The correlation of cerebral vasospasm and the amount of subarachnoid blood detected by computerized cranial tomography after aneurysm rupture. In *Cerebral arterial spasm,* Wilkins R (ed). Baltimore: Williams & Wilkins, 1980.

Fode N: Subarachnoid hemorrhage from ruptured intracranial aneurysm. *Amer J Nurse* 1988; 88(5):673–680.

George M: Neuromuscular respiratory failure: What the nurse knows may make the difference. *J Neurosci Nurs* 1988; 20(2):112–117.

Germon K: Interpretation of ICP pulse waves to determine intracerebral compliance. *J Neurosci Nurs* 1988; 20(6): 344–350.

Getting myasthenic patients through a crisis. *Emerg Med* 1986; 18:110, 112–113.

Gobiet W, Bock W, Liesegang J: Treatment of acute cerebral edema with high dose dexamethasone. In *Dynamics of brain edema,* Pappuis H, Feindel W (eds). New York: Springer-Verlag, 1976.

Gracey D et al.: Plasmapheresis in the treatment of ventilator-dependent myasthenia gravis patients: Report of four cases. *Chest* 1984; 85:739–743.

Gress D: Stopping seizures. *Emerg Med* 1990; January 15, 22–29.

Griswold K, Ropper A: An approach to the care of patients with Guillain-Barré syndrome. *Heart Lung* 1984; 13:66–72.

Gudeman S, Miller J, Becker D: Failure of high dose steroid therapy to influence intracranial pressure in patients with severe head injury. *J Neurosurg* 1979; 51:301–306.

Guyton A: *Textbook of medical physiology,* 8th ed. Philadelphia: Saunders, 1991.

Hall E et al.: Effects of the 21 aminosteroid U74006F on experimental head injury in mice. *J Neurosurg* 1988; 68:456–461.

Hatton PD, et al.: Transsternal radical thymectomy for myasthenia gravis; *Apr. Thorac Surgery* 1989, June; 47(6):838–840.

Heros R, Kistler J: Intracranial arterial aneurysm: An update. *Stroke* 1983; 18:1–5.

Herrmann C Jr.: Myasthenia gravis—Current concepts. Clinical conference, *West J Med* 1985; 142:797–809.

Higashida R et al.: Transluminal angioplasty for treatment of intracranial arterial vasospasm. *J Neurosurg* 1989; 71:648–653.

Hollingsworth-Fridlund P, Vos H, Daily E: Use of fiber-optic pressure transducer for intracranial pressure measurements: A preliminary report. *Heart Lung* 1988; 17:111–118.

Hummel SK: Cerebral vasospasm: current concepts of pathogenesis and treatment (care plan, CEU, exam questions, nursing diagnosis). *J. Neurosci Nurs.* August 21 1989; (4):216–225.

Jahnke H: Experimental Ancrod (Arvin) for acute ischemic stroke: Nursing implications. *J Neurosci Nurs* 1991; 23(6):386–389.

Jones H: Diseases of the peripheral motor-sensory unit. *Clin Symposia* 1985; 37(2):2–32.

Kassell N, Torner J, Adams H: Antifibrinolytic therapy in the acute period following aneurysmal arachnoid hemorrhage: Preliminary observations from the Cooperative Aneurysm Study. *J Neurosurg* 1984; 61:225–230.

Kess R: Suddenly in crisis: Unpredictable myasthenia. *Am J Nurs* 1984; 84:994–998.

Kneisl C, Ames S: The client with nervous system dysfunction. Unit 6 in *Adult health nursing: A biopsychosocial approach.* Menlo Park, CA: Addison-Wesley, 1986.

Leahy N: *Quick reference to neurological critical care nursing.* Maryland: Aspen, 1990.

Levin A, Duff T, Javid M: Treatment of increased intracranial pressure: A comparison of different hyperosmotic agents and the use of thiopental. *Neurosurg* 1979; 5:570.

Lothman E: The biochemical basis and pathophysiology of status epilepticus. *Neurology* 1990; 40 (suppl 2):13–23.

Lovely M, Ozuna J: Status epilepticus. In *The critically ill neurosurgical patient,* Nikas D (ed). New York: Churchill Livingstone, 1982.

MacDonald E: Aneurysmal subarachnoid hemorrhage. *J Neurosci Nurs* 1989; 21(5):313–321.

Manifold S: Aneurysmal SAH: Cerebral vasospasm and early repair. *Crit Care Nurse* 1990; 10(8):62–71.

Marshall S et al.: *Neuroscience critical care: Pathophysiology and patient management.* Philadelphia: Saunders, 1990.

Marshall L, Bowers S: Medical management of intracranial pressure. In *Head injury,* Cooper P (ed). Baltimore: Williams & Wilkins, 1982.

McGillicuddy J: Cerebral protection: Pathophysiology and treatment of increased intracranial pressure. *Chest* (Jan) 1985; 87:85–93.

McQuillan K: Intracranial pressure monitoring: Technical imperatives. In *Clin Issues Crit Care Nurs* 1991; 2(4):623–636.

Meldrum B, Brierly J: Prolonged epileptic seizures in primates. *Arch Neurol* 1973; 28:10–17.

Miller R: Guillain-Barré syndrome: Current methods of diagnosis and treatment. *Postgrad Med* (May) 1985; 77:57–59, 62–64.

Miller E, Williams S: Alteration in cerebral perfusion: Clinical concept or nursing diagnosis? *J Neurosci Nursing* 1987; 19(4):183–190.

Mitchell P: Decreased adaptive capacity, intracranial: A proposal for a nursing diagnosis. *J Neurosci Nurs* 1986; 18(4):170–175.

Mitchell P: Intracranial pressure: Dynamics, assessment and control. Chapter 2 in *The critically ill neurosurgical patient,* Nikas D (ed). New York: Churchill Livingstone, 1982.

Mitchell P et al.: Moving the patient in bed: Effects on intracranial pressure. *Nurs Res* 1981; 30:212–218.

Morgan S: A passage through paralysis. *Am J Nurs* 1991; 91(10):70–74.

Mulder D et al.: Thymectomy: Surgical procedure for myasthenia gravis. *AORN* 1986; 43:640–646.

Muizelaar J et al.: Adverse effects of prolonged hyperventilation in patients with severe head injury: A randomized clinical trial. *J Neurosurg* 1991; 75:731–739.

Muizelaar J et al.: Pial arteriolar vessel diameter and CO_2 reactivity during prolonged hyperventilation in the rabbit. *J Neurosurg* 1988; 69:923–927.

Newell D et al.: Angioplasty for the treatment of symptomatic vasospasm following subarachnoid hemorrhage. *J Neurosurg* 1989; 71:654–660.

Niedermeyer E: *The epilepsies: Diagnosis and management.* Baltimore: Urbain & Schwarzenberg, 1990.

Nikas D: The neurologic system. In Alspach J (ed): *Core Curriculum for Critical Care Nursing,* 4th ed. Philadelphia: Saunders, 1991, pgs. 315–471.

Noroian E: Myasthenia gravis: A nursing perspective. *J Neurosurg Nurs* 1986; 18:74–80.

Oertel L: The dilemma of cerebral vasospasm treatment. *J Neurosurg Nurse* 1985; 17(1):7–13.

Ohman J, Servo A, Heiskanen O: Long term effects of nimodipine on cerebral infarcts and outcome after aneurysmal subarachnoid hemorrhage and surgery. *J Neurosurg* 1991; 74:8–13.

Osorio I et al.: Phenytoin-induced seizures: A paradoxical effect of toxic concentrations in epileptic patients. *Epilepsia* 1989; 30 (suppl 2):S22–S26.

Osterman P et al.: Serum antibodies to peripheral nerve tissue in acute Guillain Barré syndrome in relation to outcome of plasma exchange. *J Neurol* 1988; 235:285–289.

Petruk K et al.: Nimodipine treatment in poor-grade aneurysm patients. *J Neurosurg* 1988; 4(6):39–42.

Pfister S, Bullas J: Acute Guillain-Barré syndrome. *Crit Care Nurse* 1990; 10(10):68–71.

Pickard J, Murray G, Illingworth R, et al.: Effect of oral nimodipine on cerebral infarction and outcome after subarachnoid hemorrhage: British aneurysm nimodipine trial. *Brit Med J* 1989; 298:636–642.

Plum F, Posner J: *The diagnosis of stupor and coma.* Philadelphia: Davis, 1980.

Restak R: *The Mind* New York: Bantam, 1989.

Rich J: Action STAT: Generalized motor seizure. *Nurs 86;* (Apr) 1986; 16:33.

Ropper A, Kennedy S: *Neurological and neurosurgical intensive care,* 2d ed. Rockville, MD: Aspen, 1988.

Seybold M: Myasthenia gravis. *Hosp Med* 1986; 22:139–140, 143, 147–148.

Simon R, Aminoff M, Greenberg D: *Clinical neurology.* San Mateo, CA: Appleton & Lange, 1989.

Toole J: *Cerebrovascular disorders,* 4th ed. New York: Raven Press, 1990.

Tsementzis S, Harris P, Loizou L: The effect of routine nursing care procedures on the ICP in severe head injuries. *Acta neurochirurgica* 1982; 65:153–166.

Vermeulen M, Lindsay K, Murray G: Antifibrinolytic treatment in subarachnoid hemorrhage. *N Engl J Med* 1984; 311:432–437.

Walleck C: Controversies in the management of the head-injured patient. *Crit Care Nurs Clin North Am* 1989; 1(1):67–74.

Walleck CA: Preventing secondary brain injury. AACN *Clin Issues Crit Care Nurs* 1992 Feb; 31(1):19–30.

Wechsler L, Ropper A: Critical care neurology. In: Shoemaker W et al. (eds): *Textbook of critical care,* 2d ed. Philadelphia: Saunders, 1989, pgs. 1369–1383.

Wittman B: Research shorts: Refractory status epilepticus. *J Neurosurg Nurs* 1985; 17:138–140.

Zubkov Y, Nikiforov B, Shustin V: Balloon catheter technique for dilatation of constricted cerebral arteries after aneurysmal SAH. *Acta Neurochir* 1984; 70:65–69.

6

Neurologic Interventions

CLINICAL INSIGHT

Domain: The teaching-coaching function

Competency: Providing an interpretation of the patient's condition and giving a rationale for procedures

The complex, high-technology world of the intensive care unit (ICU) can seem foreign and forbidding to patients and their families. The need to make crucial decisions in such an environment can be paralyzing, yet patients and families often must choose among treatment options that all seem fraught with peril. Expert nurses are committed to demystifying these choices by translating the esoteric language in which they may have been presented into understandable options. In this paradigm, the nurse demonstrates that expert teaching in the ICU is more than simply giving information. By making herself or himself available to the patient, the nurse thoughtfully helps that patient face a potentially devastating choice of

treatment, as the following exemplar shows (Benner 1984, pp. 87–88):

It was a typical morning with doctors coming and going, patients going off to tests, etc. when I walked into one of my patients' rooms. A vascular surgeon and a neurosurgeon had just come out. . . . The patient was slowly going blind due to an aneurysm at the optic chiasma. . . . The patient was quite jittery. . . .

Her first words were, "Should I have the surgery? Do you think it is safe?" She took a deep breath and began to express her many fears and concerns about the surgery. She expressed the thought that if she didn't have the surgery she would only get progressively more blind but still live. If she had the surgery she could die, she could go completely blind, she could be permanently disabled, or she could live with the remaining part of her vision. . . . I asked her if she would like me to explain what would be going on, to which she agreed. I took in Ichabod Crani—a plastic puzzle of the head with removable parts and identification of all the parts—brain, bone, veins, arteries, etc. In the next hour we played with the parts, and I answered her questions. By the end of the hour the patient had decided that since she had come all this way, she would go ahead with the surgery.

When I finally left the room, I felt that the patient had made the right decision but that she had made it on her own. I felt good because I had given her a very descriptive account, in terms she could understand, of what was to happen to her. I had tried to remain unbiased and open and answer her questions accordingly. It was a very positive experience and it seemed to be for her. . . . She eventually got better, with lots of care, and is now at a rehab hospital and recuperating remarkably well.

In order to provide the degree of teaching evidenced in this paradigm, the nurse must have a thorough understanding of various therapies. Improved neurodiagnostic imaging methods, such as computed tomography (CT) and magnetic resonance imaging (MRI), have revolutionized surgical intervention for intracranial lesions. Improved neurosurgical techniques are a result of the introduction of the operating microscope, microinstrumentation, and the surgical laser. This chapter discusses nursing care related to intracranial surgery, ventricular shunts, and carotid endarterectomy.

Intracranial Surgery

Assessment

Risk Conditions Intracranial lesions requiring surgical treatment include tumors, aneurysms, hematomas, abscesses, arteriovenous malformations, hydrocephalus, and seizure focus.

Operative Procedures The particular neurosurgical procedure performed depends on the type and location of the lesion.

Burr Hole A burr hole is a small circular opening drilled in the skull. Evacuation of extracerebral hematomas or brain biopsies may be done through a burr hole.

Craniotomy A *craniotomy* is a surgical opening or window in the skull large enough to allow for visualization of the intracranial lesion. The purpose of a craniotomy is to identify and/or remove pathology, preserve vital structures, decompress cranial contents, reduce intracranial pressure (ICP), relieve symptoms, or improve neurologic status and quality of life. The bone flap may be replaced at the end of the procedure or at a later date. Rationales for leaving the bone flap out are to provide additional room for swelling, to reduce the incidence of ischemia due to increased intracranial pressure, to prevent herniation, or to decompress the cranial contents. The bone is placed in a sterile container, labeled, and stored in a bone bank for future reimplantation. The bone flap may not be replaced if the tumor has invaded the bone or if the bone is infected. The chart, nursing care plan, and, in some institutions, the patient's dressing should be labeled clearly with the words, "BONE FLAP OUT." This is a reminder to all persons caring for the patient of the high risk for injury should the patient fall or have a seizure and hit his or her head on the furniture.

Craniotomies often are described as supratentorial or infratentorial. The *tentorium* is the dural sheath that separates the cerebrum from the brainstem and cerebellum. *Supratentorial* craniotomies provide access to the cerebral hemispheres (Figure 6–1). The brainstem and cerebellum are approached via an *infratentorial craniotomy* (Figure 6–2). This operation is usually performed in the sitting position and requires intensive monitoring due to the risk of an air embolus.

Craniectomy Removal of a portion of the skull without replacing it is a *craniectomy*. This procedure may be done to explore and debride areas underlying depressed fractures and penetrating injuries and with posterior fossa surgery, where the area is protected by large muscles.

Cranioplasty A *cranioplasty* is the insertion of bone or protective material into the area where the cranium is missing. This procedure is performed in order to reestablish the contour and integrity of the skull, provide protection to the brain, and create a cosmetically appealing appearance. A number of materials can be used to fill the skull defect, including autogenous skull from a previous surgery or the patient's rib or iliac bone. In recent years, homologous bone grafting (cadaver-donated bone) and acrylic resin have replaced the metallic plates used in the 1960s and 1970s. Methyl methacrylate, a synthetic glue, provides an excellent fit; good cosmetic results; and simple, safe application.

Operating Room Protocol Awareness of events in the operating suite provides the nurse with a more comprehensive understanding of the care of the neurosurgical patient.

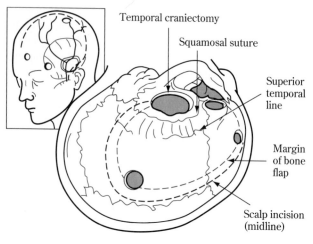

Temporal craniectomy

Squamosal suture

Superior temporal line

Margin of bone flap

Scalp incision (midline)

FIGURE 6–1

Outline of the standard craniotomy flap recommended for evacuation of acute epidural, subdural, and intracerebral hematomas and contusions. This exposure will provide access to the critical areas commonly injured in acute acceleration or deceleration "rotational" injuries. Through this flap the surgeon will be able to decompress the epidural and subdural spaces, debride contused anterior temporal and frontal lobes and orbital gyri, and control hemorrhage from midline avulsed bridging veins or the basal dural or skull areas. (Reprinted with permission from Youmans JR (ed): *Neurological Surgery,* Vol. 4. Philadelphia: Saunders, 1982, p. 206.)

Preparation Upon arrival in the operating suite, the patient is prepared as for any major surgery. Vascular access for fluid and drug administration is accomplished with insertion of peripheral and central lines. ECG and temperature are monitored continuously. Placement of an arterial line and central venous pressure line or pulmonary artery catheter is done to track hemodynamics.

Once the patient is intubated and anesthesia is initiated, the head is shaved. Great care is taken to avoid cuts, which could be a source of infection. The head is then prepped and supported in a pinned headrest (Figure 6–3). At the same time, the patient is positioned according to the surgical procedure to be performed.

Adjuncts to Surgery Measures employed to enhance the surgical repair are controlled hyperventilation, hypotension, and hypothermia. *Hyperventilation* is a quick and effective means of decreasing intracranial pressure (ICP). Moderate hypocapnia (Pco_2 between 25 and 30 mm hg) causes cerebral vasoconstriction and reduced cerebral blood flow. Intracranial pressure is further reduced with the administration of intravenous mannitol and/or furosemide (Lasix). The combined effect is to provide precious space for the neurosurgeon's work. Controlled *hypotension* is utilized when vascular lesions are being repaired. It also may be employed when unexpected bleeding occurs. Deepening anesthesia by using more enflurane (a volatile anesthetic) may lower the blood pressure. Nitroprusside may also be used to rapidly lower blood pressure. *Hypothermia* may be induced unintentionally, second-

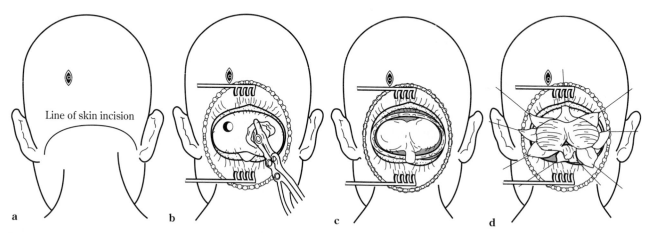

Line of skin incision

a   b   c   d

FIGURE 6–2

Suboccipital craniotomy with bone removed. **a,** Skin incision: note signs of left ventricular puncture. **b,** Scalp retracted, bone being rongeured around right burr hole. **c,** Dura exposed. **d,** Dura incised and cerebellum exposed. (From Carini E, Owens G: *Neurological and neurosurgical nursing,* 6th ed. St. Louis: Mosby, 1974, p. 335.)

ary to the cold operating room environment and anesthesia, or intentionally using a cooling blanket. In theory, each degree centigrade of temperature drop reduces oxygen consumption by the brain approximately 6%. Theoretically, intentional intraoperative hypothermia is advantageous; practically, however, it may not be employed because it causes shivering (increased muscle activity will increase tissue utilization of oxygen) and it may result in dramatic changes in electrolyte levels, cardiac rhythm, and cardiac function.

Preoperative Planning and Implementation

Fear Related to Impending Surgery Patients should be prepared for craniotomy according to established hospital protocol. This includes ensuring that the informed consent form has been signed and routine laboratory tests have been done. Markin (1986) identifies the following patient concerns prior to craniotomy: (1) loss of function, (2) return of function, (3) current disability, (4) physician's ability, (5) the

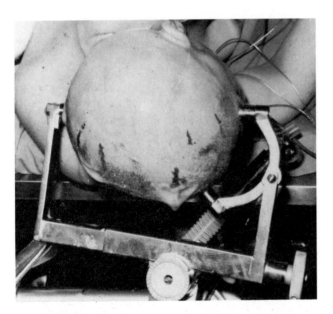

FIGURE 6–3

Head supported in pinned headrest device prior to draping. The clamp is applied to the head and tightened until the pins penetrate the outer table of the skull. (From Kaminski D: *Surgical approaches to nervous system dysfunction in adult health nursing: A biopsychosocial approach,* Kneisl C, Ames S (eds). Redwood City, CA: Addison-Wesley, 1986, p. 118.)

operation, (6) prognosis, and (7) advance directives (such as living wills, durable Power of Attorney for Health Care, Death with Dignity, and other documents). Every patient should be treated as a unique person with specific needs. Provide time for the patient to express his or her concerns. Reinforce explanations about pre- and postoperative care that will be administered. Help clarify any misconceptions the patient or family might have related to the procedure. Utilize other health team members as needed to provide emotional support.

High Risk for Altered Cerebral Perfusion Related to Intracranial Lesion Neurologic examination is an ongoing process, from admission to discharge. An in-depth neurologic assessment should be completed and documented *before* the patient goes to surgery. The preoperative and postoperative neurologic assessments should be compared to quickly establish if the patient's neurologic status is the same, improved,

NURSING DIAGNOSES

PREOPERATIVE

Two major preoperative concerns for the nurse are (1) the patient's emotional needs and (2) establishing a baseline neurologic assessment to monitor for impaired cerebral perfusion. Appropriate nursing diagnoses are:

- Fear
- High risk for altered cerebral perfusion

POSTOPERATIVE

Critical parameters to be monitored in the immediate postoperative period are airway, neurologic checks, vital signs, and fluid and electrolyte balance. Nursing diagnoses that may be identified include:

- High risk for ineffective airway clearance
- High risk for impaired gas exchange
- High risk for ineffective breathing pattern
- High risk for altered tissue perfusion: cerebral
- High risk for altered cardiac performance*
- High risk for fluid and electrolyte imbalance*
- High risk for injury

*Diagnosis developed by former contributor.

or worse. At any time, should the neurologic assessment indicate deterioration, the physician needs to be called immediately.

Postoperative Planning and Implementation

High Risk for Ineffective Airway Clearance Related to Neurologic Deficits and/or Altered Level of Consciousness

Impaired Gas Exchange Related to Altered Level of Consciousness

High Risk for Ineffective Breathing Pattern Related to Interruption of Centers Controlling Respiration The cerebral vasodilating effects of an elevated $Paco_2$ and decreased Pao_2 are discussed in Chapter 5. The nurse should be especially careful to prevent hypercapnia and hypoxemia, since the occurrence of either is detrimental to the patient. The best way to optimize gas exchange is to provide a patent airway and ensure an effective respiratory pattern. If the patient has good respiratory effort, only supplemental oxygen is needed.

Gag reflex, swallowing ability, tongue control, and ability to maintain a patent airway (mediated by cranial nerves 9, 10, and 12) must be assessed on all patients with impaired level of consciousness. Altered levels of consciousness may be accompanied by the patient's inability to maintain a patent airway or may be associated with a change in respiratory pattern. Recognition of either should prompt immediate assessment of the respiratory system, including arterial blood gases (ABGs). An artificial airway and controlled ventilation may be necessary.

NURSING TIP

Postoperative Mental Status Changes

The most common cause of altered level of consciousness in the postoperative patient is hypoxia, so the adequacy of respiration is your first concern when a change in mental status occurs. You cannot assess the patient's mental status accurately until you have corrected hypoxia.

High Risk for Altered Cerebral Perfusion Related to Intracranial Lesion, Cerebral Edema, Increased Intracranial Pressure, or Brain Herniation Refer to the sections on increased ICP and herniation syndromes in Chapter 5 for further information on these disorders. Cerebral edema reaches its peak 24–72 hours after craniotomy. It is a major cause of increased intracranial pressure. Control of cerebral edema can best be accomplished by:

- Maintaining the head of the bed at 30 degrees elevation or according to physician order. Although 30 degrees is a common elevation, the degree of elevation often must be individualized depending on the surgery (refer to Table 6–1).
- Close monitoring of intake and output
- Adhering to fluid restriction as ordered
- Administering dexamethasone (Decadron), mannitol, or furosemide (Lasix) as ordered

High Risk for Altered Cardiac Performance Related to Hypothalamic Dysfunction or a Complication of Surgery Hypothalamic dysfunction may be related to the primary lesion, surgical manipulation, or increased intracranial pressure. Sympathetic stimulation produces marked hypertension and is associated with lowering of the ventricular fibrillation threshold. Parasympathetic stimulation causes bradycardia and hypotension. Blood pressure should be monitored and measures implemented per medical orders to treat hyper- or hypotension. Cardiac monitoring may reveal dysrhythmias. Cardiac dysrhythmias are common following subarachnoid hemorrhage and have been implicated as the probable mechanism of sudden death in patients with intracerebral bleeds (Marshall et al. 1990). Whenever a change in rhythm occurs, the

TABLE 6–1

Head-of-Bed Positions at a Glance

SURGICAL PROCEDURE	HEAD-OF-BED POSITION
Supratentorial craniotomy	↑, Head and torso in neutral alignment
Infratentorial craniotomy	↓, Head and torso in neutral alignment
Transsphenoidal surgery	↑, Head and torso in neutral alignment
Shunt insertion	↓, Patient on nonoperative side

patient should be assessed for its effect on cardiac performance. Bradycardia associated with hypotension or frequent ventricular premature beats should be treated with atropine. Frequent ventricular premature beats or ventricular tachycardia should be treated with lidocaine.

The 12-lead ECG may show ST-segment elevation or depression, T-wave inversion, prominent U waves, or a prolonged Q-T interval. If a long Q-T interval is documented, the nurse should review the present drug regimen. Drugs that prolong the Q-T interval include quinidine, disopyramide, and amiodarone. If the patient is not on any of the antidysrhythmics that prolong the Q-T interval, then the prolongation is presumed to be due to the intracranial event. The patient should be closely monitored for the development of polymorphic ventricular tachycardia.

High Risk for Fluid and Electrolyte Imbalance Related to Surgery or Hypothalamic Dysfunction
Monitoring of intake and output, serum electrolytes, and osmolality is necessary to detect fluid and electrolyte imbalance. In the neurosurgical critical-care setting, electrolyte imbalances often are associated with complications of organ system failure and resuscitation. Major electrolyte imbalances may occur as a result of renal insufficiency, changes in metabolic rate, volume and solute deficit, and altered dietary intake. Dehydration and osmotic diuresis can result in hypokalemia and/or hypernatremia; iatrogenic fluid overload or low sodium intake can lead to hyponatremia; and prolonged hyperventilation can produce alkalosis

and hypocalcemia. Electrolyte dysfunction in the neurosurgical patient is usually reversible and is often avoidable with careful monitoring.

Neurosurgical procedures or diseases involving the hypothalamus and neuropophysis may precipitate neuroendocrine abnormalities. Hypothalamic dysfunction may manifest as over- or underproduction of antidiuretic hormone (ADH). *Diabetes insipidus* occurs when ADH is not secreted in sufficient quantity. Suspect this condition when urine output exceeds 200 cc per hour for 2 hours and no diuretic has been administered. Polyuria following head trauma or neurosurgery is a common occurrence. Dehydration and hypernatremia can occur unless you recognize the condition and report it to the physician (Germon 1987). Treatment consists of fluid replacement and administration of vasopressin (Pitressin). Vasopressin conserves up to 90% of water that might otherwise be excreted in urine. A number of synthetic pituitary hormones preparations are currently available. Aqueous Pitressin, a short-acting ADH preparation (duration: 3–6 hours) and Pitressin tannate in oil (duration: 24–72 hours) may be ordered. Aqueous Pitressin is generally considered more suitable for the unconscious patient. Its short duration minimizes the risk of water intoxication. Other effects of this drug include vasoconstriction of small arterioles in the gastrointestinal, coronary, skin, and muscular systems. Desmopressin acetate (1-desamino-8-D-arginine-vasopressin, DDAVP) (duration 8–24 hours) is available as a nasal spray and for parenteral use. In recent years, this drug has gained popularity due to its longer half-life, greater antidiuretic potency, and lesser risk of hypertension due to its weaker vasopressive effect (Mercer 1990; Patterson 1989).

The *syndrome of inappropriate antidiuretic hormone (SIADH)* is due to oversecretion of ADH. Urine output less than 30 cc per hour and hyponatremia suggest "water intoxication." SIADH is treated by restricting water intake. If the hyponatremia is severe, administration of hypertonic sodium chloride solution or furosemide may be necessary (Patterson 1989). For further discussion of diabetes insipidus and SIADH, see Chapter 16.

High Risk for Injury Related to Improper Positioning or Cranial Nerve Deficits

Supratentorial versus Infratentorial Craniotomy Nursing management is influenced by whether the patient has had a supratentorial or infratentorial craniotomy. Specific areas of concern deal with positioning, ambulation, and the risk of cranial nerve deficits (Hamm 1988).

NURSING TIP

Changes in Postoperative Neuro-checks

Level of consciousness is the most sensitive indicator of cerebral function. Postoperatively, stand at the foot of the bed and think about body systems. Ask yourself: "Is this finding normal or abnormal? If abnormal, was this a baseline finding prior to craniotomy or other surgery? If not, do I need to intervene or call the physician?" Remember, anesthesia and drug administration do not lead to lateralization (focal neurologic signs such as hemiparesis, aphasia, or changes in vision).

Positioning An important area of nursing responsibility for the neurosurgical patient is maintenance of appropriate positioning. Position the patient with a supratentorial craniotomy with the head of the bed raised to 30 degrees. Maintain the head in neutral position to promote venous drainage, thereby decreasing cerebral edema and intracranial pressure. Positioning after infratentorial surgery may be with the head of the bed up to 15–30 degrees or flat. This seems contradictory, but differences of opinion exist. The rationale for elevating the head of the bed is to prevent distention of venous sinuses and resultant increased pressure in the posterior fossa. Advocates for the head-flat position believe it prevents downward pressure on the brainstem and dizziness. Follow the physician's orders about position. Clearly label the head of the bed with the head position so all can see it. The patient with an infratentorial craniotomy should not flex the neck, as this puts stress on the suture line and is very painful. To prevent patient discomfort, be very gentle when turning the head. Patients with posterior fossa surgery are frequently nauseated, especially after turning. If a craniectomy has been performed, the patient should not lie on the operative site.

Vital Signs Evaluate the patient every 15 minutes until he or she is awake or stable. Vital signs may then be assessed at 1 to 4 hour intervals, depending on the patient's condition. Maintain the systemic blood pressure at least at the preoperative level or slightly higher. Obtain specific guidelines from the physician. Antihypertensive therapy should be instituted with extreme caution in order to avoid precipitating cerebral ischemia.

Ambulation Ambulation after supratentorial craniotomy generally progresses fairly rapidly, limited only by the patient's general condition and response to surgery. After infratentorial surgery, patients have problems with dizziness and ataxia, so ambulation progresses more slowly. Do not move the patient quickly. Avoid abrupt changes in position in order to prevent orthostatic hypotension due to prolonged bedrest, moderate dehydration, or autonomic dysfunction. When getting the patient up, place the patient's feet on a stool or be sure they firmly touch the floor. This stimulates the posterior columns and helps to orient the patient in space.

Collection Devices Collection devices may be placed in the ventricular, subdural, or epidural space or outside the skull in the subgalea space for continuous external drainage. Pay close attention to and accurately record the volume, color, and consistency of the drainage each shift. Theoretically, the longer the drain is in place, the more likely the patient will develop an infection. Therefore, it is common practice to put the patient on prophylactic antibiotic coverage and send samples of the drainage or cerebrospinal fluid (CSF) every several days for culture, cell count, glucose, protein, and Gram stain. The nurse's vigilance in maintaining the integrity of these systems and the sterility of the insertion site and drainage system is of utmost importance. The most serious possible complications of these collection devices are meningitis or tension pneumocephalus. Observe the patient for signs of meningeal irritation such as headache, nuchal rigidity and photophobia, and signs of increased intracranial pressure. Tension pneumocephalus may occur if CSF is drained too rapidly or air is introduced into the system. Brain compression, midline deviation, herniation, or death may occur. Symptoms of tension pneumocephalus include lethargy, unilateral or bilateral pupillary dilation, and weakness progressing to abnormal posturing.

Wound Care Check the surgical dressing frequently for signs of drainage. Usually, the dressing is not removed or changed without an order. Dressings soaked with cerebrospinal fluid and blood may encourage bacterial growth. To prevent infection, change wet dressings immediately, using strict aseptic technique. Observe the suture line for signs of infection. Do not let the patient lie directly on the sutures or bone flap where the skull has been removed. A donut made out of soft material and covered with stockinette will help support the head and reduce the pressure on the operative site. If the bone flap has been left out, protective head gear or a helmet may be ordered once the drains have been removed and the incision has healed, to prevent brain injury.

Cranial Nerve Deficits Cranial nerve deficits are more likely to occur with infratentorial craniotomies, because the cranial nerves exit through the brainstem. Lesions in the posterior fossa, surgical trauma, or edema can compromise cranial nerve function. Assess the patient's gag reflex and ability to swallow and cough. Dysarthria and dysphagia may be present. Keep suction equipment at the bedside at all times. Position the patient upright for meals. Speech, physical therapy, and dietary consultations are needed for patients with significant feeding problems. Diplopia and loss of the corneal blink reflex may occur. Establish an eye-patching routine if diplopia is present. Absence of the corneal blink reflex makes the eye vulnerable to injury. Use ophthalmic drops or ointment along with an eye shield.

Outcome Evaluation

Evaluate the patient's progress according to these outcome criteria:

- Expresses concerns regarding surgery.
- Can describe what to expect in the postoperative phase.
- Neurologic status is the same or improved.
- Normal respiratory effort.
- ABGs within normal limits (WNL) for patient.
- Vital signs WNL for patient.
- Absence of signs and symptoms of increased ICP.
- Fluid and electrolytes WNL.

Ventricular Shunts

Assessment

Risk Conditions Ventricular shunts are used in the treatment of hydrocephalus. *Hydrocephalus* is a progressive accumulation of excess CSF in the cerebral ventricular system due to congenital or acquired conditions (Grief and Miller 1991; Scott 1990). Hydrocephalus is caused by faulty reabsorption of CSF (the most frequent cause in adults), obstruction in the ventricular system, overproduction of CSF (very rare), or impaired venous reabsorption (Grant 1984).

Types of Hydrocephalus Hydrocephalus is classified as communicating vs noncommunicating, or as high-pressure vs normal-pressure.

Communicating (nonobstructive) hydrocephalus is characterized by free flow of CSF within the ventricular system and the subarachnoid space, coupled with either overproduction of CSF (Grief and Miller 1991) or inadequate reabsorption. Subarachnoid hemorrhage or exudate from meningitis commonly causes communicating hydrocephalus. Hydrocephalus occurs in 40–50% of patients several weeks after subarachnoid hemorrhage.

Noncommunicating (obstructive) hydrocephalus is characterized by an obstruction within the ventricular system or proximal to the subarachnoid space outflow tracts (the foramens of Luschka and Magendie) from the fourth ventricle (Barr 1988). Masses in or near the ventricular system (such as tumors or cysts) or congenital stenosis of the aqueduct of Sylvius commonly cause noncommunicating hydrocephalus.

High-pressure hydrocephalus is exactly what its name says: there is ventricular enlargement with elevated ICP. Obstruction of CSF flow due to tumors within the ventricular system or in the adjacent brain tissue usually causes high-pressure hydrocephalus. Other causes may be nonneoplastic masses (cysts, abscesses, hematomas), subarachnoid pathway obstruction, or congenital stricture of the aqueduct, which is symptomatic only in adults. Clinical symptoms usually start with morning, bifrontal headaches that progressively worsen until they are generalized and continuous, sometimes awakening the individual in the night. Neck pain may be present and is possibly due to protrusion of the cerebellar tonsils into the foramen magnum. Vomiting, visual disturbances, incontinence, and generally diminished mental and motor functions also may be present. As pressure increases, the person exhibits more confusion and papilledema is noted. Gait disturbances resembling ataxia or spastic paraparesis are later symptoms. Deep tendon reflexes (DTRs) generally are increased, and plantar extensor reflex is present. Cranial nerve dysfunctions or focal neurologic signs can suggest the site of obstruction. These symptoms may be gradual or acute, depending on how rapidly ICP increases.

Normal-pressure hydrocephalus (NPH) also is what its name implies. The following information draws from Meyer et al. 1985, Scott 1990, and Youmans 1990. Inflammatory processes involving the dura, arachnoid or brain tissue, subarachnoid hemorrhage, head trauma, thrombosis of the superior sagittal sinus, aqueductal stenosis, hypertensive ectasia of the basilar artery with aqueductal kinking, or tumors or cysts obstructing ventricular flow can cause NPH, or it can be idiopathic. Idiopathic NPH frequently is seen in patients over age 60. Symptoms of hydrocephalus usually occur several weeks or months later and may be due to scarring of the basal cistern or, rarely, to blockage of the major venous sinus, third ventricle, or aqueduct (Youmans 1990).

Clinical symptoms are the triad of dementia, apraxia or other gait disturbance, and urinary incontinence, which are insidious or slow to develop. The initial forgetfulness can progress to an unmanageable state. Gait disturbances start with a slowed pace, a wide base, and a zigzag step that makes the person prone to falls and trauma. Urinary incontinence, usually a late symptom, may be due to forgetfulness and lack of social inhibition. Unexplained nystagmus frequently is seen, but headache and papilledema are not. Late symptoms may include positive Babinski, grasp, and sucking reflexes. Unfortunately these symptoms frequently are misinterpreted as artifacts of the normal process of aging. NPH, however, is a reversible dementia, although when untreated it can lead to total disability and death.

Pathophysiology Regardless of the type of hydrocephalus, the basic problem is an imbalance between the production and reabsorption of CSF that results in an increase in ICP. Compensatory mechanisms will allow normal brain function, up to a point, but beyond that point the clinical signs and symptoms of increased ICP are seen (Youmans 1990). Initially the brain acts like a sponge and responds to the increasing pressure by decreasing venous capacity and extracellular space. The effective CSF pressure, or gradient between intraventricular CSF pressure and venous blood pressure, remains less than the elasticity of the brain parenchyma. As CSF accumulates and stretches the ventricles, the effective pressure rises until the brain parenchyma gives way and fluid is lost intracellularly. The periventricular region receives the greatest stress and yields as the ventricles enlarge. This is readily demonstrated on MRI or CT scan as enlarged ventricles and as decreased cerebral blood flow in the periventricular area on CT scan with xenon gas contrast.

Medical treatment of hydrocephalus may include administration of acetazolamide (Diamox), a carbonic anhydrase inhibitor, and isosorbide (Hydronol) (Aimard 1990; Youmans 1990). Both of these drugs have been shown clinically to reduce intracranial pressure by decreasing CSF production by 30–50%. Cardiac glycosides have the potential for reducing CSF production, but their systemic and cardiac effects, especially in older patients, have significant drawbacks. Recently, furosemide (Lasix) has been used to treat patients with increased intracranial pressure and has been shown to decrease CSF production by 30–70% (Marshall et al. 1990).

Rationale for Shunt Insertion Treatment of hydrocephalus is to decrease CSF pressure by unblocking the normal drainage pathways (which can happen spontaneously), opening new pathways, or improving the absorption of CSF (Youmans 1990). Currently the most reliable method of reducing CSF pressure is with a ventricular shunt. The shunt diverts excess CSF to another part of the body, where it is absorbed. The type of shunt inserted will depend on the patient's age and any previous or existing disease. Daily lumbar taps, lumbar drains, or ventriculostomies may be used to evaluate changes in mental status, to evaluate efficacy of shunting, and to help determine the type of pressure valve to insert (Youmans 1990).

Ventricular shunting is indicated when increased intracranial pressure or volume depresses normal

---

NURSING TIP

Teaching Patients About Shunts

Dolls are available from a variety of sources to use in teaching patients about surgical procedures (one source is Cordis Shunt Company). The Cordis doll, with a shunt, incision, pump, and suture, is ideal for explaining the procedure and teaching how to examine the catheter path for signs of infection. The author has found this doll beneficial for both children and adults. Coloring books and story books describing hydrocephalus and shunting procedures also are available. These teaching adjuncts are ideal for decreasing presurgery anxiety, facilitating learning, and providing emotional support to help the patient express concerns.

---

neurologic function. Occasionally, it is used as an intermittent device to lower ICP and stabilize the patient's medical or nutritional status before surgical removal of a lesion. Less commonly, shunts are used to provide access to the ventricular system for direct administration of chemotherapeutic or antibiotic agents or periodic sampling of CSF via the reservoir.

Insertion Procedure The relatively short procedure for shunt insertion is done under aseptic technique and with general anesthesia (Kneisl and Ames 1986). Minimal monitoring and preparation are needed. An intravenous line, cardiac monitor, possibly prophylactic antibiotics, and skin preparation to the head, neck and/or abdomen are all that are usually necessary preoperatively (Kneisl and Ames 1986).

The ventricular shunt is composed of a ventricular catheter, a one-way valve unit, and a distal catheter, such as a peritoneal catheter. A reservoir is added to this basic structure for some patients. The systems may be one-piece or constructed from components. The following descriptions of surgical technique and shunt function are based on Youmans (1990). The ventricular catheter usually is placed in the right lateral ventricle (frontal or occipital horn), since this is the nondominant hemisphere for most people (Figure 6–4). If a frontal approach is used, the incision is placed behind the hairline and a frontal burr hole is made. The catheter then is threaded 5–6 cm into the ventricle. With the occipital approach, the incision is made above

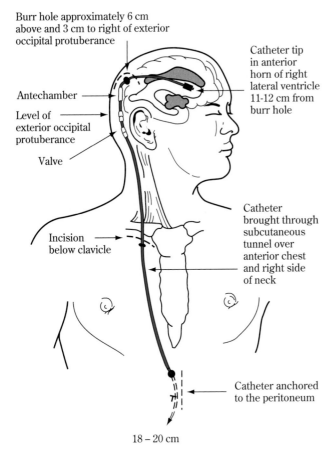

Burr hole approximately 6 cm above and 3 cm to right of exterior occipital protuberance

Catheter tip in anterior horn of right lateral ventricle 11-12 cm from burr hole

Antechamber

Level of exterior occipital protuberance

Valve

Catheter brought through subcutaneous tunnel over anterior chest and right side of neck

Incision below clavicle

Catheter anchored to the peritoneum

18 – 20 cm

FIGURE 6–4

Placement of ventriculoperitoneal shunt in the adult via an occipital burr hole. Usually a midline incision is made above the umbilicus. The peritoneal catheter is inserted for a distance of at least 18–20 cm. It is anchored at the peritoneum and placed in a subcutaneous tunnel over the anterior chest and the right side of the neck. Youmans J: *Neurological Surgery,* 3e. Vol. 2. Philadelphia: Saunders, p. 1279.

and behind the ear, where the parieto-occipital burr hole is made. The catheter then is threaded 11–12 cm into the ventricle.

The distal (peritoneal) catheter is tunneled subcutaneously from the neck toward the abdomen. Likewise, the reservoir or valve is threaded subcutaneously under the scalp behind the ear and down toward the neck. The ventricular and peritoneal catheter are connected to the valve unit and secured with suture. The valve dome is repeatedly depressed and released until fluid flows out the peritoneal catheter. If fluid flows out, the shunt is patent. Finally, an incision in the abdominal muscles is made, the peritoneum is exposed, and the catheter is threaded 18–20 cm into the peritoneal cavity and secured with suture. Positions of both ventricular and peritoneal catheters may be

verified by aspiration and analysis of CSF, as well as post-procedural CT.

Shunt Function Currently, a wide and often confusing array of valves, catheters, and other devices is available for definitive treatment of symptomatic hydrocephalus. The development of flow-regulated valves, which decrease the potential for debris and protein to accumulate around the valve, on/off devices, and numerous types of reservoirs now enable the surgeon to select the shunt that best maintains a normal intracranial pressure while arresting the progression of hydrocephalus. The valve (low, medium, or high pressure) allows unidirectional flow to prevent backflow into the ventricles. When CSF pressure falls below valve pressure, the valve closes and there is no forward or backward flow through the valve. The valve may have a reservoir attached to it. Reservoirs are used for easy sampling of CSF, injection of radiopaque or medicinal agents into the ventricles, or "pumping" the system. The reservoir is placed under the scalp, either close to the burr hole site or along the mastoid bone. Mastoid bone reservoir placement is used for "pumping" the system, to check patency, and to flush the system of exudates.

The complication rate for shunts is 10–40%, with infection being the major risk (Youmans 1990). Other complications include shunt malfunction or failure, subdural effusions, subdural or intracerebral hematoma, seizures, excess drainage of CSF, and foreign-body reaction (Youmans 1990; Scott 1990). Exposure of the peritoneal cavity may also result in the following complications: ascites, hernias, ileus, peritonitis, perforation of the small bowel, and migration of the catheter.

Effects of Insertion Patient response to shunt insertion will depend on age, type of hydrocephalus, complications, number of revisions, and any underlying disease process. The degree of improvement has no relationship to preshunt ventricular size (Scott 1990; Youmans 1990). Improvement is manifested by less dementia, incontinence, or gait disturbances; greater participation in activities of daily living; increased rates of cerebral blood flow; or decreased ventricular size.

Continence usually returns after 2 months; mental functions may return quickly or in 3–7 months (Meyer et al. 1985). Gait disturbances usually take several months to improve, depending on the preshunt severity, and may not completely disappear (Youmans 1990). However, there are patients who may have end-stage idiopathic normal pressure hydrocephalus that may not be reversible because of the extent of brain insult (Marshall 1990; Youmans 1990). A common problem in shunting for NPH is matching the valve to the patient's ventricular system (Youmans 1990). Overshunting, reducing the ventricular size, and dramatically reducing the pressure may result in chronic subdural collections. Undershunting and allowing too high a pressure may not allow the ventricles to diminish in size. In patients whose ventricular size does not diminish and who do not show clinical improvement, a lumbar puncture should be performed to assess shunt function and opening pressure. Other techniques used to assess shunt function include shunt tap, lumbar infusion testing, and instillation of indium (a dye) into the shunt system (Youmans 1990).

The response of idiopathic hydrocephalus to shunt is difficult to determine, since improvement may be spontaneous (Youmans 1990). Best results are seen when gait disturbances with or without mental changes are the symptoms. Striking improvement can occur with shunt insertion in posttrauma patients. In well-controlled studies, the improvement rate for NPH with shunt insertion is 60–85% (Meyer et al. 1985). Less improvement is noted when NPH is associated with degenerative disease, Alzheimer's disease, multi-infarct dementia, alcoholic dementia, chronic hydrocephalus, or technical complications with the shunt insertion (Meyer et al. 1985).

NURSING DIAGNOSES

The following nursing diagnoses are pertinent to the care of a patient with a ventricular shunt device.

- High risk for infection
- High risk for neurologic status deterioration*
- Knowledge deficit about signs and symptoms of shunt malfunction

*Diagnosis developed by former contributor.

Planning and Implementation of Care

The care of the postcraniotomy patient is pertinent to the ventricular shunt patient. Please review the nursing diagnoses and planning and implementation under "Craniotomy" for specific information in addition to that discussed in the following sections.

High Risk for Infection Related to Contamination
It is imperative that the nurse systematically assess the patient for signs of shunt infection. Infection is the major complication of shunting and is reported to range from 2–30% of operated cases (Youmans 1990; Scheinblum and Hammond 1990). Most infections occur within two weeks to two months following shunt insertion. The shunt may harbor an infection without signs or symptoms (Youmans 1990). Strategies to evaluate the risk of infection include: inspection of all incisions along the pathway for redness, swelling, tenderness or drainage; palpation and inspection of the subcutaneous tunnel for the catheters, valve and reservoirs; and evaluation of vital signs and laboratory data. Aseptic dressing changes immediately after surgery will reduce the chance of infection. Documenting and promptly notifying the physician of any wound drainage or other signs of infection will ensure timely therapy for the patient. The diagnosis of infection may be confirmed by the presence of increased white blood cells in the ventricular fluid and positive CSF cultures. Presence of a reservoir allows for culturing of CSF samples. The finding that most shunt infections are caused by *Staphylococcus epidermidis* suggests that contamination by the patient's skin at the time of shunt insertion may be a chief source of infection (Youmans 1990; Scheinblum and Hammond 1990). Sampling of CSF fluid from the reservoir using aseptic technique will ensure uncontaminated samples and reduce the risk of introducing infection into the shunt. Pseudocysts, peritonitis, and other infections may cause ventriculitis (Scheinblum and Hammond 1990). Although no studies conclusively demonstrate prophylactic perioperative antibiotics to be of additional value, many physicians will order vancomycin at the time of anesthesia and for one to three days postoperatively (Youmans 1990). Controversy exists over the need for shunt removal in the presence of an infection. Some physicians will choose to treat with systemic antibiotics while others advocate the removal of the shunt, antibiotic therapy, and a temporary external catheter drainage system for both CSF drainage and antibiotic instillation (Youmans 1990). If the shunt becomes occluded with necrotic cells, tissue or debris, hydrocephalus may reoccur.

High Risk for Neurologic Status Deterioration
Deterioration in neurologic status can result from shunt malfunction or failure, siphonage of CSF, or subdural hematoma, as well as from many other causes. Shunt malfunction or failure should be suspected any time symptoms recur. Malfunction can occur for a variety of reasons, including disconnection or kinking anywhere along the system, the tip of the catheter resting on the choroid plexus or in brain tissue, a blood clot, elevated protein levels in the CSF,

faulty initial placement, or decreased ventricular size after decompression (Kneisl and Ames 1986). Frequent serial neurologic checks with vital signs are important for correct assessment of the postoperative shunt patient. Immediate notification of the physician about any deterioration is mandatory. Monitor the patient for signs of increased intracranial pressure (see Chapter 5's section on increased intracranial pressure for a complete description), such as diminished level of consciousness, focal neurologic deficits, and pupillary reaction changes. Analyze the patient for subtle behavioral changes that could be clues to shunt malfunction or subdural hematoma, such as restlessness, drowsiness, lethargy, any change in orientation, or irritability. Inspect the entire length of the system pathway for swelling that would result from the system's becoming disconnected. Anticipate a return to surgery for malfunction or infection, and prepare the patient and family for this once such a decision is made by the surgeon.

To maintain patency, follow specific physician orders for pumping the shunt. Pump it only with a physician's order directing the frequency of pumping and the number of times to press the reservoir. Then use the index and middle fingers or the thumb to press and gently release the reservoir the specified number of times. Notify the physician of any change in the feel of the reservoir (which should be bouncy) or of difficulty in pumping the reservoir. Be alert to the signs of CSF overdrainage: headache, nausea, tachycardia, and diaphoresis. Unlike with most other neurosurgical patients, initially maintain the head of the bed flat until the physician orders its elevation. The rationale is to decompress the ventricles slowly and prevent siphoning of CSF. Keeping the patient flat in bed may necessitate soft restraints for the confused, disoriented, restless, or combative patient. Monitor the patient closely for signs of siphonage while gradually elevating the head of the bed. If these signs appear, halt the procedure and notify the physician of patient progress.

Knowledge Deficit About Signs and Symptoms of Shunt Malfunction Patient and family teaching concerning the signs and symptoms of increased intracranial pressure is one of the most important nursing interventions for the ventricular shunt patient. Assess the family's understanding of hydrocephalus, or "water on the brain," and address any preconceived notions they may have. Explain to the family in the immediate postoperative period about the expected gradual return of function seen with decompression of the ventricles. This will help to reduce anxiety if the patient has a slow recovery. Once the patient is able to understand, start teaching him or her and the family about the signs of

increased intracranial pressure. Supply written material for reinforcement and learning at the patient's own pace. Include a review of the signs of shunt infection, hydrocephalus, and disconnection. Review the need to have ready access to sophisticated medical care at all times in case of shunt malfunction, infection, or failure, since prompt medical care could save the patient's life. Impress on the patient the need for regular medical checkups once he or she has been discharged from the hospital (Jackson 1990). Suggest the use of a wallet card to inform medical personnel of shunt insertion. This could be helpful should the patient be alone when shunt malfunction occurs or involved in an accident and unable to communicate this information.

Generally, there are no restrictions on daily activities for patients with shunts. However, some physicians suggest shunted patients refrain from contact sports such as boxing, football, and soccer. Medical personnel, as well as members of the family, should be encouraged to allow the client to attempt to live a normal life in academic achievement and in physical activities. Include the family when teaching the signs of shunt infection or malfunction and increased ICP. Stress the need to understand that the shunt is not a cure but simply a treatment for hydrocephalus. Help the family understand that the degree of recovery may depend on the underlying disease process and general health of the patient.

Outcome Evaluation

Evaluate the patient with a ventricular shunt according to the following criteria:

- Return to normal neurologic status.
- Prevention of complications.
- Patient and family able to list the signs of increased ICP and shunt disconnection and appropriate response.

Carotid Endarterectomy

Assessment

Risk Conditions A sudden crippling stroke ranks among the most catastrophic events afflicting humanity and is the third leading cause of death in the United States (Marshall et al. 1990; Toole 1990; Johnson and Anderson 1991). Carotid endarterectomy, which was introduced in 1954, is usually viewed as preventive surgery for patients at risk for stroke (Eastcott et al. 1954; DeBakey 1975). The procedure is not of benefit in completed strok e with poor neurologic recovery or when the stenosis or thrombus extends up to the carotid siphon (hairpin turn before the carotid artery enters the skull) out of the reach of the surgeon (Toole 1990). Although some controversy exists regarding patient selection, most would agree that the surgery should be performed before the patient shows significant neurologic dysfunction.

This preventive treatment frequently is recommended for two major groups of patients: those who have significant extracranial atherosclerotic disease and progressive narrowing, and those who have had symptoms, such as transient ischemic attacks (TIAs) (Marshall et al 1990; Merrick 1986; Toole 1990). The therapeutic goal of carotid endarterectomy is to remove atherosclerotic plaque formation and thereby prevent the stroke. This surgery is performed to prevent progression of disease; re-establish normal pressure, volume and flow; remove a source for emboli; and/or bypass obstruction. Although the indications for carotid endarterectomy as a surgical intervention for stroke are subject to extensive debate in the literature, the procedure has been shown to decrease the incidence of stroke when compared with medical management of similar types of patients (Johnson and Anderson 1991). With improved radiographic imaging technics (both noninvasive and invasive), perioperative patency and flow velocity studies, and low perioperative mortality and morbidity rates, some vascular surgeons will operate on patients with asymptomatic carotid artery bruits (Park et al. 1990). (A bruit is a sound or murmur that is generated by turbulent blood flow within blood vessels due to damage or narrowing.) In this era of controversy, others believe that such prophylactic operations have demonstrated mortality and morbidity higher than the natural history of asymptomatic bruits, and therefore recommend nonsurgical interventions and close medical surveillance (Merrick et al. 1986).

Pathophysiology The brain has a very high metabolic rate and a limited storage of energy substrates such as glucose and oxygen. It is believed that under normal conditions, blood flow to a specific area in the brain is related directly to its rate of metabolism. This coupling between supply and demand often is compromised or lost in acute cerebrovascular disease. Extracranial atherosclerosis produces cerebral ischemia, the primary cause of cerebral injury and stroke, either because obstruction critically reduces cerebral blood flow or because the plaque sheds debris or emboli

(Fode 1990; Webster 1985). The signs and symptoms depend on the nature of the lesion, its location, the extent of obstruction, and the presence or absence of collateral circulation to the affected area.

Types of Symptoms Clinical presentation varies greatly, but generally speaking, the neurologic deficit of a TIA reflects the distribution of the transient ischemia.

- TIA in the carotid distribution: Monoparesis or hemiparesis, transient aphasia, dysphasia, slurred speech, clumsy "bear paw" hand, hemisensory deficit or transient blindness (amaurosis fugax). The patient may report a "shade coming down" over his or her eye.
- TIA in the vertebrobasilar distribution: Slurred speech, dizziness, ataxia, vertigo, syncope, dysphagia, numbness around lips or face, double vision and transient loss of vision in a portion of each eye (homonymous field deficit).

Other evidence of occlusion or narrowing of the carotid artery includes: a) decreased or absent pulsation of the carotid in the neck; b) a bruit over the carotid; c) Horner's syndrome (small, nonreactive pupil on the same side as the disease); d) hypertensive changes in the fundus of the eye; and e) cholesterol emboli visible in the retinal arteries on the same side as the carotid disease. Pulses in the facial arteries vary, depending on the site of the occlusion. The common carotid artery provides flow to both the internal and external carotids. When only the internal carotid artery is blocked, the extracranial obstruction of the internal carotid restricts flow to the brain. This restriction increases the volume of blood to the external carotid supplying the face and scalp, so the facial pulse increases. However, if the lesion involves portions of the common carotid proximal to the bifurcation, then both internal and external carotid pulses are decreased.

Diagnostic Procedures A detailed history, including exact symptoms and duration, as well as a precise history of hypertension, diabetes, medications, subjective bruit, and cardiac disease, is essential. New noninvasive carotid evaluation has revolutionized the diagnosis and prevention of stroke. The methods of Doppler carotid flow studies, carotid phonoangiography, and thermography are now of sufficiently high quality that they are used as routine screening procedures (Gorelick 1986; Marshall et al. 1990). CT and the unique qualities of the MRI have tremendous clinical importance and application for the evaluation of

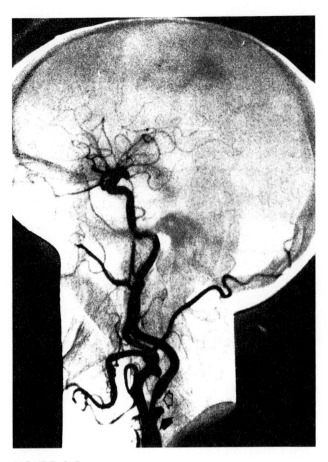

FIGURE 6–5

A left common carotid arteriogram demonstrating significant stenosis at the origin of the internal carotid artery (open arrow) with an associated ulcerated plaque (solid arrow). (From Marshall S, et al. *Neuroscience Critical Care,* Philadelphia: Saunders, 1990; p. 219.)

stroke. The main value of CT scanning is detection of hemorrhage or any unsuspected condition. However, there is no substitute for angiography in assessing cerebrovascular disease (Marshall et al. 1990). It is used to accurately diagnose stenosis, occlusions, thrombus, ulcerated plaques, multiple lesions, and bilateral abnormalities. Figure 6–5 shows an abnormal carotid arteriogram.

Operative Approach Carotid endarterectomy allows for the surgical removal of an atherosclerotic plaque by opening the carotid artery at the site of the lesion. The plaque is dissected out of the intimal wall in order to widen the vessel lumen and thus increase the flow of blood to the brain. Carotid endarterectomy may be the easiest and shortest major operation in vascular surgery, but meticulous attention to detail is necessary to minimize the possibility of transient or permanent neurologic sequelae (Webster 1985). Anesthetic management, monitoring of the adequacy of cerebral perfusion during the period of carotid occlusion, optimal oxygenation, and control of blood pressure in the perioperative period are essential.

An incision is made along the anterior sternocleidomastoid muscle. Meticulous resection of the neck in order to identify and avoid injury to the jugular vein and the accessory, vagus, facial, and hypoglossal nerves is fundamental. The carotid sheath is opened and the diseased portion of the artery exposed. Vasodilators, such as nitroprusside and nitroglycerin, and thiopental may be administered to produce a rapid and dramatic reduction in mean arterial pressure (MAP) at the time the common carotid is clamped. A shunt to bypass carotid flow during the endarterectomy may reduce ischemic cerebral injury (Johnson and Anderson 1991). There are some potential disadvantages to the routine use of a shunt, such as increased operating time, air embolus, and dislodged debris during the placement of the shunt; however, the surgeon's ability to perform an unhurried endarterectomy may outweigh these disadvantages (Webster 1985).

Clamps are placed above and below the obstruction and an arteriotomy is begun well away from the carotid body. The diseased portion of the artery is opened with a longitudinal incision and the plaque is dissected judiciously. The plaque often can be removed in one piece. The intima is examined for residual loose plaque or loose strands of media. The site is irrigated with heparinized saline and systematically closed. A final flushing to dislodge and remove any residual air is performed before final closure of the artery. The clamps are removed and a cervical drain (Penrose or Jackson-Pratt) is inserted to drain any blood and serum. A sterile dressing is applied over the incision.

The overall morbidity and mortality associated with carotid endarterectomy have been reported to be between 2–6%. The most frequent cause of death following carotid endarterectomy is myocardial infarction associated with coronary disease. The most common postoperative complications are hypertension (20–55%), hypotension (15–40%), and cranial nerve dysfunction (Grotta 1987; Lowenthal 1988; Mackey 1990; Toole 1990). The majority of neurologic complications are the result of intra- or postoperative thromboembolism (Toole 1990). Serious postoperative neurologic complications occur in 1–2% of patients (Toole 1990). However, in the hands of a skilled surgeon, the risks are small and carotid endarterectomy has provided an invaluable option in the management of patients at risk for stroke.

CRITICAL CARE GERONTOLOGY

Carotid Endarterectomy in the Aged

Generally speaking, the elderly are more often affected by stroke, with a sharp increase in frequency noted in people 65 years and older. In a 1989 study, Fisher addressed the effect of age on the operative risk of carotid endarterectomies. Fisher's population consisted of 2,171 Medicare recipients who underwent carotid endarterectomies in six New England states. He found that operative mortality increased markedly with age. In fact, older patients faced a three-fold increased risk of operative death rates compared to younger patients. Those over age 70 faced progressively increased risk, with those over age 80 facing a

four-fold increase compared to those ages 65–69. Furthermore, the operative risk was significantly higher in hospitals with a low surgical volume of Medicare/elderly patient populations. Those patients undergoing surgery at low-volume hospitals faced an additional three-fold risk of death compared to those receiving surgery at high-volume hospitals.

The special care needs of the geriatric patient are well documented in nursing literature. Nursing and medical management for these unique patients is complex and demands meticulous attention to detail. The quality of nursing care

may have a major influence on the patient's outcome in terms of complications and permanent disabilities. Systemic hypertension, coronary disease, impaired hepatic blood flow, sensitivity to drugs, and pre-existing physical impairment can turn even a relatively minor complication into a major one that can, in turn, threaten the patient's life. Studies such as Fisher's suggest that it may be reasonable to restrict carotid artery surgery for the elderly to high-volume hospitals that demonstrate low morbidity and mortality rates and good outcomes.

NURSING DIAGNOSES

The following nursing diagnoses pertain to the care of a patient following carotid endarterectomy.

- High risk for altered cerebral tissue perfusion
- High risk for neurologic deterioration*
- High risk for impaired verbal communication or swallowing
- High risk for death related to cardiovascular disease*

*Non-NANDA diagnosis.

Planning and Implementation of Care

The care of craniotomy patients, discussed earlier in this chapter, pertains to the carotid endarterectomy patient as well. Following are additional nursing care considerations specific to carotid endarterectomy.

High Risk for Altered Cerebral Tissue Perfusion Related to Blood Pressure Fluctuations Postoperative hypertension and blood pressure lability are the most frequent problems encountered in the immediate postoperative period (Johnson and Anderson 1991; Fode 1990). Manipulation of the carotid body and baroreceptors during the surgical procedure causes postoperative blood pressure and pulse changes. Manipulation of these baroreceptors may cause a short-term disruption in the feedback system the body uses to sense and maintain changes in blood pressure and thus blood flow (Johnson and Anderson 1991; Fode 1990).

It is imperative that the nurse monitor and maintain optimum systemic blood pressure and oxygenation following this surgery. Uncontrolled systemic hypertension may be associated with catastrophic sequelae such as increased incidence of intracranial hemorrhage, postoperative stroke, and postoperative neurologic deficits. (An elevation in MAP may also be a sign of increased ICP or patient discomfort.) Hypertension should be controlled aggressively to prevent stroke or bleeding at the operative site. This can usually be accomplished by the use of a vasodilator such as nitroprusside or nitroglycerin drip. An arterial line will be necessary for continuous assess-

RESEARCH NOTE

Mackey W, O'Donnell T, Callow A
Cardiac risk in patients undergoing carotid endarterectomy:
Impact on perioperative and long-term mortality.
J Vasc Surg 1990; 11(2):226–234.

CLINICAL APPLICATION

It is well known that pre-existing coronary disease is associated with increased mortality during the years following vascular surgery. But what about patients without overt disease? Is the presence of significant risk factors associated with increased mortality following this surgery?

Mackey et al. studied 614 patients with and without overt cardiac disease who underwent carotid endarterectomy and who were entered in New England Medical Center's carotid registry. The patients were divided into two groups. Group I had overt coronary disease (prior myocardial infarction, angina, or significant ECG abnormalities). The group II patients were divided into two subgroups: group IIA, with significant coronary risk factors (diabetes, cigarette smoking, or hyperlipidemia) and group IIB, without these risk factors. Perioperative (30-day) morbidity and mortality rates and late (up to 15 years) life-table survival rates were determined for each group.

The findings revealed that the risk of both perioperative and late death after carotid endarterectomy can be conceptualized as a continuum. In order of decreasing risk are patients with overt coronary disease, patients without overt coronary disease but with risk factors, and patients without risk factors.

Patients with overt coronary disease have a significantly higher risk of both perioperative (p = 0.03) and late (p < 0.0001) death than do patients without overt coronary disease. Patients without overt coronary disease but with risk factors have no greater risk of perioperative death than those without risk factors, but they do have a greater risk of late death after endarterectomy (p = 0.01). Although this study found perioperative mortality to be acceptably low (1.5%) even in patients with overt cardiac disease, late mortality due to coronary disease and related risk factors remains a significant problem.

CRITICAL THINKING

Limitations: (1) Follow-up data could be obtained on only 670 (82.2%) of the 815 patients who underwent endarterectomy at this institution since 1961. Of the 670, there was inadequate data on 56 to allow accurate group assignment. This study population of 614 patients therefore constituted 75.3% of the patients who underwent this surgery. The risk of perioperative mortality might have been different had the remaining 200 patients been included. (2) The incidence of perioperative events is much smaller than some series have reported, and the lead author was unable to explain why. (3) This was a retrospective study of one form of treatment. The authors point out that a prospective randomized study of conservative cardiac risk management versus aggressive therapy is necessary to determine the value of each approach in long-term survival.

Strengths:
This study addresses an important clinical problem and has clear implications for nurses. In this study, approximately half the patients who underwent carotid endarterectomy had clinical evidence of coronary artery disease; this finding emphasizes the importance of monitoring patients pre- and postoperatively for cardiac ischemia. Moreover, patients undergoing this surgery were more likely to die later from cardiovascular disease rather than stroke. The risk of MI was highest in the first 3 years after surgery. These findings emphasize the crucial role the nurse can play in educating patients and families about risk factor management, coronary artery disease, prompt recognition of MI, and the importance of long-term medical follow-up.

---

ment of the pressure and titration of vasoactive medication.

Bleeding from the operative site may lead to hematoma formation, which may compress the upper airway and cause respiratory difficulty. Watch the patient closely for signs indicating airway obstruction. Also, examine the operative site for evidence of swelling. Notify the physician if either occurs.

Although not as common as hypertension in the postoperative period, hypotension—sometimes caused by manipulation of the baroreceptors—can be just as detrimental (Johnson and Anderson 1991; Fode 1990). Insufficient blood pressure may decrease cerebral blood flow and perfusion. The use of vasoconstrictive drips, such as dopamine or dobutamine, may be necessary to maintain adequate cerebral perfusion and prevent cerebral ischemia. Any change from baseline vital signs is a cause for careful observation and further serial neurologic assessment.

If the carotid bodies are damaged bilaterally by the

procedure, there will be loss of ventilatory and circulatory response to hypoxia (Johnson and Anderson 1991; Fode 1990). Assessment of arterial blood gases and continuous monitoring of oxygen saturation will provide an ongoing record and may facilitate an early recognition of impending hypoxia. Restlessness, agitation, and/or changes in LOC may indicate hypoxemia.

High Risk for Neurologic Deterioration Related to Cerebral Ischemia Neurologic sequelae following carotid vascular exploration and temporary cessation of cerebral blood flow are a primary concern. Perform frequent neurologic checks and compare them to the preoperative assessment. Observe closely for the following signs of decreased cerebral function and report them immediately:

- Decreased level of consciousness
- Unequal, dilated pupils
- Motor weakness, drift, or hemiplegia
- Visual disturbances (homonymous hemianopsia)
- Respiratory pattern changes
- Dysphasia
- Widening pulse pressure
- Ipsilateral vascular-type headache

After the effects of anesthesia have worn off, examine the patient closely for evidence of diminished LOC, decreasing Glasgow Coma Scale (GCS) values, focal neurologic deficits, pupillary changes, asymmetry of lip movement, facial asymmetry, and any other changes indicative of cerebral ischemia and stroke (Fode 1990; Johnson and Anderson 1991). Immediately notify the physician of any change and anticipate CT scanning, angiography, or return to surgery.

High Risk for Impaired Verbal Communication or Swallowing Related to Cranial Nerve Impairment Assessment for dysfunction of cranial nerves VII, X, and XII is routine following this surgery (Figure 6–6). Assess the patient for facial asymmetry, mouth contraction, and impaired chewing, which indicate injury to the facial nerve (VII). Assess for loss or impairment of the gag and swallow reflexes, hoarseness, or an inability to speak clearly, which may result from injury to the vagus nerve (X). Injury to this nerve may temporarily or permanently paralyze the laryngeal nerve supplying the vocal cords (Fode 1990). The hypoglossal nerve (XII) supplies the muscles of the tongue, so check the tongue for deviation. Damage to this nerve may impair communication, ability to maintain a patent airway, and ability to swallow. Patients may not be able to eat or drink at all, or they may be able to swallow only soft foods and not liquids. These problems are not unique to the endarterectomy patient, and the nurse's plan of care is essentially the same as for stroke patients in general.

Some authors report cranial nerve palsy, a temporary (rarely permanent) dysfunction occurring in upward of 15% of patients following carotid endarterectomy (Toole 1990). The hypoglossal nerve is the most commonly injured nerve (Toole 1990). However, the meticulous skills of the vascular neurosurgeon, new noninvasive and invasive monitors, and several adjunctive maneuvers to permit high exposure of the cervical carotid artery and cranial nerves have played a key role in reducing the incidence of permanent cranial nerve damage.

Clinicians eagerly await the results of a number of trial studies currently in progress investigating balloon angioplasty for carotid stenosis. Although the use of this procedure may avoid the need for surgery, the danger of emboli or arterial dissection is worrisome.

High Risk for Death Related to Cardiovascular Disease Early recognition and correction of any condition associated with increased myocardial oxygen demands is essential. Frequently, these patients are bradycardic, with junctional or ventricular escape beats occurring due to the slow sinus rate. Atropine may be necessary to maintain a rate high enough to suppress ectopy. It is crucial that the nurse recognize that myocardial infarction is the primary cause of late death after endarterectomy (Mackey et al. 1989; Mackey et al. 1990). The nurse's role is not limited to aggressive postoperative monitoring but also includes educating the patient about overall health awareness, disease prevention, and the importance of exercise and smoking cessation or reduction. Despite the medical and technical advances in this surgery, the problem of death due to cardiovascular disease in the postoperative carotid endarterectomy patient is formidable. The need to educate the public regarding risk factors, coronary disease, cardiopulmonary resuscitation (CPR), and prompt recognition of life-threatening emergencies is critical. Patient education, CPR training, medical management of cardiac disease, and follow-up care may favorably affect long-term outcome following carotid surgery.

Outcome Evaluation

Evaluate the patient with a carotid endarterectomy according to the following criteria:

- Return to premorbid neurologic status.
- Prevention of complications.

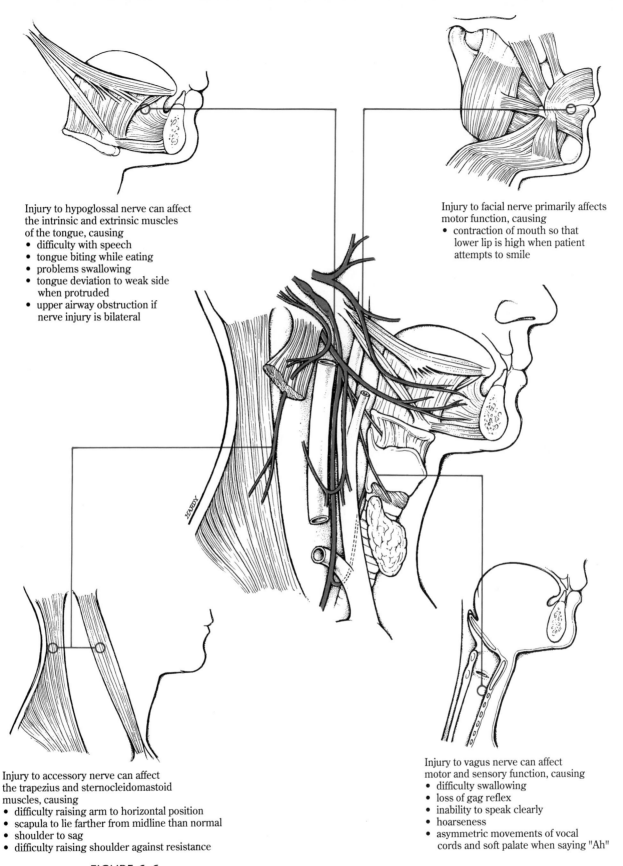

Injury to hypoglossal nerve can affect
the intrinsic and extrinsic muscles
of the tongue, causing
- difficulty with speech
- tongue biting while eating
- problems swallowing
- tongue deviation to weak side
  when protruded
- upper airway obstruction if
  nerve injury is bilateral

Injury to facial nerve primarily affects
motor function, causing
- contraction of mouth so that
  lower lip is high when patient
  attempts to smile

Injury to accessory nerve can affect
the trapezius and sternocleidomastoid
muscles, causing
- difficulty raising arm to horizontal position
- scapula to lie farther from midline than normal
- shoulder to sag
- difficulty raising shoulder against resistance

Injury to vagus nerve can affect
motor and sensory function, causing
- difficulty swallowing
- loss of gag reflex
- inability to speak clearly
- hoarseness
- asymmetric movements of vocal
  cords and soft palate when saying "Ah"

FIGURE 6–6

Signs of cranial nerve injury following carotid endarterectomy. From Webb P: Neurological deficit after carotid endarterectomy. *Am J Nurs* 1979; (Apr): p. 655.

- Psychosocial and emotional needs of patient and family met.
- Referred for rehabilitation if necessary.

REFERENCES

Aimard G et al.: Acetazolamide: An alternative to shunting in normal pressure hydrocephalus? *Rev Neurol* 1990; 146:6–7.

Benner J, *From novice to expert, excellence and power in clinical nursing practice.* Menlo Park, CA: Addison–Wesley, 1984.

Chanson P: Ultra-low doses of vasopressin in the management of diabetes insipidus. *Crit Care Med* 1987; 15(1):44–46.

DeBakey M: Successful carotid endarterectomy for cerebrovascular insufficiency: nineteen-year follow-up. *JAMA* 1975; 233:1083–1085.

Eastcott H: The beginning of carotid surgery. In *Cerebrovascular Insufficiency,* Bergan J, Yao J (eds). New York: Grune & Stratton, 1983.

Fode N: Carotid endarterectomy: Nursing care and controversies. *J Neurosci Nurs* 1990; 22(1):25–31.

Germon K: Fluid and electrolyte problems associated with diabetes insipidus and syndrome of inappropriate antidiuretic hormone. *Nurs Clin North Am* 1987; 22(4):785–795.

Gorelick R: Cerebrovascular disease: Pathophysiology and diagnosis. *Nurs Clin North Am* 1986; 21(2):275–288.

Grant L: Hydrocephalus: An overview and update. *J Neurosurg Nurs* 1984; 16:313–318.

Grief L, Miller C: Shunt lengthening: A descriptive review. *J Neurosci Nurs* 1991; 23(2):120–124.

Grotta J: Current medical and surgical therapy for cerebrovascular disease. *N Engl J Med* 1987; 317:1505–1516.

Hamm C et al.: The effects of transportation between the recovery room and intensive care unit on postoperative accoustic tumor patients. *J Neurosci Nurs* 1988; 20(5): 303–308.

Jackson P: Primary care needs of children with hydrocephalus. *J Ped Health Care* 1990; 4(2):59–71.

Johnson S, Anderson B: Carotid endarterectomy: A review. *Crit Care Nurs Clin North Am* 1991; 3(3): 499–506.

Kneisl C, Ames S: *Adult health nursing: A biopsychosocial approach.* Menlo Park, CA: Addison-Wesley, 1986.

Lowenthal A: European stroke prevention study. *Acta Neurol Belgique* 1988; 88:14–18.

Lubin M et al. (eds): *Medical management of the surgical patient.* Boston: Butterworth, 1988.

Mackey W, O'Donnell T, Callow A: Cardiac risk in patients undergoing carotid endarterectomy: Impact on perioperative and long term mortality. *J Vasc Surg* 1990; 11(2):226–234.

Mackey W et al.: Carotid endarterectomy in patients with intracranial vascular disease: Short term risk and long term outcome. *J Vasc Surg* 1989; 10(4): 132–138.

Marshall S et al.: *Neuroscience critical care.* Philadelphia: Saunders, 1990.

Mercer M: Myths and facts . . . about diabetes insipidus. *Nursing 90* 1990; 20(5):20.

Merrick N et al.: Use of carotid endarterectomy in five California Veterans Administration medical centers. *JAMA* 1986; 256:2531–2535.

Meyer J et al.: Evaluation of treatment of normal-pressure hydrocephalus. *J Neurosurg* 1985; 62:513–521.

Patterson L, Bloom S: Diabetes insipidus versus syndrome of inappropriate antidiuretic hormone. *Dimen Crit Care Nurs* 1989; 8(4):226–234.

Park Y et al.: Safety and long term benefit of carotid endarterectomy in the asymptomatic patient. *Ann Vasc Surg* 1990; 4(3):218–222.

Scott R: Hydrocephalus. In *Concepts in neurosurgery,* Vol. 3, Baltimore: Williams & Wilkins; 1990.

Toole J: *Cerebrovascular disorders,* 4th ed. New York: Raven Press, 1990.

Webster M: Carotid endarterectomy: Indications and techniques. *Surg Rounds* 1985; 8(5):57–75.

Youmans J: Hydrocephalus in adults. In *Neurological surgery,* 3d ed, Vol. 2. Philadelphia: Saunders, 1990.

7

Pulmonary Assessment

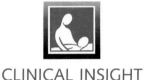

CLINICAL INSIGHT

Domain: The diagnostic and monitoring function

Competency: Assessing the patient's potential for wellness and for responding to various treatment strategies

The patient's emotional energy to help himself or herself is of paramount importance to recovery. Stunned and overwhelmed by critical illness, the patient still somehow must muster the energy to respond to treatment in order to become well again. But how do nurses assess the presence of such an ineffable state? Listen to this expert nurse (Benner and Tanner 1987, p. 25):

I am able to tune into patients. For example, a woman came in yesterday with respiratory distress, emphysema history, heart-failure problems. Her P_{CO_2} was 80 when she arrived. . . . This problem had perhaps been exacerbated by the news that her

daughter, who had been hospitalized for a heart attack, had just died. So we talked a little bit about it. . . . I was just listening, commenting, "She sounds very special."

I let her know that she didn't have to worry and that I was going to take care of her, so she could let go a little bit; she trusted me.

She did well until her family came in early in the evening. Then, she got upset because suddenly maybe she could see their grief, I guess. She was intubated about midnight. This morning she was in discomfort and scared but she looked as if she could go through it. She had some strength and energy and was willing to participate in her illness. It seemed that she was going to cooperate with what was going on. I was looking for clues: Had this lady really lost it in her grief? Was she so emotional she was not going to be able to be coached along through this illness? Was she going to be so uptight

*that we were never going to be able to get her com-
fortable or maybe achieve some things we could
in terms of rest and relaxation, and giving her
breathing treatments and suctioning today? Was she
going to be available?*

*You could see it in her eyes. She focused. She
looked at me when I said, "Good morning. It looks
as if you've had a rough night." Here is an instance
of recognizing that a patient is resourceful and going to be all right, at least in the near future. If
it's something we can get through then she can get
through it. She's got some energy there. She has
some energy to help herself and that is one of the
basic things we need, one of the predominant things
we need.*

In the Clinical Insight, the nurse eloquently describes
the process of "tuning in" to patients. Although this
patient has a pulmonary problem, tuning in applies to
all types of patients and to all stages of the nursing
process.

In addition to the assessment of coping energy, the
nurse will need to assess many other factors to judge
a patient's pulmonary function.

Gas exchange is a process that includes four major
phases. The first phase, *ventilation,* is the movement
of air into and out of the alveoli. The second phase is
the exchange of gases between the alveoli and pulmonary capillaries, called *alveolar–capillary diffusion.* The
third phase is the *transport of gases* in the blood, to
and from the cells, and the fourth is *capillary–tissue
diffusion.*

Your ability to assess the adequacy of your patient's
gas exchange is vital in assisting that patient to
maintain adequate oxygenation and ventilation. Table
7–1 suggests a format for nursing assessment of
pulmonary function.

History and Physical
Examination

The scope and depth of the nurse's history-taking in
the critical-care setting depend on the urgency of the
situation and whether the physician has already
examined the patient. Pertinent factors to note include
smoking history, exposure to inhaled toxins, chest
trauma, past respiratory illnesses, thoracic surgery,
and development of symptoms such as easy fatigability,
dyspnea, hemoptysis, or chest pain.

The physical examination provides information
about the patient's current pulmonary status. The
following sections describe in detail pulmonary physical assessment skills useful for the critical-care nurse,
beginning first with a review of pulmonary anatomy
and physiology and then proceeding through the
techniques of inspection, palpation, percussion, and
auscultation.

The Lungs and Thorax

The physical examination must be based on a clear
understanding of the relationships between external
chest landmarks and the underlying respiratory
structures. Figure 7–1 illustrates the location of the
lungs in the chest regions. The apices of the lungs
extend above the clavicles, anteriorly. The bases
extend to the diaphragm, anteriorly between the
fifth and sixth rib on expiration and posteriorly to
the level of the tenth thoracic spinous process on
expiration.

The right lung has three lobes: the upper and middle
lobes, separated by the minor fissure, and the lower
lobe separated by the major fissure. The left lung has
only an upper lobe and a lower lobe, also separated by
a major fissure. It is important to note in Figure 7–1 that
the upper lobes (and right middle lobe) are primarily
anterior structures, whereas the lower lobes are
primarily posterior structures. The lobes are further
subdivided into ten segments in the right lung and
eight in the left.

Figure 7–2 is a cast of the branching airways of the
lung without the alveoli. Figure 7–3 illustrates the way
in which human airways branch from the trachea into
the right and left mainstem bronchi and then into
bronchioles, terminal (nonrespiratory) bronchioles,
respiratory bronchioles, alveolar ducts, and alveolar
sacs. The airways from the nasal passages down to the
terminal bronchioles serve to conduct air but do not
participate in gas exchange. This area is collectively
referred to as the conducting airways. Gas exchange
occurs *only* in the primary respiratory units. A primary
respiratory unit is composed of a respiratory bronchi-
ole and its subdivisions (alveolar ducts, alveolar sacs,
and alveoli).

The lungs are perfused by two circulations: the
bronchial and the pulmonary. The bronchial circulation
provides oxygenated blood to supply the lung structures down to and including the terminal bronchioles.
The pulmonary circulation provides deoxygenated
blood to participate in gas exchange and incidentally
nourishes the structures beyond the terminal bronchi-
ole. After it is oxygenated, the blood enters a branch of
the pulmonary veins, which ultimately empty into the
left atrium.

TABLE 7–1

Pulmonary Assessment Format

1. History
   A. Chief complaint _____
   B. Usual shortness of breath _____
   C. Activity level at home _____
   D. Smoking history: pks/day: _____ Yrs smoked: _____ Yr quit: _____
   E. Childhood respiratory illnesses _____
   F. Recent travel _____
   G. Occupational history: Work/home environment _____
   H. Allergies _____
   I. Meds at home, oxygen _____
   J. Nutritional status _____
2. Physical
   A. Inspection
      Patient position _____   Sputum _____
      Thoracic shape/scars _____   Cyanosis _____
      Respirations: rate/rhythm _____   Clubbing _____
      Chest expansion _____   Use of accessory muscles _____
      Sensorium _____   Pursed-lip breathing _____
   B. Palpation
      Trachea _____   Tactile fremitus _____
      Subcutaneous emphysema (crepitus) _____   Edema _____
   C. Percussion _____
   D. Auscultation
      Breath sounds _____
      _____
      Adventitious sounds _____
      _____
      Voice and whispered sounds _____
   E. Dyspnea, chest pain, cough _____
3. Diagnostic procedures and laboratory tests
   Arterial blood gases: F_IO_2 _____ pH _____ P_aO_2 _____ P_aCO_2 _____ HCO_3 _____ $A\text{-}aDO_2$ _____
   Electrolytes: K^+ _____ Na _____ Cl _____ CO_2 _____ Mg _____ PO_4 _____
   Chest x-ray _____   Sputum _____
   Pulmonary function tests: FEV_1 _____ FVC _____ FEV_1/FVC _____ RV/TLC _____ (% pred) _____
      Maximum Inspiratory Force _____ Diffusing capacity _____ Compliance _____ V_D/V_T _____
      Other _____
   Psychosocial: _____
   Other: _____

Description of Examination Findings   Describe the location of your findings in reference to the closest intercostal space or rib and the imaginary chest reference lines. Anteriorly, it is fairly easy to number ribs and spaces by using the angle of Louis as the reference point. (See Chapter 10 if you wish to review the technique.) Remember that only the costal cartilages of ribs 1–7 attach to the sternum. Those of ribs 8–10 attach to the cartilage immediately above each of them, and ribs 11 and 12 have free anterior tips. The

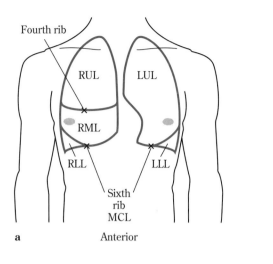

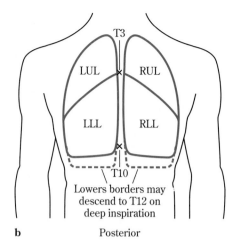

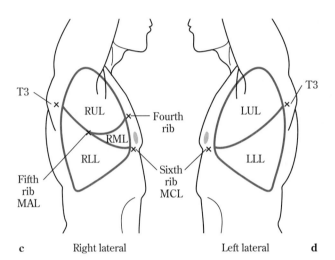

FIGURE 7–1

Lung boundaries. Locating the lobes of the lungs in anterior **(a)** and posterior **(b)** chest regions and in right **(c)** and left **(d)** lateral chest regions. *RUL,* right upper lobe; *RML,* right middle lobe; *RLL,* right lower lobe; *LUL,* left upper lobe; *LLL,* left lower lobe; *MCL,* midclavicular line; *MAL,* midaxillary line; *T,* thoracic vertebrae. (From Kersten L: *Comprehensive respiratory nursing.* Philadelphia: Saunders, 1989, p. 258, 259.)

reference lines on the anterior chest are the midsternal and midclavicular; on the lateral chest, they are the anterior, mid, and posterior axillary lines (Figures 7–4 and 7–5).

Posteriorly, numbering ribs is difficult, since the spinous processes of T_4–T_{11} overlie the vertebral body of the next lower rib (for example, the T_7 spinous process is near the attachment of the eighth rib). It is possible to number the ribs by having the patient flex the neck; the prominent bump at the base of the neck usually is the seventh cervical spinous process. From there down you can palpate and count the thoracic

spinous processes. The imaginary reference lines on the posterior chest are the vertebral and midscapular.

Inspection

Thoracic Shape   Inspect the chest for shape and symmetry. The normal thoracic shape is symmetric, with the anteroposterior (AP) diameter less than the lateral diameter. When the AP diameter is equal to or greater than the lateral diameter, the patient is said to have a

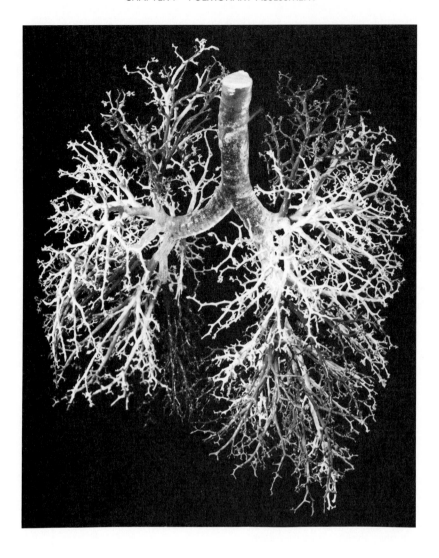

FIGURE 7–2

Cast of the airways of a human lung. The alveoli have been pruned away, but the conducting airways from the trachea to the terminal bronchioles can be seen. (From West J: *Respiratory physiology,* 4th ed. Baltimore: Williams & Wilkins, 1990, p. 5.)

barrel chest, which frequently is seen in chronic pulmonary disease. Other important observations include curvature of the spine and asymmetry of the chest wall.

Respiratory Rate and Rhythm First note the rate and rhythm of respiration. The rate and rhythm of respiration are controlled by the *respiratory center.* According to Guyton (1991), the respiratory center consists of three neuronal groups dispersed in the medulla and pons (Figure 7–6). The first group, the "dorsal respiratory group" located along the length of the dorsal medulla, is mainly responsible for inspiration. Its neurons, collectively referred to as the inspiratory area, set the basic rhythm of respiration.

Their property of intrinsic excitability allows them to stimulate inspiration with repetitive discharges. The second group of neurons, the "ventral respiratory group," is found in the ventrolateral area of the medulla and can stimulate inspiration or expiration when high levels of ventilation are needed. The third collection of neurons, the "pneumotaxic center" on the dorsal superior area of the pons, is involved in the regulation of both rate and pattern of breathing by controlling the point at which inspiration ends.

The "apneustic center," located in the lower pons, is not involved in normal ventilation. Normally overridden by the above centers, its pattern is one of excessive inspiration with short expiratory pauses. This pattern occasionally is observed in neurologic patients.

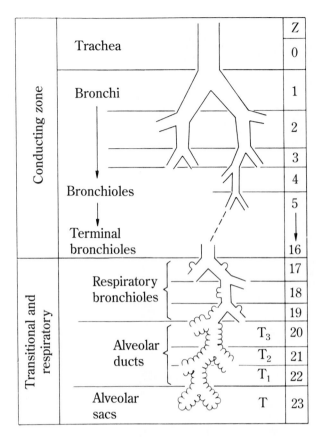

FIGURE 7–3

Idealization of the human airways according to Weibel. Note that the first 16 generations *(Z)* make up the conducting airways and the last 7 the respiratory zone (or the transitional and respiratory zone). (From Weibel E: *Morphometry of the human lung.* Berlin: Springer-Verlag, 1963, p. 111.)

Various receptors involved in the regulation of respiration include central and peripheral chemoreceptors and intrapulmonary receptors. The most potent stimulus to respiration is the partial pressure of carbon dioxide (Pco_2). This stimulus is mediated primarily by *central chemoreceptors* in the medulla and secondarily by *peripheral chemoreceptors* in the aorta and carotid bodies.

Central chemoreceptors are highly responsive to carbon dioxide (CO_2). CO_2 affects the central chemoreceptors through its influence on the acidity of cerebrospinal fluid, which bathes the medulla. CO_2 diffuses freely across the blood–brain barrier. It then combines with water to form carbonic acid, which dissociates into a hydrogen ion (H^+) and a bicarbonate ion. The increased H^+ concentration lowers the pH of cerebrospinal fluid and directly stimulates the respiratory center, causing an increase in the rate and depth of ventilation *(hyperventilation)*. Similarly, a decrease in

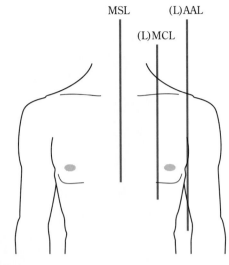

FIGURE 7–4

Vertical imaginary lines shown on the anterior chest region. *MSL,* midsternal line; *MCL,* midclavicular line; *AAL,* anterior axillary line. (From Kersten L: *Comprehensive respiratory nursing.* Philadelphia: Saunders, 1989, p. 256.)

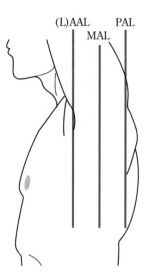

FIGURE 7–5

Vertical imaginary lines shown on the left lateral side of the chest. *AAL,* anterior axillary line; *MAL,* midaxillary line; *PAL,* posterior axillary line. (From Kersten L: *Comprehensive respiratory nursing.* Philadelphia: Saunders, 1989, p. 257.)

Pco_2 causes a decrease in ventilation *(hypoventilation)*. Peripheral chemoreceptors are mainly sensitive to changes in arterial Po_2 although they also respond to changes in arterial Pco_2 and pH.

The partial pressure of oxygen in arterial blood (P_ao_2) probably is not a strong stimulus to respiration

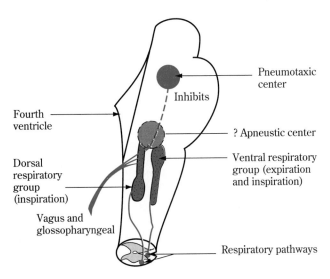

FIGURE 7-6

Organization of the respiratory center. (From Guyton A: *Textbook of medical physiology,* 8th ed. Philadelphia: Saunders, 1991, p. 445.)

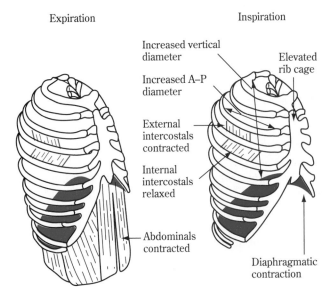

FIGURE 7-7

Expansion and contraction of the thoracic cage during expiration and inspiration, illustrating especially diaphragmatic contraction, elevation of the rib cage, and function of the intercostals. (From Guyton A: *Textbook of medical physiology,* 8th ed. Philadelphia: Saunders, 1991, p. 403.)

within the normal P_aO_2 range (80 mm Hg or above). As P_aO_2 drops, the chemoreceptors in the aortic and carotid bodies become excited and stimulate the respiratory center by reflex action. Below a P_aO_2 of about 50 mm Hg, however, the respiratory centers become hypoxic and depressed.

There are three groups of *intrapulmonary receptors:* stretch (Hering-Breuer), irritant, and "J" receptors. *Stretch receptors,* located in the walls of bronchi and bronchioles, are only stimulated with excessive inspiration (tidal volumes over 1.5 liters) and therefore do not play a significant role in normal adult respiration (Guyton 1991). *Irritant receptors* are located in the airways, and *"J" receptors* are located in the alveolar interstitium. They respond to changes such as pulmonary congestion with an increase in respiratory rate (Carrieri et al. 1984) and possibly contribute to the sensation of dyspnea (Guyton 1991).

On physical examination, the respiratory rate normally is 8–16 breaths per minute. The rhythm is regular, with inspiration slightly shorter than expiration, that is, an I/E ratio of 1:1.5 or 1:2. Abnormal rhythms and their physiologic causes are discussed in detail in Chapter 4 on neurologic assessment.

Chest Expansion Next, inspect chest expansion to evaluate symmetry and the muscular work of breathing. Muscular movement depends on the adequacy of neural impulses from the respiratory center to the muscles and on the integrity of the muscles and bones of the thorax. The chief nerves involved in inspiration

are the nerves innervating the external intercostal muscles and the nerve innervating the diaphragm (phrenic nerve). Motor stimuli from the respiratory center cause the diaphragm and intercostal muscles to contract. Contraction of the dome-shaped diaphragm causes it to flatten, thus expanding the thorax downward. (The diaphragm performs 80% of the work of breathing.) Contraction of the external intercostals elevates the ribs, expanding the chest laterally (Figure 7-7).

The lungs expand because their covering (the *visceral pleura*) closely approximates the lining of the chest (the *parietal pleura*). The space between the visceral and parietal pleurae is a potential space, with a thin layer of pleural fluid to allow gliding movement between the pleural layers. It is important to remember that each lung has a separate pouch of pleura (and pleural space) that surrounds it except at its attachment to the mainstem bronchi and pulmonary vessels (its hilum).

Observe whether the chest and abdomen rise and fall together with respiration or if breathing is primarily just chest or abdominal movement. Normally, inspiration causes both expansion of the thorax and outward movement of the abdomen. Predominantly thoracic breathing may be either normal (as in late pregnancy) or abnormal (as in abdominal pain or distention). Predominantly abdominal breathing also may be either normal (as in healthy males) or abnormal. Patients with chronic obstructive pulmonary disease (COPD) often use a mixture of thoracic and abdominal breathing, with upper thoracic effort prominent on inspiration. Expiration normally occurs passively due to the elastic recoil of the lungs. COPD patients, however, may use forceful abdominal contraction on exhalation, because the diaphragm is depressed and relatively immobile, and in some cases (emphysema), the lung has lost its elastic recoil.

Also note whether the ribs and sternum move symmetrically. One abnormal sign is *paradoxical movement;* that is, part of the chest wall moves in on inspiration and out on expiration. Such movement can be a sign of underlying pleural disease. *Flail chest,* the term for an unstable chest wall, results from double fractures of three or more adjacent ribs and causes severe respiratory distress.

The depth of chest expansion can be classified only crudely by inspection as normal, increased, or decreased. Accurate evaluation of the degree of expansion must be made with a spirometer.

Cyanosis One of the extrathoracic signs of respiratory distress is cyanosis. Cyanosis results from the presence of at least 5 g of desaturated hemoglobin (Hgb) per 100 ml of blood. In the normal person, this amount is equivalent to about one-third of the hemoglobin; however, cyanosis is due not to the proportion of unsaturated Hgb but to the absolute amount. For this reason, the anemic patient may not show cyanosis because he or she does not have enough hemoglobin to accumulate five desaturated grams; the polycythemic patient may display cyanosis even when he or she has an adequate oxygen content. Thus, cyanosis is an unreliable indicator of the degree of oxygen deficit.

There are two basic types of cyanosis: peripheral and central. In peripheral cyanosis, nailbeds and extremities appear blue-tinged, because although Hgb is saturated normally, flow to the periphery is slowed due to cold, nervousness, or low cardiac output. In central cyanosis, the lips, oral membranes, and tongue appear blue-tinged, because Hgb is inadequately saturated with oxygen in the lungs. Central cyanosis is more serious, since it indicates an oxygen saturation of about 75–80%.

Clubbing Clubbing may be seen in the terminal phalanges of the fingers and toes (Figure 7–8). To recognize it, examine the angle between the base of the nail and the skin. The normal angle is about 160°; the increase of this angle to 180° or more is called clubbing. The cause of this increase in soft tissue is a combination of proliferation of fibroelastic tissue, interstitial

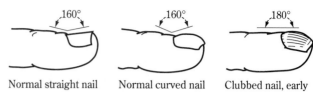

FIGURE 7–8

Normal and abnormal angles between the base of the nail and the finger. (From Cherniack R, Cherniack L: *Respiration in health and disease,* 3d ed. Philadelphia: Saunders, 1983, p. 211.)

edema, and dilatation and engorgement of the arterioles and venules (Cherniack and Cherniack 1983).

Palpation, Percussion, Auscultation

The remaining steps of palpation, percussion, and auscultation enable you to assess the vibrations transmitted by the thoracic contents. You will recall that air enters the lungs through the nose and mouth, which filter, humidify, and warm it. It then passes through the glottis to the trachea, which is highly vascular and supported by C-shaped cartilaginous rings. The trachea bifurcates into the mainstem bronchi at the carina, located anteriorly at the level of the angle of Louis and posteriorly at the level of T_4. The right mainstem bronchus is shorter, wider, and at a greater angle to the trachea than the left mainstem bronchus. The bronchi then subdivide repeatedly into the smaller airways.

In palpation, you will use your hands to feel the vibrations created by the movement of air through the airways when the patient speaks. In percussion, you will feel the vibrations created when you tap on the chest. In auscultation, you will use a stethoscope to exclude extraneous noise while you listen to the vibrations created by patient's breathing or speaking.

Sound Transmission While performing these steps, it is useful to remember some principles of sound transmission. Solid structures conduct sound better than air, unless they are too big or too compressed to respond to sound. Air in the pleural space conducts sound very poorly.

Sounds are described according to their intensity, pitch, quality, and duration. *Intensity* refers to loudness and *pitch* to the frequency of vibrations. *Quality* refers to the unique characteristics of a sound that enable you to identify it again once you have heard it, such as the quality of a fingernail scraping a blackboard.

To date, different authorities have used a bewildering array of terms to describe findings on palpation, percussion, and auscultation. This chapter presents the terms currently used by most practitioners as well as the simplified pulmonary labels recommended by the American Thoracic Society (Murphy and Holford 1980).

Palpation To continue the examination, palpate the chest to assess the position of the trachea, chest expansion, tactile fremitus, tenderness, and the presence of crepitus. The *trachea* should be midline; tracheal deviation can result from such conditions as tension pneumothorax and atelectasis. To evaluate *chest expansion* further, stand in back of the patient and place your hands on the lower rib cage so that you grasp the lateral ribs. Instruct the patient to exhale completely and then to inhale deeply (using the abdominal muscles) to try to move your hands. As the patient breathes in, note whether your thumbs move apart equally. This technique can be useful in postoperative thoracotomy patients with shallow breathing patterns.

Tactile fremitus is the name given to palpable vibrations caused by speaking. To palpate for fremitus, use the most sensitive part of your hands—either the pads of your fingertips or the part of your palm that overlies the heads of the metacarpal bones. Ask the patient to say "ninety-nine" several times while you palpate the chest wall bilaterally. Normally, you will be able to feel vibrations like the purring of a cat over the trachea and bronchi. These vibrations should be equal bilaterally, except over the heart. Since solids conduct vibrations better than air, any condition that consolidates the lung close to the chest wall increases fremitus. Decreased or absent fremitus occurs when a condition blocks the passage of air (such as an obstructed bronchus) or moves the lung tissue away from the chest wall (such as a pneumothorax). The presence of *crepitus,* or air leaking from the lung into the subcutaneous tissue, is particularly important to assess in the trauma patient or any patient with chest tubes in place. As the chest wall is palpated, a crackling sensation is felt under your fingertips.

Percussion Percussion of the chest is used to evaluate the density of structures just below the chest wall. Although percussion is used less frequently than other assessment techniques, it is included here because the concepts on which it is based are important to an understanding of various lung disorders. To percuss the chest, press the terminal phalanx of your middle finger on the chest wall and strike it on the knuckle with the tip of your other middle finger.

(Be sure to press only the terminal phalanx on the chest wall; if you allow contact between the rest of your hand and the chest, it will damp the vibrations.) Strike the phalanx quickly at almost a 90-degree angle by cocking your wrist. Begin at the apices and percuss side to side down the chest until you reach the diaphragm. Listen for the sounds and feel for the vibrations produced.

There are four sounds you may hear depending upon the absence or presence of densities and/or air in the chest. A resonant sound is heard in the normal lung fields, a hyperresonant sound is heard in emphysematous lungs or pneumothorax, and dull to flat sounds are heard in the presence of fluid or over other densities such as the heart. If you hear an abnormal percussion sound, localize the finding by percussing from an area of resonance to the abnormal area.

Auscultation Finally, use the diaphragm of a stethoscope to auscultate the upper lobes anteriorly and the lower lobes posteriorly, comparing side to side as you do so. Hold the bell of the stethoscope between your middle finger and forefinger, and press firmly on the skin surface. If possible, have the patient sit upright. In the critically ill patient, listen anteriorly and then either get assistance to sit the patient forward or turn the patient to his or her side to listen posteriorly. Ask the person to breathe through the mouth a little more deeply than normal.

Listen first for breath sounds. There are basically three types: bronchial, vesicular, and bronchovesicular. Hollow, tubular sounds are heard over the trachea and are referred to as *bronchial.* They seem close to the ear and have a short inspiration, a pause, and a longer, louder expiration. Sounds heard over smaller airways in the periphery of the lung are referred to as *vesicular.* They are soft, with a long inspiration, no pause, and a shorter, softer expiration. Sounds heard over medium-sized airways are referred to as *bronchovesicular* and have inspiratory and expiratory phases equal in loudness and length.

Any condition that solidifies (consolidates) the lung, such as pneumonia, increases sound transmission to the chest wall. Thus, it is abnormal to hear increased (bronchial or bronchovesicular) sounds over the lung fields. Decreased or absent breath sounds are caused by any condition that reduces air flow (such as an obstructed bronchus) or moves the lungs away from the chest wall (such as pneumothorax or pleural effusion). Because interpretation varies with the listener, it is recommended that breath sounds be described only as normal, decreased, absent, or bronchial.

Also listen for adventitious sounds, abnormal sounds superimposed on breath sounds (see Table

TABLE 7–2

Types of Adventitious Sounds

TYPE	GENERAL LOCATION	ASSOCIATED PROBLEM(S)	CHARACTERISTICS	GRAPHIC ILLUSTRATION
Crackles (rales)	Peripheral airways and alveoli	Atelectasis Inflammation Excess fluid Excess mucus	Group of discrete crackles or popping sounds Discontinuous sound Usually inspiratory, may be inspiratory and expiratory	fine coarse
Rhonchi (gurgles)	Large airways	Inflammation Excess fluid Excess mucus	Coarse, low-pitched sonorous sounds Continuous sound Usually expiratory, may be inspiratory and expiratory Changes in quality and timing with coughing	
Wheeze	Large and/or small airways	Bronchoconstriction (airway narrowing) from bronchospasm, fluid, mucus, inflammatory by-products, obstructive lesion Airway instability	High- (sometimes low-) pitched musical sound Continuous sound Usually expiratory, may be inspiratory and expiratory	
Pleural friction rub	Pleural surfaces	Inflamed or roughened pleural surfaces (pleuritis)	Grating sound with continuous and discontinuous qualities May appear intermittently Variable duration; usually inspiratory, may be inspiratory and expiratory Sounds the same or louder with coughing	

(From Kersten L: *Comprehensive respiratory nursing.* Philadelphia: Saunders, 1989, p. 310.)

7–2). Listen carefully to determine if the sound is continuous or discontinuous, high- or low-pitched, and during inspiration or expiration. The American Thoracic Society recommends the use of four terms: two different discontinuous sounds, referred to as coarse crackles and fine crackles (previously referred to as *rales*), and two continuous sounds—high-pitched wheeze and low-pitched rhonchus. *Crackles* (rales) result from either the sudden opening of closed alveoli, as in pulmonary fibrosis, or from air bubbling through fluid in the airway, as in pulmonary edema. Crackles may be heard during inspiration only or during both inspiration and expiration. A high-pitched continuous sound, or *wheeze,* results from air passing through a narrowed airway, as in bronchospasm, airway edema, foreign body, or tumor. If this high-pitched continuous sound is heard only during inspiration, it is called *stridor* (Kersten 1989). A low-pitched continuous sound, a *rhonchus* or gurgle, is often associated with secretions and may clear following coughing or suctioning. A pleural friction rub may also be detected as

a grating, continuous sound that results from pleural inflammation and varies with breathing.

The critical-care nurse rarely checks abnormal voice and whispered sounds in a screening examination. They are included here primarily so you will understand their significance when noted in a thorough workup. Voice sounds are the auscultatory equivalent of the vibrations palpated during tactile fremitus. The patient is asked to say "ninety-nine" repeatedly. Normally, the sounds are heard indistinctly over the large airways and are equal bilaterally. The American Thoracic Society recommends that findings be reported as voice or whispered sounds that are normal; decreased or absent; or increased in intensity or clarity. Decreased or absent voice sounds occur when air flow is blocked (as in an obstructed bronchus) or the lung and chest wall are separated (as in a pneumothorax). Increased voice sounds are due to consolidation (solidification) of the lung. Increased sounds are detected when the syllables are heard more clearly than normal although still muffled; this finding is

TABLE 7–3

Typical Assessment Findings

CONDITION	INSPECTION	PERCUSSION	PALPATION	AUSCULTATION
Emphysema	Patient sitting upright, leaning foward Pursed-lip breathing Barrel chest Using neck muscles Copious sputum (often green-tinged)	Hyperresonant ↓ diaphragm movement	↓ chest excursion	Decreased breath sounds Decreased voice sounds
Chronic bronchitis	Patient sitting upright, leaning forward Copious sputum Ankle edema	Resonant to hyper-resonant	Normal to ↓ excursion	Rhonchi Crackles Wheezes
Acute asthma	Patient sitting upright, leaning forward Sticky, thick sputum Anxious Accessory muscle use	Hyperresonant	Chest excursion ↑ then ↓ with fatigue Diaphoretic	Wheezes
Pulmonary edema	Patient sitting upright Shallow, rapid respirations Distended neck veins Copious frothy sputum	Normal to dull	↓ chest excursion	Coarse crackles (inspiration and expiration) S_3 or S_4 gallop Often, irregular heart rhythm May wheeze
Pneumothorax	Asymmetric chest excursion (if large)	Hyperresonant	Trachea midline or shifted away from pneumothorax (tension) ↓ chest movement	Absent breath sounds Absent fremitus Absent voice sounds
Consolidation (pneumonia)	Tachypnea Purulent discolored sputum	Dull		Bronchial breath sounds Increased fremitus Increased voice sounds
Atelectasis	Tachypnea (+/−)	Dull	↓ chest movement on affected side (if severe) Trachea midline or deviated toward affected side	Decreased breath sounds* Decreased fremitus Decreased voice sounds
Pleural effusion	Tachypnea	Dull	↓ chest movement on affected side (if large) Trachea deviated away from affected side	Decreased breath sounds Decreased fremitus Decreased voice sounds Some crackles

*May hear bronchial breath sounds if lobe collapsed and bronchus open.

called *bronchophony.* A related finding, also due to consolidation, occurs when the patient's spoken E is heard as A; this phenomenon is called *egophony.* Whispered sounds normally are heard only faintly over the mainstem bronchi. In consolidation they are heard clearly; this occurrence is called *whispered pectoriloquy.*

Significance of Findings To interpret the significance of the findings from inspection, palpation, percussion, and auscultation, consider them in association with each other; some of the common groupings are included in Table 7–3.

Your skill at chest diagnosis can be a valuable tool in assessing, diagnosing, planning, implementing, and evaluating the care you give patients. When you assume responsibility for a patient, it is essential to inspect and auscultate the chest so you have a basis for comparison as you later evaluate the effects of your nursing care. For instance, in your initial assessment you might note that your patient is restless and slightly tachypneic. Auscultation might reveal diffuse crackles and rhonchi. After chest physiotherapy and suctioning, you would again auscultate the chest; the absence of the adventitious sounds would indicate the effectiveness of your intervention to improve oxygenation.

Signs and Symptoms of Respiratory Distress

Your initial assessment can reveal a great deal of information about the work of breathing that the patient is having to do. Always note and investigate an increase in respiratory rate, an early indicator of respiratory distress. Use of accessory muscles in the neck or upper chest, retraction or bulging of the intercostal muscles, and active contraction of the abdominal muscles are all signs of possible respiratory distress. Another sign of respiratory muscle fatigue is asynchronous or paradoxical breathing (Figure 7–9). This sign is observed during inspiration, when the chest rises but the abdomen sinks inward, and during expiration, when the chest falls but the abdomen

NURSING TIP
Chest Assessment
In the critical-care setting, chest inspection may be difficult because of the patient's supine position. Stand at the foot of the bed to observe for bilateral anterior chest movement. Auscultation may be difficult if the patient is receiving low tidal volumes while being mechanically ventilated. By manually sighing the patient or listening while someone manually "bags" the patient, you may hear breath sounds more easily.

pushes outward. This "rocking boat" motion indicates diaphragmatic fatigue.

Other findings of respiratory failure include nasal flaring, the use of pursed-lip breathing, and an upright, leaning-forward position. If you observe them, ask the patient if he or she is feeling more breathless than usual, as some of the above findings are present in

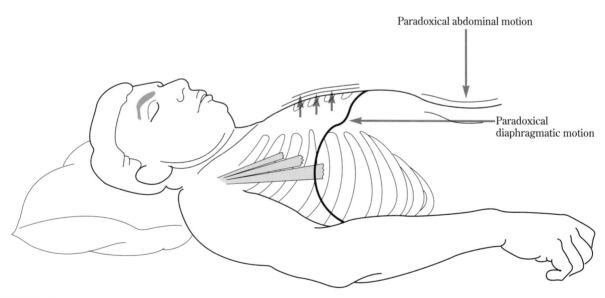

FIGURE 7–9

Paradoxical abdominal motion. In the supine position a patient laboring under a heavy work load relative to his capability often demonstrates inward (paradoxical) abdominal motion as air is drawn into the lungs. (From Wheeler A, Marini J: Avoiding the consequences of respiratory muscle fatigue. *J Respir Dis* 1985 6(9): 107–125.)

patients who have adapted to chronic breathlessness. Dyspnea, or the patient's subjective feeling of breathlessness, is experienced almost universally by patients with pulmonary and cardiovascular disease. Tables 7–4 and 7–5 summarize causes of acute and chronic dyspnea. Elicit from your patient what makes his or her dyspnea worse and what he or she does at home to decrease it.

Assess the presence, strength, and productivity of cough. Examine sputum for consistency, color, amount, and odor. Copious frothy sputum may indicate fluid overload or congestive heart failure (CHF), while sticky, difficult-to-raise secretions are classic in the patient in status asthmaticus. Chest pain may indicate viral infection, pulmonary embolism, pulmonary hypertension, pleurisy, pneumothorax, rib fractures, myocardial ischemia, pneumonia, or pulmonary infarct (Kersten 1989). Identify the location, intensity, and aggravating and alleviating factors.

Confusion and disorientation may be seen in hypoxia or CO_2 retention; drowsiness and headache may indicate CO_2 retention. Peripheral edema, jugular venous distention, and liver tenderness may be seen in cor pulmonale.

Atrial and supraventricular dysrhythmias are common in the patient with chronic obstructive pulmonary disease (COPD) due to cor pulmonale. In COPD and other respiratory disorders, hypoxia and blood-gas–related electrolyte disturbances can result in tachycardia, ectopy, and blood pressure changes.

Pulmonary Function Tests

A basic understanding of frequently performed pulmonary function tests (PFTs) is essential for the critical-care nurse. PFTs are used to diagnose the type of lung disease, monitor the rate of lung function decline, and assess airway reactivity to bronchodilators. With an increasingly older patient population, many of whom still smoke, it is not unusual to have pulmonary function tests available for the patient in chronic respiratory failure as well as the patient with COPD undergoing open heart surgery. Identifying the patient at risk for developing postoperative respiratory failure can help you plan, implement, and evaluate your nursing care. PFTs are divided into the

TABLE 7–4

Characteristics of Various Etiologies for Acute Dyspnea

DISORDER	CLINICAL FINDINGS	CHEST RADIOGRAPH
Airway obstruction:		
Laryngospasm	Stridor; possible allergic reaction; shock	
Aspirated foreign body	History of choking; gurgling respirations	
Bronchoconstriction	History of airway disease; wheezing	Hyperinflation with flattened diaphragms
Hyperventilation syndrome	Recent emotional upset; neurotic personality	Normal
Chest trauma:		
Fractured ribs	Tenderness on chest palpation; unilateral hyperresonance; diminished or absent breath sounds	Disruption of rib shadows; air in pleural space with collapse of lung; shift of mediastinum if tension
Pneumothorax		
Pneumonia	Fever; purulent sputum	Parenchymal infiltrate
Pulmonary edema:		
Cardiogenic	Frothy sputum; cyanosis; crackles	Cardiomegaly; pleural effusions
Noncardiogenic	Frothy sputum; cyanosis; crackles	Normal heart size
Pulmonary embolism	Pleuritic chest pain; predisposing risk factors	May be normal; atelectasis; oligemia; pleural effusion; consolidation
Pulmonary hemorrhage	Hemoptysis	Focal or diffuse alveolar infiltrates; may clear within 24–48 hours
Spontaneous pneumothorax	Unilateral hyperresonance; diminished or absent breath sounds	Air in pleural space with collapse of lung; shift of mediastinum if tension

(From Kersten L: *Comprehensive respiratory nursing.* Philadelphia: Saunders, 1989, p. 256.)

TABLE 7–5

Causes of Chronic Dyspnea

Respiratory

  Airway disease

    Asthma

    Chronic obstructive pulmonary disease (chronic bronchitis and emphysema)

    Cystic fibrosis

    Upper airway obstruction

  Parenchymal lung disease

    Interstitial lung disease

    Malignancy—primary or metastatic

  Pneumonia

  Pulmonary vascular disease

    Arteriovenous malformations

    Plexogenic pulmonary hypertension

    Thromboembolism

    Vasculitis

    Veno-occlusive disease

  Pleural disease

    Effusion

    Fibrosis

    Malignancy

  Chest wall disease

    Deformities (e.g., scoliosis, kyphosis, ankylosing spondylitis)

    Obesity

    Ascites

    Pregnancy

  Respiratory muscle disease and/or dysfunction

    Neuromuscular disorders (e.g., muscular dystrophy, amylotrophic lateral sclerosis, myasthenia gravis, polio)

  Malnutrition

  Thyroid disease

  Chronic primary fibromyalgia

Cardiovascular

  Elevated pulmonary venous pressure

  Decreased cardiac output

  Right-to-left shunt

Anemia

Deconditioning

Psychologic factors

(From Mahler D (ed): *Dyspnea.* Mt. Kisko, NY: Futura, 1990, p. 167.)

assessment of lung volumes, gas exchange, and mechanics of ventilation.

Lung Volumes and Capacities

The air in the lungs can be subdivided into several volumes and capacities. Figure 7–10 presents the volumes and capacities graphically and gives examples of normal values. It must be stressed that clinically, these normal values are variable and are predicted on the basis of sex, age, height, weight, activity, and barometric pressure. The "normal" values given here apply only to a healthy young male lying at rest and breathing air at sea level. They are taken from Guyton (1991).

Lung Volumes *Tidal volume* (V_T) is the amount of gas inspired or expired with a normal breath. Its normal value is 500 ml. *Inspiratory reserve volume* is the volume that can be inspired above tidal volume; the normal value is about 3,000 ml. *Expiratory reserve volume* is the amount that can be expired below tidal volume; the normal value is about 1,100 ml.

Residual volume (RV) is the amount of gas that always remains in the lungs, that is, that cannot be expelled even with a maximal expiration. It cannot be measured directly or at the bedside. A normal value is 1,200 cc; RV is increased in emphysema and acute asthma.

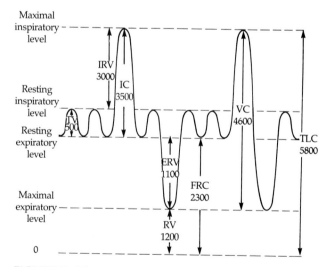

FIGURE 7–10

Lung volumes and capacities. *ERV,* expiratory reserve volume; *FRC,* functional residual capacity; *IC,* inspiratory capacity; *IRV,* inspiratory reserve volume; *RV,* residual volume; *TLC,* total lung capacity; *TV,* tidal volume; *VC,* vital capacity.

Lung Capacities Two or more volumes combine to make a lung capacity. *Inspiratory capacity* is the maximum volume that can be inspired starting from a resting expiratory level, in other words, the tidal volume plus the inspiratory reserve volume. Inspiratory capacity measures about 3,500 ml and usually represents 75% of the vital capacity.

Functional residual capacity (FRC) consists of the residual volume plus the expiratory reserve volume and represents the volume of air in the lungs at the end of a normal expiration. A usual value is 2,300 ml. The FRC functions to maintain a constant alveolar Pco_2. It increases in hyperinflation, such as in emphysema or acute asthma. An increased FRC means an increased muscular effort of breathing, because thoracic size is increased. It also means impaired ability to increase ventilation and to alter quickly the composition of alveolar gas. A decrease in FRC is seen in restrictive diseases that decrease the number of open alveoli, such as atelectasis, pulmonary edema, and pneumonia. A decrease in FRC is the primary defect in the adult respiratory distress syndrome (ARDS) that causes hypoxemia due to severe atelectasis and alveolar edema. Positive end-expiratory pressure (PEEP) increases FRC by increasing alveolar surface area for gas exchange. (ARDS and PEEP are discussed in Chapters 8 and 9.) Deep inspiratory maneuvers also aid to reexpand alveoli and increase FRC.

The total amount of air in the lungs is called *total lung capacity* and measures about 5,800 ml. It consists of FRC and inspiratory capacity.

Vital capacity (VC) equals the total lung capacity minus the residual volume. It is important clinically, because it is a measure of the person's ability to take a deep breath. Normal vital capacity is about 4,600 ml. A decreased vital capacity is a helpful but nonspecific sign, since it may be caused by depression of the respiratory center, obstructive diseases, or restrictive conditions. It is important to recognize that a normal vital capacity does not rule out the presence of pulmonary disease, such as pulmonary embolism.

Bedside Measurement of Pulmonary Function At the bedside, the critically care nurse or respiratory therapist can measure vital capacity, described above, and *maximum inspiratory force* (MIF) to assess the ability of the patient to move air and cough effectively. Bedside measurement of VC and MIF in the intubated patient can help predict the ability of that patient to cough and take deep breaths following extubation. To measure VC, the examiner tells the patient to take a deep inspiration and then expel as much air as possible. The exhaled volume is measured with a spirometer. MIF is measured by having the patient breathe in against a negative-pressure manometer while his or her airway is occluded. The normal MIF is about −60 to −100 cm H_2O pressure. If the MIF is less than −25 cm H_2O, the person probably cannot maintain a normal sigh volume or cough effectively.

NURSING TIP

Bedside Measurement of MIF and VC

Prior to measuring the MIF and VC, place the patient in a high Fowler's position to optimize the ability to take a deep breath.

Airflow Rates The degree of obstruction to airflow is measured by the forced expiratory volume in one second (FEV_1). The normal individual is able to exhale 80% of forced vital capacity in one second, or about 2–3 liters. The ratio between the forced expiratory volume and the forced vital capacity (FEV_1/FVC) is an indicator of resistance in the larger airways. In the patient with COPD, this value may be as low as 30–50%. Maximal mid-expiratory flow rates (MMEFR) represent flow in the medium-to-smaller airways and may be a more sensitive parameter of small airway disease. Peak expiratory flow rates (PEFR) are frequently measured in asthmatic patients to get a quick assessment of their degree of obstruction, for example, in the emergency department. Patients at home also can measure PEFRs, so they know their "baseline." All of the above airflow rates can be measured at the bedside of the critically ill patient.

Gas Exchange

Diffusing Capacity The ability of the alveolar-capillary membrane to exchange a gas is called its *diffusing capacity*. Guyton (1991) defines diffusing capacity as "the volume of a gas that diffuses through the membrane each minute for a pressure difference of 1 mm Hg." The diffusing capacity for a given gas is affected by the pressure gradient across the membrane, the area of the membrane, the thickness of the membrane, and the diffusion coefficient of the gas. Diffusing capacity is decreased in emphysema and fibrotic diseases due to the damage and loss of the alveolar capillary membrane.

Pressure Gradients The pressure gradients for O_2 and CO_2 are major determinants of gas exchange. In a mixture of gases, such as atmospheric or alveolar air, the pressure exerted by each gas is independent of the other gases and proportional to its percentage of the total gas (Dalton's law). The pressure exerted by each gas is called its *partial pressure*. The total pressure of the air inspired is the *barometric (atmospheric) pressure,* which varies in relation to distance above or below sea level; at sea level it is 760 mm Hg. The partial pressure of a gas is calculated by multiplying the total pressure by the percentage of the gas. Table 7–6 presents the approximate percentages and partial pressures for inspired (tracheal) air, which consists primarily of nitrogen, oxygen, carbon dioxide, and water vapor. (*Note:* To obtain the partial pressures of inspired gases, the pressure exerted by water vapor must be subtracted first. The reason for this subtraction is that gases in the airways are completely humidified; this means that at 37°C the other gases can exert a maximum partial pressure of 713 mm Hg.) The partial pressure of oxygen in inspired air is 150 mm Hg, while the partial pressure of CO_2 is 0.2 mm Hg.

Alveolar air differs somewhat from tracheal air. Nitrogen, which accounts for the greatest percentage, readily establishes equilibrium across the alveolar-capillary membrane and therefore can be disregarded. The remaining gas consists of about 14% oxygen, 5% CO_2, and 6% water vapor. Thus, alveolar air contains less oxygen and more carbon dioxide than tracheal air.

The partial pressure of O_2 in alveolar air is about 100 mm Hg. The partial pressure of CO_2 in alveolar air is 40 mm Hg. Blood in the pulmonary capillaries has P_{O_2} of 40 mm Hg and P_{CO_2} of 45 mm Hg. The resulting pressure gradients cause oxygen to diffuse from the

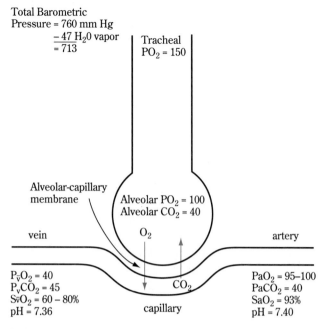

FIGURE 7–11

Alveolar-capillary gas exchange.

alveoli into the capillaries and carbon dioxide to diffuse from the capillaries into the alveoli (Figure 7–11). Although the pressure gradient for CO_2 is small, carbon dioxide diffuses faster than oxygen because its solubility is much greater.

Of the four factors affecting diffusing capacity, changes in pressure gradients are most important clinically. Pressure gradients depend on the relationship between ventilation and blood flow in alveolar-capillary units.

The relationship between ventilation ($\dot{V}$) and perfusion ($\dot{Q}$) has a critical influence on gas exchange. There is a continuum of relationships between ventilation and perfusion (Figure 7–12). At one end of the continuum is a unit that is perfused but not ventilated, the *shunt unit* discussed later in this chapter. In the middle of the continuum, the *normal unit* is both ventilated and perfused. Further along the continuum is a unit that is ventilated but not perfused, the *deadspace unit* discussed later. If a unit is neither ventilated nor perfused, it is referred to as a *silent unit*.

Even in the normal lung, the distribution of ventilation in relation to perfusion is uneven; some areas of the lung have too much ventilation in relation to perfusion, others too little. These regional ventilation to perfusion ($\dot{V}/\dot{Q}$) mismatches are unimportant in the healthy person. In the critically ill patient, improving the matching of ventilation and perfusion—by using

TABLE 7–6

Composition of Inspired (Tracheal) Gas at Sea Level

Total barometric pressure	760 mm Hg
–Water vapor at 37°C	47
Corrected barometric pressure	713 mm Hg

GAS	PERCENTAGE				PARTIAL PRESSURE
Nitrogen	79.03%	×	713	=	563.5 mm Hg
Oxygen	20.94%	×	713	=	149.3
Carbon dioxide	0.03%	×	713	=	0.2
Total	100%				713.0 mm Hg

turning, suctioning, and hyperinflation maneuvers—is one of the nurse's primary concerns.

Surface Area and Thickness of Membrane In addition to the pressure gradients, the alveolar surface area and the thickness of the alveolar-capillary membrane affect gas exchange. The alveolar surface area varies with age, body size, lung volume, presence of surfactant, and other factors. It decreases with emphysema and pneumonectomy.

The thickness of the alveolar-capillary membrane occasionally becomes clinically important, because increased thickness reduces the diffusing capacity. The membrane's thickness increases with pulmonary edema and pulmonary fibrosis.

Diffusion Coefficient The diffusion coefficient expresses the rate of gas transfer across the membrane. According to Guyton (1991), the coefficient depends on both the gas's solubility and its molecular weight. The diffusion coefficient of carbon dioxide is approximately twenty times that of oxygen.

Deadspace The total volume of air that ventilates the lungs per minute is called the *minute ventilation* ($\dot{V}_E$). It is the product of tidal volume (V_T) and respiratory rate (f).

Part of the minute ventilation merely fills the tracheobronchial tree and does not participate in gas exchange; this volume is called *deadspace* (V_E). There are two types of deadspace: anatomic and alveolar. *Anatomic deadspace* is air in the tracheobronchial tree down through the terminal bronchioles. *Alveolar deadspace* is air in the alveoli that does not participate in gas exchange, because the alveoli containing it are without adequate capillary blood flow. The sum of anatomic deadspace and alveolar deadspace is called *physiologic deadspace.*

The part of minute ventilation that reaches the alveoli and participates in gas exchange is called *alveolar ventilation* ($\dot{V}_A$). Alveolar ventilation equals tidal volume minus deadspace, times respiratory rate; that is, $\dot{V}_A = (V_T - V_D)f$. A normal value is about 5,200 ml, assuming $V_T = 500$, $V_D = 150$, and f = 15. Alveolar ventilation can be either estimated or measured. To estimate it, you must know the tidal volume, respiratory rate, and weight of your patient. Assume that the anatomic deadspace equals 2 ml/kg (1 ml/lb) of body weight, subtract that value from the tidal volume, and multiply by the rate. Note that this formula does not take into account alveolar deadspace and will be inaccurate for patients with either increased alveolar deadspace (as in pulmonary embolism) or altered anatomic deadspace (as in a tracheostomy).

Alveolar ventilation can be calculated more accurately by measuring physiologic deadspace. The patient's expired air is collected for several minutes and analyzed for expired P_{CO_2} ($P_{\bar{E}CO_2}$). The arterial P_{CO_2} (P_aCO_2*) is measured from an arterial blood sample. The values are entered into a modified Bohr equation:

$$VD = VT \times (P_aCO_2 - P_{\bar{E}}CO_2)/P_aCO_2$$

* A subscript written with a capital letter means the gas is in the gaseous phase; a lowercase letter signifies the gas in a liquid phase. Thus, P_{ACO_2} means alveolar P_{CO_2}, whereas P_aCO_2 means arterial P_{CO_2}. A dash above a symbol signifies a mean value. See Table 7–7 for a list of abbreviations and their definitions.

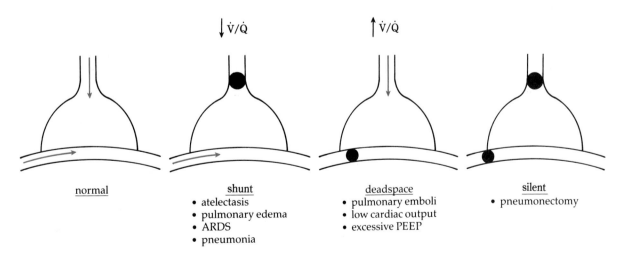

FIGURE 7–12

Types of ventilation-perfusion units.

TABLE 7–7

List of Abbreviations and Symbols for Pulmonary Function

V_T	tidal volume	P_B	atmospheric pressure
FRC	functional residual capacity	Palv	alveolar pressure
ERV	expiratory reserve volume	Ppl	pleural pressure
RV	residual volume	P_{O_2}	partial pressure of oxygen
IC	inspiratory capacity	P_{CO_2}	partial pressure of carbon dioxide
IRV	inspiratory reserve volume	P_{N_2}	partial pressure of nitrogen
TLC	total lung capacity	Pa_{O_2}	partial pressure of oxygen in arterial blood
VC	vital capacity	Pa_{CO_2}	partial pressure of carbon dioxide in arterial blood
Raw	resistance of tracheobronchial tree to flow of air into the lung	PA_{O_2}	partial pressure of oxygen in alveolar gas
C	compliance	PA_{CO_2}	partial pressure of carbon dioxide in alveolar gas
V_D	volume of dead space gas	PA_{H_2O}	partial pressure of water in alveolar gas
V_A	volume of alveolar gas	R	respiratory exchange ratio
$\dot{V}_I$	inspired volume of ventilation per minute	$\dot{Q}$	cardiac output
$\dot{V}_E$	expired volume of ventilation per minute	$\dot{Q}S$	shunt flow
$\dot{V}_A$	alveolar ventilation per minute	Ca_{O_2}	concentration of oxygen in arterial blood
$\dot{V}_{O_2}$	rate of oxygen uptake per minute	$C\bar{v}_{O_2}$	concentration of oxygen in mixed venous blood
$\dot{V}_{CO_2}$	amount of carbon dioxide eliminated per minute	S_{O_2}	percentage saturation of hemoglobin with oxygen
$\dot{V}_{CO}$	rate of carbon monoxide uptake per minute	Sa_{O_2}	percentage saturation of hemoglobin with oxygen in arterial blood
$D_{L_{O_2}}$	diffusing capacity of the lung for oxygen		
$D_{L_{co}}$	diffusing capacity of the lung for carbon monoxide		

(From Guyton A: *Textbook of medical physiology,* 8th ed, Philadelphia: Saunders, 1991, p. 403.)

The value obtained for deadspace then is subtracted from tidal volume. The resulting number is multiplied by rate to calculate alveolar ventilation.

In the normal lung, deadspace is minimized by a protective reflex. When alveolar deadspace increases, the lack of matching perfusion causes local broncho-constriction, which redirects ventilation to better-perfused areas.

V_D/V_T Ratio In the clinical setting, we are less interested in the amount of alveolar ventilation per se than in the ratio between deadspace and tidal volume. This V_D/V_T ratio indicates what proportion of tidal volume is being wasted as deadspace. As explained in further detail later, the P_{CO_2} of arterial blood is a useful indicator of tidal volume. Comparing the P_{CO_2} of arterial blood and the P_{CO_2} of expired gas indicates the amount of wasted ventilation. Rearranging the terms of the modified Bohr equation gives the equation for the V_D/V_T ratio:

$$V_D/V_T = (P_a co_2 - P_{\bar{E}} co_2)/P_a co_2$$

The usual V_D/V_T ratio is approximately 0.3; above 0.6,

it is unlikely that the person can maintain spontaneous ventilation.

Mechanics of Ventilation

In order for air to move in and out of the lungs, the work of breathing must overcome a variety of resistances. These resistances can be subdivided into three categories: airway resistance, tissue resistance, and compliance (Guyton 1991).

Airway Resistance Resistance to gas flow depends on the lumen size, velocity of air flow and gas characteristics. In normal, quiet breathing, airway resistance is slight. Airway resistance can be evaluated by measuring the relationship between pressure and air flow. It is not feasible to measure airway resistance directly in the critically ill, but indirect measurements can be obtained by measuring expiratory flow rates. Airway resistance is affected by factors such as endo-tracheal tube size, bronchospasm, airway edema, and secretions.

Tissue Resistance The tissues of the lung and thorax also have elastic resistances that must be overcome during inspiration. The lung tissues resist inspiration because they contain elastic fibers and because the fluids lining the alveoli have surface tension, as explained below. These factors make the lungs tend to recoil (deflate). The thoracic muscles, tendons, and connective tissue also have elastic properties that make them resist expansion.

Compliance The expansibility of the lungs and chest wall is called *compliance*. It can be evaluated by measuring the relationship between pressure and volume and can be expressed as the change in volume (V) per unit of change in pressure (P): $C = \Delta V / \Delta P$. In the critically ill, effective dynamic compliance equals tidal volume (V_T) divided by inspiratory peak pressure; normal is about 45 ml/cm H_2O. Since peak pressure is affected by resistance in the airway and breathing circuit, a more accurate compliance measure may be effective static compliance. It equals V_T divided by inspiratory plateau pressure (end-inspiratory pressure); normal is about 70 ml/cm H_2O. (If PEEP is used, it is subtracted from the peak inspiratory pressure or the inspiratory plateau pressure, depending on whether dynamic or static compliance is being measured.)

Compliance decreases in conditions that (a) increase the resistance of the chest wall, such as scoliosis, tight dressings, and musculoskeletal diseases such as polio, or that (b) reduce the distensibility of the lung, such as pulmonary congestion, atelectasis, restrictive diseases, and disorders characterized by decreased surfactant. The surface between the alveolar gas and alveolar wall has the property of surface tension, that is, attraction between the surface molecules of the fluid. This property tends to make the alveoli collapse, thereby making expansion very difficult. Surfactant, a lipoprotein made by special alveolar cells, counters this tendency. It progressively decreases surface tension on expiration, thus helping to control alveolar volume and prevent alveolar collapse. When surfactant decreases (as in ARDS), alveolar surface tension increases. Because of the resulting decrease in lung distensibility, compliance decreases.

Significance of Pulmonary Function Tests and Lung Mechanics Measurements

Results of PFTs characterize the patient's lung disorder as either obstructive or restrictive. Chronic Obstructive Pulmonary Disease (COPD) is characterized by decreased expiratory flow rates ($FEV_1 < 70\%$), in- creased lung volumes (FRC, RV/TLC ratio) and, in emphysema, decreased diffusing capacity due to loss of capillary bed. Flow rates are decreased in asthma and chronic bronchitis due to airway inflammation, bronchospasm, and secretions. Restrictive lung disease is characterized by decreased lung volumes as a result of chest wall, pleural, or lung tissue problems. Scoliosis, pulmonary fibrosis, pleural effusion, thoracotomy, and pneumothorax are examples of restrictive processes. Understanding the type of lung disorder and its severity is crucial to developing an individualized plan of care.

The concepts of airway resistance and lung compliance are applied clinically to the care of the mechanically ventilated patient. For example, increased inspiratory pressures might reflect increased lung water or bronchospasm. In addition, a small endotracheal tube increases airway resistance and a tracheostomy decreases deadspace (see Chapter 9). Nursing assessment is aimed at identifying the specific abnormality and implementing appropriate interventions.

Blood Gas Values

Arterial blood gas (ABG) analysis enables the critical-care nurse to evaluate the adequacy of gas exchange in the lungs. The blood sample is obtained by withdrawal from an existing arterial line or by percutaneous puncture of an artery.

Interpreting Blood Gas Values

The laboratory report of arterial blood gases states the Po_2, Pco_2, and a measure of bases in the body (either bicarbonate or base excess). A convenient progression in analyzing these values is first to analyze the partial pressures reported and then to analyze the acid–base values. This chapter reviews the interpretation of partial pressures, which are reported in mm Hg or torr (1 torr = 1 mm Hg at 0°C). Chapter 16 on metabolic imbalances presents the interpretation of acid–base values.

Relationship Among Indices of Oxygenation In order to interpret Po_2 and other indices of oxygenation, the nurse needs a clear understanding of the relationship among them. Because the distinctions among these measurements can be confusing, they are defined in the following sections.

Oxygen is carried in the blood in two ways: about 97% is bound to hemoglobin, and about 3% is dissolved in the blood. The amount of oxygen that fully saturated hemoglobin could carry is 1.34 ml O_2/g hemoglobin. Assuming a normal hemoglobin level of 15 g/100 ml, the hemoglobin could carry 15×1.34 ml = 20.1 ml O_2 in each 100 ml of blood. The amount that can be dissolved in the blood is about 0.3 ml/100 ml blood. The total amount Hgb *could* carry (20.1 ml/100 ml) plus the dissolved amount (0.3 ml/100 ml) is called the *O_2 carrying capacity*. The *actual* amount of oxygen the blood is carrying is the *O_2 content*.

Clinically, the percentage of hemoglobin's binding sites filled with oxygen is measured as *oxygen saturation* (SO_2). The oxygen dissolved in the blood is measured as the *partial pressure of oxygen* (Po_2). Po_2 is the major determinant of SO_2. SO_2 in turn provides a close estimate of O_2 content.

Oxyhemoglobin Dissociation Curve The relationship of Po_2 to O_2 saturation is expressed in the *oxygen-hemoglobin dissociation curve* (Figure 7–13). This relationship is not linear; a given amount of change in Po_2 may be associated with varying amounts of change in O_2 saturation.

It is critical for you to understand the implications of changes in a patient's SO_2 at the bedside and how these changes are reflected on the oxygen-hemoglobin dissociation curve. For example, at a high Po_2 (such as that in lung capillaries), hemoglobin becomes almost completely saturated with O_2, producing a normal O_2 saturation of 95–98% for arterial blood. This fact

enables it to carry O_2 to areas of low Po_2 such as the tissue capillaries. There, Po_2 is about 40 mm Hg; as a result, hemoglobin becomes less saturated, giving up its O_2 to the tissues, which need it for cellular metabolism. The normal saturation for venous blood is about 70–75%.

You will notice that the upper portion of the curve is relatively flat while the middle and lower parts are steep. At the upper end of the curve, a large change in Po_2 is associated with only a small change in O_2 saturation. This fact is the reason we are not very alarmed when a patient's arterial Po_2 drops from 90% to 80%; the hemoglobin still will be well saturated and therefore able to carry O_2 to the tissues. On the steep portion of the curve, however, a change in Po_2 is associated with a much greater effect on O_2 saturation. A drop in arterial Po_2 from 60% to 50%; for instance, indicates a significant reduction in the amount of O_2 carried by hemoglobin to the tissues.

Another important implication of the curve is that an arterial Po_2 over 100 mm Hg does not really benefit a patient, because hemoglobin saturation cannot exceed 100%. In other words, once all hemoglobin molecules are carrying oxygen, adding more oxygen does not increase the amount delivered to the tissues. In fact, high levels of inspired oxygen (i.e., F_IO_2 > 50–60%) can damage alveoli. The goal is to maintain a safe SO_2 or P_aO_2 with the least amount of oxygen administration.

A number of conditions can alter the oxygen-hemoglobin dissociation curve for the patient. Examples are fever and acidosis, which shift the curve to the right, indicating that hemoglobin has less affinity for O_2. With a shift to the right, since less oxygen is picked up in the lungs, O_2 content decreases. At the tissue level, although oxygen is able to dissociate from hemoglobin more easily than normal, the decreased O_2 content limits the amount of oxygen that can be delivered to the tissues. A subnormal temperature or alkalosis will move the curve to the left, causing a higher than usual O_2 saturation, which indicates that hemoglobin has more affinity for O_2. With a shift to the left, lungs pick up more oxygen than normal, so that O_2 content is increased. At the tissue level, however, it is harder than normal for oxygen to dissociate from hemoglobin so oxygen delivery to the tissues is impaired.

Oxygen saturation can be measured in a variety of ways: arterial oxygen saturation (S_aO_2), arterial oxygen saturation by pulse oximetry (S_pO_2) and mixed venous oxygen saturation ($S_{\bar{v}}O_2$). The following sections discuss interpretations of these measurements.

S_aO_2 Interpretation by Pulse Oximetry Pulse oximetry allows continuous monitoring of the critically ill patient's S_aO_2. The pulse oximeter consists of a

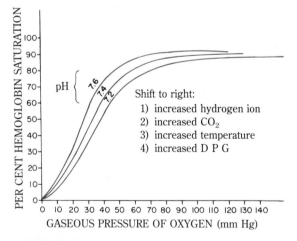

FIGURE 7–13

Shift of the oxygen-hemoglobin dissociation curve to the right by increases in *(1)* hydrogen ions, *(2)* CO_2, *(3)* temperature, or *(4)* DPG. (From Guyton A: *Textbook of medical physiology,* 8th ed. Philadelphia: Saunders, 1991, p. 438.)

sensor, containing pulsating light-emitting diodes (LEDs) and a photodetector, connected by cable to a computer (Figure 7–14). The LEDs beam lights through the tissue. Oxygenated hemoglobin and reduced hemoglobin absorb different amounts of the lights. The detector picks up arterial pulsations and measures the amounts of light absorbed. The computer uses this information to calculate S_pO_2. A continuous reading of this number is provided at the patient's bedside. The normal value for S_pO_2 is 95–100%.

Pulse oximetry provides you with a continuous measurement trend that reflects the effectiveness of interventions or a change in the patient's condition. False or inaccurate readings may occur with shock states, vasoconstriction due to vasopressors or hypothermia, compression of the artery during blood pressure measurement, dyshemoglobinemia, motion artifact, external light sources, intravenous dyes, elevated lipid levels, and elevated venous pressures (Szaflarski and Cohen 1989).

Sensors are available that can be applied to the finger, toe, nose, and ear. The sensor needs to be applied so that the LEDs are in line with the photodetector. Sometimes, the limb can be wrapped in a warm blanket to enhance circulation. Sites should be inspected and rotated regularly. Each unit also has alarm settings to alert you of falling values. Document the S_pO_2 values on the patient flow sheet, especially in conjunction with interventions such as decreasing F_IO_2, titration of hemodynamic agents, position changes, suctioning, weaning or extubation maneuvers, and diuresis. An S_pO_2 of 92–94% ensures adequate oxygenation; below these values (especially $< S_aO_2$ of 90%), oxygenation to the tissues falls off sharply and warrants immediate intervention.

Another limitation of S_pO_2 monitoring is that only oxygenation of blood is measured, not the *delivery* of that blood to the tissue or the needs of the tissue. For example, a shivering, febrile patient with a large myocardial infarction may have adequate S_pO_2 readings, but these do not ensure that the tissues are actually *receiving* adequate blood flow or that the oxygen received is enough to meet the tissue needs. The anemic patient may have 98% of his or her hemoglobin saturated with oxygen but may have a hemoglobin level of only 8 g/100 ml blood. In this situation, oxygen content also would be insufficient to meet tissue needs. In summary, *adequate tissue oxygenation depends on an adequate Po_2 for optimal hemoglo*

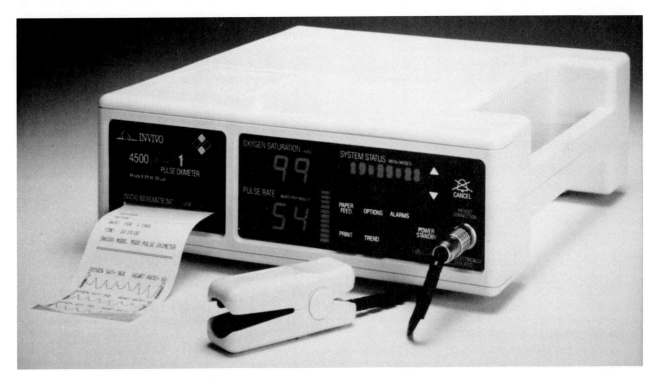

FIGURE 7–14

Invivo 4500-Plus Pulse Oximeter. Reprinted with permission from Invivo Research Incorporated, Winter Park, FL.

bin saturation, *a normal level of hemoglobin* to carry the oxygen, *and satisfactory circulation* to carry the oxygen to the tissues.

P_aO_2 Interpretation　When evaluating P_aO_2 values, make the following observations:

- Note the measured P_aO_2 and the percentage of inspired oxygen at the time the sample was obtained. This percentage usually is expressed as the fractional inspired oxygen concentration, or F_IO_2; the value is given as a decimal. An F_IO_2 of 0.4, for instance, means 40% O_2 concentration. The F_IO_2 of room air is 0.21.

- Compare the actual P_aO_2 and F_IO_2 to the desired P_aO_2 and F_IO_2 for that patient. Ideal values are P_aO_2 of 80–100 mm Hg on an F_IO_2 of 0.21 (room air).

Mixed Venous Blood Values　So far, we have been discussing analysis of arterial blood samples. As arterial blood has not yet reached the systemic tissues, it does not give a full picture of what is happening on the cellular level. In some situations, it is helpful to analyze mixed venous oxygen saturation ($S\bar{v}O_2$) levels. Mixed venous blood cannot be obtained from peripheral veins, as the amount of oxygen consumed by tissues varies in different parts of the body. The PO_2 of peripheral venous blood represents the arterial-venous O_2 difference of only that area of tissue, and varies depending on the area sampled, its metabolic activity, and the distance from the heart. True mixed venous blood is obtained from the distal port of a catheter in the pulmonary artery. By the time blood reaches the pulmonary artery, venous drainage from various peripheral areas, the coronary sinus, and Thebesian veins has become blended, so this blood reflects the state of overall tissue oxygenation.

Alveolar-Arterial O_2 Difference　Often, a critically ill person will have hypoxemia. Identification of the cause is essential for optimal therapy.

Hypoxemia can occur in two general ways: First, the alveolar PO_2 may be low, as in hypoventilation or, rarely, decreased F_IO_2 in high altitudes. Second, alveolar PO_2 may be normal but diffusion into the capillaries may be impaired, as in ventilation/perfusion mismatch, increased shunting, or, rarely, a diffusion block at the alveolar-capillary membrane.

Because the diffusing capacity of carbon dioxide is about twenty times that of oxygen, damage to the

CRITICAL CARE GERONTOLOGY

Pulmonary Assessment Findings in the Elderly

The aging process produces changes in pulmonary assessment findings (Kerston 1989; Knudson 1989). Inspection may reveal a forward bent posture secondary to demineralization of vertebrae. Gradual emphysematous changes take place, resulting in slight lung hyperinflation. Widening of the costal angle (the angle formed by the lower margin of the ribs with the xiphoid process) may occur as a result. Normally this angle is 45 degrees; however, with hyperinflation it may approach (but not reach) 90 degrees. There is a normal decline of expiratory flow rates of 20–50 cc per breath per year of age. In smokers this decline advances to 40–80 cc per breath per year. Diffusing capacity also decreases with age, as a result of gradual loss of capillary bed and fibrotic changes. The calculation for P_aO_2 based on age is: $P_aO_2 = 104.2 - (0.27 \times age)$. Based on this equation, a normal P_aO_2 for a patient 60–80 years old is from 60–80 mm Hg.

ADVANCES IN CRITICAL CARE TECHNOLOGY

$S\bar{v}o_2$ Monitoring

THE TECHNOLOGY

Current technology allows for continuous monitoring of mixed venous oxygen saturation ($S\bar{v}o_2$) values from specially designed pulmonary artery catheters (Figure 7–15). The monitoring device is used in critically ill patients to supply the nurse with information about the balance of oxygen and demand. After the blood is oxygenated in the lungs and delivered by the cardiac output, the tissues extract the oxygen that they need. What returns to the right heart (mixed venous blood) reflects the "leftover" oxygen which can be measured as $S\bar{v}o_2$ (Figure 7-16). Normal $S\bar{v}o_2$ values are 60–80% (see Table 7–8). A continuous digital reading at the bedside alerts the nurse to an imbalance between oxygen supply and demand at the tissue level. This monitoring device also has a memory and can print out trends over the previous 24 hours.

Patient Care Considerations Abnormal readings alert you to evaluate factors affecting oxygen supply and demand. On the supply side, factors that reduce the tissues' oxygen supply (producing decreased $S\bar{v}o_2$ values) are decreased arterial oxygen saturation, inadequate cardiac output (the pump or delivery system), and reduced hemoglobin level (the carrier of oxygen). On the demand side, factors that increase the tissues' need for oxygen (producing decreased $S\bar{v}o_2$ values) are fever, shivering, seizures, pain, anxiety, increased work of breathing, burns, bed weights, portable chest x-ray, turning, and chest physiotherapy (Figure 7–17). Conditions that decrease tissue oxygen needs (producing increased $S\bar{v}o_2$ values) include sedation, paralysis, anesthesia, and hypothermia. A left-to-right cardiac shunt would falsely elevate $S\bar{v}o_2$ readings due to arterial admixture on the right side of the heart.

If, for example, you have a febrile, septic patient who has suffered a myocardial infarction, the cardiac output may not be able to increase sufficiently to meet increased tissue oxygen needs. In this case, the tissue will extract more than the normal amount of oxygen, leaving the mixed venous blood less saturated, as reflected by an $S\bar{v}o_2 < 60\%$.

In this patient, you might decrease oxygen demand by treating the fever with ordered antipyretics and sedating the patient to alleviate pain and anxiety. Oxygen supply could be increased by titrating hemodynamic agents to optimize cardiac output, correcting any anemia, and assessing for signs of lung congestion and the need for diuretics. Treatments such as bedweights, turning, or suctioning might be postponed until $S\bar{v}o_2$ values rose to a safe level, thus preventing complications of prolonged tissue hypoxia (White et al. 1990).

---

alveolar-capillary membrane affects oxygen diffusion long before it affects carbon dioxide diffusion. In the clinical setting, oxygen diffusing capacity cannot be measured directly. Instead, the adequacy of diffusing capacity can be inferred from the alveolar-arterial oxygen difference (A-aDo$_2$), sometimes called the *alveolar-arterial (A–a) gradient.*

Formula for Calculation The A-aDo$_2$ can be calculated from a set of arterial blood gas values on a known oxygen percentage. A simplified version of the alveolar gas equation is used:

$$P_Ao_2 = P_Io_2 - P_Aco_2/R$$

In other words, the Po$_2$ of alveolar air equals the inspired Po$_2$, minus the alveolar Pco$_2$ divided by the respiratory exchange ratio (R). The respiratory exchange ratio is the amount of CO$_2$ produced divided by

the amount of oxygen consumed; the usual value on a mixed diet is 0.8. P_Aco_2 is assumed equal to P_aco_2, so the equation becomes:

$$P_Ao_2 = P_Io_2 - P_aco_2/0.8$$

To determine P_Ao_2, the appropriate values for P_Io_2 and P_aco_2 are entered in the equation and the alveolar Po$_2$ is calculated. Finally, the difference between the alveolar and arterial Po$_2$ (the A-aDo$_2$) is determined by subtracting the measured P_ao_2 from the calculated P_Ao_2.

Clinical Significance of Values If the blood gases are drawn on room air, the normal A-aDo$_2$ is less than 15 mm Hg. If the hypoxemic patient has a normal A-aDo$_2$, the cause of the hypoxemia probably is an inadequate alveolar Po$_2$, that is, hypoventilation. If the patient has an increased A-aDo$_2$, the hypoxemia probably results

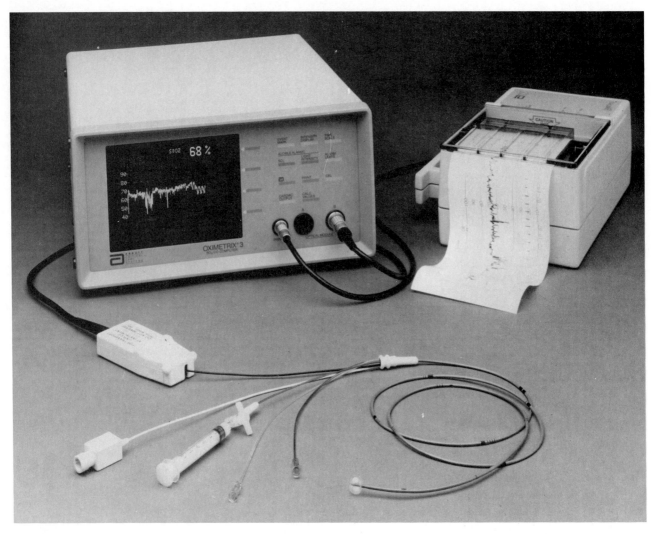

FIGURE 7–15

Oximetrix (Abbott) mixed venous oxygen saturation ($S\bar{v}o_2$) monitor with Swan-Ganz catheter attached. Reprinted with permission from Abbott Laboratories, © ACCS/ Abbott.

from a problem at the alveolar-capillary level. Although theoretically such a problem could be due to uneven ventilation, alveolar-capillary block, or shunt, using 100% O_2 almost completely eliminates the first two causes. Therefore, an increased A-aDo_2 on 100% O_2 most likely is due to an increased shunt.

Shunt and Increased A-aDo_2 *Physiologic shunt* is the percentage of CO that represents wasted perfusion because it does not exchange gas in the alveoli. It is subdivided into: (a) anatomic shunt, (b) capillary shunt, and (c) $\dot{V}/\dot{Q}$ mismatch or venous admixture (Shapiro et al. 1991).

Anatomic shunt is that portion of CO that anatomically bypasses the pulmonary capillaries and returns, unoxygenated, to the left atrium. Normally, it results from venous drainage from the bronchial, pleural, and Thebesian veins and represents 2–5% of CO. It accounts for the fact that arterial Po_2 normally is slightly lower (95 mm Hg) than alveolar Po_2 (100 mm Hg). Abnormal venoarterial communications such as right-to-left cardiac shunts increase anatomic shunt.

Capillary shunt is that portion of CO that goes through pulmonary capillaries in contact with completely unventilated alveoli. Because it does not exchange with alveolar gas, it also returns unoxygenated to the left atrium. The sum of anatomic and capillary shunt is referred to as *true shunt* or *absolute shunt*.

The third type of shunt, $\dot{V}/\dot{Q}$ *mismatch* or *venous admixture,* occurs in a unit that is well perfused but

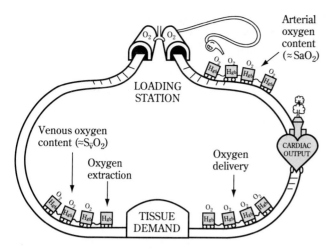

FIGURE 7–16

Mixed venous oxygen saturation (From American Edwards Labs: "Understanding continuous mixed venous oxygen saturation monitoring with the Swan-Ganz Oximetry TD system" information pamphlet, p. 8 Irvine, CA: Baxter Healthcare Corporation, © 1992.

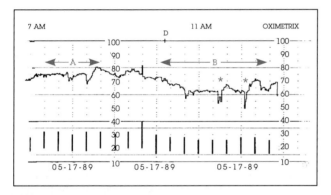

FIGURE 7–17

Svo_2 readout interpretation. **a,** normal readings from 70–80%; **b,** decreased readings during change from assist-control mode to spontaneous breathing with increased agitation and work of breathing; *, suctioning.

poorly ventilated. Blood returning to the heart from this unit has a lower Po_2 than blood returning from a normal unit. $\dot{V}/\dot{Q}$ mismatch is responsive to oxygen therapy.

Shunting is minimized in the normal lung by a protective reflex. When shunting increases, diminished or absent local ventilation causes a low P_AO_2. The local blood vessels constrict, redirecting flow to better-ventilated areas. $\dot{V}/\dot{Q}$ mismatch may be due to failure of this protective reflex or to diffuse disease of the lung or vasculature, which prevents adequate matching or compensation. Nursing interventions such as suc-

TABLE 7–8

Mixed Venous Blood Values and Arterial Blood Values Compared

	ARTERIAL BLOOD	MIXED VENOUS BLOOD
Po_2	80–100 mm Hg	35–40 mm Hg
O_2 saturation	95% or above	70–75%
O_2 content	19.8 ml O_2/100 ml blood	15.5 ml O_2/100 ml blood

tioning, repositioning, and hyperinflation maneuvers are aimed at decreasing shunting and improving oxygenation.

Evaluating P_aco_2 Carbon dioxide is produced by cellular metabolism and eliminated by the lungs. In the blood, it is carried in three forms (Guyton 1991). About 70% is converted to bicarbonate in this reaction:

$$CO_2 + H_2O \rightleftharpoons H_2CO_3 \rightleftharpoons H^+ + HCO_3^-$$

In other words, carbon dioxide combines with water to form carbonic acid, which then dissociates to a hydrogen ion and a bicarbonate ion. An enzyme called *carbonic anhydrase* facilitates the formation of carbonic acid. Because much more carbonic anhydrase is contained in red blood cells than in plasma, most of the body's bicarbonate is formed in the red blood cells. It then diffuses out of the cells into the plasma, where it is carried. About 20% of the CO_2 is carried in combination with hemoglobin and plasma proteins. About the last 10% is physically dissolved in the blood. It is the pressure of this dissolved CO_2 that is measured in P_aco_2.

Normal P_aco_2 is 35–45 mm Hg. P_aco_2 varies with both the production of carbon dioxide and its elimination by the lungs. Altered P_aco_2 levels reflect changes in alveolar ventilation. A decreased P_aco_2 indicates hyperventilation, as in hypoxia or compensation for metabolic acidosis. An increased P_aco_2 (hypercapnia or hypercarbia) indicates hypoventilation, as in respiratory center depression, increased V_D/V_T ratio, or compensation for metabolic alkalosis. The P_aco_2 is a better indicator of alveolar ventilation than is the patient's P_aO_2. Abnormal CO_2 values are caused only by abnormal ventilation; abnormal O_2 values can be caused by many factors. Continuous assessment of alveolar CO_2 can be done at the bedside of mechanically ventilated patients with end-tidal CO_2 monitors, discussed in Chapter 9.

Diagnostic Procedures

Chest X-ray

Reading the chest x-ray report is another step in assessing a patient's aeration status. A basic understanding of chest x-ray interpretation is useful in reading x-ray reports and understanding medical discussions of your patient's condition. Occasionally, too, you may be the first person to see an abnormal film; your ability to spot abnormalities needing urgent attention may enable you to obtain medical therapy immediately for your patient. The following information is based on Kersten (1989) and Jacquith (1986).

Different substances allow varying amounts of x-ray radiation to pass through them and strike the film, producing different x-ray densities. Because bone absorbs most of the radiation and allows very little to strike the film, it produces a white color. Soft tissues and blood absorb less amount of energy and appear gray. Lungs appear black because they allow most of the radiation to pass through. When the x-ray beam traverses several structures of different densities, it will produce an image combining their densities.

In examining a film, follow a logical sequence such as the one indicated in Table 7–9. The most significant principle to remember is that you can see a structure only if the density of its edge contrasts with the surrounding density.

Normal Characteristics The normal chest film has the following pulmonary characteristics (Figure 7–18). (For a diagram view of the chest and internal structures, see Figure 7–19.)

The ribs are intact and can be traced starting from their more superior attachment to the spine. The spine usually is straight and can be seen through the heart shadow in a film of good quality. The clavicles, visible in the upper thorax, are intact and equidistant, indicating the person was centered properly.

The hemidiaphragms appear rounded. The upper edge of each hemidiaphragm is visible because of the contrast between air and water densities. The right hemidiaphragm usually is slightly higher than the left because of the liver. On the left hemidiaphragm, the lower edge may be visible because the stomach often contains air. The lower edge of the right hemidiaphragm should not be visible. If it is, it signifies free air in the abdomen, such as from a perforated ulcer. The lateral angles between the diaphragm and ribs (the costophrenic angles) are clear. The pleura is not visible.

The trachea is midline, with the carina visible at the level of the aortic knob or at the second intercostal

TABLE 7–9

Chest X-Ray Interpretation

1. Look at the soft tissues of the chest wall and for the breast.
2. Examine the bony thorax, including the clavicles, scapula, ribs, humeri, and cervical and thoracic spines.
3. Look at the soft tissues of the neck.
4. Examine the width of the intercostal spaces.
5. Examine the diaphragm and the area below the diaphragm.
6. Examine the pleura and the costophrenic sulci.
7. Look at the mediastinum in both the frontal and lateral projections.
8. Look at the trachea and bronchial tree.
9. Look at the heart and the great vessels, making sure that no area is silhouetted out.
10. Look at the lung fields, being sure to compare both sides.
11. Look at the hila.
12. Look at the peripheral pulmonary vascularity.

space. The aortic knob, which is formed by the arch of the aorta, is seen as a knoblike water density to the left of the spine.

The heart appears solid, since the blood in it and its walls are the same density. The edges of the heart are clear because of the contrast with the surrounding air density of the lung.

Just above the heart, small bilateral water densities are visible. These densities mark the hila, where the pulmonary vessels and bronchi join the lungs. The left hilum usually is slightly higher than the right because the left main pulmonary artery is higher and more posterior than the right. Lesser vascular markings (also called *lung markings*) are seen out to the edge of the lung fields; they are more prominent in the lower lungs when the person is upright. Because the vascular markings are water density, they cause the lung fields to look like a wispy air density. Beyond a small amount of mainstem bronchus visible to about one inch out from the hila, the bronchi usually cannot be seen. They have thin walls, and since they are filled with air, they do not contrast with the air density of the surrounding lung.

Individual lobes of the lung can be identified because the lobes are separated by fissures (also called septa). These interlobar septa are visible in different projections. Septa between lobules (interlobular septa) normally cannot be seen.

Abnormal Signs Important signs you may see or hear discussed are the silhouette sign and the air bronchogram.

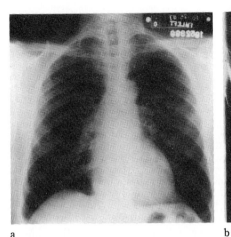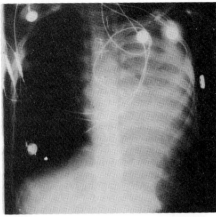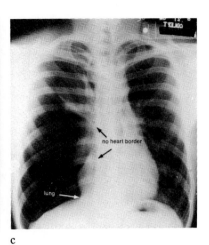

a   b   c

FIGURE 7–18

Chest x-rays. **a,** Normal posteroanterior (PA) chest film taken from 6 feet away, with the patient standing, and with as much of the anterior chest touching the plate as possible. Note that the normal heart is really quite small. **b,** A problem in the left lung is obvious in this X-ray; note the air bronchogram sign on the left indicating atelectasis. The air bronchogram clearly delineates the bronchus as it passes into the lower lobes of the left lung; left upper lobe bronchus is not visible indicating the probable presence of a mucous plug in that area. Vigorous endotracheal suctioning with ventilatory therapy produced significant clearing in 24 hours in this four-year-old girl. X-ray was taken two days post open heart surgery. Note endotracheal tube and wires used to close the sternum. **c,** The pneumothorax here is very extensive. Note that pressure in the right hemithorax must be greater than in the left, because the heart and other mediastinal structures are shifted away from the free air. This is a tension pneumothorax. Air entering the right pleural space is unable to escape because of a ball-valve effect, and each inspiration increases the intrapleural pressure. Prompt diagnosis and treatment, perhaps even with a large-bore needle at first, are essential, often lifesaving. (From Tinker JH: Understanding chest x-rays. *Am J Nurs* 1976; 7:1:54–58. Courtesy John H. Tinker, MD and *American Journal of Nursing.*)

Silhouette Sign You will recall that in order for a structure to be visible, the density of its edge must contrast with the surrounding density. The loss of contrast is called the *silhouette sign;* it indicates that the densities of the two structures have become the same and that the structures are in direct contact with one another. This sign is useful in localizing processes that increase the water content of the lung, such as pneumonia and infiltrates. For instance, since the heart is an anterior organ, the complete loss of the right cardiac silhouette implies that the pathology lies anteriorly (in the upper or middle lobes) in an area in anatomic contact with the heart. A shadow overlapping a border without obliterating a silhouette implies that the process is located in the lower (posterior) lobes, the posterior mediastinum, or the posterior pleural cavity.

Air Bronchogram Sign Another sign of a process that is making part of the lung have a water density is the *air bronchogram sign.* You will remember that the bronchi normally cannot be seen because they and the

surrounding lung are both of air density. When a process (such as pneumonia or pulmonary edema) makes the lung tissue have a water density, the contrast makes the bronchi visible, unless the bronchi themselves are filled with secretions or destroyed. The appearance of the air bronchogram sign identifies the disorder as intrapulmonary.

Easily Identified Abnormalities Differential diagnosis of chest x-ray findings is a complex science beyond the scope of this book. However, you will encounter some abnormalities so frequently that they are worth reviewing here: collapse, pneumothorax, consolidation, pleural effusion, and pulmonary edema.

Collapse Collapse of a part of the lung has many causes. One is bronchial obstruction followed by absorption of the air remaining in that area of the lung (atelectasis). Another cause is compression, such as from air in the pleural space. A third cause is contraction, such as in pulmonary fibrosis.

Collapse is diagnosed by displacement of the septa,

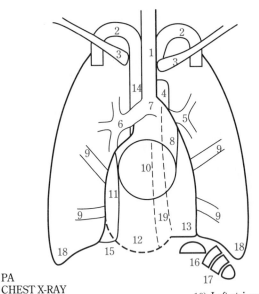

PA
CHEST X-RAY

1) Trachea
2) First rib
3) Clavicle
4) Aortic knob
5) Left pulmonary artery
6) Right pulmonary artery
7) Carina
8) Pulmonary trunk
9) Pulmonary veins
10) Left atrium
11) Right atrium
12) Right ventricle
13) Left ventricle
14) Superior vena cava
15) Inferior vena cava
16) Gastric air bubble
17) Splenic flexure air
18) Costophrenic angles
19) Descending aorta

FIGURE 7–19

Structures seen on a PA (posteroanterior) chest x-ray film. (From Gomella L (ed): *Clinician's Pocket Reference*, 6th ed. East Norwalk, CT: Appleton & Lange, 1989, p. 166.

crowding of the vascular markings or air bronchograms, and increased radiopacity of the lung tissue. Other signs sometimes seen are shift of the trachea toward the area of collapse (if the upper lobes are involved), displacement of the hilum, increased closeness of the ribs, elevation of the diaphragm on the affected side, and compensatory overexpansion of the adjacent parts of the lung causing increased radiolucency in those areas.

Pneumothorax If you see an area of clear blackness (that is, no lung markings), it probably results from a pneumothorax. As air rises, look at the apices for this sign on an upright or semirecumbent film. Other signs you may see are increased radiopacity of the collapsed lung tissue, depression of the diaphragm, and tracheal and mediastinal shift away from the pneumothorax. The findings may be more apparent on an expiratory film, because during exhalation the air-filled pleural space contrasts better with the more-solid compressed lung tissue.

Consolidation Areas of increased density (whiteness) are referred to as areas of consolidation. The numerous causes of consolidation can be broadly grouped into those that collapse the lung tissue, thereby making it more dense, and those that increase the fluid content of the lung. Increases in density due to fluid accumulation may be diffuse or localized. Diffuse increases are seen in pulmonary edema and pneumonia, as well as in other disorders. They can be differentiated on the basis of associated signs, such as air bronchograms, and the pattern of fluid distribution.

Pleural Effusion Localized increases in density due to fluid are usually pleural effusions. Fluid that causes partial or complete obliteration of the costophrenic angle on an upright film probably is *free pleural fluid*. When a film is taken with the patient on the side or back, this fluid will appear in the dependent part of the chest cavity. Fluid that does not shift with position is called *encapsulated* or *loculated*.

Pulmonary Edema Pulmonary edema results from pulmonic vascular congestion so severe that the oncotic pressure of the blood is no longer able to maintain normal fluid dynamics across the capillary membrane. The resulting edema fluid is taken up by the pulmonary lymphatics at the hilar region. The main pulmonary artery and hilar branches increase in radiologic prominence due to the increased pressure. When the edema becomes severe, alveolar flooding or "white-out" is seen.

These descriptions, although brief, will enable you to better interpret chest x-ray film reports and spot common abnormalities on chest films.

Lung Scans

Two types of lung scans can be performed: *perfusion scans* and *ventilation scans*. A *perfusion scan* is performed to evaluate arterial pulmonary blood flow and to detect pulmonary emboli. Patient preparation involves explanation of the purpose and technique of the

---

NURSING TIP

Chest X-ray

To prepare for a chest x-ray, position the patient as upright as possible without rotation. If the patient is rotated in the bed, the chest x-ray film will be distorted. Move as many tubes and monitoring lines off the chest as possible.

test. It is unnecessary to withhold food or fluids. The scan takes approximately 30 minutes to perform. A radioactive contrast agent is injected via a peripheral vein in the arm. The agent used most often is human albumin tagged with technetium. After injection, a scintillation camera records distribution of the agent while the patient is in the supine position. The procedure then is repeated with the patient in a prone position. As with cardiac technetium scans, areas with normal perfusion show high uptake of the agent. The normal scan shows complete, even distribution. Areas of low uptake appear as "cold spots" and suggest the presence of an embolus.

A *ventilation scan* is performed to evaluate the distribution of ventilation after the patient inhales a radioactive gas, usually xenon. A nuclear scanner records gas distribution during the buildup phase, equilibrium phase, and washout phase (as the gas is removed from the lungs). A normal scan shows equal distribution during all phases. Uneven gas distribution or areas of slow washout indicate poor ventilation. The ventilation scan is particularly helpful when interpreted in conjunction with a perfusion scan. In diseases of the lung parenchyma, such as emphysema or pneumonia, ventilation is diminished. In pulmonary vascular conditions, ventilation is maintained but perfusion is decreased. Comparison of ventilation and perfusion scans thus is particularly helpful in the diagnosis of pulmonary embolism. Patient preparation is the same as that for perfusion scanning. You need provide no post-procedure care beyond continuing to provide emotional support while the patient waits for the diagnosis and therapeutic strategy recommendations.

Bronchoscopy

Bronchoscopy is a diagnostic or therapeutic procedure that utilizes a rigid metal bronchoscope or flexible fiberoptic bronchoscope to provide direct visualization of the tracheobronchial tree. The *rigid bronchoscope* sometimes is used to remove foreign objects and bronchial lesions. The *fiberoptic bronchoscope* is used more frequently because it is safer, it is more comfortable for the patient, and it allows a greater viewing range because of its smaller size and flexibility. The fiberoptic bronchoscope is able to reach as far as the subsegmental bronchi. The examination and biopsy of lung nodules and identification of interstitial diseases are the most common diagnostic purposes. Broncho-alveolar lavage and transbronchial lung biopsy are also useful in the diagnosis and assessment of various infectious lung disorders. Therapeutic purposes include easing a difficult intubation, changing endotracheal tubes, reversing whole lung or lobar atelectasis,

removing secretions and mucous plugs, controlling hemoptysis, and excising endobronchial lesions (Ahmad 1988; Chan and Hyland 1989).

Patient preparation includes a brief explanation of the purpose of the procedure, the steps involved, and the sensations to expect. Food and liquids usually are withheld for 6–8 hours pre-procedure. Atropine may be administered prior to the procedure to reduce secretions and the danger of a vasovagal response. A sedative is also given.

The patient is positioned in semi-Fowler's position or sits upright. A local anesthetic is sprayed into the nose and mouth to abolish the gag reflex. The anesthetic has a bitter taste and it is useful to alert the patient that the unpleasant taste is normal. When anesthesia occurs, the patient may have the sensation that there is something caught in the back of the throat that cannot be expelled. This is an alarming sensation, and the person should be reassured that it is normal and that the airway will not be blocked during the procedure. Encourage the person to breathe through the nose, or pant, and to relax. If the patient is on a ventilator, a special adapter allows passage of the bronchoscope. During a bronchoscopy on a mechanically ventilated patient, tidal volume decreases, P_aO_2 decreases, and P_aCO_2 rises. The patient should be placed on 100% oxygen; PEEP should be discontinued and suctioning time minimized.

Nursing care during the procedure focuses on patient monitoring and emotional support. Continuous monitoring of hemodynamics and S_aO_2 is essential. Complications can include laryngospasm, bronchospasm, hypoxemia, bleeding, drug reactions, hypotension, and dysrhythmias (Ahmad 1988). To minimize hypoxemia, supplemental oxygen is administered before, during, and after the procedure. Complication rates are quite low, with minor complications at 0.2%, major complications at 0.8%, and a mortality rate of 0.01% (Ahmad 1988).

Post-procedure nursing care includes observation for the described complications. Food and fluids are withheld until the gag reflex returns, several hours post-procedure. Hoarseness, sore throat, and blood-streaked sputum are common and may subside spontaneously or be treated with local analgesics such as lozenges or throat sprays.

Pulmonary Angiography

Pulmonary angiography is an invasive diagnostic procedure in which the pulmonary vascular tree is visualized following injection of a contrast medium. It is used primarily to diagnose pulmonary embolism when scan results are equivocal.

Patient preparation includes a brief description of the technique and an explanation of its value in diagnosing disorders. Food and fluids are withheld for 6–8 hours prior to the test.

The procedure is performed in an angiography laboratory. The patient is placed supine, a cardiac monitor is attached, and an IV peripheral line is started if one is not already in place. Local anesthetic is injected into the groin, a small incision is made, and a catheter is introduced and passed up through the right atrium and the right ventricle into the pulmonary artery. The contrast agent is injected into the right and/or left pulmonary artery, depending on the results from the $\dot{V}/\dot{Q}$ scan, and x-rays are taken. At the time of the injection, the patient may experience a flushed feeling or nausea, either of which usually passes rapidly.

The normal distribution of dye through the pulmonary vascular tree is unimpeded and symmetric. Areas of narrowing may indicate stenosis, and areas of complete occlusion (cutoff) usually indicate emboli.

Complications of this procedure may include ventricular dysrhythmias from catheter stimulation of the myocardium, myocardial perforation, right ventricular failure, and allergic reaction to the dye. After the procedure, a pressure dressing is applied over the insertion site. Post-procedure complications and care are similar to those for cardiac catheterization and include monitoring for bleeding and hematoma formation, arterial occlusion, hypotension related to osmotic diureses, and delayed allergic reaction.

Thoracentesis

Thoracentesis is the procedure used to remove fluid from the pleural space. It can be done as either a diagnostic or a therapeutic modality. After receiving an explanation of the procedure, the patient is placed in the upright position and the lower posterior chest is prepared and anesthetized. A needle is introduced into the pleural space, and either a small amount of fluid is withdrawn for lab analysis or as much fluid as possible is withdrawn to evacuate the effusion. A biopsy of the pleura may also be obtained in this manner. The major complication is pneumothorax, so a post-procedure chest film should always be obtained. The patient should also be observed for any onset of respiratory distress.

Computed Tomography

Computed tomography (CT) is a newer imaging technique that allows visualization of pulmonary le-

sions not readily seen on a routine chest film. It is also useful in identifying pleural and chest wall anatomy, infective processes, and the pleural effects of occupational lung diseases. High-resolution CT enables visualization of interstitial or airway processes, such as bronchiectasis and bronchiolitis. Critically ill patients are transported to the CT area accompanied by a nurse and monitored closely during the scan.

Magnetic Resonance Imaging

Magnetic resonance imaging (MRI) has the advantage over CT of being able to differentiate lung tumors from normal tissues, particularly in the mediastinum and hilar areas. These techniques play an important role in the assessment of lung cancers. An explanation of MRI is contained in Chapter 4.

Open Lung Biopsy

In the event that a diagnosis cannot be made using the previously described techniques, it may be necessary to surgically enter the chest via thoracotomy and obtain a biopsy specimen. Care of the thoracotomy patient is covered in Chapter 9.

REFERENCES

Ahmad M: Therapeutic bronchoscopy. In *Current respiratory care* Kazmarek R (ed.) Toronto: Decker, 1988.

Benner P, Tanner C: Clinical judgement: How expert nurses use intuition. *Am J Nurs* 1987; 87:23–31.

Carrieri V et al.: The sensation of dyspnea: A review. *Heart Lung* 1984; 13:436–447.

Chan C, Hyland R: New diagnostic techniques. In *Current therapy of respiratory disease,* 3d ed., Cherniack R (ed). Decker, 1989.

Cherniak R, Cherniak L: *Respiration in Health and Disease,* 3d ed., Saunders, 1983.

Guyton A: *Textbook of medical physiology,* 8th ed. Saunders, 1991.

Jacquith S: Chest x-ray interpretation: Implications for nursing intervention. *DCCN* 1986; 5(1):8–19.

Kersten L: *Comprehensive respiratory nursing.* Saunders, 1989.

Knudson R: Aging of the respiratory system. In *Current pulmonology.* Simmons D (ed.) Chicago: Year Book, 1989.

Mahler D (ed): *Dyspnea.* Futura Publishing, 1990.

Szaflarski N, Cohen N: Use of pulse oximetry in critically ill adults. *Heart Lung* 1989; 18(5):444–453.

White K et al.: The physiology basis for continuous mixed venous oxygen saturation monitoring. *Heart Lung;* 1990; 10(5):548–551.

8

Pulmonary Disorders

CLINICAL INSIGHT

Domain: Monitoring and ensuring the quality of health care practices

Competency: Getting appropriate and timely responses from physicians

The alliance between nursing and medicine in the critical-care unit can be an awkward one at times. A nurse who knows what she or he wants from a physician can be a sight to behold—resolute and determined. There's a fine line—some might say a tightrope—between being respectful of the physician's expertise and authority and being persistent in getting medical attention in a particular situation.

To present a convincing case to physicians, nurses learn to speak the language of medicine, to be conversant with the highly physiologically oriented knowledge base traditionally within the purview only of physicians. Most physicians appreciate a nurse's alerting them to a problem, but an individual physician's recep-

tivity to a nurse's approach may be less than ideal. Remaining persistent in the face of sometimes brusque or dismissive responses requires a solid experiential base and, at times, personal courage. Nurses also learn the value of timing, of knowing a physician's idiosyncracies, and of assertiveness in dealing with touchy or inadequate responses, as the following exemplar shows (Benner 1984, pp. 142–143):

A patient was admitted with a diagnosis of thrombophlebitis. He had been on heparin therapy for about two days. . . . The report from the night shift said that he had had a difficult night. He had been having pain, more than usual. The intern on call was phoned, but did not come up to see the man. Instead Demerol was ordered I.M. Because the I.M. medication did not relieve the pain, the nurse phoned the intern again. By this time the nurse told the doctor that the patient was slightly short of breath. But the intern thought the nurse was being an alarmist and did not come up to see the man. The doctor then ordered Percodan. By 7 A.M. when I went in to see the patient, the man was clammy, cool, restless, and his vital signs were changing. He was more short of breath . . . , diaphoretic, had thready pulse, and was still in pain. I phoned the intern who regularly followed him and recounted the events of the night. He listened, paused, and then asked if I was calling to get more pain medication for the man. In a controlled manner I told him that something was going wrong with his patient and that giving him more narcotics would not solve the problem. I also said that I was calling because I wanted a doctor to see this man NOW. The intern came right up, and not a minute too soon. The man's level of consciousness was dramatically changing for the worse as were his vital signs. The patient had an infarction in his lung. Fortunately, swift action was taken and a specialist was called who, through surgery, was able to save the man's life and lung. The intern thanked me for my persistence in getting the patient seen promptly.

Persistence, like that demonstrated in the Clinical Insight exemplar, requires conviction in your understanding of the care a patient needs and confidence in your skills. This chapter is intended to help you provide nursing care that can anticipate, prevent, recognize, and alleviate various types of acute and chronic respiratory failure. *Respiratory failure* is defined as the inability of the cardiopulmonary system to provide adequate oxygenation and/or carbon dioxide removal to meet tissue metabolic needs. Respiratory failure may be further categorized as either failure of oxygenation, as in pulmonary edema, or ventilatory failure, as in chronic bronchitis and emphysema. The diagnosis is based on clinical assessment of the patient plus laboratory data.

The many respiratory disorders that can predispose or directly cause respiratory failure are divided into two primary categories. Those that affect lung expansion are classified as *restrictive* disorders, with the defect being either inside the lung tissue, as in pneumonia, or outside the lung tissue. Defects outside the lung tissue that restrict lung excursion may be pleural processes, chest wall problems, respiratory muscle problems, or other causes (Table 8–1). *Obstructive* disorders such as asthma, emphysema, and bronchitis are characterized by decreased airflow

TABLE 8-1

Classification of Restrictive Disorders

OUTSIDE LUNG	INSIDE LUNG
Pleural Processes	*Lung Tissue Restriction*
Pleural effusion	Surgical resection (thoracotomy)
Hemothorax	
Chylothorax	Atelectasis
Empyema	Pneumonia
Pneumothorax	Diffuse interstitial fibrosis
Pleuritis	Granulomatous disease (sarcoidosis)
Chest Wall Problems	Collagen disease (scleroderma)
Kyphoscoliosis	Pneumoconioses (silicosis, asbestosis)
Pectus excavatum	
Obesity	Neoplastic disease
Respiratory Muscle Problems	Vascular disease (pulmonary edema, adult respiratory distress syndrome, pulmonary hypertension)
Muscular dystrophy	
Guillain-Barré syndrome	
Myasthenia gravis	
Paralysis	
Other	
Abdominal distention	
Pregnancy	
Chest binders	
CNS disturbances	

through the bronchi and smaller airways. Pulmonary emboli are actually a result of a problem outside of the lung but are sometimes referred to as a type of pulmonary vascular disease.

The following discussions focus on the most common conditions seen in the critical-care units of each category of respiratory disease. Restrictive disorders are the most common causes of acute respiratory failure in the critical-care unit, while obstructive disorders are the most common causes of chronic respiratory failure. The patient with stable chronic obstructive pulmonary disease (COPD) may be admitted to the critical-care unit for another disorder, e.g., cardiac surgery. The COPD patient also may develop an acute restrictive defect, such as pneumonia, which exacerbates chronic respiratory failure and may precipitate superimposed acute respiratory failure.

RESTRICTIVE DISORDERS

Cardiogenic Pulmonary Edema

Pulmonary edema (excess fluid in the interstitial and/or alveolar spaces) results from two basic mechanisms. In the first, increased hydrostatic pressure in the pulmonary capillaries causes fluid to move across intact capillary membranes. This increased hydrostatic pressure can result from cardiac dysfunction and elevated left-heart pressures or from decreased pulmonary lymphatic drainage. This type of pulmonary edema sometimes is called *high-pressure pulmonary edema.* If it results from cardiac dysfunction, it may be termed *cardiogenic pulmonary edema.* In the second type of pulmonary edema, left-heart pressures are normal, but "leaky" capillary membranes (more permeable than normal) allow excessive fluid movement. This type is referred to as *normal-pressure or noncardiogenic pulmonary edema.* High-pressure pulmonary edema is discussed in the section that follows. Normal-pressure pulmonary edema is discussed in the next section (adult respiratory distress syndrome).

Assessment

Risk Conditions Recognize patients at risk for acute pulmonary edema; prevent it when possible. Conditions that increase risk include:

- Increased pulmonary capillary pressure: fluid overload, acute myocardial infarction (MI), severe mitral stenosis, advanced aortic stenosis, severe hypertension, massive pulmonary embolism.
- Decreased lymphatic drainage: pneumonia, pulmonary contusion, microemboli, and increased central venous pressure (because lymphatics empty into systemic veins).

Prevention of Risk Consider ways to prevent the above conditions. Some examples follow. Closely monitor intake and output to avoid circulatory overload. If the patient has a pulmonary artery line, closely monitor hemodynamic readings for increased pulmonary capillary wedge pressure (PCWP) and increased pulmonary artery diastolic pressure (PAD), which reflect left ventricular end-diastolic pressure. If cardiac catheterization data are available, learning the ejection fraction will help you determine the risk of pump failure (see Chapter 13). Minimize physical and emotional stress to

decrease left ventricular workload. Teach the stable patient with chronic heart disease the importance of continuing medications at home, the symptoms of congestive heart failure, and the need for prompt medical attention if symptoms occur. Prevent acute MI and shock as outlined in Chapter 13.

Signs and Symptoms The signs and symptoms of pulmonary edema are those of increased work of breathing, hypoxia, and fluid-filled alveoli. Pulmonary edema can be sudden in onset and present as a medical emergency with respiratory arrest and cardiovascular collapse.

Observe for signs of increased work of breathing due to decreased lung compliance, for example, use of accessory muscles, intercostal and supraclavicular retractions, expiratory wheeze, rapid, shallow respiratory pattern, and increased anxiety. Check for signs of hypoxia, such as tachypnea, tachycardia, hypertension, severe apprehension, diaphoresis, dysrhythmias, and peripheral vasoconstriction. Note signs of transudation of fluid into alveoli—profuse, frothy, pink sputum; cough; and crackles. Monitor for increased PCWP and/or central venous pressure (CVP).

NURSING DIAGNOSES

The most important nursing diagnoses for the patient in pulmonary edema are:

- Impaired gas exchange
- Anxiety

Planning and Implementation of Care

Take measures described in the following paragraphs to relieve symptoms as promptly as possible.

Impaired Gas Exchange Related to Excess Lung Water Decrease lung water and improve gas exchange promptly by taking action as follows:

1. While summoning the physician, elevate the head of bed 45°–90°, and lower the legs to pool blood in the periphery if possible.
2. Give IV morphine sulfate as ordered by the physician to decrease apprehension and

sympathetic stimulation (thereby decreasing peripheral arterial resistance and increasing venous capacitance). Anticipate a fall in pulmonary pressures and CVP. Assess systemic arterial pressure frequently. Morphine decreases the circulating blood volume, so be alert for early signs of shock. It also decreases respiratory center sensitivity to $P_{a}CO_2$, so watch for respiratory depression and possible respiratory arrest.

3. Administer rapid-acting diuretics as ordered by the physician. Anticipate a drop in CVP and PCWP.

4. Anticipate administration of vasoactive agents for preload and afterload manipulation.

5. To improve oxygenation and ventilation, take these steps. Administer supplemental O_2 as described in Chapter 9. The patient will need particular emotional support to accept an oxygen mask, since it often reinforces the sensation of smothering. Intubation and mechanical ventilation may be necessary if the work of breathing is excessive and exacerbates signs of myocardial ischemia and pump failure.

6. Work with the physician to alleviate the cause of the attack. For example, administer digitalis or dopamine if the problem is poor myocardial contractility; assist with cardioversion if tachycardia precipitated the attack. For a more detailed description of pharmacologic management, refer to Chapter 13.

Anxiety Related to Difficulty Breathing and to the Unknown   Take action to relieve the patient's anxiety. Stay with the patient, and try to provide a calm environment and brief, clear explanations. Also, administer morphine to relieve anxiety. For further interventions related to this diagnosis, see Chapter 13.

Outcome Evaluation

Evaluate the patient's progress according to these outcome criteria:

- Unlabored respirations 12–18 times per minute.
- Blood pressure (BP) and pulse within normal limits (WNL) for patient.
- Lungs clear on auscultation.
- Skin warm and dry (and pink if the patient is Caucasian).
- No cough or sputum.

- Ability to tolerate level of anxiety or apprehension, as indicated verbally or nonverbally (by facial expression and body posture).
- Arterial blood gases WNL for patient.

Non-Cardiogenic Pulmonary Edema: Adult Respiratory Distress Syndrome (ARDS)

Adult respiratory distress syndrome (ARDS) is a form of noncardiogenic pulmonary edema that occurs from diffuse injury to the alveolar-capillary membrane and results in stiff, wet lungs and refractory hypoxemia. This acute restrictive disorder is known by numerous other names, including *shock lung, wet lung, stiff lung, pump lung, congestive atelectasis, adult hyaline membrane disease, noncardiogenic pulmonary edema,* and *capillary leak syndrome.*

Assessment

Risk Conditions   The clinical causes of ARDS are diverse; ARDS seems to be a final result of either a direct lung injury, as in severe pneumonia, *or* a total body insult, such as sepsis. The result of either event is damage to the pulmonary capillary endothelium. Incidence is approximately 150,000–250,000 per year, with a 50–65% mortality rate (Crowley and Raffin 1991). Approximately one-third of survivors have some permanent changes in pulmonary function. Table 8–2 lists etiologies associated with ARDS (Crowley and Raffin 1991). Patients with two or more risk factors have a substantially higher chance of developing ARDS.

Preventive Measures   The critical-care nurse is in a key position to prevent this catastrophic syndrome or identify it early. Knowing that the patient is at risk is the first step—the trauma patient who is now septic, for instance. Prevention lies in meticulous monitoring of fluid administration, filtering of blood products, maintaining strict asepsis, and preventing aspiration with the use of nasogastric drainage. Aggressive pulmonary care such as turning, suctioning, and hyperinflation may allow the use of lower oxygen concentrations (below 50%) to prevent oxygen toxicity, which can exacerbate the syndrome (Brown 1990).

Pathophysiology   ARDS is a syndrome characterized by: (1) a precipitating event, (2) pulmonary edema due to capillary injury and leak, (3) marked respiratory

TABLE 8-2

Etiologies Associated with ARDS

Shock of any etiology

Trauma

    Fat embolism

    Lung contusion

    Nonthoracic trauma

    Head injury

    Burns

Aspiration

    Gastric contents

    Near drowning

Infections

    Gram-negative sepsis

    Diffuse pneumonia (bacterial, viral, Legionnaire's, *Pneumocystis carinii*)

    Radiation pneumonitis

Hematologic disorders

    Disseminated intravascular coagulation

    Massive transfusions

    Prolonged cardiopulmonary bypass

    Transfusion reactions

Inhaled toxic substances

    Oxygen

    Smoke

    Chemicals

Drug ingestion and overdose (heroin, barbiturates, methadone)

Metabolic

    Pancreatitis

    Uremia

Miscellaneous

    Paraquat ingestion

    Eclampsia

    Amniotic fluid embolism

    Fluid overload

    High altitude

    Air emboli

    Burns

    Radiation

NURSING TIP

ARDS

The first sign you may notice at the bedside is an increased respiratory rate, accompanied by visibly increased work of breathing and patient complaints of breathlessness and air hunger.

---

increased permeability of the pulmonary capillaries. In addition, "capillary leak" promotes altered hydrostatic and oncotic pressure dynamics, with transudation of fluid and plasma proteins into the interstitium. The result is frank pulmonary edema with progressive atelectasis due to surfactant dysfunction. Arterial hypoxemia and decreased compliance result.

In later stages, hyaline membranes line the alveolar ducts; and finally, fibrotic changes occur. This late stage is marked by decreased lung compliance, increased physiologic deadspace and pulmonary vascular resistance, and shunting unresponsive to positive end-expiratory pressure (PEEP). Intra-alveolar septal thickening and the decreased surface area create a diffusion defect and increased deadspace hallmarked by an increased P_{CO_2} in addition to refractory hypoxemia.

Signs and Symptoms The clinical onset of respiratory distress varies from 6–24 hours after the initial clinical disorder (Mathay 1989). Blood gas changes may or may not be present at this time; there may be only a respiratory alkalosis (P_{CO_2} 25–35) without marked hypoxemia. Chest assessment findings are extremely variable and depend upon the underlying initiating insult; the same is true for the CXR.

As the syndrome progresses, respiratory distress becomes more marked with use of all accessory muscles and respiratory rates in the 40s. The P_aO_2 falls below 50 and does not respond to oxygen therapy. Your patient may exhibit new signs of being confused and agitated. The CXR, whose changes may lag 24 hours behind the clinical onset of respiratory distress, now shows increasing diffuse infiltrates. The patient requires intubation and mechanical ventilation. Increasing lung stiffness (decreased lung compliance) is evidenced by high peak inspiratory pressures over 50 cm H_2O.

Hemodynamic instability increases, and its treatment depends on your patient's underlying problem.

distress, (4) diffuse infiltrates on chest x-ray (CXR), and (5) refractory hypoxemia. The injury to the pulmonary capillary is an integral factor in the development of the clinical presentation. Figure 8–1 illustrates the sequence of changes seen in ARDS.

Pulmonary capillary injury results in inflammation, bronchoconstriction, vasoconstriction, congestion, and

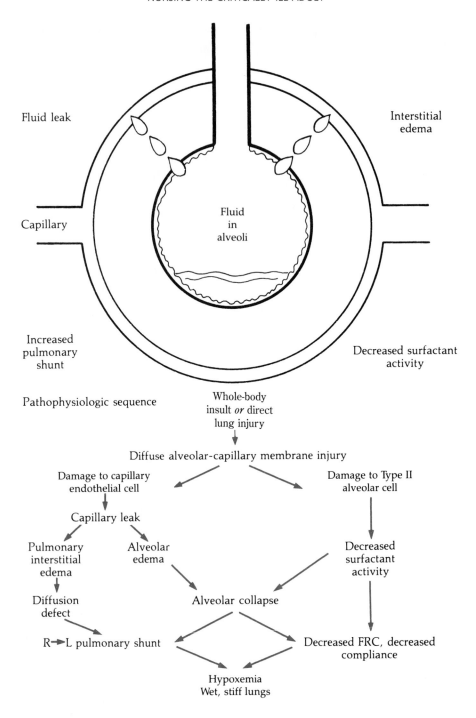

FIGURE 8–1

Pathophysiologic sequence in ARDS: a pictorial presentation.

An important hemodynamic finding is that, despite pulmonary edema, your patient's PCWP may be normal. This finding confirms that the cause of your patient's pulmonary edema is a "leaky capillary" syndrome as opposed to left-ventricular failure. Some patients, however, may have a combination of a damaged capillary membrane and pump failure.

Other hemodynamic changes include elevated pulmonary artery systolic and diastolic pressures, because alveolar hypoxia and acidemia are both potent pulmonary artery vasoconstrictors. Other mechanisms contributing to pulmonary hypertension include the release of vasoactive substances like histamine, platelets, and bradykinin and accumulation of neutro-

NURSING DIAGNOSES

A variety of nursing diagnoses can apply to the patient with ARDS, depending on the individual patient and the stage of development. The major diagnoses are:

- Impaired gas exchange
- Ineffective breathing pattern
- Ineffective airway clearance
- Anxiety

Care related to these diagnoses is discussed below.

phils and fibrin within the vessels (Crowley and Raffin 1991).

To maintain an adequate blood pressure and cardiac output, inotropic and vasopressor agents may be used. Fluid boluses are avoided in order to maintain as dry a lung as possible.

The late stages of ARDS reflect the damage to the pulmonary capillaries, which prevents not only oxygenation of the blood but also removal of CO_2 from the blood. In addition, the progressive hypoxemia is reflected by tissue hypoxia and a metabolic acidosis (decreased bicarbonate). This combination of metabolic and respiratory acidosis is a poor prognostic sign. The CXR usually has progressed to a "white-out," and sputum analysis shows that large amounts of albumin have leaked from the serum into the alveolus. Hypotension and bradycardia often follow, with death soon thereafter. Sepsis and multiple-system organ failure are usual causes of death in ARDS.

Planning and Implementation of Care

Selected aspects of nursing care are presented in the nearby Nursing Care Plan.

Impaired Gas Exchange Related to Alveolar Edema and Alveolar Collapse Gas exchange is compromised in ARDS for a variety of reasons. Shunt increases due to fluid and cellular debris filling the alveoli and also due to alveolar collapse, secondary to mechanical compression from interstitial edema and from decreased surfactant. Deadspace increases due to capillary compression and occlusion. The lung thus is characterized by mixed areas of shunt, deadspace, and

silent (nonfunctional) and functional alveolar-capillary units. A diffusion defect also is present because of the hyaline membranes, which probably are formed from transudated proteins.

Judicious fluid therapy is crucial to avoid further deleterious increases in lung water. In fact, one study demonstrated improved survival in patients with ARDS whose management during the acute phase included lowering of the pulmonary capillary wedge pressure by 25% (Humphrey et al. 1990).

Diuretics are administered cautiously to mobilize lung water. Furosemide and other rapid-acting diuretics are given in small doses, and fluid and electrolyte status and renal function are monitored closely.

Attention to ventilation and oxygenation is of paramount importance. Because of the increased shunt, simple oxygen supplementation is insufficient to achieve satisfactory P_aO_2 values. The patient is intubated and mechanically ventilated to overcome the widespread alveolar collapse and decreased compliance. Initial F_IO_2 is usually high (70–100%) to achieve a $P_aO_2 > 60$ mm Hg. Because extremely high inspired oxygen fractions are necessary in ARDS, with the concomitant risk of oxygen toxicity, the patient is placed on PEEP. By keeping alveoli constantly under positive pressure, PEEP increases functional residual capacity, allowing more surface area for gas exchange across the alveolar-capillary membrane. It thus allows the use of lower fractional inspired oxygen concentrations to achieve satisfactory levels of oxygenation.

When acceptable P_aO_2 values cannot be reached despite the use of PEEP, it may be necessary to use neuromuscular agents to paralyze and sedate the restless and hypoxic patient. This measure accomplishes two goals: First, the pressure needed to ventilate the patient is decreased by relaxing the chest wall, thus decreasing the risk of pneumothorax. Second, and more important, oxygen consumption by the respiratory muscles is decreased so that oxygen supply can better meet metabolic demand, thereby avoiding tissue hypoxia and resulting metabolic acidosis. It is **crucial to sedate** the patient, because paralytic agents do not change the patient's awareness of surroundings or discomfort.

Ineffective Breathing Pattern Related to Increased Lung Stiffness Alveolar edema and scarring of the alveolar-capillary membrane decrease lung tissue compliance, thus creating a need for more pressure to inflate the lungs. A rapid, shallow respiratory pattern increases work of breathing, oxygen consumption, and deadspace ventilation. Intubation, mechanical ventilation, and sedation are necessary to decrease oxygen consumption and enhance oxygen delivery to vital

NURSING CARE PLAN

The Patient with ARDS (Postintubation)

NURSING DIAGNOSIS	SIGNS AND SYMPTOMS	NURSING ACTION	DESIRED OUTCOMES
Impaired gas exchange related to alveolar edema and alveolar collapse	• Reduced P_aO_2 • Restlessness, agitation • Confusion, disorientation • Dyspnea • Dysrhythmias • Tachycardia • Cyanosis (in severe hypoxemia) • Crackles, bronchial breath sounds • $S\bar{v}O_2 < 60\%$	1. Maintain airway for oxygen therapy; restrain patient PRN to prevent extubation. 2. Maintain PEEP at all times; use suction adapter, manual ventilation bag with PEEP valve. 3. Continuously monitor ECG. 4. Measure VS (BP, HR, PAD/PAW, CVP) q1hr. 5. Evaluate cardiac output q4hr. Monitor $S\bar{v}O_2$ (or S_aO_2) as ordered, preferably continuously. 6. Monitor ABGs as ordered. 7. Monitor fluid balance carefully; avoid fluid overload. 8. Weigh patient daily if tolerated. 9. Adminster diuretics as ordered.	• $P_aO_2 > 60$ mm Hg on $F_1O_2 < 0.60$ • $S\bar{v}O_2 > 60\%$ • Patient is oriented • Clear CXR • Even fluid balance • No dysrhythmias
Ineffective breathing pattern related to patient breathing out of synchrony with ventilator	All the above plus: • Patient is "fighting" ventilator • Use of accessory muscles • Intercostal retractions	1. Verbally attempt to coach patient to breathe in phase with ventilator. 2. Sedate as ordered. 3. Frequently orient to time, place, and condition. 4. If coaching and sedation are unsuccessful with severe hypoxemia, consult with physician about paralyzing patient, **continuing sedation.** Explain to patient that he or she will be unable to move but you will keep him or her sedated and comfortable.	• $S\bar{v}O_2 > 60\%$ • Decreased work of breathing • Absence of inspiratory effort in the paralyzed patient
Ineffective breathing pattern related to decreased compliance	• Peak inspiratory pressures over 50 cm H_2O • Tachypnea • Elevated arterial carbon dioxide (P_aCO_2) • Dyspnea • Use of accessory muscles • Difficulty with manual ventilation	1. Check peak inspiratory pressures every 4 hours. 2. Decrease tidal volume and increase respiratory rate (RR) to decrease peak inspiratory pressures, as ordered. 3. Increase RR to decrease P_aCO_2 as ordered.	• Normal P_aCO_2 • PIPs < 40 cm H_2O • RR 8–18 • Normal CXR • Normal chest/diaphragm movement

(Continues)

NURSING CARE PLAN

The Patient with ARDS (Postintubation) (Continued)

NURSING DIAGNOSIS	SIGNS AND SYMPTOMS	NURSING ACTION	DESIRED OUTCOMES
		4. Perform chest auscultation q1–2hr to detect pneumothorax due to high inspiratory pressures and damaged lung parenchyma. 5. Paralyze patient with severe decreased compliance to facilitate ventilation, as ordered. 6. In end-stage ARDS with uncorrectable CO_2 retention signifying irreversible lung damage, discuss prognosis/plan with physican and family.	
Decreased cardiac output related to high levels of PEEP	• Cool extremities • Decreased urine output • Decreased/loss of peripheral pulses • Decreased blood pressure • Tachycardia • $S\bar{v}o_2 < 60\%$	1. Measure cardiac output, ABG 30 min after each increase in PEEP. 2. Monitor $S\bar{v}o_2$ continuously, as ordered. 3. Monitor urine output. 4. Assess for signs of decreasing peripheral perfusion. 5. Use inotropes/vasopressors as ordered to maintain BP.	• Normal cardiac output • Normal renal function • Warm periphery

organs. The need for increasing pressures to ventilate the patient, combined with the lung injury, put the patient at risk for barotrauma.

Ineffective Airway Clearance Related to Depressed Ciliary Function, Increased Mucus Production, and Increased Airway Resistance The patient with ARDS may or may not have excessive secretions, depending on the underlying etiology. Airway resistance may be increased because of early airway closure resulting from bronchoconstriction and mechanical compression from interstitial edema. To reduce retention of secretions, institute a program of vigorous pulmonary hygiene. Some extremely hypoxic patients do not tolerate turning, postural drainage, or suctioning without hypotension and dysrhythmias. Close observation of hemodynamics, ECG, S_ao_2, and $S\bar{v}o_2$ monitors is essential during position changes or interventions such as weights, CXR, central line placement, etc. Use of a continual lateral rotation bed improves gas exchange and prevents complications

such as airway loss with turning. The patient with ARDS frequently progresses to multiple organ involvement. Supporting adequate oxygenation of target organs while the lung injury heals becomes a primary goal along with the prevention of complications such as infection. Infection is prevented by meticulous attention to handwashing, care of invasive catheters, and decontamination of respiratory equipment. Nutritional needs should be closely met to ensure an anabolic state and augmented defenses against infection.

Anxiety Related to Dyspnea and to the Unknown The patient with ARDS requires skillful, compassionate nursing care to reduce anxiety. Brief mention will be made here of effective measures, as they are discussed in detail in Chapter 3. Project a calm, competent air as you care for the patient. Encourage her or him to rest as much as possible; for example, group your nursing care activities to allow for uninterrupted periods of rest. Try to maintain normal day/night cycles. Ideally, assign a primary nurse to the patient to facilitate a relationship of trust. Provide brief explanations of activities and procedures. Encourage family visits. Provide spiritual support if the patient wishes it by offering to contact a spiritual counselor. Use touch for reassurance if the patient is receptive.

Outcome Evaluation

The mortality rate in ARDS is high. For patients who survive, desirable outcome criteria are the following:

- Alert, oriented level of consciousness.
- Normal CO, as evidenced by arterial blood pressure WNL and normal thermodilution CO values.
- Good peripheral perfusion, as manifested by warm, dry skin, and bilaterally equal peripheral pulses of normal volume.
- Pulmonary Artery (PA), Central Venous Pressure (CVP), and Pulmonary Capillary Wedge Pressure (PCWP) readings WNL.
- Urinary output of 1 ml or more per minute.
- Arterial blood gases and serum electrolytes WNL.
- Normal respiratory pattern and rate.

Atelectasis

Atelectasis means absence of gas in part or all of the lung due to collapsed alveoli. Although the term may be used to refer to collapse due to compression (as with a tumor), it commonly refers to collapse caused by (a) airway obstruction followed by absorption of gas in the alveoli, or (b) decreased surfactant production.

Assessment

Risk Conditions Recognize the conditions that increase the risk of developing atelectasis: *shallow breathing* (as with pain), *dehydration, aspiration* of foreign objects, *retained secretions* (mucous plugs), *bronchospasm, ciliary depression,* and *decreased surfactant* (usually due to decreased alveolar expansion).

Preventive Measures The following measures help to prevent atelectasis:

1. Auscultate the lungs to determine the need for, frequency of, and effectiveness of the interventions that follow.

2. Establish rapport with the patient, and teach about deep breathing, coughing, turning, suctioning, and chest physiotherapy. Emphasize the importance of these techniques in maintaining pulmonary function. Praise the patient for participating in her or his own care, and inform the patient that during the stay in the critical-care unit you will assist with these measures. Encourage the patient to practice breathing and coughing exercises several times a day. Observe that she or he performs them correctly. If the exercises cause pain, give adequate analgesics before them and wait long enough for the analgesics to take effect. Then capitalize on your relationship to motivate the patient to perform breathing exercises in spite of any remaining discomfort.

3. Elevate the head of the bed to facilitate lung expansion. Avoid pronounced compression of the diaphragm.

4. Turn the patient every 1–2 hours to lessen pooling of secretions and prevent regional atelectasis.

5. Help the spontaneously breathing patient to deep breathe every 1–2 hours to reexpand closed alveoli. (Patients on continuous ventilation with high tidal volumes do not need to be sighed.)

6. Encourage oral fluids (if permitted) to reduce viscosity of secretions. If only intravenous fluids are allowed, maintain adequate hydration.

7. Mobilize secretions by performing chest physiotherapy periodically, instilling saline before suctioning, and using mucolytic agents and bronchodilators as ordered.

8. Help the patient to cough effectively by supporting abdominal or thoracic incisions by holding a pillow or folded sheet firmly against the incision. If necessary, stimulate the cough reflex by passing a nasal catheter down the trachea or by pressing over the trachea. If the patient has increased secretions and is unable to raise them, suction the trachea and bronchi.

9. Coach the patient to perform incentive spirometry hourly while awake, if ordered by the physician.

10. Administer pain medication before implementing interventions such as getting the patient out of bed or using inspiratory devices and coughing.

Signs and Symptoms Recognize the signs of developing atelectasis. If the airways to major atelectatic areas are open, bronchial breathing and increased tactile fremitus, voice sounds, and whispered sounds may be present. If the airways are plugged, these signs are absent. The chest x-ray may show patches or larger areas of consolidation, an elevated diaphragm, and a mediastinal shift, depending upon the site and extent of the collapse. Most postoperative atelectasis is microatelectasis (random alveolar collapse not detectable on chest x-ray). Signs and symptoms usually are subtle and may include restlessness, tachypnea, tachycardia, increased temperature, decreasing P_aO_2 or increasing A-aDo$_2$, or dullness on percussion over areas that should be resonant.

NURSING DIAGNOSES

The nursing diagnoses most appropriate for the patient with atelectasis are:

- Impaired gas exchange
- High risk for infection

Planning and Implementation of Care

Atelectasis results in increased physiologic shunting (explained in Chapter 7) and often in stasis pneumonia, as the retained secretions in collapsed alveoli are an excellent medium for bacterial growth.

Impaired Gas Exchange Related to Alveolar Collapse Relieve the hypoxia that results from increased physiologic shunting by taking these measures.

1. Provide supplemental O_2 as ordered by the physician.
2. If the obstruction is massive, it may be necessary for the physician to bronchoscope the patient.
3. Maintain high tidal volumes or PEEP, as ordered, in the mechanically ventilated patient to promote alveolar expansion and surfactant production.
4. Assist with mask continuous positive airway pressure (CPAP) if prescribed for the spontaneously ventilating patient.

High Risk for Infection Related to Decreased Host Defenses Prevent or treat growth of infectious organisms in the retained secretions and collapsed alveoli.

1. Monitor the patient's temperature every 2–4 hours.
2. Observe the quality of secretions and culture them as necessary.
3. Use scrupulous handwashing and sterile technique with suctioning, fluid lines, and incisions.
4. Administer prophylactic or therapeutic antibiotics as ordered by the physician. Drawing peak and valley antibiotic blood levels, as ordered, is critical to ensure their effectiveness and avoid toxicity.

Outcome Evaluation

Use these outcome criteria to judge the patient's progress:

- Respiratory rate 12–18 times per minute.
- Pulse rate 60–100 times per minute.
- P_aO_2 80–100 mm Hg and $S_aO_2 > 92\%$ on room air.
- Lung physical examination normal (no bronchial breathing over lung fields; normal voice sounds and whispered sounds; resonance on percussion; normal tactile fremitus).
- Chest x-ray normal (no consolidation, diaphragmatic elevation, or mediastinal shift).

Pneumonia

The diagnosis of pneumonia is based on CXR, physical exam, and laboratory data, including bacteriologic cultures. Infecting agents include bacteria (such as *Legionella* and *Mycoplasma*), viruses, fungi, parasites, and others. Bacterial infections, however, are most common in ICU patients who have weakened immunologic defenses and those who are being mechanically ventilated (Craven 1989). One study demonstrated that 22% of mechanically ventilated patients develop a bacterial pneumonia after a mean of 7.9 days (Rello et al. 1991). Fagon (1989) found that 9–21% of intubated and ventilated patients experiencing respiratory failure acquire nosocomial (hospital-acquired) pneumonia. Documented mortality is 40–50%. The following section will focus on nosocomial bacterial pneumonias.

Assessment

Risk Conditions Patients at greatest risk are those with compromised host defenses. Factors associated with a higher rate of nosocomial pneumonia include age, severity of illness, immunosuppression, duration of hospitalization, prior antibiotic use, major surgery, alcoholism, diabetes, coma, hypertension, and acidosis (Washington 1991). Abdominal and thoracic surgical procedures are associated with a high incidence of atelectasis and pneumonia due to decreased ventilatory muscle function. Patients with COPD are at extremely high risk for pneumonias postoperatively due to poor diaphragmatic function, decreased cough, and impaired mucociliary clearance. Oxygen and corticosteroids also depress alveolar macrophage function (Shapiro et al. 1989).

With the above risk factors, the primary mechanism of infection is colonization of the oropharyngeal mucosa with gram-negative bacilli that then are aspi-rated into the lower respiratory tract. Direct aspiration of gastric contents may also occur. A third mechanism that has been recently explored is the alkalinization of the gastrointestinal (GI) tract with antacids, which actually *promotes* growth of bacteria found in the gut. The bacteria ascend via the nasogastric (NG) tube and are then aspirated down into the lower respiratory tract (Flaherty 1988). A fourth mechanism is direct inoculation of the respiratory tract by contamination from caregivers' hands, either between patients or via cross-contamination from the GI tract to the endotracheal tube. The following section on prevention addresses these mechanisms.

Preventive Measures Most all patients in critical-care units today fall under the category of high risk for the development of pneumonia. Specific measures by the nurse can help to decrease the incidence as well as to institute early treatment. In both the surgical and medical populations, knowing the patient's preoperative pulmonary function is key in identifying appropriate postoperative pulmonary care. Frequent

CRITICAL CARE GERONTOLOGY

Pneumonia in the Elderly

The United States population over 65 is projected to double in the next 35 years. This increase, plus the fact that respiratory infection is the fourth leading cause of death among the elderly, are indications that pneumonia in the elderly will become an increasing problem (Caruthers 1990). If the older person who acquires pneumonia either in the community or while in the hospital also has underlying pulmonary disease, complications of respiratory failure are certain.

Organisms that cause pneumonia in persons over 65 are numerous. Community-acquired pneumonias are due to infection with *pneumococcus (Streptococcus), Haemophilus influenzae, Branhamella catarrhalis, Mycoplasma pneumoniae* and *Legionella pneumophila.* Pneumo-coccal pneumonia presents differently in the elderly than in younger patients, often with very few symptoms other than altered mental status and dehydration. Caregivers of younger children are most at risk for infection with *Mycoplasma pneumoniae,* with complaints of fever, nonproductive cough, malaise, and headache. Viral pneumonias in the elderly are most commonly caused by influenza A, but more troublesome are the secondary bacterial infections that often follow this virus. Nosocomial (hospital-acquired) infections are usually caused by gram-negative bacilli such as *Klebsiella pneumoniae* and *Pseudomonas aeruginosa.*

The elderly patient with pneumonia is often admitted to the critical-care unit intubated and me-chanically ventilated due to acute respiratory failure.

Pneumonia also may follow chest and upper abdominal surgical procedures that result in hypoventilation, atelectasis, and retention of secretions. With increased age, the lungs become less compliant and airways close earlier in expiration, thus increasing the risk of postoperative stasis pneumonia (Kersten 1989).

Awareness of who is at greatest risk, combined with aggressive hyperventilation and secretion mobilization, can prevent pneumonia in the vulnerable elderly. Patient education regarding a one-time pneumococcal vaccine and annual influenza vaccines in October are important preventive measures.

repositioning prevents stasis of secretions and promotes their drainage. Multiple studies of trauma patients have found a significantly lower incidence of pneumonia (and therefore shorter hospital stay) in groups of patients who were placed on a mechanical bed that continuously turns side to side (Fink et al. 1990; Sahn 1991). Assessment of respiratory pattern with appropriate pain relief prevents hypoventilation and atelectasis; both are precursors of pneumonia. Preoperative teaching of proper bronchial hygiene familiarizes the patient with equipment and routines and decreases pain and anxiety in the postoperative period. Aggressive pulmonary care can shorten the length of time the patient is intubated and in the intensive care unit, which decreases the risk of developing pneumonia.

Aspiration is prevented by nasogastric drainage plus side positioning for neurologically impaired patients (Table 8–3).

Handwashing is the cornerstone of preventing transfer of organisms between patients or cross-contamination of GI tract pathogens to the respiratory tract. Caregivers' hands are also a source of gram-negative bacilli. Vigorous mobilization of secretions, aseptic suctioning, and careful fluid management are first-line management strategies in protecting your patient from contracting pneumonia. The use of disposable and closed-system ventilator tubing and humidifiers has made this equipment a less likely source of contamination. Ventilator tubing circuits are changed every 48 hours. Careful handling of ventilator tubing to drain condensate *away* from the patient before turning or raising siderails prevents massive inoculation of the respiratory tract. Isolating patients with respiratory infections from other populations prevents cross-exposure to their bacterial flora.

Signs and Symptoms Bacterial pneumonias such as those caused by *Klebsiella* and *Pseudomonas* often begin with a rapid onset of fever; in critically ill patients, however, fever may not be present. The patient with bacterial pneumonia appears more ill than the patient with viral pneumonia. Bacterial pneumonias produce a localized infiltrate resulting in bronchial breath sounds, which contrasts with viral pneumonias that are more diffuse and produce chest findings of scattered crackles and rhonchi. Pneumonia due to infection with *Klebsiella* may be multilobar; pneumonia caused by *Pseudomonas* is also multilobar, but with a predisposition for the lower lobes. Atelectasis and small pleural effusions are common. Other pneumonias caused by gram-negative bacteria such as those caused by infection with *Escherichia coli, Enterobacter, Proteus,* and *Bacteroides,* appear similarly, though not as much in the lower lobes. These types of bacterial pneumonia are particularly severe due to their necrotizing effect on lung tissue.

Cough is a predominant symptom but may not be present in the critically ill. Sputum is purulent, although the organism identified on Gram stain may not be the one responsible for the pneumonia. When obtaining a specimen in the intubated patient, pass the suction catheter deep into the trachea, apply suction, release it, and withdraw the catheter. Tachypnea may be present due to fever and consolidation.

Planning and Implementation of Care

Impaired Gas Exchange Related to Increased Shunting Institute oxygen therapy according to the degree of hypoxemia, and monitor arterial blood gases.

TABLE 8–3

**Interventions to Prevent
Aspiration Pneumonia**

1. Elevate head of bed of unconscious patient 6–8 inches.
2. Check NG tube position with initial x-ray and then before each feeding if possible.
3. Check NG suction in patient not receiving feedings, to keep stomach empty.
4. Turn off continuous tube feedings 30 minutes before chest physiotherapy or procedures such as CT scans, etc.
5. Elevate head of bed of continuously tube-fed patient 30–45 degrees.
6. Instill food coloring in tube feeding.
7. Use small-bore, mercury-weighted tube when possible to place in duodenum.
8. Check residual amount (depending on caliber of tube) before each feeding in intermittently fed patient or every shift in continuously fed patients.

NURSING DIAGNOSES

The nursing diagnoses most appropriate for the pneumonia patient are:

- Impaired gas exchange
- Ineffective airway clearance

Obtain chest x-rays daily and correlate chest assessment findings with chest x-ray reports. Turning and deep breathing will enhance matching of ventilation and perfusion. For best matching of ventilation and perfusion, position the patient with the best lung down.

Ineffective Airway Clearance Related to Secretions and Debilitation Humidify oxygen, and observe secretions for increased viscosity. Administer antibiotics as ordered, observing for side effects, particularly of aminoglycosides, as renal function may be affected. Avoid fluid overload. Use gentle and aseptic suctioning with chest percussion, postural drainage, and position changes as tolerated by the patient. Observe sputum for changes that may indicate a superinfection, particularly in the patient on broad-spectrum antibiotics.

Outcome Evaluation

Evaluate the patient's progress according to the following desirable outcome criteria:

- Absence of fever.
- Arterial blood gas values WNL for the patient.
- Presence of normal breath sounds; absence of bronchial breath sounds.
- Absence of or normal-appearing sputum.

Pneumothorax

Whereas *pneumonia* is a process occurring in the alveolar spaces, *pneumothorax* is a collection of free air within the pleural space, thus impairing lung expansion.

Assessment

Risk Conditions Anticipate and prevent a pneumothorax whenever possible, by first recognizing patients at risk. Predisposing conditions are as follows:

1. Chest trauma, especially penetrating injuries or rib fractures.
2. Pneumonia, because it leads to lung abscesses.
3. Diseases causing degenerative changes in lungs, such as emphysema and bronchitis.
4. Airway obstruction due to bronchospasm, inflammation, or retained secretions.

5. Catheterization of the subclavian vein, because it rests on the apical pleura.
6. Thoracentesis.
7. Pericardial tap.
8. Positive pressure ventilation. Risk of a pneumothorax from positive pressure ventilation increases if additional factors are present that increase intrathoracic pressure. If the patient has chronic obstructive lung disease or is fighting the ventilator, pressure inside the thorax may rise dangerously. The risk of pneumothorax also increases if the tidal volume is over 15 ml/kg, the peak inspiratory pressure is over 40–50 cm H_2O, or positive end-expiratory pressure is applied.

The likelihood of pneumothorax escalates with increasing numbers of risk conditions. For example, the emphysematous patient on mechanical ventilation who develops retained secretions is more likely to develop a pneumothorax than the previously healthy person on mechanical ventilation whose nurses keep the airway clear. Pneumothorax also occurs in previously healthy people for unknown reasons.

Preventive Measures Take whatever steps are possible to prevent the predisposing conditions. For example, encourage turning and deep breathing and coughing exercises to clear secretions. If the patient is unable to raise secretions through these methods, stimulate the cough reflex, perform chest physiotherapy, or suction the airway as needed.

Administer bronchodilators, steroids, and antibiotics prescribed by the physician to minimize airway obstruction. During subclavian catheterization, use Trendelenburg's position and have the patient perform a Valsalva maneuver.

Signs and Symptoms Consistent and frequent chest assessment will ensure that you detect the pneumothorax promptly. Signs and symptoms vary, depending on the size and type of pneumothorax. The types are: *open,* with a continued communication between the pleural space and the outside; *closed,* with closure of the pleural tear as the lung collapses; and *tension,* with the opening acting as a one-way valve to let air in but not out (Figure 8–2). The key signs and symptoms are pain, dyspnea, hypoxia, chest x-ray changes, and sometimes mediastinal shift. Signs of decreased cardiac output and shock may occur with tension pneumothorax as air builds inside the pleural space and pushes the heart and great vessels toward the opposite side, resulting in a fall in blood pressure.

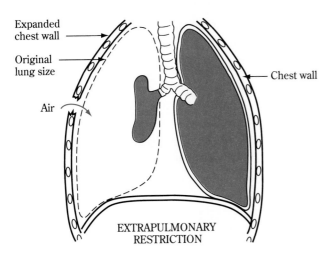

Expanded chest wall

Original lung size

Air

Chest wall

EXTRAPULMONARY RESTRICTION

FIGURE 8–2

Example of extrapulmonary restriction. A chest wall injury permits air to enter the pleural space (open pneumothorax). The lung collapses and cannot re-expand owing to surrounding atmospheric pressure. A drastically reduced lung volume results. (From Kersten L: *Comprehensive respiratory nursing.* Philadelphia: Saunders, 1990, p. 128.)

Watch for *chest pain* that is abrupt, sharp, and constant and usually unilateral. Signs of *dyspnea* and *hypoxia* include tachypnea, nasal flaring, cyanosis, accessory muscle use, retractions, and decreased P_aO_2 or S_aO_2. On physical examination, the affected side may appear larger, with decreased movement, decreased tactile fremitus, hyperresonance or tympany, depressed diaphragm, and decreased breath sounds. The *chest x-ray* may show loss of lung markings peripherally, compression collapse centrally, or possible mediastinal shift.

Observe for signs of *mediastinal shift* away from the pneumothorax (if pressure is great enough) as follows.

1. Check for tracheal deviation away from the affected side.

NURSING TIP

Pneumothorax

If your patient is receiving mechanical ventilation, a sudden rise in peak inspiratory pressures may accompany a pneumothorax.

2. Monitor for signs of decreased venous return, such as jugular venous distention and increased central venous pressure readings.

3. Observe for signs of decreased CO, such as mental confusion, angina, oliguria, tachycardia, hypotension, peripheral vasoconstriction, and diaphoresis.

4. Auscultate the precordium for deviation in heart sound locations. A crunching sound with the heartbeat (Hamman's sign, resulting from pneumomediastinum) may also be present.

NURSING DIAGNOSES

Among the possible nursing diagnoses for a patient with a pneumothorax are the following:

- Ineffective breathing pattern
- Chest pain
- High risk for decreased CO

Planning and Implementation of Care

Ineffective Breathing Pattern Related to Restricted Lung Expansion The loss of pleural integrity causes lung collapse and interferes with lung re-expansion. Measures to alleviate the ineffective breathing pattern include stabilization of the thoracic cage, relief of positive intrapleural pressure, and compensation for altered lung volumes.

Stabilization of Thoracic Cage Stabilization of the thoracic cage is essential to minimize abnormal pulmonary dynamics. For an open pneumothorax *(sucking chest wound),* cover the wound with white Vaseline gauze until a chest tube can be inserted. If, however, respiratory distress worsens after covering the wound with gauze, uncover it to allow escape of air and to avoid build-up of air inside the chest. If there is no sucking wound but there is an associated rib fracture or flail chest, paradoxical chest wall movement can be minimized initially by splinting the chest, for example, by placing your hands over the affected area. Obtain medical help for further stabilization, which is usually achieved with chest tube insertion and positive pressure ventilation.

Relief of Positive Intrapleural Pressure Reduce the positive intrapleural pressure that caused the lung collapse and interferes with its re-expansion. Methods of reducing the pressure vary with the type and size of pneumothorax.

1. For a small closed pneumothorax, the physician may prescribe bedrest and supplemental O_2. The air will be reabsorbed slowly because of the pressure gradient between it and the surrounding blood and tissue.

2. For a tension or larger closed pneumothorax, assist with emergency decompression with a large-bore needle, stopcock, and syringe; Heimlich valve; or chest tube. (See Chapter 9 for information on the technique and nursing responsibilities related to chest tubes.)

3. Elevate the head of the bed 30° to facilitate expansion of the lung and evacuation of air via the chest tube. Use a footboard to keep the patient from slipping down in bed and restricting diaphragmatic movement.

4. For recurrent pneumothoraces, the physician may elect to create adhesions between the lung and chest wall via injection of an irritating substance into the pleural cavity under local anesthesia or via parietal pleurectomy under general anesthesia.

Chest Pain Related to Nerve Irritation To reduce the chest pain, consult with the physician about type, dosage, and frequency of analgesics. If the pain persists in spite of analgesics, consult with the physician about intercostal nerve blocks.

High Risk for Decreased CO Related to Mediastinal Shift Monitor the patient for signs of mediastinal shift as described earlier under signs and symptoms. If they occur in a patient without chest drainage, call them to the physician's attention immediately—prompt decompression is mandatory. If they occur in a patient with chest drainage, immediately check the patency of the system and alert the physician.

Outcome Evaluation

Use these outcome criteria to evaluate the patient's progress:

- No chest pain.
- Unlabored spontaneous respirations 12–18 times per minute.
- Chest symmetric in size and expansion.
- Normal breath sounds.
- Involved area of chest resonant on percussion.
- Trachea midline.
- Heart sounds in normal location; no Hamman's sign.
- Venous return normal (neck veins undistended, CVP readings normal).
- BP, pulse, and urinary output WNL for patient.
- Alert and oriented.
- Skin warm and dry (and pink if the patient is Caucasian).
- Chest x-ray—normal peripheral lung markings, no central compression collapse, no mediastinal shift.
- No air leak in the water seal column of the chest drainage system.

Pleural Effusion

A *pleural effusion* is an accumulation of fluid in the pleural space. Because of the variety of etiologies resulting in fluid in the pleural space, effusions are common in the critical-care setting.

Figure 8–3 illustrates the differences in tracheal and mediastinal shift with the processes of atelectasis, pleural effusion, and consolidation.

Effusions are classified on the basis of the protein concentration in the pleural fluid. An effusion is termed *exudative* if the pleural-fluid-to-serum-total-protein ratio is greater than 0.5. *Transudative* effusions result from fluid leaking into the pleural space as a result of changes in hydrostatic pressure or oncotic pressure, as in congestive heart failure (CHF) or hypoalbuminemia. Exudative effusions usually reflect pleural disease and inflammation while transudative ones do not (Antony 1989). Thick yellow-green fluid on aspiration indicates emphysema; bloody pleural fluid may indicate malignancy.

Assessment

Risk Conditions Exudative effusions are seen in half of patients with pneumonia and may become infected. Grossly purulent pleural fluid is referred to as *empyema* or *pyothorax* if a large amount of pus is present. Empyemas may result as complications of respiratory infections, chest trauma, or chest surgery. Transuda-

a SHIFT **TOWARDS** PATHOLOGY   b SHIFT **AWAY** FROM PATHOLOGY   c TRACHEA AND MEDIASTINUM
                                                                                     REMAIN IN MIDLINE POSITION

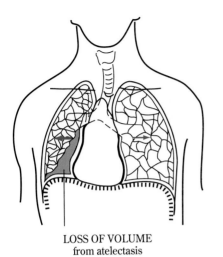
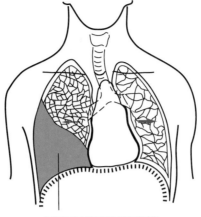
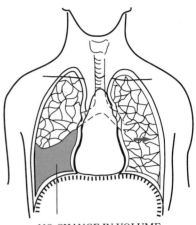

LOSS OF VOLUME   INCREASE IN VOLUME   NO CHANGE IN VOLUME
from atelectasis   from pleural effusion   from consolidation

FIGURE 8–3

Tracheal and mediastinal shift in respiratory disease. In **a** and **b,** the large arrow represents the direction of the shift and the more negative end-expiratory pleural pressures on that side. In **c,** pleural pressures remain about equal for right and left lungs. (From Kersten L: *Comprehensive respiratory nursing.* Philadelphia: Saunders, 1990, p. 2681. Adapted from Cherniack R and Cherniack L: *Respiration in health and disease,* 3d ed. Philadelphia: Saunders, 1983.)

tive effusions may be seen in patients with chronic left-sided heart failure and patients with low albumin levels due to cirrhosis and liver disease. Bloody effusions are seen following chest trauma and with some chest tumors. Serosanguinous effusions are seen after open heart surgery when the pleural space is entered. Chylous effusions are seen with obstruction of lymph flow, as in some malignancies. Malignant effusions tend to be large and to reoccur after drainage; they are a poor prognostic sign.

which it accumulated. Symptoms include complaints of dyspnea by the patient, decreased activity level, and decreased appetite. Signs include tachypnea, shallow respirations, tracheal deviation away from the side of the effusion, decreased breath sounds, and the absence of tactile and voice vibrations. A decubitus chest film helps identify free pleural fluid by a shift in the fluid level as the patient turns on his or her side. Percussion of the area results in a dull note. Arterial blood gas analysis may show hypoxemia due to compression of lung tissue and shunting.

NURSING DIAGNOSES

Nursing diagnoses that may apply to the patient with a pleural effusion include:

- Impaired gas exchange
- Activity intolerance

Signs and Symptoms The presence of symptoms depends on the size of the effusion and the rate at

Planning and Implementation of Care

Impaired Gas Exchange Related to Decreased Lung Expansion Place the patient in a position to optimize lung expansion and decrease patient feelings of breathlessness, usually by elevating the head of the bed. Avoid positions that restrict diaphragmatic movement. Assess the degree of effusion by frequent chest auscultation. Encourage deep breathing by use of incentive spirometry in the nonintubated patient. Follow blood gas analysis for hypoxemia, and observe the patient for signs of increasing hypoxia and/or hypercarbia.

Activity Intolerance Related to Inadequate Ventilation Space activities to avoid tiring the patient. Eating may be difficult due to extreme dyspnea, so encourage the patient to eat small amounts frequently. This will also avoid gastric distention and further lung restriction. Alert the physician about any decreasing activity tolerance and increasing dyspnea, as most effusions are treated based on patient symptoms, not on the quantity of fluid estimated to be present in the pleural space.

Outcome Evaluation

Judge the patient's progress according to these desirable outcome criteria:

- Arterial blood gas WNL for patient.
- CXR WNL for patient.
- Normal breath and voice sounds.
- Normal percussion note.
- Decreased levels of dyspnea and energy as noted by the patient.

OBSTRUCTIVE AIRWAY DISEASE

Acute or chronic respiratory failure can result from obstruction of either the upper or the lower airway. Examples of upper airway obstruction include epiglottitis, trauma, inhalation injury, foreign body, congenital abnormalities, tracheal stenosis, neoplasms, subglottic stenosis, and obstructive sleep apnea syndrome (Kersten 1989).

Obstructive diseases of the lower airways refer to those disorders that decrease expiratory flow rates, as evidenced by FEV_1. Chronic bronchitis, emphysema, and asthma are the most common examples of *chronic* obstructive disorders. Asthma, however, can be acute and reversible, therefore, asthmatic patients are not usually included in the diagnosis of COPD *unless* the asthma has become chronic and severe. There is an overlap among these three entities. For instance, the chronic bronchitis may also have a reversible asthmatic component, as evidenced by improved flow rates after bronchodilator therapy, or the patient may have chronic bronchitis and emphysema. Therefore, therapy for the COPD patient differs from that for the acute asthmatic whose airway obstruction is completely or partially reversible.

In 1987, COPD was responsible for 78,000 deaths in the United States and was listed as the fifth leading cause of death (National Heart, Lung, and Blood Institute 1990). It is estimated that there are 15 million persons suffering from COPD, 12.7 million with chronic bronchitis, and 2 million with emphysema (American Lung Association 1989).

Persons with COPD are often seen in the critical-care units because they have little pulmonary reserve and are at risk for developing acute respiratory failure when, for instance, they acquire pneumonia or undergo a surgical procedure.

Chronic Bronchitis and Emphysema

Assessment

Risk Conditions Cigarette smoking remains the highest risk factor for developing bronchitis and emphysema. Cigarette smoke affects three major areas in the lung. The larger airways, the *bronchi,* undergo enlargement of the submucosal bronchial glands. The smaller airways become irritated, resulting in bronchiolitis in both the terminal and respiratory *bronchioles.* Mucus cells multiply, inflammatory cells infiltrate the area, fibrotic changes occur, and smooth muscle hypertrophies, all contributing to airflow obstruction. As the effects of smoking continue, the *air spaces* are affected (emphysema) and elastic recoil is lost, causing the airways to become floppy and narrowed during expiration (Fahling and Snider 1989). Other risks of smoking include cancer of the lung, larynx, mouth, esophagus, bladder and pancreas; hypertension; coronary artery disease, and peripheral vascular disease.

Air pollution with noxious gases and particulate matter in urban areas also potentiates irritation to the lung and exacerbates COPD symptoms. Respiratory infections of childhood may also contribute to the development of COPD later in life.

Preventive Measures Measures to prevent acute exacerbations include smoking-cessation educational programs and pulmonary rehabilitation programs. Smoking-cessation education is appropriate both in the high school setting (to prevent development of COPD) and for the adult public. Components of a successful pulmonary rehabilitation program include teaching bronchial hygiene measures, energy conservation techniques, dyspnea control, medication guidelines, and exercise programs to increase activity tolerance and independence.

The most common precipitating causes of acute respiratory failure in COPD patients are infection, left ventricular failure, myocardial infarction, pulmonary emboli, bronchospasm, sedative drugs, and removal of the hypoxic drive to breathe. Care of COPD patients who undergo other procedures, such as surgery, should reflect knowledge of these risk factors. Meticulous asepsis, fluid management, positioning, and drug (including oxygen) administration can help shorten their stay in the ICU and prevent precipitating acute respiratory failure.

During resolution of an episode of acute respiratory failure, the nurse and patient together can begin to identify teaching needs. Some breathing retraining and dyspnea control techniques can be begun in the ICU postextubation in coordination with respiratory therapy personnel. Family should be included when possible. With physician guidance, referral to a pulmonary rehabilitation program may prevent future hospitalizations, increase exercise tolerance, and improve general feelings of well-being.

Signs and Symptoms *Chronic bronchitis* is characterized by inflammation of small airways and hypersecretion of mucus. It is defined as the presence of a recurrent, productive cough 3 months of the year for at least 2 successive years (American Thoracic Society 1982). Ciliary clearance is greatly impaired.

Emphysema is characterized by destructive changes of the alveoli, with resultant enlargement of the distal air spaces. The process is irreversible, causes lung tissue to lose its elastic recoil, and results in increased lung compliance. The increase in air spaces results in a large increase in residual volume.

Bronchitis and emphysema often overlap; many presenting signs and symptoms are common to both entities. Hyperinflation, or "barrel chest," is present due to air-trapping and increased residual volume, particularly in emphysema. This increased lung volume causes flattening of the diaphragm, decreasing inspiratory efficiency and increasing work of breathing, as noted by use of accessory muscles. Hyperresonance upon percussion and decreased chest excursion are also present. The respiratory rate may be reduced, with prolongation of the expiratory phase. Pursed-lip breathing may be present as the patient tries to reduce premature collapse of floppy airways and decrease air-trapping. Chest auscultation may reveal decreased breath sounds throughout in the pure emphysemic patient, or wheezing due to narrowing of airways on expiration, airway edema, and

secretions in the bronchitic patient or the patient with both entities.

Cyanosis and hypoxemia are more common in the bronchitic patient because of secretions and shunting. When hypoventilation is present, CO_2 retention occurs. Chronic hypoventilation results in chronic CO_2 retention. These patients therefore depend on hypoxemia ($P_aO_2 < 60$ mm Hg) as their respiratory stimulus.

In the emphysemic patient, destruction of the alveolar-capillary membrane results in a diffusion defect that produces hypoxemia, particularly during exercise.

As hypoxemia and CO_2 retention progress, the patient may first become agitated and combative and then lethargic and confused. Work of breathing becomes overwhelming due to increased air-trapping, secretions, and bronchospasm, and intubation and mechanical ventilation become necessary. With this chronically ill population the decision to intubate should ideally be discussed prior to its emergent need, because some patients may not be able to be weaned from such support. Following previous intubations, some patients—with family and physician support—may decide against reintubation should their condition deteriorate.

NURSING DIAGNOSES

The nursing diagnoses most applicable to the COPD patient are:

- Ineffective airway clearance
- Ineffective breathing pattern
- Impaired gas exchange
- Anxiety
- Hopelessness

Planning and Implementation of Care

Ineffective Airway Clearance Related to Ineffective Cough and Mucociliary Mechanisms Aggressive bronchial hygiene therapy is a necessity to clear secretions and decrease airway resistance as well as prevent infection. Ensure that the patient is adequately hydrated, including having inhaled gases humidified. To ensure efficient coughing, assist the patient to a semi-Fowler's position. Patients unable to sit can be turned onto their sides with knees drawn upward. In COPD patients, "huff" coughing may produce higher flow rates despite airway collapse. ("Huff" coughing is a series of small coughs done with the glottis held open while saying "huff.") Chest physiotherapy and postural drainage, discussed in Chapter 9, enhance secretion removal.

Ineffective Breathing Pattern Related to Decreased Diaphragmatic Function and Increased Lung Volumes Position your patient to augment diaphragmatic descent, i.e., high up in the bed and leaning over a bedside table if possible. Work with the respiratory therapists to determine the appropriateness of teaching diaphragmatic and pursed-lip breathing (see Chapter 9). Some COPD patients on ventilators increase air-trapping because they receive their next breath before they have finished exhaling the current one. To detect this problem, observe for increasing peak inspiratory pressures; lengthening the expiratory phase may be necessary. In addition, when manually "bagging" these patients, you must be sure to allow for complete exhalation before manually giving the next breath.

Impaired Gas Exchange Related to Destroyed Alveolar-Capillary Membrane and Increased Secretions Perform maneuvers described under "Ineffective Airway Clearance." Monitor the patient for signs of hypoxia, and check arterial blood gases for degree of hypoxemia. Check the history and physical to ascertain what is normal for your patient.

Anxiety Due to Feelings of Breathlessness Establish a relationship of trust with the patient. Do not leave the bedside of a newly intubated or extremely dyspneic, panicked patient. Talk in a quiet, clear, concise manner. Many COPD patients do not like being hovered over or confined to a semisupine position. Explain in a concise manner exactly what you are doing

or plan to do to help alleviate the feelings of breathlessness. Elicit the assistance of a respiratory therapist to "talk the patient through" dyspnea control maneuvers while you prepare an aminophylline infusion, send off lab work, etc. Broad statements such as "Just relax, Mrs. Jones" are ineffective and only serve to worsen the patient's panic.

Hopelessness Due to Irreversible Nature of Disease Dudley et al. (1980) have described the consequences of chronic dyspnea, anxiety, and depression as an "emotional straitjacket" because many patients use isolation, denial, and repression of emotions as defense mechanisms. Laughing, expressing anger, or crying all serve to increase their breathlessness. The resulting inactivity perpetuates lower levels of activity tolerance, and soon the patient is in a physically and emotionally confining world. Feelings of anger, despair, and hopelessness are common and may be taken out on caregivers. Pulmonary rehabilitation programs offer hope of increasing activity tolerance and independence. As the bedside nurse, you can be instrumental in facilitating referral to such resources. In some cases psychiatric counseling may be helpful to treat severe depression, particularly in the long-term ventilator patient.

Outcome Evaluation

Evaluate the patient's progress according to the following desirable outcome criteria:

- Arterial blood gases WNL for that patient.
- Absence of infection.
- Demonstration of bronchial hygiene maneuvers.
- Demonstration of diaphragmatic and pursed-lip breathing techniques.
- Ability to describe signs and symptoms of infection.
- Report of decreased anxiety and hopelessness.

Acute Asthma

Asthma is a *chronic* disease characterized by recurrent attacks of reversible airway obstruction. Death rates from asthma have risen 31% from 1980–1987; during that same period the occurrence of asthma has risen 29% (Sly 1988). An *acute asthmatic attack* is a self-perpetuating complex, characterized by airway

---

NURSING TIP

COPD

Using a fan at the bedside may decrease your patient's sensation of breathlessness.

obstruction, airway inflammation, and increased bronchospasm, occurring as a result of various stimuli such as allergens, cold air, inhaled particulate matter, or infection.

Inflammation has received greater attention recently, with more therapy—such as the use of inhaled steroids—being aimed specifically at this problem. Release of chemical mediators from mast cells, white blood cells, and epithelial cells also triggers bronchospasm and edema. Structural changes in the epithelial lining may allow increased permeability to irritants and allergic stimuli. Secretions are also more difficult to clear due to injury of the mucociliary blanket. Abnormalities in the neurologic innervation of the airway smooth muscle, such as elevated parasympathetic tone, may result in bronchoconstriction. This problem is treated with anticholinergic inhaled agents.

Status asthmaticus is a severe, unrelenting attack unresponsive to the patient's usual forms of therapy. Widespread bronchoconstriction affects all gas exchange units. The constriction causes air-trapping, so that functional residual capacity increases and, as a result, vital capacity decreases. The overdistension of alveoli causes increased deadspace, which results in wasted ventilation. The overinflation of the lungs, combined with the increased airway resistance, markedly increases the work of breathing. The reduced air intake and fatigue lead to hypoventilation and eventual hypercapnia.

Because asthma also is characterized by increased production of tenacious secretions, local areas of atelectasis occur. Continuing capillary flow past these areas of alveolar collapse results in increased shunting, which produces severe hypoxemia.

Assessment

Risk Conditions A number of risk conditions can precipitate an attack of status asthmaticus. Most common is respiratory infection, which typically is viral in nature. Other risk factors include failure to take prescribed medications or overuse of medications, particularly sympathomimetic agents. Weather changes, exposure to allergens, and emotional stress are other common precipitating factors. Persons at risk for death from an asthma attack include those in older age groups and those in their late teens or early 20s, African Americans, those persons having previous episodes of respiratory failure or intubation as a result of asthma, those hospitalized

in the previous year for asthma, and those whose disease severity is underestimated or denied (National Heart, Lung, and Blood Institute 1991). You should be aware of these factors in assessing the need for aggressive intervention in the patient with acute asthma.

Signs and Symptoms The clinical presentation of a patient in status asthmaticus is unforgettable. The patient presents with extreme dyspnea, exhaustion, difficulty walking, and fear. The patient or person accompanying the patient may give a history of increasing breathlessness, with increasing use of beta$_2$ agonist drugs with little or no responsiveness. Tachypnea, a compensatory response to the hypoxemia, is accompanied by accessory muscle use and often by cyanosis. Breath sounds are diminished. The patient may be wheezing markedly on inspiration and expiration. The absence of this sign is ominous, indicating that so little air is moving that a wheeze cannot occur. Coughing is almost impossible. The patient is tachycardic, diaphoretic, dizzy, and may have pulsus paradoxus. Clinical signs of dehydration usually are present. Speech is often only two to three words at a time, due to breathlessness. Most noticeable are the exhaustion and fear exhibited by the patient.

NURSING DIAGNOSES

The nursing diagnoses applicable to the patient in status asthmaticus include:

- Impaired gas exchange
- Ineffective airway clearance
- Activity intolerance
- Fluid volume deficit
- High risk for decreased CO
- Fear

Planning and Implementation of Care

Impaired Gas Exchange Related to Increased Shunting Start the patient immediately on supplemental oxygen to attain S_aO_2 over 90%. Draw arterial blood gases, on the physician's order, to determine the degree of hypoxemia; assist with arterial line placement if necessary for frequent blood gas assessments. Blood gases usually show severe hypoxemia, with P_aO_2 values of 50 mm Hg or less, and a normal pH and normal or low P_aco_2 due to hyperventilation. A rising P_aco_2 and falling pH are ominous signs, indicating that the patient is tiring in the effort to stave off impending respiratory failure. Unless checked, the continuing rise in P_aco_2 will result in acute respiratory failure and apnea.

Intubation and mechanical ventilation are used when adequate gas exchange cannot be maintained. The primary danger associated with mechanical ventilation for this patient is the increased risk of pneumothorax, due to the high inspiratory pressures necessary to overcome the increased airway resistance and the patient's tendency to breathe out-of-phase with the ventilator. The mechanically ventilated asthmatic must be sedated, and possibly paralyzed, to diminish the risk of fighting the ventilator. Expiratory retard may be used to maintain airway patency on expiration, thus allowing better emptying of lung volumes.

Ineffective Airway Clearance Related to Bronchospasm, Mucosal Edema, and Thick Secretions
After obtaining a brief history, determine the peak expiratory flow rate (PEFR) by having the patient forcefully exhale into a peak flow meter. This measure will give a rapid assessment of the severity of airway

obstruction. Administer medications as ordered by the physician. Figure 8–4 diagrams drug effects on airway obstructions. Table 8–4 describes inhaled pulmonary medications. Nebulized inhaled beta$_2$ agonist bronchodilators are the first line therapy to reverse bronchospasm in acute asthma. In a monitored setting, they may be repeated three times in 30–60 minutes. These medications may also be administered subcutaneously. If the patient is not responding to beta$_2$ agonists or is on oral corticosteroids, an intravenous line is started and a bolus of steroid may be given. Steroids diminish the nonspecific inflammatory reaction and inhibit the release of chemical mediators promoting bronchoconstriction. Sedatives are withheld because they blunt the respiratory drive. An aminophylline infusion may be ordered; the nurse should be aware of complications of dysrhythmias and seizures with this drug, especially when aminophylline is used in combination with other sympathomimetic drugs.

Anticipate orders for tests such as complete blood count, electrolytes, theophylline levels, and chest x-ray. The role of the nurse is to act quickly but with a calm and controlled manner so as not to further panic the patient. Explaining all procedures, positioning the patient, and coaching the patient to relax shoulder and neck muscles and perform pursed-lip breathing will also help to decrease work of breathing and calm the patient.

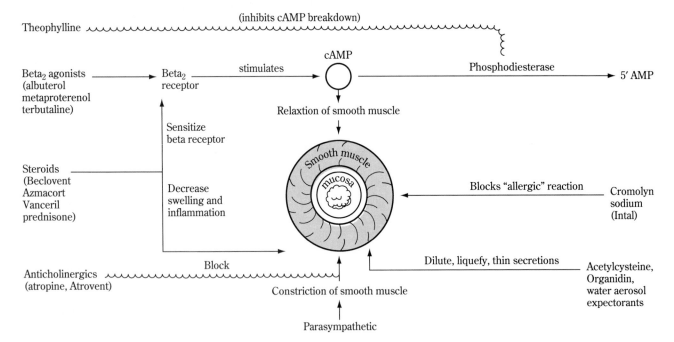

FIGURE 8–4

Drug effects on airway obstruction.

Activity Intolerance Related to Hypoxemia Promote physical and emotional rest for the patient. Allow him or her to assume a position of comfort. The typical posture chosen by the acute asthmatic is sitting up, leaning forward, with arms supported and shoulders elevated. You can make this position more comfortable for the patient by providing an over-the-bed table or pillows on which to lean.

TABLE 8–4

Nurse's Guide to Inhaled Medications

DRUG	DOSE	NURSING REMINDERS
Beta₂ agonists		

Albuterol (salbutamol)
    Proventil
    Ventolin
	0.5 ml of 0.5% in 2 ml normal saline, every 4 hours or 2 puffs 4 times per day	Monitor pulse and BP: may cause tachycardia and hypertension

Metaproterenol sulfate
    Alupent
    Metaprel
	0.3 ml in 2 ml normal saline, or 2–4 puffs 4 times per day	Same as albuterol

Terbutaline Brethaire	1–2 puffs every 4–6 hours	Same as albuterol
Pirbuterol Maxaire	1–2 puffs every 4–6 hours or 4 times a day	Same as albuterol
Isoetharine Bronkosol	0.25–1.0 ml in 2 ml normal saline or 2 puffs 4 times per day	Monitor pulse and BP: may cause tachycardia and BP fluctuations

Isoproterenol hydrochloride
    Isuprel
    Medi-haler-Iso
	0.5 ml of 1:200 in 2.5 ml normal saline, every 4 hours	Monitor pulse and BP: may cause tachycardia and hypotension

Epinephrine
    Adrenaline
    Primatene Mist
    Vaponefrin
	0.2 ml of 2.25% racemic in normal saline, every 2–4 hours, or 2 puffs 4 times per day	Monitor pulse and BP: may cause tachycardia and hypertension. Also may cause excitement or shaking

Anti-cholinergics		
Atropine sulfate	1-2 mg in 2 cc normal saline, every 4–6 hours	Use with caution with glaucoma or bladder neck hypertrophy. Use with spacer device to avoid spraying in eyes and causing blurred vision. Other side effects include dry mouth, tachycardia.
Ipratropium bromide (Atrovent)	2 puffs 4 times per day	Same as atropine
Steroids		

Beclomethasone dipropionate
    Vanceril
    Beclovent
	100 mg in 2 inhalations, 3–4 times per day	Rinse mouth after use; use as last inhaler if using more than one. Spacer device will decrease mouth and throat irritation

Flunisolide Aerobid	2–4 puffs, 2 times per day	None
Triamcinolone Azmacort	2 puffs, 2–4 times per day; up to 16 puffs daily	None
Anti-allergic		

Cromolyn sodium
    Aarane
    Intal
	20 mg 4 times per day	Not used in emergency treatment of asthma, but for long-term prevention of attacks or exercise-induced asthma

Mucolytic		
Acetylcysteine Mucomyst	1–2 ml of 10–20% instilled into trachea; or 3–5 ml of 10%, or 6–10 ml of 20%, inhaled 3–4 times per day	After opening, store in refrigerator and use within 96 hours. May cause nausea, broncho-spasm: use very cautiously in asthmatics

Fluid Volume Deficit Related to Diaphoresis, Increased Lung Water Loss, and Diuresis Due to Aminophylline Administration Administer fluids as previously described. Assist with CVP line placement, if desired by the physician, to monitor fluid therapy. Monitor BP, pulse, level of consciousness, urinary output, breath sounds, and peripheral perfusion closely. After the patient is stabilized and able to swallow safely, encourage the intake of oral fluids.

High Risk for Decreased CO Related to Right Heart Failure Monitor the patient for signs and symptoms of impending cardiac failure (see Chapter 13 for further details). Usually, the failure is right-heart failure precipitated by the high pulmonary vascular resistance (cor pulmonale).

Fear Related to Inability to Breathe Comfortably Provide emotional support by projecting a calm, competent air. If accepted by the patient, use touch to provide reassurance. Allow a loved one, if calm, to stay with the patient. For further suggestions on provision of emotional support, see Chapters 2 and 3.

Outcome Evaluation

Evaluate the patient's progress according to the following desirable outcome criteria:

- Vital signs WNL for patient.
- Arterial blood gas values WNL for patient.
- Presence of normal breath sounds.
- Absence of dyspnea and wheezing.
- Recovery of normal energy level.

PULMONARY VASCULAR DISEASE

Pulmonary Embolus

An *embolus* is an undissolved mass that travels in the bloodstream and occludes a blood vessel. Emboli to the lungs include venous thromboemboli, air emboli, fat emboli, and catheter emboli. Incidence is estimated as high as 630,000 per year, with a death rate of 200,000 annually in the United States (Stein and Levy 1991).

Assessment

Risk Conditions Anticipate and prevent emboli whenever possible. Conditions increasing the likelihood of different types of emboli are stated in the next sections to enhance your ability to identify patients at risk.

1. *Thromboemboli* may result from blood stasis, venous wall abnormalities, clotting abnormalities, or irrigation of clotted catheter tips. In 1846, Virchow identified blood stasis, venous wall abnormalities, and clotting abnormalities as factors promoting venous thrombosis. Remembering this triad can help you to recognize risk conditions for thromboemboli. For example, blood stasis may be caused by obesity, congestive heart failure, immobilization (bedrest), atrial fibrillation or standstill, or severely decreased myocardial contractility. Venous wall abnormalities can result from venous punctures or incisions, trauma, or atherosclerosis. Disorders causing abnormal blood clotting include thrombocytosis and dehydration. Ninety percent of pulmonary emboli arise from the deep veins of the leg.

   The critical-care nurse also must be aware that forceful irrigation of clotted catheter tips can dislodge the clots, creating emboli.

2. *Air emboli* may result from surgery on the peritoneal cavity, air in intravenous lines, or breakage of a pulmonary artery catheter balloon.

3. *Fat emboli* can result from long-bone fractures (especially the femur and tibia), sternal splitting incisions, use of a pump oxygenator during cardiopulmonary bypass, or trauma to subcutaneous fat. The exact mechanism of fat embolization is unclear; fat release from bones and tissues, alteration of circulating fats, and other factors have been implicated.

4. *Catheter emboli* may also occur. Many polyethylene intravenous catheters have a surrounding short steel needle to facilitate venipuncture. After venipuncture, the catheter is advanced through the needle, which is withdrawn and covered by a protective shield. If the catheter is advanced and then manipulated while the needle is unshielded, a portion of the catheter can be sliced off and embolize to the lung.

5. *Septic emboli* or *tumor emboli* also may occur.

Preventive Measures Virchow's triad of factors contributing to thromboemboli has numerous implications for preventive measures. Follow these measures to reduce risk of *thromboemboli.*

1. Decrease *venous stasis* as follows:
    (a) Consult with the physician about the use of antiembolic stockings or pneumatic sequential compression boots to maintain venous flow.
    (b) Ensure that active or passive lower extremity exercises are performed, since muscular activity promotes venous flow by alternatively compressing and releasing the veins.
    (c) Some physicians recommend elevating the supine patient's legs about 15° to aid venous flow without causing inguinal pooling. Avoid constant Fowler's position whenever not required by other conditions (such as acute pulmonary edema).
2. Reduce *venous wall trauma* as follows:
    (a) Avoid venous punctures on the legs whenever possible.
    (b) Observe vascular catheter insertion sites for inflammation and phlebitis. If they occur, discontinue the line (unless no other sites are available) and restart elsewhere.
3. If you suspect a line has become clotted, first try to aspirate blood; reposition the tip; and then irrigate gently. Do *not* irrigate forcefully.
4. Prevent dehydration to help maintain normal coagulability.
5. Administer low-dose heparin if ordered by the physician. Research has confirmed the effectiveness of mini-dose heparin in preventing fatal postoperative pulmonary emboli in major surgical procedures performed on patients over 40 years of age (Multicentre trial 1975).

Take preventive action against *air emboli.* Always remove air from vascular lines when assembling them. If you note a bubble once the line is in use, remove it with a needle and syringe without breaking continuity of the line. To prevent air embolization from breakage of a pulmonary artery catheter balloon, see Chapter 11, on cardiac assessment and hemodynamic monitoring lines.

Reduce the risk of *catheter emboli* by implementing the following measures. If it is necessary to reposition a catheter during insertion, withdraw the catheter and unshielded needle simultaneously. Once a catheter is positioned properly, withdraw the needle and cover it with the protective shield.

If a venous catheter is sliced off accidentally, it is imperative that you try to prevent it from reaching the heart. Immediately clamp your hands around the limb between the insertion site and the heart, and obtain immediate medical assistance to remove the catheter.

Signs and Symptoms Detect the occurrence of pulmonary embolism promptly. Signs and symptoms vary, depending on the type, size, and hemodynamic consequences of the embolus.

Thromboembolism A thromboembolus consists of fibrin, platelets, and red blood cells. When the platelets degranulate, they release substances that cause smooth muscle constriction in both the pulmonary arteries and bronchi. Constriction of blood vessels feeding well-ventilated lung units increases wasted ventilation. To compensate, the patient increases his or her minute ventilation to excrete CO_2. This wasted ventilation is reduced somewhat by the constriction of bronchi due to platelet degranulation and distal airways due to alveolar hypocapnia. This constriction is a protective measure, redirecting ventilation to better perfused areas. Unfortunately, it also increases airway resistance and work of breathing. Loss of surfactant may also occur, leading to atelectasis and edema (Currie 1990).

Chest Pain

Dyspnea, pleuritic chest pain, cough, hemoptysis, syncope, tachypnea, tachycardia, and crackles may all be found in the patient with pulmonary embolism (Leeper 1988). Chest pain and tachypnea are the most common findings. The cause of chest pain is unclear.

Signs of Hypoxia

Watch for signs of hypoxia resulting from the increased alveolar deadspace. The signs include tachypnea, restlessness, and irritability.

Signs of Acute Right Ventricular Failure

Monitor for signs of possible acute right ventricular failure *(cor pulmonale).* This condition results from a large embolus that occludes over 50% of the pulmonary vascular bed. An accentuated P_2 (pulmonic component of second heart sound), atrial dysrhythmias, increased CVP readings, distended neck veins, and liver engorgement all indicate right-heart failure. Mortality is 85–90% for this group. Pulmonary hypertension may also result from chronic multiple small emboli.

Signs of Decreased CO

Observe for potential indications of decreased CO. Signs resulting from decreased left ventricular filling are tachycardia, hypotension, dizziness or confusion, shock, or angina. Angina results from decreased coronary artery perfusion coupled with an increased right ventricular workload.

Air Embolism A churning noise upon auscultation of the right ventricle is a sign of air embolism to the ventricle. It is accompanied by sudden dyspnea, shock, and cyanosis.

Fat Embolism Suspect fat embolism if you see petechiae along with the signs and symptoms of increased deadspace, right ventricular failure, or decreased CO. Petechiae are most common on the anterior chest, neck, and axillary folds.

Pulmonary Infarction Be alert for symptoms of a possible pulmonary infarction. The signs are those indicated above plus fever over 39°C; transient or persistent pleuritic pain and/or pleural friction rub; cough; and hemoptysis. A chest x-ray 12–24 hours postembolization frequently will show a localized density in the periphery with a rounded edge facing the hilum.

Infarction occurs in only about 10% of the known episodes of embolization. The probable reason is the dual blood supply to the lungs. The numerous anastomoses between the bronchial and pulmonary capillaries and veins produce a network that facilitates collateral flow in the event of an embolus.

Other Diagnostic Aids Keep abreast of the results of other diagnostic maneuvers. Additional tests may or may not be helpful in detecting an embolus. The ECG occasionally shows signs of right axis deviation and right ventricular strain. The routine chest x-ray may show nothing or may show an elevated diaphragm due to pneumoconstriction, decreased or absent vascular markings, or dilatation of the main pulmonary artery and right ventricle. Evaluation of the leg veins with flow studies or radiographic scan may identify a deep vein thrombus as the source for pulmonary embolus. Ventilation/perfusion scans usually show an area of normal ventilation with decreased or absent perfusion. Blood gases may be normal or show hypoxemia and an increased A-aDo$_2$. Pulmonary angiography, in which contrast material is injected directly into the pulmonary arteries, is the most definitive diagnostic test for pulmonary embolism.

Planning and Implementation of Care

If you suspect an air embolus in the right ventricle, immediately place the patient on the left side with the head dependent. This will prevent the air from obstructing the right ventricular outflow tract or migrating to the pulmonary artery. The air will be displaced to the apex, where a physician can aspirate it.

For any type of embolus reaching the pulmonary artery, the goals of care are to relieve the hypoxia resulting from the increased alveolar deadspace, combat any significant decrease in CO, and treat shock vigorously if present.

Impaired Gas Exchange Related to Ventilation/Perfusion Mismatch Observe for signs of progressive hypoxemia and hypo/hypercapnia. Maintain bedrest, with the head of the bed elevated to promote respiratory excursion. Assist the person with bathing, eating, and other activities that increase dyspnea. Administer supplemental oxygen as ordered by the physician.

High Risk for Decreased CO Related to Increased Right Ventricular Afterload Decrease additional insults to the right ventricle by reducing its workload: provide physical rest; and reduce emotional stress by providing as calm an atmosphere as possible, administering analgesics to control pain, and relieving anxiety as much as possible.

Prevent recurrent embolization by administering anticoagulants and thrombolytic agents as ordered by the physician.

A mainstay of medical therapy for thromboembolism is anticoagulation. Heparin is the drug of choice in treating acute thromboembolism because it inactivates thrombin, thus blocking further clot formation, and also inhibits the degranulation of platelets surrounding the thrombus, thus limiting the release of substances causing smooth muscle constriction. It is administered intravenously as a continuous infusion. Therapy is monitored with Lee White clotting times or partial thromboplastin times kept at 2 to 2½ times normal. Heparin therapy is continued for several days or

---

NURSING DIAGNOSES

Nursing diagnoses that may apply to the patient with a pulmonary embolus include:

- Impaired gas exchange
- High risk for decreased CO
- High risk for knowledge deficit

longer; a transition is made to oral anticoagulants as soon as the patient is ambulatory.

Because heparin does not directly affect fibrin, it has no fibrinolytic activity. Therefore, although it can prevent further clot formation, it cannot lyse formed clots. To achieve the latter therapeutic goal, thrombolytic agents such as intravenous streptokinase and urokinase are prescribed for those patients experiencing severe hemodynamic compromise.

If shock occurs, follow measures outlined in the care plan for shock (Chapter 13). For persistent shock from a centrally located embolus, surgical embolectomy may be attempted. Mortality is high, and this procedure is reserved for the patient with cardiac and pulmonary deterioration for whom thrombolytic therapy and anticoagulation have failed (Stein and Levy 1991).

High Risk for Decreased CO Related to Bleeding Protect the patient from excessive anticoagulation and fibrinolysis by monitoring clotting and/or prothrombin times, observing for signs of internal or external bleeding, minimizing intramuscular injections, testing gastric contents and bowel movements for occult blood, and consulting with the clinical pharmacist on interactions between anticoagulants and the patient's other medications.

If anticoagulation is contraindicated or emboli persist despite anticoagulation, either the common femoral veins or the vena cava may be ligated; alternatively, a device may be inserted in the vena cava to trap further emboli.

High Risk for Knowledge Deficit When the patient's condition permits, teach him or her how to prevent, recognize, and respond to symptoms postdischarge. Emphasize the importance of exercise, hydration, measures to promote venous flow, and medical follow-up. Oral anticoagulants may be continued as long as the risk is present, permanently if necessary.

Outcome Evaluation

Judge the patient's progress according to these outcome criteria:

- Unlabored respirations 12–18 times a minute.
- Pulse, BP, and temperature WNL for patient.
- No signs of right ventricular failure (undistended neck veins, normal CVP readings, no liver engorgement).
- Alert and oriented.
- No churning noise when right ventricle is auscultated.
- No cough, hemoptysis, or pleural friction rub.
- Normal breath sounds

REFERENCES

American Lung Association. *Estimated prevalence and incidence of respiratory disease by Lung Association Territory,* Sept. 1989.

American Thoracic Society: Definition and classification of chronic bronchitis, asthma and pulmonary emphysema. *Am Rev Respir Dis* 1982; 85:762.

Antony VB: Pleural effusion. In *Current therapy of respiratory disease, Vol 3,* Cherniack R (ed). Toronto, Decker, 1989.

Benner P: *From novice to expert.* Menlo Park, CA: Addison-Wesley, 1984.

Brown L: Pulmonary oxygen toxicity. *Focus Crit Care* 1990; (17)1:66–75.

Caruthers K: Infectious pneumonia in the elderly. *Am J Nurs* 1990; 90(2):56–60.

Craven D: Nosocomial pneumonia in the ICU patient. *Crit Care Nurs Quart* 1989; 11(4):28–44.

Crowley J, Raffin T: Acute lung injury: Mechanisms and potential therapy. In *Current pulmonology,* Simmons D (ed). St Louis: Mosby/Year Book, 1991.

Currie D: Pulmonary embolism: Diagnosis and management. *Crit Care Nurs Quart* 1990; 13(2):41–49.

Dudley D et al.: Psychosocial concomitants to rehabilitation in chronic obstructive pulmonary disease. *Chest* 1980; 77:413–420.

Fagon J et al.: Nosocomial pneumonia in patients receiving continuous mechanical ventilation: Prospective analysis of 52 episodes with use of a protected specimen brush and quantitative culture techniques. *Am Rev Respir Dis* 1989; 139:877–84.

Fahling L, Snider G: Treatment of chronic obstructive pulmonary disease. *Current Pulmonology,* In Simmons D (ed). Chicago: Year Book, 1989.

Fink M et al.: The efficacy of an oscillating bed in the prevention of lower respiratory tract infection in critically ill victims of blunt trauma. *Chest* 1990; 97(1):132–137.

Flaherty J et al.: Nonabsorbable antibiotics versus sucralfate in preventing colonization in a cardiac intensive care unit. Paper read before the *28th Interscience Conference on Antimicrobial Agents and Chemotherapy,* Los Angeles, CA. October 1988.

Humphrey H et al.: Improved survival in ARDS patients associated with a reduction in pulmonary capillary wedge pressure. *Chest* 1990; 97(5):1176–1180.

Kersten L: *Comprehensive respiratory nursing.* Philadelphia: Saunders, 1989.

Ledingham M et al.: Triple regimen of selective decontamination of the digestive tract, systemic cefotaxime, and microbiological surveillance for prevention of acquired infection to intensive care. *Lancet* 1988; 1:785–790.

Leeper K et al.: Clinical manifestations of acute pulmonary embolism: Henry Ford Hospital experience, a five-year review. *Henry Ford Hosp Med J* 1988; 36:29–34.

Mathay M: The adult respiratory distress syndrome: New insights into diagnosis, pathophysiology, and treatment (Medical Staff Conference). *West J Med* 1989; 150:187–194.

Multicentre trial: Prevention of fatal postoperative pulmonary embolism by low doses of heparin. *Lancet* 1975 (July):45–51.

National Heart, Lung, and Blood Institute: *Morbidity and mortality chart book on cardiovascular, lung, and blood diseases.* U.S. Department of Health and Human Services, 1990.

National Heart, Lung, and Blood Institute: National Asthma Education Program Expert Panel Report. *Guidelines for the diagnosis and management of asthma.* U.S. Department of Health and Human Services, 1991.

Rello J et al.: Incidence, etiology, and outcome of nosocomial pneumonia in mechanically ventilated patients. *Chest* 1991; 100(2):439–444.

Sahn S: Continuous lateral rotational therapy and nosocomial pneumonia. *Chest* 1991; 99(5):1263–1267.

Shapiro B et al.: *Clinical application of respiratory care,* 4th ed. Chicago: Year Book, 1989.

Sly R: Mortality from asthma, 1979–87. *J Allergy Clin Immunol* 1988; 82:705–717.

Stein M, Levy S: Pulmonary thromboembolic disease. In *Respiratory care: a guide to clinical practice.* Burton G, Hodgkin J, Wald J (eds). Philadelphia: Lippincott, 1991.

Washington J: Infectious disease aspects of respiratory therapy. In *Respiratory care: A guide to clinical practice,* Burton et al. (eds). New York: Lippincott, 1991.

9

Pulmonary Interventions

CLINICAL INSIGHT

Domain: The helping role

Competency: The healing relationship: creating a climate for and establishing a commitment to healing

In the face of the devastation wrought by critical illness or injury, the nurse can help the patient maintain an awareness of the possibilities for recovery and a sense of optimism. Helping the patient this way requires a complex alloy of technical expertise, analytic skills, and intuition. Here, an expert nurse confidently builds on the trust established with physicians, and in doing so, achieves both an act of mercy and a victory, whose importance her patient recognizes. The following exemplar comes from Benner (1984, pp. 52–53, 512).

The patient was a 17-year-old male admitted post c-spine fracture. The patient presented to the ICU awake, alert, and quadriplegic. Within 24 hours, due to poor ventilatory effort, significant lung consolidation developed. The doctors decided to intubate him in order to provide positive airway pressure from a ventilator. The patient was extremely apprehensive about his intubation. His respiratory rate increased dramatically after the tube was passed. His respiratory rate increased into the 40s and his P_{CO_2} was dropping. The patient was unable to decrease his respiratory rate due to his high anxiety. The doctors were considering increasing his sedation enough to knock out his respiratory drive so that we could totally control his ventilation with this respirator. This increased his anxiety even more. This measure would have added to his already monumental problems with recovery and rehabilitation—something he didn't need. I just knew we could resolve this—his anxiety and thus rapid respiration rate—without using such drastic *measures. I intervened in his behalf with his multiple physicians; I explained my "gut feeling," my concerns for his recovery, and negotiated for more time to attempt to resolve this problem. Then I began reassuring him, using my calmest voice. I spoke assuredly, honestly, professionally, and yet personally. He could not speak, as he was intubated. He could not write, as he was quadriplegic, and we didn't allow him to nod his head due to his unstable neck fracture. His only communication was with his eyes and his amazing ability to mouth words clearly and understandably. It took three and a half hours before he began to relax. He needed to know that we cared about him, as an individual, not just another helpless patient. He needed to be involved, not just prescribed to, and he felt so very helpless. This incident is critical to me because it was what nursing is all about for me. The point was made by one simple statement he mouthed to me late in the day—when he had a respiration rate in the 20s, and he was no longer threatened with having the few remaining functional muscles chemically paralyzed. His words were: "Thank you. You've really helped me a lot. I don't want to imagine what would have happened to me if you weren't here and hadn't cared."*

An arsenal of interventions to improve pulmonary function lies at a nurse's fingertips. Sometimes a given intervention needs to be applied; at other times, as in the Clinical Insight, it needs to be withheld and an alternate tried instead. This chapter discusses oxygen therapy, chest physiotherapy, artificial airways, tracheal suctioning, mechanical ventilation, chest drainage, and thoracic surgery.

Oxygen Therapy

The goal of oxygen therapy is to ensure that tissue metabolic needs are met. Oxygen can be administered to prevent or reverse hypoxemia. Specific signs indicating a possible need for supplemental oxygen include decreased mental status (confusion, impaired thought processes, drowsiness, or lethargy), impaired ventilation (tachypnea, hyperventilation, respiratory depression, cyanosis, and decreased P_aO_2), and increased myocardial work (tachycardia, dysrhythmias, premature beats, hypotension). The physician is responsible for prescribing the type of therapy, its frequency and duration, F_IO_2 (fractional inspired oxygen), and liter flow. In an emergency (such as shock, severe respiratory depression, impending myocardial infarction

(MI), or serious dysrhythmias), the nurse should be empowered to start oxygen therapy under standing unit guidelines.

Guidelines for Initial F_IO_2 Selection

Although the indications for oxygen therapy vary for each person, a general guideline is that as S_aO_2 falls below 90% or P_aO_2 falls below 60 mm Hg, supplemental oxygen is indicated (Ryerson 1991).

Oxygen therapy is titrated carefully in patients who have chronically elevated carbon dioxide levels. These patients—often those with severe chronic obstructive pulmonary disease (COPD)—have a blunted response to elevated carbon dioxide levels as a stimulus to breathe and instead are driven by the "hypoxic drive," or a P_aO_2 below 60 mm Hg. Therefore, administration of high levels of oxygen (i.e., above 2 L/min or over 30–40%) may actually *suppress* their ventilation as their P_aO_2 rises above 60 mm Hg and their hypoxic drive to breathe is lost. Arterial blood gases and the patient's clinical status are monitored carefully when adjusting oxygen therapy for this group of patients.

Intubated patients on positive pressure ventilation, once stabilized, should receive the F_IO_2 that most nearly reproduces their baseline arterial blood gases (ABGs) and/or achieves a saturation of at least 90%.

It should be emphasized that the above are guidelines for selection of initial F_IO_2 only and should not replace clinical judgment. Subsequent F_IO_2 adjustment is based on arterial blood gas values and close monitoring of the patient's clinical status.

Methods of Oxygen Therapy

The following information on methods of oxygen therapy is based primarily on Shapiro et al. (1991).

The ideal O_2 delivery system would deliver a consistent F_IO_2 that could be controlled easily, allow accurate measurement of inspired F_IO_2, be comfortable for the patient, be convenient for the therapist, and be inexpensive. Unfortunately, no current method meets all these criteria. One must choose from a variety of devices the one that will best meet the patient's needs. They may be classified into low-flow and high-flow systems. Oxygen flow is *not* synonymous with oxygen concentration, because concentration depends on the relationship between O_2 flow *and* total air flow. (A low oxygen concentration is below 35%, a moderate concentration is 35–50%, and a high concentration is above 50%).

Low-Flow Systems A low-flow system is one in which the gas flow is insufficient to meet all the requirements for inspiration; room air must also be inspired. Low-flow systems have an oxygen reservoir that is diluted with room air. The cannula, catheter, and simple mask use the nose, nasopharynx, and oropharynx as an anatomic reservoir. Some cannulas have a small built-in reservoir under the nares. The mask with reservoir bag adds an additional O_2 reservoir from which the patient inspires. Without a one-way valve between this bag and mask, the system is a partial rebreathing mask. If there is a one-way valve between the bag and mask, the system is a nonrebreathing mask.

The advantages and disadvantages of low-flow systems are summarized in Table 9–1. Variations in respiratory rate or tidal volume affect the inspired oxygen concentration. The slower the rate or the lower

TABLE 9–1

Selected Options in Oxygenation (for Spontaneously Breathing Patients)

	PATIENT CRITERIA	ADVANTAGES	DISADVANTAGES	NURSING PRECAUTIONS
Low-Flow Systems				
Nasal cannula 1–6 L 24–40%	Normal V_t Respiratory rate < 25 Regular respiratory pattern	Comfortable No breathing of expired air Allows eating and taking Practical for long-term therapy Cost	Easily dislodged Cannot be used with nasal obstruction Straps irritate ears Nasal prongs irritate nose	Make sure the nares are patent. May use even with a mouthbreather, since oropharyngeal air flow creates Bernoulli effect, pulling in O_2 through nasopharynx. Do not increase L above 6 because it will not increase F_IO_2; switch to a mask.
Simple oxygen mask 5–8 L 40–60%	Same as above	Higher concentrations than cannula Cost	Tight seal may cause facial irritation, or increase anxiety in dyspneic patients Interferes with eating and talking	Do not run below 5 L, as exhaled CO_2 will not be washed out. To increase F_IO_2 above 0.60, do not increase liter flow: switch to a bag with reservoir.
Partial rebreathing mask with reservoir bag 6–15 L 35–60%	Same as above	Higher concentration because rebreathe from O_2 reservoir Cost	Tight seal, as above Interferes with eating and talking	Maintain flow rate sufficient to keep bag from completely collapsing on inspiration.
Nonrebreathing mask with reservoir 6–15 L 55–90%	Same as above	Highest concentration Cost	Seal may irritate skin Bag must be kept properly inflated Can lead to oxygen toxicity Valve can stick	Maintain flow rate sufficient to keep bag from completely collapsing on inspiration.
High-Flow Systems				
Venturi mask 4–8 L 24–40%	Patients relying on hypoxic drive, needing constant precise F_IO_2	Delivers exact concentration despite variations in respiratory pattern F_IO_2 directly analyzed	May irritate facial skin Interferes with eating and talking Cost	To increase F_IO_2, switch to a higher-concentration mask/adapter.

the tidal volume, the higher the F_IO_2; the faster the rate or the higher the tidal volume, the lower the F_IO_2.

For these reasons, monitor oxygen saturation by pulse oximetry (S_pO_2) and assess the respiratory rate, depth, and pattern every 2–4 hours. If the respiratory rate increases above 25, breathing becomes shallow, mental status changes, or the ventilatory pattern becomes irregular or inconsistent, alert the physician, who may want to switch to a high-flow system.

High-Flow Systems High-flow systems (described in Table 9–1) include Venturi masks and nebulizers using the Venturi device. This device is based on the Bernoulli principle, which states that as the velocity of gas flow increases, its lateral pressure decreases. In a device using this principle, the oxygen flows through a small orifice at a high velocity. Just after the oxygen leaves the orifice, the low lateral pressure pulls in, or "entrains," room air. By varying the size of the orifice and the flow of oxygen, one can provide a precise F_IO_2. The high-flow systems deliver a consistent, precise oxygen concentration. In addition, temperature and humidity are better controlled as the patient breathes only the system's air. Unfortunately, high-flow systems often are tolerated poorly by patients in respiratory distress, as the mask frequently is removed due to feelings of claustrophobia and needing "fresh air."

Complications

The use of 100% oxygen is indicated in certain situations, such as cardiac arrest, transport of critically ill patients, and acute cardiopulmonary instability. However, the nurse should be aware of the complications of oxygen therapy: dehydration of mucosa, hypoventilation, absorption atelectasis, and acute oxygen toxicity. Preventive measures are described in the following paragraphs.

Dehydration of Mucosa Always humidify oxygen because it is a dry gas that can quickly dehydrate the mucosa. Humidification can be achieved with humidifiers or nebulizers. Heated humidifiers deliver fully saturated water vapor, while nebulizers deliver aerosols (tiny water particles).

Hypoventilation Avoid provoking hypoventilation in chronic lung disease patients. These patients depend upon the hypoxic stimulus to ventilation rather than the normal hypercapnic stimulus, as previously discussed.

Suppression of the drive to breathe may be due to removal of this hypoxic stimulus.

To prevent this problem, use low O_2 concentrations if the patient is not mechanically ventilated. Monitor the ventilatory pattern closely and maintain S_pO_2 at 90–92% or as specified by the physician.

Absorption Atelectasis Prevent absorption atelectasis caused by oxygen "washing out" nitrogen in the alveoli. When nitrogen is replaced by oxygen, which is readily absorbed, the residual volume decreases and the alveoli collapse. Prevent this problem by limiting the duration of 100% inspired O_2; maintaining a patent airway; mobilizing secretions; sighing the patient; or providing constantly high tidal volumes. The use of positive end-expiratory pressure (PEEP) (described later in this chapter) may allow lower oxygen concentrations.

Acute Oxygen Toxicity Acute oxygen toxicity depends on both the alveolar oxygen pressure (not alveolar O_2 concentration or P_aO_2) and duration of exposure.

In a review of findings related to the manifestations of oxygen toxicity, Brown (1990) identified substernal soreness (most common), cough, sore throat, dyspnea, painful inspiration, and nasal congestion. Some of these signs and symptoms were seen after 14 hours of breathing pure oxygen. Changes in lung volumes and diffusing capacity also have been noted. After 24–48 hours, adult respiratory distress syndrome (ARDS) may occur.

Guidelines for prevention of oxygen toxicity are somewhat uncertain. The following ones represent a reasonable consensus (Shapiro et al. 1990; Brown 1990; Ryerson 1991):

1. Limit the use of 100% oxygen to brief periods in emergency situations.
2. As early as possible, reduce the F_IO_2 to the lowest possible level that provides adequate oxygenation.
3. There is little or no serious lung injury with exposure to 100% for up to 24 hours.
4. Toxicity may occur after 24 hours of exposure to 50% oxygen.
5. Prolonged use of F_IO_2s below 50% rarely causes acute oxygen toxicity.

These guidelines of course *must* be considered in light of the patient's need for relief of hypoxia. With many critically ill patients, the dangers of this therapy are outweighed by the need for high inspired oxygen concentrations over prolonged periods to maintain adequate tissue oxygenation. Above all, remember that S_pO_2 or ABG monitoring is critical for appropriate oxygen therapy.

Outcome Evaluation

Evaluate the effectiveness of O_2 therapy by using these outcome criteria:

- Improved level of consciousness, ideally alert, oriented, and relaxed.
- Blood pressure (BP), pulse rate, and cardiac rhythm within normal limits (WNL) for patient.
- Spontaneous, unlabored respirations 12–18 times per minute.
- Urinary output WNL for patient.
- Extremities warm and dry (and pink if the patient is Caucasian).
- ABGs WNL for patient.

Chest Physiotherapy

Therapeutic use of chest physiotherapy can benefit patients with respiratory depression, thoracic or abdominal incisions, atelectasis, copious or viscous secretions, pneumonia, bronchitis, or emphysema. Chest physiotherapy will provide no benefit for patients with pneumothorax, hemothorax, or pleural effusion (because the pleural space does not connect with bronchi); pulmonary edema; or congestive heart failure.

To assess the need for chest PT, examine a variety of indicators. Physical examination may reveal increased respiratory rate or effort, decreased chest excursion, decreased or bronchial breath sounds, crackles or rhonchi. Arterial blood gases may show decreased P_aO_2 and/or increased P_aco_2. The chest x-ray may show consolidation, atelectasis, or infiltration.

Prevent patient apprehension and pain. Explain to the patient the benefits and techniques of chest PT. (Demonstrate them on yourself or gently on him or her.) Administer analgesics before starting, unless they are contraindicated by the patient's pulmonary or systemic status. If the patient is receiving bronchodilator therapy, administer the drugs before chest physiotherapy to enhance secretion mobilization. In addition, to prevent aspiration, turn continuous tube feedings off for 30 minutes prior to therapy.

Techniques of Chest PT

A repertoire of chest PT techniques includes those aimed at improving respiratory muscle efficiency (or "breathing retraining") and those aimed at mobilizing secretions.

Pursed-Lip Breathing and Diaphragmatic Breathing These two techniques most commonly are used with those patients who have COPD and, due to lung hyperinflation, have inefficient respiratory mechanics and an increased work of breathing. Both of these techniques should be taught in the critical-care setting to the extubated patient who is not in respiratory distress, so that they can be used more easily during episodes of extreme dyspnea.

To teach pursed-lip breathing, instruct the patient to inhale through the nose over several seconds and then exhale gently through pursed lips for 4–6 seconds. Emphasize relaxation of the neck and chest muscles, slow rhythmic breathing and prolonging exhalation.

NURSING TIP

Pursed-Lip Breathing

If the patient is receiving mechanical ventilation, the same technique of prolonging exhalation, slowing the rate, and relaxing neck and shoulder muscles can be used without pursed lips.

Diaphragmatic breathing is aimed at strengthening the diaphragm and improving the depth of ventilation. Position the patient comfortably, either supine or sitting. Place your hand or the patient's dominant hand on his or her abdomen. Instruct the patient to relax the abdomen on inspiration and contract and pull it in on expiration.

Huff Coughing Place the patient in a comfortable upright position. Tell the patient to take a deep breath, blow part of it out in a short huff by contracting the abdominal muscles, and continue huffing until he or she must inspire.

Localized Expansion It is possible to improve the expansion of a general area of the lung, such as the apex, base, or lateral lung, with localized expansion techniques. Place one hand anteriorly and the other posteriorly over the area for treatment. Tell the patient to take a deep breath. As the patient inspires, compress the area with the anterior hand. At the height of inspiration, release the pressure suddenly.

Postural Drainage Use the diagrams in Figure 9–1 to position the patient to drain the desired segments. Patients in the critical-care setting usually will tolerate only three or four position changes for postural drainage and chest percussion.

Percussion The object of using percussion is to trap and compress air between your hand and the chest wall, thus transmitting an energy wave to the lung tissue to loosen mucous. Use the postural drainage diagrams to position the patient according to the area you want to treat. Cover the skin with a thin towel. Do not percuss over bony prominences, female breasts, or bare skin.

Cup your hands. Relax your shoulders and elbows. Move your hands from the wrists (Figure 9–2) to produce a hollow percussion note rather than a slapping sound.

Work with gravity; that is, percuss from the least dependent to the most dependent area. Do not percuss in the opposite direction, but instead return your hands to the starting position and repeat the movement.

Begin percussing slowly and gently to accustom the patient to the sensation. Increase the percussion until you are percussing vigorously about 200 times a minute. Percuss for 2–3 minutes in the same area to loosen secretions.

Commercial percussion and vibration devices that are quiet and comfortable for the patient are also available.

Vibration Place one hand over the desired area. Place the other hand on top of and parallel to the first. Flex your elbows slightly. Using your shoulder muscles, vibrate your hands on the chest wall throughout exhalation. Repeat for at least five exhalations. Aim at delivering a vibration frequency of about 200 per minute.

Coordinating Techniques and Treatment Goals
From the preceding techniques, select those appropriate to the goal of treatment and your patient's condition.

1. To improve tidal volume and exhalation, use pursed-lip breathing, diaphragmatic breathing, localized expansion, or huff coughing. To mobilize secretions, use percussion, vibration, or huff coughing in conjunction with postural drainage.

2. Do not use percussion at all if the patient has acute cardiac disease, thoracic inflammation, hemorrhage, or a very low platelet count. Percuss gently on patients who have or are prone to rib fractures, such as those with osteoporosis, bone cancer, or hypocalcemia. Do not percuss over an incision or area of pain, but percuss normally over the rest of the chest. Brace the incision or painful area with a sheet folded into a belt or with your hand.

3. Modify postural drainage for patients with increased intracranial pressure, orthopnea, or poor cardiovascular reserve.

   If the problem is increased intracranial pressure, check with the physician as to acceptable positioning. If the patient has orthopnea or diminished cardiovascular reserve, lower the head as much as tolerable.

4. Coordinate the duration and frequency of the treatments to achieve the therapeutic goal without exhausting the patient. In general, perform chest PT every 2–4 hours, rotating treatment sites. Limit treatments to 10–20 minutes. Do not perform them within 30 minutes of oral feedings. Work together with respiratory therapists to time PT with bronchodilator therapy for optimal effect. Observe the S_pO_2 monitor during treatment to assess the patient's tolerance.

Outcome Evaluation

Evaluate the effectiveness of your treatments according to these outcome criteria:

- Lungs clear on auscultation.
- Arterial blood gases WNL for patient.
- Tidal volume and tidal capacity WNL for patient.
- Chest x-ray clear.

Artificial Airways

Patients with an upper airway obstruction, profuse secretions, a need for mechanical ventilation, or a likelihood of aspirating gastric secretions can benefit from an artificial airway.

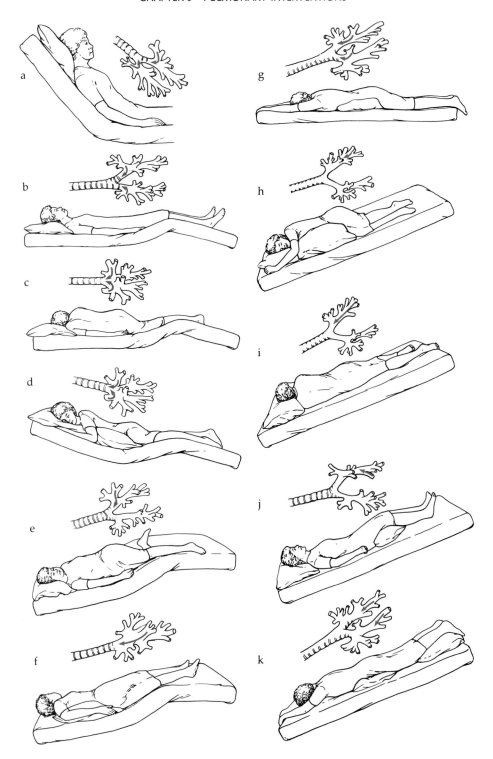

FIGURE 9–1

Postural drainage positions for specific pulmonary segments. **a,** left and right upper lobes (apical segment); **b,** left and right upper lobes (anterior segments); **c,** right upper lobe (posterior segment); **d,** left upper lobe (posterior segment); **e,** left upper lobe (lingular segment); **f,** middle lobe of right lung; **g,** lower lobe (superior segment); **h,** left lower lobe (lateral basal segment); **i,** left and right lower lobes (anterior basal segments); **j,** left and right lower lobes (anterior basal segments); **k,** left and right lower lobes (posterior basal segments). (Source: Kneisl C, Ames S. *Adult health nursing.* Menlo Park, CA: Addison-Wesley, 1986, p. 555.)

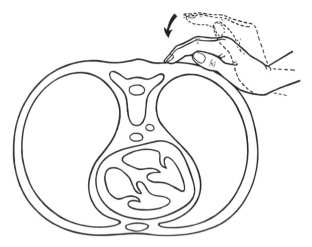

FIGURE 9–2

Chest percussion.

The most common upper airway obstruction in the nonalert patient is the tongue, which falls back and occludes the hypopharynx. For this reason, whenever possible place the nonalert patient on his or her side or prone. Do not leave such a patient unattended in the supine position, especially with a pillow under the head.

If the previously alert patient develops apnea or noisy breathing with diminished air movement, immediately open the airway, following current American Heart Association life support recommendations for initial airway establishment. For more secure maintenance, insert an artificial airway or assist a physician to do so.

Types of Artificial Airways

The three categories of artificial airways are the pharyngeal airway, the endotracheal tube, and the tracheostomy tube. Their advantages and disadvantages are summarized in Table 9–2.

Pharyngeal Airways There are two types of pharyngeal airways: the oropharyngeal and the nasopharyngeal. Often, the nurse may insert these at his or her own discretion. The oropharyngeal or oral airway extends from the lips to the pharynx and therefore displaces the tongue anteriorly. It is made of curved, rigid plastic. To insert one, select a size suitable for the patient. Open the mouth with a tongue depressor or your thumb and index finger. Turn the airway sideways and slide it along the buccal mucosa until the flange on the end touches the lips. Then turn it so the curve fits over the tongue. Tape it in position.

A nasopharyngeal airway is a soft rubber tube that extends from the nare to the pharynx. The end of the tube is funnel shaped to prevent it from entering the nostril. Select the largest-diameter tube that will fit the nostril. Choose the appropriate length by holding the tube against the patient's cheek, with the funnel-shaped end at the nostril and the other end pointing toward the back of the throat. The end of the tube should be about one inch beyond the earlobe. Lubricate the entire length with water soluble jelly and insert it gently. It should be changed every 8–12 hours to prevent occlusion with secretions.

Endotracheal Tube An endotracheal tube extends from the nose or mouth into the trachea. An endotracheal tube may be inserted at the bedside by the physician or specially trained nurse or respiratory therapist. The orotracheal route is preferred in emergencies. Although the tube can be inserted rapidly by this route, it is more difficult to stabilize the tube and kinking develops more easily than with the nasotracheal route. The nasotracheal route of insertion is more difficult, and the diameter of the tube is limited by the size of the nares. To assist with orotracheal intubation:

1. Bring the emergency cart equipped with the following to the bedside: laryngoscope with several sizes of curved and straight blades, extra bulb and battery; assorted sizes of endotracheal tubes; a stylet; topical anesthesia; Yankauer pharyngeal suction tip; suction apparatus; sterile catheters and gloves; syringes; needles; intravenous muscle relaxants (succinylcholine or pancuronium bromide); narcotics and sedatives such as morphine and diazepam; water-soluble lubricant; Magill forceps; benzoin; tape, a bite block or oral airway; and the ordered delivery system for oxygenation and/or ventilation.

2. Snap the size and type of blade preferred by the physician onto the laryngoscope handle. Make sure the light works; if not, replace the bulb or the battery in the laryngoscope handle.

3. Connect the Yankauer suction tip to the suction apparatus. Suction and preoxygenate the patient.

4. Inflate the endotracheal tube cuff to test for symmetry of the cuff and any possible leak in the cuff. Then deflate it.

5. Bend the stylet to a curve with a radius of about 30°. Insert it in the tube until it reaches

TABLE 9–2

Artificial Airways

TYPE	ADVANTAGES	DISADVANTAGES
Pharyngeal Airways		
Oral pharyngeal	Quick and easy to insert	May cause patient to gag
Nasopharyngeal	Quick and easy to insert	Clogs easily
		Kinks easily
		May cause pressure necrosis
Endotracheal		
Orotracheal	Rapid insertion	Special training needed for insertion
	Larger tube size possible than with nasotracheal	Can be bitten
	Less traumatic insertion than nasotracheal	Interferes with coughing
		Can cause pressure necrosis
		Possible tracheal damage from cuff or tube
		Kinks easily
		More difficult to stabilize position
		More uncomfortable for patient
Nasotracheal	Cannot be bitten	Special training needed for insertion
	Easier to stabilize position	Insertion more traumatic
	More comfortable for patient	Size of tube limited
		Can cause pressure necrosis of nose
		Possible tracheal damage from cuff or tube
		Interferes with coughing
		Kinks easily
Tracheostomy		
Uncuffed tube	Suitable for children due to small diameter of trachea	Danger of aspiration
	Decreased risk of tracheal damage	Cannot be used for mechanical ventilation in adults
Cuffed plastic (low pressure)	Large, low-pressure cuff reduces risk of tracheal damage	Expensive
	Cuff bonded to tube	
Cuffed plastic (high pressure)	Cuff bonded to tube	Increased risk of tracheal damage
Cuffed metal	Easy to clean because inner cannula removable	Cuff not bonded to tube; can slip off and occlude tube
		May need adapter for manual or mechanical ventilator
All	Decreased deadspace	Surgical insertion necessary, so is not suitable as method of emergency airway establishment
	Easier to suction	
	Patient can swallow	
Laryngectomy		
	Decreased deadspace	Permanent
	No risk of aspiration	Surgical procedure
		Patient unable to talk normally

half an inch proximal to the tube's end (if you protrude it past the tip, it may damage the trachea).

6. Position the head in moderate dorsiflexion. If the patient is conscious, the physician may apply topical anesthesia to the trachea and administer a muscle relaxant.

7. Lubricate only the tip of the tube; if you lubricate the whole tube, the physician will have difficulty handling it. Hand the tube to the physician.

8. The physician will insert the laryngoscope blade and visualize the vocal cords. Using the hand or the Magill forceps, the physician will pass the tube between the vocal cords, through the larynx, and into the trachea. When she or he indicates, quickly inflate the cuff. The physician will remove the stylet and laryngoscope and hold the tube in place.

9. Hand ventilate the patient until he or she is calm and tolerating the tube.

10. Connect the tube's opening to the ventilating device and begin ventilation. Auscultate the lung fields bilaterally to confirm tube placement in the trachea. Insert an oral airway or bite block, paint the skin with benzoin, and tape the tube securely. Mark the exit point of the endotracheal tube and/or chart the corresponding number of centimeters that are on the side of the tube.

11. Obtain an immediate chest x-ray to verify tube placement. Observe the monitor closely for dysrhythmias, and check BP frequently.

Tracheostomy Tube A *tracheostomy* is an artificial opening into the trachea; *tracheotomy* is the operative procedure that creates it. A tracheostomy is indicated when the anticipated time interval for an artificial airway exceeds 2–3 weeks, an upper airway obstruction prevents the use of an endotracheal tube, radical neck surgery is performed, or anatomic deadspace is excessive.

Ideally, the tracheotomy is not performed in an emergency. For emergency airway establishment, the patient should be intubated at the bedside and transferred to the operating room, where the surgeon can perform technically more difficult tracheotomy under calmer, sterile conditions. General anesthesia is administered and the head and neck extended. A horizontal incision is made between the second and third tracheal rings, and a window the size of the tracheostomy tube excised. The largest cannula that will fit the trachea is inserted. A fabric tape is placed around the neck and

tied to the flange of the tube. The tube is not sutured to the skin.

If the patient has a severe upper airway obstruction precluding intubation before tracheotomy, an emergency cricothyrotomy may be performed at the bedside. The physician palpates the thyroid cartilage and cricoid ring. He or she then uses a scalpel or scissors to incise the cricothyroid membrane. A tracheostomy tube is inserted and the patient transported to the operating room for tracheotomy and closure of the cricothyrotomy.

Prevention of Complications

The critical-care nurse plays a crucial role in forestalling possible problems with an artificial airway. Such complications include: apprehension, malposition or loss of the airway, airway obstruction, infection, and tracheal damage.

Incorporate the following guidelines into your routine care of the person with an artificial airway. Many of them apply to any type of artificial airway. When one applies only to a specific type of airway, it is so stated.

Apprehension Relieve the patient's apprehension due to fear of the unknown, discomfort, or inability to talk. Whenever possible before insertion, prepare the patient psychologically. In many cases, you will have to delay this preparation until the airway has been established. Insertion of any of these airways is uncomfortable; the conscious patient will experience an unpleasant sensation of pressure or choking. The endotracheal tube is probably the most uncomfortable. The newly tracheotomized patient may require medication for the pain of the incision. Most patients learn to tolerate an artificial airway. The patient is justifiably anxious when he realizes the airway interferes with speech and he cannot call for help. Explain that he will be able to speak again when the airway is removed. In the meantime, establish a communication system (see Chapter 3) and call it to the attention of all staff caring for the patient.

Malposition or Loss of the Airway Prevent inadequate ventilation due to the malposition or loss of the airway. Take these preventive measures:

1. After an endotracheal or tracheostomy tube is inserted, obtain an x-ray to verify placement. Also, auscultate both lung fields at least every 2 hours. Sometimes the tube is placed improperly or migrates so that it enters the right mainstem bronchus rather than remaining

above the carina as is necessary for bilateral ventilation. In this case, breath sounds will be present in only one lung.

NURSING TIP

Loss of Airway

If the tube slips forward to the hypopharynx, the patient may be able to vocalize. Mechanically ventilated patients will not receive their tidal volumes, and alarms should sound. Using a tongue blade and flashlight, check the back of the patient's throat for presence of the cuff. If you see the cuff, immediately notify the physician to advance the tube into the trachea or reintubate if necessary.

---

2. Have readily accessible within the unit a laryngoscope, extra tubes, and tracheotomy tray. At the bedside, keep an airway mask and hand-ventilation bag; in addition, for a tracheostomy tube, keep the obturator (if one was used) and a tracheal dilator.

3. Avoid accidental extubation. For a tracheostomy tube, be sure the tapes holding it in place are tied firmly. For an endotracheal tube, note the centimeter number on the tube at the point it enters the patient's nose or mouth and chart it, for reference in chest x-ray interpretation and repositioning. Restrain the hands of confused, agitated patients at risk for self-extubation, and sedate per orders.

Airway Obstruction Forestall obstruction of the airway. Follow these steps to avoid obstruction:

1. Eliminate airway obstruction due to kinking of the endotracheal tube. Position the patient's head neutrally; avoid flexing it. Support the ventilator tubing with a pillow or rolled towel. Some patients will bite an orotracheal tube, thereby occluding it. Prevent this by inserting an oral airway or bite block.

2. Prevent obstruction due to herniation of the cuff over the tip of the tube. Avoid overdistending the cuff by checking cuff pressures whenever air is inserted.

3. Prevent airway obstruction due to retained secretions. Because these tubes bypass the humidification provided normally by the upper airway, provide artificial humidification. Also maintain adequate systemic hydration. For a tracheostomy, remove the inner cannula (if there is one) at least every 8 hours, and rinse with normal saline. Tracheostomy tubes are also available with disposable inner cannulas.

    Institute a vigorous program of coughing, turning, and chest physiotherapy to mobilize secretions. Since a tube in the trachea prevents normal coughing, meticulous attention to removal of secretions is vital. See other sections of this chapter on suctioning and chest physiotherapy for details.

4. Inhibit the formation of tracheal granulation tissue. While this tissue will not cause obstruction during intubation, it may cause obstruction after extubation. To minimize the development of granulation tissue, reduce factors that irritate the trachea. Remove the secretions that accumulate above the cuff, causing chemical irritation of the trachea. Do not use aerosol sprays where the patient can inhale them. Keep cotton fibers from entering the airway by using noncotton gauze around a tracheostomy stoma. If your sterile gloves are powdered on the outside, rinse them with sterile solution before suctioning.

Infection Because the upper airway defense mechanisms are bypassed, pulmonary infection frequently occurs. Sinusitis also is a problem with nasal intubation. Follow these procedures to prevent infection:

1. Use meticulous sterile technique during suctioning and tracheostomy care. Keep the skin around a tracheostomy tube free of secretions by cleaning it with hydrogen peroxide and normal saline and applying a dry sterile dressing around the stoma. Use sterile suctioning technique with a fresh sterile catheter for each episode of suctioning.

2. Give thorough mouth care at least every 8 hours to reduce the potential of the oropharynx as a focus of infection.

3. Drain the water that condenses in the ventilator tubing by disconnecting the tubing and letting it empty into a basin or in-line drainage trap. Do *not* drain the condensed water back into the patient's lungs or the reservoir of the humidifier. Handle condensate from ventilator tubing

as infectious waste. Empty tubing before turning the patient.

4. Follow a prescribed schedule of changing ventilatory equipment. In most units, standard policy is to replace the humidifier or nebulizer and ventilatory tubing every 24–48 hours. Disposable tubing and humidifier units have decreased the risk of equipment-borne infections.

5. Tie tracheostomy tapes snugly but not tight enough to irritate the skin. Reduce chafing by tying the tape so that there are no knots at the sides of the flange and by changing the tape when it becomes soiled. To eliminate knots at the sides of the flange, loop the tape through one side of the flange, pass both ends behind the patient's neck, and loop the bottom piece of tape through the other side of the flange. Then tie a knot several centimeters away from the flange so the knot is on top of the lower piece of tape. This method provides a smooth surface against the skin. (See Figure 9–3.)

Upper Airway Damage   With a nasotracheal tube, avoid pressure necrosis of the nare by cleaning around a nasotracheal tube and observing for areas of pressure or necrosis that may necessitate changing the tube to

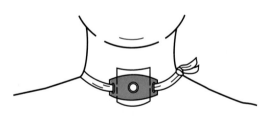

FIGURE 9–3

Tracheostomy tie procedure.

• Cut a long, 20- to 30-inch piece of tape.
• Loop the tape around the far flange. Pull tightly so the ends are equal in length and extend them around the neck.
• Loop the bottom end through the flange close to you.
• Tie in a knot to the side of the neck at a tension allowing one finger to be placed between tape and neck.

Adapted from Kersten LD, *Comprehensive respiratory nursing.* Philadelphia: Saunders, 1989, pp. 677 & 678.

the other nostril. With an orotracheal tube, prevent oral necrosis by repositioning the tube every 24 hours. Have one person hold the tube while you deflate the cuff (suction the oropharynx first) and remove the tape securing the airway. Move the tube to the opposite side of the mouth, check that the same centimeter distance (as marked on the tube) has been maintained, tape it in position, and reinflate the cuff.

Also, forestall tracheal damage from cuffed tubes. Tracheal damage may consist of necrosis, stenosis, tracheoesophageal fistula, distension, or tracheomalacia (loss of cartilage). Numerous factors have been implicated in the genesis of tracheal damage. Among them are infection; the length of intubation; improper size or placement of the tube; cuff size, pliability and shape; intracuff pressure and hypotension (Shapiro et al. 1991). The following paragraphs describe measures that reduce tracheal damage.

Minimize cuff pressure. Numerous studies have been reported on the relationship between cuff pressures over 25–30 mm Hg and increased tracheal damage. Cuff pressures in excess of 30 mm Hg impede arterial flow, causing ischemia. Cuff pressures over 50 mm Hg usually create patchy ischemic and necrotic areas within 48 hours. Tracheal mucosal damage is completely reversible unless necrosis and sloughing occur circumferentially (Shapiro et al. 1991). The ritual of deflating the cuff 5 minutes each hour does not counter mucosal damage sufficiently. Tubes are available with a "foam cuff" to allow the cuff to conform to the shape of the trachea and decrease pressure damage.

To minimize cuff pressure, take these steps:

1. Adjust cuff pressure according to the technique used in your unit: minimal occluding volume or minimal leak. In the *minimal occluding volume technique,* inflate the cuff just until an inspiratory air leak (audible with your stethoscope) disappears. In the *minimal leak technique,* once the air leak has been obliterated, withdraw a small amount of air so that there is a slight leak present at peak inspiration. With either technique, once the desired point has been reached, note the pressure on the manometer and then close the cuff inflation line. Record the measured pressure.

2. Check cuff pressure every 8 hours, according to unit protocol. Call to the physician's attention pressures over 20 mm Hg, increases in cuff pressure or volume, or a leak (other than a deliberate minimal leak).

3. Tracheal necrosis is more common when both an endotracheal or tracheostomy tube and a

large nasogastric tube are in place. If nasogastric drainage is necessary, use a nasogastric tube as small as possible.

Watch for other ways to reduce tracheal damage with a tracheostomy tube. Observe for bleeding around the tube or pulsations of the tube. Bleeding around the tube usually is minor and due to trauma. Pulsations of the tube when none were present previously may indicate imminent hemorrhage through the tube due to erosion of the tip into the innominate artery. This complication is rare but life-threatening. If you spot new pulsations, obtain immediate medical evaluation. It may be necessary to reposition the tube or replace it with a shorter or narrower tube.

Observe for the appearance of oral feedings or tube feedings in the tracheal aspirate. Their presence suggests either a tracheoesophageal fistula or, more commonly, swallowing dysfunction resulting from the tube's interference with the normal swallowing mechanism. You cannot prevent this dysfunction but can minimize it by inflating the cuff and elevating the head of the bed during feedings and for 30 minutes afterward. Both swallowing dysfunction and a tracheoesophageal fistula will cause a positive methylene blue test. When this dye is added to the feeding, its appearance in tracheal secretions confirms the connection between the esophagus and trachea. Differentiating the two causes requires radiology or endoscopy. A fistula usually takes 2–4 weeks to develop, so a positive dye test before then probably indicates swallowing dysfunction. The dysfunction usually will disappear after the airway is removed.

Watch for puffed-up tissues that crackle when palpated, indicating subcutaneous emphysema. Possible causes include air escaping from the stoma into the tissues and a bronchopleural fistula. Call this finding to the physician's attention, as it will necessitate treatment if it continues and compresses the trachea. Once the source is controlled, the air is reabsorbed slowly. If the subcutaneous emphysema is severe, the physician may decompress the tissues by inserting several 18-gauge needles or making small incisions under local anesthesia. Stroking the skin toward the needles or incisions causes the air to escape.

Treatment of Complications

The previous section stressed the role you can play in preventing the complications of an artificial airway. If complications do occur, you must recognize them promptly and respond appropriately.

Relief of Airway Obstruction Retractions, increased inspiratory pressure on a ventilator, severe apprehension, and decreased or absent air movement signify acute airway obstruction. This life-threatening problem can be caused by kinking; by placement of the end of the tube against the carina, tracheal wall, or bronchus; or by mucous plugs or herniation of the cuff over the tube's end if a cuff is overinflated.

If you suspect acute airway obstruction, (a) manipulate the head, neck, or tube slightly to eliminate kinking or reposition the tip; (b) suction the airway; and (c) deflate the cuff. If the airway is a tracheostomy with an inner cannula, remove the inner cannula. If the obstruction persists, summon medical help immediately.

Relief of Bleeding Profuse frank bleeding from the endotracheal or tracheostomy tube after the perioperative period indicates erosion of the tube into the innominate artery. Pulsation of the tube may precede this event. Summon medical assistance immediately. Hyperinflate the cuff to tamponade the bleeding. An immediate operation is necessary to suture the site of the erosion.

Response to Accidental Extubation If accidental extubation occurs, *do not panic*. For a tracheostomy, use a tracheal dilator to maintain the stoma and attempt to reinsert the tube (using its obturator if it has one). For other airways, open the airway by hyperextending the head or using the jaw-thrust maneuver and manually ventilate the patient with a bag-valve-mask device. Call a physician immediately to reintubate the patient.

Treatment of Infection Purulent or colored secretions or an elevated temperature may indicate a pulmonary infection. Culture the secretions to identify the specific organism, and consult with the physician about drug therapy.

Removal of Artificial Airways

When the airway is no longer needed, prepare the patient for its removal. Pharyngeal airways are removed in one step. An endotracheal or tracheostomy tube is removed in several steps. First, the patient must maintain spontaneous ventilation for several hours if he or she has been on a mechanical ventilator; this step is discussed in greater detail under the section on mechanical ventilation. The gag reflex and swallowing ability must be intact. When these criteria are met and it is time to remove the tracheostomy or endotracheal tube, first explain the extubation procedure to the patient. Preoxygenate the patient, suction the trachea, and then suction the pharynx. Ask the patient to take a deep breath, or inflate the lungs with a hand ventilating bag. At the peak of inspiration, the physician or nurse will deflate the cuff and remove the tube, at the same time encouraging the patient to cough up secretions. Immediately provide humidified supplemental oxygen. Observe the patient closely for signs of recurrent respiratory distress. A sore throat and hoarse voice are common after extubation and require no treatment other than an explanation to the patient and humidification. Inspiratory stridor occurring upon extubation or more commonly about 24 hours later indicates laryngeal edema. Alert the physician, who may reintubate the patient or order further observation, humidification, and local application of a steroid and vasoconstrictor (racemic epinephrine) to reduce the edema.

Outcome Evaluation

Evaluate the effectiveness of the artificial airway and your care according to these outcome criteria:

- Patient able to communicate needs to staff.
- Calm, relaxed appearance.
- Unlabored respirations within limit desired for patient.
- Arterial blood gases WNL for patient.
- Lungs clear to auscultation.
- No signs of necrosis or bleeding around the airway.
- Tracheal cultures without pathologic flora.
- No oral feedings or tube feedings in tracheal aspirate.
- Clean tracheostomy stoma without redness or drainage.

Tracheal Suctioning

Be alert for patients who need tracheal suctioning. Conditions that indicate difficulty with spontaneous clearing of secretions include the following:

1. Increased viscosity of secretions.
2. Weak or paralyzed thoracic or abdominal muscles, for example, owing to thoracic surgery or paraplegia.
3. Depressed ciliary activity such as after general anesthesia.

4. Increased production of secretions.
5. Ineffective cough; a patient is unable to cough effectively if he or she has an endotracheal or tracheostomy tube, or if vital capacity is less than 15 ml/kg or inspiratory capacity below 75% of normal (Shapiro et al. 1991).

Prevention of Complications

Suctioning is not a benign procedure. Potential complications include hypoxemia, dysrhythmias, sudden death, laryngospasm or bronchospasm, and infection.

Avoidance of Routine Suctioning Avoid routine suctioning by capitalizing whenever possible on the patient's ability to remove secretions:

1. Teach the cooperative and able patient how to cough effectively. Tell her or him to take in a deep breath and close the glottis on a count of "one," contract the thoracic and abdominal muscles on "two," and open the glottis on "three." Demonstrate the sound of an effective cough versus an ineffective one with the glottis open and no abdominal movement.
2. Maintain adequate systemic hydration (and airway humidification if an artificial airway is in place).
3. Implement a program of chest PT and postural drainage to assist the patient to raise secretions.
4. If necessary, utilize cough stimulation techniques to enhance secretion removal by the patient. Following are some methods of cough stimulation. (a) Press firmly over the lower trachea until the patient coughs. (b) If recommended in your institution, instill 2–5 ml of sterile saline down the endotracheal or tracheostomy tube to loosen secretions and initiate a cough. (c) Pass a suction catheter until it reaches the carina. In most patients, this contact will initiate a forceful cough.

   Assess the effectiveness of these techniques by auscultating the lung fields every 1–4 hours for crackles and wheezes, examining serial lung x-ray reports (looking for infiltrates or atelectatic areas), and evaluating the blood gases.

Recommended Suctioning Technique Suction when secretions are retained in spite of the measures outlined above. Prevent or minimize complications by adhering closely to these recommendations:

1. Explain to the patient the purpose, technique, and sensations involved. Warn that she or he may feel out of breath or may feel like choking. Suctioning is not a pleasant experience; patients deserve to know this, as well as that the discomfort will be brief. The properly prepared patient is less likely to panic during the procedure. Convey a positive attitude, saying, for example, "I'm going to suction you so you can breathe more easily." You may want to sedate the patient with cardiopulmonary instability before suctioning to avoid excessive coughing and agitation which could worsen hypoxemia.

2. Do not suction if you note signs of laryngospasm (crowing respirations), bronchospasm (severe wheezing), or bradycardia.

3. Bring to the bedside single sterile gloves, sterile saline in a small cup, sterile suction catheters, unit-dose packets of sterile saline, sterile water-soluble lubricant, a hand ventilating bag connected to 100% oxygen and a mask or endotracheal/tracheostomy tube adaptor, and tissues. Turn the suction apparatus on to 80–120 mm Hg.

4. Wash your hands.

5. Preoxygenate the patient. (For options, see the discussion in the next section.)

6. Open the catheter package sterilely. Designate one hand as sterile, to handle the catheter only. Place a sterile glove on it. Designate the other hand as unsterile, to connect the suction and occlude the vent. To minimize resistance and trauma while passing the catheter, leave the vent open. Apply sterile water-soluble lubricant or sterile saline to the catheter.

7. If the patient has an endotracheal or tracheostomy tube, disconnect the airway from the adapter on the hand ventilating bag with the unsterile hand. This maneuver is tricky; if you cannot do it rapidly, use an assistant to hand ventilate and to disconnect and reconnect the airway. The ventilator tubing should be either capped or placed on a sterile surface, such as on the packaging for the suction catheter or gloves.

8. If the patient does not have an endotracheal or tracheostomy tube, facilitate catheter entry into the trachea by placing him or her in Fowler's position. Put a pillow behind the shoulders and tilt the head backward. Do not automatically turn the head to the right to enter the left bronchus or vice versa; these positions are not as effective as has been thought in the past, since it is difficult to enter the more sharply angled left bronchus without a curved-tip catheter.

Grasp the tongue with a gauze square and pull it forward gently. To retract the epiglottis, have the patient cough or breathe deeply while you pass the catheter only on inhalation. When the catheter enters the trachea, the patient may become very restless and apprehensive. Talk soothingly, reminding him or her that the procedure will be over soon.

9. Advance the catheter gently and rapidly as far as it will go; then withdraw it 1–2 cm to avoid traumatizing the tracheal wall. Since the carina is very sensitive to mechanical stimulation, the patient may cough forcefully at this point.

10. Occlude the vent intermittently and suction no more than 10 seconds. Rotate the catheter gently as you withdraw it. Watch the cardiac monitor for the development of dysrhythmias.

11. Reoxygenate the patient. If secretions are thick, rinse the catheter with sterile solution.

12. Repeat the suctioning and oxygenating until the secretions are removed.

13. Next, suction the oropharynx using the same catheter. (Note: it is acceptable to use the same catheter to suction first the sterile trachea and then the oropharynx, but *not* the reverse.)

14. Discard the glove, catheter, and cup after *each* suctioning session.

Options for Preventing Hypoxemia The recommended techniques for preventing hypoxemia during suctioning are controversial, particularly for ventilator-dependent patients. Among the techniques that have been recommended are the following:

Ventilator Hyperoxygenation/Hyperinflation with Removal from the Ventilator During Suctioning Before suctioning, adjust the patient's ventilator to administer approximately 5 breaths of 100% oxygen, at a tidal volume 1.5 times larger than the maintenance volume being used to ventilate the patient. Disconnect the patient from the ventilator during suctioning. Then reconnect, maintain the increased tidal volume and 100% oxygen for another 5–8 breaths, and return the dials to their original settings.

The length of time required to reach the new F_IO_2 varies according to the ventilator type, baseline F_IO_2, and minute ventilation (Chulay 1987). In addition, in a busy critical-care unit the nurse may forget to return the dials to their previous setting, subjecting the patient to an increased risk of oxygen toxicity, barotrauma, and absorptive atelectasis.

Manual Hyperoxygenation/Hyperinflation with Removal from the Ventilator During Suctioning Before suctioning, disconnect the patient from the ventilator circuit; manually ventilate with a bag-valve device for approximately 5 breaths at 100% oxygen and a tidal volume 1.5 times larger than the patient's usual tidal volume. After suctioning, reoxygenate the same way and reconnect the patient to the ventilator.

Pierce and Piazza (1987) compared arterial Po_2 after suctioning, ventilatory sighing, and manual bagging in a convenience sample of 30 cardiac surgery patients. Compared to P_aO_2 before suctioning, P_aO_2 rose with ventilatory sighing/oxygenation but dropped with bag-valve sighing/oxygenation. In addition, blood pH and O_2 saturation were significantly lower with bag-valve postsuctioning sighing. These researchers therefore recommended that ventilatory sighing be used as a postoxygenation method whenever possible.

Hyperoxygenation/Hyperinflation with Ventilator Maintenance During Suctioning Alternatively, to allow suctioning without disconnection from the ventilator circuit, use a special swivel adapter attached to the standard endotracheal tube adapter, or use a modification of the standard adapter itself. Bodai (1982) studied use of a valve that fits commercially available respiratory circuits and contains a diaphragm to allow catheter introduction. He found the drop in P_aO_2 was significantly less with the valve system than with the standard suction technique. Adapters and valves that allow suctioning without interrupting ventilation are particularly helpful for patients who are very sensitive to routine suctioning, such as those with severe pulmonary dysfunction and those on PEEP.

Oxygen Insufflation Without Ventilator Disconnect, Preoxygenation, or Hyperinflation Bodai et al. (1987) studied a commercially available double-lumen catheter that allows simultaneous oxygen insufflation into the trachea along with suctioning. After evaluating it with 24 ventilator-dependent patients in varying degrees of respiratory failure, with diverse medical diagnoses, and a variety of suctioning protocols, they concluded that oxygen insufflation alone was as effective as preoxygenation and hyperinflation in preventing suction-related hypoxemia. They recommended that oxygen insufflation replace bagging for most

patients and that patients with severe pulmonary failure who are sensitive to suctioning be ventilated via a valve system that maintains ventilator connection and PEEP.

Treatment of Complications

During and after suctioning, observe heart rate and rhythm, respiratory rate, blood pressure, S_pO_2, $S\bar{v}o_2$, if available and skin color and moisture. Recognize and respond promptly to signs of complications. Restlessness and cyanosis usually indicate hypoxemia secondary to depletion of P_aO_2. Terminate the suctioning and oxygenate the patient. For future suctioning episodes, increase the duration of preoxygenation and decrease the duration of each suctioning episode.

Increased dysrhythmias may result from hypoxia, catecholamine release during anxiety, or mechanical stimulation of the vagal fibers innervating the trachea. Remove the suction catheter, oxygenate the patient, and calm him or her if apprehensive. Stone et al. (1991) prevented complications from postsuctioning hypoxemia by using hyperoxygenation/hyperinflation maneuvers in cardiac surgery patients. The most common changes from baseline rhythms were increases in premature atrial contractions (PACs) and heart rate that were not clinically significant. If the dysrhythmia persists, notify the physician.

Crowing, wheezing, or resistance to catheter removal indicates laryngospasm or bronchospasm. If the catheter can move freely, remove it and do not attempt to suction again; otherwise, disconnect the suction and leave the catheter in the trachea. Oxygenate the patient and summon a physician immediately.

Purulent or foul-smelling secretions suggest infection. Inform the physician and send a specimen for culture and sensitivity.

Outcome Evaluation

Evaluate the effectiveness of suctioning against these outcome criteria:

- Toleration of suctioning without panic.
- No restlessness, cyanosis, or more severe dysrhythmias during or after suctioning.
- No crowing, wheezing, or resistance to catheter removal.
- Tracheal cultures without pathologic flora.
- Improved breath sounds.
- Improved arterial blood gases.

Mechanical Ventilation

The physician's decision to institute mechanical ventilation is based not on the disease entity per se but rather on the physiologic stress it imposes on the patient. Objective signs that a person probably cannot maintain adequate ventilation for a prolonged period of time include a vital capacity less than 15 ml/kg or twice a predicted tidal volume; a maximum inspiratory force (MIF) weaker than –20 cm of water; arterial P_{CO_2} more than 10 mm Hg above the patient's normal value; a shunt greater than 30%; and/or a deadspace/tidal volume (V_D/V_T) ratio greater than 60%. The broad indications for mechanical ventilation are apnea, impending or actual acute ventilatory failure, and some cases of hypoxemia. Impending acute ventilatory failure is best documented by progressively increasing $P_{a}CO_2$ values and decreasing pH values. Mechanical ventilation may be indicated for hypoxemia without hypercapnia due to decreased functional residual capacity, severely increased work of breathing, or an inadequate pattern of breathing.

Procedure for Mechanical Ventilation

Prepare the patient psychologically. If time and the patient's condition permit, help the physician explain to both the patient and the family the purpose of mechanical assistance before it is instituted or as soon afterward as feasible. Briefly, explain the equipment involved and the care the patient will receive, for example suctioning and blood gas checks. Emphasize the sensations the patient will experience—those of having something breathe for him or her and those related to the artificial airway. Establish a system by which the patient can summon help immediately. Assure the patient that the ventilator has mechanical alarms; demonstrate the noises the alarms make, and explain how the staff will respond. Also assure the patient that a nurse will always be at the bedside or within hearing distance. This psychologic preparation will not only reduce the patient's apprehension but also will have physiologic benefits. The properly prepared patient is less likely to fight the ventilator. Fighting the ventilator is detrimental because it increases catecholamine release, oxygen consumption, and the need for paralyzing drugs.

Bring to the bedside the necessary equipment. From the respiratory therapy department, order the type of ventilator and the settings specified by the physician. Place at the bedside a hand ventilating bag, mask and oxygen tubing, and sterile suction supplies.

Types of Ventilators Ventilators can be classified in various ways. Two general categories are positive pressure ventilators and negative pressure ventilators. Negative pressure ventilators mimic spontaneous breathing in that they create a negative or sucking pressure to draw the chest outward. Examples include the iron lung, a cuirass ventilator, or the PulmoWrap, all of which operate by creating a subatmospheric pressure outside the chest wall, thereby drawing the chest outward and air into the lungs. Positive pressure ventilators, seen more commonly in the critical-care setting, operate by *pushing* air into the lungs.

Positive pressure ventilators come in two basic types: pressure-cycled and volume-cycled. Pressure-cycled ventilators include the Bird Mark 7 and Bennett PR II. With pressure-cycled ventilators, the pressure is preset and the volume of gas delivered varies. For example, when the airway is clear, the desired volume is delivered; but if it becomes obstructed, the set pressure is reached much earlier and a much smaller volume will be delivered. Volume-cycled ventilators include the Bennett 7200, MA-1, and MA-2; Ohio 560; Bear 5; and Hamilton Veolar and Amadeus ventilators. With volume-cycled ventilators, the volume is preset and the pressure varies. With the newer ventilatory mode of pressure support (discussed later in this chapter), various ventilators such as the Siemens Servo 900 C now can be either volume- or pressure-cycled. Figure 9–4 shows two ventilator models currently used.

The type of ventilator chosen depends on the patient's need and in some cases the availability of the ventilator. The patient with normal or stable compliance is a suitable candidate for the pressure-cycled ventilator, since one can be reasonably sure of the delivered volume for a given pressure. The patient with poor or variable compliance needs a volume-cycled ventilator, since it is more difficult to predict from a given pressure whether the patient will receive the desired minute ventilation, consistently. With pressure support gaining popularity in some institutions, ventilators that offer both modes are increasingly popular.

Ventilatory Modes When the decision is made to place the patient on a ventilator, the mode or pattern of ventilation must be chosen. Assist/control, intermittent mandatory ventilation, and pressure support are the three most commonly used modes.

A *control* mode also is available but is less commonly used, except perhaps in apneic patients. In this mode, the machine delivers a set number of ventilations per minute without regard to the patient's efforts. In this situation, patients usually are paralyzed or apneic, as stated above. This mode has several significant disad-

CRITICAL CARE GERONTOLOGY

Ethical Issues in Pulmonary Interventions with Elderly Patients

The critical-care nurse is in a unique position as a patient advocate for the delivery of high-quality and compassionate care. With an increasingly older population surviving to undergo procedures such as cardiac surgery, complex decisions about what available interventions may *not* be justified or desired by the patient and family will become increasingly frequent. Initiation or withdrawal of mechanical ventilation is an example of a dilemma facing the elderly.

Fundamental ethical principles include the preservation of life, alleviation of suffering, prevention of harm, respect for the autonomy of the individual patient, and fair allocation of medical resources (Ruark and Raffin 1988). The patient and his or her legal representatives have a right to control what happens to the patient. As a critical-care nurse, ensuring that your patient and his or her family receive care and explaining the consequences of any procedures *in understandable terms* are primary responsibilities. Helping the physician and family find a place away from the stress and chaos of the ICU will enhance their communication, as stress, fear, and intimidation can interfere with patient and family understanding of what is said to them. You may also be responsible for suggesting to the physician

the availability of a social worker, pastoral care person, or psychiatrist for consultation.

The initiation of mechanical ventilation in the emergency department for an 80-year-old with severe COPD presents a classic example of the above dilemma. First, if the patient is successfully weaned from mechanical support, it should be discussed with him or her whether, should the situation arise again, the patient would want to be reintubated. The nurse can, through open-ended conversation and listening, encourage the patient to discuss this issue with family or physician. If weaning is unsuccessful, goals for that patient—for example, wanting to go home even if on a ventilator—should be identified and respected.

Withdrawal of support with the understanding that the patient will not survive presents more complex issues. For instance, the APACHE study (Knaus et al. 1985) found that advanced age increased the probability of developing multiple organ system failure. Mortality for 99 patients who had at least three days of three or more organ systems in failure was 98%. (See Chapter 20 for a further discussion of multiple organ system failure.) Others have found that elderly patients are more likely to receive life support inter-

ventions and less likely to survive them (Campion et al. 1981). Quality of life if these interventions are survived is another area to be addressed. Withdrawal of life support interventions in such elderly patients draws upon guidelines from hospital ethics committees, and nursing staff should be represented on such committees.

Involving the family in regular patient care conferences and goal setting helps avoid conflicts when urgent decisions are required, as in cardiac arrest. As a critical-care nurse, facing personal feelings that arise when the act of detaching someone from the ventilator results in death is easier when communication among patient, family, nurse, and physician has been ongoing.

Communicating with a unit-based liaison to the hospital ethics committee is the best way to remain educated about hospital procedures surrounding initiating and withdrawing life support. The older population needs education regarding issues such as designation of surrogates to make critical health care decisions when they cannot do so themselves. As a critical-care nurse, you are in a position to explore these issues with patients, family, and staff.

vantages. It is important to understand that if your patient accidentally is disconnected from the ventilator in this mode, *no ventilation will occur.* If this mode is used for the nonapneic patient, the patient may become extremely anxious from making respiratory efforts without receiving a breath. The need to heavily sedate or pharmacologically paralyze the nonapneic patient when using this mode makes neurologic assessment difficult.

The *assist/control* mode provides a minimum number of breaths per minute but allows the patient to initiate the breath and to breathe at a more rapid rate if desired. Whether the breath is initiated by the patient or by the machine (if the patient fails to breathe), each breath is of the same tidal volume and delivered under positive pressure. With the assist-control mode, any increase in respiratory rate, as with anxiety or pain, greatly elevates the minute ventilation, due to an

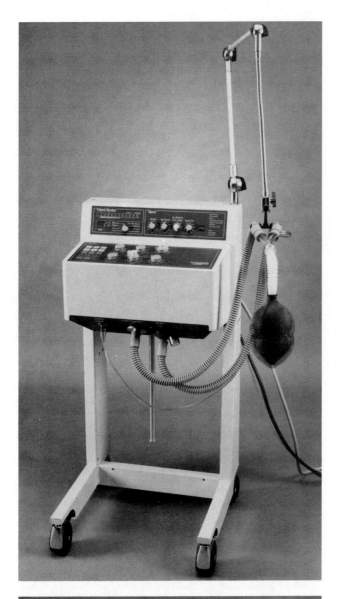

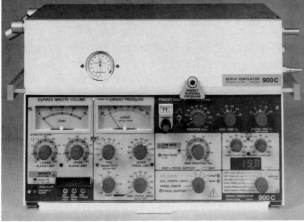

FIGURE 9–4

Positive pressure ventilators. **a,** Amadeus ventilator. Photo courtesy of: Hamilton Medical, Inc., Reno, NV. 1992; **b,** Siemens Servo 900-C ventilator. Photo courtesy of: Patient Care Systems, A Division of Siemens Medical Systems, Inc., Iselin, NJ. 1991

increase in the number of ventilator-preset volume breaths. Respiratory alkalosis may occur as a result.

Intermittent mandatory ventilation (IMV) is a mode capable of providing either full or partial ventilatory support (as may be desired during weaning). A preset number of volume-limited breaths is delivered by the machine, and in between the patient may breathe spontaneously with no machine assistance and at his or her own varying tidal volumes. *Synchronized IMV (SIMV)* allows the predetermined breath to be delivered in phase with the patient's own inspiratory efforts. If the IMV rate is set at 10, the machine is doing most of the ventilatory work; if the IMV rate is set at 4, the patient must assume part of the ventilatory work, as during the weaning process. Some of the purported advantages of IMV modes include the ability to gradually turn down the IMV rate so there is a smoother transition from ventilator-supported breaths to independent breathing without ventilator-assisted breaths. The patient also can control baseline minute ventilation by varying the rate and volume of the interspersed spontaneous breaths. Positive pressure exerted within the chest, even with the use of PEEP, is less with SIMV mode, thereby resulting in less decrease in cardiac output. In addition, SIMV is purported to prevent respiratory muscle atrophy; however, at low rates it may also result in respiratory muscle fatigue (Desautels and Blanch 1991; Hess et al. 1991).

Pressure support (PS) ventilation is a form of assisted ventilation where the patient makes an inspiratory effort and receives a preset level (3–35 cm H_2O) of pressurized inspiratory flow. The flow is cycled off either after it decelerates to less than 25% of the initial flow rate or after a time limit is reached for the length of inspiration. The tidal volume is determined by a combination of the level of pressure support, lung compliance, airway resistance, and patient effort. The amount of PS needed is determined by the respiratory rate and/or the desired tidal volume.

Breathing may be more comfortable with PS due to decreased work of breathing as well as increased patient control over respiratory rate, inspiratory flow, and inspiratory time. The work of breathing through an endotracheal tube and ventilatory circuitry also is overcome with PS.

At higher (20–30 cm H_2O) levels of pressure support, PS ventilation can provide the patient's total minute ventilation. Although PS is a pure ventilatory mode, it can also be used in combination with SIMV (see discussion on weaning) (Ashworth 1990; MacIntyre 1988; Hughes and Popovich 1989).

Inverse Ratio Ventilation (IRV) is a newer, less traditional form of ventilation in which the inspiratory phase is longer than the expiratory phase, i.e., the reverse of a normal inspiration/expiration ratio. It has been employed in patients with severe ARDS in hopes of reversing refractory hypoxemia by prolonging the duration of positive airway pressure during the inspiratory phase. The disadvantages include decreased cardiac output, excessive air-trapping, and possible lung damage resulting from overdistending alveoli (Marcy and Marini 1991; Hudson 1991).

High Frequency Ventilation (HFV) may use high rates (60–100) and small tidal volumes, "jet" pulses of gas through an airway catheter, or oscillation of small volumes of gas in the airways. All three methods are characterized by very low pressures exerted in the chest and a larger number of open gas exchange units. Patients who may benefit from a form of HFV include 1) those with ARDS at risk for barotrauma; 2) those undergoing short procedures such as bronchoscopy or surgery (e.g., lobectomy), where movement of the lung is undesirable; and 3) those with bronchopleural fistula where positive pressure ventilation prevents healing. Attention to secretion clearance is important in this mode; suctioning is done through an adaptor so that the patient is not disconnected from the ventilator during the procedure (Burns 1991).

Nasal or Face Mask Positive Pressure Ventilation uses a tight-fitting nasal or face mask. Patients who benefit from this mode are those with neuromuscular disease or chronic hypoventilation who are in an exacerbated condition that makes intubation undesirable. Meduri et al. (1991) reported success with face mask ventilation in acute hypercapnic respiratory failure. This mode was successful in avoiding intubation in 13 of 18 patients, with a 16% decrease in P_aco_2. Two patients did not tolerate the face mask. Complications of aspiration and skin necrosis occurred in 2 patients. Some patients with sleep apnea or respiratory muscle fatigue may use the nasal mask mode at night in the home setting to prevent nocturnal oxygen desaturation or to rest respiratory muscles (Burns 1991; Hess 1988).

Expiratory Maneuvers The most common expiratory adjustment or maneuver is the application of *positive end-expiratory pressure* (PEEP). PEEP can be applied to any of the above-described modes of ventilation. In addition, it can be applied to the spontaneously breathing patient via an endotracheal tube or by mask. When positive airway pressure is applied to the spontaneously breathing patient, it is called *continuous positive airway pressure* (CPAP). Figure 9–5 illustrates various ventilatory modes with PEEP and CPAP.

PEEP PEEP has several significant physiologic effects. Recall that critically ill patients often suffer

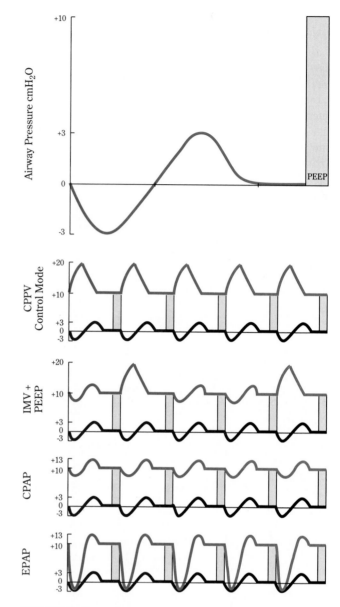

FIGURE 9–5

Airway pressure curves of various modes of positive end-expiratory pressure (PEEP). **CPPV,** continuous positive pressure ventilation, sometimes referred to as "the ventilator with PEEP"; **IMV,** intermittent mandatory ventilation; **CPAP,** continuous positive airway pressure; **EPAP,** expiratory positive airway pressure. (Reproduced with permission from Shapiro BA, Harrison RA, Kazmarek RM, Cane RD: *Clinical application of respiratory care,* 4th ed. Copyright 1991 by Year Book Medical Publishers, Inc. Chicago.)

alveolar collapse, due to the loss of surfactant, absorption atelectasis during the administration of oxygen, or early small airway closure.

When alveoli collapse, the continuing pulmonary capillary blood flow is not oxygenated; that is, increased shunting occurs. Alveolar collapse also decreases residual volume and therefore *functional residual capacity* (FRC). In addition, alveolar collapse decreases lung compliance, because it takes a higher-than-normal airway pressure to reopen the alveoli. Thus, alveolar collapse causes both hypoxia and increased work of breathing. The application of PEEP causes airways to stay open longer, decreasing shunt, increasing FRC, and improving ventilation/perfusion match. As a result, the patient's blood can be oxygenated more readily. PEEP often allows the use of a lower F_Io_2, an important consideration in preventing oxygen toxicity.

PEEP usually is instituted in any patient unable to maintain a P_ao_2 greater than 60 on less than 50% oxygen. Controversy exists regarding optimal levels of PEEP because of its potential detrimental effects, which include decreased venous return, increased risk of pneumothorax, and increased water retention due to stimulation of antidiuretic hormone (ADH) production. For these reasons, PEEP is added in 2–3 cm H_2O increments with close surveillance of the patient's BP, pulse, cardiac output, and ABGs. The usual therapeutic level of PEEP is 5–15 cm H_2O pressure (Shapiro et al. 1991).

CPAP While weaning the intubated patient, continuing some positive airway pressure (5 cm H_2O) during the trial of spontaneous breathing optimizes oxygenation. The patient may then be extubated directly from the CPAP mode, or positive pressure may be removed and the patient placed on a T-piece or blow-by and then extubated.

Mask CPAP is utilized in the unintubated patient who is suffering from severe hypoxemia without carbon dioxide retention. Mask CPAP can help reopen and expand alveoli, correct hypoxemia, and possibly alleviate the need for intubation. It can also be used in patients deemed to be at high risk for developing an acute lung injury (Shapiro et al. 1991). The mask must be tight fitting, the patient alert and cooperative. A nasogastric tube is recommended to prevent aspiration from vomiting; otherwise, the patient's arms must be free to remove the mask should vomiting occur (Hess 1988).

Ventilator Settings Initially, ventilator settings are approximate. Ideally, a slow ventilatory rate (10–14 per minute) and high tidal volume are chosen. The initial tidal volume setting usually is 10–15 ml/kg body weight. Other settings, such as F_Io_2, sensitivity, and PEEP, depend on the patient's condition. Patient observation and evaluation of blood gases must be used to refine these settings to match the patient's need.

Large tidal volumes with slow rates have several physiologic advantages. Slow rates minimize the effects of deadspace better than fast rates. They also lower mean airway pressure; as a result, venous return is diminished less. Ventilation with normal tidal volumes removes the normal sigh mechanism, which prevents collapsed alveoli and promotes surfactant production. Patients on normal tidal volumes need to be given periodic deep inflations, while large tidal volumes obviate the need for sighing and so are more effective in preventing microatelectasis.

Hemodynamic Monitoring and the Effects of Positive Pressure Ventilation During normal respiration, pressure changes occur in the thoracic cavity that cause fluctuation in pulmonary artery waveforms. Patients receiving positive pressure ventilation have additional variations in these pressure waveforms. Digital displays average consecutive waveforms over a set period of time. In the patient with marked waveform fluctuation, this averaging may lead to inaccurate pressures. Digital and graph recordings should be compared periodically to assure accuracy of digital values (Kersten 1989).

In order to obtain standardized, accurate hemodynamic readings it is recommended that values be obtained at end-expiration, or that period of the cycle preceding inspiration (Reidinger et al. 1981). The use of a graph paper recording enables the nurse to consistently identify end-expiration and its corresponding pulmonary artery pressure. Normal spontaneous breathing can be thought of as negative pressure breathing, since intrapleural pressures drop during inspiration. On observing a pulmonary artery waveform readout on such a patient, you will note that the waveform dips during inspiration. The opposite effect is seen during positive pressure breaths given by a mechanical ventilator; the waveform will rise during inspiration. After identifying inspiration on the recording, the nurse examines the preceding section of the waveform to identify end-expiration and read the pressure. Figure 9–6 shows examples of hemodynamic pressure interpretation in a spontaneously breathing or mechanically ventilated patient.

Prevention of Complications

The primary complications associated with mechanical ventilation are insufficient or excessive oxygenation and/or ventilation, water imbalances, decreased CO, pneumothorax, infection, atelectasis, and gastrointestinal hemorrhage or dilatation. Prevent them by incorporating the actions described in the

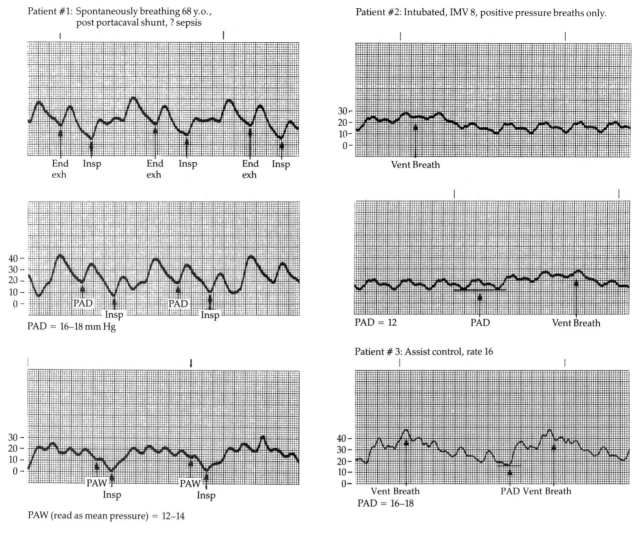

Patient #1: Spontaneously breathing 68 y.o., post portacaval shunt, ? sepsis

End exh   Insp   End exh   Insp   End exh   Insp

PAD   PAD
Insp   Insp
PAD = 16–18 mm Hg

PAW   PAW
Insp   Insp

PAW (read as mean pressure) = 12–14

Patient #2: Intubated, IMV 8, positive pressure breaths only.

Vent Breath

PAD = 12   PAD   Vent Breath

Patient # 3: Assist control, rate 16

Vent Breath   PAD Vent Breath
PAD = 16–18

FIGURE 9–6

Reading hemodynamic pressures in spontaneously breathing or mechanically ventilated patients. **Insp,** inspiration; **End exh,** end-exhalation; **PAD,** pulmonary artery diastolic pressure; **PAW,** pulmonary artery wedge pressure; **Vent Breath,** ventilator breath. Horizontal marks added to show where pressure is read.

following sections into your care of any ventilated patient.

Incorrect Ventilation Monitor the ventilator settings and the delivered values at least hourly. (Ventilator settings often are slightly inaccurate; it is important to note *both* the machine settings and the delivered values.) Make the following checks or, if the respiratory therapist performs them, keep yourself informed of the values.

1. Count the delivered respiratory rate by observing the patient's chest. Compare it to the set ventilator frequency.

2. Monitor the exhaled tidal volume. The machine's gauge estimates only the set tidal volume. Delivered tidal volume is measured with a spirometer attached to the exhalation port.

3. Read the peak inspiratory pressure (PIP) from a dial on the ventilator. Also note the maximum inspiratory pressure—the setting of the pressure pop-off valve. The pop-off usually is set about 10 cm above the pressure necessary to deliver the desired tidal volume. An increased PIP signifies obstructed flow, for example, from increased lung stiffness (decreased compliance), secretions in the airway, patient biting the tube, tube positioned low on the carina, or

right mainstem intubation. A sudden increase in PIP may indicate pneumothorax.

4. Monitor the ratio between inspiration and expiration (I/E ratio), which usually is 1:2. Inspiration must be shorter than expiration to prevent trapping air in the chest. I/E ratio may be prolonged to 1:3 or 4 in patients with COPD.

5. Keep the alarms *on*. Rather than turning them off when you need to disconnect the patient temporarily—for example, to suction or to drain condensed water from the tubing—you can safely press the alarm silence button on the ventilator to prevent the alarm from sounding for 2 minutes.

6. Check the sigh settings. Most volume-cycled ventilators have an optional "sigh" mechanism to mimic the normal deep breaths we take unconsciously. These hyperinflations help to prevent atelectasis and promote surfactant production. The sigh mechanism usually is not used when the patient is on high tidal volumes or PEEP, since these maneuvers also help to prevent atelectasis. If the sigh mechanism is selected, check its rate (usually 6 sighs per hour), volume (usually 150% of tidal volume), and pressure limit (usually the same or slightly higher than the maximum tidal volume inspiratory pressure).

Oxygen Toxicity As discussed earlier in this chapter, excessive amounts of oxygen can cause lung parenchymal damage (oxygen toxicity) and absorption atelectasis. For this reason, periodically check the F_IO_2 setting and the delivered oxygen concentration. Note the machine setting, especially after the patient has been placed on an F_IO_2 of 1.0 prior to suctioning or blood gas sampling. If you fail to reset the F_IO_2 after these procedures, the person may develop nitrogen washout (absorption atelectasis) or oxygen toxicity. The respiratory therapist usually is responsible for determining the delivered oxygen concentration, by using an oxygen analyzer with its tip placed at the patient's airway.

Patients requiring more than 40% oxygen for several hours to maintain a normal P_aO_2 customarily are considered candidates for PEEP, which reduces the risk of oxygen toxicity by allowing the use of a lower F_IO_2.

Water Imbalances The patient may develop dehydration or a positive water balance. Dehydration may result from high temperature or low humidity of the inspired gas. To prevent dehydration, be sure there is

a thermometer dial in the inspiratory tubing. Visually check it every 2 hours to maintain the temperature between 32° and 37°C. Place the patient on intake and output recording. When calculating water balance, consider both the retention of fluid normally lost and the addition of fluid from the equipment. Also monitor the patient's weight, compliance, hematocrit, serum sodium, and chest x-ray for signs of water retention.

Decreased Cardiac Output Positive pressure ventilation increases intrathoracic pressure and therefore decreases venous return to the heart. This effect is increased when control, assist-control, and/or PEEP modes are used. Most patients can tolerate this effect, increasing their peripheral venous tone to compensate. Patients with conditions that diminish sympathetic responses (for example, hypovolemia, drugs interfering with sympathetic tone, or old age) cannot compensate for increased intrathoracic pressure. Monitor the heart rate, arterial blood pressure, peripheral perfusion, and venous pressure to detect the patient's response to the increased intrathoracic pressure; notify the physician promptly if you observe signs of falling cardiac output.

Pneumothorax Pneumothorax may occur due to rupture of a bleb in the lung, disruption of lung sutures, or procedures such as central venous pressure (CVP) line insertion while the patient is on the ventilator. Its incidence is increased in the patient with PEEP. See Chapter 8 for ways to prevent, recognize, and respond to this complication.

Infection Minimize the ventilator as a source of infection. The Respiratory Therapist should follow a regular program of decontaminating equipment including changing ventilator tubing once every 24–48 hours. When water condenses in the tubing, empty it externally rather than draining it back into the patient's lungs. Handwashing is of crucial importance, both between patients as well as between care procedures with the same patient, for example, emptying Foley bags or providing wound care and then suctioning.

Atelectasis Prevent atelectasis by following the measures outlined in Chapter 8. In addition, if normal tidal volumes are being used, periodically sigh the patient to prevent microatelectasis. If the ventilator does not have a sigh button, hand ventilate the patient with a tidal volume larger than the ventilator's. Once the patient has developed microatelectasis, the sigh will not reopen collapsed alveoli. To promote reexpansion, deliver a deep breath and hold the inflation momentarily, that is, "yawn" the patient (Shapiro et al. 1991).

Some ventilators have an end-inspiratory pause or "inflation hold" button; if yours does not, hand ventilate the patient and briefly hold inspiration to mimic a normal yawn.

Gastrointestinal Complications Prevent gastrointestinal (GI) complications. Hemorrhage occurs in about 25% of patients with prolonged mechanical ventilation. Consult with the physician about administering antacids or histamine$_2$ blockers such as ranitidine or cimetidine, which have been found effective in reducing the incidence of massive GI hemorrhage in intubated, mechanically ventilated patients in respiratory failure. Test gastric and fecal matter for occult blood, and notify the physician if present. Avoid gastric dilatation (caused by air swallowing) and aspiration by consulting with the physician about using nasogastric decompression.

Treatment of Complications

Recognize and respond promptly to the problems of *loss of ventilation, cardiovascular deterioration,* and/or a *struggling patient.*

Whenever adequate ventilation fails abruptly, immediately disconnect the ventilator and hand ventilate the patient while you evaluate the problem further. A sudden increase in inspiratory pressure, often accompanied by release of the pop-off valve, signifies obstruction. Check for kinks in the tubing, and suction the airway. A falling pressure in a volume-cycled ventilator or a rapidly decreasing tidal volume in a pressure-cycled ventilator indicates a leak in the system. Check the tubing connections. If these simple actions fail to correct the problem, summon the assistance of another nurse, respiratory therapist, or physician.

The cause of cardiovascular deterioration usually is increased intrathoracic pressure. Reversal of hypotension usually is accomplished by fluid and/or sympathomimetic drug administration. If the decompensation is acute, hand ventilate the patient. Obtain immediate medical reevaluation of the therapy.

A restless or struggling patient may indicate hypoxia or emotional panic. Manually ventilate the patient while blood gases are checked; the ventilator settings may have been inadequate. If the gases are abnormal, inform the physician, who may want to alter the settings. If the gases are normal, the problem may be that the patient is terrified of the sensation of being unable to ventilate himself or herself. When this occurs, hand ventilate, starting at the person's spontaneous rate and slowly decreasing the frequency until the desired rate is reached. Then, reconnect the patient while you coach him or her to breathe in synchrony with the ventilator. The attitude you convey during this maneuver is very important. If your tone or actions are critical or demeaning, you will only increase patient anxiety. If you verbally acknowledge the fright and convey calmness, especially if the patient has developed trust in you before the episode, you will be considerably more effective in aiding adaptation to dependence on the ventilator. If the problem continues, consult with the physician about revising the ventilator settings. If all other measures fail, the physician may order the patient sedated with morphine or paralyzed with small doses of pancuronium bromide or another neuromuscular blocker along with the sedation.

Discontinuation of Mechanical Ventilation

Knebel (1991) divides the process of discontinuing mechanical ventilation into three phases: preweaning, weaning, and extubation. Table 9–3 identifies the criteria for determining the readiness of the patient to begin the weaning process. Table 9–4 lists those parameters that can be determined at the bedside to predict weaning success. Establishing a relationship of trust and support is essential in avoiding the panic and anxiety that commonly thwart weaning attempts despite "physiologic" readiness.

A patient who has been receiving PEEP must be weaned from PEEP before being weaned from the ventilator. Weaning from PEEP can begin when the P$_a$O$_2$ is acceptable on 40% oxygen. PEEP is decreased in small amounts, with arterial blood gases used to evaluate the effects of each reduction, until atmospheric pressure is tolerated or 5 cm CPAP is applied.

Once readiness to wean from the ventilator is established, there are *many* ways to approach the weaning process in terms of ventilatory modes.

The decision of which approach to pursue is dependent on many factors including ventilator capacity, physician/institutional philosophy, and patient needs. The process of weaning often is facilitated by IMV, PS ventilation, and in some cases by CPAP.

Explain the plan for the day to the patient. Allowing the patient choices when possible in the day's schedule promotes a sense of control and cooperation. Let the patient know that there may be changes in the sensation of breathing initially and that you will stay at the bedside and monitor closely. Explain that if he or she cannot tolerate weaning, ventilatory support will be increased or resumed. Place the patient in high Fowler's position to promote optimal expansion of the lung, and suction the airway.

RESEARCH NOTE

Bergbom-Engberg I, Haljamae H:
Assessment of patients' experience of discomfort during respiratory therapy.
Critical Care Medicine, 1989; 17:1068–1072.

CLINICAL APPLICATION

Prolonged mechanical ventilation presents an ethical, financial, and clinical challenge in the critical-care setting. What role does psychologic distress play in preventing successful weaning from mechanical ventilation? What are patient's perceptions during mechanical ventilation?

The issue of patient distress and discomfort while on a ventilator was addressed in this study, which questioned 304 patients who had received mechanical ventilation during their hospital stay. The patients were surveyed after discharge to home from 2 months to 4 years following their episode of ventilation in the intensive care unit.

Fifty-two percent of the sample were able to recall their experience while on the ventilator. The two most frequently recalled discomforts (50% of the sample) were 1) anxiety and fear and 2) the inability to communicate with nursing staff and relatives. Secretions and pain were reported as problems by 39% and 36% of the sample, respectively. Almost one-third of the patients described sleeping difficulties, including nightmares, while intubated. Thirty percent reported severe psychologic distress at one time during this period. There was a significant correlation between the duration of treatment (more than 7 days) and anxiety/fear, agony, panic, and nightmares. Suctioning also was reported as more distressful as the length of time on the ventilator increased. Breathing out of synchrony with the ventilator correlated with the onset of many reported emotional symptoms such as panic and fear. Patients also stated that the degree of trust they had in their caregivers determined how secure they felt.

Limitations: A major limitation of this work is its retrospective design. The ability of some patients to remember experiences 4 years prior to the interview is questionable.

Strengths: This study presents findings that are extremely relevant to critical-care practice. Suctioning, a frequently performed procedure, was identified by patients as distressful. Isolation due to inability to communicate may be alleviated by the nurse who pursues alternative communication techniques such as special adapters, pencil and paper, and word boards. Manual ventilation of the patient through periods of asynchrony can help the patient relax and not "fight" the ventilator. Establishing a caring and concerned relationship with the patient and family can increase their trust and thus the patient's feelings of security.

Results of this study demonstrating that some patients recalled unpleasant experiences 4 years after the events indicate the need to incorporate this awareness into your practice with ventilator-dependent patients.

In previously healthy patients who have received short-term ventilation, connect the airway to a T-piece rather than the ventilator. In addition to the arm that connects to the patient, another arm of the T connects to wide-bore oxygen tubing; the third arm is an exhalation port. The patient usually receives 10–20% more oxygen when the ventilator is discontinued.

Monitor pulse, blood pressure, peripheral perfusion, level of consciousness, and rate and ease of breathing for the first 15 minutes. A mild increase in pulse, respiration rate (RR), and BP is normal. Suction as necessary, and coach the patient to breathe slowly and deeply along with you.

After 15 minutes, evaluate the blood gases, vital capacity, and cardiopulmonary status. If they are satisfactory, continue oxygen, deep breathing and coughing exercises, and chest PT. If the patient remains stable for several hours, the artificial airway then may be discontinued.

When the patient cannot maintain spontaneous breathing after the ventilator is discontinued, the cause may be physical or psychologic. The possible reasons require careful evaluation by the nurse and the physician. Alternative approaches to weaning include using SIMV, gradually decreasing the set rate, or gradually shifting the workload to the patient over a period of days. Higher SIMV rates are used at night so that respiratory muscles are rested and the patient can sleep. The advent of pressure support (PS) ventilation provides another mode in which the level of support gradually is decreased

TABLE 9–3

Assessment of Physiologic Readiness for Weaning

CENTRAL NERVOUS SYSTEM	METABOLIC	CARDIOVASCULAR/ HEMODYNAMIC	PULMONARY	RENAL
No seizures	Adequate calories $1.5 \times$ REE or 3.5 kcal/kg/day	Heart rate < 120 beats/ min	Breathing pattern: $V_T > 5$ cc/kg; respiratory rate < 30/breaths/min	Intake = Output
Adequate ventilatory drive = $\dot{V}_E > 5$ L/min	Avoid excessive calories $\geq 2 \times$ REE	Systolic blood pressure > 80 or < 180 mm Hg	Lungs clear to auscultation	No edema
Able to protect airway	Afebrile	No arrythmias	Few secretions Suction < every 1–2 hr	Electrolytes: Mg 1.8–3 mg/dl PO_4 2.5–4.8 mg/dl K 3.5–5.9 mEq/L
Several hours of sleep		Hemoglobin 12–15 gm/ 100 ml Hematocrit 40–50/ 100 ml	No accessory muscle use or paradox	No inappropriate weight gain
		No angina	No mouth opening or nasal flaring $P_aO_2 > 50$ mm Hg $P_aCO_2 < 60$ mm Hg or not varying more than 33% from baseline No splinting caused by pain	pH 7.35–7.45

REE, Resting energy expenditure = 3.9 (V_{O_2}) + 1.1 (V_{CO_2}); $\dot{V}_E$, minute ventilation; V_T, tidal volume.

Source: Knebel AR: Weaning from mechanical ventilation: Current controversies. *Heart Lung* 1991; 20(4):322.

TABLE 9–4

Bedside Pulmonary Function Parameters for Predicting Weaning

		MECHANICS	
OXYGENATION	VENTILATION	Strength	Endurance
$F_IO_2 < 0.5$ to maintain $P_aO_2 > 50$ mm Hg	$\dot{V}_E$ requirement < 10 L/min $V_{DS}/V_T < 0.55$ $P_aCO_2 < 60$ mm Hg	MIP < –25 cm H_2O VC > 10 ml/kg $V_T > 5$ ml/kg	MVV > $2 \times \dot{V}_E$ Static compliance > 30 ml/cm H_2O

MIP, Maximal inspiratory pressure; *MVV*, maximal voluntary ventilation; *VC*, vital capacity; *VDS/VT*, dead space to tidal volume ratio; *$\dot{V}_E$* minute volume; *VT*, tidal volume.

Source: Knebel AR: Weaning from mechanical ventilation: Current controversies. *Heart Lung* 1991; 20(4):324.

over a period of days (or weeks). An alternative approach to the gradual withdrawal of support is the rest/exercise schedule, in which the patient is placed on blow-by for short periods at first (5–10 minutes out of each hour) and then rested on assist-control. The periods of spontaneous ventilation are lengthened gradually until extubation is deemed possible.

Outcome Evaluation

Evaluate the effectiveness of mechanical ventilation according to these outcome criteria:

- Calm, relaxed, not struggling against ventilator.
- Arterial blood gases within desired limits for patient, usually $P_{a}O_2$ 60–100 mm Hg and $P_{a}CO_2$ 35–45 mm Hg.
- No signs of dehydration or fluid overload.
- BP, pulse rate, venous pressure, and peripheral perfusion WNL for patient.
- Tracheal aspirate without pathologic flora.
- No frank or occult blood in gastric or fecal matter; hemoglobin and hematocrit levels WNL for patient.

Chest Drainage

In order for the lungs to expand properly, the pleural space must remain a potential space, with a pressure below intrathoracic pressure. In addition, for the heart to expand properly, there must be no accumulation of fluid or air in the mediastinum. When air and/or fluid accumulates in the pleural space or mediastinum, a chest tube will relieve the pressure, drain the fluid, and thereby facilitate resumption of normal cardiopulmonary dynamics.

Techniques of Chest Drainage

Recognize patients who could benefit from chest drainage, that is, those with pneumothorax causing respiratory embarrassment, hemothorax, pneumomediastinum, or hemomediastinum. Examples are the

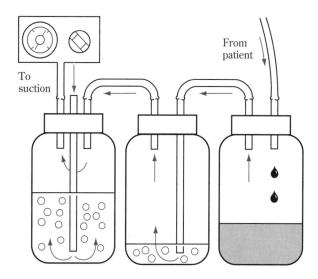
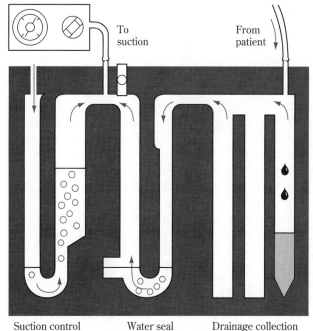

Suction control   Water seal   Drainage collection

FIGURE 9–7

Pleurevac pleural drainage system. Air vent is shown. (From Luce J et al.: *Intensive respiratory care.* Philadelphia: Saunders, 1984, p. 166.)

patient with a rib fracture and pleural tear and the thoracic surgical patient. Most hospitals use a disposable chest drainage system, such as the Pleurevac, because it is simpler to use, less cumbersome, and less prone to breakage than the older bottle system. The principles of chest drainage will be explained using the simplest type of Pleurevac; correlations with the three-bottle system will be included (Figure 9–7).

The three-bottle system and the Pleurevac have three chambers: a collection chamber, a water seal chamber, and a suction control chamber. Depending on which chambers are used, the unit can provide straight gravity drainage or drainage under low suction (from an external suction source). Fluid drainage accumulates in the *collection chamber*. The *water seal* allows displaced air from the collection chamber to escape but prevents atmospheric air from entering the pleural space. The *suction chamber* controls the amount of suction exerted on the chest. Displaced air leaves the system through a vent. Argyle manufactures a four-chamber system that includes a safety water seal chamber that allows release of pressure should the suction accidentally be disrupted or kinked (Figure 9–8). This chamber allows any build-up of air to be vented to the atmosphere, thus avoiding a tension pneumothorax (Kersten 1989).

Assisting with Chest Tube Insertion Assist with bedside chest tube insertion by acting as the unsterile person and by monitoring the patient's condition. Explain the procedure to the patient and sedate if needed. Before the tube is inserted, set up the drainage system according to the manufacturer's recommendations. Mark all fluid levels with the date and time. The physician will insert one or more tubes, depending on the problem. To evacuate air from the pleural space, the physician will insert the tube anteriorly at the second intercostal space. To remove fluid from the pleural space, the physician will insert it in the eighth or ninth intercostal space in the midaxillary line.

To evacuate air or fluid from the mediastinum, the tubes are inserted in the operating room. One tube is placed anteriorly at the base of the pericardium. The other is placed anteriorly just below the xiphoid process.

When the tube is inserted and the obturator removed, connect the tube to the drainage system. The doctor will suture the tube to the chest wall and dress the site occlusively. If suction has been ordered, turn the suction source on until you see gentle bubbling in the suction chamber. Tape connections securely in a circular fashion, except at the connection between the chest tube and the connecting tubing. There, tape longitudinally, leaving a narrow space so you can observe the drainage.

Maintenance of Chest Drainage

Once the system is established, maintain its patency and effectiveness by assessing the system from the dressing to the drainage unit to the wall suction source.

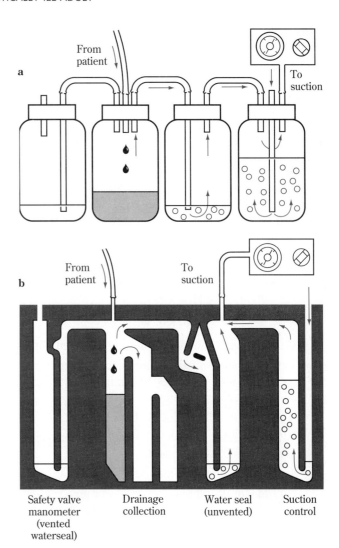

Safety valve manometer (vented waterseal) | Drainage collection | Water seal (unvented) | Suction control

FIGURE 9–8

Four-bottle (chamber) chest tube drainage systems. **a,** standard four-bottle system; **b,** Argyle double-seal drainage system. (In Kersten LD, *Comprehensive respiratory nursing*. Saunders, 1989, p. 778. Reproduced and adapted by permission from Luce J, Tyler M, Pierson D. *Intensive respiratory care*. Philadelphia: Saunders, 1984.)

Amount, Rate, and Quality of Drainage Observe the collection chamber for the amount, rate, and quality of drainage. Mark the level of drainage each hour. Call a rate over 100 ml per hour or frank bleeding to the attention of the physician.

Decreased drainage may result from obstructions in the system, pooling of secretions, or reexpansion of the lung. Keep the tubing free of kinks by taping connections to tongue blades to stabilize them. Loosely coil the tubing flat on the bed; dependent loops cause increased pressure. Unless contraindicated, place the patient in Fowler's position to facilitate both air and fluid removal. Turn the patient regularly. In some units, the nurse is expected to strip the tubes routinely every 15 minutes to one hour if fluid is being evacuated. (The usual stripping procedure is as follows. To strip the tube, lubricate about 12 inches at a time with hand cream, or use an alcohol swab. Pinch the tube shut proximal to the chest. Maintain the occlusion while you pinch the tube with your other thumb and forefinger and slide them away distally. Then, maintain the distal occlusion while you release the proximal one, creating suction. Finally, remove the distal pinch.) Strip the tube down to the collection chamber to suck fluid and clots into it. Hand-over-hand compression is another method for moving fluid and clots. To strip the tube this way, start proximally. Squeeze it with one hand, place your other hand distally and squeeze it, and then release the proximal hand. Continue hand over hand to the collection chamber.

Alternative stripping methods include fan-folding several layers of tubing and squeezing them with both hands, and hand-over-hand stripping in which each hand's compression is released before the next one is applied.

Stripping is used most commonly with mediastinal drainage tubes in cardiac surgical patients, as bleeding is more profuse and cardiac tamponade must be prevented. Even in this population, however, various studies have examined the necessity of such "routine" protocols (Duncan 1987; Knauss 1985; Lim-Levy et al. 1986; Pierce et al. 1991). A classic nursing research project by Duncan and Erickson (1982) demonstrated that, in human subjects, stripping can generate chest tube pressures far in excess of the amount of suction normally applied during drainage with suction. Stripping the entire length of the tube via the most common manual or roller method often generated pressures in excess of -400 cm H_2O! Hand-over-hand sustained compression generated up to -330 cm H_2O pressure. Fan-folding caused pressures of about -50 cm H_2O, and intermittent hand-over-hand compression created about -30 cm H_2O pressure. The length of tubing stripped was directly related to the amount of negative pressure generated.

As it is reasonable to assume that chest tube pressures are transmitted to the pleural space, these findings should give one pause and call into question the value and safety of routine stripping, particularly with regard to pleural tubes. A prudent course is to evaluate each clinical situation separately, use stripping only if fluid is not draining freely, and use whichever lowest-pressure stripping method is effective in that particular situation. Also, assess the patient's response to chest tube stripping, as the procedure can cause great discomfort.

Water Seal Fluid Level Observe the water seal chamber for the level of fluid once every 8 hours. Too little fluid may allow air to enter the chest; too much means the intrapleural pressure will have to rise excessively before air or fluid can be expelled. Add or remove water as necessary.

Water Seal Fluctuations Also observe the water seal chamber for fluctuations. The fluctuations ("tidaling") result from changes in intrapleural pressure with respiration. Normally, the Pleurevac's water seal will show fluid movement upward on inspiration and downward on expiration. In the bottle system, the fluid in the glass tube will move upward on inspiration and downward on expiration. (If the patient is on a positive pressure ventilator, the direction is reversed.) Excessive fluctuations indicate coughing or respiratory distress. Decreased fluctuations may indicate an obstruction to drainage or reexpansion of the lung. Tidaling is less marked with mediastinal tubes.

Bubbles in Water Seal Observe the water seal chamber for bubbles. Bubbles result from air leaking from the patient's lung, into the collection chamber, and through the water seal before leaving the system. Thus, they reflect the amount of air leaking from the lung into the pleural space. You should see occasional bubbles in the seal, but not continuous bubbles. Persistent continuous bubbling indicates an air leak in the system or a massive air leak from the patient. To identify which, briefly clamp the tube near the patient. If the bubbling stops, you know the leak is at the insertion site or inside the patient. (Palpate around the insertion site to see if the leak is there. If it is, notify the physician, who can put in a purse-string skin suture or reposition the tube. If the leak is inside the patient, notify the physician; surgical repair may be necessary. Pleurevacs are available with an air-leak meter to help quantify changes in the size of an air leak.) On the other hand, if the bubbling does not stop when you clamp the tube, you know the leak is in the system itself. Continue clamping along the system to localize the leak. If it is in the tubing, replace it or tape the connections more firmly. If the leak is in the bottle or Pleurevac, replace it. Chart the presence or absence of an air leak in your initial baseline assessment.

Fluid Level and Bubbling in Suction Control Chamber Observe the suction control chamber for fluid level and bubbling. Note the level of fluid in the suction control chamber and the rate of bubbling, once every 8 hours. The amount of suction depends on the amount of fluid in the suction control chamber, not the setting on the external suction source or the rate of bubbling. Maintain a gentle, constant bubbling; vigorous bubbling simply promotes evaporation of the fluid. Whenever the level of the water decreases, add more to maintain the desired suction. With a Pleurevac, minimize evaporation of fluid from the suction chamber by using the rubber cap with the small air vent to cover the large opening of the suction control chamber.

Placement of System When using bottles, place them in holders and warn visitors and staff not to kick them accidentally. Pleurevacs may be hung from the bedside or placed in a holder on the floor. Keep the system below the patient's chest, even while transporting him or her. If necessary when turning the patient, the collection chamber may be lifted over the chest momentarily.

Prevention of Complications

Utilize preventive measures described in the following sections to avoid complications.

Pneumothorax Prevent a tension pneumothorax by keeping the system vented and by clamping only when appropriate.

The drainage system must always be vented to air in order to prevent a dangerous buildup of pressure in the chest. When suction is applied with a Pleurevac, make sure the small hole in the rubber cap of the suction control chamber is not occluded. In the three-bottle system, be sure the upper end of the vent tube in the suction control chamber is not occluded. If it is necessary to interrupt the suction (to transport the patient or if the external source fails), be sure to vent the drainage system.

Keep two clamps at the bedside, and learn the principles underlying when to clamp and when not to clamp the chest tube. You may clamp the system briefly to locate the source of an air leak. You also may clamp the chest tube briefly near the thoracic wall when changing the collection chamber or when the chamber breaks, *unless* the patient has an air leak.

Ankylosis and Discomfort Prevent shoulder ankylosis and discomfort. Assist the patient with range of motion exercises several times daily. Splint the insertion site while turning or coughing.

Removal of Chest Tubes

Assist with chest tube removal when the lung has expanded or drainage has become minimal. Signs of lung expansion are cessation of bubbling in water seal fluid, normal physical examination, and a chest x-ray showing fully aerated lungs. Explain the procedure to the patient, and premedicate if possible, since removal is moderately painful. Bring to the bedside a suture removal set, sterile Vaseline gauze, dressing supplies, and a towel. Spread the towel over the bed so the tube can be placed on it after removal. Remove the dressing. The physician will cut the suture and hold the Vaseline gauze over the insertion site. The doctor will tell the patient to take a deep breath and bear down while he or she quickly pulls out the tube and covers the site firmly with the gauze, to seal it off. Secure the Vaseline gauze with gauze squares and tape. (Some physicians prefer to place a suture around the tube on insertion and have you tighten it as the tube is removed. Also, some believe Vaseline gauze is unnecessary and instead use dry gauze squares to cover the site.) A small amount of serosanguinous drainage may occur after removal. If necessary, simply reinforce the dressing for the first 48–72 hours; then it can be changed.

Outcome Evaluation

Evaluate the effectiveness of chest drainage according to these outcome criteria:

- Calm, relaxed appearance.
- Unlabored respirations WNL for patient.
- Performs range of motion and breathing exercises and moves about willingly.
- Lungs fully aerated, as manifested by chest x-ray and physical examination.

Thoracic Surgery

Patients undergoing thoracic surgery are at risk for pulmonary complications. Vital capacity is estimated to decrease 30–50% during the first 24 hours (Shapiro et al. 1991). The thoracic incision causes severe pain with resultant rapid and shallow respirations. These patients are typically middle-aged or older and frequently have a significant smoking history. The procedure itself usually involves manipulation or resection of lung tissue necessitating reexpansion of the lung during the postoperative period. All of these factors emphasize the role of the critical-care nurse in outlining a plan of aggressive, preventive pulmonary care beginning with preoperative teaching and continuing with vigilant postoperative assessment and interventions.

Preoperative Assessment

It is important for you to be able to identify the patient who is at high risk for postoperative complications such as ventilatory failure, pneumonia, and atelectasis. Even though you may not see the patient in the preoperative period, a quick review of the history and physical can provide two or three pieces of data that have been demonstrated to predict postoperative problems. A forced vital capacity less than 20 ml/kg (normal 55–85 ml/kg) and/or a FEV_1/FVC (see Chapter 7) less than 50% places the patient at greater risk for postoperative ventilatory failure (Shapiro et al. 1991). Other data, such as smoking history, nutrition, and activity level, are important to note.

Preoperative teaching of inspiratory maneuvers, splinting techniques, and, if appropriate, mechanical ventilation support should be reviewed by either the nurse or the respiratory therapist.

Operative Procedures

For most procedures involving resection of lung tissue, the patient is intubated with a double-lumen endotracheal tube to allow independent ventilation of the unaffected lung while leaving the operative lung deflated for ease of manipulation. The operative lung is inflated occasionally during the procedure. Because the patient is placed in a side-lying position with the good lung dependent, the dual-lumen endotracheal tube prevents debris, blood, or infectious material from moving into that dependent lung. Stasis of secretions in the dependent lung and atelectasis in the operative lung are primary postoperative problems, in addition to a large incision involving resection of ribs and separation of muscle. During chest closure, both lungs are maximally inflated and chest tubes are placed in positions to evacuate air and fluid and to reestablish normal negative intrapleural pressures.

Segmental Resection The most common thoracic procedures are usually for removal of malignancies. *Segmental or wedge resections* involve actual cutting into lung tissue and alveolar surfaces. Patients undergoing such procedures are more prone to air leaks of longer duration as well as atelectasis due to traumatized lung tissue. Chest tube drainage with negative suction is used to evacuate air and fluid. If lung expansion does not occur, a procedure is performed to roughen up the visceral pleura and make the lung adhere directly to the chest wall.

Lobectomy A *lobectomy* involves removal of an entire lobe; therefore, the surgical procedure involves closing of a bronchus or resecting a bronchus to maintain ventilation of distal lung tissue. Following removal of such a volume of lung tissue, the remaining lung will eventually shift and fill the space, unless atelectasis and/or an air leak persists.

Pneumonectomy Removal of an entire lung *(pneumonectomy)* results in the closure of a mainstem bronchus. Following removal of the lung, the vacated hemithorax fills with serosanguinous fluid, which eventually solidifies to form a space-occupying mass. This process aids in preventing a shift of mediastinal contents. For this reason, chest tubes usually are not placed postoperatively. If they are placed, they may be clamped but are never applied to suction. If shifting of the mediastinum does occur, fluid can be intermittently drained. Bronchopleural fistula can be a serious complication following pneumonectomy, as fluid (blood or infectious fluid) can drain into the remaining lung, producing acute respiratory failure. Another major complication is rupture of the bronchial stump, which results in a major and massive air leak due to its size.

Decortication *Decortication* is the surgical removal of the visceral pleura. This procedure is performed when other maneuvers, such as chest tube drainage, have failed to reexpand the lung, and air and/or fluid remains in the pleural space, placing the patient at risk for empyema or an infected pleural effusion.

Postoperative Complications

Hypoventilation Splinting due to pain and increased stiffness of the chest wall results in a pattern of rapid and shallow breathing. Subsequent atelectasis, secretion retention, shunting, and hypoxemia increase the risk for developing acute ventilatory failure. The nurse directly coordinates careful pain control with "stir-up" pulmonary regimes every 1–2 hours, to prevent having to intubate and mechanically ventilate a patient. The advent of epidural narcotics now enables control of pain without oversedating the patient.

ADVANCES IN CRITICAL CARE TECHNOLOGY

Capnography in the Critical-Care Unit

THE TECHNOLOGY

Capnography refers to the monitoring of exhaled carbon dioxide levels that reflect ventilation in the intubated critically ill patient. Physical assessment, vital signs, and neurologic status are common ways we assess the adequacy of ventilation, but abnormalities may not be evident until substantial CO_2 retention has occurred or may in fact not result from changes in ventilation. An arterial blood gas is the most precise measurement of your patient's ventilation, as reflected by the P_aCO_2. Capnography displays at the bedside a continuous digital and waveform readout of the patient's end-tidal CO_2 ($PetCO_2$). The difference between the P_aCO_2 and the $PetCO_2$ is usually less than 6 mm Hg, with the arterial levels being higher.

Normal CO_2 elimination occurs as venous blood enters the pulmonary capillary bed, having released oxygen to the tissues and acquired CO_2 as a by-product of cellular metabolism. As this venous blood traverses the capillary with a CO_2 of approximately 46 mm Hg, CO_2 moves from the blood across the alveolar-capillary membrane and enters the alveolus, where the CO_2 is approximately 40 mm Hg (Figure 9–9). From there, it is exhaled. In the ventilated patient, exhalation occurs through the ventilator tubing, where an analyzer is placed to measure levels of exhaled CO_2 throughout the ventilatory cycle. The digital readout displays the end-tidal CO_2 level or that last portion of gas to leave the airway during exhalation.

PATIENT CARE CONSIDERATIONS

The most dramatic changes in your patient's $PetCO_2$ level occur with changes in the matching of ventilation and perfusion that result in *decreased perfusion* to well-ventilated lung units. Examples include hypotension, high levels of PEEP, or pulmonary embolism (Figure 9–10). The result is a lung unit that is well ventilated but poorly perfused, so CO_2 is not eliminated from the blood into the alveolus and exhaled. End-tidal CO_2 values sensed in the exhalation limb of the ventilator circuit therefore are lower than normal.

Clinical examples of the usefulness of end-tidal CO_2 monitoring include observing the *shape* of the waveform. The shape of the waveform (Figure 9–11) reflects a rising $PetCO_2$ as alveolar CO_2 is exhaled. The waveform then levels off during the rest of exhalation ("alveolar plateau"). When the patient inhales, CO_2-free gas is pulled into the airway and $PetCO_2$ falls to zero. A waveform that lacks a plateau occurs in bronchitis, asthma, and emphysema, indicating airway obstruction. Bronchodilator therapy may return the waveform to normal. Erratic waveforms or those with clefts in the middle of the plateau indicate ventilatory modes poorly synchronized with patient efforts. Sedation or changing the sensitivity or mode may result in a smoother, consistent waveform as well as increased patient comfort. During CPR, rising $PetCO_2$ values indicate ineffective compressions and/or ventilation. When assessing PEEP therapy, a falling $PetCO_2$ (or increasing gradient between P_aCO_2 and end-tidal CO_2) indicates increasing deadspace, due to compression of extra-alveolar capillaries from overdistention of alveoli. In the patient who is paralyzed, the return of diaphragmatic activity will first be seen on the capnogram as dips or clefts in the alveolar plateau. During weaning trials, an increasing $PetCO_2$ value with increased respiratory rate and loss of a plateau on the waveform should alert you to weaning failure.

The system has mechanical limitations. As a nurse, you will need to learn procedures for calibration and for detecting malfunctions as well as system leaks. There are some critically ill patients (those in severe respiratory failure) in whom the gradient between P_aCO_2 and end-tidal CO_2 has been shown to vary; therefore, these values should be correlated regularly. Future research regarding the usefulness of this noninvasive monitoring of ventilation needs to be conducted to determine issues related to cost and the impact on patient outcome (Szaflarski and Cohen 1991; Peterson 1990; Skoog 1989).

Hemorrhage Close monitoring of chest tube drainage in the first 8 hours is important to detect bleeding. In general, blood loss over 100 ml/hr or a sudden increase in blood loss should be reported to the surgeon. Keeping chest tubes in view, avoiding kinking, and turning the patient side to side will allow early detection of bleeding. In pneumonectomy patients without chest tube drainage, physical signs such as

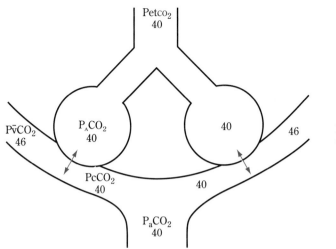

FIGURE 9–9

Carbon dioxide elimination in normal lung. P_ccO_2, partial pressure of CO_2 in capillary blood. (From: Szaflarski NL, Cohen NH: Use of capnography in critically ill adults. *Heart Lung* 1991; 20(4):364.)

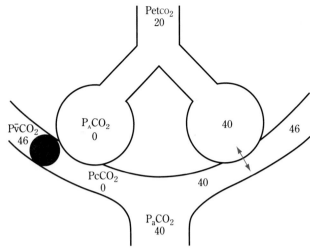

FIGURE 9–10

CO_2 elimination in the case of increased dead space ventilation caused by pulmonary emboli. Because CO_2 elimination is halted in affected lung, $Petco_2$ is significantly lowered. P_ccO_2, partial pressure of CO_2 in capillary blood. (From: Szaflarski NL, Cohen NH: Use of capnography in critically ill adults. *Heart Lung* 1991; 20(4):365.)

hypotension, tachycardia, and oliguria are used to monitor blood loss. Serial hematocrits are also followed.

Tension Pneumothorax The presence of an air leak is assessed in the immediate postoperative period by noting constant bubbling in the underwater seal of the chest drainage system. The absence of chest tubes in pneumonectomy patients places them at higher risk for the development of a tension pneumothorax. In that case, rupture of the bronchial stump allows air to pass into the chest, building up until pressure shifts the mediastinum (heart, trachea, and great vessels) toward

the remaining lung. Cardiac output is impaired, and the patient presents in shock.

Cardiovascular Complications You should be aware of any pre-existing cardiac conditions that place your patient at risk for myocardial infarction. Most commonly, supraventricular dysrhythmias such as atrial flutter and atrial fibrillation may occur. Fluid management is important to prevent overloading your patient, with resultant congestive heart failure and/or respiratory failure.

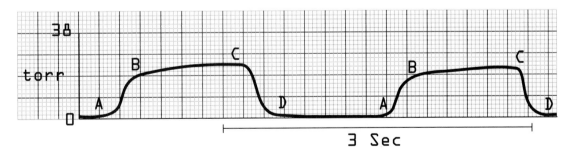

FIGURE 9–11

Phases of normal capnogram. Exhalation begins at point A and continues to point C with segment B–C representing alveolar plateau phase. Inspiration is signaled by rapid, descending limb of segment C–D, which reaches zero baseline. (From: Szaflarski NL, Cohen NH: Use of capnography in critically ill adults. *Heart Lung* 1991; 20(4):365.)

Summary

The thoracic surgical patient presents a great challenge to the ICU nurse, particularly when the patient has pre-existing pulmonary disease, as many do. Astute pulmonary care applied early and aggressively can forestall a prolonged ICU stay, with its many attendant complications.

REFERENCES

Ashworth L: Pressure support ventilation. *Crit Care Nurse* 1990; 10(7):20–25.

Benner P: *From novice to expert.* Menlo Park, CA: Addison-Wesley, 1984.

Bodai B: A means of suctioning without cardiopulmonary depression. *Heart Lung* 1982; 11:172–176.

Bodai B et al.: A clinical evaluation of an oxygen insufflation/suction catheter. *Heart Lung* 1987; 16:39–46.

Brown L: Pulmonary oxygen toxicity. *Focus Crit Care* 1990; 17(1):66–75.

Burns S: Advances in ventilator therapy. *FOCUS* 1991; 17(3):227–237.

Campion E et al.: Medical intensive care for the elderly: A study of current use, costs, and outcomes. *JAMA* 1981; 246:2052–2056.

Chulay M: Hyperinflation/hyperoxygenation to prevent endotracheal suctioning complications. *Crit Care Nurse* 1987; 7:100–102.

Desautels D, Blanch P: Mechanical ventilation. In *Respiratory care: A guide to clinical practice,* Burton G et al. (eds). Philadelphia: Lippincott, 1991.

Duncan C, Erickson R: Pressures associated with chest tube stripping. *Heart Lung* 1982; 11:166–170.

Duncan C, Erickson R: Effect of chest tube management on drainage after cardiac surgery. *Heart Lung* 1987; 16(1):1–9.

Hess D: Controversies in respiratory critical care. *Crit Care Nurse Quart* 1988; 11(3):62–78.

Hess D et al: Mechanical ventilation: Initiation, management and weaning. In *Respiratory care: A guide to clinical practice,* Burton G et al. (eds). Philadelphia: Lippincott, 1991.

Hudson L: Adult respiratory distress syndrome. In *Respiratory care: A guide to clinical practice,* Burton G et al. (eds). Philadelphia: Lippincott, 1991.

Hughes C, Popovich J: Uses and abuses of pressure support ventilation. *J Crit Illness* 1989; 4(4):25–32.

Kersten L: Hemodynamic monitoring—Respiratory applications. In *Comprehensive respiratory nursing,* Kersten L (ed). Philadelphia: Saunders, 1989.

Knauss P: Chest tube stripping: Is it necessary? *FOCUS* 1985; 12(6):41–43.

Knaus W et al.: Prognosis in acute organ-system failure. *Ann Surg* 1985; 202:685–692.

Knebel A: Weaning from mechanical ventilation: Current controversies. *Heart Lung* 1991; 20(4):321–324.

Lim-Levy F et al.: Is milking and stripping chest tubes really necessary? *Ann Thorac Surg* 1986; 42:77–80.

MacIntyre N: Weaning from mechanical ventilatory support: Volume-assisting intermittent breaths versus pressure-assisting every breath. *Resp Care* 1988; 33(2):121–125.

Marcy T, Marini J: Inverse ratio ventilation in ARDS: Rationale and implementation. *Chest* 1991; 100(2):494–504.

Meduri G et al.: Noninvasive face mask mechanical ventilation in patients with acute hypercapnic respiratory failure. *Chest* 1991; 100(2):445–454.

Peterson M: Questions and answers on capnography. *Crit Care Choices* 1990; 12–17.

Pierce B, Piazza D: Differences in postsuctioning arterial blood oxygenation values using two postoxygenation methods. *Heart Lung* 1987; 16:34–38.

Pierce J et al.: Effects of two chest tube clearance protocols on drainage in patients after myocardial revascularization surgery. *Heart Lung* 1991; 20:125–130.

Reidinger M et al.: Reading pulmonary artery and pulmonary capillary wedge pressure waveforms with respiratory variations. *Heart Lung* 1981; 10:675–678.

Ruark J, Raffin J: Initiating and withdrawing life support. *N Engl J Med* 1988; 318(1):25–30.

Ryerson G, Block J: Oxygen as a drug: Clinical properties, benefits, modes and hazards of administration. In *Respiratory care: A guide to clinical practice,* Burton G et al. (eds). Philadelphia: Lippincott, 1991.

Shapiro B et al.: *Clinical application of respiratory care,* 4th ed. Chicago: Year Book, 1991.

Skoog R: Capnography in the post anesthesia care unit. *J Post Anesth Nurs* 1989; 4(3):147–155.

Stone K et al.: Effect of lung hyperinflation and endotracheal suctioning on heart rate and rhythm in patients after coronary artery bypass graft surgery. *Heart Lung* 1991; 20:443–450.

Szaflarski N, Cohen N: Use of capnography in critically ill adults. *Heart Lung* 1991; 20(4):363–372.

10

Cardiovascular Physical Assessment

CLINICAL INSIGHT

Domain: Effective management of rapidly changing situations

Competency: Skilled performance in extreme, life-threatening emergencies: rapid grasp of a problem

In the ICU, life-threatening emergencies can occur with unnerving suddenness. The abilities to rapidly assess chaotic situations and quickly grasp life-threatening problems are hallmarks of skilled performance. In the following paradigm (Crabtree and Jorgenson 1986, p. 144), a nurse expertly orchestrates the care necessary to save a life in jeopardy.

Nurse: I was in charge; it was a Sunday morning, and it was very quiet; we didn't have any beds open. The unit was full and we had no forewarning. All of a sudden one of the cardiac surgeons, with two residents, wheeled in this cart and said, have this patient.

Interviewer: They hadn't called?

Nurse: No, nothing. Absolutely nothing. Said, we need an ICU bed, or at least an ICU nurse. One or the other. And I said, well, what is going on? They said, we just did a biopsy on this man, and he is in acute rejection. We believe he is acute rejection from a cardiac heart transplant a year and one-half ago. He needs an ICU bed. There was no time to argue with them about, why didn't you call first or do something, because this guy was obviously crashing. So, we had to move a patient out quickly, and I asked one of the nurses on the unit to go out and get a blood pressure on this guy and see if he needed to be bagged or needed to be intubated or needed anything. I said, keep him out in the hall, and watch him until we can move a patient out of the room. He was on a cart in the hall, so one of the nurses on the unit [who] wasn't busy at the time, but who had two of her own patients, went out there quickly while I wheeled a patient out bed 8. . . . That was a patient that was transferable, so we bumped that patient out to the floor. I was in charge and had to take this patient. I knew absolutely nothing about him except that he was desperately ill. The family was scared to death, and so was the patient. He had been, 24 hours earlier, in fine shape.

Rapidly, the team springs into action: the patient is intubated, the pulmonary artery cannulated, and multiple vasopressors started. Then, since the patient must be transferred back to the state in which he received the transplant, the nurse not only manages this critically ill patient but also expertly coordinates the transfer.

So, for two hours I had to monitor this guy, knowing absolutely no medical history, and knowing that he was crashing. I was calling RT saying, I need this or I need that, setting up the lines I knew he would need. And, I was trying to deal with, over the phone—with an air ambulance company. It took a lot of coordination, a lot of work with the family, to try and alleviate their anxieties and the patient's. And I think about 4 or so in the afternoon, we finally got him moved out. We took the patient on a ventilator over to the airport. When we left, when we were loading the patient up, the wife of the patient came up and told me—this was a very emotional moment, after trying so hard all day to deal with this—this woman came up and told me, it's so wonderful that there are people like you in nursing.

Astute practice of the competency illustrated in the Clinical Insight requires an extensive foundation of clinical experience built on a thorough understanding of normal and abnormal physiology. This chapter focuses on cardiovascular physical assessment. A convenient assessment format is shown in Table 10–1; each of the items in Table 10–1 will be discussed in this chapter.

History

One of the most important steps in assessing a patient is rapid, accurate symptom evaluation. One simple, easily remembered method of evaluating cardiovascular complaints is to use the PQRST mnemonic, in which each initial identifies an important aspect of symptom analysis. The PQRST approach is presented in Table 10–2.

The cardiovascular symptoms that most often trouble patients are chest pain, shortness of breath, palpitations, syncope, intermittent claudication, and abnormal sensations or temperature of the extremities.

Chest pain is the most common cardiovascular complaint. Although it most often is due to myocardial ischemia, chest pain also can indicate a variety of other disorders. The differential diagnosis of chest pain is covered in Chapter 13. Chest pain due to cardiovascular disorders can radiate anywhere within the 6-dermatome region, which ranges from the jaw area to the epigastrium. This region includes the back, neck, upper extremities, and so on.

Shortness of breath is the subjective sensation of being unable to draw in enough air to breathe. It most often is associated with congestive heart failure but also may accompany other disorders, such as myocardial infarction. Related pulmonary variants include dyspnea on exertion (DOE), orthopnea (the inability to breathe comfortably while lying flat), and paroxysmal nocturnal dyspnea (PND), in which the person has nighttime episodes of shortness of breath due to fluid movement into the lungs brought about by lying flat and thereby increasing venous return.

Palpitations are premature heartbeats or other cardiac rhythm abnormalities that the person experiences as skipping, pounding, or thumping sensations in the chest.

Syncope is a temporary loss of consciousness (fainting) from which the person recovers spontaneously. Cardiovascular causes include stenosis of the aortic valve, rhythm disturbances (most often heart block), abnormally sensitive carotid sinus, and pacemaker failure.

Intermittent claudication is leg pain on exertion due to arterial insufficiency. Decreased arterial perfusion also may cause severe pain, as in arterial thrombosis, or result in *prickling, numbness,* or *coolness of extremities.*

Assessment of Activities of Daily Living (ADLs) provides information regarding cardiac function. Patients who are limited in their ability to perform daily living activities or walking may have a cardiac disorder. For example, patients who are limited in walking due to shortness of breath may have ischemia or decreased cardiac function. Patients who complain of chest pain when performing certain activities may have atherosclerosis and narrowing of the coronary arteries.

Risk factor assessment also provides the nurse with information regarding behaviors which may place the patient at risk for a cardiac event. The major risk factors include smoking, hypertension, and hypercholesterol-

TABLE 10–1

Cardiovascular Assessment Format

1. History
   A. Chief complaint_____
   B. Activity level
      ADL_____
      Walking (approx. distance)_____
      symptoms_____
      _____

   C. Risk factors (please check)
      _____ smoking   _____ high-fat diet
      _____hypertension   _____ sedentary lifestyle
      _____hypercholesterolemia _____ stress
      _____diabetes mellitus
2. Physical assessment
   A. General appearance
      Age_____ Sex_____ Height_____ Weight_____
      General development_____ nourishment_____
      Degree of distress_____
   B. Vital signs
      Temperature_____ Pulse_____ Respirations_____ BP_____
   C. Skin: color_____ temperature_____
      trophic changes_____
      vascular lesions_____
      tenderness_____
      edema_____
   D. Arterial pulses
      carotid_____ brachial_____ radial_____
      femoral_____ popliteal_____
      dorsalis pedis_____ posterior tibial_____
   E. Bruits_____
   F. Neck veins/jugular venous pressure_____
   G. Heart
      PMI_____
      Precordial movements_____
      Heart sounds
      S_1_____ S_2_____
      S_3_____ S_4_____
      Murmurs_____
      Rubs_____
3. Diagnostic procedures and laboratory tests
   A. CBC: RBC_____ Hgb_____ Hct_____
           WBC_____ Differential_____
   B. Clotting time_____ PT_____ PTT_____
   C. Cardiac enzymes_____
   D. ECG_____
   E. Chest x-ray_____
   F. Cardiac pressures CVP_____ RA_____ RV_____ LA_____
                         LV_____ PA_____ PCWP_____ Aorta_____
   G. Other_____
4. Other relevant data_____

TABLE 10–2

PQRST Mnemonic for Symptom Assessment

LETTER	ASPECT	SAMPLE QUESTIONS
P	Precipitators	What were you doing when the _____started?
		Have you ever had this before?
Q	Quality	What does it feel like?
		On a scale of 1 to 10, where would you rate this?
R	Region Radiation	Point to where it hurts.
		Does it move anywhere?
S	Signs and Symptoms	Have you had any other symptoms?
T	Time	When did it start?
		Is it constant or does it come and go?
		Did it come on suddenly or gradually?
	Treatment	What have you done to make it go away?
		Did it help?

emia. Additional risk factors include diabetes mellitus, high-fat diet, sedentary lifestyle, and stress. Identification of these risk factors helps the nurse form a plan for patient education and risk factor reduction.

Physical Examination

Physical examination techniques elicit a significant portion of the database from which the nurse generates nursing diagnoses. The usual four techniques of physical assessment are *inspection, palpation, percussion,* and *auscultation,* and they demand refinement of the senses of sight, touch, and hearing to detect subtle indicators of patient status. In addition, critical-care nurses often use two other senses, those of smell and intuition.

This chapter presents cardiovascular assessment techniques in the order in which most nurses use them. This practical approach will enhance your ability to integrate these techniques comfortably in the daily care of your patients. The order is as follows:

- General inspection
- Assessment of vital signs
- Palpation of arterial pulses
- Auscultation of blood pressure
- Examination of skin
- Inspection of neck veins
- Inspection and palpation of precordium
- Auscultation of heart sounds

The basic equipment for cardiovascular assessment should be at hand: stethoscope, sphygmomanometer with the appropriate-size cuff, centimeter ruler, and penlight or flashlight. The stethoscope must have both a diaphragm and a bell to detect both high- and low-pitched sounds. Its tubing should be flexible and no longer than 12–15 inches, since longer tubing diminishes sound conduction.

Related anatomy and physiology are integrated in the following discussions to help you understand not only the *what* and *how* of assessment, but also the *why.*

General Inspection

Inspection of the cardiovascular system centers on the patient's general appearance. Information regarding the patient's age and sex is important, since these are considered cardiac risk factors. Cardiac disease is more common among males than females, and the incidence of cardiac disease is higher in the elderly population. Other parameters which should be assessed are the patient's height and weight. The nurse measures the patient's weight in proportion to height to assess for obesity (cardiac risk factor) or cachexia (which can be present in chronic congestive heart failure patients). The nurse also assesses the general development and overall nourishment of the patient. Since abnormalities of the cardiovascular system may be severe and life threatening, the nurse also observes the patient for the degree of distress he or she is experiencing. For example, when the patient is in discomfort with chest pain or needs to exert effort to breathe, an emergent situation is present. These are all-important observations in assessing general appearance.

Developing the skill of inspection can provide you with a great deal of information about your patient. For instance, does your patient look apprehensive? cyanotic? Is your patient gasping or doubled over in pain? diaphoretic? These signs suggest a serious illness, such as myocardial infarction or a large pulmonary embolus, and are hard to miss. Unless you look specifically for more subtle signs, however, you may not notice such clues as cyanosis of the buccal mucosa and clubbing of the fingers (Figure 10–1), both indicative of hypoxemia, or distended neck veins, indicative of right-sided heart failure.

RESEARCH NOTE

Vines S, Simmons J:
Evaluating a staff development physical assessment program.
J Nurs Staff Devel 1991; 7:74–77.

CLINICAL APPLICATION

Although many physical assessment programs are offered to nurses in staff development departments, few reveal the impact of these programs on nursing practice. The purpose of this study was to evaluate whether nursing staff who took a mandatory physical assessment course were using the information in their daily practice.

A questionnaire designed to assess clinical usage of 17 physical assessment skills was sent to the 23 nurses who completed the first four classes of an assessment course.

Frequencies and percentages were used to analyze the data.

The results showed that the majority of the nurses used only 9 of the 17 skills on a daily basis. Skills used most frequently were mental status and skin system assessments. The skills reported least used were assessments for extraocular movement, cranial nerves, and jugular vein distention.

CRITICAL THINKING

Limitations: The majority of the nurses studied were from medical-surgical units and psychiatric units.

Few were from specialty areas like critical care, where more extensive and in-depth assessments may be done.

Strengths: This study addresses an important practice issue for nurses as well as staff development personnel. These results imply that nurses may be applying only those skills required by the patient population on their particular unit. Staff development educators need to reassess physical assessment course content and tailor the course to teach the skills required for specialty patient populations.

Assessment of Vital Signs

Changes in vital signs can provide important information regarding the patient's cardiac status. An elevation in the temperature can indicate the presence of an infectious process, as in pericarditis, endocarditis, or rheumatic heart disease. The rate and regularity of the pulse also can provide important clues during the cardiac assessment. Patients who experience heart failure or low cardiac output states often have increased heart rates. Patients with chest pain due to ischemia or infarction may have irregularities of the heart rhythm and have abnormally fast or slow pulse rates. Evaluation of respirations can provide information on the adequacy of gas exchange in maintaining adequate oxygen and carbon dioxide levels. Abnormally high respiratory rates may indicate that the patient needs more oxygen delivered to the tissues. Consequently, the patient's cardiac function in delivering oxygen may not be meeting the tissues' demand. Blood pressure also can provide important information. Hypertension is a cardiac risk factor and may predispose the patient to other cardiac diseases. Hypotension is seen in conditions which cause the cardiac output to be low, such as angina or infarction. Mechanisms of blood pressure control and regulation are discussed later in this chapter.

Examination of the Skin

The skin reflects both systemic and local changes in cardiovascular status. Skin assessment signs can be grouped conveniently into three areas: acutely decreased perfusion, chronically decreased perfusion, and edema.

Acute Decreases in Perfusion   Acute decreases in perfusion can be detected by evaluation of "skin vital signs," that is, color, temperature, and moisture of the skin.

Inspect the skin for color. Color abnormalities may include pallor, mottling, cyanosis, or rubor (redness produced by reactive hyperemia when a severely ischemic limb is allowed to become dependent). Signs of bleeding include frank bleeding, hematomas, bruises, and petechiae (small, round red spots indicating an increased tendency to bleed). Also note the presence of varicose veins.

Inspect the nailbeds, too, for the presence of cyanosis or clubbing. Check capillary filling time by pressing the end of the nail and releasing it quickly. Normally, the nailbed blanches on pressure but pinks up within 3 seconds on release of pressure. A delay in return to the normal nailbed color indicates poor arterial perfusion.

CLUBBING OF THE NAILS

NORMAL	EARLY CLUBBING	LATE CLUBBING

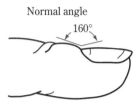 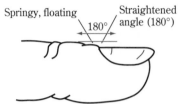 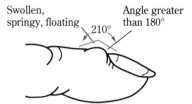

Normal angle

160°

Springy, floating   Straightened
                     angle (180°)
          180°

Swollen,   Angle greater
springy, floating   than 180°
            210°

The angle between the normal finger nail and nail base is about 160°. When palpated the nail base feels firm.

In early clubbing the angle between nail and nail base straightens out. The nail base gives a springy or floating sensation when palpated. You can simulate this by squeezing your middle finger from each side between your thumb and ring finger of the same hand, just behind the nail. Then palpate the nail base with the index finger of the opposite hand.

In late clubbing the base of the nail becomes visibly swollen and the angle between nail and nail base exceeds 180°.

Clubbing has many causes, including hypoxia and lung cancer.

FIGURE 10–1

Clubbing of the nails. (Adapted from Bates B: *A guide to physical assessment and history taking,* 5th ed. Philadelphia: Lippincott, 1991, p. 149.)

Palpate the skin for temperature, and moisture. When checking for temperature changes, use the backs of your fingers, which are more temperature-sensitive than the palmar aspects. Coldness is a reliable sign of pathologic vasoconstriction only if you examine the patient in a warm environment and the patient normally does not suffer from cold extremities. Increased warmth is of less significance than coldness in evaluating the vascular system, although it often accompanies thrombophlebitis.

Skin moisture abnormalities can include diaphoresis, the clamminess of the patient in shock, or the excessively dry skin of the dehydrated patient.

Chronically Decreased Perfusion Chronically decreased perfusion causes trophic changes and clubbing. Trophic changes, which result from prolonged tissue malnourishment, include thickened nails, hairlessness, shiny taut skin, or skin ulcers.

Edema *Edema* is the accumulation of excessive fluid in the interstitial spaces of tissues. Normally, extracellular fluid and other substances move between the capillaries and interstitial spaces because of pressure gradients and capillary permeability. Movement is thought to occur primarily by diffusion, either through pores or through the capillary membrane itself. *Diffusion* is the term that applies to the movement in one direction, *filtration* the term that describes the balance of outward and inward diffusion, that is, the net fluid movement.

Many years ago, Starling hypothesized that the direction and speed of fluid exchange across the capillary membrane depends on the interaction of pressures in the capillary fluid and interstitial fluid. The following descriptions of the mechanics of fluid exchange and edema formation are based upon Guyton (1991).

Four pressures affect filtration: two pressures exerted by fluid *(hydrostatic pressures)* and two by proteins *(colloid osmotic pressures)*. Hydrostatic pressure tends to "push" fluid out of a compartment, and colloid pressure tends to "pull" fluid into a compartment. The effective filtration pressure equals the sum of the forces tending to move fluid in one direction minus the sum of the forces tending to move fluid in the opposite direction.

At the arteriolar end of the capillary, the net force causes fluid movement out of the capillary and into the interstitial space. At the venular end, the net force causes diffusion of fluid back into the capillary. About 90% of the fluid that leaves the arteriolar end of the capillary is reabsorbed at the venular end. The remainder is reabsorbed by the lymphatic system, which also reabsorbs the small amounts of protein that leak continuously from the capillary. *Starling's law of the capillaries* states that the mean filtration forces at the capillary membrane exist in equilibrium, so that the amount of fluid that leaves the capillaries equals that returned to the capillaries and lymphatics.

The factors affecting capillary dynamics suggest the various causes of edema. Increased capillary hydrostatic pressure occurs with arteriolar dilatation (as in allergic reactions), venous obstruction (as with clots or congestive heart failure), or fluid retention (as in renal failure). Decreased plasma proteins can result from inadequate nutrition or accelerated protein loss, as in nephrosis. Increased capillary permeability occurs in capillary damage—for example, with burns or endotoxins. Finally, decreased lymphatic drainage can produce edema—for instance following surgical removal of diseased lymphatic glands.

There is a safety zone in which some of these causes can exist without producing clinically obvious edema (Guyton 1991). Interstitial hydrostatic pressure normally is negative. As it becomes more positive, it tends to produce increased lymphatic flow, which not only carries away some of the excess fluid but also some of the tissue proteins, thereby reducing their osmotic pull on capillary fluid. Edema usually is not detectable until the interstitial fluid volume is 30% above normal; it can reach several hundred percent above normal in severe cases.

Edema may be pitting or nonpitting. To determine the presence of peripheral edema, press with three fingers spread slightly apart for 10 seconds, and after release, feel for two "hills" between three "valleys" in the skin. The *severity* of edema often is graded on a 0-to-4 scale from absent to very marked: 0, absent; 1, slight; 2, mild; 3, marked; 4, very marked (Bates 1987). A depression (pit) that slowly disappears following fingertip pressure indicates that edema fluid is soft enough to be displaced by outside pressure. Nonpitting edema usually indicates that protein has coagulated in the tissues.

Frequently, you can deduce the cause of edema from its characteristics. Edema that occurs bilaterally in dependent body parts (such as the sacrum in the bedridden patient or feet in the ambulatory patient), pits on pressure, and decreases with position changes is *dependent edema,* caused by increased capillary hydrostatic pressure secondary to gravity. Unilateral or bilateral *pitting edema,* often associated with skin ulceration, is characteristic of increased hydrostatic pressure caused by venous obstruction or valvular insufficiency. Localized nonpitting swelling of the eyes, lips, tongue, hands, or genitals, or internal swelling (especially of the larynx), often associated with itching or burning sensations, typifies *allergic (angioneurotic) edema.* This type of edema results from increased hydrostatic pressure due to arteriolar dilatation following histamine release from damaged tissues.

Evaluation of Peripheral Arterial Pulses

A screening evaluation of peripheral pulses compares them bilaterally for volume, rhythm, and rate. The *pulse volume* depends on many of the same factors as arterial pressure (such as stroke volume and peripheral resistance) as well as characteristics of the vessel and its distance from the heart. Pulse volume may be described as *absent, small* (weak), *normal,* or *large* (bounding). A numeric classification is based on a 0-to-4 scale: 0, completely absent; 1, markedly impaired; 2, moderately impaired; 3, slightly impaired; 4, normal (Bates 1987).

Occasionally, you may find a decreased or absent pulse as a normal variant, particularly when checking the brachial, popliteal, and posterior tibial pulses. This finding is not a cause for alarm, providing that a more distal pulse is palpable or that other signs of adequate circulation (such as warm skin) are present.

The pulses of leg arteries sometimes can be difficult to locate. Figure 10–2 shows the location of pulses in the lower extremities. To find the popliteal artery, flex

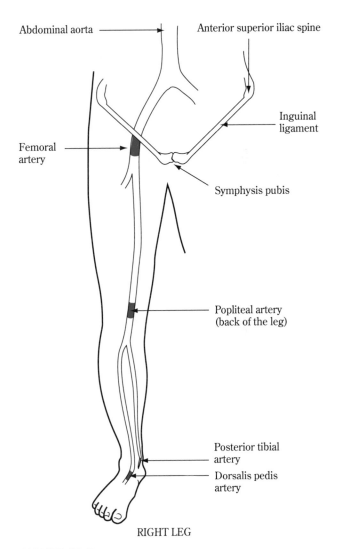

Abdominal aorta — Anterior superior iliac spine

Inguinal ligament

Femoral artery

Symphysis pubis

Popliteal artery (back of the leg)

Posterior tibial artery

Dorsalis pedis artery

RIGHT LEG

FIGURE 10–2

Location of pulses of lower extremities. (Adapted from Bates B: *A guide to physical assessment and history taking,* 4th ed. Philadelphia: Lippincott, 1987, p. 407. Susan Shapiro Brenman, medical illustrator.)

the patient's knee slightly and feel behind the knee with the fingertips of both hands. The dorsalis pedis pulse is congenitally absent or nonpalpable in about 10% of the population; however, when it is absent as a normal variant, the posterior tibial pulse usually is present. Abnormal pulses include the following:

- Loss of a previously present pulse
- Bilateral loss of radial or pedal pulses
- Unilateral pulse loss or inequality

Selected abnormalities of the arterial pulse are presented in Figure 10–3. Another abnormal pulse that can be palpated is the pulse associated with aortic stenosis, characterized by a slow rate of rise in the pulse fullness.

Blood Pressure Auscultation

Measurement of blood pressure (BP) is of vital importance in patient assessment because it is a prime indicator of the adequacy of organ perfusion.

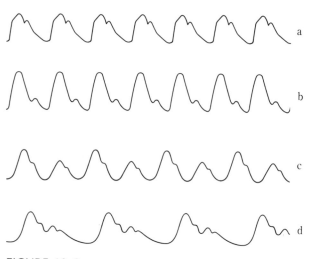

FIGURE 10–3

Abnormal arterial pulses. **a,** Normal. **b,** Large, bounding (water hammer) pulse. Characterized by rapid rise, sharp crest, rapid fall. Seen in hyperkinetic states (anxiety, fever, anemia, exercise) rapid arterial runoff (aortic regurgitation) sometimes in atherosclerosis and hypertension. **c,** Pulsus alternans. Regular alternation of pulse amplitude, due to alternation of left ventricular end-diastolic volume and contractility; seen in left ventricular failure. **d,** Bigeminal pulse. Irregular alternation of pulse amplitude, most often due to premature ventricular beats coupled to normal beats. Premature beats have small volume, normal beats larger volume due to prolonged diastolic filling after premature beats.

Technique When measuring BP noninvasively, it is essential to adhere to certain guidelines. These criteria often are overlooked in practice, resulting in the hasty recording of inaccurate pressures. The following are guidelines for accurate pressure measurement:

1. Use a sphygmomanometer cuff with a bladder that is 20% wider than the limb diameter and long enough to go halfway around the limb. Too small a cuff produces a falsely high BP, and too large a cuff a falsely low one. Usually, a cuff 12–14 cm wide is appropriate for the arm and one 18–20 cm wide is appropriate for the thigh of an average adult.

2. Identify the palpatory and auscultatory pressures. Place the limb so that the artery you will use is at the level of the heart, and palpate the arterial pulse. Center the bladder over the artery and wrap the cuff snugly. While palpating the pulse again, inflate the cuff to about 30 mm above the point at which the pulse disappears. Then lower the pressure 2–3 mm per second until you detect the pulse again. This point is the *palpatory systolic pressure,* and its importance will be explained shortly. Next, center the stethoscope over the artery and reinflate the cuff to about 30 mm above the palpatory systolic level. Auscultate the artery while you lower the pressure about 3 mm/second, noting the changes in arterial sounds (Korotkoff sounds).

The Korotkoff sounds are caused by the vibrations of turbulent flow in the partially compressed artery. The first ones occur when the cuff pressure reaches the peak systolic pressure in the artery and are characterized by clear tapping sounds of increasing intensity. As the pressure is lowered, the sounds take on a murmuring quality because of the increased volume of blood flowing through the artery. When diastolic pressure is reached, the sounds muffle suddenly and take on a blowing quality. They then gradually decrease in intensity until they disappear because the compression no longer is sufficient to cause turbulent flow. The disappearance may never be reached in high-flow states such as fever, anemia, and thyrotoxicosis.

The point at which the initial tapping sounds are heard is recorded as the *systolic* level. The muffling or disappearance of sounds represents the *diastolic* pressure.

If you are unable to hear the pressure, deflate the cuff completely and wait 2 minutes before rechecking. Failure to observe this caveat causes venous congestion, which falsely elevates the diastolic BP.

Particularly on initial evaluation, check the pressure in both arms. A difference of up to 10 mm Hg is normal. An increased difference is seen in dissection of the aorta and some congenital defects.

3. Mentally calculate the pulse pressure and mean arterial pressure. The *pulse pressure* is the difference between the systolic and diastolic readings. Pulse pressure depends primarily on stroke volume, peripheral resistance, and vessel distensibility. Increased pulse pressure is seen as a normal variant or in conditions that increase stroke volume (for example, circulatory overload or anxiety), decrease peripheral vascular resistance (fever), or decrease arterial distensibility (aging, hypertension). Decreased pulse pressure is usually not seen in normal subjects. Conditions that can cause it are decreased stroke volume (for example, shock, heart failure, hypovolemia), increased peripheral vascular resistance (shock, hypovolemia, vasoconstrictor drugs), and obstructions to ventricular ejection (mitral insufficiency, aortic stenosis).

The *mean arterial pressure* (MAP) averages out cycle-to-cycle variations in BP and therefore is the average pressure under which blood flow to the tissues occurs. A true MAP can be obtained electrically via an intra-arterial line. To approximate the MAP for patients without intra-arterial lines, add one-third the pulse pressure to the diastolic pressure; for example, for a pressure of 120/80, the mean BP is 93 mm Hg. (Note that this value is not an arithmetic mean, which would result from adding the systolic and diastolic values and dividing by 2. Because diastole is longer than systole, the mean BP is closer to the diastolic reading.)

Abnormal Findings

Auscultatory Gap In severely hypertensive patients, the sounds may completely disappear for an interval below the true systolic pressure. If you fail to establish the systolic pressure by palpation, and instead follow the common practice of inflating the cuff only a short interval above the disappearance of sounds, the point at which you stop inflation may well fall within this auscultatory gap. The first sounds you hear on deflation then will be the bottom of the auscultatory gap, rather than the true systolic pressure. Another

source of error is to raise the cuff pressure high enough to hear the true systolic pressure but release the pressure when sounds disappear; in the person with an auscultatory gap, you will be misled into interpreting the point at which sounds disappear as the diastolic level. Obviously, hasty checking may seriously underestimate the true systolic reading or overestimate the real diastolic reading. For this reason, it is wise to develop the habits of checking the systolic level by palpation before auscultating the blood pressure and continuing to auscultate until the cuff pressure is 0, particularly in patients you suspect are hypertensive. Record an auscultatory gap in this manner: "280/140 with an auscultatory gap from 250 to 220."

Pulsus Paradoxus Inspiration normally makes intrathoracic pressure more negative, causing pulmonary vessels to expand and blood to pool in the vessels. The resulting decrease in venous return to the left side of the heart decreases cardiac output. As a result, systolic arterial pressure normally drops as much as 10 mm Hg on inspiration.

Cardiac tamponade and constrictive pericarditis may cause an exaggerated drop in systolic arterial pressure because the restricted cardiac expansion causes more blood to pool in the pulmonary vessels. Severe obstructive lung disease also causes an exaggerated response, because the increased fluctuations in pulmonary pressures are transmitted to the heart and great vessels. The exaggerated systolic arterial pressure response to inspiration is known as a *paradoxical pulse,* although the name is poor because the response is merely an accentuation of the normal response rather than a paradox (an apparently absurd but true situation).

A paradoxical pulse often must be detected by auscultation rather than palpation. To check for a paradoxical pulse, instruct the patient to breathe normally. Inflate the cuff above the known systolic level. Deflate the cuff during normal expiration and note the systolic pressure. Then wait, reinflate the cuff, and check the systolic pressure when the patient inspires. A difference of less than 10 mm Hg between the two points indicates a normal response to inspiration. A greater difference indicates a paradoxical pulse. If its other causes are ruled out, this finding can be particularly valuable in confirming the presence of cardiac tamponade and the trend of readings useful in evaluating its progression.

Bruits Particularly on initial evaluation, it also is helpful to auscultate the major arteries. Auscultation normally reveals no bruits, although systolic abdominal bruits occur normally in about 25% of young people

(Daily and Schroeder 1989). In partially occluded vessels (primarily the carotid or femoral arteries), bruits indicate turbulent blood flow secondary to atherosclerosis or other pathology.

Interpretation To interpret the measurements you obtain, it is necessary to comprehend the factors that affect blood pressure and their interrelationships. These factors are presented graphically in Figure 10–4 and discussed in detail in the paragraphs that follow. The factors that affect blood pressure and their interrelationships are extremely complex and involve feedback mechanisms at many levels. The explanations presented here are simplified and are based primarily on the works of Guyton (1991) and Daily and Schroeder (1989).

Physics of Blood Flow Arterial pressure varies directly with cardiac output and peripheral resistance:

Systemic blood pressure = Cardiac output (CO)
× Systemic vascular resistance (SVR)

Cardiac output averages about 5 liters per minute. It equals the *heart rate* times the amount of blood the left ventricle ejects with each beat (the *stroke volume*). The heart rate responds primarily to nervous and hormonal stimuli. The stroke volume depends on the ventricular volume at the end of diastole and on myocardial contractility. These factors in turn depend on the venous return to the heart and on nervous and hormonal stimulation.

The degree of peripheral resistance depends on blood vessel radius, blood viscosity, and blood vessel length. Blood vessel radius and peripheral resistance are related inversely—as the radius increases, resistance decreases, and arterial pressure decreases. Even small changes in arteriolar radius can have a profound effect on arterial pressure. Changes in blood viscosity are much more important than changes in blood vessel length. As blood viscosity increases (for example, due to an increased hematocrit or serum protein level), peripheral resistance also tends to increase and so does arterial pressure.

Systemic vascular resistance (SVR) cannot be measured directly. It can be calculated, however, from mean arterial pressure (MAP), mean right atrial pressure ($\overline{RA}$), and cardiac output (CO), as follows:

$$SVR \text{ (in mm Hg/L/min)} = (MAP - \overline{RA})/CO$$

$$SVR \text{ (in dynes/sec/cm}^{-5}) = ((MAP - \overline{RA})/CO) \times 80$$

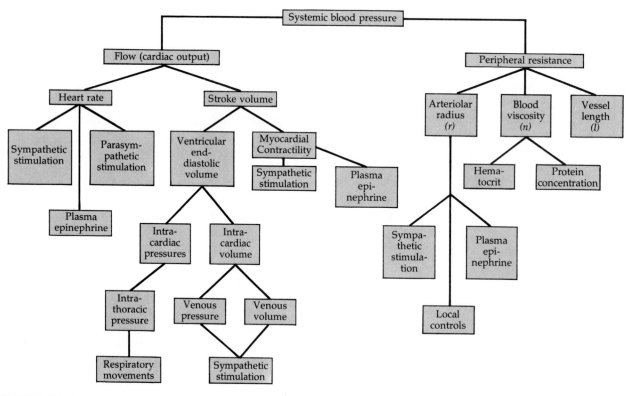

FIGURE 10–4

Multiplicity of factors affecting circulation.

Normal values for SVR are 10–15 mm Hg/L/min or 800–1,200 dynes/sec/cm^{-5} (1 mm Hg/L/min is equal to 80 dynes/sec/cm^{-5}).

Intrinsic Control of the Local Circulation Blood flow is controlled both locally and systemically. The multiple factors controlling the circulation can be grouped into intrinsic, nervous, and humoral controls (Guyton 1991). To a large degree, the vascular system is capable of functioning without outside control. The inherent mechanisms that enable it to do so are termed *intrinsic controls*. The most important intrinsic control is local control of blood flow in response to tissue demands. The following description of local control is based upon Guyton (1991).

Local control of blood flow occurs in capillary beds. Blood flows into capillary beds through arterioles. From arterioles, blood flows next into metarterioles, courses through the capillaries, and exits through the venules.

Arterioles have a continuous muscular coat. The sympathetic nervous system innervates arterioles, and to a lesser extent venules, extensively, so central nervous system stimulation controls their constriction and dilatation.

In contrast, metarterioles have an intermittent coating of smooth muscle fibers. At the point where metarterioles give rise to capillaries, smooth muscle fibers called *precapillary sphincters* surround the blood vessels. Metarterioles and precapillary sphincters are controlled not by nerves but instead almost completely by local factors.

Two major theories account for control of local blood flow: the vasodilator theory and the nutrient demand theory. According to the *vasodilator theory,* vasodilating substances may be released in response to increased tissue metabolism, decreased blood flow, or a shortage of oxygen or other nutrients. These substances may include carbon dioxide, lactic acid, hydrogen ions, histamine, adenosine, and other agents.

The *nutrient demand theory* presupposes that vessels dilate in response to a need for oxygen or other nutrients. Oxygen could control tissue flow, according to this theory, through its effect on precapillary sphincters. Normally, each individual sphincter is either completely open or completely closed at a given time and also displays intermittent contraction and relaxation, a phenomenon called *vasomotion*. Because of vasomotion, blood spurts intermittently into the capillaries. Each tissue can control its own blood flow by altering sphincter activity to influence the frequency and duration of the vasomotor cycle. In tissues that suffer a prolonged but moderate oxygen deficit, flow also is increased by dilatation of already existing bypass channels (collateral vessels) plus increases in the number and size of new blood vessels, which are laid down continuously in tissues. It is thought that the tissues have an important role in regulating CO, since they control peripheral vascular resistance and venous return, both direct determinants of cardiac output.

Nervous Control of the Circulation In addition to local controls, nervous and hormonal controls regulate tissue blood flow. Nervous control of the circulation is mediated via complex pathways, most of which are part of the autonomic nervous system. Parasympathetic control of the vascular system is relatively unimportant, affecting arterial pressure only through its ability to slow the heart rate.

In contrast, sympathetic stimuli are very important. The most important nervous regulator of the circulation is the sympathetic vasoconstrictor system, which operates through the *vasomotor center* located in the lower pons and upper medulla. The vasomotor center controls circulation chiefly by altering the degree of blood vessel constriction. From this center, impulses pass through the spinal cord to vasoconstrictor fibers, which innervate arteries and veins. These fibers secrete norepinephrine, which acts directly on the smooth muscle of blood vessels to cause constriction.

The lateral parts of the center constantly discharge stimuli that keep the blood vessels partially contracted (vasomotor tone). When stimulated to raise arterial pressure, the upper and lateral portions of the vasomotor center increase sympathetic stimulation, which increases arterial pressure in a number of ways. It constricts the veins and venous reservoirs, diminishing their capacity and thereby increasing blood volume. It accelerates the heart rate. By increasing constriction of the arteries and arterioles, it raises peripheral resistance. The center can also send impulses to the adrenal medullae, provoking secretion of epinephrine and norepinephrine, which are carried in the bloodstream and reinforce vasoconstriction. All these mechanisms raise arterial pressure.

When stimulated to lower arterial pressure, the lower and medial portion of the vasomotor center inhibits the center's release of sympathetic stimuli, thereby inhibiting vasoconstriction and decreasing the effects described in the paragraph above. The medial portion of the center also sends parasympathetic impulses via the vagus nerve to the heart, slowing its rate.

Numerous stimuli affect the vasomotor center. Higher nervous centers located throughout the cerebral cortex, diencephalon, midbrain, and pons can excite or inhibit the vasomotor center. This fact explains why circulatory changes accompany motor activity, emotional responses, and the "fight or flight" response to stress.

Humoral Control of the Circulation Humoral regulation of the circulation, the least significant of the three control types, is mediated through the actions of a number of substances in the body fluids, including both vasoconstricting and vasodilating agents. As mentioned earlier, norepinephrine release from sympathetic vasoconstrictor nerves plays an important role in nervous control of the circulation. Norepinephrine can also be secreted by the adrenal medullae in response to sympathetic stimuli from the vasomotor center, as can epinephrine. Norepinephrine vasoconstricts almost all blood vessels. Epinephrine, however, constricts some blood vessels and dilates others. Angiotensin is produced by an interplay of several chemicals in the renin-angiotensin mechanism. When blood pressure drops below physiologic levels, the kidney secretes renin. Renin activates a series of reactions that finally produce angiotensin, a stimulator of aldosterone release and a powerful arteriolar vasoconstrictor. Histamine already has been mentioned as a controller of local arteriolar dilatation. The unclear roles of other chemicals, such as bradykinin, serotonin, and prostaglandins, remain a promising area for further investigation in the understanding of vascular dynamics.

Regulation of Mean Arterial Pressure Regulation of mean arterial pressure can be subdivided into two categories: short-term (rapid-acting) control mechanisms and long-term control mechanisms.

Rapid-acting controls include three major mechanisms that respond within seconds to blood pressure changes: baroreceptor reflexes, chemoreceptor reflexes, and the central nervous system ischemic response. The following information about these reflexes is derived from Guyton (1991). Within the physiologic range of blood pressure (approximately 60—180 mm Hg), the major short-term regulators are *baroreceptors* (pressoreceptors), which sense changes in pressure. The most important ones are contained in the aortic arch and in the carotid sinuses, which are located in the internal carotid arteries just above the bifurcation of the internal and external carotid arteries. Baroreceptor response starts within seconds of a pressure change. When blood pressure drops, they transmit a decreased number of impulses to the vasomotor center.

If pressure falls below 80 mm Hg, *chemoreceptors* come into play. Chemoreceptors respond primarily to an oxygen deficit and, to a lesser extent, a carbon dioxide excess or hydrogen ion excess. The most important chemoreceptors are located in the aortic and carotid bodies (in the aortic arch and carotid bifurca-

tions). An oxygen deficit increases chemoreceptor activity and excites the vasomotor center.

A pressure fall below 50 mm Hg triggers the very powerful *CNS ischemic response*. Although the exact mechanism is uncertain, it is thought that the drop in pressure allows CO_2 to accumulate in the central nervous system, intensely stimulating the vasomotor center. An example of a CNS ischemic response is the Cushing reflex, which occurs when an extreme elevation in cerebrospinal fluid pressure cuts off the blood supply to the brain.

In addition to the three instantaneous control mechanisms mediated by the nervous system, several humoral and intrinsic control systems come into play within 20 minutes to several hours. As described above, the humoral (hormonal) mechanisms include release of norepinephrine and epinephrine from the adrenal medullae, activation of the renin-angiotensin system, and secretion of antidiuretic hormone. These hormonal mechanisms result in vasoconstriction, cardiac stimulation, and retention of sodium and water to expand blood volume. In addition, a capillary fluid shift (intrinsic control mechanism) occurs. A decreased arterial pressure alters capillary dynamics in such a way that fluid shifts from the interstitial spaces into the capillaries to reestablish equilibrium. This fluid shift also helps to increase circulating blood volume.

These reflexes are effective only temporarily (hours to days), because baroreceptors adapt to the new pressure level, the circulatory system adapts to the sympathetic stimuli, and local controls override the sympathetic response. Longer-range restoration of blood pressure is provided by the kidneys, as discussed in Chapter 15.

Examination of Neck Veins

As part of the patient examination, the nurse examines the neck veins to evaluate venous pressure noninvasively (a basic skill) and to study the waves of the venous pulse (an advanced skill).

The venous system is a low-pressure, low-resistance system. Because it is so distensible, it can easily accommodate an increase in blood volume. As it responds to a lesser degree of sympathetic stimulation than arteries and arterioles, the venous system easily shifts blood into the circulating blood volume when the need arises.

Venous reservoirs exist in all parts of the body except the heart, brain, and skeletal muscles. The most important are those in the abdominal organs, particularly the liver and spleen, and in the skin.

Among the factors affecting venous return to the heart are venous pressure (in turn affected by blood volume, venous distensibility, gravity, and right atrial pressure), venous valves, sympathetic stimulation, the contraction of skeletal and abdominal muscles, and intrathoracic pressure changes occurring during respiration.

Assessment of Venous Pressure Although venous flow is nonpulsatile, pressure changes resulting from atrial and ventricular filling are transmitted to the neck veins and can be appreciated as pulsations. Following are procedures for evaluating venous pressure by examining the neck veins:

Evaluate the *venous pressure* as normal or increased. To evaluate the venous pressure and pulse, first identify the neck veins, using the internal jugular vein on the right. Elevate the head of the bed slightly if you anticipate a relatively normal venous pressure or approximately 45° if you suspect an elevated pressure, as in congestive heart failure. Place a small pillow under the neck to relax the neck muscles. Turn the head slightly away from you.

Shine a light tangentially across the neck. Identify the carotid artery, external jugular vein, and internal jugular vein (Figure 10-5). Because the external jugular vein is superficial and engorges easily, the internal jugular vein (especially the right one) is

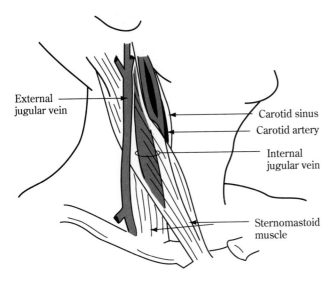

FIGURE 10-5

Great vessels of the neck. Deep to the sternomastoids run the great vessels of the neck: the carotid artery and internal jugular vein. The external jugular vein passes diagonally over the surface of the sternomastoid. (From Bates B: *A guide to physical assessment and history taking,* 4th ed. Philadelphia: Lippincott, 1987, p. 159. Susan Shapiro Brenman, medical illustrator.)

Labels on figure:
External jugular vein
Carotid sinus
Carotid artery
Internal jugular vein
Sternomastoid muscle

preferred for evaluation of venous dynamics. The inexperienced examiner easily may confuse the carotid artery with the internal jugular vein, which runs parallel to it. To distinguish them, keep these points in mind. The carotid pulse is palpable, with a single strong rapid upstroke. Respiration or position do not affect the carotid pulse, and pressure cannot obliterate it easily. The internal jugular vein lies deep, under the sternocleidomastoid muscle. Its pulsations usually are not palpable, instead being seen in gentle movements of the overlying tissue. Bates (1987) suggests looking for the internal jugular pulse beginning at the base of the neck just lateral to the juncture of the sternum and clavicle and looking upward along the sternocleidomastoid muscle to the earlobe.

In contrast to the arterial pulse, the *venous pulse* consists of two or three slower, smaller upstrokes (the *a, c,* and *v* waves discussed in a later section). The level of pulsation descends with inspiration and rises with expiration. Pressure on the vessel just above the clavicle easily obliterates the pulsations. The internal jugular pulse in a healthy person is visible only when the person is lying flat, and disappears as the head of the bed is elevated to 30-45°.

After you have identified the neck veins, use the following procedure. Vary the degree of elevation of the head of the bed until you can see the maximum pulsations of the upper level of the fluid column in the internal or external jugular veins. Then make the following observations:

1. Note the degree of elevation of the head of the bed.

2. Measure the level of the pulse. To do this, draw an imaginary horizontal line from the upper level of pulsation, and another imaginary horizontal line from the sternal angle. Measure the vertical distance between these lines. The normal measurement is 3 cm or less. Adding 4-5 cm to the measurement will give you a rough estimate of the patient's central venous pressure.

3. Note the relationship between the level of pulsation and the respiratory cycle. The normal respiratory variation is for the level to decrease on inspiration and increase on expiration. Severely increased pressure appears as a paradoxical rise in the level of distention during inspiration *(Kussmaul's sign)*.

4. Test for *hepatojugular reflux* (HJR). Ask the patient to breathe normally. If the patient holds his or her breath or bears down during the test, it is invalid. Press the right upper quadrant of

the abdomen firmly for 30 seconds while you observe the neck veins. This maneuver increases venous return from the abdomen to the heart. If this test increases venous distention 1 centimeter or less, venous pressure is normal. An increase of more than 1 cm (positive HJR) indicates increased venous pressure, such as in right heart failure or constrictive pericarditis.

If you are assessing the external jugular vein, one additional maneuver can be performed:

5. Apply pressure on the vein just above the clavicle. The vein will distend. Release the pressure suddenly and note how rapidly the vein empties. Normally, the vein immediately empties to less than 3 cm above the sternal angle (Nimoityn and Chung 1987).

Causes of increased venous pressure include right ventricular failure, fluid overload, high cardiac output states, pericardial constriction, and tricuspid valve disease.

Assessment of Venous Pulse Wave Contour The venous pulse consists of three positive waves and two descents, which are related to pressure changes during the cardiac cycle (Figure 10–6). When the right atrium contracts, forcing blood into the right ventricle during the end of diastole, the slight rise in atrial pressure produces the *a wave*. Atrial diastole causes a drop in pressure, known as the *x descent*. It is interrupted by the *c wave,* which occurs as a result of tricuspid valve closure, bulging of the tricuspid valve during ventric-

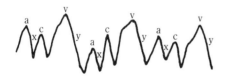

Key: *Atrial Stage*   *Ventricular Stage*
        a wave—right atrial contraction   ventricular diastole
        x descent—atrial diastole

        c wave—tricuspid bulging or im-
          pact of carotid arterial pulse;
          interrupts x descent   ventricular systole

        v wave—increased atrial pressure
          due to venous return

        y descent—tricuspid valve open-   ventricular diastole
          ing, blood entering ventricle

FIGURE 10–6
_____

Venous pulse waves.

ular systole, and/or a neck vein reflection of the nearby carotid pulse. During the last part of ventricular systole, venous return raises the atrial pressure and produces the *v wave*. The opening of the tricuspid valve and rush of blood into the ventricle create a drop in atrial pressure, the *y descent*. The cycle then repeats itself.

To identify the individual waves, look at the venous pulse while you either palpate the carotid artery on the other side of the neck or auscultate the heart. The *a* wave just precedes S_1 and the carotid upstroke. The *c* wave usually cannot be seen. The *v* wave coincides with S_2.

You may see a variety of abnormal venous pulses, which are related logically to the conditions that produce them. In atrial fibrillation, for example, effective atrial contraction does not occur, and no *a* wave is evident. Large, regular *a* waves indicate resistance to atrial emptying into the right ventricle, as in tricuspid stenosis or pulmonary hypertension. Extremely large *a* waves (cannon waves) denote atrial contraction against a closed tricuspid valve. They may occur regularly, as in junctional rhythm, or irregularly as in atrioventricular (AV) dissociation.

Examination of the Heart

External Chest Landmarks External chest landmarks serve as reference points when reporting findings from cardiac auscultation. The portion of the chest wall that overlies the heart is called the *precordium.*

Findings commonly are described in relation to the nearest rib or intercostal space (ICS) and imaginary reference line. To locate the intercostal spaces, feel for a bony ridge across the sternum about 2 inches below the suprasternal notch. This ridge is called the *sternal angle* or *angle of Louis.* It marks the attachment of the second rib and is a handy reference point from which to count the ribs and intercostal spaces. Place your second and third fingers on either side of the ridge and slide them out past the sternal border until you feel a depression under your third finger. This depression is the second intercostal space. Continue numbering the ribs and spaces by palpating downward and laterally in an oblique line. Remember that the ribs slope down at about a 45° angle from their attachment to the thoracic spine to their anterior attachment to the costal cartilages.

The imaginary reference lines on the anterior chest are the midsternal and the midclavicular. On the lateral chest, the lines are the anterior and posterior axillary lines—drawn downward from the axillary skin folds—and the midaxillary line.

The heart sits in the mediastinum, between the lungs and above the diaphragm. The sternum and ribs are anterior to the heart, and the esophagus, descending aorta, and the fifth through eighth thoracic vertebrae are posterior. The heart somewhat resembles an inverted triangle, with its narrow apex in the fifth intercostal space at approximately the left midclavicular line (MCL) and its broad base at the level of the attachments of the third ribs to the sternum. The apex is more anterior than the base. About two-thirds of the heart lies to the left of the midsternal line.

Because of the heart's oblique position in both the frontal and horizontal planes, the distance between each chamber and the chest walls varies (Figure 10–7). The right ventricle (RV) is most anterior, lying directly under the sternum. The left atrium (LA) is most posterior. The right atrium (RA) is closest to the right lateral chest wall, and the left ventricle (LV) is closest to the left lateral chest wall.

The major blood vessels enter and leave the heart at its base (Figure 10–8). The superior and inferior venae cavae (SVC and IVC) bring deoxygenated blood to the right atrium. The pulmonary artery (PA), which arises from the right ventricle and slants off to the left, carries deoxygenated blood from the right ventricle to the lungs. The four pulmonary veins return oxygenated blood to the left atrium. The aorta (Ao), which arises from the left ventricle and slants off to the right, carries oxygenated blood from the left ventricle to the systemic circulation.

The cardiac valves help control blood flow through the chambers and great vessels. The tricuspid valve (TV) lies between the right atrium and right ventricle, at the attachment of the fifth rib to the right side of the sternum. The mitral valve (MV) lies between the left atrium and left ventricle, at the attachment of the fourth rib to the left side of the sternum. The tricuspid and mitral valves sometimes are called *atrioventricular valves.* Each is anchored by chordae tendinae to the papillary muscles on its ventricular floor.

The pulmonic valve lies between the right ventricle and the pulmonary artery. The aortic valve (AV) lies between the left ventricle and the aorta. The pulmonic and aortic valves are located under the sternum at approximately the level of the attachments of the third ribs to the sternum. They are not anchored by chordae tendinae, closing instead because blood presses against their cuplike cusps. Because of their shape, the aortic and pulmonic valves sometimes are called *semilunar valves.*

Because the valves are grouped so closely anatomically, it is not possible to differentiate them with a stethoscope applied directly over their actual locations. Instead, you must listen in the auscultatory areas to which each valve's sounds are best transmitted. In general, these areas are "downstream" from the valve, along the path of blood flow through the heart; there are, however, some exceptions.

At present, there are several ways of labeling these favored sites (Figure 10–9). One way is to refer to the nearby valve; another is to refer to the nearby chamber; a third way is to give the general anatomic location; and a fourth is to give the specific anatomic location. Thus, the *aortic area* and upper right sternal border are synonymous with the second intercostal space to the

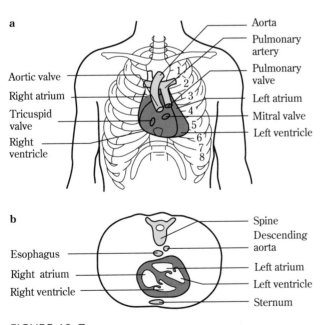

FIGURE 10–7

Position of cardiac structures. **a.** Frontal plane (numbers designate intercostal spaces); **b.** horizontal plane.

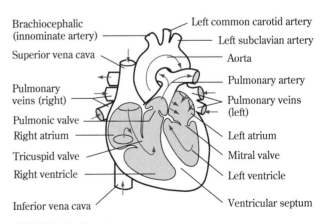

FIGURE 10–8

Cardiac structures. Arrows show direction of blood flow.

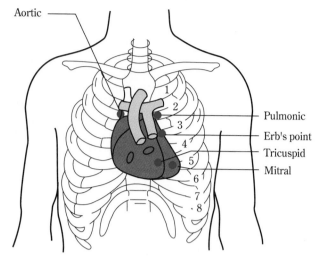

FIGURE 10–9

Auscultation sites. The second intercostal space at the right sternal border is referred to as the *aortic* area; the second intercostal space at the left sternal border is referred to as the *pulmonic* area; the third intercostal space at the left sternal border is *Erb's point;* the fifth intercostal space at the left sternal border is referred to the *tricuspid* area or lower left sternal border; the fifth intercostal space at midclavicular line is referred to as the *mitral* area or apical area.

right side of the sternum (the aorta slants off to the right of the heart). A secondary aortic area is *Erb's point,* located at the third intercostal space at the left sternal border. The *pulmonic area* and upper left sternal border are synonymous with the region of the second intercostal space to the left of the sternum (remember that the pulmonary artery slants off to the left of the heart). The *tricuspid area,* right ventricular area, and lower left sternal border all describe the same site on the chest wall, that is, the fifth intercostal space to the left of the sternum. The *mitral area,* left ventricular area, and apical area all describe the fifth intercostal space at the midclavicular line.

There are several ways to fix the preceding information in your mind. One of the most helpful is to study anatomic specimens or a three-dimensional replica of the heart. Another is to use a mnemonic to remember the areas, as shown in Table 10–3. Comprehension of the relationships between the cardiac structures and the external chest landmarks is crucial to true understanding of the possible sources of phenomena detectable at a particular chest site.

Inspection and Palpation of the Precordial Pulsations Normally, the only pulsation detectable is the apical impulse, caused by forward rotation of the heart

TABLE 10–3

Mnemonics to Help Remember Auscultation Sites

Aortic right, pulmonic left,

Tricuspid's at the sternum;

Mitral's at the apex beat—

This is how we learn 'em.*

Ape to Man:

A = aortic

P = pulmonic

E = Erb's point

To = tricuspid

Man = mitral**

*Sherman J, Fields S: *Guide to patient evaluation,* 2d ed. Garden City, NY: Medical Examination Publishing Company, 1974.
**Brykczynski K: Going ape over heart sounds. *Nurs 81* (September) 1981; 25.

at the beginning of systole. Palpate with the palm of your hand to locate the *point of maximal impulse (PMI)*. It usually is located at about the fifth intercostal space, in the left midclavicular line. The normal apical impulse is less than 2–3 cm in diameter and lasts for about a third of systole. In many patients, this impulse is not detectable. If it is, note its location, size, and character. In left ventricular hypertrophy, the impulse is displaced to the left and is larger, longer, and more forceful than normal. Also note any other abnormal precordial movement, such as a systolic parasternal lift (indicative of right ventricular enlargement), extra impulses, or vibrations (thrills).

Percussion Percussion involves striking the chest and evaluating the resulting vibrations. It was once used to estimate heart size by percussing out cardiac borders. Today, a more precise technique for estimating heart size is the x-ray film. Being of limited value in examining the heart, percussion is not discussed here.

Auscultation

Cardiac Cycle and Normal Heart Sounds Auscultation allows you to assess the sounds generated by blood flow inside the heart. Before you can understand the data it provides, you must have a thorough understanding of the relationship of the cardiac cycle to the sounds generated by the heart.

The *cardiac cycle* is that series of events between one ejection of blood from the heart and the next. During the different phases of the cycle, blood rapidly accel-

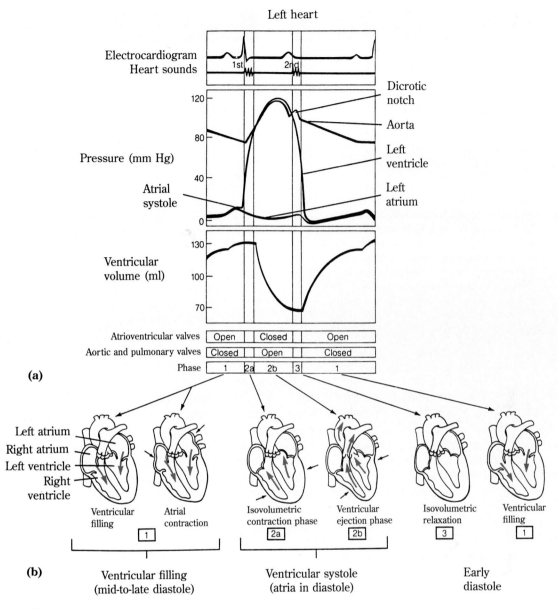

FIGURE 10–10

Summary of events occurring in the heart during the cardiac cycle. (a) Events in the left side of the heart. An ECG tracing is superimposed on the graph (top) so that pressure and volume changes can be related to electrical events occurring at any point. Time occurrence of heart sounds is also indicated. (b) Events of phases 1–3 of the cardiac cycle are depicted in diagrammatic views of the heart. (From Marieb E: *Human anatomy and physiology,* 2d ed., Redwood City, CA: Benjamin/Cummings, 1988, p. 622.)

erates or decelerates against myocardial structures. These rapid changes in blood flow cause valves and other cardiac structures to tense and vibrate. The vibrations are thought to generate sounds that can be assessed by auscultation. The events of the cardiac cycle are diagrammed in Figure 10–10, and the following description correlates with this diagram.

The cycle begins with a depolarization wave spreading across the atria (shown by the P wave on the electrocardiogram). At this time, the AV valves are open and the ventricles are slowly filling. The P wave triggers atrial systole, which fills the ventricles further, increasing ventricular volume. At the end of this time, blood entering the ventricles decelerates very rapidly because it encounters increasing pressure in the ventricles. The AV valves close, beginning ventricular systole. As they close, they produce the first heart sound.

Since both the AV and semilunar valves are now shut, the ventricles are closed chambers. The ventricles depolarize (shown by the QRS complex), and contraction begins with a tremendous increase in ventricular pressure, because the blood has no place to go (isovolumetric contraction).

The increased ventricular pressure opens the semilunar valves and ejects blood rapidly into the pulmonary artery and aorta (ventricular ejection phase). Toward the end of this phase, the increasing pulmonary arterial and aortic pressures cause rapid deceleration of blood flow. This deceleration causes the structures of the semilunar valves to vibrate just before they close, ending ventricular systole. The second heart sound is produced at this time.

The ventricles now are closed chambers again. As they relax, ventricular pressure decreases but the volume stays the same (isovolumetric relaxation). When the pressure drops sufficiently, the AV valves open, beginning the slow ventricular filling phase again. The cycle then repeats itself.

The rapid acceleration and deceleration of blood creates vibrations of the valves and surrounding structures. Authorities differ as to whether these vibrations or actual valve closure produce heart sounds. The first heart sound, S_1, occurs at the time the AV valves close. The second heart sound, S_2, occurs at the time the semilunar valves close. From this description, you can tell that S_1 marks the beginning of ventricular systole and S_2 its end. The time between S_2 and the next S_1 marks ventricular diastole. Because systole is usually shorter than diastole, the pause between S_1 and S_2 is shorter than that between S_2 and S_1.

Characteristics of S_1 and S_2 S_1, the sound associated with closure of the mitral and tricuspid valves, is heard best with the diaphragm at the apex. It forms the "lub" in the "lub-dub" sound of the normal heartbeat. Usually, S_1 is heard as one sound; however, a normal variant in adolescents and young adults is two closely associated sounds, a *split* S_1 caused by closure of the mitral valve slightly before the closure of the tricuspid valve. The split is heard best at the tricuspid area. Because S_1 signifies the onset of systole, it is heard just before the carotid arterial pulse is palpable.

S_2, the sound associated with closure of the aortic and pulmonic valves, is heard best with the diaphragm at the aortic area. S_2 is higher pitched and shorter than S_1, forming the "dub" in the normal "lub-dub" sound of the heartbeat.

Normally, the aortic valve closes slightly before the pulmonic, creating two components of S_2: the aortic sound (A_2), which is heard first, and the pulmonic sound (P_2). Usually, A_2 is louder and heard all over the precordium, while the softer P_2 is heard only in the pulmonic area. Therefore, a split S_2 is best heard at the pulmonic area. The reason for the split of S_2 is as follows.

As just mentioned, A_2 usually occurs before P_2. On inspiration, the split between these sounds widens. Although the exact cause is uncertain, many cardiologists believe that the increased negativity of chest pressure during inspiration causes different amounts of blood to be delivered to and ejected from each ventricle. The negativity may cause more blood to pool in the pulmonary vasculature, so that less blood enters the left ventricle. Because the left ventricle ejects less blood, the aortic valve closes a little early. At the same time, the increased negativity produces a suction effect on the systemic veins, causing more blood to enter the right side of the heart. Because the right ventricle ejects more blood, the pulmonic valve closes a little later than on expiration. As a result of the early A_2 and late P_2 on inspiration, the split between the sounds widens. Physiologic split S_2's are heard most often in children and young adults.

Among the abnormalities of S_1 and S_2 that may be detected are increased, decreased, or varying intensity of either sound. It also is possible to detect an abnormal relationship between the components of the second heart sound.

A number of conditions may cause S_2 to have no variation (a *fixed split*) or reversed *(paradoxical)* split, in which P_2 occurs before A_2 and widens on expiration. Physiologic mechanisms and clinical examples of conditions characterized by abnormal S_1's and S_2's are shown in Table 10–4.

Characteristics of S_3 and S_4 Occasionally, as you auscultate the precordium, you will hear extra heart sounds. Often these are *gallop rhythms,* so called because they supposedly resemble the galloping of a horse. Gallop rhythms result from an extra ventricular sound during diastole, usually generated by the rapid deceleration of blood as it enters against elevated ventricular pressure. Some gallop rhythms result from an extra sound in early diastole. The sound is called S_3, and the rhythm is called a *ventricular gallop,* or *protodiastolic gallop.* An S_3 is normal in children and in adults under age 30 years. It is almost always pathologic in adults over 30 years of age. An S_3 usually signifies volume overload in the ventricle. It is heard in

patients with congestive heart failure (CHF), valvular disease, and cardiomyopathy.

S_3 is low-pitched, so it is most audible with the bell of the stethoscope. Because it most often originates from the left ventricle, it is heard best in the mitral area, with the patient turned on the left side. It occurs so early in diastole that it immediately follows the end of systole. The pattern of S_1–S_2–S_3 sounds like "lub-*dub*-duh" or "Ken-*tuc*-ky."* Another helpful hint: S_3 is heard just after the carotid pulse wave disappears.

Another gallop rhythm results from an extra sound in late diastole, during the phase of rapid ventricular filling (which results from atrial contraction). The sound is called S_4, and the rhythm is called an *atrial gallop* or *presystolic gallop.* A physiologic S_4 may be heard in infants, small children, and healthy adults over 60 years of age (Bates 1987). An abnormal S_4 is thought to result from increased resistance to ventricular filling during atrial contraction.

S_4 is heard best with the stethoscope bell at the mitral area. The sound occurs so late in diastole that it immediately precedes systole. The pattern of S_4–S_1–S_2 sounds somewhat like "de-lub-*dub*" or "Ten-nes-*see*."* S_4 is heard just before the carotid pulse wave is felt. S_4 occurs so close to S_1 that it may be difficult at first to differentiate it from a split S_1. The key differentiating feature is the area in which the sounds are heard—a split S_1 is heard best at the tricuspid area, whereas a left-sided S_4 is heard best at the apex.

An S_4 implies decreased ventricular compliance or a "stiff" left ventricle. It is heard in hypertension, myocardial infarction, aortic or pulmonic stenosis, and cardiomyopathies, for example, and frequently is not accompanied by ventricular failure. It is a normal variant in people age 65 years or older.

In a patient with a severely failing heart, both an S_3 and an S_4 may be heard. Occasionally, during a run of tachycardia or in prolonged atrioventricular conduction, they may combine in a mid-diastolic sound called a *summation gallop.*

Physiologic mechanisms and clinical examples of disorders characterized by abnormal S_3's and S_4's are included in Table 10–4.

Other abnormal sounds are *snaps* and *clicks.* Opening *snaps* occur as stenotic AV valves open. Mitral and tricuspid opening snaps are high-pitched diastolic sounds heard shortly after S_2 and often followed by rumbles. *Clicks* are systolic sounds. Systolic ejection clicks are high-pitched sounds heard in early systole,

---

* The accented syllable in *Kentucky* and *Tennessee* corresponds with S_2.

TABLE 10–4

Abnormal Heart Sounds

SOUND	ABNORMALITY	MECHANISM	EXAMPLES
S_1	Louder than normal	1. Valve wide open	Short PR interval, premature beats, tachycardia, mitral or tricuspid stenosis
		2. Prolonged ventricular filling	Left-to-right shunts
	Softer than normal	1. Valve partly closed	First degree AV block
		2. Valve prematurely closed	Severe hypertension
		3. Normal tensing	Mitral or tricuspid insufficiency
		4. Damping of sound	Thick chest, pericardial effusion
S_2	Persistent or paradoxical split	1. Asynchronous ventricular activation	
		A. Block of bundle branch	RBBB (persistent split), LBBB (paradoxical split)
		B. Ectopy	Left ventricular (persistent), right ventricular (paradoxical)
		2. Prolonged ejection on one side of head	
		A. Systolic overload	Pulmonary stenosis or hypertension (persistent), aortic stenosis or systemic hypertension (paradoxical)
		B. Diastolic overload	Pulmonary insufficiency (persistent), atrial septal defect (persistent), ventricular septal defect (persistent), aortic insufficiency (paradoxical), patent ductus arteriosus (paradoxical)
		C. Other	Right ventricular failure (persistent), left ventricular failure (paradoxical), myocardial infarction (paradoxical), angina (paradoxical)
		3. Two outlets for ventricular ejection	Mitral insufficiency (persistent), ventricular septal defect (persistent), tricuspid insufficiency (paradoxical)
S_2	Single sound	1. One component decreased	Severe aortic or pulmonic stenosis
		2. Aortic valve anterior	Tetralogy of Fallot
		3. Murmur obscuring A_2	Atrial septal defect, patent ductus arteriosus, pulmonic stenosis
S_3	Presence	1. Diastolic overloading of ventricles	Valvular insufficiency, atrial septal defect, left-to-right shunts (RV), high output states (LV)
		2. Decreased ventricular compliance and/or increased ventricular diastolic pressure	Ventricular failure, ischemic heart disease, constructive pericarditis, cardiomyopathies
S_4	Presence	1. Systolic overloading of ventricles	Aortic or pulmonic stenosis, hypertension (systemic or pulmonary)
		2. Systolic overloading of right atrium	Tricuspid stenosis
		3. Decreased ventricular compliance and/or increased ventricular diastolic pressure	Mitral insufficiency, ventricular failure, ischemic heart disease, cardiomyopathies
		4. Systemic diseases	Severe anemia, severe infections
		5. First degree AV block	

RV, right ventricular overloading; LV, left ventricular overloading; RBBB, right bundle branch block; LBBB, left bundle branch block.

Source: Adapted from Marriott H: *Differential diagnosis of heart disease,* Oldmar, FL: Tampa Tracings, 1967.

CRITICAL CARE GERONTOLOGY

Cardiovascular Assessment in the Elderly

In people over 65 years of age, most organ systems follow the 1% rule. That is, most organ systems lose function at roughly 1% a year beginning around the age of 30. The critical difference in this loss of function lies not in the performance of the organ at rest, but rather how the organ adapts to external stress.

At rest, the physiologic changes of aging often work together to keep parameters normal. Under increased physiologic demand, however, an elder's body may not respond effectively. For example, the ability of the heart to speed up in response to orthostatic hypotension is diminished with age (Day et al. 1982). Furthermore, with age the reserve capacity for responding to stress such as exercise drops. During exercise, there is a decrease in peak heart rate, stroke volume and ejection fraction with increase in pulmonary capillary wedge pressure (Murphy and DeMots 1984). Understanding these changes in the elderly can help you in the assessment of the cardiovascular system. The following is a list of some of the physiologic changes that occur in the elderly:

1. Rigidity of arteries contributes to coronary artery disease (CAD) and to hypertension.
2. Calcification of the valves, found in one third of patients over 75 years of age, contributes to murmurs such as aortic stenosis, which is frequently found in the elderly (see Chapter 13).
3. Blunting of the baroreceptor reflex may lead to postural hypotension as well as syncope.
4. Loss of sinus node cells leads to slowing of the heart rate and irregularity of the heart rhythm, resulting in bradydysrhythmias and sick sinus syndrome.

An S_4 on auscultation, an abnormal sign consistent with decreased compliance of the left ventricle, is observed in patients with myocardial infarction and resulting necrosis and "stiffness of the left ventricle" (Canobbio 1990). However, in the elderly (older than 65 years) an S_4 is considered a *normal* variant consistent with the decrease in ventricular compliance observed as a normal aging process.

Valvular changes also occur with age. In the elderly, the murmur of aortic stenosis is common. Although some investigators report the incidence of systolic murmurs in the elderly to be as high as 80%, the true rate of prevalence is probably closer to 30% (Duthie et al. 1981). Most systolic murmurs originate from the aortic area and are attributed to a dilation of the ascending aortic cusp, usually without a hemodynamically significant stenosis. The murmurs may be best heard at the base. The murmur is usually grade 1 or 2 out of 6 in intensity, peaks early, and is of short duration. It usually radiates poorly toward the carotid artery. The most important differential diagnostic consideration is hemodynamically significant valvular aortic stenosis.

In evaluating the meaning of abnormal heart sounds in the elderly, consider other clinical findings as well as the ECG, chest x-ray, and echocardiogram (Murphy and DeMots 1984).

---

just after S_1. Systolic ejection clicks result from movement of stenotic semilunar valves or expansion of the great blood vessels. Thus, they may be heard with aortic or pulmonic stenosis and with systemic or pulmonary hypertension. Mid-systolic clicks usually are associated with mitral valve prolapse.

Murmurs A *murmur* is a long series of audible vibrations generated by turbulent blood flow. A murmur usually results from an obstruction to blood flow, flow into a dilated vessel, a high rate of flow across a normal valve, forward or backward flow across an abnormal valve, or flow through an abnormal arteriovenous communication.

A murmur is identified on the basis of its timing, location, radiation, loudness, pitch, intensity (shape), quality, and response to respiration, position changes, and pharmacologic agents. *Timing* in the cardiac cycle may be systolic, diastolic, or continuous. A systolic murmur may be described further as holosystolic (lasting throughout systole) or systolic ejection (midsystolic) murmur. The chest site where the murmur is loudest is its *location,* while *radiation* describes its transmission to other chest sites, the neck, or extremities. *Loudness* is graded on a scale from 1 to 6. A grade 1 murmur can barely be heard; a 2 is faint, but detectable; 3, moderately loud; 4, loud; 5, louder; and 6 is so loud it can be heard with the stethoscope just above but not in contact with the chest wall. *Pitch* is produced by the number of vibrations per second; high-frequency sounds are high-pitched, low-frequency ones are low-pitched. The *shape* of a murmur is described as crescendo (increasing), decrescendo (decreasing), crescendo-decrescendo (diamond-shaped), or plateau (constant). The *quality* depends on the mixture of pitches creating the sound and usually is described as harsh, blowing, rumbling, or musical. The characteristics of murmurs vary considerably; only the most common are included here (Table 10–5).

The timing of murmurs is easier to understand if you recall the events of the cardiac cycle. For instance, S_1 occurs at the time of mitral and tricuspid valve closure and marks the onset of systole. At this time, the aortic and pulmonic valves still are closed. S_2 is heard at the time of aortic and pulmonic valve closure, marking the end of systole. A *holosystolic murmur* occurs when blood flows from a chamber with a continuously higher pressure during systole into one with a lower pressure; thus it logically may result from mitral or tricuspid insufficiency or a ventricular septal defect. It usually is

high-pitched and blowing, harsh, or musical. The murmur of mitral insufficiency is best heard at the apex, tricuspid insufficiency at the lower left sternal border, and ventricular septal defect at the left sternal border.

Systolic ejection murmurs occur after S_1, the phase of isovolumetric contraction, and the opening of the aortic and pulmonic valves. These murmurs, typical of aortic and pulmonic stenosis, have a crescendo-decrescendo shape due to the blood ejection increase and decrease. They end before their respective component of S_2 (A_2 or P_2) marks the closure of the valve. They usually are harsh and medium-to-high-pitched. The murmur of aortic stenosis is heard best at the upper right sternal border; it often radiates to the apex and carotid arteries. The murmur of pulmonic stenosis is loudest at the upper left sternal border. Systolic ejection murmurs also occur with flow into a dilated vessel (as in systemic or pulmonary hypertension) or increased flow across the valve (as in aortic or pulmonic insufficiency).

In diastole, the semilunar valves should be closed and the AV valves open. *Early diastolic murmurs*

TABLE 10–5

Simplified Characteristics of Murmurs

TIMING		LOCATION	PITCH	QUALITY	TYPE
Holosystolic					
		Apex	High	Blowing	Mitral insufficiency
		LLSB	High	Blowing	Tricuspid insufficiency
		Left sternal border	High	Blowing	Ventricular septal defect
Systolic ejection					
		URSB	Medium	Harsh	Aortic stenosis
		ULSB	Medium	Harsh	Pulmonic stenosis
Early diastolic					
		URSB and Erb's point	High	Blowing	Aortic insufficiency
		ULSB	High	Blowing	Pulmonic insufficiency
Mid- to late diastolic					
		Apex	Low	Rumbling	Mitral stenosis
		LLSB	Low	Rumbling	Tricuspid stenosis

Key: LLSB = lower left sternal border; URSB = upper right sternal border; ULSB = upper left sternal border.

logically may result from aortic or pulmonic insufficiency (manifesting itself soon after closure of the valve, which is marked by S_2). They are soft, blowing, high-pitched, decrescendo murmurs. The murmur of pulmonic insufficiency is heard best at the upper left sternal border, that of aortic insufficiency at the upper right sternal border or Erb's point.

Mid- to late diastolic murmurs occur during the phase of rapid ventricular filling as blood rushes across the AV valves. They are heard in mitral and tricuspid stenosis. They cause low-pitched rumbles. A murmur of tricuspid stenosis is appreciated best at the lower left sternal border, that of mitral stenosis at the apex.

Be particularly alert for the sudden appearance of the following murmurs. A new holosystolic murmur along the left sternal border may indicate rupture of the ventricular septum following myocardial infarction, while a new holosystolic murmur at the apex may result from rupture of the papillary muscles, which anchor the mitral valve. These murmurs are accompanied by sudden, severe biventricular heart failure. In a patient with a suspected aneurysm or descending aortic dissection, the onset of a murmur of aortic insufficiency may herald additional proximal dissection.

REFERENCES

Bates B: *A guide to physical assessment and history taking,* 4th ed. Philadelphia: Lippincott, 1987.

Brykczynski K: Going ape over heart sounds. *Nurs 81* (September) 1981; 25 (Innovations in nursing: personal communication).

Canobbio M: "Assessment." *In Cardiovascular Disorders.* St Louis: Mosby, 1990.

Crabtree A, Jorgenson M: Exploring the practical knowledge in expert critical-care nursing practice. Unpublished master's thesis, University of Wisconsin, Madison, 1986.

Daily E, Schroeder J: *Techniques in bedside hemodynamic monitoring,* 4th ed. St Louis: Mosby, 1989.

Day S, Cook F, Funkenstein H, Goldman L: Evaluation and outcome of emergency room patients with transient loss of consciousness. *Amer J Med* 1982; 73:15–23.

Duthie E, Gambert S, Tresch D: Evaluation of the systolic murmur in the elderly. *J Am Geriatr Soc* 1981; 29:498–502.

Guyton A: *Textbook of medical physiology,* 8th ed. Philadelphia: Saunders, 1991.

Marriott H: *Differential diagnosis of heart disease.* Oldsmar, FL: Tampa Tracings, 1967.

Murphy E, DeMots H: "Cardiology." In *Geriatric Medicine* ed. by Cassel C, and Walsh J. New York: Springer-Verlag, 1984.

Nimoityn P, Chung E: History taking and physical diagnosis of the cardiovascular system. In *Quick references for cardiovascular diseases,* 3d ed, Chung E (ed). Philadelphia: Lippincott, 1987, pp. 1–22.

Vines S, Simmons J: Evaluating a staff development physical assessment program. *J Nurs Staff Devel* 1991; 7: 74–77.

11

Cardiovascular Diagnostic Procedures

CLINICAL INSIGHT

Domain: The diagnostic and monitoring function

Competency: Detection and documentation of significant changes in a patient's condition

The critical-care nurse functions with a constant, almost subconscious awareness of impending doom barely being held at bay by aggressively applied technologies. The expert nurse can provide care in the here and now despite this awareness; an important component of socialization into the role of critical-care nurse involves learning not to be paralyzed by this feeling or blinded to what is occurring moment to moment.

The nurse functions as the patient's first line of defense in the critical-care unit; when a harmful situation develops, it is the expert who first recognizes "something is wrong here." The ability to interpret a particular finding depends on a carefully crafted alloy of both nursing and medical knowledge, as well as

recognition that the significance of a particular change is highly dependent on its context. It is only after considering multiple possibilities in the context of the moment that the nurse's knowledge, analytic thinking, and intuition coalesce into pattern recognition. The importance of honing perceptual abilities and staying attuned to the nuances in a given situation is reinforced, sometimes painfully, in the crucible of clinical practice, as can be seen in the following words of a nurse with 9 years' critical-care experience (Benner and Tanner, 1987, p. 28).

They tried to do a cardiac catheterization and were not successful. It was a clinical situation where I didn't look for certain things I should have looked for. I was more tuned to the fact that he was in pulmonary edema. I was treating that, giving a lot of drugs and a lot of different IV drips.

264

I completely forgot to look at the things you routinely look at after cardiac catheterizations, like pedal pulses. They had injured his artery when they attempted the cardiac catheterization, and he had clotted off the arteries in his feet. All through the night he had said to me that his feet were hurting and cold. My response was to get a warm blanket for his feet.

I was just so lost in the fact that he was in acute pulmonary edema. It was very apparent in the morning that there was something horribly wrong with his feet.

I can't believe that I overlooked this. When someone has a cardiac catheterization, you always check pulses. You always document them every 15 minutes, then every half hour and so on. But he hadn't had the bona fide catheterization done, and I wasn't thinking in terms of that.

This chapter presents the cardiac diagnostic techniques you are most likely to encounter in the bedside care of patients. At the end of this chapter, you will have the theoretical knowledge necessary for (1) interpretation of selected laboratory data, (2) nursing care related to selected diagnostic procedures, and (3) management of hemodynamic monitoring lines.

Laboratory Tests

Laboratory measures of serum enzymes are helpful adjuncts to the patient's history and physical examination.

Evaluation of Serum Enzymes

Organs contain enzymes, substances that accelerate metabolic reactions. When cells are damaged, they release enzymes into the interstitial fluid and thence into the serum. Serial determinations of serum levels of selected enzymes thus can be a valuable adjunct to the history and physical exam. Analysis of characteristic patterns of elevation can be very helpful in evaluating the presence and degree of organ damage. Both the trends of values and the amounts of increases are significant. As with other laboratory tests, the normal values vary among institutions and authorities. The values and time intervals included in Table 11–1 are guidelines you should evaluate for applicability in your clinical setting.

TABLE 11–1

Characteristic Serum Enzyme Changes In Acute Myocardial Infarction

	ELEVATION		
ENZYME	**Onset**	**Peak Time**	**Duration**
CPK	4–6 hrs	12–24 hrs	3–4 days
CPK$_2$(CPK-MB)	4–6 hrs	12–24 hrs	2–3 days
LDH	8–12 hrs	24–48 hrs	10–14 days
LDH$_1$ > LDH$_2$	12–24 hrs	48 hrs	Variable; for most patients, less than 7 days

Key: CPK = creatine phosphokinase; CPK-MB = creatine phosphokinase, muscle-brain subunits; LDH = lactic dehydrogenase

In the setting of cardiac disease, the enzyme tests most frequently ordered include measurement of isoenzymes. *Isoenzymes* are alternate molecular structures of an enzyme. Isoenzyme specificity is significantly greater than total enzyme specificity.

Creatine phosphokinase (CPK) is found in the brain, the myocardium, and skeletal muscle. A normal CPK level is less than 99 units per liter (U/L) for males and less than 57 U/L for females. In myocardial infarction (MI), CPK begins to increase after 4–6 hours and peaks at 5–10 times normal by 24 hours. The elevation lasts 3–4 days. In addition to an elevated total CPK value, myocardial infarction causes significant changes in the levels of CPK isoenzymes.

Three CPK isoenzymes have been identified: the brain (CPK-BB or CPK$_1$), cardiac (CPK-MB or CPK$_2$), and skeletal muscle (CPK-MM or CPK$_3$) fractions. A normal CPK serum isoenzyme profile shows 100% of CPK from skeletal muscle and none from the heart or brain; that is, CPK$_3$ = 100%. CPK measurement is highly sensitive but relatively nonspecific. CPK elevations occur in cardiac disorders (cardioversion, angina, infarction), skeletal muscle injury (vigorous exercise, intramuscular injections, trauma, major surgery), and neurologic disorders (stroke, convulsions, head injuries). Being able to distinguish the source of CPK elevations as skeletal, cardiac, or cerebral obviously is of great diagnostic value. In the heart, most CPK is of the cardiac variety and the remainder is skeletal. In acute myocardial infarction, both the skeletal muscle and cardiac levels increase.

Numerous studies have shown CPK-MB to be the most specific and sensitive enzyme indicator of myocardial damage. Utilization of CPK isoenzymes has provided a means for quickly determining myocardial damage. It has been extremely beneficial and cost effective because it permits prompt implementation of appropriate therapy.

In assessing myocardial infarction with plasma CPK isoenzymes, it is important to sample blood on admission and every 8 hours × 3. Cardiac fraction elevations occur in all myocardial infarction patients within the first 48 hours. The serum cardiac fraction begins to rise 4–6 hours after the onset of chest pain, peaks at 12–24 hours, and lasts up to 2–3 days. As a result, CPK isoenzyme levels are most useful in the early diagnosis of myocardial infarction. If the patient is admitted to the critical-care unit more than 36 hours after onset of symptoms, analysis of CPK isoenzymes may not provide the necessary data; one should rely instead on other isoenzyme analysis.

Lactic dehydrogenase (LDH) is present in almost all tissues. The normal serum level is less than 115 IU/L. LDH has five isoenzymes, labeled according to the speed with which they migrate toward the anode in an electrophoretic field. Each isoenzyme is found in a variety of tissues. The normal LDH isoenzyme values are: LDH_1, 18–29%; LDH_2, 29–37%; LDH_3, 18–26%; LDH_4, 9–16%; and LDH_5, 5–13% (Kelber 1986). The relationship between fractions is very important in evaluating LDH isoenzyme results. Normally, LDH_2 is the largest percentage, followed, in decreasing order, by LDH_1, LDH_3, LDH_4, and LDH_5. The heart contains primarily LDH_1, with a slightly lesser amount of LDH_2 and decreasing amounts of LDH_3, LDH_4, and LDH_5. Liver and skeletal muscle tissue have the opposite pattern, that is, no LDH_1 and increasing amounts of the isoenzymes up to LDH_5. Because LDH is so widely distributed in the body, LDH elevations occur in numerous conditions, including pulmonary embolism, liver disease, renal infarction, and neoplastic conditions. For this reason, an LDH elevation by itself would not necessarily indicate myocardial injury, but LDH isoenzymes would help to pinpoint the source. An elevated LDH_5, for instance, points to skeletal muscle or hepatic damage rather than cardiac damage.

Following an infarction, the LDH level begins to rise within 8–12 hours, peaks at 24–48 hours, and persists for up to 14 days. In addition to LDH elevation, the LDH isoenzyme profile often changes. As mentioned above, the serum normally contains slightly more LDH_2 than LDH_1. An LDH_1 greater than LDH_2 is called a *flipped LDH* pattern. Eighty percent of acute MI patients show

this pattern within 48 hours post infarct. (Although other conditions—such as renal infarction—can cause the flipped LDH profile, they are rarer and readily differentiated from acute MI.) Therefore, when patients present longer than 24 hours after the onset of MI symptoms, LDH isoenzyme analysis is more revealing than CPK-MB analysis.

To summarize, the presence of myocardial infarction should be assessed with isoenzymes measured on admission and every 8 hours × 3. CPK and LDH isoenzymes are highly sensitive. In conjunction with the clinical history and electrocardiogram, isoenzyme analysis provides a powerful tool for detecting myocardial infarction. A normal CPK cardiac fraction indicates that myocardial infarction has not occurred. An elevated CPK cardiac fraction and flipped LDH indicate that a myocardial infarction definitely has occurred. An elevated CPK cardiac fraction without a flipped LDH may or may not indicate an MI.

In addition to acute myocardial infarction, isoenzyme analysis can provide clues that confirm the presence of other disorders common in acute MI patients. LDH_5 can be monitored to evaluate hepatic damage following infarction or congestive heart failure. LDH_2 and LDH_3 elevate with lung injury. The patient with acute chest pain, an elevated LDH_2 and LDH_3, normal LDH_1:LDH_2 ratio, and normal CPK-MB probably has suffered a pulmonary rather than myocardial infarction.

Because red blood cells contain LDH, hemolysis can significantly distort this test's value in diagnosing MI. When collecting blood samples for enzyme determination, perform the venipuncture as nontraumatically as possible, avoid shaking the container, and promptly send the specimen to the laboratory. Also, remember to draw the samples on time and note on the laboratory slip the date and time of drawing; when possible, also note the date and time of the suspected MI. These actions will help to ensure that results are arranged chronologically and peak elevations are detected.

Diagnostic Procedures

The critical-care nurse should read the reports and understand the significance of the wide variety of procedures available to the physician in diagnosing cardiac disorders. The diagnostic maneuvers reviewed here are chest roentgenology, echocardiography, Doppler ultrasonography, radionuclide studies, electrophysiologic studies, cardiac catheterization and coronary angiography, and arteriography.

Chest Roentgenology

This diagnostic technique utilizes an x-ray beam directed through the patient's chest to expose film placed against the opposite chest wall.

The differing densities of chest structures allow differing amounts of radiation to pass through the thorax and strike the exposed film. As a result, it is possible to differentiate on the developed film the shadows cast by the various structures. Air, which is the most radiolucent, appears black. Fat appears dark gray. Water appears light gray. Bone, which is the most radiopaque, appears white.

Because of the anatomic positions of the chambers, individual chambers are seen best on different projections. These projections are obtained by placing the chest in various positions in relation to the x-ray beam and film. In the preferred method, the patient stands and holds a deep breath while the film is taken with a beam 6 feet away.

In the *posteroanterior* (PA) view, the film is placed against the anterior chest so the beam travels from the back to the front of the thorax. The *lateral* view positions the film against the right or left lateral chest wall. The *right* or *left anterior oblique* (RAO or LAO) view positions the plate against the right or left chest so the beam traverses the thorax obliquely from the opposite portion of the posterolateral chest wall.

Since critically ill patients cannot tolerate being transported to the x-ray department or being positioned upright, the films most commonly seen in the critical-care unit are portable chest films. The patient is supine or sitting up. The x-ray beam traverses the chest from about 2 feet away, in an *anteroposterior* (AP) projection. Although the AP view is more distorted than the PA view, it nonetheless provides useful information in patient care. For example, it can indicate whether an endotracheal tube is positioned properly and whether there is a collection of air or blood in the pleural space.

In analyzing the cardiac significance of chest films, the interpreter considers heart size, signs of chamber enlargement, calcifications of myocardial structures, and evidence of altered pulmonary blood flow.

Echocardiography

In this procedure, ultrasonic waves are beamed into the heart and their echoes recorded. It is a safe, noninvasive procedure for following the mechanical activity of intracardiac structures that can be repeated as often as needed. The procedure usually is performed by a physician or specially trained technician, either at the bedside or in a laboratory.

The patient is positioned supine or on the left side. A transducer is placed in various positions on the chest, avoiding the lungs and bones. Common locations are the left sternal border at the fourth intercostal space, the right sternal border, and the suprasternal notch. The transducer emits sound waves, which bounce back from the interfaces of dissimilar materials, such as blood and muscle. By aiming the transducer in different directions, the operator picks up echoes from different cardiac structures. Correct positioning of the transducer beam is difficult and time-consuming, so the procedure usually takes 30–60 minutes. Figure 11–1 shows a schematic representation of the cardiac structures traversed by two echo beams. Figure 11–2 shows a normal echocardiogram sector scan of the left ventricle.

When the beam encounters substances with different acoustic properties (such as cardiac muscle and blood), a portion of it is reflected. The returning sounds (echoes) are recorded as one-dimensional or two-dimensional views on a strip chart or on a video recorder. The acoustic characteristics of the substances determine the intensity of the echo. Blood is recorded as a black (echo-free) space, whereas tissue appears white. The length of time before the echo returns indicates the structure's distance from the transducer. By comparing the echocardiogram to a simultaneously recorded electrocardiogram, the physician can interpret the timing of various mechanical events.

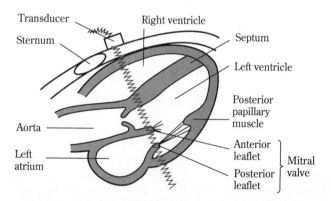

FIGURE 11–1

Echocardiography. With the transducer directed as shown, the echocardiogram will record echoes from the chest wall, right ventricular wall, ventricular septum, anterior and posterior leaflets of the mitral valve, and posterior left ventricular wall.

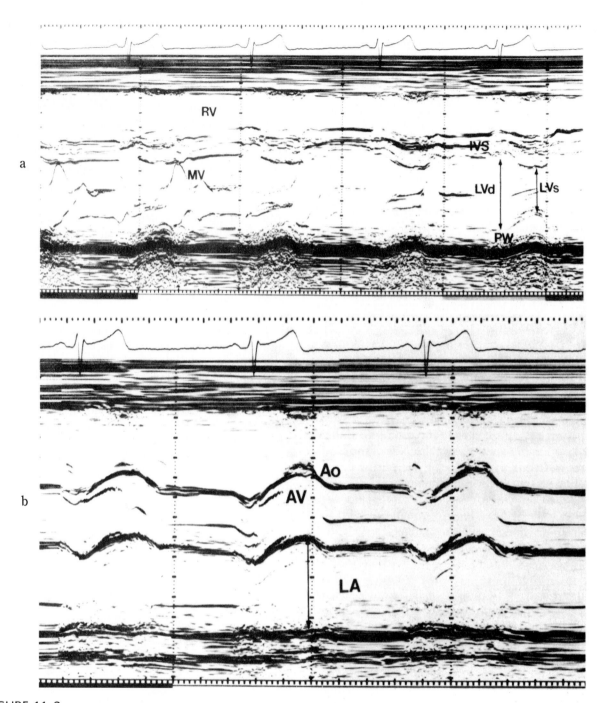

FIGURE 11–2

a. M-mode echocardiogram. The M-shaped wave in the center is made by movement of the mitral valve. **b.** Normal M-mode echocardiogram at the level of the aorta (Ao), aortic valve (AV) leaflets, and left atrium (LA). IVS, interventricular septum; LVd, left ventricular diastolic dimensions; LVs, left ventricular systolic dimensions; PW, posterior wall; RV, right ventricle; MV, mitral valve. (From Andreoli K et al.: Comprehensive cardiac care, 6th ed. St. Louis: Mosby, 1987.)

Echocardiography has matured over the years. Initially, only *motion-mode (M-mode)* echo techniques were available. Although these were extremely useful, several limitations became apparent, including the lack of spatial resolution and the inability to examine large areas of the ventricular myocardium. Thus, *two-dimensional (2-D)* echo has become the mainstay of ultrasound imaging. Today, the combination of M-mode and 2-D echo affords the best possible use of ultrasound. The strengths of 2-D echo are in terms of location and spatial orientation, while the strength of the M-mode is in allowing more precise measurement of wall thickness and valvular motion (Horowitz et al. 1980).

M-mode Echocardiography Among the conditions that can be diagnosed from an M-mode echocardiogram are disorders of mitral or aortic valve motion, left atrial tumors, pericardial effusion, septal defects, and aortic aneurysms. In addition, it is possible to calculate chamber size and blood volumes, including cardiac output. In the setting of acute myocardial infarction, the M-mode can provide certain types of additional information, allowing the cardiologist to estimate the extent of tissue damage due to the infarct; evaluate overall left ventricular function; assess for various complications of myocardial infarction, such as heart failure, papillary muscle dysfunction, myocardial rupture, thrombus formation, and pericarditis; and provide prognostic information of value in planning overall approach to the patient.

Two-Dimensional Echocardiography Left ventricular function can be accurately and reproducibly estimated at the bedside in patients by using the 2-D echo. It is a more precise technique than M-mode for identifying, quantifying, and evaluating global and regional left ventricular wall motion abnormalities in patients with acute myocardial infarction. Abnormal wall motion occurs in infarcted as well as noninfarcted zones. Patients with large infarctions and individuals with left ventricular failure demonstrate reduced left ventricular function, compared with individuals with smaller infarcts or patients without heart failure. Using this technique it is possible to delineate alterations in right ventricular chamber size and wall motion abnormalities in cases of right ventricular infarction. Of additional therapeutic importance is the ability to identify mural thrombi in all four chambers. Echocardiography can provide most of the information necessary for assessing congestive cardiomyopathy, including overall left ventricular function. It is also an extremely useful way to detect idiopathic hypertrophic cardiomyopathy and to assess the degree of outflow tract obstruction (Bommer 1985a). Finally, two-dimensional echo is useful in detection and management of the serious and often catastrophic complications of acute infarction, which include ventricular septal rupture and subsequent left-to-right shunting; mitral regurgitation due to papillary muscle dysfunction or rupture; and flail mitral leaflets with subsequent severe acute mitral regurgitation.

There are no complications of echocardiography. Postprocedure nursing care involves resuming interventions, including providing emotional support as the patient tries to cope with concern about an impending or confirmed diagnosis.

CRITICAL-CARE GERONTOLOGY

Dobutamine Echocardiograms

In elderly patients who are unable to adequately perform a stress exercise treadmill test, dobutamine echocardiograms are performed. Dobutamine, which acts on the beta$_1$ and beta$_2$ receptor sites, is infused into an intravenous line. The resulting beta$_1$ stimulation increases heart rate and contractility. An echocardiogram is done to evaluate cardiac function during such an episode of "stress." Wall motion and cardiac indices are obtained to evaluate cardiac function during the "stress" response.

You can help in identifying patients who cannot perform a standard stress test, due to arthritis or other functional impairments, and who thus may be candidates for dobutamine echocardiograms. If your patient is scheduled for this test, explain why and how the procedure will be done.

Doppler Ultrasonography

Traditionally, a Doppler ultrasonic probe has been used to evaluate arterial flow when a patient's pulse is impalpable. There is increasing interest in the use of Doppler techniques to measure blood-flow velocity in the great vessels and through the heart valves.

In *Doppler ultrasonography,* a hand-held transducer is placed over the patient's artery after a small amount of conductive jelly has been put on the tip of the transducer. The transducer emits sound waves that bounce off moving red blood cells. These sound waves can be heard through the stethoscope attached to the transducer. Normally, you can hear phasic sounds with systolic and diastolic components. If blood flow in the vessel is decreased, the sounds will be decreased also. If partial obstruction is present, you will hear a high-pitched sound at the obstruction and weaker sounds distal to it. If complete obstruction is present without collateral flow, the sounds may be completely absent.

Blood pressure readings can be taken using the Doppler probe in patients whose blood pressures are not audible using traditional auscultatory methods.

In addition to evaluation of arterial flow, the Doppler can be used to evaluate venous flow. Normal venous sounds are lower-pitched than arterial sounds, vary with respiration, and increase after the vessel is occluded proximally and the pressure then is released. If these normal signs are absent, venous thrombosis may have occurred.

According to Mauldin (1986), the Doppler is 95% accurate in detecting significant impairment of arteriovenous flow but may fail to detect small thrombi and plaques and usually fails to detect major thrombosis of the calf veins.

Doppler techniques have become part of the routine echo examination in many laboratories. Doppler *color-flow mapping* (CFM) is the newest and probably the most exciting addition to cardiac ultrasound. CFM is a type of *pulsed-wave* (PW) Doppler. In conventional pulse wave, a sample volume is positioned in a two-dimensional image to collect Doppler-shifted information from a small, discrete area. In contrast, the CFM instrument automatically gathers Doppler-shifted information from multiple sample volumes along the scan line. Color-flow mapping is a combination of Doppler-flow information and 2-D imaging. Mean velocities are calculated and blood flow is color coded for direction and velocity. The resulting colors are superimposed on the image of blood flow. These create a "noninvasive angiogram": a 2-D image of cardiac anatomy, with color representation of blood as it flows through the anatomy. It can simultaneously locate abnormal blood flow and identify the spatial extent and direction of the flow (DeMaria et al. 1985).

Radionuclide Studies

Radionuclide studies use radioisotopes to evaluate myocardial blood flow and to determine the location and extent of myocardial infarction. They are relatively safe, noninvasive procedures that can be repeated as often as necessary for serial evaluation. Several kinds of radionuclide studies are available: myocardial infarction imaging, myocardial perfusion imaging, cardiac blood pool imaging, computed tomography, magnetic resonance imaging, and positron-emitted tomography.

Myocardial Infarction Imaging In myocardial infarction imaging *(technetium pyrophosphate or "hot spot" scan),* the patient is given an intravenous injection of technetium-99 pyrophosphate and the chest is scanned with a special detector a few hours later. Pyrophosphate is taken up by bone and also selectively concentrated in recently infarcted tissue, probably because it is attracted to the calcium in destroyed mitochondria (Zeluff et al. 1980). The infarcted tissue appears as a "hot spot" on the scan due to the uptake of the radioisotope by dying cells. The infarct can be localized by comparing scans taken in various views and its size estimated by correlation with the area of uptake. Pyrophosphate scans can detect infarction as early as 12 hours after it occurs, although they are most sensitive 24–72 hours after, and are likely to be negative by 4–7 days postinfarction.

Myocardial Perfusion Imaging In contrast to myocardial infarction imaging studies, which can detect only acute infarctions, myocardial perfusion imaging *(thallium or "cold spot" scan)* can detect both acute and chronic infarctions. Thallium-201 chloride is a potassium analog that is actively transported into normal cells following injection (Pantaleo et al. 1981). In the normal scan, thallium is equally distributed throughout the myocardium because perfusion is equal. In ischemic, injured, or infarcted tissue, abnormal perfusion or abnormal uptake causes less thallium to be transported into cells, so the area appears as a "cold spot."

Thallium scans can be performed as resting or exercise scans. On a resting scan, a "cold spot" can result from a new infarct, an old infarct, or an area of ischemia. In an exercise scan, thallium is injected in the stress-testing laboratory while the patient exercises, and scans are taken immediately and 4 hours later. Comparison of the scans can help differentiate between an infarct, which shows up as a persistent "cold spot," and ischemia, in which the "cold spot" fills in on the later scans. Thallium scans thus are a powerful tool for evaluating regional myocardial perfusion.

Cardiac Blood Pool Imaging *Cardiac blood pool imaging* evaluates regional and global ventricular performance after IV injection of human serum albumin or red blood cells tagged with the isotope technetium-99m pertechnetate. A scintillation camera records the radioactivity emitted by the isotope. Blood pool imaging is more accurate and involves less risk to the patient than left ventriculography in assessing cardiac function. The purposes of this test are:

1. To evaluate left ventricular function.
2. To detect aneurysms of the left ventricle and other myocardial wall motion abnormalities (area of akinesis or dyskinesis).
3. To detect intracardiac shunting.
4. To determine prognosis in left ventricular dysfunction post MI.
5. To follow patients with valvular disease and determine left ventricular deterioration.

Several imaging methods exist. In *first-pass imaging,* the camera records the isotope's radioactivity in its initial pass through the left ventricle. The portion of the isotope ejected during each heartbeat can then be calculated to determine the ejection fraction. The presence and size of intracardiac shunts can also be determined.

Gated cardiac blood pool imaging, performed after first-pass imaging or as a separate test, utilizes a signal from an electrocardiogram (ECG) to trigger the scintillation camera. In two-frame gated imaging, the camera records left ventricular end-systole and end-diastole for a total of 4 minutes and superimposes these gated images. Comparison of end-systolic and end-diastolic images allows assessment of left ventricular contraction in order to find areas of dyskinesia or akinesia.

In *multiple-gated acquisition (MUGA) scanning,* the camera usually records 16 frames (or 14–64 points) of a single cardiac cycle, yielding sequential images that can be studied like motion picture film to evaluate regional wall motion and determine the ejection fraction and other indices of cardiac function. In the stress MUGA test, the same test is performed at rest and after exercise to detect changes in ejection fraction and cardiac function. Stress is placed on the myocardium by having the patient ride a stationary bicycle. A normal response is for ejection fraction to increase. If cardiac function is impaired, the ejection fraction decreases during exercise. In the nitro MUGA test, the scintillation camera records points in the cardiac cycle after sublingual administration of nitroglycerin, to assess its effect on ventricular function (Bentley 1987).

Advanced Diagnostic Imaging Techniques *Computed tomography (CT), magnetic resonance imaging (MRI)* (also called nuclear magnetic resonance [NMR] imaging, and *positron-emitted tomography (PET)* are three imaging techniques that have revolutionized medical diagnosis. Each "scanning" technique presents information in the form of a "tomograph," which is simply the Greek word for cross-sectional slice (Oldendorf and Oldendorf 1985). CT has been in clinical use for more than a decade. MRI scanners are also used in the clinical setting to assess a variety of cardiovascular disorders. PET scanners have been used in clinical research for several years and have been useful in evaluating myocardial metabolism.

CT, MRI, and PET exploit different physical properties of the atoms and molecules making up the tissues of the human body. It is important to understand that the picture produced by each of these techniques represents some particular characteristic of the tissue density, water concentration, or metabolic rate (Oldendorf and Oldendorf 1985). Consequently, each technique has its place in cardiac evaluation (Table 11–2). For example, PET has been used to evaluate the metabolism of ischemic areas of the heart, while MRI has been used to evaluate the presence and extent of congenital abnormalities. The three

TABLE 11–2

Advanced Diagnostic Imaging Techniques

TYPE	METHOD	CLINICAL USE
Computed tomography (CT)	Conventional x-rays (with contrast media)	—Patent coronary artery bypass grafts
		—Sizing of MI
		—Aortic aneurysms
		—Congenital heart disease
		—Pericardial disease
		—Cardiac measurements
Magnetic resonance imaging (MRI)	Magnetic field	—Valvular heart disease
		—Ischemic heart disease
		—Congenital heart disease
		—Pericardium/ myocardium
Positron emission tomography (PET)	Isotopes	—Cardiac metabolism
		—Ischemia/infarction

procedures differ also in the form of radiation employed to provide the information about the tissue. CT uses conventional x-rays, which are emitted and recorded in a new and unique fashion. PET scanners measure isotopes, which are injected intravenously. In MRI, a magnetic field is applied and the response of nuclei against the magnetic field studied (Pohost and Canby 1987).

Details of physical preparation for radionuclide tests vary among institutions. In general, no physical preparation is needed, except for the exercise scans, for which the patient must fast for a few hours before the procedure. Emotional preparation involves explanations that the procedures are relatively safe and essentially painless, as well as specific details about when, where, and how the procedures will be performed. MRI is discussed in detail in Chapter 4.

Electrophysiologic Studies

Much has been learned about cardiac dysrhythmias from clinical electrophysiologic studies (EPS) that use intracardiac recording and stimulation techniques. Recordings of local activity can be obtained from portions of the heart that are electrically silent on the body-surface electrocardiogram. It is possible to map the sequence and time of activation of the atria and ventricles and to separate atrioventricular conduction into the atrioventricular (AV) node and His-Purkinje system.

When recordings from selected sites are used in conjunction with pacing and programmed stimulation sequences, much can be learned about automaticity, conduction, refractoriness, and the origin of dysrhythmias. These techniques not only have enhanced our understanding of dysrhythmias and conduction defects but also have improved the ability to select and evaluate therapy for these disorders.

The clinical uses of electrophysiologic studies include:

1. Evaluating the mechanism, site, and extent of the ventricular or supraventricular dysrhythmia or conduction defect.

2. Evaluating syncope: determining covert defects in impulse formation or conduction.

3. Evaluating the efficacy of antidysrhythmic therapy.

Electrophysiologic studies are conducted in cardiac catheterization laboratories or a special procedure room. The equipment includes a fluoroscope, a magnetic tape recorder, a programmable stimulator, a multichannel recorder, and a defibrillator. Electrode catheters are introduced through the femoral and antecubital veins. The number and type of catheters depend on the conduction pathway being investigated. A recording is always taken from the bundle of His, along with other parts of the conduction system. In addition, intervals of activation time are recorded from each area. A catheter first is advanced to the right ventricle and then withdrawn to the area of the tricuspid valve, where the His bundle electrogram is recorded. A catheter with four electrodes then is introduced and placed against the lateral wall of the upper right atrium. The distal part of the electrode is used to stimulate the atrium. Additional electrode catheters are often placed in sites such as the coronary sinus and right ventricular apex.

Intracardiac electrograms are displayed on an oscilloscope along with tracings from several surface electrocardiographic leads and time markers. Recordings are made on a magnetic tape to ensure that transient events do not escape detection. Spontaneous rhythms are recorded. In addition, programmed stimulation is applied with a timed pacing impulse so that patterns of either atrial or ventricular dysrhythmias can be recorded. After the dysrhythmia has been induced and recorded, programmed pacing is used to terminate it. If this is unsuccessful, defibrillation or cardioversion is applied. In addition, various antidysrhythmic drugs may be given during an EPS to evaluate their efficacy in dysrhythmia control.

Nursing care prior to the procedure includes an explanation of the events of the procedure and assurance that the patient will be given medication to relax. It is important that the patient know he or she will be awake during the procedure. Encourage the patient to verbalize fears and concerns regarding the procedure. Since these patients most often have a life-threatening dysrhythmia, they need a lot of nursing support and reassurance. Postprocedure care involves assessments similar to those after cardiac catheterization. The extremity involved should be checked for bleeding, pulses, temperature, and color. In addition, the patient's cardiac rhythm should be noted.

Cardiac Catheterization and Coronary Angiography

Catheterization and coronary angiography are invasive diagnostic procedures designed to study anatomic and mechanical aspects of cardiac function. They are used to evaluate the patient with atypical chest pain or inadequate response to medical therapy, to identify anatomic lesions and associated conditions in order to plan drug or surgical therapy, and to evaluate postoperative hemodynamic status.

During catheterization of the left side of the heart, hemodynamic pressure measurements are taken in the aortic root, the left ventricle and left atrium. Radiopaque contrast medium (dye) is used to visualize the size of the heart chambers (angiogram) and the coronary arteries (arteriogram). Catheterization of the right side of the heart is performed using a thermodilution pulmonary artery catheter. Information obtained includes hemodynamic pressure measurements in the right atrium, right ventricle, pulmonary artery and pulmonary capillary; measurement of cardiac output, calculated hemodynamic values, and oxygen saturation; and an angiogram of the right heart chambers.

Patient Preparation Collaborate with the physician and catheterization laboratory staff in emotionally preparing the patient and the family. Before the procedure, the patient should have a clear idea of its benefits and risks, pre- and postprocedure care, and the steps of the procedure. In discussing the steps, focus on the sensations the patient may expect and on how the patient can interact effectively with the team.

Among the sensations the patient may experience are stinging as the local anesthetic is injected, the sense of pressure as the catheter is inserted or advanced, palpitations as the catheter is positioned in the heart, and intense warmth, a headache, and nausea as the dye is injected. These sensations are unpleasant but last only a minute or two. Let the patient know that in the room there will be many personnel in surgical dress. The patient should report if he or she experiences discomfort or does not understand what is being done.

Catheterization is a frightening experience to many patients. Assisting the patient to verbalize and cope with fears not only will contribute to equanimity during the procedure but also may reduce the likelihood of such complications as catecholamine-induced dysrhythmias and vasovagal reaction (hypotension and bradycardia resulting from massive discharge by the autonomic nervous system).

Physical preparation includes several steps. Blood is drawn for coagulation studies. If the patient is on anticoagulants, they may be discontinued several hours before the procedure. The patient usually is not permitted anything by mouth (except oral medications) for 8 hours prior to the procedure. Prophylactic antibiotics may be administered. Catheter insertion sites are scrubbed and shaved. The patient usually is premedicated with diazepam or another relaxation medication. Glasses or dentures may be worn to the laboratory.

In the laboratory, preparation consists of the application of ECG electrodes, insertion of an arterial line, skin preparation, and draping with sterile sheets. The patient will be positioned supine on a narrow cradle that can be tilted sideways to facilitate various x-ray projections, since the procedure is performed under image-intensification fluoroscopy with television monitoring and videotape playback.

Catheterization Procedures The catheterization proceeds according to a protocol determined individually for each patient. The approach to the vascular system may be percutaneous (favored for femoral vessels) or by cutdown (favored for the brachial artery or basilic vein). Among the factors that influence the choice of site are the presence of obesity or peripheral vascular disease.

Catheterization of the right heart is achieved from the basilic or femoral vein most commonly. The usual approach to the left side of the heart is a retrograde arterial approach across the aortic valve; other approaches are via a trans-septal puncture from the right atrium across the fossa ovalis, or via direct puncture through the chest wall.

Generally, the right heart is catheterized first. The catheter is left in place while the left heart is catheterized. Once that catheter is positioned, the peripheral arterial, left ventricular, and pulmonary capillary pressures are measured simultaneously.

Data Recorded During the catheterization the *pressures* are measured and the *pressure waveforms* are recorded for further study.

Oxygen contents and saturations are measured at several sites. These can be studied to determine the presence of shunts (abnormal blood flows within the heart). The usual oxygen saturation on the right side of the heart is 75%; on the left it is about 95%. Oxygen content varies from 14–15 volumes percent on the right side of the heart to 19 volumes percent on the left. An abnormal increase in oxygen content or saturation on the *right side* is called a *step-up* and is a clue to the presence of a shunt. For instance, an abnormally high oxygen content or saturation in the right atrium suggests that better-oxygenated blood is mixing with venous blood in the right atrium. Among the conditions that might cause this finding are a defect in the atrial septum and a pulmonary vein returning to the right atrium instead of the left.

Cardiac output (CO) also is calculated. CO is the amount of blood ejected by the heart each minute. It is a product of the heart rate and stroke volume, which is the amount of blood pumped out with each ventricular contraction. During catheterization, the CO may be measured both at rest and after exercise with a hand-grip or bicycle wheel mounted at the end of the table.

CO can be calculated in several ways. The most common in the catheterization laboratory is the *Fick method*. It is based on the theory that the amount of oxygen the body consumes equals that used by the tissues times the blood flow to the lungs. Oxygen consumption is measured by occluding the nose, having the patient breathe in a known concentration of oxygen, and analyzing the concentration in the air expired. The amount of oxygen used by the tissues is measured by taking simultaneous arterial and mixed venous blood samples, and subtracting the venous oxygen content from the arterial to obtain the arterio-venous (AV) oxygen content difference. The values then can be entered into the Fick equation:

$$\frac{\text{Oxygen consumption (ml/min)} \times 100}{\text{AV oxygen content difference (ml/100 ml blood)}}$$
$$= \text{Cardiac output (CO) (ml/min)}$$

CO also may be calculated by the indicator-dilution technique. In the catheterization laboratory, the indicator commonly used is a dye. A known amount of dye is injected centrally, and its concentration is measured continuously at a peripheral arterial site. A dye-dilution curve is recorded, and the cardiac output can be calculated by computing the area under the curve.

The value obtained for CO is more meaningful when related to the patient's size—specifically, the patient's body surface area. The resulting value is the *cardiac index*; its normal range is 2.5–4.0 L per minute per square meter of body surface (2.5–4.0 L/min/m^2). Similarly, the volume pumped out with each stroke is more meaningful when related to the patient's size. The normal stroke index is 30–65 ml/beat/m^2.

The volume of blood in each chamber also can be measured. From the left ventricular volumes at end-systole and end-diastole, it is possible to calculate the *ejection fraction*. This value indicates the percentage of ventricular diastolic volume that the ventricle is able to eject with each beat. A normal ejection fraction is 50–70%.

Myocardial metabolites such as lactate can be measured to evaluate oxygen supply to the myocardium. Valve orifice areas and gradients (pressure differentials) across the valves also can be determined.

Vascular resistance also can be calculated. Normal total systemic vascular resistance is 800–1,200 dynes-sec-cm^{-5}; usual total pulmonary vascular resistance is 100–300 dynes-sec-cm^{-5}.

Contrast media may be injected to opacify various cardiac structures. The general term for this procedure is *angiography. Ventriculography* is the injection of dye into the left ventricle to assess its contractility. *Aortography* is the use of contrast media to examine the function of the aorta and aortic valve. *Coronary arteriography* is the injection of dye into the coronary arteries to assess their patency. These studies are filmed for further analysis.

At the completion of the catheterization (which may last 2–4 hours), the catheters are removed. The vessels may be stripped proximally and distally to remove clots. If a cutdown was performed, the vessel is sutured. If a percutaneous approach was used, pressure is applied at the site. The site then is covered with an antibiotic ointment and an occlusive dressing applied. As it is difficult to apply an occlusive dressing at the groin, a sandbag may be placed over the dressing at the femoral site.

Complications Among the complications that may occur during catheterization are cardiac arrest, acute myocardial infarction, dysrhythmias, vasovagal reaction, anaphylactic shock, dye injection into the myocardium or pericardium, emboli to the lungs or brain, and sudden fluid shift due to the hypertonicity of contrast media.

After catheterization, potential complications include thromboemboli, hemorrhage or hematoma, renal failure, and hypotension because excretion of the hypertonic dye causes an osmotic diuresis. The patient usually is on bedrest until the next day and on intravenous fluids until oral intake equals fluid output.

When the patient first returns from catheterization, the nurse checks blood pressure, pulse rate, and urinary output. The nurse also performs an *arteriocheck* by assessing hemostasis at the insertion site and pulse and perfusion distal to the site. Arteriochecks should be performed every 15 minutes until the patient is stabilized and then gradually decreased over the first 24 hours. Transient diminution of the arterial pulse is common, but any pulse decrease should be reported promptly to the physician, because it may signal impending arterial occlusion. If you are unable to monitor the patient constantly at the bedside, be sure to teach the patient and family to alert you to any coolness, numbness, or paresthesias distal to the insertion sites. Instruct the patient to keep the extremity straight and to rotate the ankle and flex and extend the foot while on bedrest.

A sound understanding of the above information will reinforce your comprehension of cardiac anatomy and physiology. In addition, your knowledge of the normal values will help you use catheterization reports on your patients to predict nursing problems. For instance, you might note that your patient had extremely high left atrial and pulmonary arterial pressures. This knowledge would alert you that your patient was at high risk for developing pulmonary edema; you then would know to monitor the patient closely for the onset of signs and symptoms and to take such preventive measures as close attention to fluid balance.

Arteriography

Arteriography is an invasive diagnostic procedure in which arterial systems are radiographically evaluated following injection of a contrast medium. Arteriography is performed to evaluate areas of hemorrhage, obstruction, aneurysm, or vascular abnormalities.

Preprocedure care is similar to that for cardiac catheterization. During the procedure itself, a catheter is placed in the femoral, brachial, or carotid artery and passed under fluoroscopic control to the desired vessel. The dye then is injected, the vessel visualized, and x-ray films taken for diagnostic evaluation. Postprocedure care is analogous to that for cardiac catheterization.

Hemodynamic Monitoring

The Cardiac Cycle and Pressure Waves

As blood flows from chamber to chamber, as valves open and close, and as the myocardium contracts and relaxes, pressures are generated in various parts of the heart. (Refer to Chapter 10 for a review of the cardiac cycle.) These cardiovascular pressures can be measured and monitored through catheters whose tips are placed in the atria, pulmonary artery, or systemic arteries.

Uses of Hemodynamic Lines

Hemodynamic lines have several uses. They enable sampling of venous and arterial blood without repeated vascular punctures. They provide a way to monitor various waveforms, which can provide clues to patient status. The thermodilution pulmonary arterial catheter can be used to measure cardiac output. Most important, these lines enable monitoring of various cardiac pressures. Interpretation of these pressures can guide the nurse and the physician in planning and evaluating therapy in shock, fluid overload or deficit, cardiac failure, and other conditions.

Theoretical Concepts of Hemodynamic Monitoring

Cardiac output is an important measure of the functional ability of the heart. The heart is a pump. If the blood supply to the heart is sufficient, a healthy heart generally will produce enough output to meet the body's metabolic needs. When the pump is damaged, cardiac output may drop and a form of failure ensue. Determining cardiac output is a way of measuring how well the heart is performing. As reviewed in Chapter 10, cardiac output (CO) is defined as the amount of blood ejected by the ventricles during a one-minute period. The equation for determining CO is as follows:

$$CO = \text{heart rate (HR)} \times \text{stroke volume (SV)}$$

Using normal values at rest:

$$\text{HR (60–100 beats/min)} \times \text{SV (60–130 ml)}$$
$$= \text{CO (4–6 L/min)}$$

Many factors can alter CO, such as increased or decreased heart rate or changes in stroke volume. Stroke volume (SV), the amount of blood ejected by the ventricle each time it contracts, is:

$$SV = \text{CO in ml/min/HR in beats/min.}$$

Stroke volume is determined by preload, afterload, and contractility.

Preload is the volume of blood in the ventricles at the end of diastole. It is determined by the amount and distribution of intravascular volume, venous return, and atrial contraction. Preload determines the initial stretch on the ventricles. Preload of the right ventricle is measured by the central venous pressure (CVP)—normal (N) = 2–6 mm Hg—and preload of the left ventricle by the pulmonary capillary wedge pressure (PCWP)—N = 4–12 mm Hg.

Afterload is the pressure the ventricles must pump against to eject blood. The degree of afterload depends on the condition of the semilunar valves, the patency of the outflow tracts, the mass of volume in the left ventricle and the resistance in the pulmonary and systemic circulation. Constricted blood vessels increase afterload, and dilated blood vessel decrease afterload. Left ventricular afterload is determined by systemic vascular resistance (SVR):

$$SVR = \frac{MAP - RA}{CO} \times 80$$

where MAP = mean arterial pressure and RA = right atrial pressure in mm Hg. Normal SVR is 800–1,200 dynes-sec-cm^{-5}.

Contractility, or the inotropic state of the heart, is the shortening ability of cardiac muscle fibers that determines the pumping ability of the heart. This basic principle of contractility is an inherent property of cardiac muscle and independent of the Frank-Starling law of the heart.

The Frank-Starling law, which affects contractility but is not synonymous with it, states: The more the cardiac muscle fibers are stretched during diastole, the stronger the next contraction will be. This relationship is true within limits. Fibers can be stretched only so far before they lose resiliency and the ability to return to their prestretched length. Therefore, increased preload in a healthy heart will increase cardiac output, while increased preload in a heart that has lost its elasticity may result in elevated CVP and pulmonary artery pressure (PAP) and decreased cardiac output.

The sympathetic nervous system exerts a positive inotropic effect on the heart, whereas the parasympathetic nervous system has a negative inotropic effect. Therefore, drugs that increase contractility, used to treat ventricular failure, have a positive inotropic effect. Drugs that decrease contractility have a negative inotropic effect by blocking the action of the sympathetic system or the action of calcium.

Heart rate is an additional determinant of CO. The autonomic nervous system largely controls the heart rate in response to metabolic demands. Stimulation of the parasympathetic nervous system decreases heart rate, whereas sympathetic stimulation increases heart rate.

Pressure Measurements

The most important cardiac pressure is that of the left ventricle, because it is a major determinant of systemic perfusion. The pressure in the left ventricle at the end of diastole is called the *left ventricular end-diastolic pressure* (LVEDP). This pressure reflects the compliance of the left ventricle, that is, its ability to receive blood from the left atrium during diastole. When left ventricular compliance decreases, the LVEDP rises. Myocardial infarction and left ventricular failure are two examples of conditions in which left ventricular compliance decreases and LVEDP rises. Direct monitoring of LVEDP would be very helpful in detecting changes in the patient's condition and in guiding optimal fluid therapy in shock. Unfortunately, left ventricular pressure cannot be monitored directly at the bedside owing to the high potential for thromboembolization directly to the brain or other vital organs.

Correlation of Pressures There is a close correlation between LVEDP and other cardiac pressures. In the presence of a normal mitral valve, LVEDP is reflected by *left atrial pressure* (LAP). In the person with a normal mitral valve and normal lungs, the LVEDP also is reflected by the pressure in the pulmonary capillary bed (*pulmonary capillary wedge pressure,* PCWP) and the pressure in the pulmonary artery at the end of diastole, the *pulmonary artery end-diastolic pressure* (PAEDP).

This correlation is best understood if one visualizes the left ventricle, left atrium, pulmonary capillary bed, and pulmonary artery as one chamber at certain points in the cardiac cycle (see Figure 11–3). When the left ventricle is filling, the mitral valve is open and the left ventricle and left atrium form a common chamber. Therefore, LVEDP and mean LAP should be similar. Moving backwards in the blood circuit, one realizes that since there are no valves between the left atrium and the pulmonary capillary bed, their pressures should be similar, too. Continuing backwards in the vascular circuit, one realizes that when the pulmonic valve is closed, pressures in the pulmonary capillary bed should approximate PAEDP; and in fact, they do, with PAEDP normally less than 5 mm Hg higher than wedge pressures (Albarran-Sotelo et al. 1987). This "unichamber concept" is clinically useful, because it justifies the constant monitoring of PAEDP rather than frequent wedging of the balloon to obtain intermittent PCWPs, which increases the risk of balloon rupture and pulmonary artery trauma. One should note, however, that this unichamber concept holds true only for patients with normal mitral valve function and no pulmonary disease.

Left atrial pressure can be monitored at the bedside, but a LAP line can be dangerous because it provides a direct path for air or clots to enter the left ventricle and become systemic emboli. The pulmonary capillary and pulmonary arterial pressures can be monitored at the bedside with a balloon-tipped catheter placed in the pulmonary artery. With the balloon deflated, one can measure pulmonary artery systolic, diastolic, and mean pressures with the catheter. When the balloon is inflated, it wedges the catheter in a small distal branch of the pulmonary artery. The pressure recorded is that reflected back from the left atrium through the pulmonary capillary bed. This pressure is the PCWP.

Central venous pressure (CVP) is monitored at the bedside through a catheter whose tip is located at the juncture of the superior vena cava and right atrium, or through one lumen of the balloon-tipped pulmonary artery catheter that opens in the same location. The CVP reflects the pressure in the right atrium and systemic veins. It is affected primarily by changes in right-sided heart pressures and only secondarily by changes in left-sided pressures, so the CVP may be the last cardiac pressure to reflect increased LVEDP.

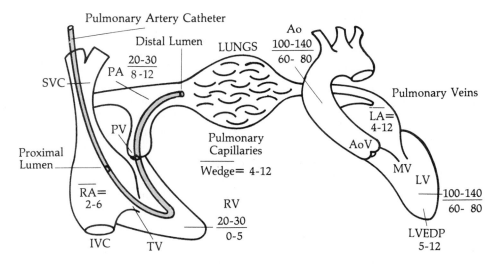

FIGURE 11–3

Unichamber concept with normal cardiac pressures. Adapted with permission from unpublished figure, NSI Educational Systems, Inc., Beverly Hills, CA.

Moreover, because the CVP can be affected by pulmonary disease, pulmonic or tricuspid stenosis, and other right atrial or ventricular abnormalities, an elevated CVP is not necessarily an accurate indication of an elevated LVEDP. The CVP line is safer than the LAP and PA lines. It is used to measure venous pressure, estimate blood volume, obtain venous blood samples, and administer fluids and some medications. It may also be used to monitor the patient in heart failure when PA monitoring is unavailable.

Systemic arterial pressure can be monitored directly through a catheter (arterial line) placed into a major systemic artery.

Values for normal resting cardiac pressures are listed below. The following, slightly modified from Daily and Schroeder (1989), may be considered normal values in millimeters of mercury (mm Hg):

- Superior vena caval or right atrial (RA) pressure: 2–6 mean
- Right ventricular (RV) pressure: 20–30 systolic and 0–5 diastolic
- Pulmonary artery (PA) pressure: 20–30 systolic, 8–12 diastolic, 10–20 mean
- Pulmonary capillary wedge pressure: 4–12 mean
- Left atrial (LA) pressure: 4–12 mean
- Left ventricular (LV) pressure: 100–140 systolic and 60–80 diastolic; left ventricular end-diastolic pressure (LVEDP): 5–12
- Aortic (Ao) pressure: 100–140 systolic, 60–80 diastolic, and 70–90 mean

There are several principles to remember in interpreting pressure data:

1. Compare the values obtained to the patient's normal values rather than an arbitrary standard. If the patient has undergone cardiac catheterization within the past few months, pressures obtained at that time may be used as baselines. If not, you must predict general values on the basis of your knowledge of the so-called normal values and your patient's pathology. For example, you would expect the patient with a narrowed tricuspid valve to have an elevated CVP. The patient with chronic obstructive lung disease probably would have both high PA pressures and CVP.

2. Remember that the consistency of measuring technique and the trend of values are much more important than individual values in assessing the patient's clinical picture.

3. Consider hemodynamic pressures in relation to each other. If one pressure is measured with a manometer and another with a transducer, you may want to convert them to the same scale. To convert millimeters of mercury (Hg) to centimeters of water, multiply by 1.36. Remember that abnormal values are not always due to primary pathology of the monitored chamber. For example, an elevated CVP in association with normal or low PA pressures suggests that the cause lies between these two sites, that is, with the pulmonary valve, right ventricle, or tricuspid valve. In contrast, an elevated CVP in

conjunction with elevated PA pressures suggests that the cause is pulmonary disease, left-sided heart disease, or fluid overload.

4. Remember that a normal value does not necessarily indicate an absence of pathology. For instance, a patient may have a normal CVP but be intensely vasoconstricted due to hypovolemia.

Central Venous Pressure (CVP) Lines

Insertion The CVP line can be inserted at the bedside by a physician. It usually is inserted percutaneously in the antecubital, internal jugular, or subclavian vein.

The nurse has three primary responsibilities related to insertion of a CVP line: preparing the patient and family, preparing equipment, and assisting and observing.

Preparing the Patient and Family Prior to insertion, whenever possible, explain to the patient and immediate family how the procedure will help in the patient's care. Tell the patient what sensations to expect. Reassure the patient that you will be observing and that you should be told promptly of any discomfort. Consult with the physician before giving an analgesic or sedative, since such drugs can alter baseline pressure measurements. Obtain baseline vital signs. Mark on the patient's chest the reference point for measurements, the *phlebostatic axis.* This point usually is at the fourth intercostal space on the lateral chest wall, midway between the anterior and posterior chest. It is important to mark it so that readings are taken at a consistent level. If they are not, variations in readings may be attributed to changes in the patient's condition when they actually result from changes in the recording technique.

Preparing the Equipment Monitoring equipment usually consists of a specific type and size of catheter, a device to measure pressures, a flush solution and related tubing, and a carpenter's level. Insertion equipment includes local anesthetic, skin preparatory solution, sterile gloves, dressing supplies, and a cutdown tray if indicated.

The measuring device may be a water manometer, discussed here, or a pressure transducer and oscilloscope, discussed along with pulmonary artery lines. The water manometer, commonly used for CVP measurement, is suitable for low pressures (under 40 cm of water), when it is not necessary to see the waveforms. A *transducer* (Figure 11–4) is an instrument that converts pressure waves to electrical energy, which then can be displayed on an oscilloscope. It usually is used for pressures too high for the water manometer or in situations where depiction of the waveform is useful, such as with pulmonary or systemic arterial pressures.

Flush systems consist of a solution (such as heparinized normal saline) and a method of irrigating the line. The least desirable irrigation method is a syringe inserted in a stopcock port because of the potential for infection and excessively high flushing pressures. The most desirable method is a continuous low-flow flush device, which is a closed system that infuses solution at a constant slow rate. For a rapid flush, the device can be activated and the system flushed without breaking sterility.

Details of the equipment and setup procedure vary from unit to unit. In general, before the procedure begins, the nurse connects the equipment (except for the catheter itself) together sterilely and securely. The nurse then flushes air out of the system and labels the system with tags at several points: the solution bag or bottle, the tubing near the rate control clamp, and the tubing near stopcocks or medication ports. Critically ill patients often have several hemodynamic and fluid infusion lines. When they are unlabeled, it is easy to confuse them and accidentally alter the flow rate or inject medication into the wrong line.

Assisting and Observing To assist the physician, first position the patient as necessary. If the subclavian or internal jugular vein is used, place the patient in Trendelenburg with the face turned away from the insertion site. Doing so maximizes ease of entry into the vein and minimizes the danger of air embolism. Also, act as the unsterile person to pour prep solution, hold the bottle of local anesthetic, and open the catheter package. As the line is inserted, observe the patient for pain and cardiopulmonary distress. As soon as blood drips out the end of the catheter, connect it to the system. The physician will dress the site of insertion while you obtain the initial measurement.

Obtaining Accurate CVP Measurements Each time you measure the pressure, follow these steps:

1. Place the patient in the baseline position, that is, the position in which all readings are taken. The usual position is supine with the bed flat. If necessary for a particular patient, the head of the bed may be elevated, but it should be placed at the same degree of elevation for each reading. If the patient is on a ventilator, you may leave it connected during the reading. Be sure

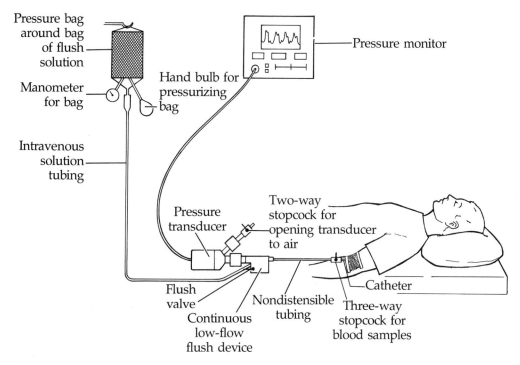

Pressure bag
around bag
of flush
solution

Manometer
for bag

Hand bulb for
pressurizing
bag

Pressure monitor

Intravenous
solution
tubing

Pressure
transducer

Two-way
stopcock for
opening transducer
to air

Flush
valve

Continuous
low-flow
flush device

Nondistensible
tubing

Three-way
stopcock for
blood samples

Catheter

FIGURE 11–4

Pressure monitoring with transducer. Pressure transducer and continuous flush device enlarged to show detail.

to note "on ventilator" when you record the pressure.

2. Check the level of the measuring device. Use a carpenter's level to make sure the "0" on the manometer is level with the reference mark on the patient's chest.

3. Look for and remove any air bubbles in the line; they can cause a damped, distorted reading or failure to get any reading.

4. Check the patency of the line by observing fluctuations in the manometer when it is opened or by aspirating blood from the line.

5. Measure the pressures. Turn the stopcock on the manometer so that fluid flows from the fluid source into the manometer. Let the manometer fill several centimeters above the expected reading, but do not let the upper end of the manometer become contaminated with fluid.

Then turn the stopcock to open the line between the manometer and the patient. The fluid level should fall and then fluctuate with respirations. The average level of the fluid represents the reading. After noting the value, turn the stopcock so the fluid again can flow from the fluid source to the patient.

There are other nursing actions to maintain accurate pressure measurements:

6. To ensure that the catheter is positioned properly, immobilize the extremity.

7. Prevent kinking of the tubing. You will not only increase the accuracy of pressure readings but will also protect your patient from fluctuating dosages of any drugs being administered through the line.

8. To ascertain whether the tip is in the correct location, obtain a chest x-ray after insertion.

Analyzing the Pressures Critically The normal CVP when measured by the manometer method is 2–8 cm H_2O.

The central venous pressure is affected by the amount of blood in the right ventricle just before systole *(preload)*, right ventricular *contractility*, and the amount of resistance against which the right ventricle must eject blood *(afterload)*.

A low CVP indicates inadequate preload, that is, inadequate venous return caused by either true hypovolemia secondary to actual fluid deficit or relative hypovolemia due to excessive vasodilatation.

A high CVP can reflect one or more problems: increased preload, decreased contractility, or increased afterload.

Increased RV Preload When preload is increased, the ventricle may be unable to pump out the excess fluid efficiently. Preload can be increased by fluid overload, such as in excessive administration of IV fluids, fluid retention in cardiac or renal disease, valvular insufficiency, and left-to-right cardiac shunts—for example, a ventricular septal defect.

Decreased RV Contractility Contractile force can be diminished in right ventricular infarction, myocarditis, or restrictions to expansion such as cardiac tamponade.

Increased RV Afterload Right ventricular afterload increases whenever pulmonary vascular resistance increases due to pulmonary obstruction or pulmonary vasoconstriction. Examples include chronic obstructive lung disease, pulmonary embolism, and other pulmonary disorders. Right ventricular afterload also increases in the presence of mitral or pulmonic stenosis.

Prevention of Complications Anticipate and prevent complications by taking the appropriate nursing measures. The most common complications associated with CVP catheters are pneumothorax, infection, fluid overload, and poor infusion of fluid.

Pneumothorax Pneumothorax may occur during insertion of the CVP line into the subclavian or jugular vein. The reason for this complication is that the apex of the lung extends above the clavicle. Because it is in close proximity to these veins, it may be punctured accidentally during insertion. For information on the recognition and treatment of pneumothorax, see Chapter 8.

Infection Maintain scrupulous sterile technique. Observe the insertion site every 8 hours for signs of inflammation. Clean the site and change the dressing at least daily. Check the patient's temperature at least once every 8 hours, and call unexplained elevations to the physician's attention.

Fluid Overload Fluids commonly are administered via the CVP line. To prevent accidental fluid overload via a CVP line, use measuring chambers and small-drop infusion sets.

Poor Infusion of Fluid This problem occurs most commonly because of partial obstruction of the catheter tip due to fibrin deposition, but it may also occur due to kinking of the catheter. If the catheter is not kinked, try to aspirate fluid from the line or to irrigate it gently. Do not attempt to clear the line by a forceful manual flush, because you may cause a thrombus on the tip of the catheter to embolize to the pulmonary vessels.

Pulmonary Arterial (PA) Lines

PA and pulmonary capillary wedge (PCWP) pressures can be monitored at the bedside through a balloon-tipped, flow-directed catheter placed in the pulmonary artery. This type of catheter sometimes is referred to generically by the name of one specific brand of catheter, the *Swan-Ganz* pulmonary artery catheter.

A variety of catheters is available. The double-lumen catheter has two openings, one at the distal end and one for balloon inflation. With it, one can record PA pressures and PCWP only. The *triple-lumen catheter* has an additional lumen (proximal lumen) that opens in the right atrium, so it has the additional capability of recording CVP. The *thermodilution cardiac output catheter* has a fourth lumen, which connects with a temperature-sensitive thermistor on the end of the catheter. With this catheter, one can record the pressures in the pulmonary artery, pulmonary capillaries, and right atrium, as well as measure CO by the thermodilution method. Other catheters available include a multipurpose catheter, which enables not only pressure recordings but also electrical pacing of the right heart, and an $S\bar{v}o_2$ monitoring catheter, which allows continuous monitoring of mixed venous oxygen saturation ($S\bar{v}o_2$), a sensitive indicator of tissue oxygen balance. ($S\bar{v}o_2$ monitoring is discussed in detail in Chapter 7.)

Insertion The catheter is inserted by a physician, percutaneously or via cutdown. The usual insertion site is the subclavian, internal jugular, brachial, or femoral vein. Preparation of the patient and family is similar to that for CVP line insertion. Preparation of the equipment is more elaborate, as each pressure-monitoring lumen must be attached to a heparinized, pressurized, calibrated monitoring system. Details of this setup vary, depending on how many pressures will be monitored with how many transducers and depending on the protocol for setup used in the unit. The general steps involved in setup include maintaining a sterile connection of the components of the monitoring system, flushing air from the tubing and transducers, balancing the system to zero, and calibrating it to a known calibration factor. (Opening the transducer to air and balancing to zero negates the influence of atmospheric pressure so that only cardiovascular pressures will be measured. Calibration is accomplished by introducing a known pressure into the system and verifying that the value measured by the machine is correct, to ensure that the cardiovascular pressures will be recorded accurately.) Finally, the balloon on the catheter is submerged in sterile fluid in a basin and inflated to check for leaks, then deflated. The catheter is then filled with the heparinized solution and connected to the monitoring system. Most protocols call for lidocaine at the bedside because of the risk of ventricular irritability.

After the vessel is entered, the catheter is usually advanced under fluoroscopic and ECG observation, with the balloon deflated until it reaches the right atrium. At that point, the balloon is partially inflated, and blood flow inside the heart carries it through the tricuspid valve into the right ventricle and through the pulmonic valve into the pulmonary artery. The balloon is then inflated to float the catheter through the pulmonary arterial tree until it wedges itself in a small pulmonary artery. The balloon then is allowed to deflate. Figure 11–5 shows the change in pressure and waveform as the catheter advances through the right atrium, right ventricle, and pulmonary artery into a pulmonary wedge position.

During insertion, the nurse's primary responsibility is to observe the patient for complications, which can include: ventricular dysrhythmias due to irritation of the heart by the catheter tip, especially when the tip is located in the right ventricle; hematoma at the insertion site; and pneumothorax if a subclavian approach is used and the lung is punctured. An additional responsibility is to observe the waveforms appearing on the monitor screen as the catheter passes through each chamber. Each chamber has a distinct waveform that indicates the catheter's exact location and progress.

Once the line is inserted, it is the nurse's responsibility to secure a portable chest x-ray to ensure correct placement of the catheter tip, to obtain accurate measurements, and to prevent or minimize complications.

Right Atrial (RA) Pressure RA pressure (which is the same as CVP pressure) can be monitored by using a transducer connected to the proximal lumen of a flow-directed, balloon-tipped catheter in the pulmonary artery. In this situation, the nurse is able to record RA pressure by setting the pressure monitoring switch on "mean." The normal RA pressure is 2–6 mm Hg. The normal waveform includes three ascending and two descending waves (Figure 11–6), which correlate with the phases of the cardiac cycle. The *a wave* is produced by atrial contraction. The *x descent* occurs as atrial pressure drops during atrial diastole. It is possible that the onset of ventricular contraction contributes to this

descent by tugging downward on the atrioventricular valve. The *c wave* may result from closure of the tricuspid valve or bulging of the valve into the atria during early ventricular contraction. The *v wave* occurs as the atria fill and their pressure increases while the last part of ventricular systole is occurring. The *y descent* shows the rapid drop in atrial pressure after the atrioventricular valve opens and rapid ventricular filling ensues.

Changes in waveforms can be clues to malposition of the catheter tip, obstructions in the line, or changes in the patient's clinical state. Causes of abnormal pressure readings are reviewed in the previous section on CVP lines.

Right Ventricular (RV) Pressure RV pressure normally is monitored only during PA catheter insertion. Normal RV pressure is 20–30 mm Hg systolic, with an end-diastolic pressure of 0–5 mm Hg.

The RV waveform demonstrates a gradually increasing pressure during ventricular filling, with a small bulge at the time of atrial contraction (Figure 11–7). After the tricuspid valve closes, the pressure increases sharply during systole until it causes the pulmonic valve to open. Then it peaks and drops rapidly, until the pulmonic valve closes and diastole begins.

There is one other situation in which the nurse should be alert to the appearance of an RV waveform, and that is once the PA catheter has been placed in the pulmonary artery. In that situation, the appearance of an RV waveform signifies that the catheter has migrated backwards into the right ventricle. When this happens, the catheter can flip around inside the ventricle, irritate the ventricular wall, and precipitate ventricular ectopy. At times, in fact, the catheter may slip forward into the pulmonary artery and backward into the right ventricle, alternately producing PA and RV waveforms.

PA Pressures When the catheter is in the pulmonary artery with the balloon deflated, the nurse can monitor systolic, diastolic, and mean PA pressures. Normal PA pressures are: 20–30 systolic and 8–12 diastolic, both measured in mm Hg. It is important to realize that pulmonary artery pressures normally fluctuate in critically ill patients. According to research by Nemens and Woods (1982), a change of 5 mm Hg in PA systolic or mean pressure or a change of 4 mm Hg in PA diastolic pressure is likely to be clinically significant for most patients.

The pulmonary arterial waveform has a characteristic appearance (Figure 11–8). After the beginning of systole, the wave form shows a rapid upstroke during ventricular ejection, followed by a more gradual

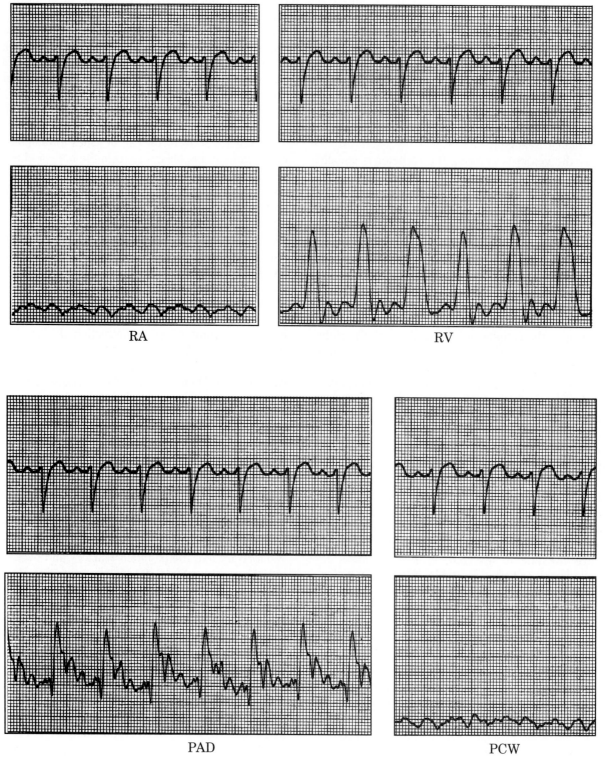

RA

RV

PAD

PCW

FIGURE 11–5

Changes in pressure as the PA catheter advances through the heart. Each set of strips shows the ECG in the upper strip and the simultaneously recorded waveform in the lower strip. RA, (right atrial pressure); RV, (right ventricular pressure); PAD, (pulmonary artery pressure); PCW, (pulmonary capillary wedge pressure).

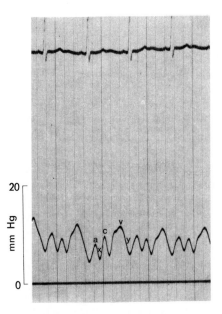

FIGURE 11–6

RA pressure waveform showing *a, c,* and *v* waves with *x* and *y* descents. Note that the recorded waveforms are delayed from the corresponding electrical event in the P-QRS-T. This delay occurs because of the delay in recording pressure events through a long catheter. (From Daily E, Schroeder J: *Techniques in bedside hemodynamic monitoring,* 4th ed. St. Louis: Mosby, 1989.)

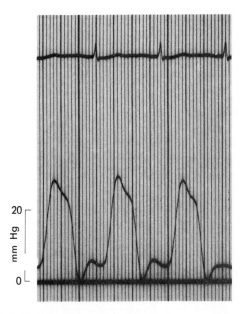

FIGURE 11–7

Normal right ventricular pressure tracing. (From Daily E, Schroeder J: *Techniques in bedside hemodynamic monitoring,* 3d ed. St. Louis: Mosby, 1985.)

downstroke. The downstroke is interrupted by the dicrotic notch, signifying the closure of the pulmonic valve and the onset of diastole.

PA pressures reflect both pulmonary blood volume and pulmonary vascular resistance. Low PA pressures indicate hypovolemia due to either fluid loss or vasodilation. Elevated PA pressures can reflect increased pulmonary blood volume or increased pulmonary vascular resistance.

Increased Pulmonary Blood Volume This situation can occur in fluid overload, intracardiac shunts, mitral valve disease, left ventricular failure, or cardiac tamponade or constrictive pericarditis.

Increased Pulmonary Vascular Resistance This situation can occur when there is an obstruction to blood flow, such as in pulmonary embolism, when pulmonary hypertension is present in cardiac or pulmonary disease, or when pulmonary vessels vasoconstrict due to hypoxemia or hypercapnia.

PCWP When the balloon on the tip of the pulmonary artery catheter is inflated, the catheter tip is moved along by blood flow until it wedges in a small pulmonary artery. The inflated balloon in effect

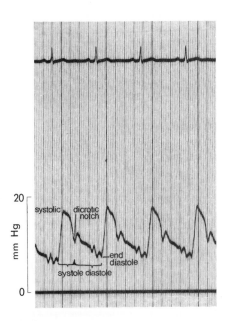

FIGURE 11–8

PA pressure waveform showing phases of systole, dicrotic notch (pulmonic valve closure), and diastole. Normally, PA end-diastole closely represents LVEDP. (From Daily E, Schroeder J: *Techniques in bedside hemodynamic monitoring,* 4th ed. St. Louis: Mosby, 1989.)

"blocks" the recording of pressure behind it in the pulmonary artery and allows recording only of pressures forward from it, that is, the pressures in the pulmonary capillaries themselves. As there are no valves between the pulmonary capillaries and the left atrium, PCWP reflects mean LAP. The normal PCWP is 4–12 mm Hg.

The wedge pressure waveform (Figure 11–9) is similar to the LA waveform (Figure 11–10) in that it displays the typical *a* and *v* waves of atrial contraction and ventricular systole. Normally, the *c* wave, which reflects bulging of the mitral valve during early ventricular systole, is so small it cannot be seen.

Decreased PCWP values are seen in hypovolemia due to true fluid loss or vasodilatation. Increased PCWP values can indicate increased preload, decreased contractility, or increased afterload.

Increased LV Preload   When more blood returns to the left ventricle than it can pump out, left ventricular end-diastolic volume and LVEDP increase. This increase is reflected in an elevated wedge pressure. This situation can occur in volume overload due to excessive intravenous solutions, fluid retention in cardiac or renal failure, aortic or mitral valvular disease, or intracardiac shunts.

Decreased LV Contractility   Decreased left ventricular (LV) contractility can occur in myocardial ischemia or infarction, ventricular aneurysms, myocarditis, acid–

base imbalances, cardiomyopathy, or restrictions to filling, such as cardiac tamponade.

Increased LV Afterload   Resistance to LV ejection (increased systemic vascular resistance) elevates wedge pressure. Situations in which this can occur include systemic hypertension, administration of vasoconstricting agents, and outlet obstructions such as coarctation of the aorta and aortic stenosis.

Measures to Obtain Accurate PA and Wedge Pressures   As with a CVP line, the nurse ensures that the transducer is leveled and the line patent before attempting to record PA and wedge pressures. The reference point on the patient's chest (the phlebostatic axis, at the fourth intercostal space, mid-axillary line) should be leveled with the air–fluid interface in the transducer. Patency of the line can be checked by inspecting for kinks in the catheter and observing the normal waveform on the oscilloscope before recording the pressures.

To measure systolic, diastolic, and mean pressures from the monitor's digital readout, place the monitor switch on the appropriate settings. To measure pulmonary capillary pressure, place the switch on "mean" and inflate the balloon with no more than the specified amount of air for that size catheter. Insert the air until the characteristic PCWP wave form (containing *a* and

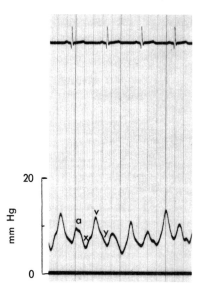

FIGURE 11–9

Normal pulmonary artery wedge pressure waveform showing *a* and *v* waves and *x* and *y* descents. (From Daily E, Schroeder J: *Techniques in bedside hemodynamic monitoring,* 4th ed. St. Louis: Mosby, 1989.)

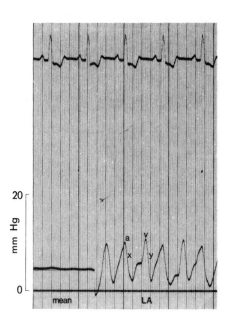

FIGURE 11–10

LA pressure waveform demonstrating similarity to PA wedge waveform. This pressure is normal. (From Daily E, Schroeder J: *Techniques in bedside hemodynamic monitoring,* 4th ed. St. Louis: Mosby, 1989.)

v waves) appears on the oscilloscope. To keep the balloon inflated while you read the pressure from the monitor, hold the syringe in place or use the lever on the catheter's end to lock the air in place. Do not inflate the balloon longer than 3 seconds. After taking the reading, be sure to remove the syringe or release the lock so the balloon can deflate.

Nursing Considerations When caring for a patient with a PA catheter, the nurse monitors the PA tracing continuously. A significant component of the nursing assessment involves evaluation of the PA waveform to ensure that the catheter has not migrated forward into the wedge position, since a segment of the lung can be infarcted if the catheter occludes a small pulmonary artery for a prolonged period. Other factors that affect PA measurement include head-of-bed position and lateral body position relative to transducer height placement. If the transducer is placed at the level of the phlebostatic axis, a head-of-bed position up to 45° is appropriate for most patients in the supine position. In the lateral position, the fourth intercostal space and midsternum are suggested as the reference level. However, some patients, such as those with low cardiac output, can have marked changes in their hemodynamics in the lateral position. Therefore, the supine position is generally recommended. Other nursing considerations include troubleshooting techniques for problems such as damping, inappropriate high or low pressures, catheter fling, and respiratory variation.

Numerous systems problems can occur to interfere with the recording of accurate pressures. Among the most common are damping, inappropriately high or low pressures, catheter whip artifact, and respiratory fluctuations. *Damping* results from poor transmission of the pressure wave to the oscilloscope and is recognized by decreased amplitude of the waveform. Possible causes include partial occlusion of the catheter tip by a clot, placement of the catheter tip against the vessel wall, and air bubbles in the line or transducer. To avoid damping, use a pressurized, heparinized, low-flow flush system, periodically rapid-flushing it. If damping occurs, try aspirating the line for blood, having the patient cough, changing the patient's position, checking the system for air bubbles and removing them, and/or flushing the line. If none of those measures works, the line may need to be repositioned by the physician.

Inappropriately high or low pressures can be caused by improper leveling, loose connections, or migration of the catheter tip. To prevent them, always level the transducer before measuring pressures, and connect the system components securely. If inappropriate pressures occur, it helps to double-check the patient's

position relative to the transducer, check the connections and tighten them if necessary, and alert the physician if inappropriate waveforms indicate the catheter tip has migrated from the pulmonary artery so it can be repositioned.

Catheter fling (Figure 11–11) is an artifact of excessive movement of the catheter. To compensate for it, record only average (mean) pressures or ask the physician to reposition the catheter.

Respiratory variation (Figure 11–12) results from transmission of normal respiratory pressure fluctuations to the monitoring system. For greatest accuracy, record pressures at end-expiration (see Chapter 9 for details). If the patient is on a ventilator, record the pressures with the patient on the ventilator. Off-ventilator pressures are somewhat irrelevant, since the on-ventilator pressures represent the actual pressures under which the cardiovascular system is functioning the majority of the time.

Cardiac Output (CO) Determinations At the bedside, the most common method of measuring CO is the thermodilution method, using a balloon-tipped, flow-directed thermodilution catheter. A known amount of solution, at a known temperature, is injected into the right atrial port of the catheter. A thermistor in the pulmonary artery measures the resulting temperature change of the blood. A computer then calculates cardiac output.

To measure CO, attach a thermodilution output computer to its connector on the end of the thermodilution catheter. Prepare the injectate by drawing sterile solution, usually 5% dextrose in water, into plastic syringes. The best syringes to use are those that have finger rings on the barrel and a thumb ring on the plunger, because they allow you to hold the syringe without handling the barrel and therefore transmitting your body heat to the injectate. The injectate used may be either cold or at room temperature. The temperature of the injectate is fed into the computer.

To inject the solution, attach an injectate syringe to the three-way stopcock connected to the proximal (right atrial) port of the catheter. Turn the stopcock to shut off the routine drip to this port. Inject the solution evenly and within 4 seconds. Then read the CO measurement shown by the computer. Usually, three CO determinations are made and the values averaged to obtain the measurement.

Normal cardiac output is 4–8 liters per minute. As these values do not take into account body size, however, a more meaningful measurement is cardiac index. The *cardiac index* equals the cardiac output divided by the body surface area, which can be determined using a Dubois body surface chart. The

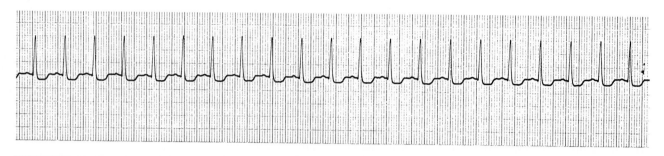

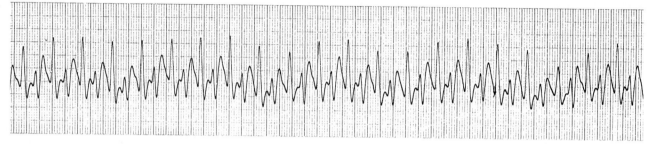

FIGURE 11–11

Catheter fling in PA waveform. Upper strip shows ECG; lower strip shows PA waveform.

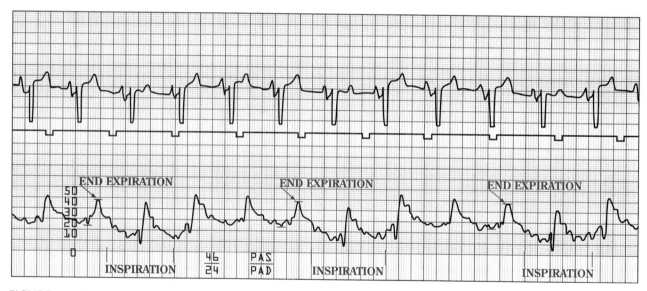

FIGURE 11–12

Respiratory variation of PA waveform. Upper strip shows ECG; lower strip shows PA waveform. Horizontal marks indicate end-expiration points for reading systolic and diastolic pressure. Pressure here is 46/24.

Dubois body surface area chart is a nomogram used to determine body surface area (BSA) from the patient's height and weight. The normal cardiac index is 2.5–4.0 liters/minute/meter^2.

If the individual measurements vary more than 10% from each other, suspect an error in measurement. Possible sources of error include varying injectate temperatures, due to touching the barrel of the syringe

RESEARCH NOTE

Doering L, Dracup K:
Comparisons of cardiac output in supine and lateral positions.
Nurs Res 1988; 37: 114–118.

CLINICAL APPLICATION

Considerable evidence exists to suggest that pulmonary artery pressures and cardiac output (CO) do not vary significantly with modest backrest position elevation. However, there is little data on whether cardiac output differs between supine and lateral positioning. This study compared cardiac output measurements in the supine and lateral positions.

A convenience sample of 51 adult post cardiac surgical patients were studied. To control for sequence effects, patients were assigned by coin toss to one of two position sequences: supine-right-left or supine-left-right. Twenty-six patients were studied using the former sequence and 25 using the latter. Cardiac output measurements were taken with the patients in supine and lateral positions. Two cardiac outputs were measured with 10 ml iced saline at each position.

Statistical analyses were conducted using one-way analysis of variance with repeated measures to compare cardiac output values in all three positions. Results showed there was a significant difference in cardiac output among the three positions. Patients with the greatest difference in cardiac output were those who had a low cardiac index (<2.3 L min/m^2), had vasoactive drips, and were mechanically ventilated.

CRITICAL THINKING

Limitations: The average of three successive cardiac output measurements is recommended as the standard of practice, but only two measurements were averaged in this study. Research demonstrates that the first CO measurement can vary considerably, and if it is more than 10% the second and third CO should be averaged.

Strengths: This study addressed an important practice issue and provides valuable information for critical-care nurses. Characteristics of patients who may be at risk for changes in CO measurement in the lateral position include low CO, mechanical ventilation, and vasoactive therapy. This study's data supports consistent use of the supine position when measuring CO in these patients.

---

or injecting more slowly than 4 seconds; varying injectate amounts, due to inaccurate filling of the syringes; and improper catheter tip placement in the right ventricle or wedge position rather than in the pulmonary artery.

Complications of PA Catheters Complications of PA catheters include ventricular dysrhythmias, pulmonary infarction, thromboemboli, air emboli, and balloon rupture, as well as the problems of hemorrhage, infection, and patient discomfort common to any hemodynamic monitoring line.

Ventricular Dysrhythmias Ventricular dysrhythmias can be caused by displacement of the PA catheter into the right ventricle. This displacement will cause a change in the contour of the waveform, from the typical PA tracing to a right ventricular (RV) tracing. This problem again emphasizes the need to keep an eye on the waveforms displayed on the oscilloscope. Inflate the balloon to see if it will float back up into the pulmonary artery. Repositioning the patient on the left side also may help the catheter float back into the pulmonary artery. If it does not, the physician will need to reposition the catheter. After repositioning, get a new chest x-ray to verify catheter placement.

Pulmonary Infarction Pulmonary infarction may result if the PA catheter balloon is left inflated or if the deflated balloon spontaneously wedges itself. Adhere to the safety precautions described below under the problem of balloon rupture. You may be able to dislodge a spontaneously wedged catheter by having the patient cough or turn. If these measures are unsuccessful, notify the physician promptly.

Thromboemboli To minimize the risk of thromboemboli, utilize a continuous low-flow flush system whenever possible. Flush lines after blood samples are drawn, including flushing the stopcock port from which the sample was obtained. Also flush promptly if the tracing becomes damped. If you are unable to aspirate blood or infuse fluid, the line may be clotted. Do not attempt to clear the line by a forceful manual flush because you may cause a thrombus to embolize.

Air Emboli Air emboli can be prevented in several ways. Be sure that air is flushed from the line before initial use. During insertion of the PA line in the subclavian vein or jugular vein, place the patient's head below the level of the thorax. If you spot air bubbles in the line, remove them with a needle and syringe or shut the line off to the patient and flush it. Whenever it is necessary to open the transducer to air (as in balancing it), first turn off the stopcock to the patient.

Balloon Rupture Breakage of the balloon used to obtain the PCWP presents another source of potential air emboli. Minimize the risk of breakage by inserting no more air than appropriate for the specific size catheter (usually a maximum of 1.5 ml), and by releasing the air after the reading. You should feel a slight resistance to inflation of the balloon. If the balloon breaks, you will know because the air will enter with minimal resistance, no wedge tracing will appear, and blood may leak out of the balloon lumen. If you suspect breakage, turn the lumen off to the patient and notify the physician. The small amount of air in the balloon is not dangerous, but repeated injections of air by well-meaning misinformed staff can be unsafe.

Right Ventricular Ejection Fraction Catheters A new catheter is available which is used to evaluate right ventricular ejection fraction and cardiac output. The ejection fraction is the percentage of blood ejected from the ventricle in one beat. Normal ejection fraction is 50–70%. When myocardial fibers are stretched to the point where the increase in stroke volume is not proportional to the increase in end-diastolic volume, the ejection fraction decreases. Clinical evaluation of the right ventricular ejection fraction can help to optimize the preload delivered to the left ventricle and thus optimize cardiac function.

Arterial Lines

Arterial lines are catheters placed in systemic arteries to facilitate recording of continuous, accurate data about BP in the patient who has an unstable hemodynamic status, and to allow frequent sampling of arterial blood gases without the need for repeated arterial punctures. Arterial lines commonly are placed percutaneously in the radial, brachial, or femoral arteries.

To assist with insertion, prepare the patient as described in the section on CVP lines and set up a pressurized, heparinized pressure monitoring system. If the site chosen is the radial artery, either you or the

physician should perform an *Allen's test* of the patency of the ulnar artery. To perform this test, have the patient make a fist, and then occlude both the radial and ulnar arteries. Have the patient open her or his hand, and release the pressure on the ulnar artery. If the hand pinks up quickly, you can assume that good collateral blood flow is available to the hand in the event the radial artery becomes occluded.

Once the line is inserted, recording of pressures and observation of the arterial waveform become nursing responsibilities. Normal arterial pressures vary widely; a general range of aortic systolic pressure is 100–140 mm Hg, with diastolic pressures of 60–80 mm Hg, and mean pressures of 70–90 mm Hg. Catheters terminating more distally than the central aorta will show higher systolic pressures. Systolic pressure in the femoral artery, for example, may be as much as 20 mm higher than aortic pressure, due to the amplification of the pulse pressure wave during systole (Daily and Schroeder 1989).

The normal arterial waveform has a sharp upstroke and a more gradual downstroke with an evident dicrotic notch, due to a small rise in pressure that occurs at the time of aortic valve closure (Figure 11–13). End-diastole should be clearly seen.

To ensure accurate recordings, balance and calibrate the transducer according to the manufacturer's recommended procedure at least every 8 hours. Also

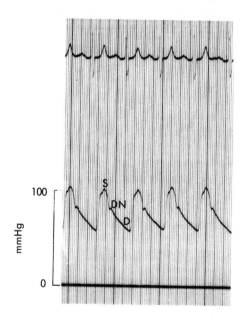

FIGURE 11–13

Normal arterial pressure tracing. S, systole; DN, dicrotic notch; D, diastole. (From Daily E, Schroeder J: *Hemodynamic waveforms: Exercises in Identification and Analysis,* 2d ed. St. Louis: Mosby, 1990.)

NURSING TIP

Artifact in Arterial Pressure Recordings

Artifact can occur in arterial pressure waveforms from excessive catheter movement or damping. One way to determine if artifact exists in an arterial tracing is to compare the timing of the ECG components to the simultaneously recorded waveform. The systolic peak usually occurs after the QRS complex. Peak systolic values that occur later than the T wave probably represent artifact.

NURSING TIP

Inaccurate Arterial Pressure

A dampened arterial pressure can cause inaccurate arterial pressure. Damping can be due to a clot at the end of the catheter, kinks in the catheter or tubing, or air bubbles in the system. If there is any doubt about the accuracy of the arterial waveform, take a cuff blood pressure reading. As part of the routine nursing assessment, take a cuff blood pressure every shift and correlate it with the intra-arterial pressure.

compare the recorded measurement to the blood pressure obtained with a sphygmomanometer at least every 8 hours. Remember that many factors can give you discrepancies between the cuff BP and arterial line. Among the most common are wrong cuff size, dysrhythmias, peripheral vasoconstriction or vasospasm, and unbalanced or uncalibrated equipment.

Arterial lines share with PA lines the problems of damping, spurious readings, thrombosis, and infection. Exsanguination also can occur with arterial lines if a stopcock port is accidentally left open after an arterial blood sample is drawn. The blood in the artery is under such high pressure that a patient can lose a significant amount of blood if this occurs or if connections in the system are loose. For this reason, the limb with the arterial line should always remain uncovered and

pressure alarms should be set to alert you if accidental disconnection occurs. In addition, when the line is removed, maintain firm pressure on the site for at least 5 minutes to prevent hematoma formation due to the high intravascular pressure.

REFERENCES

Albarran-Sotelo R et al.: *Textbook of advanced cardiac life support.* Dallas: American Heart Association, 1987.

Benner P, Tanner C: Clinical judgment: How expert nurses use intuition. *Am J Nurs* 1987; 87:23–31.

Bentley L: Radionuclide imaging techniques for the diagnosis and treatment of coronary heart disease. *Focus Crit Care* 1987; 14(6):27.

Bommer W: Analyzing blood flow with echocardiography. *Diagnostic Imaging* 1985a; 5:76–79.

Bommer W: Basic principles of flow imaging. *Echocardiography* 1985b; 11:501–509.

Chen J: Chest roentgenography. In *The heart, arteries, and veins,* 6th ed, Hurst J et al. New York: McGraw-Hill, 1986.

Daily E, Schroeder J: *Techniques in bedside hemodynamic monitoring,* 4th ed. St Louis: Mosby, 1989.

DeMaria A et al.: Doppler flow imaging: Another step in the evolution of cardiac ultrasound. *Echocardiography* 1985; 2(6):495–500.

Horowitz S et al.: Complementary roles of cardiac ultrasound and cardiovascular nuclear medicine. *Sem Nuclear Med* 1980; 10:94–105.

Kelber M Sr: Cardiac enzymes. In *Diagnostics,* pp. 99–133. Springhouse, PA: Intermed Communications, 1986.

Mauldin N: Doppler ultrasonography. In *Diagnostics,* pp. 939–943. Springhouse, PA: Intermed Communications, 1986.

Nemens E, Woods S: Normal fluctuations in pulmonary artery and pulmonary capillary wedge pressures in acutely ill patients. *Heart Lung* 1982; 11:393–398.

Oldendorf W, Oldendorf JR: CT, NMR and PET: Modern diagnostic imaging techniques in medicine. *Am J Cont Ed Nurs* 1985; 1:26–30.

Pantaleo N et al.: Thallium myocardial scintigraphy and its use in the assessment of coronary artery disease. *Heart Lung* 1981; 10:61–70.

Pohost G, Canby R: Nuclear magnetic resonance imaging: Current application and future prospects. *Circ* 1987; 75(1):88.

Sanderson R, Kurth C (eds): *The cardiac patient,* 2d ed. Philadelphia: Saunders, 1983.

Shellock F, Riedinger M: Reproducibility and accuracy of using room-temperature vs. ice-temperature injectate for thermodilution cardiac output determination. *Heart Lung* 1983; 12:175–176.

Strong A: Cardiac radiography. In *Diagnostics,* pp. 900–902. Springhouse, PA: Intermed Communications, 1986.

Zeluff G et al.: Evaluation of the coronary arteries and myocardium by radionuclide imaging. *Heart Lung* 1980; 9:344–348.

12

Dysrhythmias
and Conduction Defects

CLINICAL INSIGHT

Domain: Administering and monitoring therapeutic interventions and regimens

Competency: Administering medications accurately and safely: Monitoring untoward effects, reactions, therapeutic responses, toxicities, and incompatibilities

With patients in precarious physiologic status, the ability to titrate multiple pharmacologic agents to maintain vital functions within normal limits often becomes a determining factor in patient survival. Often—but not always—medication administration falls within prescribed protocols; at other times, the nurse may be functioning in uncharted seas with new or experimental therapies.

Potent medications with a slim margin of safety are the rule rather than the exception in critical care, and a patient's life may depend on the nurse's knowledge of appropriate use of these powerful agents. In the fol-

lowing exemplar, from Crabtree and Jorgenson (1986, pp. 158–159), a nurse challenges a physician to expand his tunnel vision and reconsider an order for a medication, which, given the patient's history, could be lethal to her.

This lady came in with an MI, and this resident after working with these people liked to push IV propranolol with anybody who has an acute cardiac event. He felt that the woman was having an acute MI, but he was not seeing the multiple problems associated with this. He was seeing an acute MI; he was really treating acute MI's, with this IV Inderal, which was contraindicated for various reasons. I think that it's a good drug in its right use. And I think that they've shown, . . . studies have shown propranolol in acute infarcts can limit the infarct size, but you can't use it on somebody that has severe COPD, who has heart block, and is in pulmonary edema. I think those are all strong contraindication to its use. He didn't look at the patient, because in this case, he was telling me to give this woman 1 mg of propranolol. The woman was bolt upright in bed and gasping. And she would just shake her head yes or no; she just didn't have enough air to say more than that. And I was trying to tell the resident, don't do that, because she was obviously in pulmonary edema. She was a terrible smoker. She had lung problems. And when she first came in, she had a prolonged PR interval, and as I was sitting there disagreeing with this doctor, she started going into a 2:1 and by the time I'm done giving my little dissertation . . . she's going into third-degree heart block. I said I could not do these things because—and I listed the reasons why I felt uncomfortable being forced to give this drug.

And I said, legally I am . . . responsible if I would inject this, and I had drawn up the medication and I said, if you feel strongly, you can do it.

Critically ill patients are subject to a wide variety of dysrhythmias, which range from inconsequential to lethal. Since the inception of electrocardiographic monitoring, nurses have assumed increasing responsibility for accurate recognition and rapid termination of life-threatening dysrhythmias. And, as illustrated in the Clinical Insight, nurses also play a key role in preventing complications of antidysrhythmic medication administration.

This chapter shows you the mechanics of analyzing the electrocardiogram (ECG). It also assists you in recognizing and responding appropriately to the dysrhythmias and conduction defects you are most likely to encounter in clinical practice.

Dysrhythmia Diagnosis

ECG Recording

Contraction of the cardiac chambers is provoked by an electrical stimulus. The initiation and propagation of this stimulus can be recorded on an ECG.

12-Lead Electrocardiogram The standard electrocardiogram consists of six limb leads and six precordial leads, each of which has a slightly different orientation toward the heart. The limb leads are I, II, III, AVR, AVL, and AVF. They are oriented toward the frontal plane of the heart. The six precordial leads are V_1 through V_6. They give a transverse view of cardiac activity.

Leads I, II, and III, called *standard limb leads,* create Einthoven's triangle (Figure 12–1). In lead I, the ECG machine reads the right arm (RA) electrode as negative and the left arm (LA) electrode as positive. In lead II, it reads the RA electrode as negative and the left leg (LL) as positive. In lead III, it reads the LA as negative and the LL as positive. Each of these leads measures the difference in potential between two electrodes. The standard limb leads therefore are called *bipolar* leads. Leads I, II, and III form an equilateral triangle whose apices are the right arm, left arm, and left leg electrodes. These electrodes are considered to be electrically equidistant from the heart, which is at zero potential.

In contrast, the remaining limb leads and the precordial leads are *unipolar* leads, that is, they measure the actual potential under one electrode. If the electrodes from which these leads are recorded are connected to a common terminal, its potential is zero.

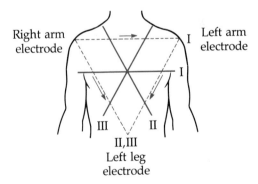

FIGURE 12–1

Standard limb leads, demonstrating Einthoven's triangle. The three dashed lines represent the leads as recorded and are labeled to show the direction of current, from negative to positive poles. The solid lines represent the shifting of these axes (without altering their direction) so that they intersect at the zero point, the heart. The lines are labeled at their positive poles.

For the augmented limb leads (AVR, AVL, and AVF) (Figure 12–2), the machine reads one electrode as positive and combines the remaining two electrodes to create the neutral electrode. For example, to record

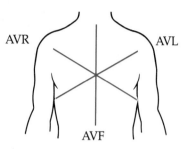

FIGURE 12–2

Augmented limb leads. Leads are labeled at their positive poles.

AVR, the right arm electrode is read as positive and the left arm and left leg electrodes are joined to form the neutral electrode. Each augmented lead measures the difference in potential between the center of the heart and the limb wearing the positive electrode.

The remaining six leads (V_1 through V_6) also are unipolar leads (Figure 12–3). A separate exploring electrode is placed at different positions on the precordium, and the right arm, left arm, and left leg electrodes collectively serve to produce a zero potential reference point at the center of the heart.

The twelve leads intersect at the heart, thus providing twelve views of the heart—six frontal and six transverse (Figure 12–4). Occasionally the exploring electrode is moved to positions on the right chest for additional lead placements when a right ventricular infarction is suspected (V_3R–V_6R). Each of the 12 leads of the ECG views the electrical activity of the heart

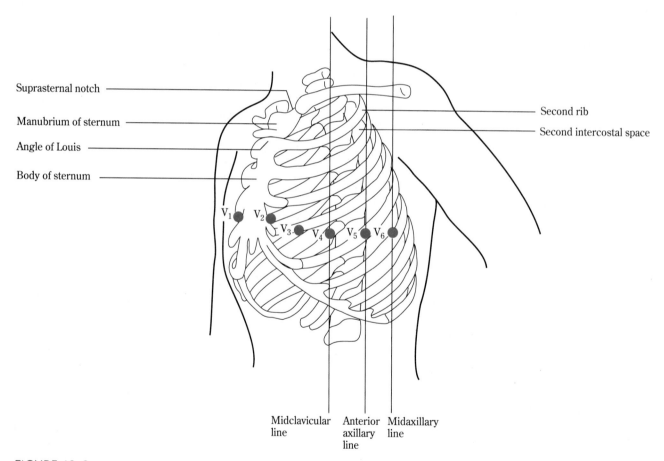

FIGURE 12–3

Placement of precordial (chest) leads. Positions of the precordial electrode: V1, fourth intercostal space at the right sternal border; V2, fourth intercostal space at left sternal border; V3, midway between V2 and V4; V4, fifth intercostal space at midclavicular line; V5, directly lateral to V4, at anterior axillary line; V6 directly lateral to V5 at midaxillary line.

from a different vantage point, and thus will record the same electrical activity but with a different pattern or morphology.

Bedside Cardiac Monitoring Modifications of the standard 12 leads are used for routine cardiac monitoring at the bedside. Specifics of monitors vary from manufacturer to manufacturer. The following general guidelines will help you work with a variety of models.

The bedside monitor consists of a monitor console, a patient cable, and electrode wires that can be connected to disposable electrodes. The console contains an oscilloscope screen to display the tracing and various buttons and switches to obtain the tracing. In most units, the bedside monitors also are connected to displays at the nurses' station or central monitoring area.

When you are notified of an admission, turn the monitor on with the power switch to let it warm up. Connect electrodes to the electrode wires. Connect the electrode wires to the patient cable and plug the cable into the monitor itself. Check that the following switches are on their standard settings. The *sweep speed switch* controls the rate at which the beam traverses the screen; its usual setting is 25 mm per second. The *filter switch* controls the amount of external interference in the tracing. It has two settings, "diagnostic" and "monitor." The usual setting for routine monitoring is "monitor" because it filters out most of the muscle artifact.

When the patient arrives, take these steps:

1. Explain to the patient why and how you will monitor cardiac rhythm. Depending on the patient's condition, you may need to modify or delay this explanation.

2. Prepare the electrode sites. If they are hairy, clip the hair with scissors. Rub the skin briskly with an alcohol sponge (let the freshly clipped patient know that the alcohol may sting). Allow the sites to dry. Use an abrasive ECG preparation pad to wipe the skin surface (1–5 times). Peel the electrodes off their backing without touching the gel or the adhesive surface.

3. Position the electrodes. Placements of the electrodes will vary, depending on the lead you want to monitor (Figure 12–5) and the number of electrodes used. The most common routine monitoring leads are lead 2 and MCL_1. Lead 2 provides the same view of cardiac activity as standard lead II; the difference is that lead 2 electrodes are placed on the chest, whereas lead II electrodes are placed on the limbs. Lead 2, however, is not the ideal lead for visualizing atrial activity or ventricular activity. A superior lead is the right chest lead, V_1, because it clearly records the sequence of ventricular depolarization. It thus facilitates differentiation of right from left premature ventricular beats; right from left bundle branch block; and premature

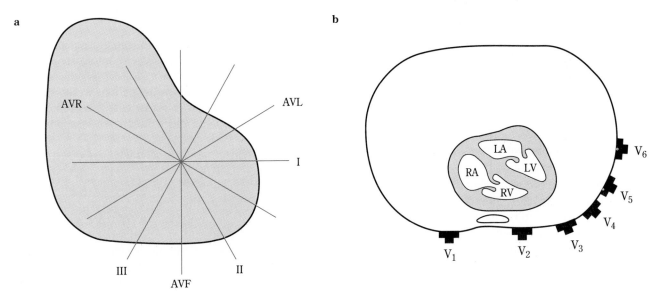

FIGURE 12–4

ECG views of the heart. **a,** Frontal plane (hexaxial reference system). Leads are labeled at their positive poles. **b,** Horizontal plane (precordial leads). *RA,* right atrium; *RV,* right ventricle; *LA,* left atrium; *LV,* left ventricle.

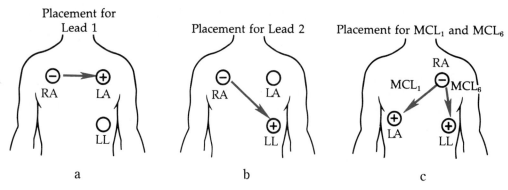

FIGURE 12–5

Placement of electrodes for routine monitoring. **a,** For lead 1, place electrode marked ⊖ or RA under right clavicle, electrode marked + or LA under left clavicle, and electrode marked ground or LL at sixth or seventh intercostal space in anterior axillary line. Place selector switch on lead 1. **b,** To monitor lead 2, place electrodes as in lead 1 and set switch on lead 2. The machine will read the RA electrode as negative and the LL electrode as positive. **c,** To monitor MCL$_1$ or MCL$_6$, place electrode marked – or RA under left clavicle, electrode marked + or LA in V$_1$ position, and electrode marked ground or LL in V$_6$ position. Then switch selector to lead 1 position to obtain MCL$_1$ and lead 2 position to obtain MCL$_6$.

left ventricular beats from premature right bundle aberrant beats. Unfortunately, routine monitoring in this lead is mechanically inconvenient, since it requires four limb electrodes plus a precordial electrode. MCL$_1$ is a lead developed to overcome the diagnostic disadvantages of lead 2 and the mechanical disadvantages of lead V$_1$. Using MCL$_1$ in combination with an additional MCL$_6$ electrode will provide additional dysrhythmia diagnostic data.

4. After placing the electrodes and setting the selector knob, observe the ECG pattern on the screen. Adjust the position of the baseline with the position knob. If the complexes are not tall enough to be counted by the machine's rate meter, increase them with the sensitivity knob. (This knob sometimes is labeled "gain" or "size.")

5. Next note the rate being displayed on the rate readout. Set the rate alarms according to the limits at which you want to be alerted. For the patient with a satisfactory rate, these limits usually are ±20 beats from the patient's normal rate. For patients with abnormally slow or fast rates, you may wish to narrow the limits to deviations of 10 beats per minute in the abnormal direction. For example, for a patient with a heart rate of 60, you might place the low-rate alarm at 50 and the high-rate alarm at 90.

6. Trigger a printout of the rhythm by pressing the appropriate button or switch on the monitor. Analyze the rhythm and mount it in the patient's chart along with your admission nursing assessment.

7. Many monitors will also store additional patient information, such as the patient's name, age, or weight, which requires keypad entry.

Monitoring Problems Common monitoring problems include muscle artifact, 60-cycle interference, and wandering baseline (Figure 12–6). *Muscle artifact* appears as random, narrow deflections in the tracing. Make sure the patient is warm and in a comfortable position. Position the electrodes over less muscular areas.

The baseline may appear thickened due to poor electrode contact or electrical interference with the machine. Reposition the electrodes over more bony areas and make sure the straps are tight enough to hold them securely. With *60-cycle interference,* you actually may be able to see 60 tiny peaks per second in the baseline due to electrical interference. If the patient's bed is electric, unplug it. Also check for broken electrode wires or cable. Ground other electrical equipment in the immediate vicinity.

When the baseline does not remain centered on the paper but instead moves up and down, it is said to be wandering. *Wandering baseline* is due to respiratory or muscle movement. Reposition the electrodes.

RESEARCH NOTE

Drew B, Ide B, Sparacino P
Accuracy of electrocardiographic monitoring: A report on current practices of critical care nurses.
Heart Lung 1991; 20:597–608.

CLINICAL APPLICATION

Lead selection and accuracy of lead placement are important variables in analyzing electrocardiographic monitoring data. Diagnostic criteria for dysrhythmia interpretation are frequently "lead specific." Are nurses selecting the appropriate lead for monitoring a particular patient? Once the lead is selected, are the electrodes correctly placed to obtain reliable data from this lead?

A random sample of 1,000 staff nurse members of the American Association of Critical-Care Nurses (AACN) was surveyed by questionnaire to elicit this information, with a response of 302 nurses. The questionnaire asked respondents to demonstrate the usual admission lead placement on a diagram and requested similar demonstration of MCL_1 or MCL_6. Additionally, the questionnaire queried respondents regarding selection of a particular lead, use of simultaneous leads, routine assessment of more than one lead in tachycardias, and resources for technical information. The chi-square test was used to determine the statistical significance of factor differences.

Data analysis indicated that 74% of these responding selected Lead II for single-channel monitoring. Eighty-seven percent of the nurses selected Lead II plus V_1 or MCL_1 for dual-channel monitoring. The low correct lead placement rate (37% for single lead and 13% for dual lead) is a cause for concern. Findings showed that the left leg electrode frequently was placed too high on the chest. Of even more importance was the imprecise positioning of the chest electrode of V_1 or MCL_1. This error could invalidate QRS pattern criteria for distinguishing ventricular tachycardia from supraventricular tachycardia with a wide complex.

CRITICAL THINKING

Limitations: The sample size was small with a low (30%) response rate. The sample reflected a motivated subgroup of critical-care nurses (members of AACN who took the time to respond) and may therefore represent above average nursing practice. One wonders if the same practices would be verified by another study method.

Strengths: The study raises concerns about inappropriate lead selection, inaccurate lead placement, and ineffective monitoring practices by nurses. If these concerns are verified by observation of practice, this study may document generalizable nursing education needs. These needs are for increased understanding of the goals of monitoring a particular patient, the lead specificity of diagnostic monitoring criteria, and the value of correct lead selection and placement.

ECG Analysis

ECG analysis is most meaningful when you comprehend the relationship between the electrical forces in the heart and the recording obtained at the chest surface.

Membrane Potentials and the ECG   All heart cells have a membrane potential, which is simply a difference in electrical charge across a semipermeable cell membrane. There are two types of potentials: the *resting membrane potential* (RMP), and the *action potential,* which has two stages, depolarization and repolarization. These potentials and their relationship to ionic movement are depicted in Figure 12–7, which diagrams the recording from a microelectrode inserted inside a *ventricular* (nonpacemaker) cell.

Three channels allow ions to move across cell membranes: *fast* channels, *slow* channels, and *potassium* channels. Their characteristics are presented in Table 12–1.

Membrane potentials are affected by both the permeability of the cell membrane to sodium (Na^+), calcium (Ca^{++}) and potassium (K^+) ions and the rate at which these ions pass across the membrane. In the resting state, no electrical activity is occurring. Sodium and potassium each establishes its own equilibrium across the cell membrane. Relatively more sodium is outside the cell. Relatively more potassium is inside the cell. Although the cell contains many positively charged potassium ions and fewer positively charged

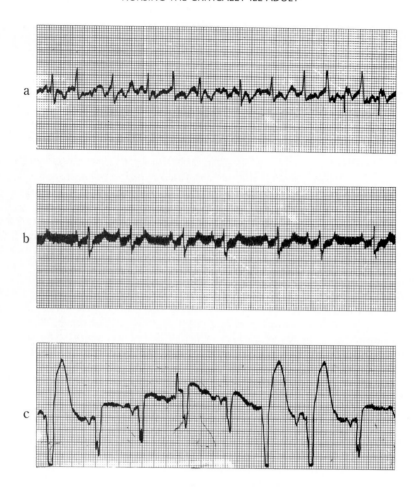

FIGURE 12–6

ECG artifacts. **a,** Muscle movement; **b,** 60-cycle interference; **c,** wandering baseline.

sodium ions, these positive charges are exceeded by negatively charged ions, primarily proteins and phosphates. As a result, the cell is polarized with more negative charges inside and more positive charges outside. This stage is represented by an isoelectric (flat) line on the ventricular action potential diagram at –90 mV.

When a sufficient stimulus occurs, membrane permeability changes. This stimulus may be electrical, chemical (as in hypoxia), or mechanical (as in chamber dilatation). If the stimulation is strong enough, the membrane will reach a certain point at which its potential changes significantly. This point is called the *threshold.* If the membrane reaches threshold, an action potential occurs on an all-or-none basis—that is, either the whole membrane changes its potential or none of it does. The action potential results from the movement of ions into and out of the cell according to the membrane's permeability for each ion and the gradient of each ion across the cell membrane.

When stimulation occurs and threshold potential is reached, the complex *fast-channel* gating mechanism opens, allowing the membrane to become much more permeable to sodium. It allows such a large amount of sodium ions to rush into the cell, carrying their positive charges with them, that the inside of the cell rapidly becomes positive. Because the cell now is more positive inside than outside (the reversal of the polarized state), this process is called *depolarization.* On the action potential diagram, depolarization is seen as a rapid upstroke (phase 0). It ends with a spike on the action potential diagram (phase 1), representing early *repolarization* as the fast channels close.

The cell remains with little or no voltage change during a plateau period (phase 2), as the slow channels open and calcium leaks in. Because calcium ions are positive, they sustain the positivity inside the cell, which provides time for the release of intracellular calcium stores and contraction of the car-

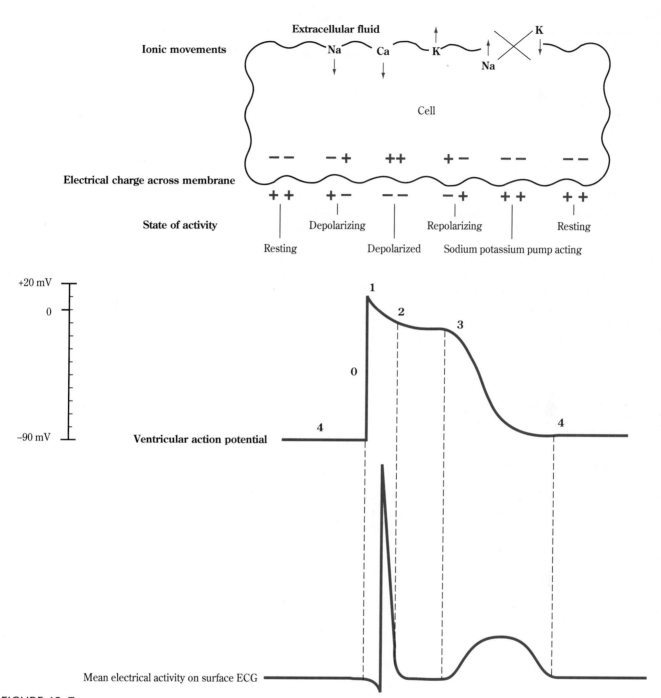

FIGURE 12–7

Ionic movements related to ventricular action potential.

diac muscle fiber. The plateau ends abruptly with final repolarization (phase 3) as the slow channels close and the potassium channels open (Guyton 1991). As potassium diffuses out of the cell, the potential becomes progressively more negative until it returns to resting potential (phase 4). Although the overall balance of positive versus negative charges is restored, the distribution of most of the sodium and potassium is the reverse of what it was in the original polarized state. Using energy, the sodium-potassium pump in the cell membrane transports sodium out of the cell and potassium back in to restore the correct balance. This restoration does not disrupt the phase 4 baseline.

TABLE 12–1

Depolarization Channels

CHANNEL	MEMBRANE POTENTIAL	IONIC MOVEMENT	RESULT
Fast	–90 mV	Sodium into cell	Rapid depolarization of muscle cells
Slow	–60 mV	Calcium-sodium into cell	Pacemaker activity of SA node, AV junction, and possibly ectopic sites
			Prolongation of phase 2 in nonpacemaker cells (follows fast-channel activity
Potassium	——	Potassium out of cell	Speedy repolarization (follows slow-channel activity)

Refractory Periods During phases 0, 1, and 2, the myocardial cells cannot respond to another impulse. This time is called the *absolute refractory period*. During phase 3, repolarization, the cell may respond to an impulse. This period is called the *relative refractory period*. During the relative refractory period, a stimulus must be stronger than usual to evoke a response. At the end of phase 3, however, there is a temporary increase in excitability, during which a weaker than normal impulse can provoke repetitive depolarization; this time is called the *vulnerable period*. During phase 4, no refractoriness is present, so excitability is normal.

Conduction System Changes in membrane potential spread more rapidly along the heart's conduction system than through other cardiac cells. Figure 12–8 shows the major components of the conduction system. They are not nerves but rather specialized muscle

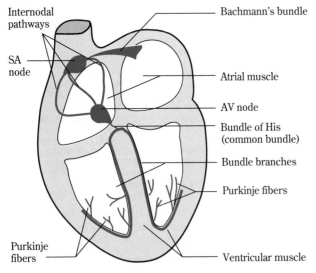

Internodal pathways — Bachmann's bundle
SA node
Atrial muscle
AV node
Bundle of His (common bundle)
Bundle branches
Purkinje fibers
Purkinje fibers — Ventricular muscle

FIGURE 12–8

Cardiac conduction system.

tissue. Normally, impulses arise in the *sinoatrial (SA) node* at the juncture of the right atrium and superior vena cava. From the sinus node, they spread across the atria and over preferential pathways to the *atrioventricular (AV) node* and left atrium. The preferential pathways to the AV node are the anterior, middle, and posterior internodal bundles. Bachmann's bundle, a branch of the anterior internodal bundle, is the preferential pathway to the left atrium. The AV node is located just to the right of the base of the interatrial septum and above the tricuspid valve. The impulses next travel to the *bundle of His,* which extends leftward from the AV node into the upper membranous part of the interventricular septum. (The AV node and bundle of His sometimes are referred to as the AV junction.) The bundle of His, also called the common bundle, splits into *right and left bundle branches* that travel down the muscular interventricular septum. The left bundle branch has two major divisions to the left ventricle, the anterior-superior branch and the posterior-inferior branch. The bundle branches split into the terminal part of the conduction system, the network of *Purkinje fibers,* which spreads the impulses from the endocardium to the epicardium.

Cells in the conduction system have different transmembrane potentials from cells outside the system (Figure 12–9). The most important difference relates to the resting phase. The phase 4 of cells outside the system is stable; they must wait for a stimulus to depolarize them. In contrast, the resting phase of cells inside the system shows a gentle positive slope. These cells are able to reach threshold potential spontaneously, thus depolarizing themselves. SA nodal fibers, for example, have a resting potential of approximately –60 mV. This level allows only slow calcium-sodium channels to be open, not the fast sodium channels, so the action potential develops and recovers more slowly than with ventricular cells; in addition, SA nodal fibers are "leaky" to sodium ions, which allows the resting

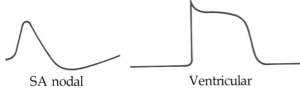

SA nodal   Ventricular

FIGURE 12–9

SA nodal versus ventricular action potentials.

RE-ENTRY

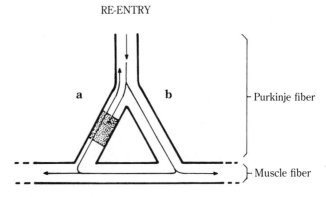

a   b   Purkinje fiber

Muscle fiber

FIGURE 12–10

Diagrammatic representation of mechanism of re-entry. Branches of Purkinje fiber which join muscle fiber are represented by **a** and **b**. Shaded area in **a** represents area of unidirectional block. (From Albarran-Sotelo R et al.: *Textbook of advanced cardiac life support.* Dallas: American Heart Association, 1987, 1990, p. 48. Reproduced with permission. © American Heart Association.)

potential to rise slowly until the calcium-sodium channels open and the action potential ensues (Guyton 1991). This property of spontaneous diastolic depolarization is called *automaticity*. These cells also have the property of *rhythmicity;* that is, they can depolarize themselves rhythmically. The ability to transmit electrical impulses from one cell to another is called *conductivity.*

Because cells in the conduction system can depolarize themselves, they can function as pacemakers to depolarize the rest of the heart. Pacemaker cells are of two types, dominant and latent. Although *latent* pacemakers exhibit diastolic depolarization, they usually become excited by an impulse transmitted from higher up in the system before they reach threshold spontaneously. A latent pacemaker may become a *dominant* pacemaker if it speeds up, a higher pacemaker slows down, or impulses from a higher pacemaker become blocked. Normally, the SA node is the dominant pacemaker because it can depolarize itself faster than the other potential pacemakers, 60–100 times a minute. If it slows down, fails, or becomes blocked, the next pacemaker to take over is the AV junction, at 40–60 beats per minute. If the Purkinje fibers are not depolarized by the SA node or AV junction, they will depolarize spontaneously at 20–40 beats per minute.

The two major mechanisms of impulse formation are automaticity and re-entry. *Normal automaticity,* described earlier, is present in pacemaker cells. *Abnormal automaticity* may result from impulse formation related to abnormal slow-channel activity. The other mechanism of impulse formation is *re-entry,* which can occur inside or outside the conduction system. For re-entry to occur, there must be branching conduction pathways. One pathway must have a unidirectional *(antegrade)* block or a longer refractory period than the other pathway.

Figure 12–10 diagrams one type of re-entry. It shows a Purkinje fiber that branches in two and serves a ventricular muscle fiber. The impulse from the Purkinje fiber starts to travel down both branches but is blocked in one branch. It travels down the other branch, through the muscle fiber, and arrives at the bottom of the first branch. From there, it spreads retrograde (backward up the branch) to the original starting point, which by now has repolarized. From that point, it can travel through the rest of the conduction system, creating an isolated ectopic beat or a series of fast, repetitive beats, which appear as tachycardia. In the atria, for example, this mechanism is thought to be responsible for producing atrial tachycardia.

Impulse formation and propagation are affected by many stimuli discussed elsewhere in the text. Briefly, sympathetic nerves (from the cervical and upper thoracic sympathetic ganglion chain) innervate the SA node, AV node, and ventricles. When sympathetic stimulation is increased, impulses are formed and conducted more quickly, and the ventricles contract more forcefully.

Parasympathetic control is provided by the vagus nerves from the medulla. Parasympathetic fibers innervate the SA and AV nodes. When parasympathetic stimulation is increased, impulses are formed and conducted more slowly.

Refer to Chapter 10 for detailed discussion of cardiovascular dynamics and hormonal and chemical influences on cardiac impulses. The blood supply to the conduction system is discussed in detail in the myocardial infarction section of Chapter 13.

Vectors and the ECG To interpret an ECG, you must have a clear mental picture of the relationship between the 12 leads and the heart's position in the frontal and transverse planes. If this is unclear, review the previous sections of this chapter dealing with those topics before proceeding with the following sections on ECG analysis.

At a given point in time, numerous cardiac cells' individual membrane potential changes interact to form an electrical force. This force, called a *vector,* has both direction and magnitude. It can be recorded by an ECG electrode on the chest surface.

It is important to recognize that the ECG records only the heart's electrical activity, not its mechanical activity, which follows electrical activation. It thus can record depolarization and repolarization, but not chamber contraction and relaxation nor valvular motion. Since the ECG can record electrical activity even in the absence of mechanical response, a rhythm can occur without a pulse. This uncommon event is called electromechanical dissociation (EMD).

The surface ECG is able to record the relatively large vectors of the atria and ventricles but not the smaller vectors of individual parts of the conduction system. Whenever it is unable to detect electrical activity, it records a straight line, called the *baseline* or *isoelectric line.* When it detects a vector, it records a deflection from the baseline.

The direction and magnitude of the deflection depend on (a) the distance between the force's starting point and the lead, and (b) the relation between the force's direction and the lead's axis, the imaginary line between the poles of the lead (Figure 12–11). If the force's direction is toward the lead's positive pole, a positive deflection is recorded. If it is directed away from the positive pole, a negative deflection is recorded. The more parallel the force is to the lead, the larger the recorded deflection; the more perpendicular, the smaller the deflection. If the force and lead are completely perpendicular to each other, no deflection is recorded. When the positive and negative forces are equal, a diphasic (part negative, part positive) deflection is recorded. In this case, the mean vector is perpendicular.

Labeling Deflections By convention, the deflections are labeled with the letters P through U (Figure 12–12). Atrial depolarization, as impulses travel from the SA node through both atria to the AV node, produces the *P wave.* Ventricular depolarization, as impulses travel from the bundle branches through the ventricles, causes the *QRS complex.* Ventricular repolarization is seen as the *T wave.*

Intervals including or between these deflections are labeled as follows. The *PR interval* is from the start of atrial depolarization (the P wave) to start of ventricular depolarization (the QRS). It represents the length of time for an impulse to depolarize the atria and travel

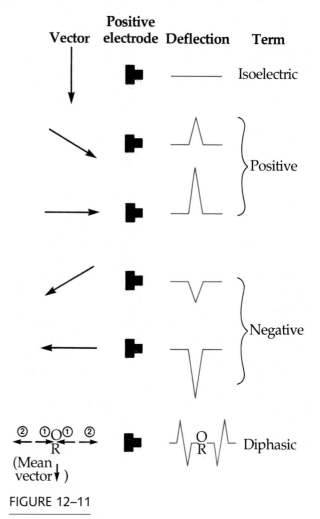

FIGURE 12–11

Vectors and associated ECG deflections.

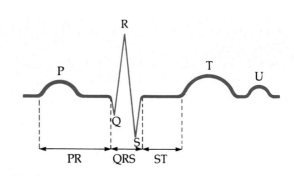

FIGURE 12–12

ECG deflections and intervals.

through the AV junction and bundle of His to the bundle branches. The *ST segment* is the interval between the end of ventricular depolarization (QRS) and the T wave. The end of the S wave and start of the

Examples of P waves

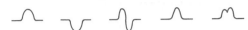

Positive Negative Diphasic Peaked Notched

Examples of QRS complexes

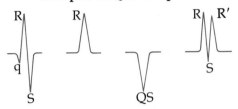

Examples of T waves

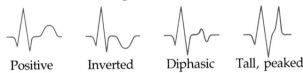

Positive   Inverted   Diphasic   Tall, peaked

FIGURE 12–13

Labeling ECG deflections.

ST segment sometimes is referred to as the J point. The *QT interval* is the duration of ventricular depolarization and repolarization. It is measured from the beginning of the QRS to the end of the T wave.

P and T waves are called those whether they are positive, negative, or diphasic. In contrast, the letters used to label the QRS complex vary with the polarity and sequence of the deflections. *QRS complex* is a generic term applied to any ventricular depolarization; combinations of these letters are used to designate specific ventricular configurations (Figure 12–13). The first negative deflection after the P wave is called a *Q wave*. The first positive deflection after the P wave is called an *R wave*. The first negative deflection after the R wave is called an *S wave*. If the QRS complex consists of only one negative wave, it is called a QS configuration. Other variations include the notched R, when the negative deflection after the R wave does not reach the baseline, and the RSR', when it does. The relative size of the ventricular deflections can be indicated by using small letters for small waves and capital letters for large ones.

Correlation with Action Potential The QRST complex corresponds approximately to the phases of the ventricular action potential described earlier. The QRS corresponds with ventricular depolarization and early repolarization (phases 0 and 1). The ST segment represents phase 2, the plateau. The T wave corresponds with final repolarization during phase 3. The

---

NURSING TIP

Premature Beats

An atrial premature beat (APB) falling during the ventricles' absolute refractory period cannot depolarize them. A ventricular premature beat (VPB) occurring during the vulnerable period of the T wave (R-on-T phenomenon), however, can provoke lethal ventricular tachycardia or ventricular fibrillation. For this reason, keep an eagle eye on the distance between T waves and ventricular premature beats!

---

baseline between complexes corresponds with phase 4, the resting potential.

The QRST complex also corresponds with the refractory periods mentioned earlier. The QRS and ST segment correspond roughly with the absolute refractory period. The T wave corresponds with the relative refractory period, with the T wave's downstroke corresponding with the vulnerable period.

Plotting Vectors Vectors can be plotted on reference systems to determine their normality. Although plotting is an advanced skill that you may not perform yourself, it is valuable to understand the vector concept for two reasons: axis deviation is determined by vector analysis, and comprehension of normal vectors will help you spot whether a given deflection is normal for the lead in which it appears.

Frontal plane vectors can be plotted on the hexaxial reference system (Figure 12–14). This reference system is formed by the intersection of the six frontal leads, which divide the frontal plane into 30° units. By convention, all degrees in the upper half of the figure are negative and all those in the lower half are positive. This convention is unrelated to the positive and negative poles of a lead. For example, AVL's positive pole is at –30°, while AVR's negative pole is at +30°.

The hexaxial reference system is divided into quadrants by leads I and AVF. Lead I divides the body into superior and inferior parts, and lead AVF, into right and left sides. By examining deflections in those leads, you can determine the quadrant of the reference figure into which the vector falls and the direction of the vector in the heart.

For instance, suppose you found a patient's QRS complex to be positive in both leads I and AVF. You could refer to Figure 12–14 and note that the quadrant in which both of these leads have a positive QRS is the quadrant of normal axis. Alternatively, you could reason out the axis. If the QRS is positive in lead I, the electrical activity must be traveling toward the positive pole of lead I, that is, the left side of the body. If it is positive in lead AVF, it must also be traveling toward AVF's positive pole, that is, the foot. Thus, the vector is leftward and inferior.

It is possible to locate the vector more precisely. For details of the technique, consult a cardiology text. Horizontal plane vectors also can be plotted on a precordial reference figure formed by the six precordial leads.

Axis Deviation The most important vectors are the mean frontal P, QRS, and T vectors and the initial QRS vector. The mean frontal P, QRS, and T vectors of the normal electrocardiogram lie within the quadrant bounded by the positive sides of leads I and AVF (0° to +90°). This signifies that the mean direction of atrial depolarization, ventricular depolarization, and ventricular repolarization is leftward and inferior. Since this is the normal direction, the person is said to have a normal axis. If the vectors fall outside the quadrant, axis deviation is present. Axis deviation can result from different positions of the heart within the chest cavity, cardiac disease (such as hypertrophy or conduction disturbances), or disease of other chest

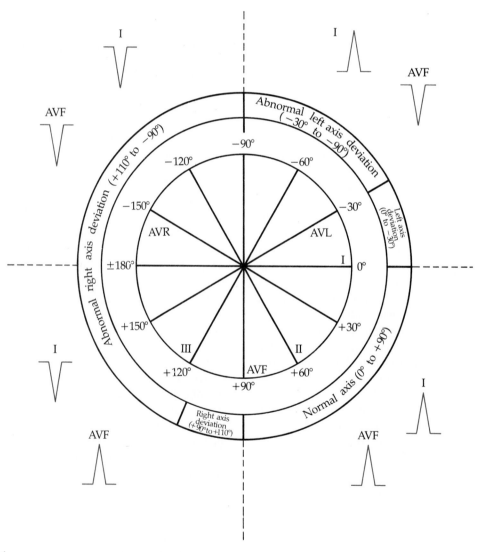

FIGURE 12–14

Hexaxial reference figure for determination of mean frontal QRS vector.

organs that alters their ability to conduct electrical impulses.

A mean QRS vector between +90° and −90° to the right of the axis of lead AVF indicates right axis deviation. That within the range of +90° to +110° may be normal. Right axis deviation from +110° to −90° is abnormal and usually results from right ventricular hypertrophy or right bundle branch block. A mean QRS vector between 0° and −90° represents left axis deviation. The range from 0° to −30° may be normal. Abnormal left axis deviation (−30° to −90°) suggests left ventricular hypertrophy or left anterior hemiblock.

Vectors and Related ECG Deflections The next section discusses the P, QRS, and T wave vectors and the ECG complexes they produce. The vectors are shown diagrammatically in Figure 12–15.

The *P wave* represents right atrial depolarization followed by left atrial depolarization. Sinus P waves usually are rounded and symmetric, with a low amplitude or voltage. The normal mean frontal P wave axis is about +60°. Looking on the hexaxial reference figure, you can see that the leads closest to this vector are II and AVR, with the vector moving toward the positive pole of lead II and away from the positive pole of AVR. You can anticipate, then, that in normal sinus rhythm, II and AVR are the leads which will best display atrial activity, and the P wave will be positive in II and negative in AVR. The P wave normally is positive in the remaining limb and precordial leads. Occasionally, however, the normal P wave is negative, flat, or diphasic in III or AVL.

Following atrial depolarization, an isoelectric line is recorded as the impulse travels through the AV node, the bundle of His, and bundle branches. The interval from the start of the P wave to the end of this isoelectric line (that is, to the start of the QRS) is known as the *PR interval*.

Atrial repolarization usually is not recorded because it is obscured by ventricular depolarization.

The *QRS complex* represents ventricular depolarization. The frontal plane QRS axis normally lies from 0° to +90° and varies with age. It is about +60° to +90° in the young adult and moves leftward (more horizontally) with increasing age. Ventricular depolarization normally starts on the left side of the interventricular septum and initially moves to the right across the septum and anteriorly to the tip of the right ventricle. This initial QRS vector also moves either inferiorly or superiorly. The inferior orientation is more common in the person with a more horizontal mean QRS vector.

Small negative deflections *(normal Q waves)* may be present in some leads. These normal Q waves represent septal depolarization. In addition to the patient's axis and lead in which Q waves are seen, normal Q waves are defined by width and depth. These criteria

LEAD II

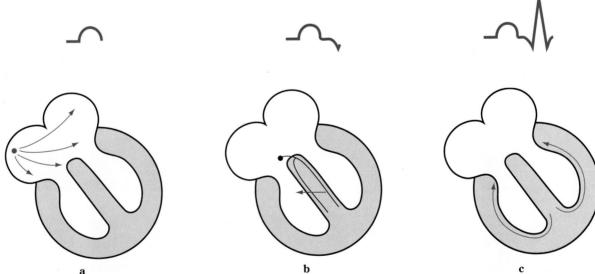

a   b   c

FIGURE 12–15

ECG deflections and sequence of depolarization. **a,** Atrial depolarization—P wave vector is leftward, inferior, and anterior. **b,** septal depolarization—initial QRS vector is rightward, anterior, and either inferior or superior. **c,** free ventricular wall depolarization—mean QRS vector is leftward, inferior, and posterior.

vary with leads, but in general a Q wave is abnormal if it (1) appears in a lead where it was not present earlier, (2) is more than 0.04 second wide, (3) is greater than one-fourth the height of the R wave, or (4) accompanies a left bundle branch block in leads I, AVL, AVF, V_4, V_5, or V_6. The reason for the latter criterion is that left bundle branch block usually causes the loss of normal Q waves in leads oriented toward the left ventricle; therefore, the appearance of even a small Q wave in these leads usually indicates an infarction in addition to the bundle branch block.

Depolarization next spreads through the right and left free ventricular walls, from endocardium to epicardium. Because the muscle mass of the left ventricle is larger than that of the right ventricle, the ECG reflects primarily left ventricular vectors, which are oriented leftward and inferiorly. They progress from the initial anterior orientation toward a strongly posterior orientation, because the bulk of the left ventricle is posterior.

The posterior base of the ventricles is the last area depolarized. This vector is posterior, superior, and rightward.

The changing QRS vectors are reflected in the ECG (Figure 12–16). They cause increasingly positive waves (R waves) in leads toward whose positive poles they are traveling and increasingly negative waves (S waves) in leads away from whose positive poles they are traveling. Thus, lead II normally is characterized by a small Q wave (of septal depolarization) and large R wave, while AVR displays a normal deep, wide QS wave. V_1 normally is characterized by either a large wide Q wave or a small R wave and large S wave. The R wave becomes progressively larger and the S wave progressively smaller from V_1 to V_6.

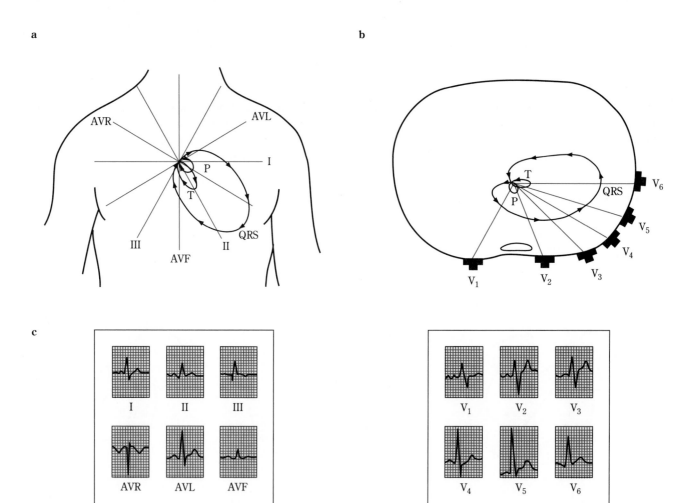

FIGURE 12–16

Normal patterns of depolarization and related deflections on 12-lead ECG. **a,** Frontal plane; **b,** transverse plane; **c,** order of appearance on 12-lead ECG.

The *ST segment* is isoelectric because early ventricular repolarization is very slow. The ST segment should be level with the PR interval line. Abnormal elevation is 1 mm or more above the line and abnormal depression 1 mm or more below it. ST segment deviations may indicate myocardial ischemia and injury. They are discussed in greater detail in Chapter 13.

The *T wave* represents ventricular repolarization and is evaluated by vector, size, and shape. Normally, the T wave is positive when the QRS is predominantly positive and negative when the QRS is negative. If the T wave's polarity is opposite to that of the QRS, the T wave is called *inverted*. The T wave usually is rounded and symmetric. A T wave greater than 0.3 mV (3 mm) tall in a precordial lead is abnormally high or deep.

The *QT interval* represents the length of time for ventricular depolarization and repolarization. Measured from the beginning of the QRS to the end of the T wave, this interval varies with heart rate, and needs to be rate-corrected by calculating the QT_c ($QT_c = QT/\sqrt{RR \text{ interval}}$). The QT is lengthened by certain antidysrhythmics (e.g., quinidine, disopyramide, and procainamide), hypokalemia, and some psychoactive drugs. A lengthened QT may precipitate torsades de pointes.

NURSING TIP

T Waves

Tall, narrow, peaked T waves are seen in hyperkalemia. Giant inverted T waves commonly appear with myocardial infarction and ventricular premature beats.

Sometimes, a small wave is recorded after the T wave. This *U wave* is poorly understood but may represent the very end of ventricular repolarization.

ECG wave configuration or interval lengths may be altered by numerous factors. These factors include metabolic imbalances and pharmacologic effects, as presented in Table 12–2.

Analyzing the ECG   Train yourself to use a systematic approach to ECG analysis so that you do not overlook important data. The exact sequence is not as

---

TABLE 12–2

Metabolic and Drug Influences on the ECG

Hyperkalemia	Mild to moderate (K = 5–7 mEq/L): Tall, symmetrically peaked T waves with a narrow base
	More severe (K = 8–11 mEq/L): QRS widens, PR segment prolongs, P wave disappears; ECG resembles a sine wave in severe cases
Hypokalemia	ST depression
	T wave flattening
	Large positive U wave
Hypercalcemia	Shortened QT interval due to a shortened ST segment
Hypocalcemia	Prolonged QT interval due to a prolonged ST segment; T wave duration normal
Hypothermia	Osborne or J waves: J point elevation with a characteristic elevation of the early ST segment. Slow rhythm, baseline artifact due to shivering often present.
Digitalis	ST depression
	T wave flattening or inversion
	Shortened QT interval, increased U wave amplitude

Quinidine
  procainamide
  disopyramide
  phenothiazines
  tricyclic antidepressants
	Prolonged QT interval, mainly due to prolonged T wave duration with flattening or inversion
	QRS prolongation
	Increased U wave amplitude

CNS insult (e.g., intracerebral hemorrhage)	Diffuse, wide, deeply inverted T waves with prolonged QT

(From Andreoli T et al. Cecil Essentials of Medicine. Philadelphia: Saunders, 1986)

important as your consistency in using it. The following approach integrates analysis of the timing of cardiac events and waveform configurations. It requires the use of a measuring device called *calipers*.

1. *Note ventricular regularity and measure ventricular rate.* The rate can be determined in relation to the measurements on the ECG paper (Figure 12–17). By convention, horizontal measurements represent time and vertical measurements represent electrical voltage. At the standard recording rate of 25 mm/sec, each small box measured horizontally equals 0.04 second. By remembering this value, you can figure out that each large box (five small boxes) equals 0.20 second, and 30 large boxes equal 6 seconds.

   If the rhythm is regular, there are several ways to calculate rate. Since 300 boxes equal one minute, you can count the number of large boxes between the same point on two consecutive R waves and divide into 300. This method is accurate only if each of the R waves falls on the edge of a big box. Since 1,500 small boxes also equal one minute, another way is to count the number of small boxes between two consecutive R waves and divide into 1,500. A third method is that recommended by Dubin (1988):

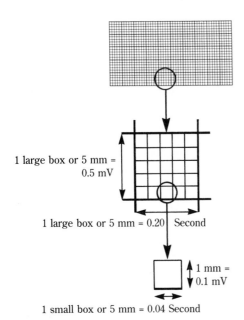

1 large box or 5 mm = 0.5 mV

1 large box or 5 mm = 0.20 Second

1 mm = 0.1 mV

1 small box or 5 mm = 0.04 Second

FIGURE 12–17

Time and voltage measurements on ECG paper (when recording speed is 25 mm/sec.)

A. Find a deflection occurring on a heavy black line. For instance, to calculate ventricular rate, look for a QRS on a heavy black line. Use the distance between it and the same point on the next QRS to calculate the rate. If there is no QRS falling exactly on a heavy line, measure the distance between two QRSs with your calipers by placing one caliper point on the first QRS and the other on the same point on the next QRS. Without changing the relative position of the points, lift the calipers to the edge of the strip and place the first point on a heavy line, as shown in Figure 12–18. Then count to the second caliper point to determine the rate.

B. Count out the rates represented by each heavy black line until you reach the ones closest to the second caliper point. The rates represented by each heavy line are shown in the figure and may be memorized easily. You can see that the rate of the strip in the figure lies between 60 and 75. (The rates shown in the figure were derived this way: A deflection occurring on each heavy line is occurring at a frequency of 1 per 0.2 second, or 300 per minute. One occurring every other black line equals a frequency of 1 per 0.4 second, or 150 per minute. The remaining rates were calculated in a similar fashion.)

C. Pinpoint the rate using the values represented by the small black lines. Although they are not as easy to remember, frequent practice with them will make them second nature. The precise ventricular rate of the strip in the figure is 65. These smaller rate divisions also were determined logically, by dividing frequencies into 60. For example, the rate 65 was obtained by adding 0.8 seconds (the frequency of the next highest heavy line) to the 0.12 second (the frequency represented by two additional small boxes), and dividing the sum 0.92 into 60 to get 65 beats per minute.

   If the rate is irregular, you can get an estimate by counting the number of R waves in a 6-second (30 large boxes) strip and multiplying it by 10.

2. *Note atrial regularity and measure the atrial rate.* Use the above methods, but calculate the distance between the same point on two consecutive P waves.

3. *Examine the P waves* to identify the source of atrial activity. What is their contour, width, and

amplitude? Do all the P waves resemble each other? Do they occur before, during, or after the QRS? Is their polarity normal for the lead you are examining?

4. *Measure the PR interval* to evaluate conduction through the atria, AV junction, and bundle of His. To do this, measure from the onset of the P wave to the onset of the first ventricular deflection (it may not always be an R wave). Multiply the number of small boxes between these points by 0.04 seconds to get the measurement. The normal PR interval is 0.12–0.20 second and constant. Is the patient's measurement normal, shortened, or prolonged? Is the PR interval constant, irregular with a consistent pattern, or completely irregular?

5. *Examine the QRS* to analyze the length and sequence of ventricular depolarization. Measure from the onset of the first ventricular deflection from the baseline to the end of the last ventricular deflection, that is, the return to the baseline. (If the demarcation between the baseline and the deflections is not clear, the onset and termination of the QRS may be difficult to detect. Sometimes, you will be able to see the change from a thick line, caused by slow electrical activity, to a thinner line result-

ing from the faster ventricular depolarization.) Multiply the number of small boxes by 0.04 seconds to get the measurement. The normal QRS interval is 0.06–0.10 second and constant. Is the patient's value normal or prolonged? Is it constant, variable with a consistent pattern, or completely variable?

Examine the QRS deflections to assess the direction of ventricular depolarization. Are the deflections appropriate to the lead? If a Q wave is present, is its presence normal for that patient and lead? Is the appearance of the QRS similar for all complexes in a given lead?

6. *Examine the ST segment and T wave* to evaluate ventricular repolarization. Is the ST segment normal (isoelectric and level with the flat part of the PR interval), elevated above the baseline, or depressed? Is the T wave normal or abnormal?

7. *Measure the QT interval, and rate-correct it* using a nomogram. Is the QT_c normal, short, or prolonged?

In summary, the normal ECG has the following characteristics. The impulse originates in the SA node at a rate of 60–100 beats per minute. It produces a P wave that is symmetric and rounded and that precedes ventricular activity. It travels across the atria, the AV

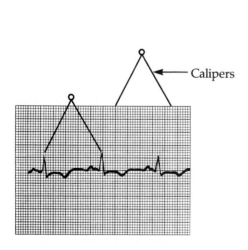

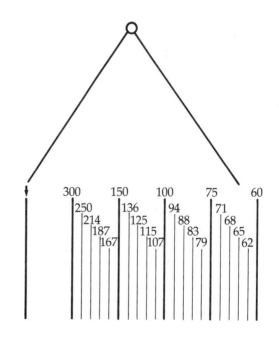

FIGURE 12–18

Rapid rate calculation for regular rhythms. (Adapted from Dubin D: *Rapid interpretation of EKG's,* 4th ed. Tampa, FL: COVER Publishing Co. 1989, pp. 68 and 281. Used with permission of Dale Dubin, M.D. and COVER Publishing Co.)

node, and the bundle of His in 0.12–0.20 second. It produces a QRS complex that lasts 0.06–0.10 second. The complex is followed by an isoelectric ST segment and a T wave that is symmetric, rounded, and of the same polarity as the QRS. The vectors of the P wave, QRS complex, and T wave are appropriate for the lead being examined. The rate-corrected QT interval is appropriate for the heart rate.

Common Dysrhythmias

Rhythms traditionally are classified on the basis of their origin and their underlying mechanisms. The origin of a dysrhythmia may be the sinus node, atria, AV junction, or ventricles. Mechanisms usually are grouped into disturbances of impulse formation and disturbances of impulse conduction (blocks). Definitions of disturbances of impulse formation follow.

A *bradycardia* is any rhythm with a regular ventricular rate under 60 beats per minute (bpm).

A *tachycardia* is any rhythm with a regular ventricular rate over 100 bpm. Not all interpreters use this terminology. For instance, a spontaneous ventricular rhythm usually has a rate between 20 and 40 bpm. If the rate exceeds 40, some interpreters call it ventricular tachycardia; similarly, a junctional rhythm over 60 bpm may be called a junctional tachycardia. You can see how confusing this usage is, since "tachycardia" used this way can refer to a ventricular rate above 40, 60, or 100 bpm. For clarity, restrict the term *tachycardia* to rates over 100. Rates less than 100 bpm, but above normal for their sources, are best called *accelerated*.

Flutter is a regular rhythm, more rapid than tachycardia, with a saw-toothed appearance. The term usually is applied only to an atrial dysrhythmia, although an occasional author calls ventricular tachycardia with this contour ventricular flutter.

Fibrillation refers to chaotic depolarization. It produces an irregular, wavy baseline in which complexes cannot be distinguished clearly. Fibrillation may occur in either the atria or the ventricles.

The disturbances of impulse formation are named by combining their source with their mechanism—for example, *sinus bradycardia*. To enable you to compare and contrast the basic sinus, atrial, junctional, and ventricular rhythms, their characteristics are presented in tabular form and illustrated with ECG strips. Table 12–3 presents sinus rhythms; Table 12–4, paroxysmal supraventricular tachycardias; Table 12–5,

atrial rhythms; Table 12–6, junctional rhythms; and Table 12–7, ventricular rhythms.

Conduction Defects

Disturbances of impulse conduction also may occur. These are called *blocks* and are subdivided into sinus blocks, atrioventricular (AV) blocks, bundle branch blocks, and hemiblocks (block of a subdivision of the left bundle branch). AV blocks, bundle branch blocks, and hemiblocks are the most common and are presented in this chapter.

A block may be superimposed on any disturbance of the cardiac rhythm; thus, a patient might have an atrial tachycardia with AV block or a normal sinus rhythm with bundle branch block. Labeling of AV blocks can be confusing. To label an AV block, count the number of P waves per QRS. For example, if a rhythm had two P waves for each QRS, it would be described as a 2:1 block. Occasionally, an atrial wave may be obscured by the QRS deflections. To detect a hidden wave, use your ECG calipers to measure the P–P interval on visible waves. If the distance between the P waves just before and just after a QRS is twice the measured P–P interval, you can deduce that a P wave is being obscured by the QRS. Atrioventricular blocks are shown in Table 12–8.

AV dissociation is a term that means the atria and ventricles are beating independently, that is, dissociated. Because AV dissociation can occur with many different dysrhythmias, it is not a primary dysrhythmia. Whenever you use the term, you also must state the primary rhythms causing atrial and ventricular beating—for example, AV dissociation with sinus bradycardia and ventricular rhythm. AV dissociation may occur in three different ways. If the primary pacemaker slows, a latent pacemaker may escape from a lower site. An example is the sinus bradycardia and ventricular rhythm mentioned above. AV dissociation also may occur if the primary pacemaker discharges at a normal rate but an ectopic pacemaker accelerates. An example of this category is sinus rhythm and ventricular tachycardia. The third way that AV dissociation may occur is if impulses from the primary pacemaker become completely blocked (third-degree AV block). This type of dissociation is detected easily if the atrial rate is greater than the ventricular. If the ventricular rate is greater than the atrial, however, you cannot tell just from the ECG strip whether a third-degree block is present. It is possible, however, that a third-degree block occurred followed by acceleration of a rhythm from a junctional or ventricular focus. In order to diagnose the cause of the dissociation in this case, the physician will attempt to accelerate the rhythm driving the atria to see whether a block is in fact present.

In the first two types of dissociation, AV conduction is normal. Occasionally, then, when a P wave is far enough away from a QRS, it may conduct to the ventricles, thus capturing (depolarizing) them. Such a beat is called a *capture beat.* It occurs because the impulse reaches the ventricles at a time when they can respond, that is, when they are not already refractory from the impulses otherwise driving them.

Bundle branch blocks (BBB) are a type of conduction disturbance in which the right or left bundle branch fails to conduct impulses. To understand the ECG patterns that result from BBBs, it is helpful to understand the relationship between the sequence of ventricular activation and the corresponding ECG

TABLE 12–3

Sinus Rhythms

REGULARITY AND RATE			AV CONDUCTION		
Ventricular	**Atrial**	**P Waves**	**P:QRS Ratio**	**PR Interval**	**QRS**
Normal Sinus Rhythm (NSR)					
Regular, 60–100	Same as ventricular	Symmetric, rounded	1:1	0.12–0.20 sec	0.06–0.10 sec

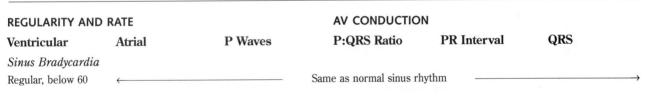

CAUSES Normal heart
SIGNIFICANCE Normal rhythm
TREATMENT None

REGULARITY AND RATE			AV CONDUCTION		
Ventricular	**Atrial**	**P Waves**	**P:QRS Ratio**	**PR Interval**	**QRS**
Sinus Bradycardia					
Regular, below 60	←————————		Same as normal sinus rhythm		————————→

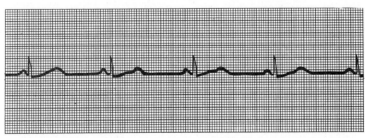

CAUSES Normal heart; athletic heart; sleep; vagal stimulation; myocardial infarction; increased intracranial pressure
SIGNIFICANCE Significance depends on rate. If moderate, allows for increased ventricular filling and decreased myocardial oxygen
                demand; if too slow, inadequate cardiac output
TREATMENT None if asymptomatic; if symptomatic, atropine, isoproterenol, or artificial pacemaker

(Continues)

TABLE 12–3 (Continued)

Sinus Rhythms

REGULARITY AND RATE			AV CONDUCTION		
Ventricular	**Atrial**	**P Waves**	**P:QRS Ratio**	**PR Interval**	**QRS**
Sinus Tachycardia					
Regular, above 100 (usually up to 180)	←		Same as normal sinus rhythm		→

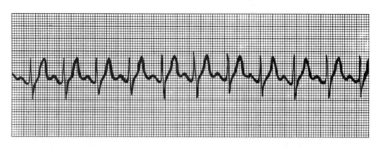

CAUSES   Normal heart: tea, coffee, tobacco, alcohol; physical or emotional stress; inflammatory heart disease; coronary artery disease
SIGNIFICANCE   Usually not significant except in patient with heart disease; then may cause angina, infarction, congestive heart failure, shock
TREATMENT   If asymptomatic, none; if symptomatic, treat the cause

REGULARITY AND RATE			AV CONDUCTION		
Ventricular	**Atrial**	**P Waves**	**P:QRS Ratio**	**PR Interval**	**QRS**
Sinus Arrhythmia					
Irregular, 60–100	←		Same as normal sinus rhythm		→

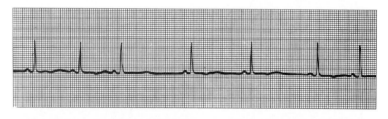

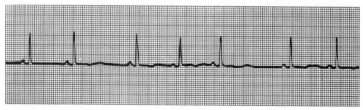

(continuous strips)

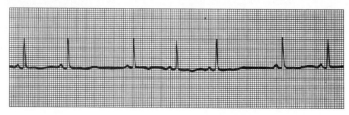

COMMENTS   Rate increases with inspiration, decreases with expiration, in cyclic fashion
CAUSES   Normal heart (variation in sympathetic and parasympathetic stimulation during respiration)
SIGNIFICANCE   Normal variant
TREATMENT   None

TABLE 12-3 (Continued)

Sinus Rhythms

REGULARITY AND RATE			AV CONDUCTION		
Ventricular	Atrial	P Waves	P:QRS Ratio	PR Interval	QRS
Sinus Arrest					
Regular but with occasional absence of entire PQRST complex; any rate	←		Same as normal sinus rhythm		→

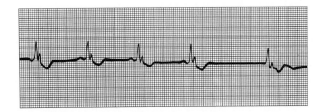

COMMENTS   Cycle containing missed beat is not a multiple of the basic sinus cycle
CAUSES   Failure of sinus node (owing to infarction), increased vagal tone, fibrosis, digitalis toxicity
SIGNIFICANCE   May be transient or prolonged. If transient, no significance; if prolonged, patient develops asystole unless escape rhythm
           occurs.
TREATMENT   If prolonged, atropine, isoproterenol, or artificial pacemaker

deflections (Table 12–9). Normally, ventricular depolarization occurs in two major steps. Septal depolarization proceeds rightward, followed by free ventricular wall depolarization. The right ventricle depolarizes rightward; simultaneously, the left ventricle depolarizes leftward. Because left ventricular muscle mass exceeds that of the right ventricle, the ECG normally reflects primarily left ventricular depolarization. This normal sequence of ventricular depolarization can be seen clearly in ECG recordings from V_1, an electrode over the right ventricle, and V_6, an electrode over the left ventricle. The wave of septal depolarization travels toward V_1 (which records a small positive or R wave) and away from V_6 (which records a small negative or Q wave). The wave of free ventricular wall depolarization travels in the opposite direction—away from V_1 (which records a large negative or S wave) and toward V_6 (which records a large positive or R wave). As a result, normal bundle branch conduction produces an rS pattern in V_1 and a qR pattern in V_6.

When the right bundle branch is blocked, right ventricular stimulation is delayed. Septal depolarization proceeds normally, rightward. The ventricles, however, no longer depolarize simultaneously; instead the left ventricle depolarizes before the right ventricle. Left ventricular depolarization proceeds normally, leftward. Because the right bundle branch cannot conduct the

impulse to the right ventricle, though, right ventricular depolarization occurs via spread of the impulse from the left ventricle. This spread occurs slowly because the impulse travels outside the conduction system; as a result, the QRS measures greater than 0.12 second. Although the length of right ventricular depolarization is prolonged, the direction remains normal, rightward. The three steps of ventricular depolarization are reflected in the ECG. Instead of the normal rS, a V_1 electrode records a triphasic (rSR') deflection: a small positive wave of septal depolarization, a large negative wave of free left ventricular wall depolarization, and a large positive wave of free right ventricular wall depolarization. The V_6 electrode also records a triphasic deflection, but it is a qRS; the q wave reflects septal depolarization, the R wave reflects left free ventricular wall depolarization, and a wide S wave reflects the slow free right ventricular wall depolarization. Due to abnormal ventricular repolarization, the T wave that follows a right BBB is inverted.

When the left bundle branch is blocked, the pattern of depolarization is disrupted to a greater extent. Septal depolarization no longer proceeds rightward; its direction is reversed. The right ventricle depolarizes next, in its normal direction (rightward). Left ventricular stimulation is delayed and occurs via spread of the impulse from the right ventricle, again outside the conduction

TABLE 12–4

Paroxysmal Supraventricular Tachycardias

REGULARITY AND RATE			AV CONDUCTION		
Ventricular	**Atrial**	**P Waves**	**P:QRS Ratio**	**PR Interval**	**QRS**
Paroxysmal Atrial Tachycardia (PAT)					
Regular, 150–250	Same as ventricular	Contour slightly different from sinus P waves	1:1	Normal or prolonged or shortened	Normal

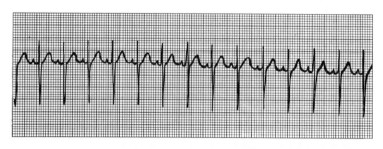

COMMENTS Onset and termination sudden
CAUSES Normal heart; stimulation from coffee, tea, tobacco; coronary artery disease; hyperthyroidism; rheumatic heart disease
         Mechanism: re-entry at AV node
SIGNIFICANCE May produce heart failure, shock, angina, dizziness
TREATMENT Depends on patient's tolerance, cause, and history of previous attacks; vagal stimulation, verapamil, cardioversion, propranolol, procainamide, digitalization, sedation

REGULARITY AND RATE			AV CONDUCTION		
Ventricular	**Atrial**	**P Waves**	**P:QRS Ratio**	**PR Interval**	**QRS**
Supraventricular Tachycardia					
Regular, 150–250	←—————————		Not detectable	—————————→	Normal

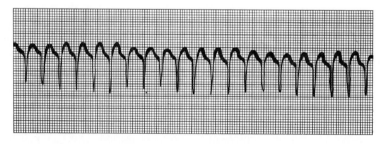

CAUSES See sinus, atrial and junctional tachycardia (Tables 12–3, 12–5, and 12–6, respectively)
SIGNIFICANCE Global term indicating rhythm originating above ventricles but whose source cannot be identified (because P waves are not clearly visible)
TREATMENT Differentiation requires additional maneuvers such as carotid sinus massage, study of a waves in jugular venous pulse, and assessment of S_1 intensity and S_2 splitting

system. The left ventricle therefore depolarizes last, but in the normal direction, leftward.

The ECG patterns again reflect the ventricular activity clearly. V_1 records a small negative wave of septal depolarization, sometimes a small positive wave of right ventricular depolarization, and a large negative wave of free left ventricular wall depolarization. These deflections usually are seen as a monophasic QS wave, sometimes with a small positive notch. The deflections may also present as a small R wave followed by a large wide S wave. The V_6 electrode records a small positive wave, sometimes a small negative wave, and a large positive wave, resulting in a wide, monophasic R wave, occasionally with a small negative notch. The

TABLE 12–4 (Continued)

Paroxysmal Supraventricular Tachycardias

REGULARITY AND RATE			AV CONDUCTION		
Ventricular	Atrial	P Waves	P:QRS Ratio	PR Interval	QRS
Supraventricular Tachycardia With Aberration					
Regular 150–250	←		Not detectable	→	Wide RBBB or LBBB pattern

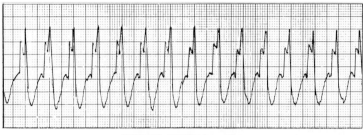

SVT with RBBB aberration

CAUSES See sinus, atrial and junctional tachycardia (Tables 12–3, 12–5, and 12–6, respectively)
SIGNIFICANCE Same as in sinus, atrial and junctional tachycardia (Tables 12–3, 12–5, and 12–6, respectively); temporarily abnormal conduction through bundle branches because supraventricular impulses fall when one branch still refractory; easily confused with ventricular tachycardia
TREATMENT As for supraventricular tachycardia

T wave usually is inverted, due to abnormal ventricular repolarization.

Because the initial forces in the right bundle branch block are not changed, ECG signs of myocardial infarction can be detected on the patient's ECG. In contrast, left BBB does alter the initial forces; when myocardial infarction occurs in the patient with left BBB, its characteristic ECG signs often are obscured.

Hemiblocks (a type of *fascicular block*) are blocks in one of the two divisions of the left bundle branch, which subdivides into an *anterior/superior fascicle* and an *inferior/posterior fascicle*. Hemiblocks are caused by the same factors that cause left BBB, which represents the block of both fascicles. The block of only one fascicle causes frontal axis deviation with a normal or slightly prolonged QRS duration.

Left anterior hemiblock (LAH) occurs more often than *left posterior hemiblock (LPH)*. The anterior fascicle is more vulnerable to injury than the posterior fascicle, because it is thinner and supplied only by the left coronary artery. LAH thus is seen in anteroseptal and anterolateral myocardial infarctions, which result from blockage of the left coronary artery. The ECG signs of LAH include left axis deviation (–45° or greater). Lead I shows an initial Q wave (qR configuration), while leads III and AVF show predominantly negative complexes (rS configurations) rather than the predominantly positive complexes normally seen in those leads.

LPH is seen less often, probably because the posterior fascicle is less vulnerable to injury due to its thickness and its dual blood supply from both the right and left coronary arteries. When LPH is seen, it usually indicates a worse prognosis than LAH, because disease extensive enough to damage the posterior fascicle often damages the anterior fascicle and right bundle branch as well. ECG signs of LPH include an axis of +120° or greater (right axis deviation). Leads I and AVL show a negative (rS) complex instead of the positive complex usually seen, while leads III and AVF have an initial Q wave (qR configuration).

No therapy is available for hemiblocks. Nursing care involves close monitoring for progression to more advanced degrees of block using a lead such as 1 or 3 to detect axis shifts. LPH is more likely than LAH to progress to more severe forms of block. Be particularly alert to the danger of progression to second- or third-degree heart block if the patient has right BBB with LAH or LPH, because only one unblocked fascicle remains to conduct impulses to the ventricles. Monitoring the patient in lead MCL$_1$ would be helpful in detecting the onset of right BBB. Also be especially

TABLE 12–5

Atrial Rhythms

| REGULARITY AND RATE | | | AV CONDUCTION | | |
Ventricular	Atrial	P Waves	P:QRS Ratio	PR Interval	QRS
Atrial tachycardia with block					
Regular if block is constant; irregular if block is variable; any rate	Regular, 150–250. If block is constant, atrial rate is multiple of ventricular rate	Contour slightly different from sinus P waves	More than 1:1	Normal or prolonged on conducted beats	Normal

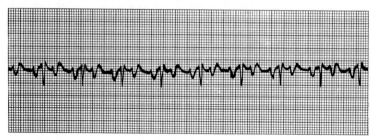

Atrial tachycardia with 2:1 block

COMMENTS If atrial rate above 200, block usually is physiologic owing to arrival of some atrial impulses at AV node during its refractory period

If atrial rate below 200, nonparoxysmal tachycardia, or block greater than 2:1, block usually due to pathology

CAUSES Coronary artery disease; digitalis intoxication

SIGNIFICANCE Symptoms depend on ventricular rate

TREATMENT If asymptomatic, observation; if digitalis is cause, discontinuation of drug, administration of potassium chloride; if digitalis not cause, digitalis to slow ventricular rate

| REGULARITY AND RATE | | | AV CONDUCTION | | |
Ventricular	Atrial	P Waves	P:QRS Ratio	PR Interval	QRS
Atrial flutter					
Regular or irregular, depending on constancy of block; any rate	Regular, 200–350. If block is constant, atrial rate is multiple of ventricular rate	Sawtooth	More than 1:1. Usually constant, even block—2:1, 4:1, etc.	Normal on conducted beats	Normal

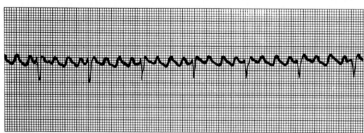

COMMENTS Mechanism probably re-entry in atria

CAUSES Coronary artery disease; mitral or tricuspid valvular disease; cor pulmonale

SIGNIFICANCE Carotid sinus massage increases degree of block temporarily but does not terminate dysrhythmia

TREATMENT Cardioversion; verapamil; digitalis; propranolol; quinidine; overdrive pacing

TABLE 12–5 (Continued)

Atrial Rhythms

REGULARITY AND RATE			AV CONDUCTION		
Ventricular	Atrial	P Waves	P:QRS Ratio	PR Interval	QRS
Atrial fibrillation					
Irregular; rate varies, but averages 160–180	Unmeasurable	Chaotic (fine or coarse) fibrillatory (f) waves, seen as wavy baseline	Very variable; numerous f waves per QRS	Variable	Normal

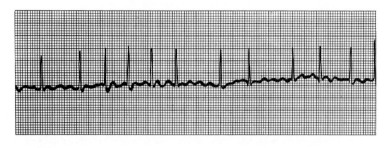

COMMENTS If ventricular rate becomes regular in digitalized patient, clue to digitalis intoxication
         Chronic or paroxysmal
CAUSES Normal heart; mitral stenosis; thyrotoxicosis; pericarditis; coronary artery disease; hypertensive heart disease
SIGNIFICANCE No effective atrial contraction; predisposes to pulmonary or systemic thromboemboli (about one-third of patients
         develop). May precipitate or exacerbate congestive heart failure
TREATMENT Cardioversion; digitalis; quinidine; verapamil; propranolol

---

alert to the development of Mobitz II block, which represents intermittent trifascicular block and heralds the development of constant trifascicular block (complete heart block). Because of the danger of progression, the patient with an acute myocardial infarction who develops a hemiblock usually will undergo prophylactic pacemaker insertion.

Wide Complex Ectopy

Often when you examine an ECG strip you will notice "funny-looking" wide QRS complexes. These usually are *ectopic depolarizations* (beats that arise outside the SA node). Because ectopic complexes vary in significance, it is important to use a logical method to analyze a funny-looking complex. A good method of analysis is the following:

1. Determine whether a complex is early or late by comparing the interval between it and the preceding complex to an R–R interval of the dominant rhythm. If it is late, it is escape ectopy. *Escape ectopy* occurs when the dominant pacemaker fails to fire and depolarize slower sites of impulse formation. Escape beats appear "late," that is, after the next-expected dominant complex. If the funny-looking complex is an escape beat, you can identify it further as an *escape junctional* or *escape ventricular ectopy* by looking for a P wave and measuring the QRS.

A complex that occurs early (before the next-expected dominant complex) is a *premature complex.* Supraventricular premature complexes may be blocked, conducted normally, or conducted aberrantly. This last term means the impulse is conducted down the bundle branches, although abnormally. *Aberration* is a transient conduction abnormality that occurs because the premature impulse reaches the bundle branches before they are fully repolarized. Since the bundle branches have unequal refractory periods, a premature impulse may find one branch still refractory (usually the right). The impulse still can travel the conduction pathway, but in a temporarily abnormal manner. At first glance, a premature supraventricular beat with aberration somewhat resembles a ventricular premature beat. It is important to differentiate them because their

TABLE 12–6

Junctional Rhythms

| REGULARITY AND RATE | | | AV CONDUCTION | | |
Ventricular	Atrial	P Waves	P:QRS Ratio	PR Interval	QRS
Junctional escape rhythm					
Regular, 40–60	0 or same as ventricular	Absent; before QRS and inverted; during QRS; or after QRS	0 or 1:1	If present, less than 0.12 second	Normal

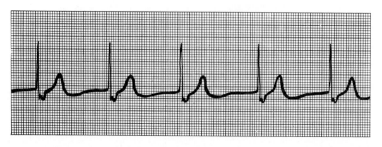

COMMENTS If P waves are present, junctional stimulus has been conducted retrograde to atria; usually seen best as negative P waves in leads II, III, and AVF
CAUSES Failure of sinus node
SIGNIFICANCE Protects patient from asystole
TREATMENT Treatment of failure of sinus node; atropine, isoproterenol to increase junctional rate; or artificial pacemaker

| REGULARITY AND RATE | | | AV CONDUCTION | | |
Ventricular	Atrial	P Waves	P:QRS Ratio	PR Interval	QRS
Accelerated junctional rhythm					
Regular, 60–100	0 or same as ventricular	Same as junctional escape rhythm	Same as junctional escape rhythm	Same as junctional escape rhythm	Same as junctional escape rhythm

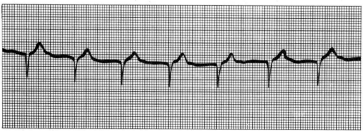

COMMENTS Also known as nonparoxysmal AV junctional tachycardia
CAUSES Digitalis intoxication, inferior infarction, myocarditis, postcardiotomy
SIGNIFICANCE Same as junctional escape rhythm; in addition, produces near-normal cardiac output
TREATMENT Treatment of cause

significance and treatment differ. Continue to follow a logical consistent approach to analyzing the complex.

2. Measure the QRS duration. A normal duration means the impulse's origin is supraventricular. A wide QRS (when the dominant QRS is normal) can mean either supraventricular ectopy with aberration or ventricular ectopy.

3. Look for a P wave related to the premature complex. Its presence strongly suggests the impulse is supraventricular.

TABLE 12–6 (Continued)

Junctional Rhythms

REGULARITY AND RATE			AV CONDUCTION		
Ventricular	**Atrial**	**P Waves**	**P:QRS Ratio**	**PR Interval**	**QRS**
Junctional tachycardia					
Regular, over 100	0 or same as ventricular	Same as junctional escape rhythm	Same as junctional escape rhythm	Same as junctional escape rhythm	Same as junctional escape rhythm

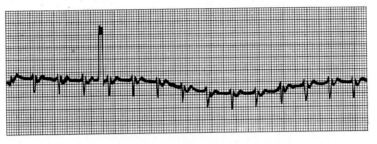

COMMENTS Same as junctional escape rhythm. Upright deflection in strip is standardization mark.
CAUSES Digitalis intoxication, myocardial infarction, myocarditis, postcardiotomy
SIGNIFICANCE Depends on patient's tolerance; usually stops spontaneously if tolerated well
TREATMENT If asymptomatic, treatment of cause
  If symptomatic, discontinuation of digitalis (if cause); cardioversion, digitalis (if not cause)
  If paroxysmal junctional tachycardia, see "Paroxysmal atrial tachycardia," Table 12–4

4. Analyze the pause after the premature complex. To do this, compare the interval consisting of two dominant cycles to the interval between the two dominant complexes surrounding the premature complex (see Figure 12–19). If the interval containing the premature complex is shorter than the interval containing two dominant cycles, the pause is called *noncompensatory*. It occurs because the premature impulse has depolarized the SA node, causing it, and therefore the ventricles, to pause. If the interval containing the premature complex is equal to or longer than twice the dominant cycle, the pause is called *compensatory*. It occurs because the impulse has not depolarized the SA node but instead has made the ventricles refractory to the next sinus impulse. That is, the SA node does not pause but the ventricles do—until the second sinus impulse after the premature complex, which arrives at a time when they can respond.

5. Compare the coupling intervals. The *couple* is the premature complex and the dominant complex immediately preceding it. Compare the interval between these R waves to that of other couples in the strip. Constant (fixed) coupling is a characteristic of ventricular premature ectopy.

6. Compare the R–R interval immediately preceding the premature complex to others in the dominant rhythm. A sudden lengthening just before the premature complex predisposes to aberration. The reason for this is that the refractory period of the bundle branches depends on the length of the preceding R–R interval—when the interval is long, the refractory period is long.

7. Examine the pattern of QRS deflections compared to the dominant QRS and to other premature beats:

   A. Initial deflections similar to those of dominant complexes suggest the impulse is traveling the usual conduction system; that is, it is supraventricular.

   B. A pattern of deflections similar to that of other premature complexes suggests that you probably are seeing a premature ectopic impulse from the same source.

   C. A BBB pattern may indicate supraventricular aberration or ventricular ectopy.

TABLE 12–7

Ventricular Rhythms

REGULARITY AND RATE			AV CONDUCTION		
Ventricular	Atrial	P Waves	P:QRS Ratio	PR Interval	QRS
Ventricular rhythm					
Regular, 20–40	Absent; or if present, unrelated to ventricular activity				Greater than 0.12 second

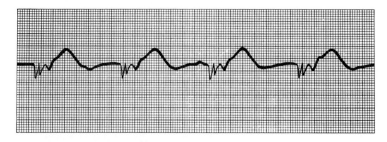

CAUSES Failure of higher pacemakers or complete AV block
SIGNIFICANCE Escape rhythm; if this rhythm occurs with no pulse or an insufficient pulse, treat as electromechanical dissociation
        (EMD)
TREATMENT Atropine, isoproterenol, artificial pacemaker; if EMD, CPR and epinephrine

REGULARITY AND RATE			AV CONDUCTION		
Ventricular	Atrial	P Waves	P:QRS Ratio	PR Interval	QRS
Accelerated ventricular rhythm					
Regular, 40–100	Absent; or if present, unrelated to ventricular activity				Greater than 0.12 second

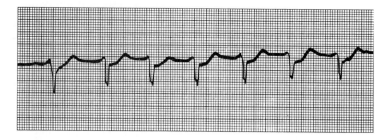

COMMENTS Transient episodes
CAUSES Acute myocardial infarction; digitalis intoxication
SIGNIFICANCE Ectopic ventricular pacemaker accelerates to rate approximating normal sinus rhythm
TREATMENT Close observation; treatment of cause; rarely, atropine; lidocaine

Aberration produces a BBB pattern when the early impulse reaches the ventricles while one bundle branch is still refractory. Since the refractory period of the right bundle branch usually is longer than that of the left bundle branch, aberration usually appears as a right BBB configuration.

Ventricular ectopy also may cause a BBB pattern. You will remember that in BBB, the impulse must spread cell to cell from the normally stimulated ventricle to the blocked one. As a ventricular premature beat arises outside the conduction system, it also spreads cell to cell to the other ventricle. For this reason, premature ectopy from the left

TABLE 12–7 (Continued)

Ventricular Rhythms

REGULARITY AND RATE			AV CONDUCTION		
Ventricular	**Atrial**	**P Waves**	**P:QRS Ratio**	**PR Interval**	**QRS**
Ventricular tachycardia					
Regular, 100–220	Absent; or if present, unrelated to ventricular activity				Greater than 0.12 second

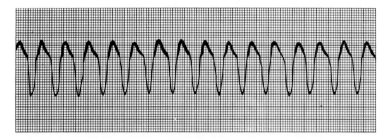

CAUSES Acute myocardial infarction; coronary artery disease; premature ventricular beat (R on T phenomenon)
SIGNIFICANCE Ominous as may progress to ventricular fibrillation; symptoms depend on underlying heart disease, rate, and duration of VT; may cause angina, cardiac failure, shock
TREATMENT If pulseless, treat as ventricular fibrillation; if with pulse and hemodynamically stable, lidocaine, procainamide, cardioversion; if with pulse but hemodynamically unstable, cardioversion, lidocaine, procainamide, bretylium

REGULARITY AND RATE			AV CONDUCTION		
Ventricular	**Atrial**	**P Waves**	**P:QRS Ratio**	**PR Interval**	**QRS**
Ventricular fibrillation					
400–600	Absent; or if present, unrelated to ventricular activity				None

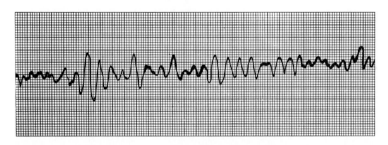

COMMENTS Chaotic depolarization produces grossly irregular, bizarre ECG deflections
CAUSES Acute myocardial infarction; coronary artery disease; electrical shock; premature ventricular beat (R on T phenomenon); dying heart
SIGNIFICANCE Lethal within 4–6 minutes; symptoms include loss of consciousness, pulse, heart sounds and respirations; and absent blood pressure
TREATMENT Precordial thump; immediate defibrillation; if ineffective, cardiopulmonary resuscitation; epinephrine, lidocaine, bretylium, sodium bicarbonate may be considered

(Continues)

ventricle may form the same QRS configuration as a right BBB, while right ventricular premature ectopy may simulate a left BBB.

Certain QRS configurations are more likely to represent ectopy than others. Clues to whether a QRS is ectopic or aberrant are presented in Figure 12–20 and Table 12–10.

TABLE 12–7 (Continued)

Ventricular Rhythms

REGULARITY AND RATE

AV CONDUCTION

Ventricular	Atrial	P Waves	P:QRS Ratio	PR Interval	QRS

Torsades de pointes (polymorphous ventricular tachycardia)

| 0 | Absent | | | | Greater than 0.12 second, varying morphology, twists around baseline |

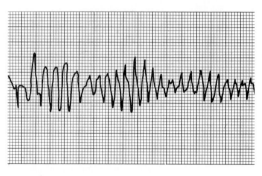

COMMENTS Frequently initiated with R-on-T phenomenon; associated with long QT interval
CAUSES Hypokalemia; quinidine-like drug toxicity; hypomagnesemia
SIGNIFICANCE May progress to ventricular fibrillation or spontaneously convert
TREATMENT Temporary pacing; lidocaine, magnesium sulfate

REGULARITY AND RATE

AV CONDUCTION

Ventricular	Atrial	P Waves	P:QRS Ratio	PR Interval	QRS

Ventricular asystole

| 0 | | Absent, or if present, unrelated to ventricular activity | | | None |

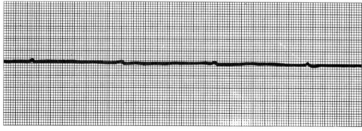

Ventricular standstill

COMMENTS In illustration, deflections are P waves
CAUSES Acute myocardial infarction; coronary artery disease; complete heart block; dying heart
SIGNIFICANCE Same as ventricular fibrillation
TREATMENT Immediate cardiopulmonary resuscitation; epinephrine, atropine, sodium bicarbonate may be considered; pacemaker

Premature complexes may be classified in many ways in addition to the designations ectopic and aberrant. When classified by site of origin, they are identified as atrial, junctional, or ventricular. Another classification refers to the number of foci (sites) from which they arise, impulses from one site with constant morphology being called *unifocal* and those from more than one site (or with different shapes) being called

TABLE 12–8

Atrioventricular Blocks

REGULARITY AND RATE			**AV CONDUCTION**		
Ventricular	**Atrial**	**P Waves**	**P:QRS Ratio**	**PR Interval**	**QRS**
First degree AV block					
Regular, any rate	Same as ventricular	Sinus or atrial	1:1	Constant, but greater than 0.20 second	Normal

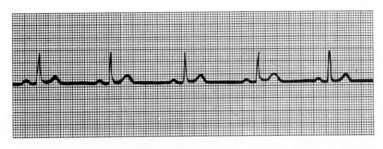

COMMENTS All impulses are conducted through AV node, but slower than usual
CAUSES Normal heart; coronary artery disease; digitalis intoxication; conduction system fibrosis; myocarditis; cardiac surgery
SIGNIFICANCE Relatively benign; may progress to second- or third-degree blocks
TREATMENT None necessary

REGULARITY AND RATE			**AV CONDUCTION**		
Ventricular	**Atrial**	**P Waves**	**P:QRS Ratio**	**PR Interval**	**QRS**
Second degree AV blocks: (1) Mobitz I (Wenckebach)					
Irregular but consistent pattern (group beating); any rate	Regular, faster than ventricular	Sinus or atrial	1:1 except for non-conducted P wave	Lengthens progressively until one P wave not conducted; cycle then repeats itself	Normal

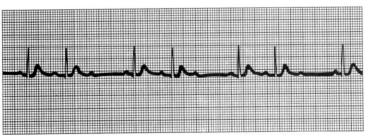

Mobitz I second degree AV block

COMMENTS In second-degree blocks, some impulses are not conducted; in Mobitz I, impulses are delayed progressively until one reaches AV node while it is absolutely refractory, so it cannot conduct that impulse
Block usually at level of AV node
CAUSES Increased parasympathetic tone; digitalis intoxication; acute inferior myocardial infarction
SIGNIFICANCE Relatively benign: does not diminish cardiac output, usually transient, does not usually progress to greater degree of block
TREATMENT Usually, none necessary; if symptomatic, atropine; discontinue digitalis if cause

(Continues)

TABLE 12–8 (Continued)

Atrioventricular Blocks

REGULARITY AND RATE			AV CONDUCTION		
Ventricular	**Atrial**	**P Waves**	**P:QRS Ratio**	**PR Interval**	**QRS**
(2) Mobitz II					
Irregular but with no consistent pattern, any rate	Regular, faster than ventricular	Sinus or atrial	1:1 except for non-conducted P wave	Constant on conducted beats, normal or prolonged	Wide with bundle branch block (if block infranodal) or normal (if block at AV node)

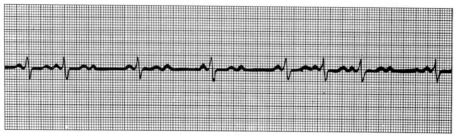

Mobitz II second degree AV block

COMMENTS Impulses are conducted normally until one is suddenly blocked
 Block usually infranodal (below AV node), commonly at bundle branch level or uncommonly at bundle of His
CAUSES Necrosis or fibrosis of conduction pathway; acute anterior myocardial infarction
SIGNIFICANCE More ominous than Mobitz I; often precedes sudden complete heart block
TREATMENT Atropine, isoproterenol, prophylactic artificial pacemaker

REGULARITY AND RATE			AV CONDUCTION		
Ventricular	**Atrial**	**P Waves**	**P:QRS Ratio**	**PR Interval**	**QRS**
Third degree (complete) AV block					
• with junctional escape rhythm					
Regular	Regular, faster than ventricular	Sinus or atrial	0; no relationship between Ps and QRSs	Appears variable, but P waves actually not conducted	Normal (due to junctional escape rhythm)

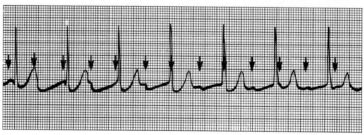

COMMENTS In third degree blocks, no impulses are conducted through AV node
 Narrow QRS in this rhythm indicates block high in AV node (in illustration, arrows point to P waves)
CAUSES Increased parasympathetic tone; drug effect; AV node damage; acute inferior MI
SIGNIFICANCE Transient; favorable prognosis
TREATMENT Atropine; temporary pacemaker

TABLE 12–8 (Continued)

Atrioventricular Blocks

REGULARITY AND RATE			AV CONDUCTION		
Ventricular	**Atrial**	**P Waves**	**P:QRS Ratio**	**PR Interval**	**QRS**
• with ventricular escape rhythm					
Regular or absent	Regular, faster than ventricular	Sinus or atrial	0; no relationship between Ps and QRSs	Appears variable, but P waves actually not conducted	Wide (due to ventricular escape rhythm) or absent

COMMENTS Wide QRS indicates block at both bundle branches or bundle of His (infranodal block)
CAUSES Extensive conduction system disease; extensive anterior MI
SIGNIFICANCE Poor prognosis; likely to progress to asystole
TREATMENT Atropine, pacemaker

• with no escape rhythm:					
Absent	Regular	Sinus or atrial	None	None	None

COMMENTS Causes ventricular standstill
CAUSES Extensive conduction system disease; extensive anterior MI
SIGNIFICANCE Cardiac arrest
TREATMENT CPR; epinephrine, pacemaker

---

multifocal (or multiformed). These and other characteristics of premature complexes are summarized and illustrated in Tables 12–11 and 12–12.

Differentiation of General ECG Patterns

So far, rhythms have been grouped primarily according to site of origin. You undoubtedly have noticed that different specific rhythms may have a similar general effect on the ECG. For instance, tachycardias from several sites have the same effect of a rapid, regular rhythm. When you first scan an ECG strip, it is the overall pattern that catches your eye, so your first impression is that of a tachycardia, bradycardia, or so on. Then, you proceed to differentiate the rhythms that could cause that effect.

Nursing Care Related to Dysrhythmias

Assessment

To improve your ability to spot dysrhythmias promptly, develop good dysrhythmia detection habits. Auscultate the apical pulse for rate and regularity. Monitor the cardiac rhythm constantly with an oscilloscope. Ob-serve the scope for changes in rate, rhythm, P wave, PR interval, QRS duration and configuration, ST segment, QT interval, and T wave. Analyze the rhythm strip, and mount it in the patient's record every 1–8 hours, depending on the stability of the patient's condition. When significant changes occur, document them with a rhythm strip or 12-lead ECG. Read the 12-lead ECG reports (or the ECGs themselves) to keep informed about the progression of ECG changes.

Risk Conditions

Learn to anticipate and prevent dysrhythmias by recognizing the conditions that increase the patient's risk of developing a dysrhythmia. The risk conditions are numerous: major categories include myocardial hypoxia, electrolyte imbalances, catecholamine stimulation, vagal stimulation, and trauma or structural interruption of the conduction system. Myocardial hypoxia can result from systemic hypoxia, inadequate coronary artery filling time (for example, in severe tachycardia), insufficient coronary artery perfusion pressure (for example, in shock), coronary artery disease, aortic valve disease, ventricular hypertrophy or dilatation, or anemia. In some cases, the patient with coronary artery disease may have an oxygen supply that is sufficient at rest or for minimal exertion, and may develop myocardial hypoxia only when myocardial workload increases (such as in tachycardia) because oxygen demand exceeds oxygen supply. Local areas of

TABLE 12–9

Bundle Branch Blocks

REGULARITY AND RATE

AV CONDUCTION

Ventricular	Atrial	P Waves	P:QRS Ratio	PR Interval	QRS

Normal conduction

| Regular or irregular, any rate, depending upon basic rhythm | | Sinus or atrial | Normal or abnormal, depending on basic rhythm | | 0.06–0.12 second V₁: rS; V₆: qR |

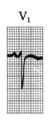 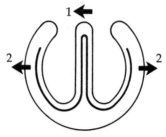 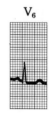

Normal sequence

COMMENTS Not a bundle branch block; included for comparison
CAUSES Normal heart
SIGNIFICANCE Normal conduction
TREATMENT None necessary

REGULARITY AND RATE

AV CONDUCTION

Ventricular	Atrial	P Waves	P:QRS Ratio	PR Interval	QRS

Right bundle branch block

| Regular or irregular, any rate, depending on basic rhythm | | Sinus or atrial | Normal or abnormal, depending on basic rhythm | | Greater than 0.12 second; V₁: triphasic rSR′; V₆: triphasic QRS, with wide S wave |

RBBB

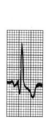 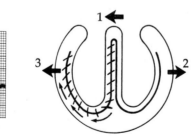 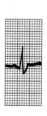

COMMENTS Does not affect recording of initial QRS waves; therefore, does not prevent ECG signs of myocardial infarction
CAUSES Normal heart; coronary artery disease; right ventricular hypertrophy; premature supraventricular beats (aberration)
SIGNIFICANCE Does not affect cardiac output
TREATMENT None necessary, unless accompanied by block of one division of left bundle branch; in that case, prophylactic artificial
            pacemaker

TABLE 12–9 (Continued)

Bundle Branch Blocks

REGULARITY AND RATE		P Waves	AV CONDUCTION		QRS
Ventricular	**Atrial**		**P:QRS Ratio**	**PR Interval**	**QRS**
Left bundle branch block					
Regular or irregular, any rate, depending on basic rhythm	Sinus or atrial		Normal or abnormal, depending on basic rhythm		Greater than 0.12 second; V_1: monophasic QS; V_6: monophasic wide R wave

LBBB

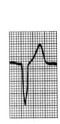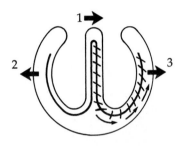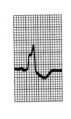

COMMENTS Block prevents recording of normal initial QRS waves, so can obscure ECG signs of myocardial infarction
CAUSES Normal heart; coronary artery disease; valvular heart disease; hypertension
SIGNIFICANCE More serious than right bundle branch block because results from more serious disorders and often accompanied by cardiomegaly
TREATMENT None

---

myocardial hypoxia may be present in myocardial infarction.

Electrolyte imbalances, particularly those of potassium and calcium, may contribute to dysrhythmias. These imbalances are discussed in Chapter 16.

Catecholamine stimulation, which predisposes toward tachydysrhythmias and premature beats, may occur in hypotension, hypertension, emotional excitement, increased muscular work, and administration of certain drugs, such as vasoconstrictor agents. Vagal stimulation, which contributes to bradydysrhythmias and heart block, may occur with digitalis intoxication, Valsalva maneuvers, or tracheal stimulation. A *Valsalva maneuver* is a forced expiration against a closed glottis; it often occurs when a patient is pushing himself up in bed or during bowel movements. Tracheal stimulation resulting in bradycardia or heart block may occur during tracheal suctioning, intubation, or vomiting.

Other factors that may provoke dysrhythmias are trauma to the conduction system (such as during cardiac surgery), structural defects (such as a ventricular septal defect), myocarditis, and stretching of myocardial fibers due to volume overload.

Planning and Implementation of Care

Prevention Whenever possible, plan to prevent dysrhythmias. One of the key goals of critical-care nursing is to develop the skill of taking preventive measures to avoid complications whenever possible. The following nursing measures are examples of planning to prevent dysrhythmias.

- Reduce catecholamine stimulation, which can produce tachycardias and premature ectopy. Minimize the patient's anxiety and pain and avoid hypotension. Promote physical and emotional rest.
- Avoid vagal stimulation, which can produce bradycardia and blocks. Take the following actions:
  1. Teach the patient to avoid Valsalva maneuvers. Also consult the physician about using stool softeners to reduce straining during bowel movements.
  2. When suctioning the trachea, watch the cardiac monitor for the onset of bradycardia

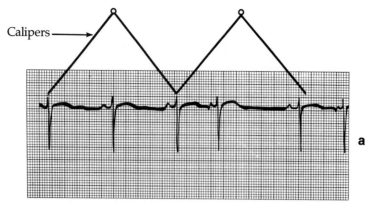

Noncompensatory pause

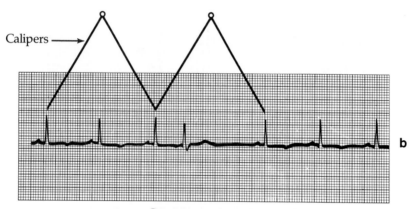

Compensatory pause

FIGURE 12–19

Noncompensatory versus compensatory pauses. To determine whether the pause following a premature beat is noncompensatory or compensatory, use your calipers to measure an interval consisting of two dominant cycles, as shown by the calipers on the left above each strip. Then, without changing the relative position of the caliper points, place the left point on the R wave preceding the premature beat, as shown by the calipers on the right above each strip. **a,** If another dominant QRS falls *before* the right point, the two cycles surrounding the premature beat are less than two dominant cycles; that is, the pause is *noncompensatory.* **b,** If the dominant QRS falls on or after the right caliper point, the cycles surrounding the premature beat are equal to or longer than two dominant cycles; that is, the pause is *compensatory.*

and observe recommended time limits for suctioning. (The trachea is innervated with vagal fibers.)

- Monitor patients on digitalis, beta-blockers, or calcium-channel blockers to detect intoxication promptly.

- Avoid or alleviate fluid and electrolyte imbalances by taking the measures listed in Chapter 16.

Intervention

The actions the nurse takes when a dysrhythmia occurs depend on the nurse's judgment about its significance and on the nurse's authorized scope of practice.

Significance of the Dysrhythmia Once the rhythm has been identified, its significance must be evaluated

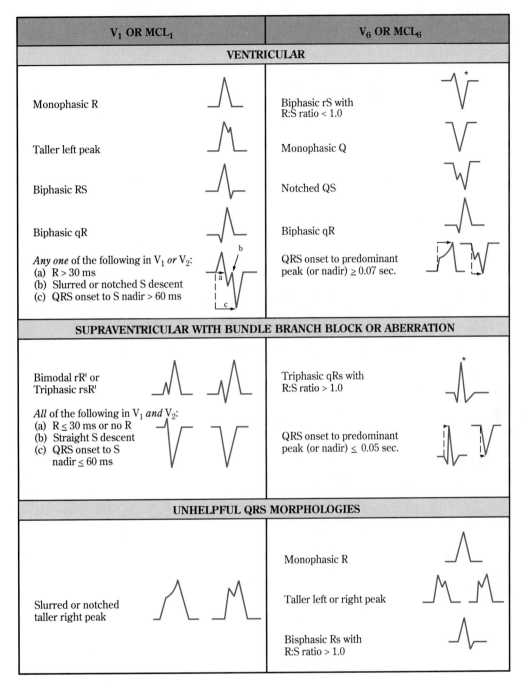

| V₁ OR MCL₁ | V₆ OR MCL₆ |

VENTRICULAR

Monophasic R

Taller left peak

Biphasic RS

Biphasic qR

Any one of the following in V₁ *or* V₂:
(a) R > 30 ms
(b) Slurred or notched S descent
(c) QRS onset to S nadir > 60 ms

Biphasic rS with R:S ratio < 1.0

Monophasic Q

Notched QS

Biphasic qR

QRS onset to predominant peak (or nadir) ≥ 0.07 sec.

SUPRAVENTRICULAR WITH BUNDLE BRANCH BLOCK OR ABERRATION

Bimodal rR' or Triphasic rsR'

All of the following in V₁ *and* V₂:
(a) R ≤ 30 ms or no R
(b) Straight S descent
(c) QRS onset to S nadir ≤ 60 ms

Triphasic qRs with R:S ratio > 1.0

QRS onset to predominant peak (or nadir) ≤ 0.05 sec.

UNHELPFUL QRS MORPHOLOGIES

Slurred or notched taller right peak

Monophasic R

Taller left or right peak

Bisphasic Rs with R:S ratio > 1.0

* Tachycardias with a right bundle branch block pattern in V₁ only

FIGURE 12–20

Summary of morphologic clues in V₁ or MCL₁ (left column) and in V₆ or MCL₆ (right column) that are valuable in distinguishing supraventricular tachycardia with bundle branch block or aberration from ventricular tachycardia. If wide complex tachycardia with taller right peak pattern (i.e., unhelpful morphology) develops in a patient monitored with a single MCL₁ lead, the nurse should change the lead to determine whether the wide complex falls into one of diagnostic patterns in MCL₆. (From Drew B: Bedside electrocardiographic monitoring: State of the art for the 1990's. *Heart Lung* 1991; 20:610–623.)

TABLE 12–10

Additional Criteria for Differentiating Supraventricular Tachycardia (SVT) with Aberration and Ventricular Tachycardia (VT)

FACTORS FAVORING SVT	FACTORS FAVORING VT
• Normal axis	• AV dissociation
• QRS less than 0.14 sec.	• –90 to –180 axis
• Preceding atrial activity	• Precordial concordance
• Premature P wave before run of tachycardia	• QRS wider than 0.14 sec.
• Anomalous second-in-the-row beat	• Capture beats
	• Fusion beats

Note: Age and hemodynamic status are unreliable criteria

Data from: Marriott H, Conover M: *Advanced concepts in arrhythmias,* 2d ed. St. Louis: Mosby, 1989; Rowlands D: *Clinical electrocardiography.* Philadelphia: Lippincott, 1991.

in terms of both its etiology and its consequences. Consequences fall into two main categories: the rhythm's effect on cardiac output and its tendency to become more serious.

Effect on Cardiac Output (CO) CO equals heart rate times stroke volume. Normal sinus rhythm is the optimal rhythm because it provides enough time for atrial and ventricular filling, proper coordination of valve openings and closings, and coronary artery filling during diastole. The coordination of AV valve movements is important because it permits the active phase of ventricular filling. During this phase, atrial contraction contributes about 30% of ventricular filling volume. Patients with poor myocardial reserve are particularly dependent on this mechanism to maintain CO. When it is lost (as in sudden atrial fibrillation), the resulting drop in CO may produce signs of shock.

Bradycardia decreases CO if its onset is sudden. If its onset is gradual, a compensatory increase in stroke volume may occur to maintain a normal CO.

Tachycardia increases CO up to the point at which it infringes seriously on ventricular filling time. At that rate (which varies from patient to patient), cardiac output drops because of the limited filling time. The patient's ability to tolerate a tachycardia depends not on its source but on its rate, the heart size, and additional insults (such as systemic hypoxia).

Tendency to Become More Serious A dysrhythmia may progress to more serious dysrhythmias. It is good

nursing practice to watch for such a tendency, and take appropriate measures when changes occur. Following are examples of some possible progressions to more serious problems.

Tachycardia predisposes to the development of faster rhythms by decreasing coronary artery filling time at the same time it increases myocardial oxygen demand. The resulting myocardial hypoxia alters the resting membrane potential of cardiac cells, enhancing the likelihood of spontaneous depolarization.

Premature beats indicate cellular irritability. They predispose toward rapid, repetitive depolarization, that is, tachycardia, flutter, and fibrillation.

Bradycardia encourages beats to escape from lower sites of impulse formation. It does so by failing to depolarize those sites and by decreasing coronary artery perfusion pressure. These escape beats may accelerate and become the dominant rhythm.

Lower degrees of block may progress to more complete blocks.

Treatment Treatment, in both emergency and non-emergency situations, depends on identification of the etiology of the dysrhythmia and selection of a therapeutic modality. The most frequently used options for treatment of each dysrhythmia are indicated in the tables throughout this chapter (Standards and Guidelines for CPR and ECC 1986). The types of therapy are discussed in Chapter 14 and in the Appendix.

Scope of Practice Selection of the treatment modality is the prerogative of the physician. As some dysrhythmias require immediate treatment and consultation with a physician may be delayed, many units have standing medical orders to guide the nurses and protect them legally in these situations.

General Principles Governing Treatment The general principles governing treatment instituted by the nurse under standing medical orders are as follows:

1. Do not initiate treatment of a dysrhythmia if the patient is stable hemodynamically and if the rhythm is unlikely to worsen.

2. Immediately treat life-threatening dysrhythmias causing pulselessness. These rhythms are ventricular asystole, ventricular fibrillation, and ventricular tachycardia.

3. Promptly terminate tachydysrhythmias that are causing hemodynamic deterioration or are likely to accelerate.

   For monitored ventricular tachycardia causing pulselessness, a precordial thump may be done; if this maneuver is not effective, then countershock immediately. For monitored ven-

TABLE 12–11

Premature Beats

QRS Duration	P Wave	PR Interval	Pause	Coupling	QRS Deflections
Atrial premature beat (APB)					
Normal	Atrial	Normal	Usually noncompensatory	Variable	Normal width; pattern same as dominant QRS

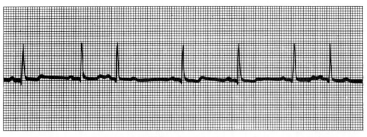

Atrial premature beat

COMMENTS Wandering atrial pacemaker (WAP) might be mistaken for sinus rhythm with ABPs because of the varying shape and rate of P waves; but in WAP the ventricular rate remains essentially regular
CAUSE Normal heart; caffeine, tobacco, alcohol stimulation; stress; myocarditis; myocardial ischemia; digitalis intoxication
SIGNIFICANCE Ectopic atrial focus; usually benign but may precede atrial tachycardia, flutter or fibrillation
TREATMENT Usually, none necessary; if very frequent, treat the cause; sedation; propranolol; digitalis (if not cause)

QRS Duration	P Wave	PR Interval	Pause	Coupling	QRS Deflections
Blocked or nonconducted APB					
Absent	Atrial	Absent	Usually noncompensatory	Variable	Absent

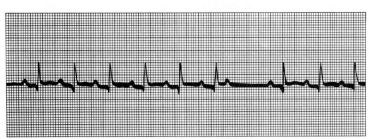

Blocked atrial premature beat

CAUSE Same as APB
SIGNIFICANCE Same as APB
TREATMENT Same as APB

(Continues)

TABLE 12–11 (Continued)

Premature Beats

QRS Duration	P Wave	PR Interval	Pause	Coupling	QRS Deflections
Aberrantly conducted APB					
Wide	Atrial	Normal	Usually noncompensatory	Variable	Wide QRS. Usually, initial deflection same as dominant QRS; usually, right bundle branch block pattern

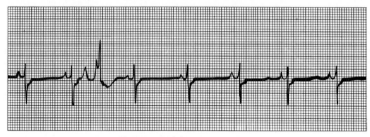

Aberrant atrial premature beat

COMMENTS Prolonged preceding R–R interval may be present
CAUSE Same as APB
SIGNIFICANCE Same as APB
TREATMENT Same as APB

QRS Duration	P Wave	PR Interval	Pause	Coupling	QRS Deflections
Junctional premature beat (JPB)					
Normal	Absent; before, during, or after QRS	Absent or less than 0.12 second	Usually noncompensatory	Variable	Normal width. Pattern same as dominant QRS

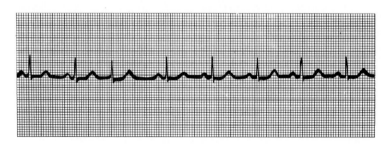

COMMENTS Retrograde atrial depolarization, so P wave negative in II, III, AVF
CAUSE Normal heart; caffeine, tobacco, alcohol stimulation; stress; myocarditis; myocardial ischemia; digitalis intoxication
SIGNIFICANCE Ectopic junctional focus; usually insignificant, but may precede junctional tachycardia
TREATMENT Usually, none necessary; if very frequent, treat the cause; sedation; propranolol; digitalis (if not cause)

TABLE 12–11 (Continued)

Premature Beats

QRS Duration	P Wave	PR Interval	Pause	Coupling	QRS Deflections
Aberrantly conducted JPB					
Wide	Absent; before, during, or after QRS	Absent or less than 0.12 second	Usually noncompensatory	Variable	Wide QRS. Usually, initial deflection same as dominant; usually, right bundle branch block pattern

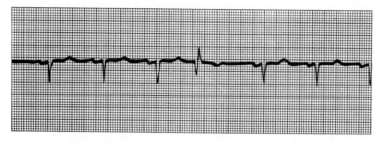

COMMENTS Prolonged preceding R–R interval may be present
CAUSE Same as JPB
SIGNIFICANCE Same as JPB
TREATMENT Same as JPB

QRS Duration	P Wave	PR Interval	Pause	Coupling	QRS Deflections
Ventricular premature beat (VPB)					
Wide	Unrelated	Absent	Usually compensatory	Depends on type	Wide QRS. Bizarre pattern; initial deflection usually opposite to dominant QRS

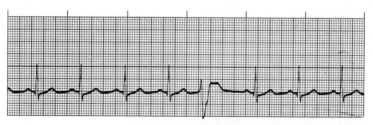

COMMENTS Followed by large inverted T wave; numerous subcategories shown in Table 12–12
CAUSE Normal heart, myocardial ischemia or infarction; electrolyte imbalances; others as in JPB
SIGNIFICANCE Ectopic ventricular focus; may progress to ventricular tachycardia or fibrillation, especially if more than 3 in a row, more than 6 per minute, multifocal, or falling on or near preceding T wave
TREATMENT None if infrequent; if frequent, lidocaine bolus IV followed by lidocaine infusion; procainamide; bretylium; treat the cause

(Continues)

TABLE 12–11 (Continued)

Premature Beats

QRS Duration	P Wave	PR Interval	Pause	Coupling	QRS Deflections
Fusion beat (shown by arrows)					
Intermediate between dominant and ectopic durations	Yes, but may be hidden in QRS	Normal or no more than 0.06–0.08 second less than dominant beat	Variable	Constant	Intermediate between dominant and ectopic contours

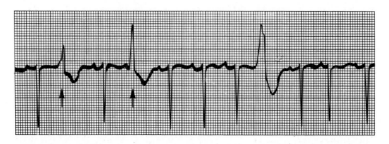

CAUSE As in other premature beats

SIGNIFICANCE Simultaneous depolarization of atria or ventricles by one normal and one ectopic focus (normal sinus beat and artificial pacemaker; normal sinus beat and APB; or supraventricular beat and VPB)

TREATMENT None necessary

---

tricular tachycardia not causing pulselessness, give a precordial thump, or lidocaine 1 mg/kg as an IV bolus. If unsuccessful, consult the physician about using procainamide or bretylium tosylate. Recurrent or persistent ventricular tachycardia may warrant amiodarone, atrial pacing, cardiac catheterization, myocardial revascularization, cardiac sympathectomy, or automatic implantable defibrillator.

4. Promptly relieve bradycardia causing hemodynamic deterioration. For sinus bradycardia and AV blocks, give 0.5 mg atropine as an IV bolus. If unsuccessful, repeat this dose to a total of 2 mg, or contact the physician about the use of isoproterenol or artificial pacing.

5. Immediately suppress premature beats if they are dangerous. Supraventricular beats rarely are; keep the physician informed of their presence, and follow his or her therapeutic plan. If premature ventricular beats are more than six per minute, more than three in a row, multifocal, or falling on or near the T wave, administer an IV bolus of lidocaine 1 mg/kg.

NURSING DIAGNOSES

The nursing diagnoses appropriate for a patient with a dysrhythmia may include one or more of the following:

- Decreased cardiac output
- Altered tissue perfusion
- Activity intolerance
- Anxiety

Outcome Evaluation

Evaluate the patient's progress according to the following outcome criteria. Ideally, the dysrhythmic episode will be terminated and the patient will develop a normal sinus rhythm. The ideal may not occur, however, particularly in the critically ill patient with preexisting heart disease. Realistic outcome criteria in the absence of normal sinus rhythm are spontaneous, drug-controlled, or artificially paced rhythms with the following characteristics:

TABLE 12–12

Subcategories of VPBs

CHARACTERISTICS   **EXAMPLES**

Unifocal VPB

Fixed coupling, constant QRS contour

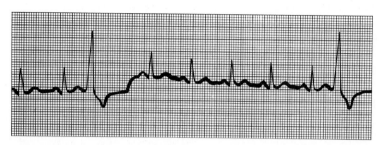

Multifocal (multiformed) VPB

Variable coupling, variable QRS contour

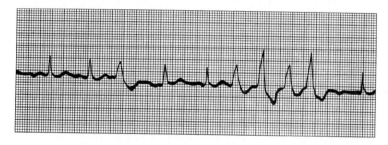

Interpolated VPB

No pause, "sandwiched" between dominant beats

Left ventricular VPB

Right bundle branch block pattern or primarily positive deflection in
leads oriented toward right ventricle (V$_1$, V$_2$)

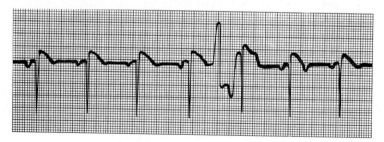

(Continues)

TABLE 12–12 (Continued)

Subcategories of VPBs

CHARACTERISTICS

Right ventricular VPB

Left bundle branch block pattern or primarily positive deflection in
leads oriented toward left ventricle (V$_5$, V$_6$)

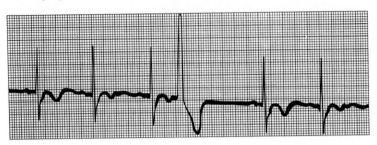

Isolated VPB

Occurring infrequently

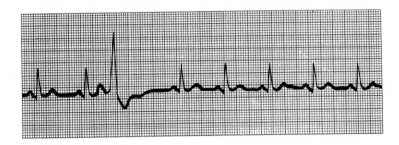

Bigeminy (ventricular)

VPB alternating with dominant beat

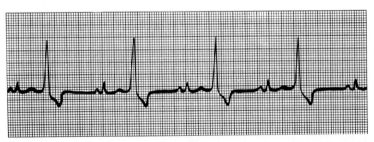

CRITICAL CARE GERONTOLOGY

Common Dysrhythmias in the Geriatric Patient

The aging process may impair the effectiveness of conductivity and contractility in the heart. Many patients, because of ischemic changes or degeneration, will experience decreased sinus node automaticity resulting in bradycardic rhythms. The effect of poor myocardial contractility, hypertension, or valvular disease may cause decreased ventricular emptying and increased filling pressures. This increased atrial pressure causes abnormal stretching of the atrial walls, increasing their irritability.

The result of decreased sinus node efficiency or increased atrial pressure may be atrial fibrillation. This common dysrhythmia seen in the elderly is frequently associated with congestive heart failure, either as the cause or the result. Uncontrolled atrial fibrillation usually produces rapid, irregular ventricular response. Coupled with loss of atrial contraction or "kick," this rhythm produces a decrease in cardiac output and an increase in intracardiac pressures. The increased pressure when reflected back into pulmonary circulation may result in congestive heart failure.

- Ventricular rate 60–100 beats per minute.
- Ventricular rate adequate to perfuse core organs and periphery, as manifested by alert mental state; absence of angina; urinary output within normal limits for patient; warm, dry skin; peripheral pulses bilaterally equal and of normal volume for patient.
- Infrequent atrial or junctional premature beats, if any.
- Six or fewer ventricular premature beats (VPBs) per minute.
- No more than three VPBs in a row.
- No multifocal VPBs.
- No VPBs falling on or near T waves.

REFERENCES

Albarran-Sotelo R et al: *Textbook of advanced cardiac life support*, 2d ed. Dallas: American Heart Association, 1987.

Crabtree A, Jorgenson M: Exploring the practical knowledge in expert nursing critical-care practice. Unpublished master's thesis, University of Wisconsin, Madison, 1986.

Drew B: Bedside electrocardiographic monitoring: State of the art for the 1990's. *Heart Lung* 1991; 20:610–623.

Drew B, Ide B, Sparacino P: Accuracy of bedside electrocardiographic monitoring: A report on current practices of critical care nurses. *Heart Lung* 1991; 20:597–608.

Dubin D: *Rapid interpretation of EKG's,* 4th ed. Tampa, FL: COVER Publishing Company, 1989.

Guyton A: *Textbook of medical physiology,* 8th ed. Philadelphia: Saunders, 1991.

Marriott H: *Practical electrocardiography.* 8th ed. Baltimore: Williams & Wilkins, 1988.

Marriott H, Conover M: *Advanced concepts in arrhythmias.* 2d ed. St. Louis: Mosby, 1989.

Rowlands C: *Clinical electrocardiography.* Philadelphia: Lippincott, 1991.

Standards and guidelines for cardiopulmonary resuscitation (CPR) and emergency cardiac care (ECC). *JAMA* 1986; 255:2915–2954.

13

Cardiovascular Disorders

CLINICAL INSIGHT

Domain: The diagnostic and monitoring function

Competency: Detection and documentation of significant changes in a patient's condition

Time is of the essence in many of the diseases and disorders considered in this chapter. On occasion a patient's fate lies literally in our hands as we speed to implement life-saving interventions. In this paradigm from Benner (1984, pp. 98–99) an expert nurse speaks of the difficulty in obtaining collegial response to an urgent patient problem.

I received a patient from CCU at about noon. She was an alert woman, in her 50s. I received a report from the CCU nurse stating that she was a post-MI, vital signs stable: pulse in the 80s, normal sinus rhythm, blood pressure between 120 and 130 (I don't recall the diastolic pressures). We made her comfortable in bed and checked her vital signs

which were stable. About 30 minutes later, the patient had vague complaints of "not feeling well." Her blood pressure dropped to 110. Pulse was in the 90s, regular.

I paged the intern and resident with no response. I finally reached the resident and reported my observations and told her the patient must be examined right away. She informed me she would be on her way to see the patient. I took another set of vital signs. The blood pressure had dropped to 104. Pulse remained the same. I noted that the patient was becoming "scared" by her facial expression. I had reassured her when she first complained that the doctor would be in to see her soon. During the whole episode, I asked an LVN to stay with the patient.

I stopped the resident who was walking by and reported the drop in blood pressure and the patient's condition. She said she would be right back. I told her firmly to examine the patient now. She examined the patient and immediately paged another resident to check the patient. They stood outside the patient's room conferring on their findings. One said he heard a murmur; the other said she didn't hear it.

While they were having their conference, I became very concerned about the patient's welfare. Time was slipping by since the onset of her complaints, and being a fresh post-MI, I felt she should be transferred back to CCU immediately. Since the onset of the patient's complaints to the time we transferred her back to CCU, it took 45 minutes. It was about 1:15 pm when we transferred her. At the end of my shift, I went to CCU to inquire about the patient. The nurses said they were still doing some tests to determine what was going on. Next morning I found out that the patient had died of a cardiac tamponade.

The critically ill patient is at high risk for developing a number of cardiovascular disorders. This chapter helps you recognize the most important cardiovascular disorders, identify appropriate nursing diagnoses, and understand the nursing and medical measures used to treat such problems. Such knowledge provides the foundation on which to build the clinical expertise illustrated in the Clinical Insight.

Acute Chest Pain

Assessment

The critical-care nurse often is called on to perform a rapid, accurate assessment of a patient who has acute chest pain and to institute emergency stabilization of that patient. The patient's symptomatology can be assessed quickly yet thoroughly using the PQRST mnemonic. As explained in Chapter 10, each letter represents an area to be evaluated:

P   Precipitating factors
Q   Quality
R   Region and radiation
S   Associated symptoms and signs
T   Time and response to treatment

The most common causes of acute chest pain can be grouped into five categories: cardiac, pulmonary, musculoskeletal, gastrointestinal, and psychosomatic. Table 13–1 presents the most common subcategories

of acute chest pain, analyzing each according to the PQRST format.

In addition to assessing the patient's symptoms, perform a quick evaluation of blood pressure, pulse, monitor rhythm, respirations, level of consciousness, and peripheral perfusion.

NURSING DIAGNOSES

Nursing diagnoses for the patient who has acute chest pain include:

- Pain
- Anxiety
- High risk for decreased cardiac output
- High risk for altered tissue perfusion

Nursing measures for each of these diagnoses are discussed elsewhere in the text; this section focuses on emergency stabilization.

Emergency Stabilization

Emergency stabilization of the patient with acute chest pain is accomplished using the following measures.

1. Place the patient in high Fowler's position to facilitate diaphragmatic expansion.

2. Start high-flow oxygen, usually 6 liters/minute via nasal cannula. If the patient has chronic lung disease, give oxygen via nasal cannula at 2–3 liters/minute.

3. Institute cardiac monitoring if not already in use.

4. Establish an intravenous (IV) lifeline, if one is not already in place. The usual fluid is 5% dextrose in water, administered at a "keep open" (very slow) rate via a microdrop infusion set.

5. Provide pain relief, per medical orders, with sublingual nitroglycerin, intravenous nitroglycerin, or intravenous analgesics.

6. Obtain diagnostic studies, as ordered. They usually include a stat chest x-ray, 12-lead electrocardiogram (ECG), and cardiac isoenzymes (particularly creatine phosphokinase-MB [CPK-MB]), as well as a routine complete blood count (CBC) and electrolyte panel.

TABLE 13–1

Chest Pain Profiles

P PRECIPITATING FACTORS	Q QUALITY	R REGION AND RADIATION	S ASSOCIATED SYMPTOMS AND SIGNS	T TIME AND RESPONSE TO TREATMENT
Cardiac				
Angina				
Physical exertion	Pressure	Substernal	Diaphoresis	Gradual onset
Emotional stress	Tightness	Unable to pinpoint	Nausea, vomiting	Duration < 30 min
Environmental factors	Squeezing	Radiates to arms, throat, jaw, back, upper abdomen	Dyspnea	Relief with rest or nitroglycerin
Eating	Burning		Syncope	
	Mild to moderate pain		Uneasiness	
Acute Myocardial Infarction				
Same as angina; more likely to occur with no precipitators	Same as angina	Same as angina	Same as angina	Sudden onset
	Severe pain		Severe apprehension	Duration > 30 min
	Worsened by fear and movement		Extra heart sounds	No relief with rest, nitroglycerin, or change in posture
			Pulmonary congestion	Relief with narcotics
Dissecting Aortic Aneurysm				
Hypertension	Tearing sensation	Substernal	Dyspnea	Sudden onset
	Excruciating pain worse at onset	Radiation to back and abdomen	Apprehension	No relief with rest or nitroglycerin
		"Traveling" sensation	Diaphoresis	Relief with narcotics
			BP differences between arms	
			Absence of pulse unilaterally	
			Hemiplegia or paraplegia	
			Murmur of aortic regurgitation	
Pericarditis				
Myocardial infarction	Sharp	Precordial	Dyspnea	Sudden onset
Uremia	Stabbing	Retrosternal	Friction rub	Continuous
Trauma	Knifelike	Radiation to neck, arms, or back		No relief with rest or nitroglycerin
Infections	Mild to severe			Relief with sitting forward or aspirin
	Deep or superficial			
	Worsened by inspiration, coughing, muscle movement, lying on left side			
Pulmonary				
Pulmonary Embolism				
Prolonged sitting or lying down	Crushing	Lateral chest (over lung fields)	Dyspnea	Sudden onset
Phlebitis	Deep ache	Radiation to shoulder, neck	Pallor or cyanosis	No relief with rest or nitroglycerin
Long-bone fracture	Shooting		Syncope	Relief with narcotics
	Increased by deep inspiration or coughing		Cough with hemoptysis	
			Apprehension	
			Sinus tachycardia	
			Pleural rub	
			Fever	

TABLE 13–1 (Continued)

Chest Pain Profiles

P PRECIPITATING FACTORS	Q QUALITY	R REGION AND RADIATION	S ASSOCIATED SYMPTOMS AND SIGNS	T TIME AND RESPONSE TO TREATMENT
Spontaneous Pneumothorax				
Chronic obstructive pulmonary disease (COPD)	Tearing Increased by breathing	Lateral chest	Dyspnea Decreased breath sounds Tachycardia Agitation	Sudden onset
Pneumonia				
Respiratory infection	Moderate ache Increased by coughing, inspiration, movement	Over lung fields Radiation to shoulder, neck	Dyspnea Tachycardia Pleural rub Fever Productive cough	Gradual onset Continuous duration Relief with sitting up
Musculoskeletal (chest wall)				
Neck or arm strain Reproducible with movement	Soreness, tenderness Increased by movement	Localized to side of midline Able to pinpoint	None	Gradual or sudden onset Continuous or intermittent No relief with nitroglycerin Relief with rest, analgesic, heat
Gastrointestinal				
Food intake Alcohol	"Heartburn" Increased by eating or lying down	Lower substernal Upper abdominal Midline Radiation to upper abdomen, back, shoulder	Dysphagia Belching Vomiting Diaphoresis	Gradual or sudden onset Continuous or intermittent Relief with antacids or sitting up
Psychosomatic				
Emotional stress Fatigue	Dull ache to sharp stabbing Superficial	Precordium rather than center of chest Pinpoint localization No radiation	Palpitations Hyperventilation Dizziness Dyspnea Fatigue Frequent sighing	Gradual or sudden Variable duration Relief with rest or sedation

These measures, particularly the first four, can be accomplished simultaneously with evaluation of the chest pain by the PQRST method. In addition, they can be accomplished simultaneously with nursing measures to relieve the patient's fear and anxiety, such as projection of a calm, competent persona, brief explanations of procedures, and therapeutic use of touch.

Definitive treatment of acute chest pain depends on its cause. For further details, consult other sections of this text that discuss cardiac and respiratory disorders, the most common causes of acute chest pain.

Acute Myocardial Infarction

Because of the prevalence of coronary artery disease in the general population and because of the stresses imposed by being critically ill, your patients have a significant risk of developing an acute myocardial infarction (MI).

Assessment

Risk Conditions   Be alert for factors associated with an increased risk of MI. Among those implicated by epidemiologic studies are these:

- Middle or old age
- Male sex
- Female sex after menopause
- Elevated serum cholesterol or triglycerides
- Hypertension
- Manifestations of coronary atherosclerotic heart disease before the age of 50 in patient's parents or sibling
- Cigarette smoking
- Diet high in calories, sugar, salt, cholesterol, total fat, and/or saturated fat and low in fish
- Diabetes, fasting blood sugar over 120 mg/100 ml, abnormal glucose tolerance test
- Sedentary lifestyle
- Constant emotional tension
- Type A behavior

In the patient with suspected or confirmed coronary artery disease, the additional following factors are associated with an increased risk of MI:

- Previous MI
- Any factor reducing coronary artery perfusion or oxygenation (for example, systemic hypoxia, hypotension)
- Any factor increasing ventricular workload (for example, physical stress, emotional stress, hypertension, aortic stenosis)

Decrease the risk factors whenever possible. Following are some examples of ways to decrease coronary risk factors. Educate patients, their families, and the general public about the risk factors and ways to reduce them. (For specific recommendations, consult the most recent literature from the American Heart Association.) Administer antihypertensive or antilipi-demic drugs if prescribed by the physician. Reduce dietary fat intake, particularly saturated fats. Maintain adequate systemic oxygenation and coronary arterial perfusion. Reduce physical stress by limiting ambulation and self-care during acute ischemic attacks. Reduce emotional stress by the measures outlined in Chapters 2 and 3.

Signs and Symptoms   Be alert to the various signs and symptoms of acute myocardial infarction.

Note the *characteristics of pain.* Acute infarction pain is usually substernal. The patient may describe it as crushing, "like a weight on my chest," and when asked to localize it will place a clenched fist on the sternum. Frequently, the pain will radiate down the left arm, down both arms, or up into the neck. Less common sites of pain for which you should be alert are the jaw, back, and abdomen. Typically, the pain is constant and unrelieved by rest or by sublingual nitroglycerin (1 tablet q5min × 3).

Observe for *increased sympathetic stimulation.* Most patients develop increased sympathetic stimulation during an infarct. This stimulation produces tachycardia, slight hypertension, diaphoresis and clammy skin, and nausea or vomiting. Some patients suffer cardiovascular depression, possibly due to reflexes from the ischemic area. These people display bradycardia and hypotension.

Check for *additional findings:* On auscultation, you may hear an S_3, S_4, or paradoxically split S_2 due to decreased left ventricular compliance. The patient usually is short of breath. Blood gases show a metabolic acidosis (due to inadequate tissue perfusion)

NURSING TIP

MI in the Elderly

MI in the adult often manifests itself with the symptoms of chest pain, sweating, nausea and vomiting, and anxiety. In the elderly individual (>65 years), symptoms of MI have been found to be atypical from those in younger adults. In the elderly, shortness of breath is often the major symptom, followed by sweating, vomiting, syncope, confusion, weakness, giddiness, and stroke (Bayer 1986). Because mortality from MI is higher in the elderly, early recognition is extremely important.

and respiratory alkalosis (due to hyperventilation). Severe apprehension is common.

Diagnostic Procedures

Causes of Infarctions Infarctions may occur for a variety of reasons; the exact cause may be difficult for the physician to diagnose. Most commonly, MI results from occlusion of a coronary artery. In the past, thrombosis was believed to cause all infarctions. This concept has been proven erroneous. Although thrombosis precedes most infarctions, other causes have been identified. The occlusion may be due to atheromatous narrowing, spasm of the artery, or embolization of thrombi, fatty plaques, air, or calcium. In some cases, the infarct may result not from occlusion but from a great disparity between myocardial oxygen demand and coronary arterial supply.

Types of Infarctions Infarctions can be classified according to the myocardial layers they affect. *Transmural (Q-wave)* infarction involves 50–75% or more of the total thickness of the ventricular wall and is characterized by abnormal Q waves and ST–T changes. It usually

CRITICAL CARE GERONTOLOGY

Cardiovascular Disease in the Elderly

Cardiovascular disease is the most prevalent medical problem in the elderly. It is the leading cause of death in patients 65 years of age or older, with 80% of these deaths due specifically to ischemic heart disease (Wei and Gersh 1987). The aged population is growing at a rapid rate and it is estimated that by the year 2030, 21% of our population will be over the age of 65, almost double what it is now (Kern 1991).

Several anatomic and physiologic changes take place during the aging process. Compliance in the blood vessels decreases due to atherosclerosis. Isolated systolic hypertension (systolic blood pressure > 160 mm Hg, diastolic blood pressure < 90 mm Hg) is common and has been found to be a risk factor for myocardial infarction and stroke. Exertional hypertension and the time it takes for the BP to return to normal are increased in the elderly. Fibrosis and sclerosis of the conduction system results in heart block and conduction delays. Sick sinus syndrome, which is related to these aging changes, is a common cause of syncope in the elderly.

Cardiac output decreases with age and the heart has a diminished ability to handle fluid volume changes. With exercise, there is little increase in cardiac output, unlike in the younger heart.

The heart also becomes less responsive to sympathetic stimulation. In a stressful situation, the heart rate may not rise, cardiac contraction may not increase, and the elderly ventricle may be unable to tolerate or compensate for volume changes.

Manifestations of heart disease in the elderly also will differ from symptoms in younger individuals. Angina may not present as chest pain, but rather as dyspnea, syncope, and exertional diaphoresis. When the elderly patient has a myocardial infarction, the first sign may be confusion, accompanied by heart failure, dysrhythmias, dyspnea, syncope, weakness, or abdominal pain (Kern 1991).

Aortic stenosis is the most common valvular abnormality seen in the elderly. The lesion usually is calcified and fixed, which results in a fixed cardiac output and poor tolerance for fluid volume changes.

The elderly patient who must undero surgery is always at high risk. Fifty five percent of the elderly have at least two major existing medical conditions (Wei and Gersh 1987). For example, heart disease frequently is accompanied by diabetes, cerebrovascular disease, or peripheral vascular disease, all of which create a high risk venue for surgery.

Nursing implications in caring for the critically ill gerontology patient include the following:

- The elderly person's decreased ability to respond to stress means that pain, stressful procedures, fever, etc. may not produce an increased heart rate, so you will need to be especially alert for other signs and symptoms.

- Syncope and hypotensive syndromes are more common in the elderly, so you will need to monitor the elderly carefully when there is fluid volume loss or when they are started on vasodilator drugs.

- Fifty percent of healthy elderly have complex ventricular dysrhythmias, and the elderly are more prone to side effects of drugs. Therefore, do not be in a hurry to treat multiple ventricular premature beats (VPB's) in the elderly.

is due to atherosclerosis and arterial occlusion. The terms *subendocardial, nontransmural,* and *non-Q-wave* have been used to describe infarcts with abnormal ST–T changes but no abnormal Q waves. Since these criteria also are consistent with small infarcts, the existence of subendocardial infarction is controversial. Infarcts limited to the subendocardium probably result not from arterial occlusion but rather from microemboli or a disparity between oxygen demand and supply. The subendocardium is particularly vulnerable to ischemia because of a combination of factors. Because it has the longest myofibrils in the heart, its O_2 need is greatest. Since coronary arteries lie on the epicardium, the epicardium is oxygenated better than the endocardium. As a result, at the same time the subendocardium needs more O_2 than other cardiac cells, the blood perfusing it has the lowest Po_2 in the heart. In addition, during systole the high pressure in the subendocardium and the wringing effect of contraction preclude perfusion of the subendocardium. Once subendocardial injury has occurred, it is particularly likely to progress to infarction and extension. The swelling of damaged cells and clotting combine to compress surrounding tissue. These factors also increase coronary arterial resistance, which further decreases flow both to the injured area and to the areas distal to it.

Coronary Blood Supply An understanding of the distribution of the coronary blood supply is helpful in comprehending the results of infarcts. The heart is supplied by three coronary arteries: the right coronary artery and two branches of the left main coronary artery (the left anterior descending and the circumflex coronary arteries) (Figure 13–1). The right and left main coronary arteries arise from sinuses of Valsalva, recesses located on the aorta just above the aortic valve. The arteries lie on the epicardial surface and send small branches into the endocardium (Figure 13–2).

The *right coronary artery* (RCA) courses along the anterior groove or sulcus between the right atrium and ventricle, giving off a branch (the marginal artery) to the apex. It continues along the posterior atrioventricular groove and in most cases descends along the posterior groove in between the ventricles, creating the posterior descending artery. In its course, the right coronary artery supplies the right atrium, right ventricle, posterior third of the septum, and the inferior (diaphragmatic) and posterior left ventricle.

The left main coronary artery splits into its two branches soon after arising from the aorta. The *left anterior descending (LAD) coronary artery* passes behind the pulmonary artery and travels down the

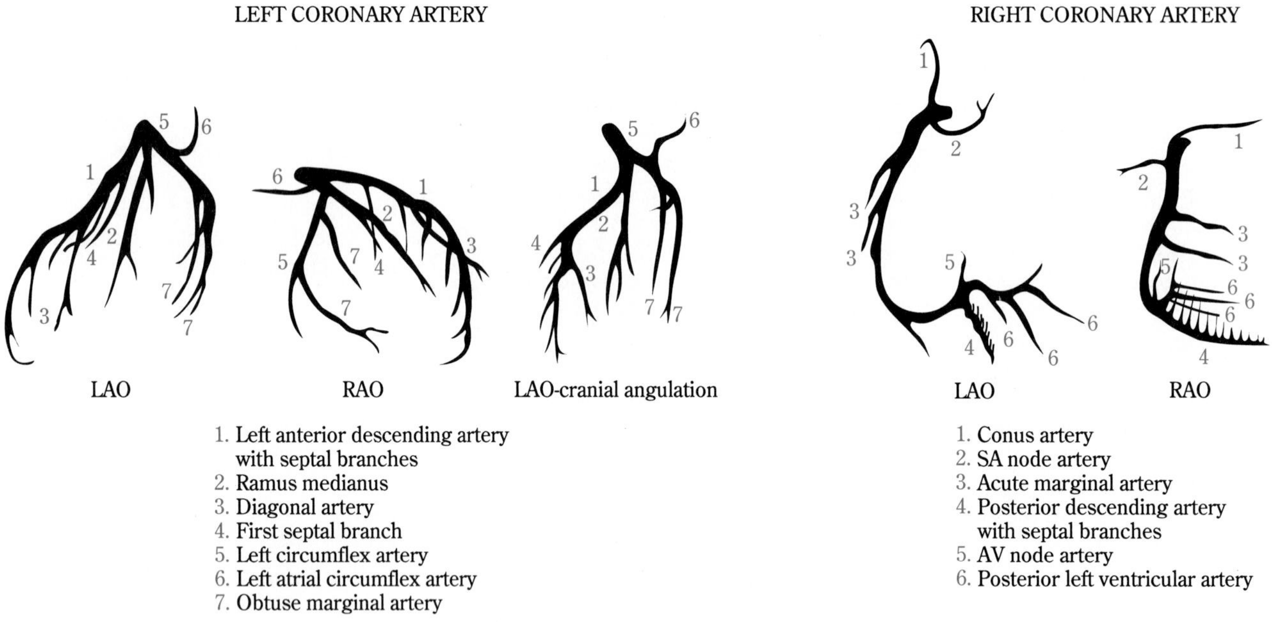

LEFT CORONARY ARTERY

LAO   RAO   LAO-cranial angulation

1. Left anterior descending artery with septal branches
2. Ramus medianus
3. Diagonal artery
4. First septal branch
5. Left circumflex artery
6. Left atrial circumflex artery
7. Obtuse marginal artery

RIGHT CORONARY ARTERY

LAO   RAO

1. Conus artery
2. SA node artery
3. Acute marginal artery
4. Posterior descending artery with septal branches
5. AV node artery
6. Posterior left ventricular artery

FIGURE 13–1

Angiographic anatomy of the right and left coronary arteries in standard left and right anterior oblique (LAO and RAO) projections. The appearance in the LAO projection with cranial angulation is also shown. (From Grossman W: *Cardiac catheterization and angiography,* 2d ed. Philadelphia: Lea & Febiger, 1980, p. 153. Reproduced with permission.)

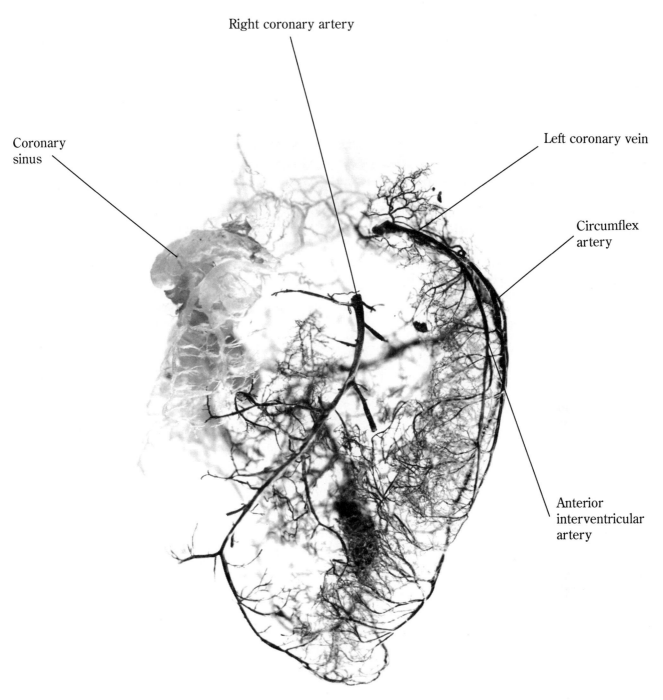

FIGURE 13–2

Cast of blood vessels of the heart. This photograph of a cardiac cast shows the network of vessels that carry blood from the chambers of the heart to the heart muscle and back again to the heart chambers. The thick, dark, branchlike structure on the left is the right coronary artery. On the right is the left coronary artery, which branches into two different arteries: the circumflex artery, which appears slightly out of focus at the back of the heart, and the anterior interventricular artery. The large white structure on the left is the coronary sinus, which drains blood into the right atrium from several of the vessels supplying the heart. (From Spence A: *Basic human anatomy,* 2d ed. Redwood City: Benjamin/Cummings, 1989, p. 284. Photograph © Carroll H. Weiss, 1973.)

anterior interventricular groove (so it sometimes also is called the anterior inter-ventricular artery). In its course, it supplies the anterior two-thirds of the septum and the anterior and apical portions of the left ventricle, as well as portions of the right ventricle.

The *left circumflex (LCX) coronary artery* traverses the left atrioventricular groove from anterior to posterior. It sometimes ends as a descending artery along the posterior left ventricle. The LCX nourishes the left atrium, lateral left ventricle, and in some cases the posterior left ventricle and posterior ventricular septum.

All three coronary arteries supply parts of the conduction system. The sinoatrial (SA) node is nour-

ished by the right coronary artery in about 60% of the population and by the circumflex artery in 40%. The internodal tracts are supplied by the right coronary artery. The atrioventricular (AV) node and bundle of His are supplied by the right coronary artery (90%) or circumflex artery (10%). The bundle branches are nourished primarily by the LAD and secondarily by the RCA.

Knowledge of the arterial blood supply will help you to understand the ECG signs of the infarction and predict specific patient problems that may occur.

ECG Indicators of Infarction If you suspect an infarct, obtain immediate medical help while you record a

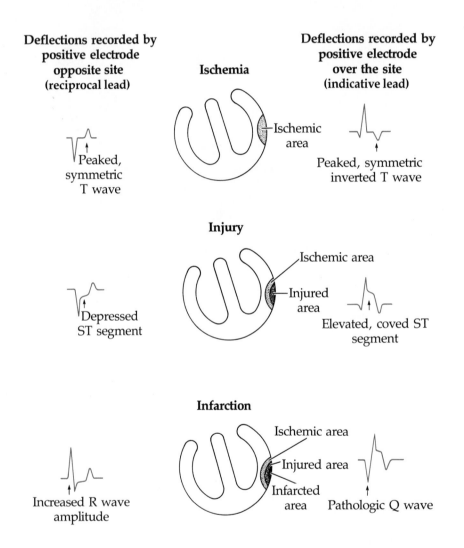

FIGURE 13–3

ECG patterns of myocardial ischemia, injury, and infarction. Note that as damage progresses, signs are superimposed on earlier changes. For example, the pattern of infarction includes the pathologic Q wave (produced by the infarcted area) and elevated ST segment (from the surrounding injured area) and an inverted T wave (from the surrounding ischemic area).

12-lead ECG. If an infarct is diagnosed, obtain further recordings each of the next three days and thereafter as determined by the physician. Follow the serial 12-lead ECGs for the location and resolution of the infarct.

Myocardial ischemia, injury, and infarction usually produce characteristic changes on the ECG (Figure 13–3). These changes are detectable in leads whose positive poles overlie the involved area (indicative leads), as well as in leads whose positive poles overlie the opposite side of the heart (reciprocal leads). *Ischemia* impairs repolarization and therefore inverts the T wave. *Injury* to the myocardium prevents cells from becoming fully polarized; it therefore alters the ST segment. Indicative leads will show ST elevation,

reciprocal leads ST depression. *Infarction* produces absence of electrical activity, creating in effect an "electrical window." Leads whose positive poles are closest to this window look "through" it, recording electrical activity on the other side of the heart as abnormal Q waves and loss of R-wave progression. (The normal R-wave progresses in size through the precordial leads, from a small R-wave in V_1 to a large R-wave in V_6.)

Consider a V_6 electrode, whose positive pole overlies the lateral left ventricle. You will recall that this lead normally displays a large R wave; it does not record right ventricular depolarization because that is obscured by the large positive wave of left ventricular depolarization. When the lateral left ventricle infarcts,

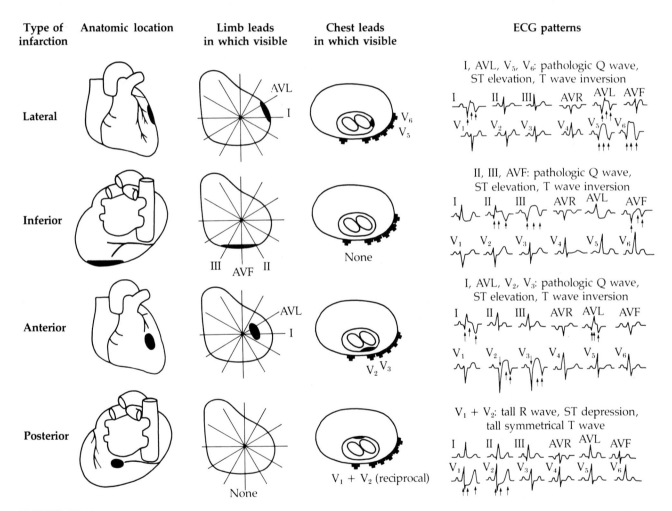

FIGURE 13–4

Localization of infarcts. *Lateral infarct* results from occlusion of the left coronary artery, circumflex branch. *Inferior infarct* usually is due to occlusion of the right coronary artery, posterior descending branch. *Anterior infarct* results from occlusion of the left coronary artery, anterior descending branch. *Posterior infarct* usually is due to occlusion of the right coronary artery.

its cells no longer transmit current, so no R wave is recorded. Without the positive wave coming toward it, the electrode is free to record electrical activity on the other side of the heart. Because this current is moving away from it, the electrode records a significant negative deflection, that is, an abnormal Q wave. Now consider a V_1 electrode, whose positive pole is opposite the infarct. It normally records a small R wave of septal depolarization. Then it records a large S wave, because the combined effect of right and left ventricular depolarization causes a current moving away from it. When the lateral left ventricle infarcts, V_1 records an initial R wave as it usually does. Now, however, there are no negative left ventricular forces to oppose right ventricular depolarization. V_1 therefore continues to inscribe a positive wave, producing a large R wave. Similar changes in other precordial leads produce the loss of normal R-wave progression.

Location and Evolution of Infarction The location of the infarct on the myocardial wall may be determined by noting in which leads the characteristic changes appear (Figure 13–4). The positive poles of leads I, AVL, and V_4–V_6 overlie the lateral left ventricular (LV) wall, and those of leads II, III, and AVF overlie the inferior LV wall. The lateral and inferior walls are opposite each other anatomically. When indicative changes occur in I, AVL, and V_4–V_6, reciprocal changes occur in II, III, and AVF, and vice versa.

The positive poles of chest leads V_1 through V_3 overlie, or "look at," the anterior LV wall. Although the anterior and posterior LV walls are opposite anatomically, the 12-lead ECG contains no leads whose positive poles overlie the posterior wall. If an anterior infarction occurs, indicative changes are seen in leads V_2 and V_3, but there are no leads that display reciprocal changes. If a posterior infarction occurs, there are no leads that demonstrate indicative changes, but V_1 and V_2 may show reciprocal changes. For this reason, it is difficult to diagnose a posterior infarct from a 12-lead ECG; other techniques, such as vectorcardiography, are more informative.

These ECG changes can be used to identify the acuteness or evolution of an infarction (Figure 13–5). As the zone of infarction may be surrounded by a zone of injury, which in turn is enclosed by a zone of ischemia, signs of all three zones may be visible simultaneously on the ECG of a patient with a fully evolved fresh infarction. Alternatively, ECG changes may occur sequentially in an evolving MI. In the

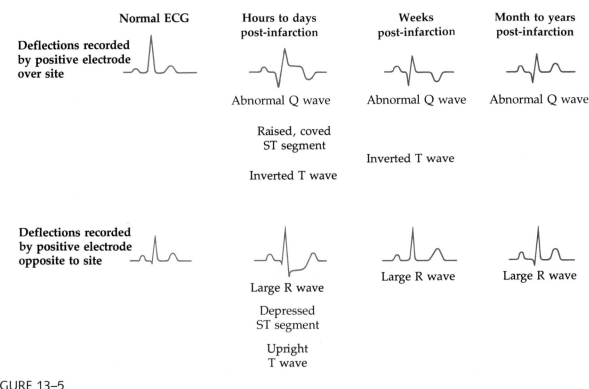

FIGURE 13–5

Evolutionary changes in myocardial infarction.

earliest hours post-MI (the *hyperacute phase*), the ECG is characterized by ST elevation merging into giant, upright T waves. T wave inversion begins within 8–24 hours post-MI; abnormal Q waves develop within several days after MI.

A few weeks post-MI, the ST segment becomes isoelectric. The T waves return to normal in anywhere from a few months to years post-MI. Typically, after 2–3 months the signs of a chronic or old infarction are apparent. The ST and T waves are normal, but the significant Q waves and the loss of R wave progression remain.

When examining the ECG for signs of ischemia, injury, and infarction, it is important to remember that changes in the T wave, ST segment, and QRS can be caused by conditions other than myocardial infarction.

NURSING CARE PLAN

Uncomplicated Myocardial Infarction

Nursing Diagnosis	Signs and Symptoms	Nursing Actions	Desired Outcomes
Behavioral responses observed in patients admitted to CCU to rule out MI:			
a. Anxiety/fear related to CCU admission	Appears restless Appears hostile, withdrawn Talks incessantly Has difficulty concentrating Muscular tenseness Watchful, frightened appearance	1. Introduce self to patient and family. 2. Limit nursing personnel caring for patient for continuity (Primary Care Nurse). 3. Stress that frequent assessments are part of the preventive purpose of unit and do not necessarily imply a deteriorating condition. 4. Inform patient/family of nurses' specialty training, if necessary. 5. Maintain a confident manner. 6. Repeat information PRN because of reduced attention span. 7. Use minor tranquilizers (e.g., Valium) judiciously. 8. Educate patient about illness. 9. Encourage family visiting.	Decreased signs and symptoms of anxiety in patient/family.
b. Fear of death, and anxiety over unfinished business	Verbalizes fatalism or acts extremely emotional, as if in grieving process Verbalizes need to contact people, cancel appointments, "put affairs in order"	1. Allow patient/family to verbalize fears. 2. Answer questions when possible; don't avoid questions. 3. Facilitate the resolution of outside stressors by use of Social Services. Discuss alternatives.	Patient/family verbalize plans for activity progression upon discharge.

(Continues)

NURSING CARE PLAN

Uncomplicated Myocardial Infarction (Continued)

Nursing Diagnosis	Signs and Symptoms	Nursing Actions	Desired Outcomes
c. Fear of the unknown: medical/nursing procedures; changes in lifestyle; expectations of performance as a patient/family	Watches procedures with apprehension Asks questions about procedures Patient/family displays confusion/anxiety as to what actions are safe	1. Provide brief and quiet explanation of admission procedure and rationale for: 　a. Placing in position of comfort (raise head of bed) and initially limiting activity to bedrest with commode privileges (activity plan). 　b. ECG monitor—purpose, alarm system, avoid tangling in wires, why continuous monitoring. 　c. Vital signs (BP, P, R, T) 　d. IV (meds, fluids) 　e. Labs (enzymes, electrolytes, UA, ECG, CXR). 　f. History-taking and cardiovascular assessment using Admit Summary. 2. Orient family and patient to environment: 　a. How bed works, telephones, TVs 　b. How to call for RN 　c. Symptoms to notify RN of, including: chest pain, shortness of breath, palpitations, IV pain. 　d. Visiting hours	Patient/family verbalizes understanding of procedures.

ST–T changes are nonspecific; tachycardia, hyperventilation, cerebral disorders, electrolyte imbalances, pericarditis, pulmonary embolism, and digitalis administration are common causes. QRS alterations also may result from left ventricular hypertrophy, pulmonary embolism, and complicated congenital heart defects, to name a few. These facts emphasize the importance of evaluating the ECG only in conjunction with other patient data.

Serum Enzymes and Radionuclide Imaging Additional measures used in the diagnosis of MI include evalua-tion of serum enzymes and radionuclide imaging. Serum enzymes show a pattern of characteristic changes, with elevations of CPK-MB and the abnormal lactic dehydrogenase ("flipped LDH") pattern most diagnostic of acute MI. With Q-wave infarction CPK-MB elevations are detected 4 hours post-MI and peak in 24 hours. In non–Q-wave infarction, there is more rapid release of CPK-MB, peaking in 17 hours. For further details on normal values, onset and duration of elevations, and significance of abnormal values, please consult Chapter 11.

Radionuclide imaging enables imaging of the infarc-

NURSING CARE PLAN

Uncomplicated Myocardial Infarction (Continued)

Nursing Diagnosis	Signs and Symptoms	Nursing Actions	Desired Outcomes
Chest pain related to myocardial ischemia/necrosis	Typically substernal, described as a heaviness, tightness, pressure, or aching. Radiation to arms (especially left) is common. May also c/o jaw, neck, throat, shoulder, back, or arm pain. Associated signs and symptoms: nausea/vomiting diaphoresis weakness anxiety shortness of breath dysrhythmias palpitations indigestion	1. Check vital signs. 2. Note monitor rhythm. 3. Administer medications to relieve pain: nitroglycerin MS (drug of choice) *or* Demerol IV 4. Administer oxygen 3–8 L/min. 5. Perform 12-lead ECG. 6. Stay with patient until discomfort is relieved, offering reassurance and explanations of care. 7. Administer thrombolytic therapy, as ordered. 8. Prepare for IABP insertion, if unrelieved by drug therapy.	Patient is free of pain. Limitation of myocardial infarction size.
Impaired gas exchange related to decreased cardiac output	Increased or decreased HR Decreased blood pressure Dusky color Decreased temperature Impaired capillary refill Restlessness Reduced arterial Po_2 Dyspnea	Administer oxygen at 3–8 liters per cannula for 24–48 hours	Normal vital signs. Good skin color. Absence of dyspnea. $Po_2 \geq 100$ mm Hg.
High risk for decreased cardiac output related to dysrhythmias	Dysrhythmias	1. Monitor ECG constantly (alarms on at all times). 2. Consider prophylactic use of antidysrhythmic drugs. 3. Monitor for side effects of antidysrhythmic drugs: hypotension, dizziness, nausea, vomiting.	Absence of life-threatening dysrhythmias.
Decreased activity and exercise due to healing myocardium	See Cardiac Rehabilitation Manual.		

Elevated enzymes confirming MI diagnosis	CPK > 100 U/L*
	CPK_2 > 6 U/L
	LDH > 290 U/L
	LDH 1 > 82
	    2 > 119
	    3 > 87
	    4 > 68
	    5 > 85
		1. Ascertain approximate time of onset of pain.
		2. Draw enzymes as ordered. Ideally enzymes drawn 12 and 24 hours after onset of acute symptoms will confirm diagnosis. If not, draw again in 36 hours after acute MI symptoms.
			Enzymes within normal limits.*
			CPK_2 < 6 U/L
			CPK < 100 U/L
			LDH < 290 U/L
			    1 ≤ 82
			    2 ≤ 119
			    3 ≤ 87
			    4 ≤ 68
			    5 ≤ 85.

*Values cited are those in use at University of Washington.

(Continues)

NURSING CARE PLAN

Uncomplicated Myocardial Infarction (Continued)

Nursing Diagnosis	Signs and Symptoms	Nursing Actions	Desired Outcomes
Constipation related to bedrest	Straining at stool Subjective feeling of fullness	1. Ensure adequate bulk in diet and adequate fluid intake. 2. Prevent straining: administer stool softeners or laxatives PRN. 3. Give bedside commode privileges—ensure privacy. 4. Progress activity as tolerated.	Elimination achieved without straining
Ineffective individual coping related to behavioral responses commonly observed in patients who experience myocardial infarction: a. Acute anxiety	Decreased verbalization Inability to concentrate, understand, or retain information Restlessness or insomnia Muscular rigidity Palmar sweating Tremulousness Tachycardia	1. Maintain consistent, continuous nurse–patient contact. 2. Give repeated orientation to CCU routines, equipment, and procedures to patient and family. 3. Assess the patient's prior experience with illness, hospitalization, and severe stress and how it relates to current condition. 4. Solicit expressions of concern and questions from patient and family. 5. Prepare patient and family for each change or move in the patient's physical environment. 6. Allow at least 6 hours of uninterrupted sleep during night. 7. If not on a tranquilizer, assess need and discuss with physician. 8. Teach progressive relaxation. 9. Encourage patient to listen to soothing music.	Verbalizations and behaviors that demonstrate decreased emotional stress. Identifies primary nurse. Verbalizes "slept all night."

NURSING CARE PLAN

Uncomplicated Myocardial Infarction (Continued)

Nursing Diagnosis	Signs and Symptoms	Nursing Actions	Desired Outcomes
b. Denial	Avoids discussing the heart attack or its significance Minimizes the severity of the condition and its consequences Describes condition by quoting others (the doctor says . . .) May verbally acknowledge having had a heart attack, but disregards activity and diet restrictions	1. Assess whether denial is inhibiting the treatment plan: is it verbal or active denial? 2. If verbal, listen but do not reinforce the denial or force acceptance of a fact patient is not ready to cope with. 3. If active (i.e., disregards activity restrictions), assess consequences of patient's actions. Are they detrimental? Conveying concern and allowing more control of the environment are more successful than "threats." 4. If necessary, consult psychiatric clinical nurse specialist.	Demonstrates adherence to activity and exercise program. Chooses foods based on restrictions. Verbalizes appropriate modifications in lifestyle.
c. Depression	Appearance, verbalizations, and behavior exhibiting depression	1. Verbally reflect your observations. 2. Solicit and listen to the patient's feelings; assess how he or she perceives the illness. 3. Allow and encourage tearfulness or crying. 4. Be "matter of fact" about patient's expressions of anger. 5. If patient becomes extremely hostile or angry, do not try to clarify or reason at that time. 6. Manipulate environment. 7. Educate patient about the illness.	Expresses feelings of anger.

Anterior Myocardial Infarction
See Uncomplicated MI, plus:

Nursing Diagnosis	Signs and Symptoms	Nursing Actions	Desired Outcomes
Anterior MI due to left anterior descending artery occlusion	ST segment elevation > 1 mm T wave inversion Possible Q wave in leads I, AVL, V_1–V_4.	Obtain 12-lead ECG every morning for 3 days.	Return of the ST segment to baseline in leads 1, AVL, V_1–V_4 within 1–6 weeks.

(Continues)

NURSING CARE PLAN

Uncomplicated Myocardial Infarction (Continued)

Nursing Diagnosis	Signs and Symptoms	Nursing Actions	Desired Outcomes
Potential bundle branch block due to septal involvement	Widened QRS complex > 0.12 sec. RBBB evidenced by: (1) rSR' in V_1; (2) Rs in $V_6(MCR_5)$ Complete LBBB evidenced by: (1) rS in V_1; (2) large monophasic R wave; no septal Q wave in $V_6(MCR_5)$ Left anterior divisional block (hemiblock) (1) Left axis deviation (axis > −60°) (2) Negative QRS deflections in I, III, and MCR_5	1. Observe monitor closely, and document width of QRS. 2. Observe daily ECG closely for axis deviation. 3. Observe for development of biventricular block.	Sinus rhythm with QRS width within normal limits. Normal QRS axis on 12-lead ECG.
Potential second degree AV block-Mobitz Type II with progression to complete heart block due to occlusion of left anterior descending coronary artery	Dizziness Syncope Alteration in LOC Mean arterial pressure (MAP) <80 mm Hg Second-degree AV block evidenced by: (1) nonconducted P waves; (2) constant PR interval of conducted beats Complete heart block evidenced by: (1) ventricular rate below 40/min;(2) atrial rate > ventricular rate; (3) QRS width > 0.12 sec.	1. Observe monitor carefully for progression of heart block. 2. Notify physician of progressive block. 3. Observe: (1) vital signs; (2) skin for color, temperature, and moisture; (3) urinary output every 2 hours. 4. Correlate heart rate and rhythm with patient's clinical status. 5. See CCU Standing Orders re: Isuprel administration 6. Prepare equipment for possible pacemaker insertion.	HR > 50/min. MAP > 80 mm Hg. Clear mentation. Absence of dizziness and syncope. Urine output > 30 cc/hr.
Potential ventricular ectopy	Ventricular ectopy (PVBs, ventricular tachycardia, and ventricular fibrillation)	1. Observe monitor for ventricular ectopy. 2. Initiate therapy according to CCU Standing Orders. 3. Monitor for side effects of antidysrhythmia drugs.	Absence of ventricular ectopy.
Potential interventricular septal rupture due to necrosis and scarring	Paradoxical pulse Distant heart sounds Holosystolic murmur at the apex and left sternal border MAP < 80 mm Hg Significant HR change Decreased level of consciousness Sudden cardiac death	1. Observe and assess patient each hour: (1) vital signs; (2) breath sounds; (3) heart sounds (S_3, S_4 systolic murmur). 2. Initiate CPR if necessary. 3. Prepare patient for surgery.	Absence of pardoxical pulse. MAP > 80 mm Hg. HR > 50/min. Clear mentation. Skin warm and dry. Urinary output > 30 cc/hr. Absence of holosystolic murmur.

Uncomplicated Myocardial Infarction (Continued)

Nursing Diagnosis	Signs and Symptoms	Nursing Actions	Desired Outcomes
Potential ventricular aneurysm	Ventricular ectopy Paradoxical pulse Distant heart sounds MAP < 80 mm Hg Significant HR change Decreased level of consciousness Sudden cardiac death	1. Initiate activity progression and monitor patient's tolerance. 2. Observe monitor for ventricular ectopy. 3. Initiate therapy for ventricular ectopy according to CCU Standing Orders. 4. Initiate CPR if necessary.	Absence of ventricular ectopy. Absence of hemodynamic changes.
Potential dysfunction or rupture of papillary muscle	Abrupt onset of holosystolic murmur caused by mitral regurgitation Presence of S_3 and/or S_4 Mid-systolic ejection click Crackles in lung field	1. Assess heart sounds, lung sounds, and vital signs q2hrs. 2. Administer vasodilator drugs as ordered. 3. Prepare patient for IABP insertion. 4. Prepare patient for surgery.	Absence of holosystolic murmur. Absence of S_3, S_4, and mid-systolic ejection click. Absence of crackles. MAP > 80 mm Hg.
Potential acute congestive heart failure	See the nursing care plan for congestive heart failure, later in this chapter.		
Potential cardiogenic shock.	See section on shock in Chapter 20.		
Potential extension into lateral wall of myocardium.	See Lateral MI.		

Diaphragmatic/Inferior MI
See Uncomplicated MI, plus:

Nursing Diagnosis	Signs and Symptoms	Nursing Actions	Desired Outcomes
Inferior MI due to occlusion of the right coronary artery	ST segment elevation > 1mm in leads II, III, and AVF T wave inversion in leads II, III, and AVF Q waves in leads II, III, and AVF	1. Obtain 12-lead ECG every morning for 3 days. 2. Observe for ST segment evolution in leads II, III, and AVF. 3. Observe for ST segment changes in other leads.	ST segment returns to baseline in leads II, III, and AVF.
Potential ischemia of SA node	Sinus bradycardia (< 60 beats per minute)	1. Assess patient for hypotension, mentation changes, pallor, fatigue, and pain. 2. Observe for junctional or ventricular escape rhythms. 3. With significant hypotension, lower head of bed and elevate legs. 4. If symptomatic, give atropine 0.6 mg IV as per Standing Orders (maximum of 2.0 mg over 2½ hrs).	Heart rate > 60 beats per minute.

(Continues)

NURSING CARE PLAN

Uncomplicated Myocardial Infarction (Continued)

Nursing Diagnosis	Signs and Symptoms	Nursing Actions	Desired Outcomes
Potential ischemia of AV node resulting in second-degree AV heart block, Mobitz Type I (Wenckebach)	Second-degree AV block (Type I), evidenced by: (1) progressive lengthening of PR interval with each successive beat until a P wave appears without a QRS; (2) irregular R–R intervals	1. Observe rhythm carefully for progression of block. 2. If symptomatic, give atropine 0.6 mg IV as per Standing Orders (maximum of 2.0 mg over 2½ hrs).	Absence of second-degree AV block, Mobitz Type I.
Potential pain related to extension to lateral or posterior myocardial wall	See Lateral MI Standard. See Posterior MI Standard.		
Pain related to inflammation of pericardium. a. Epistenocardia (focal pericarditis) within 4–5 days b. Dressler's syndrome (generalized pericarditis) within 10–14 days	Chest pain differs from myocardial pain in that it increases with deep inspiration or with movement. Fever Tachycardia Paradoxical pulse Accentuated S_2 in pulmonic area Pericardial friction rub: (1) focal pericarditis shows ST segment elevation in II, III, and AVF; (2) generalized pericarditis shows ST segment elevation in limb and precordial leads ST segment elevation is concave in pericarditis versus convex in an infarction. Elevated sedimentation rate Leukocytosis	1. Reassure patient/family that disease is an inflammatory process rather than an MI. 2. Administer steroids/antiinflammatory agents/salicylates as ordered. 3. Monitor for signs and symptoms of cardiac tamponade. 4. Monitor for potential dysrhythmias. 5. Administer antipyretics for relief of fever. 6. Place in postition of comfort. Usually if patients sits up and leans forward, pain may be somewhat relieved.	Absence of chest pain. Absence of paradoxical pulse. Absence of pericardial friction rub. Return of ST segment to baseline.
Potential right ventricular infarction	See Right Ventricular MI.		

Lateral MI
See Uncomplicated MI Standard, plus:

Nursing Diagnosis	Signs and Symptoms	Nursing Actions	Desired Outcomes
Lateral MI due to occlusion of the left circumflex artery	ST segment elevation, T wave inversion, and possible Q wave in leads, I, AVL, MCR_5, and V_6	Obtain a 12-lead ECG every morning for 3 days.	Return of ST segment to baseline in leads I, AVL, MCR_5, and V_6 within 1–6 weeks.
Potential acute congestive heart failure	See the nursing care plan for congestive heart failure, later in this chapter.		
Potential ventricular ectopy Potential ventricular rupture Potential ventricular aneurysm	See Anterior MI.		

NURSING CARE PLAN

Uncomplicated Myocardial Infarction (Continued)

Posterior MI
See Uncomplicated MI Standard, plus:

Nursing Diagnosis	Signs and Symptoms	Nursing Actions	Desired Outcomes
Posterior MI due to occlusion of circumflex branch of left coronary artery or occlusion of right coronary artery	Tall and slightly widened R wave in V_1 and V_2 Tall, upright symmetric T waves in V_1 and V_2 Depressed, concave, upward sloping ST segment or possibly isoelectric ST segment in V_1 and V_2	1. Refer to Diaphragmatic/ Inferior MI Standard and Lateral MI Standard as posterior MI is usually an extension of either one and rarely stands alone.	Normal R wave progression in the precordial leads beginning in V_1 and V_2.

Right Ventricular MI
See Uncomplicated MI Standard, plus:

Nursing Diagnosis	Signs and Symptoms	Nursing Actions	Desired Outcomes
Right ventricular infarction due to occlusion of the right coronary artery	Presence of inferior/ diaphragmatic MI Elevated cardiac enzymes History of chest pain Pallor Possible hypotension Absence of pulmonary congestion Anxiety	1. Control pain with analgesics as per order. 2. Anticipate Swan-Ganz catheter insertion.	Absence of chest pain. Uncomplicated inferior MI.
Right ventricular failure due to decreased contractility secondary to muscle damage	Elevated jugular venous pressure (neck vein distention) Elevated central venous pressure (CVP) with normal to low pulmonary capillary wedge (PCW) pressure Hypotension Pallor Lungs clear S_3 on inspiration	1. Administer fluid challenge to increase cardiac output by passive filling of left ventricle (as per order). 2. Avoid administering diuretics and nitrates, which decrease right ventricular filling volume and further decrease left ventricular filling. 3. Measure and record hemodynamic parameters.	Cardiac output 4–8 liters/ min. Absence of neck vein distention. Normal CVP. Palpable peripheral pulses. MAP > 80 mm Hg.
Potential second-degree AV block, Mobitz Type I (Wenckebach)	See Inferior MI.		

From University of Washington Critical Care Unit: Nursing care plan for MI patients. *Crit Care Nurse* (July/Aug) 1982; 79–84. Adapted with permission.

RESEARCH NOTE

Futrell A, Forst S, Harrell J, Adams L
Effects of occupied and unoccupied bedmaking on myocardial work in healthy subjects.
Heart Lung 1991; 20(2):161–167.

CLINICAL APPLICATION

It is common practice for patients who have sustained an MI to be placed on strict bedrest in order to reduce myocardial work. Bedrest is not without complications, however, and can create physical and psychologic illness. This study questioned whether or not occupied bedmaking would increase myocardial workload when compared with unoccupied bedmaking.

Twenty-two healthy individuals (10 male and 12 female) with a mean age of 48 years old (range 34 years–69 years) served as the sample for this study. Cardiovascular responses (CO, SV, HR, systolic blood pressure (SBP), diastolic blood pressure (DBP), MAP, SVR, and the ratio of pre-ejection period to left ventricular ejection time) were measured during occupied bedmaking with the nurse using a side-to-side technique, during unoccupied bedmaking with patient sitting in a chair, and during a rest period after each bedmaking procedure. Noninvasive instrumentation was used to obtain cardiac function measures: the Cardiac Output program and the Hutchison Impedence Cardiograph I 100 with a built-in A to D converter (BioMedical Technology, Inc.); and a Dinamap vital signs monitor (Critikon, Inc.). Cardiovascular data were collected every minute during the bedmaking activity.

To examine differences between bedmaking procedures, a repeated measures analysis of variance was performed by using change scores from baseline for each variable. Cardiovascular responses to occupied and unoccupied bedmaking differed significantly for most variables, whereas the rest periods showed no significant differences for all variables. While a difference was found between the two techniques, the investigators did not feel the difference was clinically significant and they recommend that further studies be performed on individuals with acute MI. The differences seen in these healthy subjects were felt to represent transient reflexive responses to posturally induced changes in venous return rather than substantial increases in myocardial work.

CRITICAL THINKING

Limitations: The study was performed on healthy individuals and therefore cannot be generalized to other populations. Sample size is also small (22).

Strengths: The study's finding that lateral rotation resulted in increased cardiac output and increased stroke volume supported previous research. Nurses in critical care have often questioned how lateral positioning affects cardiac hemodynamics. This study has added to the body of knowledge in this area. Clearly, additional research into this question would be extremely helpful to guide the clinical practice of keeping MI patients on bedrest.

---

tion and myocardial perfusion and provides indices of left ventricular function. Imaging is particularly valuable because it facilitates serial evaluation of infarction that can be repeated as often as necessary (see Chapter 11).

Planning and Implementation of Care

Nearby are presented plans of care, developed by the nursing staff of the University of Washington Critical Care Unit, for patients with uncomplicated MIs. They include specific problems and nursing actions for patients with particular types of infarcts.

Outcome Evaluation

Evaluate the patient's progress and the effects of your nursing interventions according to these outcome criteria:

- Heart rate and rhythm normal for patient.
- Cardiac output adequate, as manifested by: blood pressure (BP) within patient's normal limits; alert, oriented state; absence of refractory angina or serious dysrhythmias; urinary output above 30–60 ml/hr; warm, dry skin; peripheral pulses within normal limits (WNL).

NURSING DIAGNOSES

Nursing diagnoses that may apply to the patient suffering from an acute MI include:

- Anxiety
- Fear
- Chest pain
- Impaired gas exchange
- High risk for decreased cardiac output
- Activity intolerance
- Constipation
- Ineffective individual coping

- Realistic plans made by patient and family for coping with changes in lifestyle and for return to a satisfying lifestyle after discharge.

Heart Failure

Heart failure is a syndrome in which cardiac dysfunction is associated with reduced exercise tolerance, a high incidence of ventricular dysrhythmias, and a shortened life expectancy (Stevenson and Perloff 1988). Heart failure is the most common admitting diagnosis in hospitals today, and approximately 400,000 new cases are diagnosed each year (Faxon 1988).

Myocardial failure is a primary cardiac defect that decreases the intrinsic contractility of the myocardium. There is a general or focal loss of functioning myocardium or a change in myocardial wall dynamics (e.g., hypertrophy). *End-stage heart disease* is heart failure which is irreversible and associated with myocardial failure. The patient with end-stage heart disease usually has an ejection fraction of less than 20% and is in the New York Heart Association Classification level III or IV.

Theoretical Concepts Related to Heart Failure

In heart failure, the primary problem for the body is that the heart's output of oxygenated blood (cardiac output) is inadequate to meet the tissues' metabolic demands. A brief review of cardiac output is presented here; refer to Chapter 11 for further information.

Cardiac Output *Cardiac output* (CO) is the amount of blood ejected by the ventricle per minute. The normal cardiac output is 4–6 L/min. CO equals the product of the heart rate and stroke volume. Therefore, abnormalities of the heart rate or stroke volume can result in a change in cardiac output. The heart rate can be assessed by the radial pulse or the apical pulse or by evaluation of the ECG. When assessing heart rate, consider the normal cardiac response to varying stroke volumes. For example, the patient who is hypovolemic or in cardiac failure should develop a tachycardia. This normal response may be impaired by drug therapy, such as beta-blockers, or intrinsic atrial-ventricular conduction defects. Other dysrhythmias that may contribute to altered cardiac output are junctional rhythm and atrial fibrillation, where the atrial component of cardiac output is lost.

Determinants of Cardiac Output

Stroke Volume. *Stroke volume,* the amount of blood ejected per heartbeat, depends on myocardial preload, afterload, and contractility.

Preload. *Preload* refers to the length of ventricular fibers at the end of diastole. It is directly dependent on the volume of blood in the ventricle; as the volume increases, preload—and therefore stroke volume—increases (Frank-Starling mechanism). Preload depends upon conditions of both the heart and vascular system. This compensatory mechanism for regulating stroke volume will fail if the ventricular volume load becomes excessive. Because ventricular volume is in turn determined primarily by venous return to the heart, "preload" commonly is used as a synonym for "venous return." Preload is measured at the bedside with a pulmonary artery (PA) catheter, which enables the nurse to determine the right ventricular preload (by measuring the right atrial pressure, RAP) and left ventricular preload (by measuring the pulmonary capillary wedge pressure, PCWP). An *elevated* preload may indicate cardiac failure or hypervolemia; a *decreased* preload may indicate hypovolemia (fluid volume deficit). Both problems can lead to an alteration in cardiac output.

Afterload. *Afterload* refers to the tension and stress that develops in the wall of the ventricle during systole. It is determined by the peripheral resistance, the compliance of the arteries, the volume of the blood contained in the arterial system, and the status of the aortic valve. Since the major determinant of afterload is peripheral resistance, clinicians use peripheral resistance measurements as their guide for afterload. The normal systemic vascular resistance (the measure of left ventricular afterload) is 800–1,200 dynes/sec/ cm^{-5}. The normal pulmonary vascular resistance (the measure of right ventricular afterload) is 100–300 dynes/sec/cm^{-5}.

Contractility. *Contractility* is a property intrinsic to the cardiac muscle. It is initiated by cellular depolarization. The change in ionic balance triggers a series of events causing movement of the very fine fibers of the myocardial muscle bundle (excitation-contraction coupling) (Guyton 1991). In a resting state, these fibers are only slightly overlapping. In a contractile or shortened state, they almost totally overlap. The efficiency of this mechanism is optimal within only a narrow range of myofibril stretch. When the ventricles are distended excessively, the myofibrils are pulled too far apart to permit effective coupling of their cross-bridges, and failure ensues. Although contractility cannot be measured directly, changes can be inferred when there is a fall in cardiac output and another reason for this fall is not identified.

Assessment

Risk Conditions   Risk conditions for heart failure can be grouped conveniently into those that affect blood volume, those that affect the heart, and those that affect the periphery.

Risk conditions affecting blood volume alter the *preload.* With increased preload, the ventricles are unable to contract with maximum efficiency because the excessive end-diastolic volume disrupts the optimal relationship between cardiac fiber length and force of contraction. Valvular stenosis or regurgitation, intracardiac shunts, severe bradycardia, fluid overload, and dysfunction or rupture of chordae tendineae are examples of conditions that cause increased preload.

Risk conditions directly affecting the heart are those that alter the heart's *contractility.* Contractility may be impaired by depressant drugs (such as propranolol), myocardial ischemia, acidosis, electrolyte abnormalities, decreased area of functional myocardium (as in myocardial infarction, ventricular aneurysm, or ventricular dyskinesis), myocarditis or cardiomyopathy, and ventricular fibrillation or asystole. In addition, because of the Frank-Starling relationship, contractility is decreased when the ventricles are not sufficiently distended due to obstructions to filling. Examples of filling impediments are cardiac tamponade, tricuspid or mitral stenosis, and restrictive cardiac diseases. Severe tachycardia, although not an actual physical obstruc-

tion, also limits CO by sharply decreasing ventricular filling time.

Risk conditions affecting the periphery are primarily those that increase *afterload.* Increased afterload can precipitate failure when the heart becomes unable to expel blood efficiently against the increased resistance. Increased right ventricular afterload occurs with pulmonary hypertension and massive pulmonary embolism; increased left ventricular afterload occurs with systemic hypertension or intense vasoconstriction.

In addition to increased afterload, the periphery can cause the heart to fail because of *increased metabolic demand.* When metabolic demand is increased, cardiac output is high but is still insufficient for the body's needs. This high-output failure may be seen in fever, anemia, hyperthyroidism, or severe physical or emotional stress.

When you can identify risk factors, you may be able to take steps to reduce them. For example, follow the measures to prevent and/or relieve dysrhythmias (Chapter 12), myocardial infarction, and cardiac tamponade. Also observe the patient for other risk states, and call them to the physician's attention.

Signs and Symptoms

Pathophysiology   Signs and symptoms of heart failure vary with the ventricle involved and the acuteness of the process. When the heart starts to fail, numerous compensatory mechanisms are called into play. Recall that *increases in heart rate* are an immediate compensatory response, but, particularly in the patient with decreased myocardial reserve, they are a costly way to increase CO. Because coronary artery perfusion occurs primarily during diastole, the shortened perfusion time can seriously compromise coronary artery blood flow. In addition, with tachycardia, ventricular diastolic filling time decreases, so that at high heart rates ventricular filling volume actually can decrease. Finally, tachycardia increases myocardial oxygen demand. These three factors—decreased coronary artery perfusion time, decreased ventricular filling time, and increased myocardial oxygen demand—can interact in an already weakened heart to provoke myocardial ischemia or even MI.

Stroke volume can be increased by altering preload, increasing contractility, or decreasing afterload. A normal acute compensatory mechanism to increase preload is accomplished by vasoconstriction resulting from increased sympathetic nervous system stimulation. Longer-range compensatory mechanisms to increase preload include *sodium and water retention* by the kidneys.

Sympathetic nervous system stimulation also increases myocardial contractility, as does *ventricular dilatation* resulting from the increased preload, via the Frank-Starling mechanism. Ventricular dilatation is limited as a compensatory mechanism, however; when myocardial fibers are stretched too far apart, they are no longer able to contract as forcefully as when the ends of the actin and myosin myofibrils overlap sufficiently. A final mechanism by which contractility can increase is *muscular hypertrophy*. This compensation can occur only if cardiac failure develops slowly—for example, in systemic hypertension. Hypertrophy increases contractility, unless it becomes so severe that the increased muscle mass outstrips coronary artery perfusion capability, in which case ischemia will decrease contractile force.

Changes in afterload also occur in response to decreased CO. The normal physiologic response when cardiac failure begins is *vasoconstriction,* which increases afterload. While vasoconstriction helps to maintain blood pressure, it also increases the resistance against which the ventricle must pump to eject blood. Therefore, excessive vasoconstriction, or lesser degrees of vasoconstriction confronting an already weakened ventricle, can actually worsen cardiac failure. Afterload reduction does not occur naturally in response to decreased cardiac output but instead is a therapeutic maneuver used in refractory heart failure. By capitalizing on the interrelationships between CO and afterload, afterload reduction therapy enhances CO by decreasing the resistance to ventricular ejection.

Types of Heart Failure The right or left ventricle may fail independently, or left ventricular failure may lead to right ventricular failure. At times, the left ventricle may fail so severely that the patient goes into *cardiogenic shock.*

Cardiogenic shock may result from myocardial ischemia or infarction or from abnormal cardiac muscle or valves. Mortality in cardiogenic shock exceeds 80% (Albarran-Sotello et al. 1987).

Right Ventricular Failure When the right ventricle is unable to pump out blood adequately, blood inexorably backs up into the right atrium and then into the systemic veins. Right ventricular failure thus produces increases in right ventricular pressure, right atrial pressure, and systemic venous pressure. The elevated right ventricular pressure causes the following manifestations:

- S_3 heart sound due to filling against an already distended ventricle. The appearance of an S_3 is an important early sign of ventricular failure. An S_4 also may be present.
- Increased myocardial oxygen consumption.
- Pansystolic murmur at the lower left sternal border owing to stretching of the tricuspid ring (relative tricuspid insufficiency).

The increased right atrial pressure may produce atrial fibrillation or other atrial dysrhythmias. Elevated venous pressure causes the following signs and symptoms:

- Increased central venous pressure (CVP) reading
- Distended jugular veins
- Prominent jugular venous pulsations
- Liver engorgement and tenderness
- Positive hepatojugular reflux (momentary pressure over the liver produces increased jugular venous distention)
- Dependent edema
- Ascites due to fluid accumulation in the peritoneal space
- Decreased appetite, nausea, or vomiting due to pressure on the stomach and bowel from venous engorgement of abdominal vessels
- Increased arterial-venous O_2 difference

Because right ventricular output is decreased, the patient may also show nonspecific weakness or easy fatiguability.

Left Ventricular Failure In left ventricular failure, the left ventricle is unable to pump out blood into the systemic circulation efficiently. Initially, the right ventricle is unaffected and continues to pump blood into the pulmonary circuit. Left ventricular failure thus causes increases in left ventricular pressure, left atrial pressure, and pulmonary pressures. The left ventricular pressure elevation produces the following manifestations:

- S_3 and sometimes S_4, due to filling against an already distended ventricle. The appearance of an S_3 is an important early sign of ventricular failure.
- Increased myocardial oxygen consumption.
- Pansystolic murmur at the apex caused by relative mitral insufficiency.

Atrial fibrillation or other atrial dysrhythmias may result from left atrial distention.

Elevated pulmonary pressures cause transudation of fluid into the pulmonary interstitium and alveoli, reflected by the following signs and symptoms:

- Crackles or wheezing
- Dyspnea (which may appear as dyspnea on exertion, dyspnea at rest, orthopnea, or paroxysmal nocturnal dyspnea)
- Frequent cough
- Hyperventilation and respiratory alkalosis
- Frank pulmonary edema

Because left ventricular output is decreased, the patient may also manifest:

- Dizziness or syncope, because of decreased CO to the brain
- Fatigue, because of diminished oxygenation of skeletal muscles and loss of cardiac reserve
- Metabolic (lactic) acidosis, because of insufficient oxygen for normal cellular aerobic metabolism
- Generalized edema
- Pulsus alternans (alternating volume of arterial pulse), for which the exact cause is unknown. One explanation is that the ventricle does not empty fully with the first contraction. The resulting increase in volume provokes a stronger contraction for the next beat (according to the Frank-Starling mechanism), emptying the ventricle more completely. As a result, the end-diastolic volume for the third beat resembles that for the first, and the cycle repeats itself.

If the ventricular failure is severe enough, blood will back up from the pulmonary vessels into the right side of the heart. In that case, signs and symptoms of right heart failure also will be present.

Cardiogenic shock Cardiogenic shock is present when the following signs occur:

- Systolic blood pressure falls below 80 mm Hg in a previously normotensive person or drops 70 mm Hg or more in a previously hypertensive person.
- Cardiac index falls below 1.8 L/min/m^2.
- Left ventricular filling pressure (wedge pressure) climbs above 18 mm Hg.
- Peripheral perfusion is decreased, as shown by clinical signs such as oliguria, tachycardia, and decreased level of consciousness (Albarran-Sotelo et al. 1987).

Planning and Implementation of Care

Nearby is presented a plan of care for the patient with congestive heart failure. This plan utilizes the nursing diagnoses identified above and addresses

NURSING DIAGNOSES

Nursing diagnoses that may apply to the patient with heart failure or cardiogenic shock include:

- Decreased cardiac output
- Impaired gas exchange
- High risk for fluid volume deficit
- High risk for injury: dysrhythmias
- Activity intolerance

the nursing interventions to be used in the acute phase.

Pharmacologic Therapy A wide variety of pharmacologic agents can be used to promote cardiac output in patients in severe failure or cardiogenic shock. To understand the rationale for use of various agents, it is helpful to recall related physiologic concepts.

Physiologic Concepts The key determinants of left ventricular performance are heart rate and stroke volume. Increasing the heart rate is a physiologically costly way to increase cardiac output because of tachycardia's effects on myocardial oxygen consumption and coronary artery filling time. To date, therefore, the major therapeutic efforts have been directed toward improvement of stroke volume.

Preload, contractility, and afterload all are affected by sympathetic nervous system stimuli, as well as other factors. Within the cardiovascular nervous system, three major types of sympathetic receptors exist: alpha, beta, and dopaminergic. *Alpha receptors* are located primarily in vascular smooth muscle. When stimulated, they produce vasoconstriction. *Beta receptors* are located primarily in the heart, vascular smooth muscle, and bronchi. Stimulation of beta$_1$ receptors, found in the heart, causes increased heart rate and contractility. Stimulation of beta$_2$ receptors, found mostly in vascular smooth muscle and bronchi, causes vasodilatation and bronchial dilatation. The third type of receptors, *dopaminergic receptors,* are found in renal and mesenteric blood vessels. When stimulated, they increase blood flow to the kidneys and mesentery.

Vasoconstrictors The major pharmacologic agents used in pump failure can be classed broadly into vasoconstrictors, positive inotropes, and vasodilators. Vasoconstrictors, such as norepinephrine (Levophed), are primarily alpha stimulators. Although widely used

NURSING CARE PLAN

Congestive Heart Failure, Acute Phase

Nursing Diagnosis	Signs and Symptoms	Nursing Actions	Desired Outcomes

Decreased cardiac output related to decreased myocardial contractility	Decreased measured cardiac output
	Hypotension
	Increased systemic vascular resistance (>1,200 dynes/sec/cm^{-5})
	Decreased urine output
	Cool, clammy skin
	Decreased mental alertness
	Metabolic acidosis
	Increased arterial-venous oxygen saturation difference
	Diminished peripheral pulses
	Fatigue
	Decreased exercise tolerance
	Restlessness
	Anxiety
	With left ventricular failure:
	  crackles
	  orthopnea
	  elevated pulmonary capillary wedge pressure (PCWP)
	With right ventricular failure:
	  elevated right atrial pressure (RAP)
		1. Administer supplemental oxygen.
		2. Position patient with head of bed elevated if BP stable.
		3. Administer positive inotropic agents as ordered:
		  dopamine
		  dobutamine
		  amrinone
		4. Monitor BP, heart rate, and hemodynamic measures every 15 minutes until stable, then every hour.
		5. Monitor urine output every hour.
		6. If patient is normovolemic, administer vasodilators as ordered:
		  nitroprusside
		  nitroglycerin
		  captopril
		  hydralazine
		  isosorbide dinitrate
		7. Administer diuretics as ordered.
		8. Monitor electrolytes, arterial blood gases every 6 hours until stable.
		9. Administer volume, as ordered for right ventricular failure.
		10. Provide for a quiet environment.
		11. Provide for periods of uninterrupted sleep.
		12. Instruct patient in relaxation techniques.
		13. Avoid the use of myocardial-depressing drugs, such as propranolol.
			Cardiac output within normal limits.
			Absence of the signs and symptoms of decreased cardiac output.

Decreased cardiac output related to increased afterload	Decreased measured cardiac output
	Hypotension
	Increased systemic vascular resistance
		1. Administer vasodilators as ordered:
		  nitroprusside
		  nitroglycerin
		  captopril
			Afterload within normal limits.

(Continues)

Congestive Heart Failure, Acute Phase (Continued)

Nursing Diagnosis	Signs and Symptoms	Nursing Actions	Desired Outcomes
	Decreased urinary output Cool, clammy skin Decreased mental alertness Metabolic acidosis Increased arterial-venous oxygen saturation difference Diminished peripheral pulses Fatigue Decreased peripheral pulses Fatigue Decreased exercise tolerance Restlessness Anxiety Normal or elevated PCWP, RAP Normal heart rate	hydralazine Isosorbide dinitrate 2. Monitor BP every 15 minutes until stable; monitor SVR every hour, CO every hour. 3. Administer pain medication as needed. 4. Instruct patient in relaxation techniques. 5. Provide for a quiet environment. 6. Encourage patient to listen to soothing music. 7. Provide sedation as needed.	
Impaired gas exchange related to ventilation-perfusion imbalance	Confusion Somnolence Restlessness Irritability Inability to move secretions Hypercapnea Hypoxia	1. Administer supplemental oxygen as ordered. 2. Position patient with head of bed elevated if BP stable. 3. Monitor arterial blood gases every 4 hours until stable. 4. Assess breath sounds every 2 hours. 5. Instruct patient in relaxation techniques that utilize deep breathing. 6. Monitor fluid balance to maintain normovolemic—i.e., daily weights, hourly I & O. 7. Monitor hemoglobin and hematocrit daily for anemia. 8. Treat fever as ordered. 9. Provide for adequate rest and periods of uninterrupted sleep.	Normal arterial blood gases. Absence of respiratory distress.

High risk for fluid volume deficit related to excessive diuresis	*Early:*
	  precipitous weight loss
	  output greater than intake
	Late:
	  tachycardia
	  hypotension
	  thready pulse
	  confusion
	  weakness
	  oliguria
	  decreased RAP, PCWP
		1. Monitor urinary output every hour.
		2. Monitor response to diuretic.
		3. Monitor hourly I & O.
		4. Monitor daily weights.
		5. Instruct patient on importance of measuring all fluids and urine.
		6. Instruct patient on rationale for fluid restrictions/fluid encouragement.
			No signs of fluid volume deficit.

NURSING CARE PLAN

Congestive Heart Failure, Acute Phase (Continued)

Nursing Diagnosis	Signs and Symptoms	Nursing Actions	Desired Outcomes
		7. In late phase, terminate diuretic therapy, give volume, and administer vasopressor agents, as ordered.	
High risk for injury: dysrhythmias, related to electrolyte imbalance	Hypokalemia Hyperkalemia Hyponatremia Metabolic alkalosis Metabolic acidosis ST segment depression T wave tenting U wave prominence U wave/T wave flattening Ventricular extrasystoles Complete heartblock Junctional rhythm Atrial tachycardia with block	1. Monitor electrolyte/ acid–base balance. 2. Administer potassium as ordered while patient on diuretic therapy. 3. Monitor I & O. 4. Monitor ECG for signs of hypo/hyperkalemia and digitalis toxicity. 5. If suspected dysrhythmias occur, check electrolytes, arterial blood gases, and digitalis level. Consult with physician regarding treatment.	Absence of dysrhythmias.
Activity intolerance related to generalized weakness and imbalance between oxygen supply and demand	Increased heart rate (over 20 beats/min above resting) with activity Increased BP with activity Verbal reports of fatigue or weakness Exertional discomfort or dyspnea ECG changes with activity, reflecting dysrhythmias or ischemia	1. Maintain supplemental oxygen during activities. 2. Space out activities and encourage rest periods. 3. Instruct patient in energy conservation methods. 4. Encourage patient to use assistive devices with activities, e.g., walker. 5. Monitor patient response to exercise and gradually increase activities according to response. 6. Instruct patient in relaxation techniques to be used during exercise. 7. Assist patient with activity as needed.	Increased level of activity without fatigue, weakness, discomfort, or other abnormal response.

in the past, they are used less frequently now because of their troublesome side effects and the availability of other agents. Their major disadvantage is an extension of their therapeutic action: in addition to causing peripheral vasoconstriction, they cause renal vasoconstriction. The resulting decrease in blood flow to the kidneys contributes to the very real risk of acute renal failure (specifically acute tubular necrosis) in patients on these drugs. In addition, alpha stimulators used in patients who already are vasoconstricted (as most shock patients are) can significantly decrease tissue perfusion.

Inotropes Inotropes are drugs that alter cardiac contractility; positive inotropes improve contractility. Currently, the intravenous inotropes most commonly used in acute pump failure are dopamine, dobutamine, and amrinone.

Dopamine is used in cardiogenic shock, hemodynamically significant hypotension, and refractory severe congestive heart failure. Its complex pharmacologic actions are dose-related. In the low-dose range (1–2 mcg/kg/min), its major action is stimulation of dopaminergic receptors, increasing urinary output. The resulting diuresis lowers preload, thus decreasing the workload of the heart. In the mid-dose range (2–10 mcg/kg/min), dopamine's major action is beta receptor stimulation, in addition to the dopaminergic stimulation. The target organ most affected is the heart; contractility increases significantly, with relatively little increase in heart rate. In the high-dose range (above 10 mcg/kg/min), dopamine's major effect is alpha receptor stimulation. Because the drug is a precursor of norepinephrine, administration in this range causes peripheral vasoconstriction. The vasoconstriction produced can become so intense that it can counteract the dopaminergic effect of increased renal blood flow and increase afterload. Side effects that may occur with dopamine include hypotension, especially in hypovolemic patients; tachydysrhythmias or ectopic beats; excessive vasoconstriction; and tissue necrosis and sloughing, similar to that seen with Levophed, if the infusion infiltrates.

Dobutamine (Dobutrex) is a synthetic catecholamine that is a direct beta$_1$ stimulator. It is indicated in refractory congestive heart failure, cardiogenic shock, and significant hypotension. It has a stronger inotropic effect than chronotropic effect, so it causes a marked increase in contractility with relatively little increase in heart rate. Renal and mesenteric blood flow increase indirectly, due to the improved cardiac output. Its most significant side effects are tachycardia and dysrhythmias. The usual dose range is 2.5–10 mcg/kg/min as an IV infusion.

Amrinone (Inocor) is an inotropic agent that acts directly on the contractile fibers of the myocardium, unlike digitalis or the catecholamines. It also has vasodilator properties, decreasing afterload and preload. Hemodynamically, it produces an increased CO, decreased left-ventricular end-diastolic pressure (LVEDP), decreased PCWP, and a slight decrease or no change in mean arterial pressure (MAP). It is administered as 400 mg/250 ml of normal saline, at a rate of 5–10 mcg/kg/min. Possible side effects include: dysrhythmias, thrombocytopenia, gastrointestinal (GI) effects (nausea, vomiting, abdominal pain, anorexia), and hypotension.

Vasodilators Vasodilators are drugs that can improve cardiac output by reducing resistance to ventricular ejection. Their use in shock may seem paradoxical at first but is based on a sound physiologic rationale. Recall that blood pressure equals the cardiac output times systemic vascular resistance ($BP = CO \times SVR$). Dilating peripheral vascular vessels reduces their resistance to flow. By reducing resistance to flow, these drugs reduce impedance to left ventricular ejection. Afterload reduction thus increases cardiac output, ultimately improving tissue perfusion.

The intravenous vasodilators most often used in severe heart failure or cardiogenic shock are sodium nitroprusside and nitroglycerin. *Sodium nitroprusside* (Nipride) is indicated in pump failure as well as in hypertensive crisis. It is a direct peripheral vasodilator with no direct inotropic or chronotropic activity. It acts on both the arterial and venous circuits, thus reducing both afterload and preload. As a result, systolic emptying increases, pulmonary congestion lessens, myocardial oxygen consumption decreases, and cardiac output increases. The most significant side effects are hypotension, altered ventilation-perfusion relationships due to reversal of compensatory pulmonary vasoconstriction in areas of local hypoxemia, thiocyanate toxicity, and inhibited platelet aggregation. The drug is photosensitive, so solutions must be protected from light. The usual dose range is 0.5–8.0 mcg/kg/min as an IV infusion.

Intravenous *nitroglycerin* (Tridil, Nitrostat) is used in unstable angina, congestive heart failure complicating myocardial infarction, perioperative hypertensive episodes, and induced hypotension during surgery. It appears to be particularly helpful in management of angina due to vasospasm and may help to preserve ischemic myocardium in acute myocardial infarction. It affects both the arterial and venous circuits, thus reducing both afterload and preload, but its greater effect is on the venous side. It thus lessens venous return, pulmonary congestion, myocardial workload, and oxygen consumption. The mechanism by which it relieves angina is controversial, and probably includes a combination of its effects on the peripheral vascular system, redistribution of myocardial blood flow, and relief of coronary vasospasm. The most significant side effect is hypotension, especially in patients with borderline hypovolemia. Because the drug is absorbed by the plastic used in ordinary intravenous solution bags and tubing, it may be administered using special plastic tubing. The initial IV infusion dose is 5 mcg/min, with subsequent increments titrated to the patient's clinical response.

Captopril (Capoten) is an oral vasodilator that may be used to decrease preload and afterload. It has been found to reduce postinfarction ventricular dilatation, and it improves exercise tolerance in chronic congestive heart failure. Major side effects include hypotension and bradycardia, which may occur with the first dose.

Inotrope/Vasodilator Combination Therapy When caring for patients in severe heart failure or cardiogenic shock, you may find yourself nursing a patient receiving both an inotrope and a vasodilator, typically dopamine and sodium nitroprusside. Managing a patient on such combination therapy can be confusing, because these drugs have synergistic effects on some determinants of cardiac output and opposing effects on other determinants. The following information to guide you is abstracted from Dracup et al. (1981). The goals of combination therapy are to increase cardiac output, lessen pulmonary congestion, and improve myocardial oxygen supply/demand balance. It is easiest to comprehend the effects of combination therapy by grouping them according to preload, contractility, afterload, and oxygen balance.

Nitroprusside and dopamine both decrease preload. Nitroprusside reduces preload by two mechanisms: increasing venous capacitance and improving ejection fraction. Dopamine reduces preload indirectly, by increasing urinary output and increasing ejection fraction (percentage of ventricular volume ejected during systole). Together, these agents provide greater reduction in LVEDP (leading to lessened metabolic demand) and lower wedge pressure (leading to lessened pulmonary congestion) than either drug does alone.

Nitroprusside has no direct effect on contractility but can improve it indirectly by reducing myocardial ischemia. Dopamine improves contractility directly through beta receptor stimulation. Together, the agents provide better augmentation of ejection fraction than nitroprusside alone, with less demand on the left ventricle than if dopamine were used alone.

Nitroprusside directly reduces afterload. If the reduction in afterload does not cause a sufficient compensatory increase in cardiac output, however, blood pressure falls and tissue perfusion suffers. Dopamine has no effect on afterload in low- to mid-dose ranges but increases cardiac output, so its addition to nitroprusside is distinctly advantageous. In high-dose ranges, dopamine can counteract nitroprusside's afterload reduction and thus defeat its use. As long as high-dose dopamine is not used, the combined use of the two drugs can reduce afterload, improve cardiac output, and better maintain blood pressure and tissue perfusion than if the agents were used separately.

Nitroprusside may decrease oxygen supply if it markedly decreases diastolic pressure and therefore coronary perfusion pressure. Adding dopamine can overcome this problem by increasing cardiac output and therefore coronary arterial perfusion. On the other hand, dopamine may decrease oxygen supply if it increases vascular resistance or causes tachycardia. As each drug may decrease oxygen supply, be especially alert for signs of increased ischemia when combination therapy is used.

Nitroprusside probably reduces oxygen demand by decreasing left ventricular end-diastolic volume and vascular resistance. Dopamine, on the other hand, can increase oxygen consumption by increasing heart rate and contractility. The advantage of using the two agents together, therefore, is that their effects on oxygen demand can cancel each other out. As a result, dopamine can be used more safely in the setting of myocardial ischemia than it could by itself.

In summary, simultaneous use of these agents reduces preload, reduces afterload, increases contractility, and may improve myocardial oxygen supply/demand balance. They thus can increase cardiac output, improve systemic perfusion, and may preserve ischemic myocardium.

NURSING TIP

Flagging Emergency Lines

In critical-care units, patients often have multiple IV infusions: vasodilators, antiarrhythmics, inotropic agents, antibiotics, all infusing simultaneously. In an emergency situation, such as cardiac arrest, the nurse is usually anxious and cannot take the time to trace over each IV line to its source. When emergency drugs are needed, the nurse needs to find a line quickly, one without medications—or one where it is safe to temporarily stop such medications infusing through it. One way to avoid a mix-up during a cardiac arrest is to assess your lines at the beginning of the shift. Pick the one you could safely inject emergency drugs through, and flag it with a fluorescent IV drug label. Write on the label "emergency drug line." Put the label near the injection sites where drugs could be infused. This way, if the patient arrests, you know immediately where the drugs can go.

Surgical Intervention Patients in cardiogenic shock who fail to respond to pharmacologic interventions may require mechanical support of the circulation with an intra-aortic balloon pump (IABP) or ventricular assist device (VAD), both discussed in Chapter 14. Surgical treatment of an underlying heart problem is indicated when cardiogenic shock persists despite the above interventions. Surgical procedures include aneurysmectomy, coronary bypass, valve replacement, valve repair, or septal rupture repair. Cardiac surgery is also discussed in Chapter 14.

Cardiomyopathy The interplay of pathophysiology and clinical management considerations is exemplified by *cardiomyopathy,* the second leading cause of heart failure. The term "cardiomyopathy" literally translates to "heart muscle disease." The World Health Organization defines it as a "primary disease process of heart muscle in the absence of a known underlying etiology" (Stedman's 1990).

Three anatomic types of cardiomyopathy have been identified: (1) dilated, (2) hypertrophic, and (3) restrictive (Figure 13–6). Table 13–2 shows the distinguishing features of each type. The etiologies for cardiomyopathy vary for each of the anatomic types and often are not identified. The structural abnormalities result in varying physiologic abnormalities of cardiac function, and therefore each type requires different treatment approaches.

Dilated Cardiomyopathy. Dilated cardiomyopathy (DCM), also called congestive cardiomyopathy, is characterized by dilatation of all four cardiac chambers, contractile dysfunction, impaired systolic function, and symptoms of heart failure. Ejection fraction is low, less than 40%, and biventricular volume is high. In addition, with the volume overload and the stretching of the myocardial walls, mitral regurgitation (MR) develops. This MR further adds to the problem of volume overload and myocardial failure.

The clinical manifestations of DCM reflect the forward failure and backward failure which are present. *Forward failure* refers to the fall in cardiac output which results in decreased blood flow to the body and the resulting signs and symptoms: decreased BP, decreased pulses, decreased urine output, and decreased mental alertness. *Backward failure* refers to the backup of blood into the lungs and right ventricle and the resulting signs and symptoms: shortness of breath, abdominal tenderness, liver enlargement, neck vein distension, nausea, and leg edema. While all causes of heart failure result in the signs and symptoms discussed earlier, it is important to note that in patients with end-stage or chronic heart disease, mechanisms that compensate for the body congestion may have developed. For example, in chronic heart failure, lung crackles may not be heard if the body has developed collateral lymphatic circulation in the lungs (Stevenson and Perloff 1988).

DCM can be palliated medically but often requires heart transplantation. Therapeutic goals focus on hemodynamic management of the failing heart, prevention of systemic emboli, and control of dysrhythmias. If the patient is awaiting transplantation, then prevention of malnutrition and infection become especially important.

Tailored medical therapy with oral vasodilator drugs (to reduce afterload) and diuretics (to reduce blood volume) is the best approach for these patients (Stevenson 1991). By reducing afterload, vasodilators

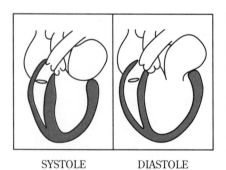
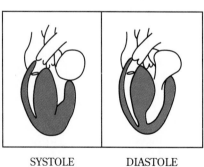
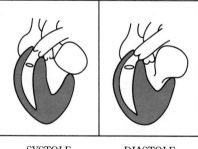

| SYSTOLE | DIASTOLE | SYSTOLE | DIASTOLE | SYSTOLE | DIASTOLE |

Dilated cardiomyopathy   Hypertrophic cardiomyopathy   Restrictive/obliterative cardiomyopathy

FIGURE 13–6

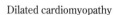

Types of cardiomyopathy. (From Purcell J: Advances in the treatment of dilated cardiomyopathy. *Clin Issues Crit Care Nurs* 1990; 1:32–33.)

lessen the work of the heart and the ventricle can empty more effectively. Wall tension also is reduced, which in turn decreases myocardial oxygen consumption. Reduction of preload reduces intraventricular volume and myocardial dilatation, and therefore lessens the amount of mitral regurgitation present. In addition, the smaller blood volume decreases venous return to the heart and therefore reduces the excess volume that contributes to the failure overall. The patient is sent home on a drug regimen combining an oral vasodilator, nitrates, and diuretics. The type of oral vasodilator used depends on the patient's response to the drugs, but research has proven the efficacy of captopril (Capoten) in reducing 1-year mortality and episodes of sudden cardiac death in these patients (Foronow 1991).

The problem of systemic emboli with DCM remains unsettled. Systemic emboli arising from intracardiac thrombi occur in up to 30% of patients with DCM and may be more common in the setting of chronic or paroxysmal atrial fibrillation (Stevenson and Perloff 1988). Use of anticoagulants carries many risks, especially in DCM patients whose venous congestion is often accompanied by liver dysfunction.

In DCM patients with an ejection fraction of less than 25%, the 1-year mortality is over 50%. In these cases, heart transplantation offers the only chance for survival. Currently, heart transplant recipients have a 1-year survival rate of 85% and a 5-year survival rate of 70%. While heart transplantation offers patients a significant improvement of life expectancy, it is available only to a limited few because of the small donor supply.

Hypertrophic Cardiomyopathy. Hypertrophic cardiomyopathy (HCM) is characterized by one or more of the following: left-sided septal enlargement, biventricular hypertrophy, or cellular fibrotic changes. The pathophysiologic effects of this disorder are obstruction to blood flow and stiffening of the ventricular wall. Although a cause for HCM is unknown, there appears to be some familial association, originating perhaps during embryonic development. Manifestations of the disease appear most often in young adulthood but may not be seen until the patient is elderly.

Early recognition of HCM is extremely important since death is often sudden and unexpected (Braunwald 1988). This is particularly true if the individual participates in competitive athletic activity, in which syncope and sudden death can occur. The most common symptom is dyspnea, seen in 90% of individuals with HCM. Angina pectoris, fatigue, and syncope are also common. Less frequently observed are: palpitations, paroxysmal nocturnal dyspnea, overt congestive heart failure (CHF), and dizziness. Exertion may exacerbate these symptoms. On auscultation, a

TABLE 13–2

Features of Cardiomyopathy

TYPE OF CARDIOMYOPATHY	PRIMARY ANATOMICAL FEATURES	TREATMENT GOALS
Dilated cardiomyopathy (formerly congestive)	Dilated atrial/ventricular chambers Usually normal thickness ventricular walls (rarely time for hypertrophy to develop)	Optimize contractility. Reduce workload. Evaluate for transplant.
Hypertrophic cardiomyopathy	(One or more of following:) Left-sided septal enlargement Idiopathic hypertrophic subaortic stenosis (IHSS) Biventricular hypertrophy Cellular fibrotic changes	Avoid sudden drop in preload, i.e., sweating, diuretics, vasodilators. Avoid excessive vasoconstriction (extreme physical exertion). Give beta-blockers to decrease contractility (especially if biventricular bulk leads to decreased outflow). Evaluate risk for sudden death/consider transplant only if high risk.
Restrictive/obliterative	Reduced ventricular cavity due to scaring of endocardium (Loeffler's eosinophilia) or amyloid deposition	Maintain good ventricular filling (avoid diuretics, sweating/dehydration, etc.). Give inotropes only if poor left ventricular function.

Source: Purcell JA: Advances in the treatment of dilated cardiomyopathy. *Clin Issues Crit Care Nurs* 1990; 1:32–33.

loud S_4 may be heard along with a harsh, crescendo-decrescendo systolic murmur. On palpation of the precordium, a systolic thrill can be palpated at the apex or left lower sternal border. The ECG will show nonspecific ST–T wave abnormalities and left ventricular hypertrophy. While these signs and symptoms are clues to the possibility of HCM, a more thorough cardiac examination is necessary to make a diagnosis.

Treatment of HCM is aimed at minimizing its consequences (Hurst et al. 1990). Any situation which increases the obstruction to blood flow or increases resistance to ventricular filling must be avoided. Therefore, these patients must be protected from competitive sports, tachycardia, sudden hypotension, sudden hypovolemia, and fainting. Positive inotropic drugs (such as digitalis, dopamine, dobutamine, amrinone, and epinephrine) should be avoided, as should vasodilator drugs (such as nitroprusside, nitrates, captopril, hydralazine, and enalapril). Beta-blockers may be used to improve hemodynamics. Because sudden death is the most common hazard of HCM, antidysrhythmic drug therapy is important. Verapamil and amiodarone have been used (Hurst et al. 1990). Use of an automatic implantable cardiac defibrillator (AICD) is sometimes necessary (see Chapter 14 for details). Antibiotic prophylaxis is important because about 5% of patients develop infective endocarditis. When dental or surgical procedures are performed, antibiotics should be prescribed before and after the procedure.

Some types of HCM can be treated surgically, although surgery is used only in severely symptomatic patients. Myotomy or myomectomy of the septum is performed and portions of the hypertrophic tissues resected. This procedure carries the risks of major heart surgery but has had good results, with a 93% 5-year survival rate (Hurst et al. 1990).

Restrictive Cardiomyopathy. Restrictive cardiomyopathy (RCM) consists of endocardial, subendocardial, or myocardial lesions that limit ventricular filling, leading to high ventricular pressures and abnormal diastolic function. The most common cause is endomyocardial fibrosis, but another leading cause is amyloid heart disease. Findings with restrictive cardiomyopathy include reduced wall motion and hypertrophy in the absence of dilatation or problems with contractility. Diastolic dysfunction (decreased distensibility) is present, while systolic function is normal or near normal. Clinical manifestations of RCM include: exercise intolerance, weakness, dyspnea, chest pain, elevated central venous pressure, peripheral edema, enlarged liver, and ascites. The general prognosis for this class of disorders is poor. The treatment will vary according to the etiology. Prevention of sudden cardiac death remains important, as well as prevention of systemic emboli. Inotropic agents may be used in special cases. Depending upon the etiology, heart transplantation may or may not be indicated. When an underlying systemic disorder is the cause of the cardiomyopathy, heart transplantation is contraindicated.

Outcome Evaluation

Evaluate the patient's progress and the effect of therapeutic measures according to these outcome criteria:

- Arterial pressure, pulmonary artery, and wedge pressures WNL for the patient.
- When thorax elevated 45°, jugular venous distention and hepatojugular reflux absent; normal jugular venous pulsations.
- Heart rate and rhythm normal for the patient; preferably normal sinus rhythm.
- No edema, ascites, or liver enlargement or tenderness.
- Lungs clear to auscultation.
- Blood gases WNL for patient.
- No dyspnea, orthopnea, or cyanosis.

Acute Cardiac Tamponade

The heart is surrounded by the pericardial sac, which fits loosely around it and protects it against friction. The sac attaches to the great vessels, diaphragm, sternum, and posterior mediastinal structures. The inner layer of the sac (the part in direct contact with the heart) is the visceral pericardium or epicardium. The outer layer, the parietal pericardium, is fibrous. Both layers are lined with serous tissue. The space between the layers, the pericardial space, normally contains only 10–20 ml of pericardial fluid but can accommodate up to 2 liters of fluid without hemodynamic changes.

Cardiac tamponade results when increased intrapericardial pressure interferes with diastolic filling of the heart. The pressure may rise because of a space-occupying lesion, such as a tumor, or more commonly because of bleeding into the pericardial sac. Etiologies for cardiac tamponade are listed in Table 13–3.

Assessment

Risk Conditions   Certain conditions increase the likelihood of tamponade. Be on the alert for these conditions.

ADVANCES IN CRITICAL CARE TECHNOLOGY

Heart Transplantation

Heart transplantation is indicated when cardiac disease is irreversible and the patient is without other medical or surgical options. A patient will undergo this procedure because of continuing symptoms, unacceptable quality of life, or high risk for early death (Stevenson and Miller 1991). While the mortality rates from this procedure were high in the past, current rates have proven that cardiac transplantation can be associated with improved survival. One-year survival now is at 88% and 5-year survival at 70% (Stevenson and Miller 1991).

The Technology The heart transplantation procedure is surgically simple. Three suture lines connect the new organ to the posterior atrial walls of the recipient's native heart, the aorta, and the pulmonary artery. Cardiopulmonary bypass supports the body's circulation during the surgery, and the patient recovers in an ICU in the same way as any heart surgery patient. Complications of the procedure are the same as those experienced by the bypass patient, with the exception that early rejection may occur. One feature unique to the transplant patient's electrocardiogram is the presence of two P waves. The SA node of the recipient's heart is always left intact, and the patient receives the graft organ with its SA node intact.

Patient Care Considerations The long-term problems associated with heart transplantation include rejection, infection, and accelerated graft atherosclerosis. Research now is directed toward finding improved medications to prevent and treat rejection. At this writing, cyclosporine, OKT3, RATG, and steroids remain the mainstay in rejection therapy. While these agents are effective, they suppress the entire immune system. Two new agents under investigation, FK-506 and RS-61443, are selective immunosuppressive agents that target only the rejection cells.

Heart transplantation, while improving longevity, does cause a major change in the patient's life. The medication regimen is extensive because it includes not only drugs to prevent rejection but also drugs to fight the side effects of the antirejection medications. The patient must have frequent laboratory tests to monitor liver and kidney function. A heart biopsy is performed yearly for the rest of the individual's life. Over time, the new heart may develop disease of the coronary vessels, and the disease process may begin again. Some patients have even required a second heart transplant. When asked, however, if they wished they had not undergone the operation, few patients would say yes. Most are extremely grateful for a second chance at life.

- Pericarditis, especially in an anticoagulated patient
- Cardiac trauma, penetrating or nonpenetrating, such as: cardiac surgery, cardiac biopsy, perforation by a transvenous pacing wire, myocardial infarction, stabbing or impalement
- Rupture of heart or great vessels

Prevent or alleviate high-risk conditions whenever possible. For instance: consult with the physician about discontinuing anticoagulants when a patient develops pericarditis; maintain the patency of mediastinal chest tubes postcardiotomy and decrease cardiac workload for the patient with a recent myocardial infarction.

Signs and Symptoms Recognize the signs of developing tamponade. They vary with the amount of fluid and the rapidity of its accumulation.

Precordial chest pain can vary from mild to severe. The pain is stabbing and knifelike, and is worsened by breathing, coughing, swallowing, moving, or lying supine. A pericardial friction rub is present in pericarditis, due to the movement of the two inflamed pericardial surfaces rubbing against each other.

Observe for signs of *systemic venous congestion* due to restricted venous return to the heart. These include distended neck veins, liver enlargement, elevated CVP or right atrial pressure readings, and/or dyspnea. A paradoxical arterial pulse (pulsus paradoxus) is an important finding in tamponade as well as in certain other cardiac disorders. Its etiology and assessment are presented in Chapter 10.

Observe for signs of *decreased CO*. Especially watch for a falling systolic blood pressure. Other signs include agitation, cyanosis, poorly palpable apical pulses, tachycardia, and sometimes muffled heart sounds.

TABLE 13–3

Etiologies of Cardiac Tamponade

Cardiovascular causes:
  chest trauma
  heart surgery
  aneurysm
  coronary angiography
  insertion and removal of pacing wires
  insertion of central venous catheter
Neoplasms
Purulent pericarditis:
  bacterial
  viral
  tubercular
Myxedema
Collagen diseases
  rheumatoid arthritis
  systemic lupus erythematosus
Uremic pericarditis
Radiation pericarditis
Hypersensitivity states
Anticoagulants

Source: Estes ME: Management of the cardiac tamponade patient: A nursing framework. *Crit Care Nurse* 1985; 5:17. © 1991 by Cahners Publishing Company.

Follow the results of diagnostic procedures. The ECG may be normal or show nonspecific signs of pericarditis. Alternating voltage (electrical alternans) of all P, QRS, and T deflections is thought to be diagnostic of tamponade; however, it is an infrequent finding. The echocardiogram will show an echo-free zone. The chest x-ray usually shows a widened mediastinum.

NURSING DIAGNOSES

Nursing diagnoses for a patient suffering from cardiac tamponade include:

- Pain
- Fear
- Decreased cardiac output
- Altered tissue perfusion

Planning and Implementation of Care

Relieve the *pain related to pericardial inflammation* by allowing the patient to assume the most comfortable position; preferably sitting up or leaning forward. Administer salicylates, analgesics, and/or steroids as ordered by the physician.

Relieve the *fear related to the unknown*. Using language appropriate to the patient's condition, explain that the symptoms are temporary and will be relieved by treatment. Inform the patient about the diagnostic and therapeutic procedures used.

Relieve the *decreased CO* and *altered tissue perfusion related to impaired ventricular filling*. As a temporary measure, the physician may want you to infuse intravenous fluids rapidly to raise ventricular filling pressure above pericardial pressure. Definitive treatment for acute cardiac tamponade is removal of the pericardial fluid, as explained below.

Assisting with Pericardiocentesis

If the symptoms are progressing rapidly, obtain *immediate* medical help and prepare for a pericardial tap *(pericardiocentesis)* or emergency sternotomy (discussed in Chapter 14). Following are the steps to take in assisting with pericardiocentesis:

1. Elevate the head of the bed about 60°.

2. Monitor the cardiac rhythm, CVP, and BP before and during the procedure. Have an emergency cart and defibrillator nearby. Ventricular fibrillation or accidental laceration of a coronary artery or the myocardium can cause shock and death.

3. Obtain a pericardiocentesis tray, sterile gloves, prep solution, and ECG machine and sterile "alligator" clips and wires. Act as the unsterile person to unwrap the tray and add to it the alligator clips and wire. The physician will connect the clips to the sterile needle and pass you the end of the wire. Connect it to the precordial lead wire of the ECG machine.

4. The physician will insert the needle at the cardiac apex or in the angle between the left costal margin and the xiphoid. As he or she does so, watch the pattern on the ECG machine and report immediately when the PR segment or ST segment elevates. These elevations indicate the needle has reached the myocardium, producing a local current of injury. They therefore warn the physician to withdraw the

needle a few millimeters to avoid myocardial laceration.

5. After the fluid is aspirated, the physician will withdraw the needle and apply pressure on the site.

6. Send the aspirated fluid for diagnostic studies ordered by the physician.

Aspiration usually will cause dramatic hemodynamic improvement, with stabilization of the BP and pulse and disappearance of the paradoxical pulse. Continue monitoring the patient for recurrent tamponade. Repeated tamponade may necessitate surgical creation of a "pericardial window" to allow continuous fluid drainage.

Outcome Evaluation

Use these outcome criteria to evaluate the patient's progress:

• Heart rate and rhythm normal for patient.

• CO sufficient, as evidenced by arterial blood pressure, mental status, urinary output, peripheral pulses, skin temperature and color normal for patient.

• Heart sounds as loud as before the tamponade.

Aortic Dissection

Aortic dissection occurs when the medial layer of the aortic wall degenerates over time. Why this degeneration occurs is unclear, but arterial hypertension clearly is a factor in its development. The degeneration weakens the arterial wall and decreases the cohesiveness between the medial and intimal layers. The dissection may or may not be associated with an intimal tear (Hurst et al. 1990). The hematoma which forms within the medial layer is usually longitudinal and in two thirds of all cases is located in the ascending aorta. Figure 13–7 illustrates the pathogenesis of acute aortic dissection.

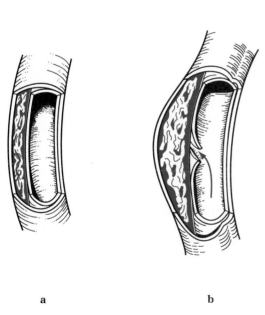
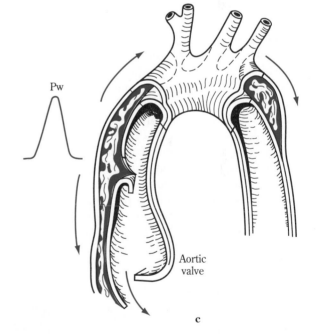

a   b   c

FIGURE 13–7

Diagrammatic representation of the pathogenesis of acute aortic dissection. **a.** Degenerative changes in medial layer of aorta set the stage. **b.** Combination of forces produces intimal tear, permitting arterial blood to enter weakened media. **c.** Resulting dissecting hematoma is propagated in one or both directions by the pulse wave (Pw) produced by each myocardial contraction and the blood pressure. (From McGoon D, McCauley K, Brest A: *McGoon's cardiac surgery: An interprofessional approach to patient care.* Philadelphia: Davis, 1985, p. 178.)

Assessment

Signs and Symptoms The clinical symptoms of aortic dissection are distinct but may vary depending on the site of the injury and the progression of the dissecting hematoma. The patient, often a middle-aged man, suddenly develops *excruciating pain that is described as sharp, tearing, knifelike, or ripping.* The pain may be unrelieved by opiates. It usually originates in the chest and then spreads down the back into the abdomen or lower extremities. Pain that subsides and then occurs again is an ominous sign, indicating perhaps the impending lethal rupture of the dissecting segment. Finally, while the pain is abdominal, nausea and vomiting do not occur. This is helpful to know in distinguishing aortic dissection from other abdominal emergencies.

Clinical signs include a precordial systolic murmur, diastolic murmur of aortic regurgitation, possible blood pressure difference between arms, loss of pulses to one or both lower extremities, strokelike symptoms, pallor, sweating, peripheral cyanosis, syncope, and decreased level of consciousness due to decreased cerebral bloodflow. Blood pressure may be very high or low, depending on the amount of blood loss. Pulse deficits in the upper extremities indicate thoracic dissections, while pulse deficits in the lower extremities often indicate an abdominal dissection.

Other clinical findings which may prove helpful are laboratory, ECG, and roentgenographic findings. With active bleeding, the red blood cell count and hematocrit will be low. Usually the white blood cell count is moderately elevated. The ECG will be negative for signs of myocardial ischemia or infarction, but it will demonstrate left ventricular hypertrophy related to the chronic hypertension. The chest x-ray is an important part of the assessment. The mediastinal image of the heart and great vessels will be widened, and pleural effusion may be present, especially if there is a leak from the dissection. Definitive diagnosis can be made with an aortogram, which will show the details of the dissection.

NURSING DIAGNOSES

Nursing diagnoses for an individual suffering from aortic dissection include:

- Altered tissue perfusion
- Pain

Planning and Implementation of Care

Altered Tissue Perfusion Related to Blood Vessel Dissection Monitor cardiovascular status at least hourly, checking pulses and BP, bilateral skin color and temperature, and cardiac murmurs. Also monitor the ECG for ST–T changes, indicating ischemia, and dysrhythmias. Monitor neurologic status hourly, including decreased level of consciousness (LOC), syncope, and pain.

Implement emergency treatment to lower the blood pressure (if patient is hypertensive) and control pain. Administer intravenous vasodilators, as ordered. Drugs which may be used include sodium nitroprusside, propranolol, trimethaphan, and guanethidine. Once the blood pressure is stabilized, the patient is taken to a cardiac catheterization laboratory, with surgical stand-by, for angiographic evaluation of the location and extent of the dissection. Dissections can be treated both medically and surgically. The surgical techniques are (1) resection and graft replacement of the aorta (Figure 13–8), (2) repair and end-to-end anastomosis of the aorta, (3) resuspension or replacement of an insufficient aortic valve, or (4) local procedures to restore flow in major branches of the aorta.

Postoperatively, prevent stress on the suture line and monitor the patient for leakage of the suture line. Control blood pressure with vasodilators, keeping systolic pressure less than 130 mm Hg. Monitor peripheral pulses closely for any change in pulse volume. Obtain daily chest x-rays to detect a widening mediastinum (indicating possible leak at the site of repair) or pleural effusion, and obtain complete blood counts to detect blood loss. Implement pulmonary exercises to prevent pneumonia.

Pain Related to Ischemia Monitor pain levels and watch especially for subsiding and then recurring pain, which may presage a rupture. Consult with the physician about appropriate analgesics; administer analgesics cautiously to minimize masking of signs of further dissection.

Outcome Evaluation

Use these outcome criteria to evaluate the patient's progress:

- Relief of pain.
- Peripheral pulses bilaterally equal and of normal volume; normal coloring of extremities.

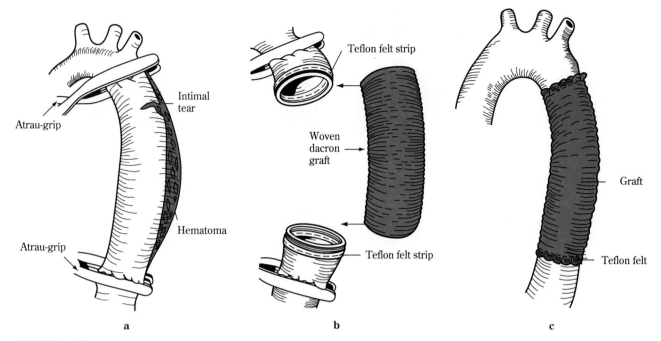

a   b   c

FIGURE 13–8

Illustration showing **a.** Acute dissection isolated; **b.** section of descending
thoracic aorta reinforced with Teflon felt strips; **c.** tightly woven crimped Dacron
graft which has been coated with heparinized blood and autoclaved for 3 minutes
(technique absolutely prevents any leakage of blood through pores in graft), rinsed,
and sewn in place. (From McGoon D, McCauley K, Brest A: *McGoon's cardiac
surgery: An interprofessional approach to patient care.* Philadelphia: Davis, 1985,
p. 193.)

- Systolic blood pressure less than 130 mm Hg or
  within range ordered by physician.
- Urine output > 30 ml/hr.
- Presence of bowel sounds.
- Absence of any signs of bleeding (no hematuria,
  melena, abdominal pain, or hematemesis).

REFERENCES

Albarran-Sotelo R et al.: *Textbook of advanced cardiac life
support.* Dallas: American Heart Association, 1987.

Bayer A et al.: Changing presentation of myocardial infarction
with increasing old age. *JAGS,* 1986; 34(4):263–266.

Benner P: *From novice to expert.* Menlo Park, CA: Addison-
Wesley, 1984.

Braunwald C: *Heart disease: A textbook of cardiovascular
medicine.* Philadelphia: Saunders, 1988.

Dracup K et al.: The physiologic basis for combined
nitroprusside-dopamine therapy in post-myocardial infarction heart failure. *Heart Lung* 1981; 10:114–120.

Faxon D: ACE inhibition for the failing heart: Experience
with captopril. *Am Heart J* 1988; 115:1085–1093.

Foronow G: Personal communication, 1991.

Guyton A: *Textbook of medical physiology,* 8th ed. Philadelphia:
Saunders, 1991.

Hurst J et al.: *The heart.* New York: McGraw-Hill, 1990.

Kern L: The elderly heart surgery patient. *Crit Care Nurs
Clin North Am* 1991; 3(4):749–756.

Stedman's Medical Dictionary, 25th ed. Baltimore: Williams &
Wilkins, 1990.

Stevenson L: Tailored therapy before transplantation for
treatment of advanced heart failure: effective use of
vasodilators and diuretics. *J Heart Lung Transplantation*
1991; 10:468–476.

Stevenson L, Miller L: Cardiac transplantation as therapy for
heart failure. *Curr Prob Cardiol* 1991; 16:219–305.

Stevenson L, Perloff J: The dilated cardiomyopathies. *Cardiol
Clin* 1988; 6:187–218.

Wei J, Gersh B: Heart disease in the elderly. *Curr Prob Cardiol*
1987; 12:7–26.

14

Cardiovascular Interventions

CLINICAL INSIGHT

Domain: The teaching-coaching function

Competency: Providing an interpretation of the patient's condition and giving a rationale for procedures

Patients in the surreal world of the intensive care unit, their minds blurred by medications, physiologic imbalances, and psychologic stress, may interpret their ordeals in bizarre ways. Often, these are recollections of profoundly disturbing episodes. Nurses can help such distraught patients make sense of their memories, thus eliminating the power of those memories to haunt them. In the following exemplar, from Benner (1984, pp. 88–89), a physician gives an account of his experience as a patient in an ICU.

All nurses coming on duty tried to make their own assessments of their patients' emotional level as well
as their physical status. At times I would try to be falsely cheerful, and they would see through it. On one memorable Monday, I was obviously depressed, and my nurse, coming on duty, asked me gently what was wrong. I didn't have a clue. I wept buckets, something I don't usually do. I felt unashamed but puzzled. She said with some confidence: "We'll figure this out," and then went on to ask a few questions. She wanted to know, "Is the sound outside disturbing you?" I realized that it was. After a little further thought she said: "You didn't hear this noise Saturday and Sunday, but you did hear it Friday when your aortic balloon came out. That was a bad time. You remember not only how painful that was but you also remember how the balloon sounded inside you during all those rough days. I bet you are remembering all that pain." My distress disappeared.

An understanding of the interventions commonly used for patients with cardiovascular disorders will enhance your ability to implement a treatment plan, evaluate its effectiveness, and protect the patient from harmful side effects. In addition, such an understanding will enable you to interpret treatment measures for the patient and family, as demonstrated in the Clinical Insight. This chapter presents information on common treatments for cardiac ischemia, rhythm disturbances, and cardiac failure. Included are cardiac drug therapies, pacemakers, percutaneous transluminal coronary angioplasty (PTCA), cardiac surgery: coronary artery bypass grafting, intra-aortic balloon counterpulsation, and ventricular assist devices.

Emergency Cardiac Drug Therapy

Sudden Cardiac Death

Sudden cardiac death (SCD) is defined as a cardiac-related death within 24 hours of the onset of symptoms. Approximately 450,000 episodes of SCD occur annually in the United States, and at least 80% of these patients die. Patients experiencing this syndrome have been shown to have a high incidence of coronary artery disease (but not necessarily acute myocardial infarction [MI]), which contributes to death from a lethal dysrhythmia or, less frequently, from myocardial failure. The precipitating abnormality is a tachydysrhythmia in 75–80% of these patients, with bradydysrhythmias and acute cardiogenic shock seen much less frequently.

While 75% of ventricular fibrillation survivors have evidence of coronary artery disease, only 19% of these events are associated with an acute MI. The typical survivor of a SCD episode is a 60-year-old male with a history of cardiovascular disease, who has not been exercising or taking antidysrhythmic medications, and who experiences no warning symptoms whatsoever prior to the event (Greene 1990). Thus, the majority of patients experiencing SCD have a disorder of electrical conduction as a result of ischemic heart disease. Because symptoms are typically absent prior to the onset of SCD, identification of high-risk patients is of paramount importance.

Risk factors for SCD include previous MI, congestive heart failure, left ventricular ejection fraction below 40%, prior SCD episode, unexplained syncope, and frequent ventricular premature beats (VPB's) (> 5 per hour). As the number of risk factors increases, survival rapidly declines. A patient with two of the above risk factors has a 76% chance of surviving 6 months, while three risk factors carry only a 38% 6-month survival rate (DiCarlo 1985). Smoking has been identified as an additional risk factor for SCD. In one study, patients who quit smoking after a SCD event decreased the recurrence of cardiac arrest from 27–19% within the following 3 years (Greene 1990). Additional factors that have been shown to increase the risk of dysrhythmias include hypokalemia, hypomagnesemia, prolongation of the QT interval, and cocaine abuse. While the presence of VPBs on Holter monitoring indicates increased risk of SCD, 90% of patients with ischemic heart disease experience some degree of ventricular ectopy (Greene 1990). Diagnostic evaluation that includes electrophysiologic testing may be indicated to evaluate patients at highest risk for SCD and to assist in treatment decisions. The automatic implantable cardioverter defibrillator (AICD) has resulted in a dramatic reduction in mortality to only 2–3% annually after implant. This treatment is discussed in the Advances in Critical Care Technology Box.

Rapid initiation of cardiopulmonary resuscitation (CPR) is the greatest determinant of outcome following SCD events. Greene (1990) found that when bystanders initiated CPR at the scene, survival increased from 21–43% and adverse neurologic sequelae following successful resuscitation were dramatically reduced. Treatment for the patient in cardiac arrest includes CPR, advanced cardiac life support techniques, and management of specific dysrhythmias. The following section reviews emergency cardiac drugs as well as medications used to support cardiac function in critically ill patients following initial resuscitative efforts.

Emergency Cardiac Drugs

Key points for the most commonly used emergency drugs are presented here. The Appendix also contains information on numerous antidysrhythmic agents that are not considered emergency drugs. The acronym L-E-A-D has been used as a tool for remembering the most common first-line code drugs: lidocaine, epinephrine, atropine, and dopamine (Jones and Bagg 1988).

Lidocaine (Xylocaine) Lidocaine is particularly useful in suppressing ventricular dysrhythmias. Its effects include a decreased rate of spontaneous phase 4 depolarization as well as local anesthetic effects on ventricular myocardium and depressed conduction via re-entrant pathways. Lidocaine has different actions in normal and ischemic tissue; it reduces the difference in

ADVANCES IN CRITICAL CARE TECHNOLOGY

Automatic Implantable Cardioverter Defibrillator (AICD)

THE TECHNOLOGY

Patients who survive an episode of sudden cardiac death may be candidates for an automatic implantable cardioverter defibrillator (AICD). This device, first used clinically in 1980, is designed to recognize malignant ventricular dysrhythmias and deliver an electrical countershock in order to restore an effective heart rhythm. AICDs are indicated for patients who have had one or more episodes of cardiac arrest not associated with an acute myocardial infarction, as ventricular dysrhythmias are common during an acute ischemic event but do not necessarily recur following recovery. Electrophysiologic studies are performed to identify an inducible ventricular tachycardia or fibrillation despite optimal antidysrhythmic therapy. Candidates should have a life expectancy of at least 6 months, be emotionally stable enough to cope with the device, and be able to participate in indefinite medical follow-up care.

An AICD system monitors the heart rate and, once programmed criteria indicating a dysrhythmia have been met, delivers an electrical countershock via electrodes that have been surgically placed on the heart. The system is usually implanted via a median sternotomy or lateral thoracotomy. It includes a pulse generator/defibrillator, which is placed in an abdominal pocket and connected to various configurations of epicardial or transvenous rhythm sensing leads and patch electrodes, which are placed anteriorly and posteriorly on the heart. After the device has been activated, it assesses the need for countershock delivery via a programmed heart rate function. If the patient's heart rate exceeds this cut-off rate, the device charges and delivers a 26–30 joule shock within 10–35 seconds. If the rhythm does not convert, up to four more shocks may be delivered. The device is capable of monitoring for up to 5 years, and can deliver up to 300 shocks before the generator must be replaced (Teplitz 1991c).

PATIENT CARE CONSIDERATIONS

Following insertion, postoperative care consists of routines normally provided to patients undergoing cardiac surgery with emphasis on avoiding hypoxia, electrolyte imbalance, or other factors that may precipitate a dysrhythmia. Although the device may or may not be activated in the immediate postoperative period, life-threatening dysrhythmias in AICD patients should always be treated as if the device were not present. Emergency resuscitation and prompt external defibrillation are initiated in the usual manner. Should the device fire while you are touching the patient, no more than a slight tingling sensation will be felt. An external doughnut magnet held over the device turns it on and off; beeping tones will be heard for 30 seconds when a magnet is applied to a device that is activated. Patients should be instructed that if they hear these tones, they are near a strong magnetic field and should leave the area immediately to avoid inactivation of their device.

Prior to hospital discharge, patients usually are taken to the electrophysiology lab for a final evaluation of the device, and it is triggered to fire while the patient is awake but sedated. Patients are usually relieved once they have experienced this sensation for the first time. Patient and family education focuses on avoiding close contact with magnetic fields (a list is included in the patient education booklet), carrying a Medic Alert ID, what to do if the device fires, and follow-up care. Because patients have often experienced an episode of sudden cardiac death, family members are encouraged to learn CPR. Many facilities offer support groups for these patients, as emotional adjustments to living with the device may seem overwhelming.

action potential duration between normal and ischemic myocardium and prolongs conduction in ischemic tissue. Lidocaine also raises the fibrillation threshold, especially in ischemic tissue, at higher plasma levels (American Heart Association 1987). It has minimal effects on contractility, blood pressure, or atrial dysrhythmias.

Lidocaine is the drug of choice for suppressing ventricular ectopy including ventricular tachycardia, ventricular fibrillation, and frequent (more than six per minute) VPBs. It is also used for multiformed VPBs, for bursts of two or more VPBs, and for potential R-on-T phenomenon (when VPBs appear close to the preceding T wave). While prophylactic lidocaine has been advocated in acute MI to prevent ventricular fibrillation, a review article of previous randomized trials has questioned this practice (MacMahon et al. 1988). No beneficial effects were seen with lidocaine prophylaxis, and the early mortality rate was 33% higher than in control patients, presumably due to a higher incidence of asystole in patients treated with lidocaine.

The appropriate route and dose for lidocaine administration depends on the setting. An initial intravenous (IV) bolus of 1 mg/kg is followed by 0.5 mg/kg every 8–10 minutes if ectopy persists, up to a total of 3 mg/kg. If IV access has not yet been established in an intubated patient, the above dose may be instilled into the endotracheal tube (ET) followed by lung inflations with an Ambu bag to distribute the drug to the tracheobronchial tree. Recommendations specific to the ET route include dilution of drug to at least 5 cc and the possible need for larger doses than with the IV route (Hasegawa 1986). Once resuscitated (by either route), the patient should receive an infusion of 2–4 mg/min. To avoid lidocaine toxicity, serum lidocaine levels should be assessed after 48 hours of therapy. Elderly patients are particularly susceptible to toxic effects, and half the standard lidocaine dose, or 1–2 mg/min, may be prescribed (American Heart Association 1987). Lidocaine toxicity results in central nervous system disturbances including lethargy, disorientation, and possible hallucinations or seizure activity.

Epinephrine Epinephrine is an endogenous catecholamine with both alpha and beta adrenergic stimulating properties. Its complex pharmacologic actions depend in part on dose and in part on the body's reflex circulatory adjustments to this drug. In cardiac emergencies, epinephrine can be expected to increase heart rate, myocardial contractility, and systemic vascular resistance (SVR). Blood pressure increases, resulting in improved coronary and cerebral perfusion. In asystole and electromechanical dissociation (EMD), epinephrine may generate a spontaneous contraction. It also makes ventricular fibrillation more susceptible to defibrillation efforts.

Epinephrine is indicated in asystole, EMD, pulseless ventricular tachycardia, and ventricular fibrillation. Current dosage recommendations are 0.5–1.0 mg (5–10 cc of a 1:10,000 solution) every 5 minutes, as needed (American Heart Association 1987). Studies have indicated that IV doses in the range of 2–5 mg may be even more effective in cardiac arrest situations, and such high-dose epinephrine is being advocated by some investigators (Guerci and Chandra 1991). Epinephrine usually is given as an IV bolus, but it may also be administered via an ET tube for absorption by the pulmonary vascular bed.

The major side effects of epinephrine are an exaggeration of its therapeutic properties, including tachycardia and ventricular irritability. As a result of increased heart rate, contractility, and SVR, myocardial oxygen demands increase and may precipitate myocardial ischemia.

Atropine Atropine blocks the transmission of parasympathetic impulses from the vagus nerve. It does so by competing with acetylcholine (the usual parasympathetic chemical mediator) for receptor sites. Because stimulation of the vagus nerve inhibits impulse initiation by the sinoatrial (SA) node and impulse conduction through the AV node, blocking the vagus nerve results in increased impulse initiation and conduction. Atropine is indicated for symptomatic sinus bradycardia, atrioventricular (AV) block, and asystole. The usual dose is a 0.5–1.0 mg bolus, repeated every 5 minutes as needed until a total dose of 2 mg has been given (American Heart Association 1987). Complete parasympathetic blockade occurs at this dose, and additional doses (though not harmful) will not have any further beneficial effects. Atropine is contraindicated in heart transplant patients, as denervation of the transplanted heart removes parasympathetic influences on cardiac function. Atropine may be given endotracheally if IV access is not yet established. Possible side effects include tachydysrhythmias with increased myocardial workload and ischemia, as well as paradoxical bradycardia at doses less than 0.5 mg.

Dopamine Dopamine is an endogenous catecholamine with dose-dependent alpha, beta, and dopaminergic stimulating properties. In low doses (1–2 mcg/kg/min), stimulation of dopaminergic receptors results in vasodilatation of renal and mesenteric arteries, resulting in increased urine output with little cardiac or blood pressure effect. Beta$_1$ and alpha effects occur at doses of 3–10 mcg/kg/min, resulting in increased heart rate, contractility, and SVR. At doses exceeding 10 mcg/kg/min, alpha effects predominate, resulting in vasoconstriction.

Low-dose dopamine is used to increase urine output in situations of low renal perfusion. Moderate doses are used for shock, low cardiac output (CO) states, and hypotension. They result in increased CO, blood pressure, SVR, and filling pressures. Doses exceeding 10 mcg/kg/min are generally avoided but may be used in profound shock states. Dopamine is administered only as a continuous infusion (never an IV bolus) at a rate of 2–20 mcg/kg/min, using the lowest dose that results in the desired hemodynamic response.

Infusion sites should be assessed carefully for signs of infiltration, as severe tissue necrosis can occur with

CRITICAL-CARE GERONTOLOGY

Drug Complications in the Elderly

The elderly compose the fastest growing segment of the population, with over 30 million persons over age 65 living in the United States. Patients in this age group take an average of 4.5 different medications—mostly cardiovascular and diuretic agents—daily. It is not surprising that 10% of all hospital admissions for this age group are related to drug toxicity, most commonly because of digoxin, diuretics, anticoagulants, hypotensives, and antidysrhythmics (Beers and Ouslander 1989; LeSage 1991).

Several physiologic changes associated with aging place elders at risk for drug complications. Compromised renal function is the most important factor leading to adverse drug effects in all patients (Jones 1989). Renal function falls by 10% per decade after age 40, but serum creatinine values remain stable because of decreased creatinine production. The following formula can be used to estimate creatinine clearance, a more accurate predictor of renal function, which is normally 100 cc/min (Kain, Reilly and Schultz 1990):

$$\text{creatinine clearance} = \frac{(140 - \text{age}) \times \text{body weight (kg)}}{\text{serum creatinine} \times 72}$$

The addition of potentially nephrotoxic medications, such as aminoglycoside antibiotics, can cause a further decline in renal function and result in the rapid development of drug toxicities. Impaired hepatic blood flow and declining hepatic metabolism lead to reduced drug elimination rates and contribute to renal effects in potentiating toxicity. Lidocaine and propranolol exhibit high levels of hepatic clearance,

warranting a 50% dose reduction to avoid adverse effects. Beta blockers, verapamil, and hydralazine are inadequately metabolized in the older patient and dosage reductions are indicated (Jones 1989). Both cimetidine and ranitidine can be rapidly toxic to the older patient if standard doses are used.

Drug distribution is altered in the elderly as a result of decreased body water, decreased albumin levels, and increased adipose tissue. Water-soluble medications will be diluted in less volume; therefore, serum concentrations will rise. The half-life of lipid-soluble medications such as benzodiazepines and lidocaine will be prolonged due to increased storage of drug in adipose tissue. These alterations in drug distribution result in elevated serum concentrations for most drugs. For example, aminophylline and theophylline, which are water-soluble, require a 50% dosage reduction in the elderly to avoid toxic effects.

Altered drug effect on target organs is also seen in elderly patients with a variety of medications. Beta receptors become less sensitive with age; therefore, "heart rate slows less with propranolol and speeds less with adrenaline" (Beers and Ouslander 1989, p. 107). The older brain is highly sensitive to narcotics, and decreased morphine requirements with equal pain relief have been demonstrated in a classic study (Bellville et al. 1971). Because standard doses often result in oversedation, respiratory depression, and confusion, initially decreased narcotic doses are merited in elder patients. Laxatives should be routinely given to patients receiving narcotics to avoid constipation, which is common in this age group.

Digitalis preparations are the most frequently prescribed medication for patients over 75, yet this drug has a very narrow safety margin in this population. Toxicities are common, even at normal serum digoxin levels, and may be evidenced by subtle findings such as anorexia, syncope, or weakness (Jones 1989). Moreover, patients may experience these toxic effects prior to achieving a therapeutic drug response.

Several guidelines for drug administration in the elderly exist. Unless a rapid increase in plasma concentration is needed, some authors recommend initiating all medications at 50% of the standard dose (Beers and Ouslander 1989). Watch closely for central nervous system (CNS) effects; virtually any drug can be psychoactive in this population. Special consideration should be given to recently introduced medications. Because drug testing often involves relatively small numbers of healthy subjects prior to market introduction, adverse effects may occur that have not been previously cited by the manufacturer.

Iatrogenic drug reactions in the elderly often present as hypotension, serious dysrhythmias, or altered mental status. The incidence of these complications rises dramatically with age and results in increased length of stay as well as untold morbidity and mortality. To promote effective drug therapy in elderly patients, be alert for subtle signs of medication toxicity and notify the physician promptly of adverse effects. Paying attention to drug doses and monitoring patients closely will help to reduce iatrogenic complications of pharmacologic therapy in this population.

dopamine extravasation. While peripheral infusions are commonplace, a central line is preferable to avoid this complication. Major side effects include tachycardia and dysrhythmias, as well as increased myocardial oxygen demand and coronary ischemia at higher doses.

NURSING TIP

Dopamine Extravasation

Following extravasation of dopamine or other vasoconstrictors, administration of the vasodilator drug phentolamine (Regitine) may prevent severe tissue necrosis. After obtaining a physician's order (many institutions have a standing protocol for drug extravasation therapy), reconstitute 5–10 mg of phentolamine with 10 cc of normal saline. Administer phentolamine into the subcutaneous tissue via multiple 1 cc injections in a circle around the area of infiltration. This therapy should be initiated promptly, preferably within 12 hours, for maximum effectiveness (Hill 1991).

Antidysrhythmics

Adenosine (Adenocard) Adenosine is a naturally occurring metabolite, important in many biochemical pathways. As a drug, adenosine has been shown to have "both diagnostic and therapeutic value with respect to supraventricular tachycardias" (Berne, DiMarco and Belardinelli 1984). Adenosine depresses SA node activity and delays impulse conduction through the AV node, terminating supraventricular tachycardia (SVT) within seconds after injection. It does not terminate atrial fibrillation, atrial flutter or ventricular tachycardia. However, its ultrashort half-life (<10 seconds) and minimal adverse effects make it useful in the differential diagnosis of wide complex tachycardia. Following adenosine administration, atrial flutter waves may become apparent, or ventricular tachycardia will continue unchanged.

Adenosine is administered as a rapid IV bolus of 6 mg peripherally or 3 mg centrally, immediately followed by a saline flush for complete drug delivery (McIntosh-Yellin and Drew 1992). Several seconds of sinus arrest and/or AV block often occur, followed by

conversion to sinus rhythm or resumption of SVT. Repeat doses of 6–12 mg may be administered if the initial dose is ineffective. Adverse effects include facial flushing, dyspnea, and chest pressure lasting less than 60 seconds. Adenosine should be administered cautiously, if at all, in patients with high-grade AV block or sick sinus syndrome, and dosage reductions are required in heart transplant patients or individuals taking dipyridamole (Lerman and Belardinelli 1991).

Procainamide (Pronestyl) Procainamide is a second-line agent for suppression of ventricular dysrhythmias if lidocaine has been ineffective, and is also indicated for suppression of supraventricular dysrhythmias. It decreases automaticity by reducing phase 4 depolarization, as well as the slope of phase 0 of the action potential. The loading dose for IV procainamide is 100 mg every 5 minutes at a rate of 20 mg/min until one of the following is reached: (1) dysrhythmia suppression, (2) hypotension, (3) increase of 50% in QRS width, or (4) total dose of 1 g administered (American Heart Association 1987). A maintenance infusion of 1–4 mg/min should follow the initial loading dose.

Verapamil Hydrochloride (Isoptin, Calan) Verapamil is a slow-channel calcium blocker, which functions by inhibiting calcium ion influx into cardiac and smooth muscle cells. As these channels play a significant role in the electrical activity of the AV node, verapamil is useful in prolonging AV conduction. Its ability to interrupt re-entrant AV nodal mechanisms makes it particularly useful in terminating episodes of SVT. By blocking calcium ion influx in myocardial cells, verapamil depresses myocardial contractility. Calcium blockade in smooth muscle cells results in peripheral vasodilatation and interruption of coronary vasospasm. Myocardial oxygen requirements are reduced as a result of decreased contractility and afterload.

Verapamil is indicated for paroxysmal SVT, atrial flutter, and atrial fibrillation. It terminates AV nodal re-entrant tachycardias in almost 90% of patients, and slows ventricular response in atrial fibrillation and flutter. Verapamil is contraindicated in patients with impaired AV conduction or congestive heart failure. Its most significant adverse effect is hypotension. Verapamil must be used with caution in Wolff-Parkinson-White syndrome, as it can accelerate the heart rate in some forms of this disorder. The recommended dose of verapamil is an initial 5 mg IV bolus over 1–2 minutes, and it may be repeated as a 5–10 mg bolus if needed. The antidote for calcium channel blocker overdose is calcium chloride injection.

Inotropes

Amrinone (Inocor) Amrinone is an inotropic agent and vasodilator that acts via phosphodiesterase inhibition rather than adrenergic stimulation. At a cellular level, amrinone increases myocardial energy stores in the form of cyclic adenosine monophosphate (c-AMP), resulting in improved cardiac contractility as well as peripheral vasodilatation. Its hemodynamic effects are similar to those of dobutamine, with greater vasodilation and less effect on heart rate at normal doses.

Amrinone is indicated for congestive heart failure in patients with an adequate blood pressure. A loading dose of 0.75 mg/kg is given as an IV bolus over 2–3 minutes, followed by a continuous infusion of 2–20 mcg/kg/min, using the minimal dose that delivers the desired response. Side effects include hypotension and dysrhythmias, as well as thrombocytopenia after prolonged infusion. Platelet counts rarely fall below 70,000 and are restored within 5–10 days after stopping the infusion (Mancini, LeJemtel and Sonnenblick 1985).

Dobutamine (Dobutrex) Dobutamine is a synthetic catecholamine with primarily $beta_1$ and $beta_2$ receptor activity, resulting in increased myocardial contractility coupled with decreased vascular resistance. It has less effect on heart rate than dopamine and has no effect on dopaminergic receptors.

Dobutamine is indicated for low cardiac output states and congestive heart failure. It results in increased CO, decreased SVR, and decreased filling pressures, with less augmentation of blood pressure and urine output than with dopamine. Dobutamine is administered as a continuous infusion from 2–20 mcg/kg/min, again using the lowest possible dose that results in the desired hemodynamic response. Side effects include tachycardia and dysrhythmias at higher doses.

Isoproterenol (Isuprel) Isoproterenol is a synthetic sympathomimetic with almost pure beta agonist activity. Its stimulation of $beta_1$ receptors results in increased heart rate and contractility, accompanied by peripheral and pulmonary vasodilation due to its $beta_2$ properties. Because of its potent chronotropic and inotropic effects, CO usually increases. Its effects on blood pressure vary, but a fall in blood pressure may be seen as a result of vasodilatation. Isoproterenol is used primarily to treat symptomatic bradycardias until pacemaker therapy can be initiated, and it is also the preferred inotrope following cardiac transplantation. It is administered as a continuous infusion at a rate of 2–10 mcg/min, titrated to the desired heart rate. Side effects include increased automaticity, leading to tachycardias and ventricular irritability, and increased oxygen consumption which may precipitate myocardial ischemia.

Vasodilators

Nitroglycerin Nitroglycerin relaxes smooth muscle of the coronary vasculature and venous system, resulting in direct coronary vasodilatation and decreased preload. Myocardial perfusion is enhanced as a result of increased coronary blood flow combined with reduced left ventricular workload.

Indications for IV nitroglycerin include acute myocardial ischemia, infarction, and congestive heart failure. A continuous infusion is initiated at 10–20 mcg/min, and increased by 10 mcg every 5–10 minutes until the desired effect is achieved. The usual dosage range is 50–200 mcg/min, but doses up to 500 mcg/min have been used for chest pain relief without adverse effects (Kaplan, Finlayson and Woodward 1980).

As a result of venous dilatation, nitroglycerin may precipitate hypotension, warranting careful blood pressure monitoring. If hypotension occurs, it usually responds to leg elevation or volume administration. Headache occurs in response to dilatation of cerebral vessels, and it is treated with analgesics as needed.

Nitroprusside (Nipride) Nitroprusside relaxes both venous and arterial smooth muscle, resulting in potent antihypertensive effects as well as reduced preload and afterload. Cardiac output rises in response to reduced SVR. A reflex tachycardia may be seen in patients with pre-existing hypovolemia. Indications for nitroprusside administration include emergency treatment of hypertension or congestive heart failure. A continuous infusion is initiated at 0.5 mcg/kg/min and titrated to achieve the desired hemodynamic endpoint. Severe hypertension may require doses of up to 8 mcg/kg/min. Solutions are protected from light to avoid loss of potency.

The most serious adverse effect of nitroprusside is hypotension, which may be quite severe and warrants continuous blood pressure monitoring to avoid this complication. Due to the drug's short half-life, discontinuance of the infusion should reverse the hypotension within minutes. With prolonged infusions, nitroprusside metabolites can accumulate, resulting in thiocyanate or cyanide toxicity. Thiocyanate levels can be monitored in patients at risk for cyanide toxicity, for example, patients on high doses for prolonged periods or patients with renal insufficiency.

Defibrillation and Cardioversion

A direct-current electrical countershock may be successful in terminating both atrial and ventricular tachydysrhythmias. Cardioversion and defibrillation are similar in that each involves a countershock that depolarizes the myocardial cell mass simultaneously, thereby allowing the SA node to resume its dominance. They differ in that cardioversion uses a lower wattage and requires synchronization of the shock with the R wave (achieved by depressing a SYNCH button on the defibrillator, which delays energy release from the paddles until an R wave occurs). Synchronization is necessary so that the shock will not fall on the T wave, during the vulnerable period of repolarization, which could result in repetitive depolarization (i.e., ventricular fibrillation). Cardioversion usually is not an emergency procedure; defibrillation is. Cardioversion usually is performed by a physician, defibrillation by the nurse if no physician is immediately available.

Defibrillation Defibrillation is the definitive treatment for ventricular fibrillation. As the duration of ventricular fibrillation increases, the likelihood of successful defibrillation rapidly decreases. Thus, prompt defibrillation is critical to patient survival.

The optimal energy dose for defibrillation is not yet established. There is no clear-cut relationship between the size of the patient and the amount of energy necessary for defibrillation. The ideal dose probably varies considerably, depending on the duration of fibrillation, previous electrical shocks, the metabolic state of the myocardium, and other factors.

American Heart Association (1987) standards recommend three rapid, consecutive shocks. The initial attempt at defibrillation should be made with 200 joules of delivered energy. If unsuccessful, defibrillation should be repeated at 200–300 joules immediately. If still unsuccessful, third and subsequent attempts should be made at 360 joules.

Cardioversion Prior to cardioversion, food and fluids are restricted and digitalis is held for up to 24 hours before the procedure. (Cardioversion is contraindicated in patients with digitalis toxicity, as refractory ventricular tachycardia may occur). The patient is anesthetized with midazolam (Versed) or thiopental sodium, and a synchronized countershock is delivered. Maintaining a patent airway and assessing for respiratory compromise is critical through all phases of the procedure.

Following cardioversion or defibrillation, monitor the ECG, blood pressure, and neuromuscular activity.

Transient hypotension and dysrhythmias (especially premature beats and sinus bradycardia) are common. Neurologic assessment is particularly important in patients who have been in atrial fibrillation prior to cardioversion. During fibrillation, thrombus can form along the wall of the atria. With restoration of synchronized atrial contractions, thrombus may break free and embolize. Potential complications from emboli are not limited to the cerebrovascular bed. Thrombus can also embolize to the coronary arteries and renal or splanchnic vascular beds, causing end-organ ischemia from small vessel occlusion. Assessment of neurologic and gastrointestinal (GI) status, ECG changes, and urine output is initiated after the procedure to detect signs of impaired organ perfusion.

Pacemakers

Artificial cardiac pacemakers are used for electrical stimulation of the heart in patients experiencing conduction abnormalities that result in impaired cardiac output. The goal of cardiac pacing is to increase heart rate to a level that will maintain organ perfusion, with minimal adverse effects. Over 300,000 permanent cardiac pacemakers are inserted annually throughout the world, making care of the pacemaker patient a reality in virtually any critical-care setting (Greatbatch 1991). Clinical assessment for these patients includes evaluation of the pacemaker circuit, ECG rhythm, and the hemodynamic response to cardiac pacing.

Indications

Current applications for artificial pacemaker support are expanding with the advent of external, noninvasive devices. Pacemakers may be used for temporary or permanent support, either therapeutically in situations of impaired electrical conduction or prophylactically when conduction defects are anticipated. Table 14–1 lists current indications for use of artificial cardiac pacemakers.

Cardiac Pacing Systems

All pacemaker systems contain two essential components: a generator that initiates electrical impulses, and an electrode that delivers these impulses to the heart, resulting in myocardial contraction. However, it should be noted that impulse conduction does not guarantee

TABLE 14–1

Potential Indications for Temporary Cardiac Pacing

Bradydysrhythmias

Asystole

Atrial fibrillation with slow ventricular response

Idioventricular rhythm

Junctional rhythm

Sick sinus syndrome

Sinus arrest

Sinus bradycardia (symptomatic)

Heart Block

Alternating bundle branch block

Right bundle branch block with hemiblock

Second-degree block

Third-degree block

Prophylactic Applications

Cardiac catheterization/PTCA

Cardiac surgery

Cardioversion

Electrophysiologic testing

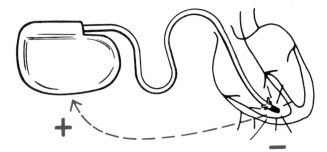

Unipolar generators

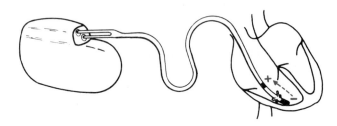

Bipolar generators

FIGURE 14–1

Unipolar **(top)** versus bipolar **(bottom)** pacemaker systems. (Reprinted with permission from Medtronic, Inc. Copyright Medtronic, Inc. 1991.)

myocardial contraction, as the heart muscle must be able to respond to an electrical stimulus. Even when a pacing system is intact and functional, massive myocardial infarction, tamponade, hypoxia, or other situations of impaired muscle function may preclude an effective cardiac output, resulting in EMD.

Cardiac pacing may be initiated with electrodes placed transcutaneously, inserted transvenously, or sewn directly onto the epicardium. Transvenous and epicardial pacing leads may contain one (unipolar) or two (bipolar) electrodes at their distal tip, in contact with the heart. Current flows from the negative electrode to the positive electrode, thus completing the electrical circuit. With a *unipolar system,* the negative electrode is in contact with the heart, and the positive electrode is contained within the pacemaker generator (Figure 14–1). *Bipolar systems* are advantageous in that both electrodes are in contact with the heart. In bipolar function, one electrode acts as a negative electrode and the other as a positive electrode. Each electrode can act as the negative electrode, so if bipolar pacing fails, the system quickly can be converted to a unipolar system. Almost all permanent and temporary electrodes inserted today are bipolar and can operate in either asynchronous or synchronous modes of pacing.

Modes of Pacing

In the *asynchronous (fixed-rate)* mode, a pacemaker stimulus is delivered at a set rate regardless of the patient's spontaneous ECG rhythm. In this mode, a pacemaker stimulus could arrive during the vulnerable period of the ECG, triggering ventricular fibrillation. Therefore, asynchronous pacing is usually reserved for patients in asystole who lack a competing, intrinsic cardiac rhythm. In the *synchronous (demand)* mode of pacing, the pacemaker is capable of sensing intrinsic electrical activity, resulting in inhibition or triggering of the pacemaker as needed. The pacemaker delivers an impulse only after a preset interval has passed with no spontaneous ECG activity, thus avoiding competition between the pacemaker and the patient's native ECG rhythm.

Pacemaker systems may allow *sensing* (recognition of ECG activity) and *pacing* (delivery of an electrical impulse) in the atria, the ventricles, or both chambers. Therefore, it is important to identify expected pacemaker function for any system. A three-letter pace-

TABLE 14-2

The NASPE/BPEG Generic Pacemaker Code for Antibradyarrhythmia and Adaptive Rate Pacing and Antitachyarrhythmia Devices

POSITION	I	II	III	IV	V
Category	Chamber(s) paced	Chamber(s) sensed	Response to sensing	Programmability, rate modulation	Antitachy-arrhythmia function(s)
	0 = None	0 = None	0 = None	0 = None	0 = None
	A = Atrium	A = Atrium	T = Triggered	P = Simple Programmable	P = Pacing (antitachyarrhythmia)
	V = Ventricle	V = Ventricle	I = Inhibited	M = Multiprogrammable	S = Shock
	D = Dual (A + V)	D = Dual (A + V)	D = Dual (T + I)	C = Communicating	D = Dual (P + S)
				R = Rate modulation	
Manufacturers' designation only	S = Single (A or V)	S = single (A or V)			

Note: Positions I through III are used exclusively for antibradyarrhythmia function.

Reprinted with permission from: Bernstein AD et al.: The NASPE/BPEG generic pacemaker code for antibradyarrhythmia and adaptive-rate pacing and antitachyarrhythmia devices. *PACE* 1987; 10:795.

maker identification code was developed as a shorthand method to describe pacemaker function, but expansion to a five-letter code has been necessary to include advances in pacemaker technology (Table 14-2). In clinical practice, pacemakers continue to be described by the first three letters of this code.

The first letter of the identification code denotes which cardiac chambers are being paced, while the second letter identifies which chambers possess sensing capability. The third letter identifies how the pacemaker responds to sensed electrical activity. In the *inhibited* mode, the pacemaker will sense intrinsic activity and will not fire. In the *triggered* mode, an impulse is delivered after an appropriate time delay, based on an absence of sensed ECG activity.

The fourth letter in the expanded, five-letter code describes permanent pacemaker characteristics regarding programmability and rate-responsiveness. *Multiprogrammable pacemakers* allow adjustments in more than two of the following functions: rate, output, sensitivity, refractory periods, hysteresis, and possibly other parameters (Teplitz 1991a). *Rate-responsive pacemakers* are capable of increasing their rate in response to physiologic cues that a faster heart rate is needed, such as increased body temperature, respiratory rate, or activity (Fabiszewski and Volosin 1991).

The fifth letter in the code signifies antitachyarrhythmia pacemaker functions, including overdrive pacing and/or internal defibrillation.

Most temporary and permanent pacemakers seen in the critical-care setting are one of three types: VVI, DVI, or DDD. *VVI pacemakers* are capable of sensing and pacing in the right ventricle only. Loss of a synchronized atrial contraction occurs with VVI pacing, resulting in a 20-30% fall in cardiac output. This mode of pacing may be poorly tolerated in some patients with impaired cardiac reserve. However, this is the only mode of pacing available to patients in atrial fibrillation, as pacemaker capture of a chaotic rhythm is not possible. *DVI (A-V sequential) pacemakers* allow for A-V synchrony by pacing both the atria and ventricles, but they do not sense atrial activity. *DDD pacemakers* have pacing and sensing capabilities in the atria and ventricles. They can pace the atria only, the ventricles only, both chambers, or neither chamber, in response to the native ECG rhythm. A new temporary DDD pacemaker is now available. Its potential advantage over DVI temporary pacing is avoidance of atrial competition via its atrial sensing capabilities.

Pacemaker Insertion

Temporary pacemaker systems include an external pulse generator connected to transvenous or epicardial electrodes. Transvenous electrodes make contact with the endocardial or inner surface of the heart, while epicardial leads are sewn to the outer myocardial surface. The epicardial approach is reserved for patients undergoing cardiac surgery. Epicardial electrodes are sutured to the heart and brought out through the chest wall, for connection to the generator via a connecting cable. The pacemaker wires are discontinued when artificial pacing is no longer potentially necessary, usually 3–7 days postoperatively. The physician gently tugs on the wire to dislodge it from the epicardium, then pulls it out through the chest wall.

Transvenous electrodes are usually placed under fluoroscopic guidance via cannulation of the femoral, subclavian, internal jugular, or brachial vein. During subclavian or jugular insertion, the patient should be positioned with the head down to increase venous filling and minimize the possibility of air embolism. Once the electrodes have been positioned in the right atrium or ventricle, the two poles of the catheter that exit the patient are connected to the pacing generator via a connecting cable. These poles, the generator, and the cable are labeled either (+) or (−) and should only be joined with positive to positive and negative to negative connections.

Electrical safety is an important aspect of care following temporary pacemaker insertion, because the pacing catheter provides a direct pathway for electricity to reach the heart and induce ventricular fibrillation. Precautions include protecting the pacemaker and leads from moisture and ensuring that electrical equipment is well grounded and judged to be electrically safe by the biomedical department. Pacemaker wires that are disconnected from the generator should be insulated by capping them with plastic tubing or needle covers, and latex gloves should be worn when handling pacemaker wires directly.

Permanent pacemakers are usually implanted under local anesthesia, with the patient awake, in either the

operating room or the cardiac catheterization lab. The generator is tunneled into the subcutaneous tissue in the chest or abdomen and connected to either transvenous or epicardial leads. Both types of leads have electrodes at their distal tip and are secured to the right atrium or ventricle. Most permanent pacemakers have lithium batteries that last 8–12 years; battery depletion results in a slowing of the preprogrammed heart rate.

Temporary Pacemaker Settings

The external DVI pulse generator (Figure 14–2) contains an on/off switch, two milliamperage (mA) output dials labeled atrial and ventricular, a millivolt (mV) sensitivity dial, an A-V interval setting, a rate setting, and pace/sense indicator lights. The amount of energy delivered by the generator is regulated via the *mA dial,* after the pacing threshold is determined. Starting with 100% atrial or ventricular pacing at the highest (20 mA) output setting, either the atrial or ventricular output is slowly decreased until the pacemaker spike is *not* followed by a paced QRS complex (loss of ventricular capture) or P wave (loss of atrial capture). This point is the pacing threshold, and the mA should be increased to 2–3 times this value for a margin of safety to ensure pacing.

The *sensitivity dial* determines the size of a spontaneous cardiac impulse, in mV, that will be recognized by the pacemaker and inhibit its firing. At its lowest setting (1.0 mV), the pacemaker is at its highest sensitivity; firing is inhibited for any sensed ECG complex ≥ 1.0 mV in height. This means that a tall P wave could potentially inhibit pacemaker firing, resulting in ventricular asystole. At its highest setting (20 mV) the pacemaker is least sensitive and operates asynchronously from the patient. No atrial or ventricular impulse is tall enough to inhibit the generator, resulting in 100% firing of the device. The sensitivity is usually set at 2–3 mV and adjusted as needed.

The *A-V interval setting* is equated with the P-R interval of the native ECG; it represents the time delay between an atrial paced event and ventricular activity. If a native QRS of sufficient voltage occurs within this interval, the ventricular output is inhibited and only atrial pacing occurs. If no QRS is sensed by the end of the A-V delay, a ventricular output is released and A-V sequential pacing occurs. If the intrinsic ventricular rate exceeds the pacemaker rate setting, atrial and ventricular outputs are both inhibited and no pacing occurs.

The *rate setting* determines the number of times per minute that the generator will fire. The patient's pulse rate may be higher than this rate, indicating inhibition

---

NURSING TIP

Covering Temporary Pacemaker Wires

Pressurized monitoring tubing can be cut into short (1½–2 inch) segments for protection of pacemaker wires that have been disconnected from a generator. The exposed wires fit snugly into the lumen of the tubing, eliminating the need for tape. In the event that emergency pacing must be reinstituted, the tubing quickly pulls off and prompt connection to the generator is facilitated.

of the pacemaker. However, a heart rate below the pacemaker rate indicates a malfunction of the generator and warrants switching to another generator. The A-V interval and atrial output settings are absent from VVI temporary pacemakers, which otherwise contain identical controls.

The DDD temporary pacemaker shown in Figure 14–3 has a liquid crystal display, instead of the dials seen on older models, as well as additional programmable functions. Additional settings with this model include:

- Lower Rate Limit: the lowest rate the pacemaker will pace
- Upper Rate Limit: the highest rate the pacemaker will pace
- Pulse Width: the duration of time the pacemaker stimulus is emitted

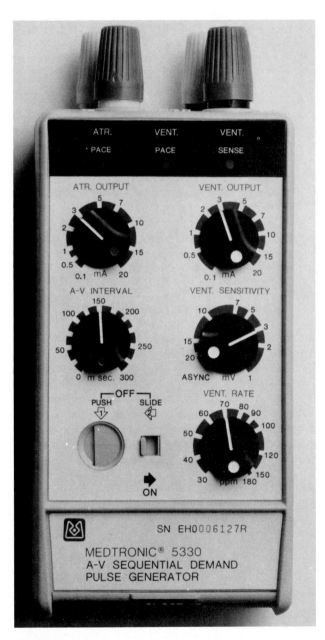

FIGURE 14–2

Medtronic Model 5330 DVI temporary pacemaker. (Reprinted with permission from Medtronic, Inc. Copyright Medtronic, Inc. 1991.)

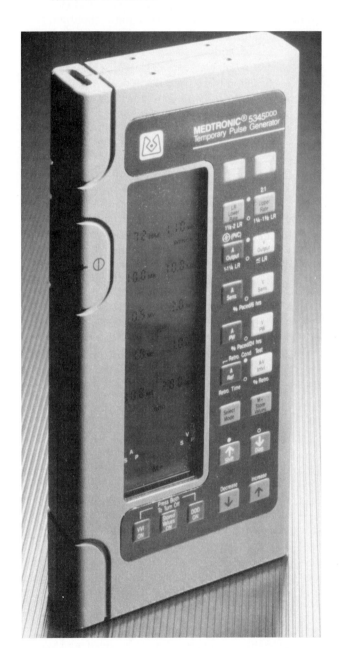

FIGURE 14–3

Medtronic Model 5345 DDD temporary pacemaker. (Reprinted with permission from Medtronic, Inc. Copyright Medtronic, Inc. 1991.)

- Refractory Period: the length of time following a paced or sensed event that the pacemaker is unresponsive to any stimulus

The lower rate limit represents the demand pacing rate, while the upper rate limit represents the fastest rate that ventricular pacing will track spontaneous atrial activity. The upper rate limit on this device may be increased as high as 800 beats per minute to pace-terminate atrial dysrhythmias. The pulse width feature, used in situations of noncapture at highest output, may result in capture by prolonging the duration of impulse delivery. Atrial and ventricular output and sensitivity settings are adjusted separately with this device. A memory function will store a set of desired parameters and return to these settings at the press of a button, even after the device has been turned off (Bartecchi and Mann 1990).

Monitoring Paced ECG Rhythms

Patients with temporary or new permanent pacemakers should receive continuous ECG monitoring to assess the appropriateness of pacemaker function. A rhythm strip should be analyzed every shift and as needed for changes, noting these characteristics:

- The appearance of pacemaker artifacts (spikes) in relation to the P wave and QRS. A spike indicates that the pacemaker fired; it should be immediately followed by a P wave (atrial capture) or a QRS (ventricular capture) to verify a myocardial response to the electrical stimulus. For example, Figure 14–4, upper strip, shows an atrial spike followed by a P wave and a native QRS, a normal pattern with a DVI generator when ventricular activity is sensed before the end of the A-V delay. Figure 14–4, middle strip, shows an atrial spike followed by a P wave and a ventricular spike followed by a QRS, a normal pattern with a DVI generator when no ventricular activity is sensed.

- The appearance of the paced QRS. Because pacemaker impulses travel via abnormal pathways, they require more time for conduction than normal and are therefore wide (>10 msec). However, if the pacemaker fires simultaneously with an intrinsic impulse, a fusion beat occurs that looks like a combination of a paced and native QRS (Figure 14–4, bottom strip).

- Whether the pacemaker rate calculated from the ECG matches the set pacemaker rate. With 100% pacing, these rates are identical. In the demand

Appropriate Pacemaker Function

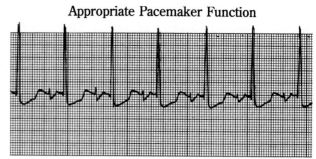

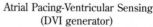

Atrial Pacing-Ventricular Sensing
(DVI generator)

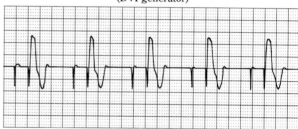

Atrial and Ventricular Pacing
(DVI generator)

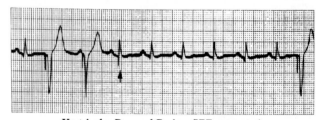

Ventricular Demand Pacing (VVI generator)
(Arrow points to fusion beat)

FIGURE 14–4

Pacemaker rhythm strips documenting normal DVI and VVI pacing.

mode, intrinsic ECG activity may lead to a heart rate that exceeds the pacemaker rate.

- The timing of the paced beats. In a demand mode, paced beats should occur only in the absence of an intrinsic ECG rhythm. Count backwards from a pacemaker spike to the previous QRS; this interval should equal the programmed pacemaker rate.

- The relationship between atrial and ventricular activity. The distance from the atrial spike (or native P wave in a DDD system) to the ventricular spike (or native QRS) should be ≤ the A-V interval.

Malfunction of a pacemaker can be a life-threatening situation and requires prompt troubleshooting by the nurse. Permanent pacemakers can be reprogrammed at the bedside with hand-held programmers, usually by a physician. Malfunction of temporary pacemakers may warrant adjustment of previous settings by a nurse or physician, depending on the clinical area. Rhythm strip analysis is used to detect pacemaker malfunctions. Examples of the following problems are included in Figure 14–5.

Failure to Pace Failure to pace is indicated by absent pacemaker spikes and bradycardia or asystole (depending on the patient's underlying rhythm), often accompanied by decreased cardiac output. There are numerous possible causes. Check that the generator is on and the dials are on the correct settings. If neither the pace nor sense indicator lights are flashing, the battery is dead and needs to be replaced. Check the sensitivity dial; if it is set too low and is mistaking P waves for QRSs, the sense indicator light will flash instead of the pace light. If the pace indicator light is flashing but spikes are not present, perhaps the output is too low or a connection is loose. If none of these interventions works, the problem could be the electrode itself. If all other measures fail, changing polarity of a bipolar electrode may restore pacing in an emergency situation. By removing the pacemaker poles from the connecting cable and reconnecting them negative to positive, and positive to negative, the proximal electrode will become negative and initiate impulse formation. If this electrode is intact, pacing will be restored.

Failure to Capture Failure to capture the myocardium is indicated by spikes that are not immediately followed by paced atrial or ventricular complexes. Loss of capture results in bradycardia, asystole, and loss of cardiac output. Failure to capture could be caused by an mA output setting that is below threshold. Increase the mA until capture is resumed, and set the output at 2–3 times this value. If the problem persists at the highest output setting, the catheter could be dislodged from the heart. To prevent catheter displacement, the patient's activity level often is restricted, and movement at the insertion site is avoided. If a transvenous catheter is floating free within the right ventricle, ventricular irritability may be noted on the ECG. Moving the patient's arm or turning the patient onto the right side may reestablish contact between catheter and endocardium.

If troubleshooting measures are ineffective for failure to either capture or pace, the physician should be called immediately and emergency resuscitative efforts instituted as needed to maintain cardiac output.

Failure to Sense (Competition) Failure to sense is indicated by pacemaker spikes appearing when they should not occur, thus competing with the native ECG rhythm. This may be caused by a sensitivity setting that is too high, making the device asynchronous with the patient. Turn the sensitivity setting clockwise to a lower number (away from the ASYNCH portion of the dial), to make it more sensitive. Catheter dislodgement is another possibility, especially if sensing and pacing problems are seen simultaneously. Failure to sense can lead to ventricular fibrillation if a pacemaker impulse falls within the vulnerable portion of the ECG. If the underlying rhythm is adequate to maintain cardiac output, the physician may order the pacemaker turned off.

Transcutaneous Pacing

Transcutaneous or external cardiac pacing is noninvasive and delivers current from an external generator to two large anteroposterior skin electrodes (Figure 14–6). Pacing occurs as current passes between the two electrodes, in either an asynchronous (fixed rate) or synchronous (demand) mode. For demand pacing, ECG leads from the generator must be connected to the patient so the system can sense intrinsic ventricular activity. Large pacemaker outputs (50–200 mA) and prolonged impulse duration (20–40 msec) are required to overcome transthoracic resistance and effectively pace the heart.

To initiate pacing, the anterior electrode should be positioned over the chest in the V_3 or V_5 position, avoiding potential defibrillator paddle sites (some machines are able to pace and defibrillate from the same electrode patch). The posterior electrode is positioned somewhere between or below the scapulae. Research has indicated that exact placement of this electrode is not critical (Falk and Ngai 1986). The electrodes then are connected to a pacing cable from the generator. ECG patches are placed on the chest in standard fashion and connected to the pacemaker ECG leads. The machine is turned on to monitor the rhythm in a lead with an upright ECG complex. The rate (beats per minute) and output (mA) are set based on the clinical situation. In an emergency, pacing is initiated at highest output and decreased until loss of capture occurs; then the mA setting is adjusted to maintain pacing above this threshold. With an alert patient in a nonemergency setting, start with the lowest output and increase in increments of 10 mA until capture is achieved. Although systems can provide outputs up to 200 mA, effective pacing is usually achieved with 55–90 mA (Teplitz 1991b).

The two major problems seen with transcutaneous pacing include patient discomfort and difficulty in assessing the ECG rhythm. Most alert patients experience some discomfort from the large outputs

Failure to Sense

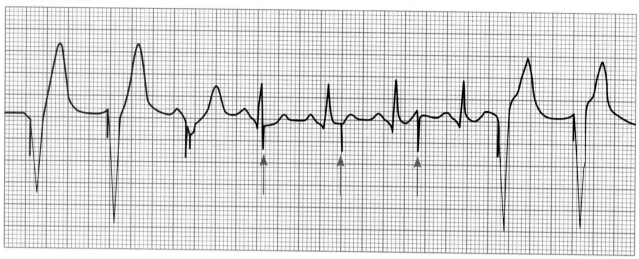

Failure to Capture

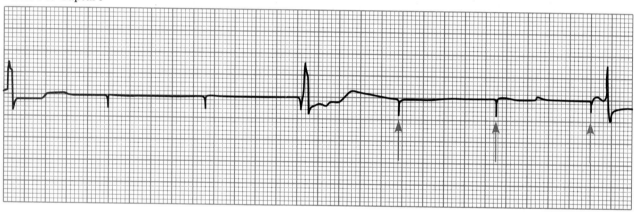

Failure to Pace

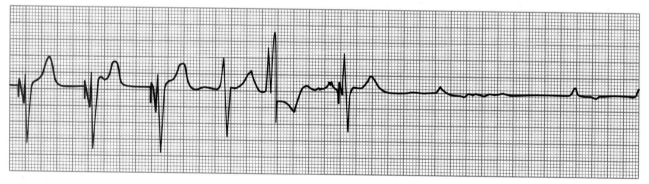

FIGURE 14–5
_____

Inappropriate pacemaker function: failure to sense, capture, and pace appropriately.

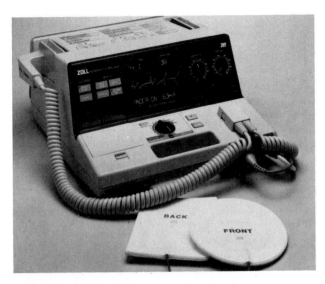

FIGURE 14–6

Zoll transcutaneous pacemaker electrodes and generator. Photo courtesy of ZMI, Inc.

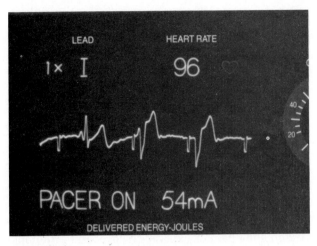

FIGURE 14–7

Pacemaker rhythm strip documenting normal transcutaneous pacing. Photo courtesy of ZMI, Inc.

required for external pacing. Discomfort can be minimized by positioning the electrodes away from major muscles, which avoids excessive musculoskeletal stimulation, and by administering analgesic medications. Artifact created by muscle stimulation can make it difficult to evaluate ventricular capture on the ECG. Assess for a combined pacing spike and QRS duration greater than 14 msec that is followed by a T wave, with overriding of the patient's native ECG rhythm as shown in Figure 14–7 (Persons 1987). Usual causes of failure to pace include an interrupted cable connection, drying of the pacing electrodes, or severe hypoxia and acidosis. Emergency resuscitation procedures should be initiated if pacing failure occurs without an adequate underlying rhythm.

Patient Teaching

Any patient who requires pacemaker therapy should receive education about the need for artificial pacing, safety measures, and specifics appropriate to the equipment being used. All patients and their families should receive a brief review of cardiac anatomy, emphasizing the purpose of the pacing system in supporting the patient. Patients should also be told to report symptoms to the nurse that could indicate a pacemaker-related problem, such as dizziness, syncope, or palpitations. For transcutaneous systems, inform the patient that uncomfortable chest sensations are expected with this type of pacing and pain medication is available. Families should be informed

that they will not receive an electric shock if pacing occurs while they are touching their loved one. For temporary systems, emphasize electrical safety requirements and the need to avoid tension on the pacemaker connections that may be caused by patient movement.

More extensive education is required for patients with a permanent pacemaker. The patient and a family member should be able to demonstrate checking the pulse, which should be performed daily after hospital discharge. The physician should be notified of a pulse rate above or below the programmed pacemaker rate by 10 beats or more, dyspnea, dizziness, palpitations or signs of angina or heart failure. Electrical interference from appliances is no longer a problem with current devices. Encourage the patient to resume normal activities and to carry a pacemaker identification card or Medic Alert ID.

Percutaneous Transluminal Coronary Angioplasty (PTCA)

Balloon catheter dilation of a coronary artery was first performed by Gruentzig in 1977 (Gruentzig and Kumpe 1979). This nonsurgical technique uses a double-lumen catheter with an expandable balloon to dilate stenotic coronary arteries and increase blood flow to myocardial tissue. Approximately 211,000 of these procedures were performed in the United States in 1988 (American Heart Association 1991). This represents tremendous growth, in PTCA procedures, primarily as a result of expanding technology that has enabled wider applications for PTCA intervention.

Candidates For PTCA

Early criteria for PTCA candidates were quite rigid and included only patients with angina of recent onset that was refractory to medical care, single vessel disease, proximal subtotal stenoses and good left ventricular (LV) function, who were also candidates for coronary artery bypass grafting (CABG) if an emergency situation arose (Sipperly 1989). Advances in catheter design and operator experience have led to the rapid expansion of these criteria to include patients with multivessel disease, total occlusions, stenotic bypass grafts and previously angioplastied vessels, as well as evolving MIs (Lynn-McHale 1989). While these complex patients now account for nearly 60% of all PTCA procedures, primary success rates have risen from 68% to over 90% (Sipperly 1989).

PTCA is indicated for some, but not all, patients with coronary artery disease. Recommendations for medical, surgical, or PTCA therapy are made after carefully weighing anticipated risks versus benefits of these procedures. Absolute contraindications to PTCA include severe and diffuse atherosclerosis, or a left main coronary lesion with ≥ 50% stenosis (Ryan et al. 1988). Factors known to decrease the likelihood of successful angioplasty include calcified lesions, right coronary artery disease versus other vessels, and increasing severity of stenosis (Savage et al. 1991). Potential risks of PTCA include bleeding, hypersensitivity reactions, infection, MI, stroke, death, and either coronary or peripheral vessel obstruction (Ryan et al. 1988).

Emergency cardiac surgery following unsuccessful PTCA occurs in approximately 3.4% of patients, therefore patients must be suitable candidates for CABG operation and a surgical team remains on "stand-by" during the procedure (Ryan et al. 1988). Complications leading to emergency surgery include sudden occlusion or rupture of the artery, dissection of the vessel, or persistent and irreversible spasm of the vessel. Abrupt vessel closure is the most frequent cause for emergency CABG, and carries a 25–40% risk of nonfatal MI and a 10–12% mortality rate (Ryan et al. 1988). Coronary perfusion or "bail-out" catheters can be used to maintain blood flow past the area of obstruction until a surgical team is mobilized, and such catheters may decrease these complications in coming years (Hui and Yock 1989).

Restenosis occurs in 25–30% of PTCA patients, usually within the first 3–4 months after the procedure, and remains the critical problem plaguing this therapy. Predisposing factors for restenosis include unstable angina, large residual stenosis after initial PTCA, and disease of the left anterior descending vessel. Repeat angioplasty has proven successful in a majority of these cases, with higher success rates and fewer complications than initial PTCA (Ryan et al. 1988). The pathology of vessels that restenose includes hyperplasia of the intima, collagen deposition, and only small amounts of lipid material, in contrast to primarily lipid and thrombus deposits seen in acutely stenotic vessels (Hui and Yock 1989). Aspirin and calcium channel blockers are routinely given for several months following PTCA to prevent this complication.

PTCA Procedure

PTCA is performed in the cardiac catheterization laboratory using fluoroscopy equipment. Premedication with aspirin, a calcium channel blocker, and a mild sedative is routine to promote patient comfort and prevent coronary artery spasm. A double-lumen PTCA catheter allows for injection of contrast medium and recording of vessel pressures through one lumen, and inflation of a sausage-shaped balloon via a second lumen (Figure 14–8). The catheter is inserted percutaneously into the femoral artery and advanced retrograde through the aorta into the coronary ostium of the vessel to be dilated. Heparin is initiated, and a temporary pacing catheter may be placed if bradycardia is anticipated. Baseline coronary angiograms are performed prior to balloon vessel dilation.

Once the balloon is properly positioned across the stenosis, the balloon is inflated for up to 90 seconds (possibly longer, if tolerated) using pressures up to 11 atmospheres (Lynn-McHale 1989). During this time, the coronary artery is totally obstructed, and the patient may experience chest pain. Repeat inflations are performed as needed, until a successful result is obtained or the procedure is abandoned. Successful PTCA is defined as ≥ 20% increase in vessel diameter, without complications, and is confirmed by improved flow on repeat angiograms. Failure to dilate a vessel may occur from inability to maneuver the balloon across the lesion, rigidity of the plaque due to calcium deposition, or previously described complications. It appears that the primary mechanism of dilatation is not compression of plaque, as was previously believed, but actual stretching of the vascular media and adventitia

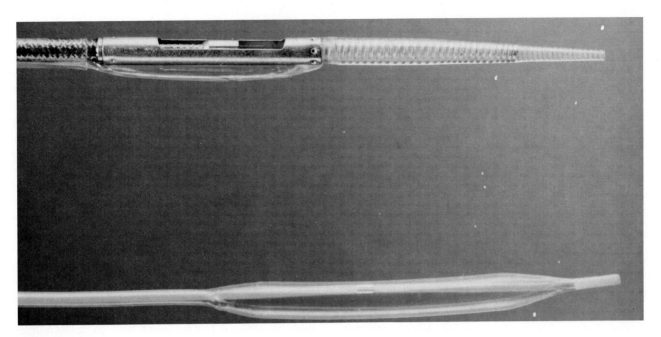

FIGURE 14–8

Atherectomy (top) and angioplasty (bottom) catheters. Photo courtesy of Advanced Cardiovascular Systems, Inc.

along with disruption of the intimal lining of the vessel (Sipperly 1989).

Lasers, Atherectomy, and Stents

A number of techniques have been developed that may be used in combination with PTCA to promote vessel patency, including intracoronary lasers, atherectomy, and stent devices. *Lasers* have been used alone and in combination with PTCA to improve flow through stenotic and occluded vessels. They can be used via a free-beam or hot-tip catheter to create an opening in an obstructed vessel, which permits placement of an angioplasty catheter for dilation. Lasers have also been used to thermally weld or glaze the inner lumen of the vessel, fusing disrupted tissue elements and creating a smooth, less thrombogenic surface (Halfman-Franey and Coburn 1990). Clinical trials with laser devices are continuing in a number of centers around the country.

Atherectomy devices allow for the extraction of atheromatous material via a rotational cutting blade located within a cylindric housing unit attached to a double-lumen balloon catheter (Figure 14–8). The catheter is positioned across the stenosis, and balloon inflation stabilizes the cutting window to surround the plaque. The cutter is slowly advanced, shaving off material that protrudes into the window and storing it in the end of the catheter. Multiple cuts are made to increase vessel patency, and care is taken to avoid cutting deeper than the vessel intima. It is believed that less vessel damage occurs with atherectomy than with PTCA, because significant stretching of the vessel wall is avoided (Halfman-Franey and Coburn 1990). Studies report an 85% success rate with atherectomy, and complications are similar to those seen with PTCA (Pinkerton et al. 1989). Limitations of atherectomy are related to the large catheter size (11–12 Fr) of current devices, which reduces the ability to reach distal or tortuous lesions and creates a potential for increased bleeding at groin sites.

Intracoronary stents are used following PTCA or atherectomy to prevent restenosis and maintain vessel patency. These devices oppose the elastic recoil of dilated vessels, and provide a scaffold that offers support to the vessel wall. A variety of stents is being investigated. Composition and method of detachment from a balloon catheter differ somewhat among various types of stents. Issues of concern when using stents include visibility (current devices cannot be seen under fluoroscopy) and endothelialization. Some degree of fibrin deposition must occur on the stent surface in order for endothelial cells to attach to the device, thus creating a smooth surface, but allowing excessive thrombus formation will lead to occlusion of the vessel lumen (Halfman-Franey and Coburn 1990). Care of patients with stents differs from routine PTCA care in that Dextran and coumadin may be incorporated into the antiplatelet regimen for these patients.

Nursing Care of PTCA Patients

Patients are often admitted only a short time before PTCA and are discharged within 24 hours after the procedure, leaving limited time for patient teaching. Nurses can minimize patient anxiety by preparing them for what they will see, hear, and feel in the cardiac catheterization laboratory. Patients should be prepared to see large numbers of people in surgical gowns and masks, with extensive monitoring equipment in a darkened room. Patients will be covered with sterile drapes for most of the procedure. They will hear loud noises and alarms, and may feel pressure in the groin as the catheters are changed. Patients should be informed that angina often occurs during balloon inflations and that pain medication is available. They will be asked to remain still during the procedure, and will be awake and informed throughout. Patients should also receive some preoperative instruction regarding cardiac surgery and sign a written surgical consent because of the risk of emergency CABG.

Following PTCA, patients will require monitoring in a coronary care or intermediate care unit. Femoral arterial and venous sheaths remain in place overnight, allowing for IV access and arterial pressure monitoring. Sheaths also facilitate prompt repeat PTCA in the event of acute vessel reocclusion. Nitroglycerin and heparin infusions are continued following the procedure; heparin is discontinued prior to sheath removal, while nitroglycerin is usually continued until after the sheaths are removed. Frequent assessments are made of vital signs, intake and output, and perfusion of the cannulated extremity.

NURSING DIAGNOSIS

Nursing diagnoses that are of particular importance include:

- High risk for decreased cardiac output
- Fluid volume deficit
- Altered tissue perfusion
- Knowledge deficit.

A patient care plan for the PTCA patient is included nearby.

High Risk for Decreased Cardiac Output Myocardial ischemia, dysrhythmias, and fluid deficits can contribute to impaired cardiac output following PTCA. Patients should be instructed to notify the nurse immediately if chest pain occurs. Angina must be distinguished from pleuritic chest discomfort that often occurs for several hours after the procedure. Following PTCA, the selection of ECG monitoring leads should take into consideration which vessels were dilated. The lead(s) that demonstrated the greatest ST segment changes *during* balloon inflations should be monitored post-procedure (Drew 1991). The presence of anginal pain or ECG rhythm changes, including ST segment elevation or depression, may signal vessel reocclusion. A 12-lead ECG should be obtained and the physician notified immediately if this complication is suspected. Cardiac isoenzymes are also assessed every 8 hours to further identify the presence of myocardial damage. Ventricular dysrhythmias may occur following PTCA and, if sustained, can contribute to a significant decrease in CO. Antidysrhythmic therapy may be initiated to control ventricular ectopy.

High Risk for Fluid Volume Deficit IV contrast medium acts as an osmotic diuretic, and significant diuresis can occur following PTCA. Excessive bleeding from the groin cannulation site also can contribute to a fluid deficit. Hypovolemia is a serious problem, as inadequate coronary flow could precipitate vessel reocclusion or vasovagal episodes during sheath removal. The patient is encouraged to drink fluids, and a maintenance IV is continued for several hours until the contrast has been excreted and volume status is stabilized. Before the patient gets out of bed after sheath removal, orthostatic vital signs should be checked to assess for a persistent fluid deficit. Although serum potassium levels are not routinely followed, they should be evaluated in patients with excessive diuresis or patients with a history of impaired potassium regulation.

High Risk for Altered Tissue Perfusion Bleeding may occur at the femoral artery insertion site as a result of anticoagulation therapy (since heparin is not reversed at the end of the procedure), resulting in a fluid deficit as well as impaired perfusion of the extremity. Patients are instructed to keep the bed elevated to < 30° and keep the affected extremity immobilized, avoiding groin flexion. Frequent assessment of the activated clotting time (ACT) or partial thromboplastin time (PTT) allows for titration of anticoagulants to an acceptable range. The hematocrit (HCT) is also assessed, and a fall in the HCT may signal internal bleeding.

The dressing over the insertion site is checked frequently for signs of bleeding or hematoma formation, both before and after sheath removal. The presence of a catheter in the femoral artery may precipitate thrombus formation, which could embolize to the distal extremity. Frequent assessment of peripheral pulses, color, temperature, capillary filling, and sensation is performed to detect signs of impaired perfusion of the extremity. Following sheath removal, pressure is applied manually or with a compression clamp for at least 20–30 minutes. The site is covered with a pressure dressing in some institutions, while others prefer only a small band-aid to allow for prompt visualization of bleeding. If no signs of bleeding occur, the patient may ambulate after 6–8 hours.

Knowledge Deficit Decreasing length of stay following PTCA leaves little time to educate patients and their families about cardiac risk factors, pathophysiology of coronary artery disease, and medication guidelines for aspirin and calcium channel blockers. Written materials and videotapes may be useful in initiating the education process, and patients are encouraged to participate in an outpatient cardiac rehabilitation program to obtain additional information. It is important that patients know angioplasty has not "cured" them of coronary artery disease; the need for continued risk factor modification must be emphasized. Patients should be advised to assess the groin site for bleeding, hematoma formation, or signs of infection and contact their physician if these complications occur.

NURSING CARE PLAN

Percutaneous Transluminal Coronary Angioplasty (PTCA)

Nursing Diagnosis	Signs & Symptoms	Nursing Actions	Desired Outcomes

High risk for decreased cardiac output related to myocardial ischemia and/or dysrhythmias.	Signs of decreased CO:
	↓ BP
	↓ LOC
	↓ UO
	↓ tissue perfusion
	Signs of myocardial ischemia:
	chest pain
	ST segment elevation or depression
	elevated CPK isoenzymes
	ventricular dysrhythmias
		1. Monitor vital signs (VS) frequently per unit protocol.
		2. Continuously monitor ECG lead which showed greatest ST–T wave changes during previous ischemic episodes (if known).
		3. Obtain CPK isoenzymes per unit protocol & PRN chest pain.
		4. Instruct patient to notify nurse for chest pain or discomfort. If present:
		  a) Obtain STAT-12-lead ECG
		  b) Notify MD
		  c) Titrate IV nitroglycerin as ordered.
			No chest pain.
			Cardiac output adequate for tissue perfusion.
			Sinus rhythm without ST–T wave abnormalities.

High risk for fluid volume deficit related to osmotic diuresis and potential bleeding.	↓ BP ↓ UO orthostatic VS changes: BP < 20 mm Hg and HR > 10 bpm 1 min. after position change from supine to sitting.	1. Administer IV fluids as ordered until sheaths removed. 2. Encourage PO fluid intake. 3. Assess intake & output q1hr. 4. Assess serum K$^+$ values as ordered.	Intake > output. BP stable. Volume status maintained. Serum K$^+$ 3.5–5.5 mEq/L

(Continued)

NURSING CARE PLAN

Percutaneous Transluminal Coronary Angioplasty (PTCA) (Continued)

Nursing Diagnosis	Signs & Symptoms	Nursing Actions	Desired Outcomes
High risk for altered tissue perfusion related to presence of sheaths and potential bleeding.	Cannulated extremity reveals: absent/decreased DP pulse coolness pallor/cyanosis pain/paresthesia delayed capillary refill Evidence of bleeding: groin dressing saturated oozing from IV sites back pain ↓ hematocrit ↓ BP	1. Assess dressing and perfusion to extremity with every VS check. 2. Notify MD of altered perfusion or bleeding. 3. Titrate heparin infusion as ordered based on PTT/ACT results. 4. If bleeding at groin site occurs: Reinforce sterile dressing and apply manual pressure for at least 10 minutes; decrease heparin infusion as ordered. 5. Instruct patient to maintain bedrest with head of bed < 30°, cannulated extremity straight (restrain PRN), and only log-roll turns permitted.	Adequate perfusion of extremities. No evidence of bleeding. PTT/ACT/HCT maintained within acceptable limits.
Knowledge deficit about PTCA procedure and cardiovascular disease.	Patient and family ask questions about procedure, or unable to state risk factors for CAD.	1. Instruct patient/family about PTCA procedure, including anticipated events in catheterization lab, effects of PTCA on coronary anatomy, and potential for CABG with anticipated lines/ nursing care if surgery occurs. 2. Begin instruction about risk factor modification using instructional books and/or videotapes ASAP. 3. Prior to hospital discharge review: a) opportunities for outpatient cardiac rehabilitation b) discharge medications c) notification of MD for hematoma formation or bleeding at groin	Patient and family verbalize understanding of PTCA procedure, post-PTCA care requirements, risk factors for CAD, and discharge medications.

Cardiac Surgery

Coronary Artery Bypass Grafting

Approximately 353,000 patients underwent coronary artery bypass graft (CABG) operations in the United States in 1988, and another 58,000 required valve procedures (American Heart Association 1991). Patients with ischemic heart disease that is not amenable to medical therapy or PTCA may be candidates for a CABG operation. This procedure does not open up blocked vessels, but uses a native artery or vein to bypass blood flow around the area of obstruction. The *saphenous vein* is the most commonly used vein graft. This vessel is carefully removed from the lower (and sometimes upper) leg and cut into small segments for grafting. The proximal end is sewn to the aorta and the distal end is anastomosed just past the obstruction, bringing arterial blood to the jeopardized area of myocardium (Figure 14–9).

The *internal mammary artery (IMA),* which normally supplies blood to the chest wall, is "the graft of choice" for CABG procedures because of its superior patency rates (Jansen and McFadden 1986). Veins that are exposed to arterial blood flow develop accelerated atherosclerosis, resulting in an occlusion rate of 50% after 10 years. The IMA graft is less susceptible to these changes; only 10% of these vessels will be occluded after 10 years (Ryan et al. 1988). There is also only one anastomosis, as the proximal end of the vessel is already connected to the arterial circulation (Figure 14–9). Disadvantages of IMA grafts are related to the extensive chest wall dissection that is required to free the vessel for use. These include increased blood loss and pleural effusion formation, as well as increased musculoskeletal pain postoperatively (Jansen and McFadden 1986).

The effectiveness of the CABG procedure has been studied in more detail than any other operation in history, yet indications for surgical intervention in ischemic heart disease remain controversial. Guidelines have been established by the American College of Cardiology and American Heart Association that rely on an analysis of risk factors, yielding probabilities that the procedure will be effective in a given clinical situation (American College of Cardiology and American Heart Association 1991). Variables affecting these risk/benefit ratios include the number and location of obstructed vessels, ejection fraction, and results of treadmill stress testing. For example, CABG is always indicated for patients with a significant left main stenosis, but may not be indicated for patients with multivessel disease if only a small area of myocardium is jeopardized.

Valve Disorders

Surgical repair or replacement of heart valves is indicated for patients experiencing symptoms as a result of valves that do not open or close properly. Valve disease may occur as a result of rheumatic fever or other infections that destroy the valve components, congenital defects, ruptured papillary muscles following acute MI, or degenerative changes such as calcium deposits or torn leaflets that occur with advanced age. Valves that do not close properly allow blood leakage *(regurgitation)* during the cardiac cycle. This results in fluid overload and dilatation of the left atrium, if the mitral valve is affected, or the left ventricle, if the aortic valve is diseased. Fluid congestion in the lungs occurs, as well as reduced cardiac output. Atrial fibrillation is common as a result of distension and irritability of this chamber.

Valves that resist opening are *stenotic* and lead to increased pressure within the heart as it tries to overcome this high resistance and open the valve. Mitral stenosis results in high left atrial pressures, pulmonary congestion, and decreased left ventricular output. Aortic stenosis results in increased left ventricular mass (hypertrophy), which can precipitate angina if myocardial oxygen supply is inadequate. The hypertrophied ventricle resists diastolic filling, resulting in elevated left atrial pressures and pulmonary congestion. Cardiac output is preserved as long as adequate volume and atrial contraction (i.e., sinus rhythm) are maintained. A valve that is severely stenotic may become fixed in an open position, leading to symptoms of regurgitation in addition to those of stenosis. While the tricuspid and pulmonic valves are sometimes affected by these disorders, the low pressure requirements of the right heart allow for compensation and require surgical correction less frequently.

Valves may be repaired or replaced, depending on the degree of dysfunction present. A *commissurotomy* is a method of repairing a stenotic valve by surgically cutting areas where the valve leaflets have fused together, or inserting a finger or instrument into the valve to break it open. An *annuloplasty* is a method of repairing a regurgitant valve by using sutures or an artificial ring to pull together the valve annulus, allowing the leaflets to close normally. Procedures that repair a valve are considered palliative, and although replacement is avoided, it is usually required at a later time.

Three major categories of artificial heart valves are currently available for replacement: tissue, mechanical,

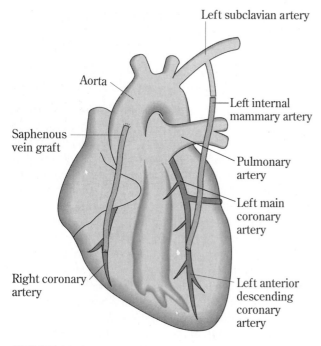

Left subclavian artery

Aorta

Saphenous
vein graft

Left internal
mammary artery

Pulmonary
artery

Left main
coronary
artery

Right coronary
artery

Left anterior
descending
coronary
artery

FIGURE 14–9

Saphenous vein and internal mammary artery grafts for coronary revascularization.

and homograft valves. Tissue valves are harvested intact as porcine aortic valves or constructed from bovine pericardium. They must undergo a preservation procedure which increases durability and allows for prolonged storage prior to implant. Despite this preservation, these valves are fragile and usually need to be replaced within 8–10 years. This limited life-span is the major disadvantage of tissue valves. Their major advantage is that because they resist clot formation, anticoagulation is rarely required (Seifert 1987).

Mechanical valves are constructed in a variety of configurations from different metals, in an attempt to create a device that closely resembles normal valve function. The ideal mechanical valve should open with minimal obstruction to blood flow during systole and close completely to prevent regurgitation during diastole. Other desirable characteristics for artificial valves include ability to open and close effectively at rapid heart rates, minimal trauma to blood cells, and absence of clot formation on the device. Unfortunately, all mechanical valves will develop thrombus if anticoagulation is omitted. Mandatory anticoagulant therapy is the greatest disadvantage of mechanical valves. They offer an advantage over tissue valves in their durability: some have been in place over 20 years and continue to function normally.

Homograft valves are obtained from hearts excised from patients receiving a heart transplant or from human cadavers within 12 hours of death. After

TABLE 14–3

Artificial Heart Valves

TYPE	DESCRIPTION
Tissue Valves	
Carpentier-Edwards	Aortic porcine valve mounted on stent
Hancock	Aortic porcine valve mounted on stent
Ionescu-Shiley	Trileaflet valve constructed from bovine pericardium
Mechanical Valves	
Bjork-Shiley	Single tilting disc
Medtronic-Hall	Single tilting disc
Omniscience	Single tilting disc
St. Jude	Bileaflet-tilting discs
Starr-Edwards	Caged-ball
Homograft Valves	
CryoLife, Inc.	Cryopreserved human aortic valve from cadaver or heart transplant recipient

immediate preservation using specialized freezing techniques, these valves then can be stored indefinitely. This processing gives homograft valves greater durability than conventional tissue valves, and anticoagulation is not required. While homografts are considered nonantigenic, case reports of rapid valve failure in children have raised the question of possible tissue rejection in certain patients. Homografts are not in great supply at present and require expertise with cryopreserved tissue. They generally are reserved for situations where a combination of durability and freedom from anticoagulation are paramount, such as in women of childbearing age or children. They are also used for patients with pre-existing infective endocarditis when placement of tissue valves carries a high risk of reinfection (Pearl et al. 1991). Several types of valves currently available for implant are categorized in Table 14–3.

Principles of Cardiopulmonary Bypass

In order to perform surgery on the heart, it is necessary that the heart be in an arrested state, with rare exceptions. It is also desirable to collapse the lungs so they are not inflating over the surgical field. The role of the cardiopulmonary bypass (CPB) machine is to support blood pressure, systemic perfusion, oxygenation, and carbon dioxide removal during the time the heart is arrested and the lungs are not ventilated, thus preserving tissue perfusion and organ function.

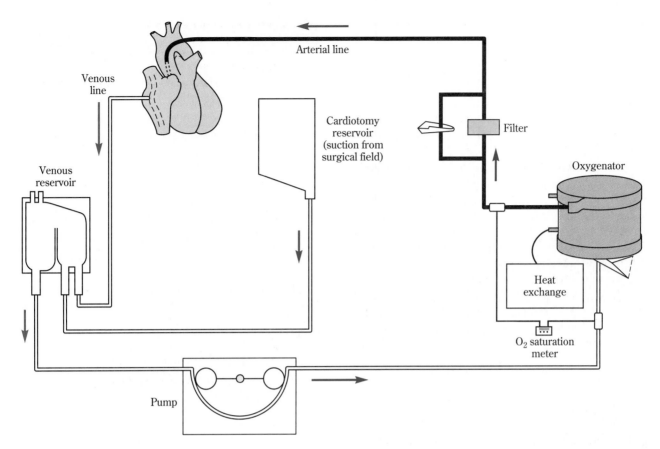

FIGURE 14–10

Cardiopulmonary bypass circuit used for heart-lung support during open heart surgery. Illustration courtesy of Circulatory Support Dept. California Pacific Medical Center, San Francisco.

The three basic components of CPB are the plastic circuitry carrying the blood, the pump, and the oxygenator. The components of a CPB circuit are illustrated in Figure 14–10. One or two cannulae are placed in the right atrium or vena cavae to bring venous blood to the CPB apparatus, essentially eliminating all blood flow through the native heart and lungs. Venous blood travels to the oxygenator for the addition of O_2 and removal of CO_2. A heat exchange element allows for cooling of blood (and body temperature) at the start of CPB, and rewarming at the end of the operation. Blood then is filtered to remove air and debris and is pumped back to the body via a cannula placed in the ascending aorta.

Roller pumps compress the blood-filled circuitry, continuously propelling blood through the oxygenator and back to the patient during the operation. Some damage to red cells, platelets, and plasma proteins occurs during this process. By adjusting how fast the rollers turn, the perfusionist can adjust pump flow. Flow rates of 1.8–2.4 L/min allow for adequate tissue perfusion while avoiding bleeding and pump problems

seen at higher rates (Furst 1989). However, these flow rates are lower than a normal CO and result in a state of mild shock, with release of endogenous catecholamines. Some degree of metabolic acidosis and vasoconstriction is seen routinely in the initial postoperative period. Three principles that allow for effective CPB are hemodilution, hypothermia, and anticoagulation (Weiland and Walker 1986).

The CPB circuit can be thought of as additional vascular space that has to be primed with fluid (such as an electrolyte and albumin solution). *Hemodilution* occurs by the addition of these nonblood fluids, decreasing blood viscosity and improving flow to the capillaries. Hematocrits during surgery typically drop to 20–25% and are raised at the conclusion of the operation by reinfusing the patient's own blood salvaged during the procedure. The effects of hemodilution include prevention of blood sludging that might result in poor capillary perfusion and microthrombus (although clot also can form in the CPB circuit itself). Hemodilution also lowers the plasma oncotic pressure, which results in body fluid shifts and accumulation of interstitial fluid.

It is not unusual for a patient to gain 2–8 kg of weight from fluid accumulation during surgery.

Hypothermia during CPB is necessary to decrease metabolic demand, consumption of oxygen, and production of carbon dioxide. Patients typically are cooled to a temperature of 28°C. By lowering oxygen requirements, this cooling provides major organs with protection from ischemia during surgery at low flow rates. Hemodilution prevents the increase in blood viscosity that would normally occur with hypothermia. Patients are rewarmed to 36°C prior to the termination of CPB but continue to lose heat from the open chest, and core temperature is lowered by restoration of perfusion to the periphery. Patients often return to the critical-care area with body temperatures below 35°C, which contributes to vasoconstriction, increased SVR, and postoperative hypertension.

In order to protect the heart from ischemia, which could result in a perioperative MI, topical cooling and cold cardioplegia are used in addition to systemic hypothermia. The myocardial cavity is packed with iced sterile saline, which further lowers the temperature (and metabolic rate) of the heart. But the greatest protection comes from the infusion of a cold (4°C) cardioplegia solution directly into the coronary arteries. This solution contains a high concentration of potassium, which aids in arresting the heart, as well as a variety of other electrolytes and medications often individualized to the surgeon's preference. Cardioplegia solution is reinfused throughout the procedure to maintain myocardial cooling as needed. With these protective maneuvers, the incidence of perioperative MI is below 2% (Thompson, Hayden and Tyers 1991).

High levels of *anticoagulation* are required intraoperatively to prevent clotting of blood in the CPB circuit. Heparin is given as a 20,000–30,000 unit IV bolus at the start of heart-lung bypass, followed by additional boluses to maintain the activated clotting time (ACT) 4–6 times greater than normal. At the conclusion of CPB, heparin is reversed with protamine sulfate, a heparin antagonist. Inadequate heparin reversal is a potential cause of postoperative bleeding abnormalities, as is heparin rebound. Rebound occurs when heparin that had been sequestered in tissues is released into the circulation. Both situations are seen within the first few hours after arrival in the ICU and are corrected with additional protamine.

While the use of heart-lung technology allows for surgical procedures that would otherwise be impossible, it should be remembered that CPB is an extremely unnatural physiologic state that can result in many potential postoperative problems. A generalized inflammatory reaction results in increased capillary permeability and edema, as well as fever and elevated white blood cell count for up to 48 hours after surgery (Furst 1989).

NURSING DIAGNOSIS

Nursing diagnoses related to CPB include the following:

- High risks for fluid volume deficit
- Injury (excessive bleeding or cardiac tamponade)
- Ineffective airway clearance
- Impaired gas exchange
- Decreased cardiac output
- Knowledge deficit

Nursing Care of Cardiac Surgery Patients

High Risk for Fluid Volume Deficit Patients who have undergone cardiac surgery with CPB may experience a fluid deficit from blood loss, osmotic diuresis, inadequate replacement, and shifting of fluid from the vascular to the interstitial space. These fluid shifts may persist for up to 6 hours postoperatively, warranting vigorous fluid administration to keep up with losses into the interstitium (Weiland and Walker 1986). Peripheral edema occurs as a result of this capillary leak syndrome and often is associated with an intravascular fluid deficit.

Osmotic diuresis also contributes to a fluid volume deficit. Mannitol is given on CPB to preserve renal blood flow and reduce myocardial edema. The diuresis induced by mannitol can result in urine outputs exceeding a liter per hour. This occurs regardless of the underlying fluid status, preventing a compensatory oliguria that might otherwise be seen with a fluid deficit. Thus, urine output is an inaccurate indicator of fluid status for the first 4–6 hours postoperatively. Many patients also develop hyperglycemia following CPB, contributing to the osmotic diuresis, as a result of epinephrine release and impaired insulin secretion (Weiland and Walker 1986). Serum glucose levels may reach 300–500 mg/dl but rapidly normalize with diuresis, and they rarely require insulin administration in patients without pre-existing diabetes mellitus.

During this phase of diuresis, fluid and electrolyte abnormalities are a primary concern. Urine potassium losses can be very high initially, warranting frequent assessment of serum potassium values. In addition to urine losses, potassium shifts into the cells during surgery, further lowering serum values. Almost all patients will require potassium replacement postoperatively, and many ICUs have protocols that allow for ongoing replacement by the nursing staff. Hypokalemia is a common cause of myocardial irritability and dysrhythmias in the postoperative period. A serum potassium value should be checked for any patient experiencing ventricular ectopy after cardiac surgery, regardless of urine output.

Adequate assessment of the fluid status may be hampered in the initial postoperative period due to excessive vasoconstriction from hypothermia and catecholamine release. This increase in SVR may result in hypertension and elevated cardiac filling pressures, masking a true intravascular fluid deficit until rewarming and vasodilation occur. Vasodilators such as nitroglycerin or nitroprusside are indicated for severe hypertension that impairs CO. Controlled vasodilation and ongoing fluid resuscitation is the goal of treatment. As rewarming occurs, vasodilation may be abrupt and result in acute hypotension if a severe mismatch occurs between the size of the vascular compartment and the intravascular fluid volume. A decreased preload will limit the patient's ability to generate an adequate cardiac output, and can even precipitate cardiac arrest.

NURSING TIP

Rewarming After Cardiac Surgery

A variety of rewarming methods is used after cardiac surgery, including lights, blankets, head coverings, and airway warming. Regardless of the method used, temperature overshoot can be anticipated. Discontinue warming techniques when the patient's temperature reaches approximately 36–36.5°, in order to avoid hyperthermia and hemodynamic instability from excessive vasodilatation.

A key component of postoperative nursing care is volume assessment and supplementation according to the individual needs of the patient. A great deal of debate exists as to the choice of fluid, crystalloid or colloid, for volume loading. Colloid solutions differ from crystalloids because they contain molecules that are too large to exit the vascular compartment. By primarily increasing intravascular volume, they have been reported to be superior in this patient population (see Research Note on page 400). Guidelines for the amount of fluid required often include fluid administration until an optimal filling pressure is reached. A pulmonary capillary wedge pressure (PCWP) of 8–10 mm Hg is adequate for most patients, although a PCWP of 14–18 mm Hg may be required by patients with ventricular dysfunction or valve disease who are accustomed to larger cardiac volumes (Ley 1988). Remember that maintenance of an adequate cardiac output is the primary goal of volume supplementation, and filling pressures are less reliable indicators of fluid status. Fluids are administered to optimize CO and tissue perfusion, but the nurse should avoid chasing an arbitrary number with fluid challenges if recovery is progressing satisfactorily.

High Risk for Injury: Bleeding and/or Cardiac Tamponade Postoperative blood loss may be due to a surgical problem resulting from small vessels that were not cauterized or from disruption of a major suture line. Although philosophies vary from institution to institution, persistent mediastinal chest tube bleeding over 200 cc/hr for more than 2 hours warrants notification of the surgeon, and may require a return to the operating room for re-exploration if coagulation studies are normal. A patient who is bleeding excessively also should be monitored closely for decreased cardiac output as a result of cardiac tamponade. Blood can accumulate and clot around the heart, resulting in impaired cardiac filling. This can occur even when chest tubes are patent, if they are not in the area of accumulation.

Cardiac tamponade occurs after cardiac surgery when there is bleeding into the pericardial space or mediastinum, with compression of the heart. This bleeding does not always occur circumferentially, and therefore clots can form on one side of the heart and not the other. The result of this uneven cardiac compression is that one heart chamber pressure (e.g., right atrial) may rise while another (e.g., left atrial) remains normal. Typically, both left- and right-sided filling pressures will rise, often becoming equal. Sinus tachycardia and hypotension are hallmarks of this problem after cardiac surgery, as is decreased CO and impaired tissue perfusion. Emergency exploratory sternotomy is the treatment of choice for tamponade and should be performed as early as possible to prevent the onset of electromechanical dissociation.

Nonsurgical causes of bleeding include inadequate reversal of heparin and heparin rebound, which were discussed previously, as well as abnormal clotting

RESEARCH NOTE

Ley S, Miller K, Skov P, Preisig P
Crystalloid versus colloid fluid therapy after cardiac surgery.
Heart Lung 1990; 19:31–40.

CLINICAL APPLICATION

Patients undergoing cardiac surgery with cardiopulmonary bypass experience a postoperative fluid deficit as a result of blood loss, diuretics, and increased capillary permeability. Several types of IV replacement fluid currently are available for clinical use: blood products, balanced salt solutions (crystalloids), and solutions containing oncotically active molecules (colloids). This study compared crystalloids to colloids after cardiac surgery with respect to: (a) IV fluid requirements, (b) hemodynamic stability, and (c) edema formation.

Twenty-one patients undergoing CABG or valve operations were randomized to receive either crystalloid (normal saline, NS) or colloid (hetastarch, HES) for postoperative fluid resuscitation. The algorhythm used was designed to maintain a cardiac index greater than 2L/min/m², with a gradual downward titration of the infusion rate. During the study period, hourly hemodynamic and intake/output data were collected.

Fluid data revealed that the NS group required 2.4 times more re-placement fluid than the HES group during the 8-hour study period: 4,655 versus 1,918 cc (p < 0.001). Because urine output did not differ, NS patients experienced a significantly (p < 0.01) greater weight gain after arrival in intensive care: 2.32 versus 0.26 kg. No difference in chest tube output or blood requirements was noted.

Hemodynamic stability was greater in the HES group, as evidenced by a significantly (p < 0.05) higher systolic blood pressure, cardiac output, and cardiac index during the study period than the NS group, although cardiac filling pressures were initially lower in the HES group. There was a 0% incidence of pulmonary edema in both groups, as evidenced by the first morning chest x-ray. Peripheral edema was present in all patients but was not significantly different between groups, as measured by thigh and ankle circumference measurements. A significantly (p < 0.001) shorter intensive care stay was noted in the HES group: 49.5 versus 68.1 hours, presumably due to less need for diuresis prior to transfer.

CRITICAL THINKING

Limitations: The relatively small sample size limits the ability to generalize these findings. Also, patients requiring multiple inotropes or an IABP were excluded, further limiting generalization to include only patients without severe postoperative cardiac dysfunction.

Strengths: Because critical-care nurses are responsible for the administration and regulation of postoperative fluid resuscitation, these results have important nursing implications. This study revealed that when nurses administer colloids postoperatively to this patient population, less IV volume will be required and hemodynamics may stabilize more quickly than with crystalloids. By lessening volume administration, diuretic requirements and length of intensive care stay may be reduced.

---

factors. Cardiopulmonary bypass results in consumption and destruction of multiple blood clotting elements, including platelets. The roller pump and suction apparatus are especially traumatic to blood cells. The longer the patient has been on the CPB machine, the greater the bleeding tendency. Correction of a consumption coagulopathy includes replacement of deficient clotting factors with blood products. Fresh frozen plasma will correct an abnormal prothrombin time (PT) and partial thromboplastin time (PTT), cryoprecipitate is given for decreased fibrinogen levels, and platelets are given even for low-normal counts if there is a suspicion of platelet dysfunction.

Nursing guidelines for managing both surgical and nonsurgical bleeding include maintaining CO via adequate volume resuscitation, as well as avoiding factors which contribute to postoperative bleeding. Rapid fluid administration helps to maintain hemodynamic stability but synthetic volume expanders such as dextran or hetastarch can worsen a coagulopathy, and are therefore avoided. By maintaining the patient in a state of "controlled hypotension," pressure on suture lines is reduced and excessive bleeding minimized.

Emergency Exploratory Sternotomy Emergency exploratory sternotomy (EES) is defined as the urgent reopening of a median sternotomy incision in the early postoperative period (<24 hours) for a life-threatening condition that is unresponsive to standard therapy. The reasons this procedure may be necessary include tamponade, hemorrhage, acute profound hypotension, coronary artery spasm, clotted grafts, refractory dysrhythmias, and cardiac arrest (Kern 1990).

Acute profound hypotension and cardiac arrest are two unexpected complications of cardiac surgery which necessitate EES. In these situations, the etiology of cardiac compromise may not be apparent. Basic Life Support (BLS) and Advanced Cardiac Life Support (ACLS) protocols, including external cardiac compressions, are first-line therapies. If they prove ineffective in promptly restoring the circulation, the chest is opened and internal cardiac massage is initiated by the physician.

EES may also be indicated for acute massive hemorrhage. Rarely, a patient suddenly develops a massive hemorrhage—usually due to a disrupted suture line—and goes into shock or suffers a cardiac arrest. EES may help in this situation, allowing the surgeon to open the chest quickly and correct the problem without the delay of returning to the operating suite.

EES Procedure Whenever possible, the nurse informs the patient and family about the need for the procedure. This procedure requires special equipment which is brought to the bedside immediately:

1. Surgical gowns, masks, gloves, hats

2. Skin antiseptic

3. An EES tray with appropriate surgical instruments, including a scalpel to cut skin sutures and wire cutters for removal of sternal wires (Scalpel and wire cutters are often kept in a separate place *outside* the EES tray, as they will be needed *first* to initiate internal cardiac massage promptly.)

4. Suction equipment, including sterile tube and sterile Yankauer tip

5. Emergency cart and defibrillator

6. Sterile internal defibrillator cable and paddles (Be sure cable and paddles are for your particular defibrillator; different models of defibrillators require their own cable and paddles.)

7. A surgical-quality light to illuminate the field

8. Surgical electrocautery machine

9. Surgical headlamp for surgeon

10. Screens to isolate the bedside, if the patient is not in a private bed space

11. Suture material and sternal wires

The nurse's primary role is to assemble the equipment, stay with the patient, and monitor the patient's vital signs during the procedure. Other personnel who are called include the pharmacist, respiratory therapist or anesthesiologist, and the patient's cardiologist. All personnel in the room are required to wear caps and masks during this sterile procedure. Depending upon hospital policy, an operating room nurse may be called to assist. During the procedure, suction, defibrillation equipment and instruments are handed to the surgeon using sterile technique. A record is kept of the patient's vital signs and response to the procedure. When the surgeon has completed the surgical repair, the incision is closed again and a new dressing applied. The nurse then assesses the patient fully for any complications and to ensure that he or she is hemodynamically stable.

High Risk for Ineffective Airway Clearance or Impaired Gas Exchange As mentioned before, the lungs are collapsed while the patient is on the CPB machine. As a result, some degree of alveolar collapse occurs, secretions are retained, and poor lung perfusion may result in microthrombus formation (Sladen 1982). Therefore, all patients will have some degree of atelectasis and pulmonary shunting. An ineffective cough may result from excessive pain, leading to further retaining of secretions and possibly pneumonia. Care is directed at increasing ventilation of alveoli with mechanical ventilation and positive end-expiratory pressure. Nursing care focuses on techniques to enhance the ventilation/perfusion ratio, such as frequent turning and suctioning. Despite the potential dysfunction induced by CPB, a majority of patients are extubated within 12–24 hours after surgery. Mobilization proceeds rapidly, and most patients will tolerate sitting up in a chair on the day after operation. Coughing and deep breathing are encouraged every 1–2 hours and are facilitated by the administration of adequate pain medication.

High Risk for Decreased Cardiac Output Myocardial depression may be seen following cardiac surgery due to hypothermia, anesthesia, myocardial edema, electrolyte imbalance, and possible perioperative ischemia (Sladen 1982). Conduction defects and bradycardia contribute to further declines in cardiac output, but they usually can be corrected with temporary pacing. Decreased myocardial contractility following cardiac surgery usually is transient, lasting less than 24 hours, but may require the addition of inotropes to maintain a CO that is adequate for tissue perfusion. It is not uncommon to administer a vasodilator such as nitroprusside for elevated SVR, in combination with an inotrope such as dopamine or dobutamine to augment CO.

Any depression of cardiac output should alert the nurse to assess for altered tissue perfusion, which may begin during CPB and persist postoperatively. Signs of impaired organ perfusion may be noted in the renal, neurologic, or GI assessment. Evidence of abnormalities include oliguria, altered sensorium, abdominal distension and tenderness, metabolic acidosis, decreased peripheral pulses, or cool and dusky extremities. Alterations in tissue perfusion also may result from embolic events during surgery. Sources of emboli include thrombus in the heart, atherosclerotic plaque, calcium or vegetations on abnormal valves, or air. Emboli may travel anywhere in the circulation, causing MI, stroke, renal failure, or mesenteric ischemia.

For patients with severe impairment of CO, weaning from bypass may be impossible without the addition of an intra-aortic balloon pump (IABP) or rarely, the placement of a ventricular assist device (VAD), described below.

Knowledge Deficit Patient education for the cardiac surgery patient begins before surgery with explanations of the anticipated postoperative course and therapies needed for recovery. The patient is informed of the purpose and anticipated duration of invasive lines and tubes, with special emphasis on awakening with an endotracheal tube (ET) in place. The importance of the ET and nonverbal methods of communication are discussed. Postoperative routines for pulmonary hygiene, early mobilization, and avoidance of pressure on the sternum are reviewed in terms of patient participation in these activities.

Postoperatively, instruction for patients with coronary artery disease focuses on modification of risk factors, while valve patients receive information about anticoagulation therapy and antibiotic prophylaxis prior to invasive procedures (including dental work). All patients receive instruction in basic cardiac anatomy and physiology and are given home care guidelines. Problems warranting notification of the physician are reviewed, including signs of infection (fever, wound drainage, etc.) or recurrence of cardiac symptoms. Written instructions are provided to address questions that will inevitably occur after discharge.

Cardiac surgery is a major life event for these patients. Depression and mood swings are common, and attention to spiritual and emotional needs are vitally important for recovery. Nurses need to be alert for signs of depression or withdrawal and can provide appropriate reassurance to patients and families. Referrals to the chaplain or a social worker may also be helpful, in order to assist patients and their loved ones in coping with the emotional upheaval of this procedure. See Chapters 2 and 3 for further guidelines.

Intra-Aortic Balloon Counterpulsation

Intra-aortic balloon counterpulsation is a method of augmenting a patient's CO and increasing coronary artery perfusion during periods of transient myocardial depression. This is achieved through the placement of a balloon device in the descending thoracic aorta either percutaneously or, less frequently, via a femoral cutdown or transthoracic approach. Because the balloon deflates when the heart is in systole and inflates when the heart is in diastole, its pumping action is counter to that of the heart—thus the term *counterpulsation*.

Physiologic Effects

The coronary arteries receive most of their blood flow during diastole, due to direct vessel compression and obstruction of the coronary ostia during systole. The *coronary perfusion pressure* (CPP) is the difference between the driving force for coronary filling (diastolic blood pressure or DBP) minus the resistance to filling offered by pressure within the heart (PCWP). Efforts to improve coronary perfusion focus on optimizing the CPP by raising the DBP and lowering the PCWP. When the intra-aortic balloon inflates during diastole, it raises diastolic pressure. This *diastolic augmentation* improves coronary blood flow and displaces blood into the peripheral circulation as well. Additional benefits are obtained by rapid deflation of the balloon just prior to systole, resulting in *afterload reduction*. Pressure in the aorta falls upon deflation, and the heart can then eject against reduced pressure, thus lowering myocardial workload (Quaal 1984).

Indications

The intra-aortic balloon pump (IABP) is a mechanical circulatory support device that has been useful in stabilizing critically ill patients with a variety of cardiac disorders. Indications for placement of an IABP include post-infarction cardiogenic shock, pre-infarction angina, and intractable ventricular dysrhythmias. The device is also used for mechanical cardiac defects such as mitral regurgitation and ventricular septal defects, which can improve dramatically with afterload reduction. The IABP can be used for cardiac surgical patients having difficulty weaning from CPB, allowing time for recovery from transient myocardial depression associated with surgery. The device also has been used prophylactically during difficult angioplasty procedures or prior to anesthesia induction in high-risk surgical patients, allowing for cardiac protection when a large portion of myocardium is in jeopardy.

Use of the IABP is reserved for patients with a competent aortic valve and a healthy aortic wall. Absolute contraindications include: (a) aortic valve insufficiency, which would permit blood to flow backward into the ventricle during diastolic augmentation; and (b) aortic aneurysm or dissection, as inflations potentially could cause further aortic wall damage and even vessel rupture. Relative contraindications include: (a) severe peripheral vascular disease, as further compromise of blood flow to the cannulated extremity could result in tissue ischemia; and (b) coagulation disorders that may result in uncontrolled bleeding. The risks of IABP use in these situations must be weighed against the potential benefit to the patient.

Equipment and Insertion

The balloon pump consists of two components: the balloon itself and the console that regulates balloon inflation and deflation. The most commonly used adult balloon has a 40 cc inflation chamber, although sizes of 20, 30, and 50 cc are also available. The balloon is mounted on a catheter that ranges in size from 8.5–11 Fr. The IABP console regulates the pumping of helium gas into the balloon chamber. Helium is used because its light weight allows it to be displaced rapidly in and out of the balloon. While a bolus of helium may be life-threatening, patients have survived helium-filled balloon rupture without apparent consequences (Quaal 1984). The console controls allow the operator to regulate triggering and timing of the balloon. A variety of ECG or arterial pressure signals can be used to regulate the balloon trigger, or what event the pump should recognize as systole and rapidly deflate. The operator can then fine-tune the balloon timing, including both inflation and deflation, to optimize hemodynamic parameters.

The balloon is usually inserted in the critical-care unit, cardiac catheterization laboratory, emergency department, or operating room. Prior to insertion, ECG monitoring and an IV line are established. The femoral artery is the most common insertion site used. The balloon usually is inserted percutaneously, although a femoral cutdown approach may be required in some patients. Rarely, a surgeon will place the balloon directly into the aorta when the chest is open during surgery. This approach requires a return to the operating room for balloon removal upon discontinuing IABP support. Regardless of the initial approach, the balloon is positioned in the thoracic aorta approximately 1–2 cm distal to the left subclavian artery and above the renal arteries (Figure 14–11).

During percutaneous insertion, local anesthesia is administered and the artery is punctured with a large-bore needle. A guidewire is then threaded into the vessel, the needle is removed, and the opening is enlarged with an introducer threaded over the guidewire. The deflated balloon comes wrapped around the IABP catheter to make it smaller and easier to insert through the introducer. Once positioned, the catheter is connected to the gas line of the IABP console and pumping is started. With initiation of pumping, the balloon unwraps itself immediately.

Balloon Timing and Triggering

Optimal timing of balloon inflation and deflation in concert with native cardiac events requires console adjustments by a specially trained nurse or IABP technician. The goal of optimal hemodynamic benefits with counterpulsation relies on careful timing of balloon events using the ECG and arterial pressure waveform, realizing that there is a slight delay between the electrical and mechanical events of the heart. A variety of triggering modes is available with current IABP technology, but the R wave of the ECG continues to be utilized in most situations. In this mode, the IABP automatically deflates upon sensing an R wave, thus avoiding balloon inflation during systole. Balloon inflation is timed to occur with the dicrotic notch of the arterial waveform, which signals the onset of diastole.

IABP timing adjustments allow for fine-tuning beyond basic triggering and are made with the IABP inflating every other beat (1:2 augmentation). This allows for comparison of augmented versus nonaugmented beats on the arterial waveform. Evaluation of IABP timing requires assessment of the following reference points (Figure 14–12): (a) peak systolic pressure (PSP); (b) balloon inflation point (IP); (c) peak diastolic pressure (PDP); (d) balloon aortic end-diastolic pressure (BAEDP); (e) assisted peak systolic pressure (APSP); and (f) patient aortic end-diastolic pressure (PAEDP) (St. Jude Medical Inc. 1987). Balloon inflation at IP produces a diastolic pressure higher than systole, while balloon deflation occurs at BAEDP and reflects the pressure drop created by afterload reduction.

Optimal augmentation occurs if balloon inflation begins as early in diastole as possible, immediately

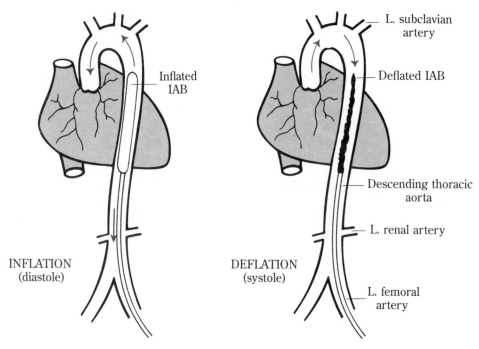

FIGURE 14–11

Position of the intra-aortic balloon (IAB) catheter during inflation and deflation. (Reprinted with permission from: Bullas J: Percutaneous intra-aortic counterpulsation balloon. *Crit Care Nurse* [July/August] 1982; 41.)

after the aortic valve closes. Proper timing of IABP inflation is noted by a V-shaped appearance at the IP, rather than a U (Quaal 1984). This should result in a PDP that exceeds all other reference points on the arterial tracing. Balloon deflation, represented by the BAEDP, is adjusted to occur just before systole. With proper timing, afterload reduction occurs and the following waveform criteria are met: (a) BAEDP is lower than PAEDP; and (b) APSP is lower than PSP.

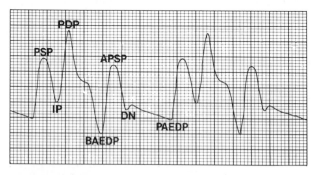

FIGURE 14–12

Arterial pressure tracing showing IABP timing reference points during 1:2 augmentation. Photo courtesy of St. Jude Medical, Inc., Cardiac Assist Division.

Improper IABP timing can result in less cardiac support than intended, at best, or severely compromise cardiac ejection, at worst. Therefore, proper timing is critical to managing the patient with an IABP, and didactic instruction in IABP timing is essential prior to accepting patient care responsibilities for this function.

Nursing care of the IABP patient is much like that of any critically ill patient. Most IABP patients, for instance, require intubation and mechanical ventilation. Because these patient care issues have been discussed elsewhere, this section will address only those aspects of care specific to the IABP.

High Risk For Decreased Cardiac Output Patients who require IABP support are at risk for impaired CO,

---

NURSING DIAGNOSIS

Nursing diagnoses for the IABP patient include:

- High risk for altered cardiac output
- High risk for altered tissue perfusion
- Knowledge deficit

as a result of continued progression of their underlying cardiovascular disease or balloon-related problems. The nurse must assess hemodynamic parameters frequently to evaluate the patient's response to treatment. Anticipated benefits of IABP counterpulsation include increased CO and mean arterial pressure, decreased SVR and filling pressures, and improved end-organ perfusion. Failure to achieve these parameters may be due to improper IABP timing, dysrhythmias, or damage to the balloon catheter.

IABP timing should be assessed at least every 8 hours and reassessed for the following situations: a change in cardiac rhythm, a heart rate change of >10 beats per minute, and hemodynamic deterioration. Dysrhythmias affect the efficiency of IABP pumping and are a potential cause of decreased CO. Specific antidysrhythmic therapy is initiated to promote sinus rhythm. While most current IABP systems can track irregular R–R intervals and tachycardias, the trigger mode may need to be changed to correct for wide QRS complexes or pacemaker artifacts.

The balloon catheter may be damaged by excessive flexion of the leg or thrombus formation. Patients are instructed not to flex the hip or raise the bed higher than 30°, and only log-roll turns are permitted. Leg restraints and sedation may be required to prevent catheter movement. Anticoagulant therapy with low-dose heparin is administered routinely to IABP patients to prevent thrombus formation on the balloon surface, warranting bleeding precautions as well.

High Risk for Altered Tissue Perfusion Use of the IABP may result in altered perfusion of the kidneys, left arm, or cannulated extremity. The urine output is assessed hourly as an indicator of adequate renal perfusion. An abrupt cessation of urine flow may indicate downward balloon migration with obstruction of the renal arteries. Upward balloon displacement can result in obstruction of the left subclavian artery, resulting in impaired arm perfusion. Correct IABP position can be evaluated with a daily chest x-ray, as the catheter tip is radiopaque.

Cannulation of the femoral artery may result in impaired perfusion of the extremity below the IABP insertion site. Limb ischemia is the most frequent complication of IABP therapy, with most studies reporting a 10–20% incidence of this complication. Ischemia can occur as a result of: (a) direct catheter obstruction of the vessel; (b) arterial injury during insertion; or (c) thromboembolism (Funk et al. 1989). Multiple risk factors have been identified for the development of vascular complications including female sex, pre-existing peripheral vascular disease,

prolonged duration of use, transthoracic placement, and diabetes mellitus (Goran 1989).

The quality of peripheral pulses should be assessed before and after balloon placement to note changes from baseline. Asymptomatic loss of distal pulses occurs frequently after IABP insertion and often does not progress to severe limb ischemia. Signs of more severe obstruction to blood flow include pain, pallor, cyanosis, decreased sensation, and loss of motor function in the affected extremity. The physician should be notified of these findings, and intervention may include removal of the IABP (if tolerated) or emergency embolectomy.

A rare but devastating complication of IABP counterpulsation is acute aortic dissection. Evidence of dissection may appear shortly after insertion or much later, and includes severe hemodynamic compromise and impaired perfusion of the kidneys and lower extremities, which is often associated with mottling of the lower body. Immediate surgical intervention is indicated to repair the aorta and restore tissue perfusion.

Knowledge Deficit Few people outside the critical-care arena will have heard of an IABP or its effects on cardiac function; therefore, educational interventions are warranted. A recent study examining family perceptions of the IABP experience revealed that 13 of 27 family members (48%) had the device explained by a nurse (Goran 1989). In the same study, all families understood the device "helped the heart," but many confused the IABP with an angioplasty balloon. These families requested information about the anticipated duration of IABP use, its complications, if the patient can feel it, how the pump is removed, and if the patient can go home with the pump in place. Additional information about cardiac anatomy and intra-aortic balloon placement was deemed very helpful for these families.

Weaning from the IABP

Weaning from the IABP is initiated once hemodynamics stabilize on minimal inotropic support, usually within 24–48 hours after insertion. Weaning is achieved by decreasing the frequency of augmentation from every beat (1:1 augmentation) to every second, fourth, or eighth beat (1:2, 1:4, or 1:8). During the weaning process, the nurse assesses for signs of intolerance to weaning as indicated by decreased CO, increased filling pressures, ventricular ectopy, or other signs of impaired cardiac function. If weaning is tolerated, the physician will remove a percutaneous

IABP in the critical-care unit. Upon removal, blood is allowed to pulsate from the artery for several beats to clear any clots that may have formed on the balloon; manual pressure is then applied. Careful assessment of perfusion to the extremity is important after IABP removal, as distal embolization can occur.

Ventricular Assist Devices

While IABP support can augment CO by approximately 10–15%, ventricular assist devices (VADs) are capable of taking over 100% of cardiac pumping function (Smith and Cleavinger 1991). These mechanical devices are intended for temporary support of a failing ventricle that has been unresponsive to IABP and pharmacologic therapy. The three patient categories for VAD support include cardiogenic shock following acute MI, postcardiotomy heart failure, and bridge-to-transplant in patients who deteriorate prior to location of a suitable organ donor. Contraindications for this technology include active malignancy, recent stroke, sepsis, multiple organ failure, or massive hemorrhage (Ley 1991). Patients should also have a reasonable chance of recovery prior to inserting the device, unless the patient is a transplant candidate. Infarction of > 40% of the myocardium will generally lead to irreversible heart failure and inability to wean from the device (Mulford 1987).

Over a dozen types of mechanical support systems are undergoing clinical trials in the United States. The Medtronic-Biomedicus centrifugal pump is a readily available system that is used for CPB support during open heart surgery in many institutions. This device uses centrifugal force to propel blood through the circulation. A large-bore cannula diverts blood from the left atrium into a pumphead, where rotating blades then propel it back into the aorta via a second cannula (Quaal 1991). Biventricular support can be provided by cannulating the right atrium and pulmonary artery in a similar fashion and using an additional pump for right ventricular support.

Results following VAD placement vary with patient category. When used in patients recovering from acute MI or cardiac surgery, 30–50% of patients can be weaned from the device, with long-term survival approaching 50% at some centers (Pennington et al. 1988). The best results have been obtained when VADs are used as a bridge-to-transplant. Approximately 60–70% of these patients are able to be transplanted, with 80–87% survival rates following transplant (Abou-Awdi 1991; Ley 1991; Shinn 1991). These survival rates are identical to cardiac transplant survival rates in

patients who did not require the device. When one considers that these same patients have a 100% mortality without VAD support, this represents a significant step forward in the management of severe cardiac failure.

Nursing care for the VAD patient focuses on supporting the patient until myocardial recovery or transplantation can occur. The reader is referred to additional sources for detailed information regarding nursing care guidelines for these challenging patients (Quaal, 1991).

NURSING DIAGNOSIS

Nursing diagnoses that are common to VAD patients include high risk for:

- Injury related to bleeding
- Impaired gas exchange
- Infection
- Inadequate nutritional intake
- Alteration in mobility
- Knowledge deficit
- Decreased cardiac output

Outcome Evaluation

Evaluate the patient's response to cardiovascular interventions according to the following outcome criteria. Ideally, the patient will develop a sinus rhythm and generate a cardiac output that is adequate for tissue perfusion. While medical and nursing interventions cannot guarantee that outcome criteria will be met, they serve as a goal toward which our interventions are directed.

Cardiac rhythm:

- Ventricular rate 60–100 beats per minute.
- Absent or infrequent premature contractions.
- Absence of cardiac dysrhythmias.

Hemodynamic status:

- Cardiac output 4–8 L/min.
- Cardiac index 2.5–4 L/min/m^2.
- Filling pressures WNL for patient.
- SVR 800–1,200 dynes/sec/cm^{-5}.

Tissue perfusion:

- No alterations in level of consciousness.
- Urine output > 30 cc/hr.
- Absence of chest pain.
- Skin warm, dry, with adequate peripheral pulses.
- Laboratory values WNL for patient.

Psychologic status:

- Absence of pain.
- Absence of anxiety.
- Asks appropriate questions.
- Verbalizes understanding of specific interventions used.

REFERENCES

Abou-Awdi N: Thermo Cardiosystems left ventricular assist device as a bridge to cardiac transplant. *AACN Clin Issues Crit Care Nurs* 1991; 2:545–551.

American College of Cardiology and American Heart Association: Guidelines and indications for coronary artery bypass graft surgery: A report of the ACC/AHA task force on assessment of diagnostic and therapeutic cardiovascular procedures. *J Am Coll Cardiol* 1991; 17:543–589.

American Heart Association: *Textbook of advanced cardiac life support,* 2d ed. Dallas, 1987.

American Heart Association: *1991 Heart and stroke facts.* Dallas, 1991.

Bartecchi C, Mann D: Pacemaker generators. Pages 291–303 in *Temporary cardiac pacing.* Bartecchi C, Mann D (eds). Chicago: Precept Press, 1990.

Beers M, Ouslander J: Risk factors in geriatric drug prescribing: A practical guide to avoiding problems. *Drugs* 1989; 37:105–112.

Bellville J et al.: Influence of age on pain relief from analgesics: A study of postoperative patients. *JAMA* 1971; 217:1835–1841.

Benner P: *From novice to expert.* Menlo Park, CA: Addison-Wesley, 1984.

Berne R, DiMarco J, Belardinelli L: Dromotropic effects of adenosine and adenosine antagonists in the treatment of cardiac arrhythmias involving the atrioventricular node. *Circ* 1984; 69:1195–1197.

Bernstein A et al.: The NASPE/BPEG generic pacemaker code for antibradyarrhythmia and adaptive-rate pacing and antitachyarrhythmia devices. *PACE* 1987; 10:795.

DiCarlo L: Cardiac arrest and sudden death in patients treated with amiodarone for sustained ventricular tachycardia or ventricular fibrillation: Risk stratification based on clinical variables. *Am J Cardiol* 1985; 55:372–374.

Drew B: Bedside electrocardiographic monitoring: State of the art for the 1990's. *Heart Lung* 1991; 20:610–623.

Fabiszewski R, Volosin K: Rate-modulated pacemakers. *J Cardiovasc Nurs* 1991; 5(3):21–31.

Falk R, Ngai S: External cardiac pacing: Influence of electrode placement on pacing threshold. *Crit Care Med* 1986; 14:931–932.

Funk M, Gleason J, Foell D: Lower limb ischemia related to use of the intra-aortic balloon pump. *Heart Lung* 1989; 18:542–552.

Furst E: Extracorporeal blood pumping during heart-lung bypass. *J Cardiovasc Nurse* 1989; 3(3):71–86.

Goran S: Family perceptions of the intra-aortic balloon pumping experience. *Crit Care Nurse Clin North Am* 1989; 1:475–477.

Goran S: Vascular complications of the patient undergoing intra-aortic balloon pumping. *Crit Care Nurse Clin North Am* 1989; 1:459–467.

Greatbatch W: Origins of the implantable cardiac pacemaker. *J Cardiovasc Nurs* 1991; 5(3):80–85.

Greene H: Sudden arrhythmic cardiac death-mechanisms, resuscitation and classification: The Seattle perspective. *Am J Cardiol* 1990; 65:4B–12B.

Gruentzig A, Kumpe D: Technique of percutaneous angioplasty with the Gruentzig balloon catheter. *Am J Roentgenol* 1979; 132:547–552.

Guerci A, Chandra N: Cardiopulmonary resuscitation. Pages 1–4 in *Current therapy in critical care medicine,* 2d ed. Parrillo J (ed). Philadelphia: Decker, 1991.

Halfman-Franey M, Coburn C: Techniques in cardiac care: Lasers, stents, and atherectomy devices. *AACN Clin Issues Crit Care Nurs* 1990; 1:87–109.

Hasegawa E: The endotracheal use of emergency drugs. *Heart Lung* 1986; 15:60–63.

Hill J: Phentolamine mesylate: The antidote for vasopressor extravasation. *Crit Care Nurse* 1991; 11(10):58–61.

Hui P, Yock P: Coronary angioplasty: Current update. *Comp Ther* 1989; 15(5):47–55.

Jansen K, McFadden M: Postoperative nursing management in patients undergoing myocardial revascularization with the internal mammary artery bypass. *Heart Lung* 1986; 15:48–54.

Jones J: Drugs and the elderly. Pages 41–60 in *Clinical aspects of aging,* Reichel W (ed). Baltimore: Williams & Wilkins, 1989.

Jones S, Bagg A: LEAD drugs for cardiac arrest. *Nurs 88* (Oct) 1988; 18:34–41.

Kain C, Reilly N, Schultz E: The older adult: A comparative assessment. *Nurs Clin North Am* 1990; 25:833–848.

Kaplan J, Finlayson D, Woodward S: Vasodilator therapy after cardiac surgery: A review of the efficacy and toxicity of nitroglycerin and nitroprusside. *Canad Anaesth Soc J* 1980; 27:254–258.

Kern L: Emergency exploratory sternotomy: the nurse's role. *Clin Issues Crit Care Nurs* 1990; 1:148–157.

Lerman B, Belardinelli L: Cardiac electrophysiology of adenosine: Basic and clinical concepts. *Circ* 1991; 83:1499–1509.

LeSage J: Polypharmacy in geriatric patients. *Nurs Clin North Am* 1991; 26:273–289.

Ley S: Fluid therapy following intracardiac operation. *Crit Care Nurs* 1988; 8(1):26–36.

Ley S: The Thoratec ventricular assist device: Nursing guidelines. *AACN Clin Issues Crit Care Nurs* 1991; 2:529–544.

Ley S et al.: Crystalloid versus colloid fluid therapy after cardiac surgery. *Heart Lung* 1990; 19:31–40.

Lynn-McHale D: Interventions for acute myocardial infarction: PTCA and CABGs. *Crit Care Nurs Quart* 1989; 12(2):38–48.

MacMahon S, et al.: Effects of prophylactic lidocaine in suspected acute myocardial infarction: An overview of results from the randomized, controlled trials. *JAMA* 1988; 260:1910–1916.

Mancini D, LeJemtel T, Sonnenblick E: Intravenous use of amrinone for the treatment of the failing heart. *Am J Cardiol* 1985; 56:8B–15B.

McIntosh-Yellin N, Drew B: Safety and efficacy of central vs peripheral adenosine for termination of supraventricular tachycardia. In press: Circulation, 1992 (Abstract).

Mulford E: Nursing perspectives for the patient receiving postoperative ventricular assistance in the critical care unit. *Heart Lung* 1987; 16:246–255.

Pearl J et al.: Management of complications of extracardiac conduits. Pages 212–223 in *Complications in cardiothoracic surgery*. Waldhausen JA, Orringer MB (eds). St Louis: Mosby, 1991.

Pennington D et al.: Seven years' experience with the Pierce-Donachy ventricular assist device. *J Thorac Cardiovasc Surg* 1988; 96:901–911.

Persons C: Transcutaneous pacing: Meeting the challenge. *Focus Crit Care* 1987; 14(1):13–19.

Pinkerton C et al.: Percutaneous coronary atherectomy: Early experiences of a multicenter trial. Presented at the 38th Annual Scientific Sessions of the American College of Cardiology; Anaheim, CA. March 19–23, 1989.

Quaal S: *Comprehensive intra-aortic balloon pumping*. St Louis: Mosby, 1984.

Quaal S: Centrifugal ventricular assist devices. *AACN Clin Issues Crit Care Nurs* 1991; 2:515–526.

Ryan T et al.: Guidelines for percutaneous transluminal coronary angioplasty: A report of the ACC/AHA task force on assessment of diagnostic and therapeutic cardiovascular procedures. *Circ* 1988; 78:486–502.

Savage M et al.: Clinical and angiographic determinants of primary coronary angioplasty success. *J Am Coll Cardiol* 1991; 17:22–28.

Seifert P: Surgery for acquired valvular heart disease. *J Cardiovasc Nurs* 1987; 1(3):26–40.

Shinn J: Novacor left ventricular assist system. *AACN Clin Issues Crit Care Nurs* 1991; 2:575–588.

Sipperly M: Expanding role of coronary angioplasty: Current implications, limitations, and nursing considerations. *Heart Lung* 1989; 18:507–513.

Sladen R: Adult cardiac surgery. Pages 502–512 in *Acute cardiovascular management: Anesthesia and intensive care*. Ream A and Fogdall R (eds). Philadelphia: Lippincott, 1982.

Smith R, Cleavinger M: Current perspectives on the use of circulatory assist devices. *AACN Clin Issues Crit Care Nurs* 1991; 2:488–499.

St. Jude Medical, Inc. Cardiac Assist Division. *Principles of counterpulsation.* 1987; 1–52.

Teplitz L: Classification of cardiac pacemakers: The pacemaker code. *J Cardiovasc Nurs* 1991a; 5(3):1–8.

Teplitz L: Transcutaneous pacemakers. *J Cardiovasc Nurs* 1991b; 5(3):44–57.

Teplitz L: Nursing diagnoses for automatic implantable cardioverter defibrillator patients. *Dimen Crit Care Nurs* 1991c; 10:188–2201.

Thompson A, Hayden R, Tyers G: Complications related to myocardial preservation in adults. Pages 75–81 in *Complications in cardiothoracic surgery*. Waldhausen J, Orringer M (eds). St Louis: Mosby, 1991.

Torrence J: Nursing management of patients with temporary pacemakers. Pages 249–267 in *Temporary cardiac pacing*. Bartecchi C, Mann D (eds). Chicago: Precept Press, 1990.

Weiland A, Walker W: Physiologic principles and clinical sequelae of cardiopulmonary bypass. *Heart Lung* 1986; 15:34–39.

15

Renal Disorders

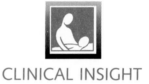

CLINICAL INSIGHT

Domain: Organizational and work-role competencies

Competency: Building and maintaining a therapeutic team to provide optimum therapy

The multiple specialty services in a critical-care unit present a complex web of interrelationships within which the nurse sometimes must negotiate to meet patients' needs. Even though specialty teams may have little contact with each other and may have conflicting goals, the nurse knows they must work well together for the patient to benefit. Often, the nurse assumes a primary role in coordinating care. In the following paradigm, from Crabtree and Jorgenson (1986, pp. 168–169), Tracy, the nurse, intervenes in a situation in which care is poorly coordinated for a dialysis patient whose only kidney recently has been removed for a cancerous tumor. Although the patient has two medical teams—nephrology and surgical trans-

plant—no one really is in charge. The patient is threatening to leave because she has been denied satisfaction of the most basic of human needs—food and water.

She was getting no fluids, nothing, no diet, no fluids. And there was nobody to really go to. This was through the time when all the fellows, the nephrology fellows, were gone. And so there was one staff person on and they came in once, early in the morning, and nobody would really make a decision as to what to do with her. And her reaction was, if they don't give me anything to drink, I'm leaving, you know. And somebody would say, well, you know, you need to have a dialysis. And she'd say, I don't care, you know, I can't live like this. And you know, it makes sense, she's right. So she was in limbo between the two teams. And so I guess I had talked to her a little bit. I felt

409

really frustrated because I thought, she's right, I mean I would be angry too, to go two days without anything at all. And you know, even dialysis patients get stuff to drink and they don't have kidneys that work, you know. She went down to dialysis and I talked to the nurse that was taking care of her and said, you know, I would call somebody and tell them how she feels and what her feelings are and that really there was no reason she shouldn't be able to have a diet. And that it would be important for her to have a diet. So, anyway, she did call and finally they came over and talked to her a little bit and she said, you know, she'd leave. I think she would have. And, they said she could have a little bit of ice chips.

Ice chips may not seem like much, but for this patient, caught in a frustrating no-man's-land between the teams, the nurse's obtaining them was an act of good nursing practice.

Caring for the renal failure patient poses unique nursing challenges. This chapter will review the causes and treatment of acute and chronic renal failure and the complications that may occur with either of these states.

Renal Anatomy and Physiology

Human kidneys have excretory, regulatory, and endocrine functions. Not only are they the major organs of excretion of metabolic waste products, they also regulate extracellular fluid volume and osmolality, maintain electrolyte balance, and assist in the control of acid–base balance. The kidney's endocrine functions include secretion of renin for regulation of blood pressure, secretion of erythropoietin for stimulation of red blood cell production, and conversion of vitamin D to its most active form.

The kidneys, which are elongated, flattened organs, measure approximately 6 by 12 cm and lie retroperitoneally on either side of the vertebral column. The left kidney is slightly higher than the right, with its upper border lying between the eleventh and twelfth ribs (Figure 15–1). The right kidney extends downward from the twelfth rib. Their lower borders are at the level of the third lumbar vertebrae. The kidneys are enclosed within a layer of perirenal fat (Figure 15–2). Both their location and their fatty protection protect them to some extent from direct trauma.

Gross Structure

The kidneys are covered by a relatively indistensible collagenous layer of tissue known as the *renal capsule.* This capsule adheres to the underlying tissue of the kidney. The inner macroscopic structures of the kidney consist of the cortex, medulla, renal pyramids, calyces, and renal pelvis (Figure 15–3). The solid tissue is delineated as the cortex, medulla, and renal pyramids, while the calyxes and renal pelvis are hollow structures which collect formed urine. The *cortex* of the kidney is the outer, most dense layer of tissue. The *medulla* contains 10–15 wedge-shaped pyramids; the apices (papillae) of these pyramids empty into the fingerlike calyces which join and extend inward to form the *renal pelvis.* From the renal pelvis, the ureter transports urine into the bladder via peristaltic movement. Urine is excreted from the bladder via the urethra.

Blood flow to each kidney is via the renal artery, which arises from the abdominal aorta; blood flow leaves the kidney via the renal vein, which empties into the inferior vena cava. Blood flow to the kidneys is at a rate of approximately 1,200 cc/min or approximately 20% of cardiac output. This high-pressure, high-flow vascular system to and within the kidney is essential to maintenance of renal function.

Microscopic Structure

The microscopic structural and functional unit of the kidney (for urine formation) is the *nephron.* There are approximately 1 million nephrons in each kidney; each of these nephrons functions independently. Each nephron is composed of a vascular and tubular system (Figure 15–4). Blood flow to the nephron arises from renal arterial branching (interlobar, arcuate, and interlobular arteries). The nephron is composed of the glomerulus, proximal convoluted tubule, loop of Henle, distal convoluted tubule, and collecting tubule. Most nephrons are located in the cortex of the kidney, although some extend into the medulla (these are known as juxtamedullary nephrons).

Blood enters the *glomerulus,* the first portion of the nephron, via the *afferent arteriole,* which subdivides into a capillary tuft (Figure 15–5). Blood exits from this capillary tuft via the *efferent arteriole.* This blood flow structure (arteriolar-capillary-arteriolar) is anomalous and partially responsible for maintaining glomerular function.

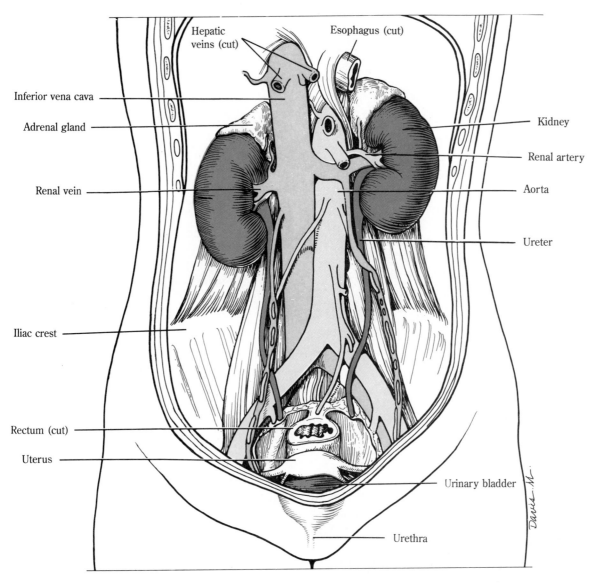

FIGURE 15–1

Organs of the urinary system. The anterior abdominal wall and most of the abdominal organs have been removed. (From Spence A: *Basic human anatomy,* 3d ed. Redwood City, CA: Benjamin/Cummings, 1990, p. 568.)

Glomerular Function

Filtration of blood is the primary function of the glomerulus. Within the capillary bed of the glomerulus, an ultrafiltrate of plasma is formed by filtration across the semipermeable capillary wall. This ultrafiltrate consists of water, end products of metabolism (waste products or toxins), electrolytes, and glucose. Because molecular size and weight determine particle movement across the capillary wall, the large mole-

cules of red and white blood cells and plasma proteins normally are not filtered.

Water moves out of the glomerular capillary bed via hydrostatic and oncotic pressure gradients. Hydrostatic pressure within the capillary tuft averages 60 mm Hg. Since the opposing hydrostatic pressure in the surrounding Bowman's capsule is 10 mm Hg, the net outward hydrostatic pressure is 50 mm Hg. In addition, normal oncotic pressure(s) preventing fluid movement from this capillary bed is 30 mm Hg. Thus, the net pressure across the glomerular capillary tuft is 20 mm

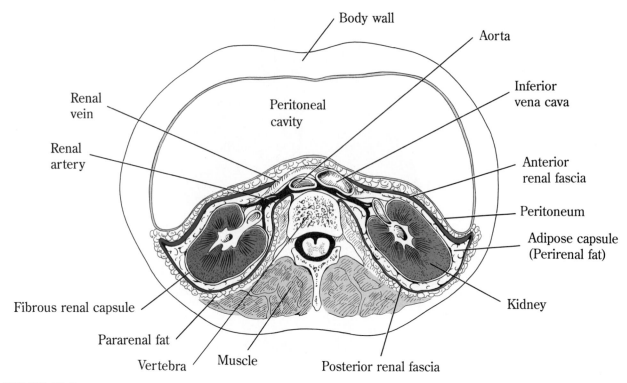

FIGURE 15–2

Transverse section of the body trunk showing the retroperitoneal location of the kidneys and the renal fascia that surrounds them. (From Spence A: *Basic human anatomy,* 3d ed. Redwood City, CA: Benjamin/Cummings, 1990, p. 570.)

Hg. This pressure gradient allows the ultrafiltrate to move out of the capillary bed of the glomerulus and to flow into the surrounding cuplike structure of *Bowman's capsule.* The rate of production of this ultrafiltrate by all of the glomeruli, the *glomerular filtration rate* (GFR), is approximately 125 cc/min. Thus, a volume of 180 L/24 hours is filtered through the glomeruli.

The glomerular filtration rate may be maintained in a remarkably steady state even when there are changes in systemic blood pressure, volume, or both. Mean arterial pressure changes in the range of 80–250 mm Hg will be tolerated by the glomerulus of the kidney, because of its ability to autoregulate the pressure within the capillary tuft. While this mechanism is not completely understood, it is known that the afferent arteriole is able to dilate or constrict to maintain the blood flow and volume entering the capillary bed. Thus, the afferent arteriole dilates to increase blood flow when a clinical situation of hypotension or hypovolemia occurs. It constricts when there is an increase in blood pressure, to maintain normal pressure within the capillary bed. Similarly, the efferent arteriole is able to constrict and dilate to maintain the

hydrostatic pressure gradient across the capillary bed and aid in maintenance of normal glomerular filtration.

Tubular Function

The *proximal convoluted tubule* receives the flow of ultrafiltrate from Bowman's capsule. The primary function of this segment of the nephron is selective reabsorption of water, electrolytes, and other solutes. Approximately 70% of the filtered water and 65% of solutes are reabsorbed in this segment of the nephron. Sodium is transported actively through the cell wall, while other positively charged ions also move out of the tubular space. Negatively charged ions also move across the tubular cell wall to maintain neutrality of charge. From the surrounding cortex, particles can also move into the proximal convoluted tubules; these include hydrogen (H^+) ions, organic acids, urea, and some metabolized medications. Amino acids and glucose are almost completely reabsorbed from the proximal convoluted tubule. Glycosuria occurs when the load of glucose filtered by the glomerulus is too much to be reabsorbed; this load and its excretion

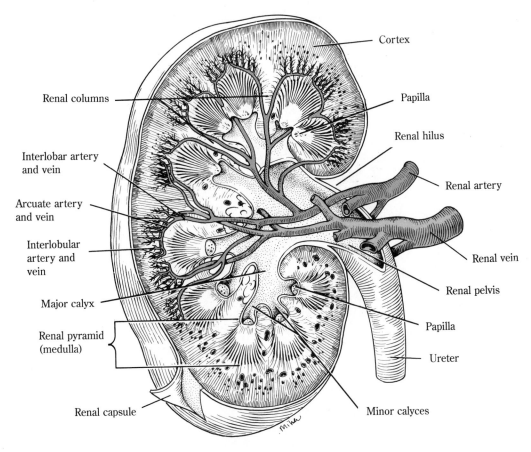

FIGURE 15–3

Longitudinal section of a kidney illustrating its internal structure. (From Spence A: *Basic human anatomy,* 3d ed. Redwood City, CA: Benjamin/Cummings, 1990, p. 571.)

exemplify the concept of the *renal threshold* of a substance (the concentration at which further reabsorption cannot be accomplished). Because of the amount and ratio of reabsorption of water and sodium, as well as other solutes, the fluid remaining in the proximal convoluted tubule is normally isotonic and iso-osmotic. No metabolic end products (e.g., urea and creatinine) are reabsorbed from this segment of the nephron. The reabsorbed solutes and water move into the surrounding vascular structure and thus return to the systemic circulation.

The loop of Henle receives this isotonic, iso-osmolar fluid into its descending limb. The countercurrent multiplier system is involved in fluid and solute shifts from the loop of Henle (Figure 15–6). The cell wall of the descending portion of the limb is freely permeable to water. The interstitial tissue surrounding the loop of Henle is increasingly hypertonic and hyperosmolar at the tip of the loop of Henle. Thus, water easily moves from the descending limb into the surrounding tissue

and vasculature *(vasa recta)*. At the tip of the loop of Henle, the fluid inside the tubule also becomes hypertonic and hyperosmolar (1,400 mosm/L).

As fluid inside the tubule flows upward through the ascending limb, the cell wall is impermeable to water; sodium chloride is actively transported from the intratubular space into the interstitial tissue and absorbed into the vasa recta. Calcium and magnesium ions also are transported out of the ascending limb of the loop of Henle. The transport of sodium chloride is so efficient that the fluid becomes hypotonic and hypo-osmotic at the top of the ascending limb. The reabsorption of both water and sodium chloride in the loop of Henle maintains systemic salt and water balance.

The *distal convoluted tubule* maintains or corrects systemic water and electrolyte balance by allowing for reabsorption of water as well as sodium chloride, particularly when the cell wall is influenced by aldosterone. Potassium ions may be exchanged

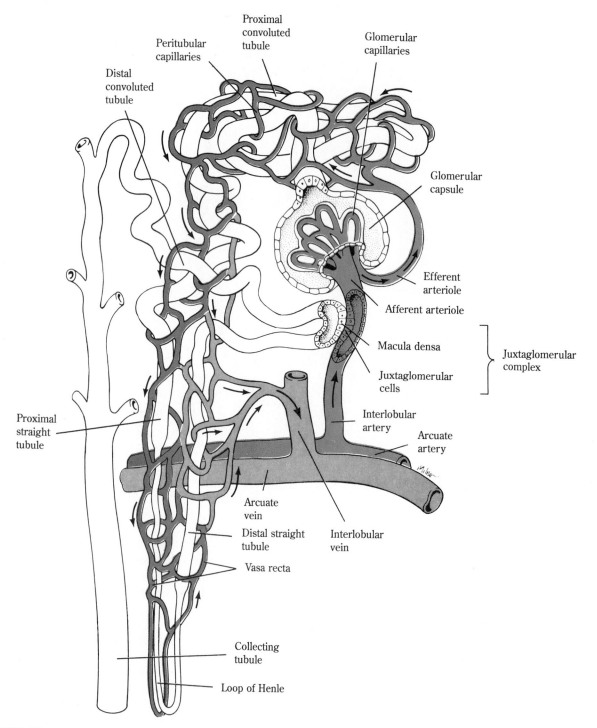

FIGURE 15–4

A juxtamedullary nephron and its blood supply. (From Spence A: *Basic human anatomy,* 3d ed. Redwood City, CA: Benjamin/Cummings, 1990, p. 576.)

for sodium ions, for reabsorption or excretion, in response to aldosterone secretion. In addition, H⁺ ions enter the tubular space from the surrounding interstitium.

The *collecting tubule* of the nephron receives this hypotonic, hypo-osmolar fluid (urine) from the distal convoluted tubule. The cell wall of the collecting tubule is permeable to the movement of urea into the

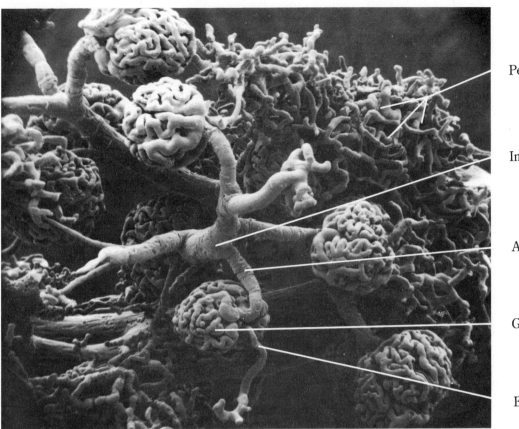

Peritubular capillaries

Interlobular artery

Afferent arteriole

Glomerulus

Efferent arteriole

FIGURE 15–5

Scanning electron micrograph of the blood vessels associated with glomeruli (×206).
(From Kessel R, Kardon R: *Tissues and organs: A text-atlas of scanning electron microscopy.* Freeman, © 1979. Reprinted with permission.)

surrounding interstitium, but it is impermeable to other solute movement. The cell wall can become permeable to water moving out of the tubule when antidiuretic hormone is present. When this free water is reabsorbed from the collecting tubule, it is absorbed into the surrounding vasculature and returned to the systemic circulation. The collecting tubules of multiple nephrons join together forming the macroscopic structure of the renal pyramids. The urine that has been formed in these nephrons enters the calyces and the renal pelvis of the kidney.

With normal fluid and food intake, the final urine volume produced in a 24-hour period is approximately 1.5–2 liters. It contains metabolic waste products and electrolytes, as determined by the dynamic filtration and reabsorption which occurred throughout the nephrons. Because the volume of fluid and concentration of solutes in urine depends on the individual's intake of nutrients and fluids and metabolic state including other organ system function, the interpreta-

tion of renal function via urine and other testing is important but inconclusive.

Endocrine Function

The kidney functions both as an endocrine organ and as a target organ for other endocrine organs. These hormonal influences affect physiologic functioning both acutely and on an ongoing basis.

Renin-Angiotensin System   The *renin-angiotensin system* has direct influence on the kidney as well as other systemic effects. *Renin* is an enzyme that is secreted from the *juxtaglomerular apparatus* (Figure 15–7). The *juxtaglomerular apparatus,* a special structure in the nephron, is composed of specialized cells, known as the macula densa in the wall of distal convoluted tubule, that are in juxtaposition to the afferent and efferent arterioles of the glomerulus.

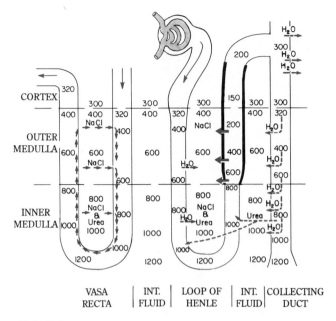

FIGURE 15–6

Countercurrent mechanism for concentration of urine. Values in mOsm/L. (From Guyton A: *Textbook of medical physiology*, 8th ed. Philadelphia: Saunders, 1991, p. 310.)

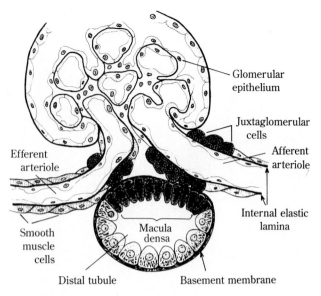

FIGURE 15–7

Structure of the juxtaglomerular apparatus, illustrating its possible feedback role in the control of nephron function. (From Guyton A: *Textbook of medical physiology*, 8th ed. Philadelphia: Saunders 1991, p. 294, as modified from Ham: *Histology*. Philadelphia: Lippincott, 1971.)

It is believed that this apparatus responds as a baroreceptor to pressure changes in these arterioles and also as a chemoreceptor to changes in the sodium concentration in the fluid in the distal convoluted tubule. Either (or both) of these changes is created by decreased blood flow into the glomerulus. When the juxtaglomerular apparatus is stimulated by these conditions, renin is secreted. In the peripheral circulation, renin converts angiotensinogen (which is synthesized and secreted by the liver) into angiotensin I. As angiotensin I circulates through the lungs, the angiotensin converting enzyme (ACE) converts angiotensin I to angiotensin II, the active form of the hormone. Angiotensin II acts on vascular smooth muscle to cause generalized peripheral vasoconstriction, thus increasing blood flow to the kidneys; it also stimulates the secretion of *aldosterone,* which acts upon the distal convoluted tubule to increase reabsorption of sodium and water. There is evidence that angiotensin II is converted to a form known as angiotensin III prior to its elimination; this form apparently is especially potent in stimulating aldosterone secretion from the adrenal cortices (Schrier 1986). Angiotensin II also stimulates the release of *antidiuretic hormone* (ADH) from the posterior pituitary gland, thus increasing the reabsorption of free water from the collecting tubule into the sys-

temic circulation. The effect of this stimulation of the renin-angiotensin system is an increase in effective vascular volume, due to peripheral vasoconstriction, shunting of blood flow to core organs (particularly the kidneys), and reabsorption of sodium and water in various segments of the nephron. The increased volume increases systemic blood pressure and renal blood flow, thus correcting glomerular function and filtration to maintain nephron function.

Prostaglandins and kinins are also thought to play a role in the maintenance of renal hemodynamics by their vasoactive effects (both dilatation and constriction), as well as their role in sodium excretion. The actions of both prostaglandins and kinins are under investigation.

Erythropoietin *Erythropoietin* is a hormonal substance apparently produced within the kidney, although the exact site has not been determined. Erythropoietin production is stimulated by decreased systemic oxygen saturation. After release from the kidney, erythropoietin is transported to bone marrow to stimulate increased red blood cell formation. When erythropoietin is not produced by the kidney (as occurs in most renal diseases), a normochromic, normocytic anemia develops.

Calcium and Phosphorus Metabolism The kidney also plays a vital role in the maintenance of calcium and phosphorus metabolism and thus the maintenance of bone matrix and various other enzyme or metabolic activities which depend on normal serum calcium levels. The kidney converts the vitamin D produced by the liver into its metabolically active form of 1,25 dihydroxycholecalciferol to allow calcium absorption from the GI tract. The parathyroid gland is stimulated to secrete parathormone (PTH) when there is a decreased serum calcium level. PTH stimulates the reabsorption of bone to increase serum calcium levels. The kidney also excretes phosphorus as an end-product of metabolism.

(For a more detailed review and discussion of renal anatomy and physiology, consult a current anatomy and physiology or nephrology text.)

Assessment of Renal Function

The loss of renal function may be an insidious and almost symptomless process, occurring over varying periods of time, and may result in conditions ranging from diminished function to total failure.

Acute renal failure is a complication of another primary disease or medical condition which develops quite rapidly. The lesions caused are generally reversible. For reasons that remain elusive, the damaged tissue is able to regenerate, with restoration of renal function.

Chronic renal failure is a progressive, irreversible process. Because the physical symptoms of uremia (to be reviewed later) occur so late in the progression of disease, patients may or may not seek medical care for potential renal problems. Patients may seek care for other reasons, only to discover that their kidneys are failing.

Because nephrons function independently of each other to form urine (as previously described), renal disease/failure depends on the amount of nephron loss. As renal disease progresses, functional hypertrophy of remaining nephrons occurs; these nephrons will maintain adequate renal function to continue life for varying periods of time. The loss of 75% of all nephrons must occur before there are evident changes in blood tests measuring renal function. The loss of 90% of nephrons creates the clinical state of *uremia,* which requires replacement therapy (dialysis, or transplantation) to maintain life. Total loss of renal function without replacement therapy is a terminal condition.

History

Medical history is important to identifying the risk for the development of renal disease. Family history is important for the diagnosis of inherited renal diseases. Other systemic diseases such as systemic lupus erythematosus (SLE), diabetes mellitus (types I and II), and hypertension have a high incidence of renal failure as a complication; thus, regular surveillance of renal function for these patients is essential.

Patients may seek care for changes in urinary output (frequency and volume) that might indicate renal changes. In older males, changes in urine flow (in force of stream) may be related to prostatic disease, which when untreated may lead to renal involvement due to obstruction.

Pain associated with kidney disease occurs primarily in inflammation and/or infection. Acute flank pain, which occurs with kidney infections, is usually severe. The pain of inflammatory processes such as glomerulonephritis may be more dull and constant. Pain which is more intermittent and sharp may indicate the presence of urinary tract stone(s); intrarenal stones cause less pain and can be a totally painless condition. The most severe pain occurs during stone movement or presence in the ureter; patients experience severe spasmodic pain until the stone is removed or passed into the bladder.

Physical Examination

Routine physical examination of the kidneys provides little information about disease states. Because of their size and placement, kidneys are difficult to palpate directly. The lower edge of the right kidney is most easily palpated when the patient is in a supine position. Enlarged kidneys (e.g., hydronephrosis or polycystic disease) obviously are palpated more easily.

Physical examination also should include auscultation for presence of a bruit in the renal artery. For patients with hypertension, this is especially important to diagnose the presence of a renal artery stenosis. The presence of pain can be identified on physical examination by applying pressure in the flank area (at the costovertebral angle).

Laboratory Tests

The most common tests of renal function performed routinely are urinalysis and blood studies of blood urea nitrogen and creatinine levels.

Routine Urine Studies *Routine Urinalysis* Routine urinalysis evaluates urine color, clarity, concentration, acidity (pH) and presence of abnormal substances. A bedside urinalysis includes visual evaluation of urine color and clarity, measurement of specific gravity, and dipstick measurement of acidity (pH), and the presence of blood, protein, and glucose. Visual observation identifies the color of urine, which is usually yellow or amber, due to the presence of urobilin. Color may be affected by diet or medications and should be correlated with patient history. Color is a general indicator of concentration and dilution but does not quantify it. Urine should be clear without the presence of sediment. Cloudiness indicates the presence of white blood cells or tissue. and is most commonly associated with infection. The odor of freshly voided urine should be assessed by the nurse and recorded and reported appropriately. Freshly voided urine should be aromatic, not odoriferous or offensive. Odors may develop when urine stagnates and are not necessarily relevant to patient condition.

Urine pH may be acidotic or alkalotic (normal range is 4.50–7.50). It is affected by the excretion of metabolic waste products or intake of certain foods or medications. Urine osmolality can vary from 75 to 1,200 mOsm/Kg. Specific gravity, which measures urine concentration as compared to water, ranges from 1.010–1.025. Both osmolality and specific gravity measure solute concentration of urine; both of these results should vary depending on renal changes in excretion of solutes and water. Fixed specific gravity or osmolality measurements indicate that the kidney is unable to concentrate or dilute urine.

The presence of blood may indicate bleeding within the urinary tract or may be a result of contamination from a woman's menstrual cycle. It will be measured as protein both on dipstick and in quantitative analysis.

The presence of glucose (glycosuria) may identify hyperglycemia in the diabetic, with the renal threshold having been exceeded; it may be the first indicator of the development of diabetes. Glycosuria may also occur after very high glucose loads (oral intake or hyperalimentation) without the presence of diabetes.

Microscopic urinalysis will identify and quantify the types of cells present, including red and white blood cells, bacteria, epithelial cells, or sperm. Crystals or casts also may be present; both are abnormal and assist in the diagnosis of location and type of the renal lesion. The most diagnostic aspect of casts is what type of cell or tissue is enclosed inside the cast (e.g., red cell casts, hyaline casts).

Protein should be absent from a normal voided urine specimen because the molecule is too large to be filtered by the glomerulus. Protein may "spill" across the glomerulus due to a high dietary intake; intense, protracted physical exercise also increases proteinuria. In these cases, the proteinuria is transitory; a repeated study should be negative. When proteinuria is always present, it is diagnostic of glomerular disease. Protein losses should be quantified by 12- or 24-hour collections, which measure the total amount of protein excreted. Normal amounts should be less than 150 mg/24 hours. In severe glomerular pathology, protein excretion can be as great as 6–7 g/24 hours. With such losses, body protein stores are lost, and the patient becomes protein depleted (negative nitrogen balance).

Electrolyte excretion (e.g., sodium, potassium, chloride) and other solutes (urea nitrogen, creatinine) can be measured in single urine samples as well as in timed collections. Such studies may be performed to determine acute changes in renal function or to measure progression of specific renal diseases.

Culture and Sensitivity Urine cultures are performed on aliquots of urine collected in an aseptic fashion. Cleaning of the exterior tissues around the urethra prevents contamination of the specimen with other organisms. A mid-stream collection also eliminates contamination that may occur at the initiation of the urine stream. These urine samples should be tested immediately to prevent overgrowth or opportunistic growth of organisms; they should be kept cool (refrigerated or on ice) until received in the laboratory. This type of study should be completed with the performance of drug sensitivities to determine the most effective antibiotic for use if the culture is positive.

Blood Studies *Blood Urea Nitrogen* (BUN) is measured frequently. Urea is an end product of protein metabolism, coming from endogenous (body muscle or red blood cells) and/or exogenous (dietary) sources. Urea nitrogen is formed from amino acid degradation, in which large amounts of ammonia are formed in the gut, absorbed into the bloodstream, and converted to urea in the liver. Urea is filtered almost completely by the glomerulus, and only small amounts are reabsorbed from the tubules into the interstitium of the kidney; this reabsorption does not affect blood and urine measurements. The normal BUN value is 10–20 mg/dl but varies depending on laboratory standards (check the normal ranges for your own medical laboratory).

Most of the urea produced is excreted by the kidney (several grams per day). Production of urea nitrogen, however, is primarily dependent on oral protein intake.

In the healthy individual, increased production is balanced by increased excretion, thus maintaining normal blood levels. Speculation that increased protein intake has adverse effects on kidney function remains unproven in humans (Anderson and Brenner 1986).

Serum creatinine results from muscle mass metabolism. The production of creatinine is determined by a person's skeletal muscle mass and thus is fairly constant. A severe catabolic state can increase creatinine production; increasing muscle mass via bodybuilding exercise and use of anabolic steroids might also increase production. Blood levels remain normal even in such altered states if glomerular filtration remains normal. Interpretation of the single value of serum creatinine requires familiarity with the patient's body structure (height, weight, muscle mass). Normal serum creatinine values range from 0.5–1.5 mg/dl; approximately 1–1.5 g is excreted in 24 hours by the normal healthy adult.

The *blood urea nitrogen/serum creatinine (BUN/ creatinine) ratio* can be calculated easily from the blood values; the ratio should be 10:1 in a steady healthy state. However, this ratio may be altered by changes in an individual's protein intake, hemolysis (due to protein released from red blood cells), septic states, and extracellular and vascular volume changes.

All serum electrolyte concentrations may be affected by loss of renal function. Specific concerns will be reviewed later in this chapter. For a complete discussion of electrolyte balance, review Chapter 16.

Renal Function Measurement In addition to the studies already described, other quantitative renal function measurements can be performed. The most diagnostic study is one which can measure the glomerular filtration rate. This study determines blood flow into the nephron and the ability of the capillary bed to filter solutes and water from the blood. Clinical measurement of the glomerular filtration rate can be performed by measuring clearance of a substance from a given amount of fluid. *Clearance* can be defined as the amount of blood (plasma) per minute from which a substance is totally removed. In the kidneys, the area in which clearance occurs is the glomerulus of the nephron.

The clearance of a given substance is a clinically useful indicator of glomerular filtration rate if the substance is filtered freely by the glomerulus but neither reabsorbed nor secreted into the tubular portion of the nephron. Creatinine is such a substance in the human body; it is almost completely filtered by the glomerulus but is not reabsorbed from the tubular system of the nephron. While minute amounts of creatinine may be secreted into the tubule, the quantity is insufficient to affect the total amount excreted. Therefore, *creatinine clearance* is the most precise test of glomerular filtration that can be performed with a minimum of difficulty in a clinical setting.

Clearance is determined by measuring the plasma concentration of a substance, the urine concentration of the same substance, and the urine flow rate (total volume of urine divided by time of production). The classic equation for this test is:

$$\text{CLEARANCE} = \frac{\text{URINE CONCENTRATION OF SUBSTANCE} \times \text{URINE FLOW RATE (volume} \div \text{time)}}{\text{PLASMA CONCENTRATION OF THE SUBSTANCE}}$$

Using creatinine as the substance cleared by healthy adult kidneys, the result of this equation is clearance of 100–150 cc/min for men and 85–125 cc/min for women. Comparison to 125 cc/min as the normal GFR verifies that this test is an adequate clinical measure of glomerular function.

Performance of this clinical test requires that all urine be collected for a given period of time. The total volume of urine is measured and divided by the time period of collection to determine urine flow rate. The traditional 24-hour period of urine collection is not necessary; collections of 2 hours or more can also give accurate results of glomerular function when indicated. A serum sample for creatinine measurement must be drawn, preferably during the urine collection time period; drawing the serum sample at the end of the collection period is also traditional and practical. Finally, for accurate calculation of creatinine production and excretion for the clearance equation, the patient's body surface area should be calculated to estimate actual muscle mass. The patient's height, weight, gender, and age allow for this calculation.

Errors in collection of samples can be identified fairly easily if the results are not logical. For example, if one's serum creatinine is normal, one must have a normal creatinine clearance. If the creatinine clearance is low in the face of a normal serum creatinine, it is fairly clear that the urine collection is inaccurate. Thus, the relationship between serum creatinine and creatinine clearance is inverse; as the serum creatinine rises, less is being filtered by the glomerulus. Serial creatinine clearance measurements are most accurate in identifying subtle changes in renal function.

Inulin is an inert substance which can be intravenously injected to measure GFR even more accurately than the clinical measure of creatinine clearance. However, inulin clearance is more difficult and invasive to perform and thus is rarely indicated in the clinical setting.

Diagnostic Procedures

The need to perform various diagnostic studies to determine the patient's renal function status or diagnose the specific type of renal disease varies. The diagnosis more often depends simply on medical history or circumstances and the nature of the symptoms. The performance of such studies is more useful and diagnostic in the early period of renal disease, which often is when the patient is not aware of the problem and not seeing a physician. Because glomerular diseases can be treated with immunosuppressive medications that stabilize or reverse imminent renal failure, diagnostic studies are critical when glomerular diseases are suspected.

Acute renal failure that develops in the hospital following a major trauma or insult requires few, if any, diagnostic studies to identify its existence. Clinical findings make this diagnosis relatively simple and highly accurate. In addition, diagnostic studies would not cause any change in treatment, since treatment is essentially standard for most types of acute renal failure. The following is a brief review of diagnostic studies and their indications for use.

1. KUB: A plain radiographic film showing the shadows of the kidneys, ureters, and bladder. Identifies presence of structures and normal or abnormal shapes. Study is painless and noninvasive.

2. Ultrasound: Use of sound waves to identify the structure of a solid organ. Identifies echogenicity of the area/organ of testing. Identifies presence or absence and shape of kidneys, ureters, and bladder (if all structures are imaged). Painless and noninvasive.

3. Computed tomography (CT) scan: Radiologic study that produces multidimensional multiple images through the organ/tissue being studied. Excellent images of structure of kidneys and urinary tract. May or may not require oral and/or intravenous (IV) contrast agents to enhance tissue contrast. IV injection may cause pain; reaction to contrast agent is possible. Kidneys may be visualized adequately during CT studies of other abdominal organs.

4. Magnetic resonance imaging (MRI): Use of magnetic field which creates images by measurement of radiofrequency energy of electrons in the body. Images resemble photographs and are multidimensional. Identifies structure of kidneys and urinary tract. May require contrast agents to enhance images. Contraindicated for patients with any metal implant, e.g., pacemakers, artificial hips, or other joints because of potential displacement due to strength of magnetic field.

5. Intravenous pyelogram (IVP): Radiographic visualization of the entire renal collecting system using an intravenously injected iodinated contrast agent. Sequential films taken over a period of time follow the progression of the contrast agent through the system. Usually all structures are well defined on the series of films. Requires intravenous injection of contrast agent; allergic responses to iodine-based agent or precipitation of acute renal failure in high-risk patients are possible.

6. Retrograde pyelogram: Radiographic imaging of renal collecting system by injection of contrast agent via catheter placed into ureter(s). Allows for more specific imaging of ureters, especially when there is a possibility of obstruction. Allergy to contrast agent is possible. An invasive study with risk of infection or trauma to renal system.

7. Renal arteriography: Radiographic assessment of renal vasculature (from renal artery throughout kidney to renal vein). Requires placement of catheter into each renal artery for images of each kidney. Iodinated contrast agent is injected into catheter at initiation of x-ray imaging. Patient experiences burning, hot flash sensation. Allergic reaction to contrast agent is a risk. Complications of catheter placement include hematoma at puncture site, arterial bleeding at puncture site, thrombosis of vessel with loss of distal blood flow, emboli from puncture site or vessel walls, and infection.

8. Renal scan (radionuclide imaging): Intravenous injection of a radioactive isotope to identify vascular and tubular structures of kidney. Radiation detection equipment measures uptake and excretion of isotope. Is dynamic, so identifies functional activity of the kidney and also outlines ureter and bladder during excretion. Pain from intravenous injection is possible. Multiple isotope injections of radioactive iodine may suppress thyroid function.

9. Cystoscopy: Direct visualization of interior of the bladder via a scope. Bladder is filled with fluid to facilitate visualization. After study,

bladder spasms may occur due to distention. Bleeding or slight hematuria are possible. Bladder perforation by cystoscope is a risk, as is urinary retention or bladder infection. Patients are usually sedated; the lithotomy position is uncomfortable.

10. Renal biopsy: Removal of a piece of renal tissue for microscopic analysis to determine type of disease process. Section should include entire nephron and interstitium. May be performed by surgical removal of small section of kidney under direct visualization. Needle biopsy may be performed at bedside; may also be done with visualization by ultrasound or CT imaging. Aching pain may occur from incision or needle puncture. Hematoma or bleeding from site may occur. Hemorrhage may occur within kidney, requiring emergent surgical intervention often resulting in removal of the kidney.

Acute Renal Failure

Acute renal failure is the sudden diminution of renal function causing fluid and electrolyte imbalances, retention of waste products of metabolism, and potential complications in other organ systems. The acute loss of kidney function secondary to an illness or insult is seen frequently in the critical-care unit and provides a major challenge to the nurse's assessment and intervention skills.

Acute renal failure (ARF) is a nonspecific term used to describe multiple specific problems that compromise normal renal function. Acute renal failure has three unique features: 1) it is always a complication of another primary illness or process, 2) it is "potentially" preventable, and 3) it is potentially and usually reversible.

Assessment

Categories of Acute Renal Failure Three categories of ARF are used to describe this disease process; these categories also reflect the anatomic area of dysfunction in the renal system. They are characterized by different clinical findings. The nurse who is aware of these differences and assesses the patient carefully can be instrumental in preventing further progression of his or her kidney dysfunction.

Prerenal causes diminish renal perfusion and de-

TABLE 15–1

Causes of Acute Renal Failure: Prerenal Causes

1. Hypovolemia due to actual fluid loss (for example, hemorrhage, burns, or dehydration) or third-spacing (internal fluid shift).

2. Decreased cardiac output due to ventricular failure (for example, congestive heart failure) or cardiogenic shock, causing decreased renal perfusion.

3. Septic shock.

4. Abdominal aortic aneurysm.

5. Renal artery thrombosis or stenosis.

6. Drugs: ACE inhibitors and nonsteroidal anti-inflammatory drugs (NSAIDs).

---

crease glomerular filtration rate. Thus, any actual reduction in circulating blood volume or any lesion which causes decreased blood flow to the kidneys is considered prerenal. Prerenal renal failure may be caused by the conditions listed in Table 15–1.

Intrarenal (parenchymal) causes of acute renal failure result in damage to the glomeruli and/or tubules of the nephron. In addition, damage to the interstitial tissue in the kidney surrounding the nephrons may occur. When this damage occurs, renal function is altered clinically.

Glomerular damage accounts for approximately 25% of cases of intrarenal failure, while tubular damage accounts for about 75%. This latter type of acute renal failure is more usually described by the term *acute tubular necrosis (ATN)*. Table 15–2 lists conditions that may cause intrarenal renal failure.

Postrenal causes of acute renal failure arise from lesions or obstruction in the collecting system or lower urinary tract (ureters and bladder). When these are unrelieved, they lead to increased pressure and stasis of urine in the kidney, causing damage or destruction of the functioning nephrons. This condition, known as hydronephrosis, may or may not be reversible. Usual causes of postrenal acute renal failure are shown in Table 15–3.

Risk Factors The critical-care nurse is responsible for monitoring the patient's renal function. Your first responsibility is to identify factors that put the patient's renal system at risk so you may implement protective care.

Because hypovolemia and shock are the leading causes of ARF and ATN, trauma patients often are considered the most likely to develop acute renal failure. Nursing surveillance for alterations in renal function can prevent renal failure (Wilkes and Mailloux

TABLE 15–2

Causes of Acute Renal Failure: Intrarenal Causes

1. Acute tubular necrosis (affects basement membrane of tubules)
   A. Severe, prolong prerenal changes (severe ischemia).
   B. Crush syndrome.
   C. Severe allergic reactions (e.g., transfusion reactions).
   D. Nephrotoxic agents including heavy metals, some insecticides, ethylene glycol, iodine-based radiographic contrast agents, and antibiotics (e.g., aminoglycosides, amphotericin B, gentamycin).
2. Glomerulonephritis (affects basement membrane of glomerulus)

TABLE 15–3

Causes of Acute Renal Failure: Postrenal Causes

1. Benign prostatic hypertrophy.
2. Prostatic carcinoma.
3. Bilateral ureteral stones (or unilateral if the patient has only one functioning kidney).
4. Obstruction of the ureters due to other lower abdominal tumors or fibrosis.
5. Large stones in the renal pelvis causing obstruction.
6. Uncorrected congenital malformations of the lower urinary tract and/or bladder.

1986; Spurney et al. 1991; Myers and Moran 1986; Gornick and Kjillstrand 1983).

Besides trauma, other factors increase patients' risk of developing ARF. The most common of these factors are primary hypertension, diabetes mellitus, and advanced age. Other risk factors include specific treatment for other medical conditions which may have compromised renal function. Examples of these treatments include cisplatin chemotherapy or gold therapy for rheumatoid arthritis. Underlying renal disease also must be considered and assessed on admission or as early as possible in the course of hospitalization. Angiotensin-converting enzyme (ACE) inhibitors may precipitate prerenal changes due to a decrease in glomerular perfusion pressure, although they also may cause intrinsic renal injury. Similarly, nonsteroidal anti-inflammatory agents may cause either prerenal or intrarenal damage. The inhibition of prostaglandins may produce hemodynamic alterations, while allergic reactions cause interstitial damage.

Diabetes mellitus (DM) poses special risk factors for the development of acute renal failure. Type I DM causes systemic microvascular changes which may require assessment and intervention. Cardiac microvessel disease is common, resulting in angina and ischemic damage. For diagnosis, these patients may be subjected to coronary angiography, which requires use of radiocontrast agents that may precipitate acute renal failure. Other contrast studies in the diabetic patient also may cause renal damage. These patients are at great risk of developing acute renal failure during this diagnostic and intervention period; close assessment and management may prevent or minimize this problem (Wish and Moritz 1990).

The patient with diabetes (type I or type II) also may suffer prerenal insult during periods of hypovolemia; a

severely elevated blood glucose with increased diuresis, infections, or vomiting due to any cause can result in changes in renal function.

Patients with long-standing hypertension (known or unknown) may have pre-existing renal microvessel damage, with renal perfusion being further compromised during periods of hypovolemia or hypotension. Careful assessment of fluid status and recognition of signs and symptoms of shock in presumably normotensive patients may help you identify patients with hypertension who currently are hypovolemic or relatively hypotensive and who are therefore at risk of changes from decreased renal perfusion.

Pathophysiology of Acute Renal Failure A variety of morphologic changes can occur throughout the kidney, particularly in the various segments of the nephron, which explain the patient's clinical findings in acute renal failure. Animal models frequently have been used to determine the cellular injury and functional alterations that occur in acute renal failure. The schematic in Figure 15–8 identifies the location of the changes that result in acute renal failure.

Vasoconstriction of Afferent Arteriole The first and most frequent cause of loss of renal function is decreased blood flow into the afferent arteriole, reducing flow through the entire glomerulus and resulting in decreased GFR. The vasoconstriction of the afferent arteriole can reduce effective blood flow into the glomeruli for periods extending to 24–48 hours, resulting in severe attenuation of the entire renal cortical circulation. The resistance created by vasoconstriction of the afferent arteriole decreases glomerular plasma flow, hydraulic pressure in the glomerulus, and glomerular transcapillary ultrafiltration pressure. This vasoconstriction is thought to be mediated by either neurogenic or hormonal stimuli.

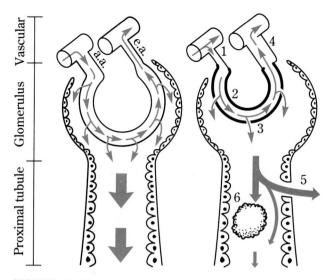

FIGURE 15–8

The nephron in acute renal failure. Left, normally, blood enters the afferent arteriole *(a.a.)* and flows through the glomerular capillary where ultrafiltration occurs *(small curved arrows)*. The filtrate then flows through Bowman's space into the proximal tubule *(large arrows)* for further processing along the nephron. Right, in acute renal failure, there are many potential sites for abnormalities. *(1)* Afferent arteriole vasoconstriction can limit blood flow to the glomerulus. There may be a pathologic decrease in the filtering properties of the glomerulus due to either *(2)* a reduction in capillary surface area or *(3)* a decrease in its intrinsic filtering properties. *(4)* Efferent arteriole *(e.a.)* vasodilatation could result in decreased hydrostatic forces for filtration. *(5)* Necrosis of cells lining the tubule could result in backleak of filtrate into the renal interstitium and systemic circulation, or cell debris may inspissate and *(6)* obstruct the flow of filtrate through the nephron. Some or all of these mechanisms may be important in various forms of acute renal failure. (From Wilkes B, Mailloux L: Acute renal failure: Pathogenesis and prevention. *Am J Med* 1986; 80:1129–1136.)

The renin-angiotensin system has been implicated as the cause of this extended renal vasoconstriction; however, there is also evidence that high levels of circulating angiotensin do not cause acute renal failure. Similarly, it has been hypothesized that norepinephrine mediates this renal vasoconstriction; it has induced such vasoconstriction in experimental models. However, the role of norepinephrine in the development of acute renal failure in humans remains unproven (Cronin 1978).

Glomerular Damage   The structure of the glomerulus also is altered in acute renal failure. Either the actual surface area or the filtering properties of the glomerulus may undergo changes which result in the loss of adequate glomerular filtration. Studies have shown that the glomerular epithelial cell bodies are flattened and the foot processes are widened, resulting in a significant reduction in the functional capillary surface area. Such changes would reduce the ability of the nephron to maintain glomerular filtration (Wilkes and Mailloux 1986). Both these cellular and vascular changes in the glomerulus can affect renal function, reducing glomerular filtration dramatically during this acute insult.

Less frequently, an acute immunologic response can also alter the glomerular capillary cells. Acute glomerulonephritis and systemic lupus erythematosus cause glomerular damage from the antigen-antibody responses of these autoimmune diseases. The suppression of this immune response may limit the damage that occurs during these episodes.

Tubular Damage   The tubular system of the nephron also is damaged both by renal ischemia and by toxic insults. The result is renal tubular cell necrosis. Lesions can occur anywhere in the tubular segment, depending on the nature of the insult. Damage to tubular cells apparently results in two specific types of functional alterations; one is the *backleak* of filtrate through the tubular cell wall and the other is the *obstruction* of the tubular lumen with cellular or pigment debris. Because of the backleak of filtrate, waste products and water are reabsorbed into the circulation. Obstruction creates a back pressure, which results in equalization of pressure with that of Bowman's space. This pressure equilibration prevents glomerular filtration from occurring (Myers and Moran 1986; Wilkes and Mailloux 1986).

Postrenal causes of renal dysfunction damage tubules from retained urine in the bladder, ureters, or collecting system of the kidney. The glomerular damage caused is usually less severe than in other types of acute renal failure. Early relief of obstruction minimizes the damage that could result from this type of acute renal failure.

The processes of injury and changes in both the vascular and tubular portions of the nephron are usually present in all forms of acute renal failure (ischemic prerenal, parenchymal, and postrenal). Specific areas of injury have been found to occur with different clinical conditions, indicating that these processes affect nephron function differently. The resulting loss of renal function creates the clinical conditions of azotemia or uremia (Wish and Moritz 1990; Reusch and Anderson 1990; Gornick and Kjillstrand 1982).

Nonoliguric Acute Renal Failure   Nonoliguric acute renal failure appears to be an attenuated form of ARF created by clinical interventions and the use of "protective agents," which are given to prevent or minimize damage to the renal system (Myers and Moran 1986; Anderson et al. 1977). Studies show that mannitol (one of these protective agents) increases renal blood flow and thus restores the glomerular filtration rate, by maintaining the hydraulic pressure gradient in the glomerulus and tubular structures, as well as decreasing fluid reabsorption in the proximal convoluted tubule. This increased flow of fluid through the tubule washes out the cellular debris that would otherwise cause obstruction of the tubule.

Signs and Symptoms   The signs and symptoms of acute renal failure vary depending on the primary cause of the patient's illness as well as on the severity of the damage to the kidneys. Patients may have minimal alteration in renal function, as determined by slight elevations in serum values of urea nitrogen, creatinine, and other waste products; this state is known as *azotemia*. The azotemic patient experiences no clinical complications and does not feel the effects of the compromised renal function. *Uremia* is the complete loss of renal function, which includes fluid and electrolyte imbalance as well as marked elevations of metabolic waste products.

Urine Volume   Urinary output may vary with both the cause and duration of failure. Oliguria (volume < 400 cc/24 hours) is common and occurs early in the course of failure. Anuria (volume < 100 cc/24 hours) is less common and may indicate the severity of ATN or the presence of total obstruction of the urinary tract (postrenal). Nonoliguric failure (output > 400 cc/24 hours) is increasingly common.

Urine Osmolality and Specific Gravity   If the cause of failure is diminished perfusion, the urine osmolality and specific gravity will be elevated, due to the increased reabsorption of free water during the kidney's response to decreased blood flow and GFR. If tubular damage (ATN) has developed, the nephron's ability to concentrate urine has been lost; urine osmolality will be normal to decreased, and urine specific gravity will be low.

Urinary Sodium Levels   The urinary sodium level usually is decreased in prerenal causes of failure, due to the avid ability of the nephron to reabsorb sodium in response to decreased volume. In ATN, the urinary sodium level is increased because of the tubules' failure to reabsorb sodium.

BUN and Creatinine   The BUN and serum creatinine will be elevated. Their levels will vary based on the severity of renal damage (azotemia to uremia) as well as on the pathophysiology caused by the primary illness or injury. Body size and muscle mass as well as crush injuries or massive bleeding with resorption of protein from red cells will increase BUN and creatinine levels. In addition, catabolic states increase BUN and creatinine generation.

BUN/Creatinine Ratio   In renal hypoperfusion, the BUN may rise more rapidly than the plasma creatinine. In the hypoperfused kidney, urine flows slowly through the tubule, resulting in increased urea reabsorption. Creatinine is not appreciably reabsorbed, thus increasing the ratio above 10:1. In ATN, the ratio remains at approximately 10:1 due to back diffusion of both urea and creatinine through the damaged tubules.

Phases of Acute Renal Failure   Acute oliguric renal failure progresses in three phases: oliguric, diuretic, and recovery. The *oliguric phase* is when urinary output is < 400 cc/24 hours. It usually begins within 48 hours of the insult and lasts for approximately 2 weeks, although it may extend up to 6–12 weeks. Depending on the severity of the failure, dialysis may be required during this period to maintain life.

The *diuretic phase* is when urinary output increases but BUN and creatinine levels remain elevated or even continue to rise. This period, in which tubular regeneration is occurring, lasts approximately 1–2 weeks. Because of rapid increases in urine output, maintaining fluid balance with increased intake is a challenge to nursing care.

The *recovery phase* is characterized by the stabilization and return of laboratory values to normal. This period can last from several months up to a year. During this period, no specific medical intervention is required.

NURSING DIAGNOSES

During the oliguric phase of ATN, the following diagnoses may apply to your patient:

- High risk for fluid volume excess
- High risk for injury
- High risk for infection
- High risk for altered nutrition: less than body requirements
- High risk for fear and anxiety

Planning and Implementation of Care

Nurses caring for the critically ill patient are confronted with multiple concerns about the patient's renal function or loss of function. You will need to determine the patient's current level of renal function, implement measures to prevent or minimize renal dysfunction or failure, provide care to the patient during the course of acute renal failure and minimize or prevent other complications. In collaboration with the physician and other members of the health care team, you will need to direct your care to the prevention or successful treatment of these problems. In addition, your nursing care includes the management of the patient's primary illness or injury, including other complications of his/her primary condition.

Oliguric Phase ATN is often characterized by oliguria, although nonoliguric renal failure appears to be increasingly common. This discussion of nursing care will focus on the oliguric patient but will also make some references to the management of the nonoliguric acute renal failure patient. Nursing diagnoses for oliguric acute renal failure are shown in the nursing care plan nearby.

High Risk for Fluid Volume Excess Related to Fluid Retention The most basic assessment of fluid volume is the accurate daily weight of the patient. Accurate intake and output records will verify any gains or losses. Include estimates of insensible losses from pulmonary, integumentary, or skin losses; these average 500 ml/day. In patients losing large amounts of fluid via the gastrointestinal (GI) tract (from diarrhea or gastric suctioning), these losses will be greater and can be at least partially quantified. Excessive perspiration associated with increased body temperatures (e.g., in septicemia) may also increase fluid loss.

NURSING TIP

Estimating Fluid Gains or Losses

Fluid gains or losses can be easily calculated because 1 Kg of weight corresponds to 1 L of fluid.

Institute fluid restrictions as appropriate to minimize excess fluid volume. As a general guideline, replace urinary output and other measurable losses plus an additional 500 ml for insensible losses. The critically ill patient will rarely receive this volume as oral intake. When appropriate, provide ice chips orally to satisfy thirst; include the volume of ice chips in total fluid intake, quantified by melting chips or cubes dispensed. IV intake, the more frequent route of fluid intake, must include all intake from infusions, line flushes, and antibiotic administration.

If the patient is able to take oral fluids, allocate them over a 24-hour period, with a smaller quantity at night. The patient with diabetes mellitus will experience increased thirst with elevations in blood glucose; assess and control blood sugars via insulin administration to minimize thirst and uncontrolled fluid intake.

NURSING TIP

Gaining Patient Cooperation with Fluid Restrictions

Include the patient in planning for oral intake allocations to diminish both the thirst he or she may be experiencing at various times and the increased anxiety and anger secondary to fluid deprivation. Provide continuing education to the patient about his or her weight and fluid balance to enhance understanding of and cooperation with these restrictions.

Monitor blood pressure carefully to identify the development of hypertension associated with fluid overload. Examine the patient for edema, including signs and symptoms of congestive heart failure and pulmonary edema. For the bedridden patient, tissue edema is more likely to be found as sacral edema rather than as lower leg and ankle edema. Assessment of edema should also include review of the serum albumin level and plasma oncotic pressure (edema is more likely to occur when plasma oncotic pressure is reduced).

Be sure to include on the intake and output record the amount of fluid removed by dialysis treatment. Hemodialysis losses are measured by weight change before and after treatment and recorded on the treatment record. Peritoneal dialysis fluid losses are quantified by measurement of excess fluid in the outflow (effluent) of the dialysis exchange and are recorded on the peritoneal dialysis treatment record.

Acute Renal Failure, Oliguric Phase

Nursing Diagnosis	Signs and Symptoms	Nursing Actions	Desired Outcomes
Fluid volume excess related to fluid retention	Oliguria Elevated CVP Peripheral edema Pulmonary edema Hypertension	1. Monitor and record intake and output. 2. Maintain fluid restriction. 3. Observe for increase in body weight. 4. Observe for peripheral edema, tachycardia, hypertension, elevated CVP, and distended neck veins. 5. Perform dialysis to remove excess fluid as prescribed.	Patient does not exhibit signs of fluid volume overload.
High risk for injury related to electrolyte imbalance	Hyperkalemia Acidemia Dysrhythmias Lethargy Nausea/vomiting Hypocalcemia	1. Restrict potassium intake in food/fluids. 2. Monitor electrolytes, BUN, and creatinine. 3. Monitor ECG for peaked T waves and other dysrhythmias. 4. Administer phosphate binders as prescribed. 5. Monitor for mental status changes. 6. Perform dialysis to correct uremia and electrolyte imbalance.	Patient exhibits electrolyte levels within expected limits.
Altered nutrition: less than body requirements related to dietary restrictions and uremia	Loss of appetite Nausea/vomiting Decreased lean body mass	1. Provide adequate protein, high-calorie diet. 2. Monitor BUN and electrolytes to evaluate response to diet. 3. Offer small, frequent meals. 4. Help patient to maintain good oral hygiene. 5. Administer antiemetics as prescribed. 6. Monitor for hyperglycemia if patient is receiving total parenteral nutrition.	Patient maintains adequate nutritional intake.
High risk for infection	Temperature elevation Purulent sputum/drainage	1. Monitor temperature for elevations. 2. Provide frequent pulmonary care. 3. Assess pulmonary secretions, wound drainage, and urine for indications of infection. 4. Use aseptic technique during dressing changes, insertion of lines, and catheterization. 5. Minimize use of in-dwelling catheters. 6. Perform skin care and oral care on a regular basis.	Patient remains free of infection.

High Risk for Injury Related to Electrolyte Imbalance
Sodium imbalances (hypernatremia or hyponatremia) may result from the administration of fluids and electrolytes during the early period of treatment; they also may reflect the patient's current hydration status. Sodium balance is corrected through management of IV fluids, dialysis, or both.

The most critical electrolyte imbalance that threatens the ARF patient is hyperkalemia. Careful assessment of your patient's risks for developing hyperkalemia may prevent this. Measure serum potassium levels daily (or more frequently). Be aware of these levels as quickly as the results become available. Monitor the electrocardiogram (ECG) for signs of hyperkalemia: tall, peaked T waves, absent P waves, and broadened QRS complexes. Your patient may complain of symptoms of fatigue, shortness of breath, or cramping, although the critically ill patient may not be able to identify the onset of such symptoms. Notify the physician promptly when you identify early ECG changes to allow for rapid treatment and reversal of this complication. Have glucose and regular insulin available for infusion along with calcium chloride and sodium bicarbonate. This IV "cocktail" will return potassium to the intracellular space, preventing further cardiac deterioration. Also administer sodium polystyrene sulfonate (Kayexalate), as ordered, to remove excess potassium through the GI tract; the route of administration will depend on the patient's condition. Oral administration is most effective; administration as a retention enema may be required if your patient is unable to tolerate oral medications. When Kayexalate is given with sorbitol, diarrhea develops, thus maximizing the removal of potassium via the GI tract. (Refer to Chapter 16 for a more complete discussion of potassium imbalances and treatment). Dialysis is also effective for the removal of potassium; a relative hypokalemic state may exist after hemodialysis but requires minimal intervention.

You will observe hypokalemia less frequently in the patient with acute renal failure. It usually results from losses through the GI tract caused by vomiting, nasogastric suction, or protracted diarrhea. If your patient has been receiving diuretic therapy without adequate potassium intake through supplements or diet, he or she may be relatively hypokalemic. If your patient is receiving digitalis therapy, the development of hypokalemia can result in digitalis toxicity.

Acid–base imbalances are usually not life-threatening to the ARF patient and are easily corrected with the IV administration of sodium bicarbonate or dialysis. The most common imbalance is metabolic acidosis, which can exacerbate hyperkalemia (refer to Chapter 16 for more complete discussions of acid–base disturbances).

Your patient may have imbalances in both serum calcium and phosphorus due to acute renal failure. Phosphate binders may be administered if the patient is able to tolerate oral medications. Because of the short-term nature of your patient's ARF, calcium and phosphorus imbalances are not usually critical to your patient's well-being.

High Risk for Altered Nutrition: Less than Body Requirements Related to Dietary Restrictions and Uremia   The patient with acute renal failure may become nutritionally compromised for a number of reasons. Your patient may require a restriction of oral protein intake to prevent increased urea nitrogen formation. Your patient's caloric requirements might be very high due to the primary injury or medical problem and attendant problems of infection, septicemia, or previous poor nutrition. Increased carbohydrate intake will supply adequate nutrition, will spare the production of ketones from fat metabolism, and will prevent gluconeogenesis from body protein utilization. If your patient can tolerate oral intake, his or her appetite may be diminished by the uremic state as well as by the selection of foods and seasonings. Your patient may experience nausea at the sight or aroma of food. Maximize intake by providing good oral hygiene, especially prior to meals, serving food as hot and fresh as possible, and providing small portions. If the family can provide special foods which your patient enjoys and which can be calculated into the dietary prescription, these should be allowed in order to enhance intake.

For critically ill patients who cannot tolerate oral intake, hyperalimentation is the best source of both caloric and essential amino acid intake. The volume of hyperalimentation requires dialytic removal of the excess fluid in the oliguric patient. Refer to Chapter 19 for a more complete discussion of nutrition in the critically ill patient.

High Risk for Infection Related to Decreased Immunologic Function and Increased Exposure to Pathogens
Your patient is at high risk for infection from a variety of sources, including a decreased immunologic response caused by uremia. Sources of infection may include trauma wounds, surgical incisions, and invasive catheters, tubes, or needles. Provide meticulous aseptic care to all of these sites. Minimize the number of invasive catheters and tubes that are placed in your patient. Provide vigorous pulmonary hygiene to prevent your patient from developing pneumonia. Because the patient with renal failure has a blunted temperature response, observe for minimal changes in temperature which may indicate infection.

Maintain excellent skin care via good positioning and turning. Your elderly, cachectic patient may be more susceptible to skin breakdown. Peripheral vascular disease makes the elderly and the patient with diabetes more prone to infections in small distal lesions or ulcers. Your daily assessment of skin and tissue integrity can prevent such infections from developing.

The need for antibiotics puts your patient's renal system at greater risk due to nephrotoxicity. Preventing opportunistic infections in your patient will further protect his or her renal function and its recovery.

High Risk for Fear and Anxiety Related to Seriousness of Illness The critically ill patient who is cognizant of his or her medical condition may have great fear, not only about his or her illness but also specifically about the need for dialysis. Many individuals interpret their need for this acute treatment as an indication it must be continued for the rest of their lives; this is often untrue. However, other patients (because of their underlying medical conditions or illnesses) may need to remain on dialysis on a more chronic basis.

You will need to understand the potential outcome of this episode of renal failure based on your patient's primary conditions and risk factors so that you can provide the patient with accurate and appropriate information about his or her current need for dialysis as well as its possible continuation after recovery from the acute illness. Giving the patient false hope about not needing continued dialysis may be inappropriate, just as giving information that it will need to continue may be misleading.

As noted in an earlier chapter (Chapter 3), the patient may have little awareness of or few concerns about his or her outcome from acute renal failure. You may need to direct nursing care more to family or significant others, who are more aware of the patient's acute renal failure and need for dialysis. Determine what their impressions and experiences with dialysis are prior to answering questions about the use of this treatment both acutely and chronically. It is clear that patients and families whose family members or friends have received dialysis will have very different fears about this treatment than will those who have never had such an experience (Pfettscher 1991).

Pain is an unusual or uncommon feature of the acute renal failure syndrome. The patient may experience pain secondary to placement of vascular access. The complications of pericarditis or pulmonary edema, which may cause pain, should be seen rarely if the patient's acute renal failure is treated appropriately.

Diuretic Phase The diuretic phase is marked by improving renal function. During the diuretic phase and thereafter during hospitalization, assess for the following hallmarks of this phase:

1. Urine volumes increase. Continue to assess the patient's volume status carefully to prevent repeated episodes of hypovolemia. Increase fluid intake to replace losses.

2. BUN and creatinine levels stabilize and then decrease. You may need to have blood values drawn daily to assist in determining whether the patient needs dialysis treatment on that day.

3. Electrolyte balance is maintained by the kidney. You will observe that edema decreases with increased excretion of sodium; potassium levels will be normal, and the patient will not require other methods of potassium removal (such as dialysis or Kayexalate).

4. GFR progressively improves. If the patient's renal function is measured by the performance of creatinine clearances, collect these specimens accurately and carefully.

5. Dialysis treatment is discontinued. Assist in the removal of the temporary access that the patient has had in place for dialysis. After this catheter is removed, observe the site for bleeding, hematoma formation, or any signs of infection.

Outcome Evaluation

Your care of the acute renal failure patient can have a positive impact on his or her outcome, even though morbidity and mortality remain high due to major illnesses and complications. If patients fully recover renal function, they seem to be at no increased risk for future complications from this episode. In patients with underlying renal disease, an episode of ARF may further compromise their renal function. Some patients' renal function may not return to normal, so that they remain azotemic; other patients may not regain enough function to be free of continued dialysis.

The greatest risk for ARF patients, however, is survival of the major illness or trauma that they have sustained. Morbidity and mortality associated with acute renal failure remains high but usually is due to the primary problem or other complications. Patients who develop acute renal failure secondary to surgical complications or trauma have a relatively high mortality rate of 50–60% despite treatment; those cases resulting from medical causes have a mortality rate of approximately 25% (Spurney et al. 1991; Gornick and Kjillstrand 1983). Critical care and hospital stays for

TABLE 15–5

Complications of Chronic Renal Disease by Body Systems (Continued)

ORGAN SYSTEM ASSESSMENT	SELECTED INTERVENTIONS
Fluid and Electrolytes	
Edema	Adequate dialysis
Hypernatremia/hyponatremia	Fluid restriction, removal
Hyperkalemia/hypokalemia	Plasma protein-osmolar pressure
Hypermagnesemia/hypomagnesemia	Adequate dietary intake/restriction
Metabolic acidosis	Treatment of hyperkalemia-IV drugs, Kayexalate
	Avoidance of drugs with Na$^+$, K$^+$
	Avoidance of magnesium gels, magnesium-containing laxatives
Nutrition	
Adequate caloric intake (protein, carbohydrates, fats)	Maintenance/correction of serum albumin level
Vitamin replacement	Prevention of catabolism
Carbohydrate intolerance/insulin sensitivity	Hyperalimentation, diet supplements
Hyperuricemia	Adequate oral intake
Hyperlipidemia	Reduction of insulin dose in diabetics
	Restriction of foods high in uric acid
Skeletal	
Hypocalcemia	Calcium carbonate/acetate binders
Hyperphosphatemia	Phosphate binders (aluminum hydroxide gels) to excrete via gut
Renal osteodystrophy	Administration of Rocaltrol® (active vitamin D)
Metastatic calcification	Prevention of hypercalcemia
Secondary hyperparathyroidism	Subtotal parathyroidectomy
	Administration of Calcijex® (IV vitamin D)
Ocular	
Hypertensive retinopathy	Blood pressure control
Red eye syndrome	Treatment of diabetic retinopathy
Band keratopathy	Calcium/phosphorus balance
	Detection of cataract formation
	Decreased anticoagulation in diabetics to prevent hemorrhage
Dermatologic	
Uremic frost	Adequate dialysis therapy
Pruritus	Moisturizers
Dry skin	Antipruretic medication (Benadryl, etc.)
Pallor	Good skin care
Pigmentation	
Ecchymosis/tissue fragility	
Calcium deposition	*(Continues)*

Your nursing interventions will address the immediate relief of the patient's respiratory and cardiac distress. Use oxygen therapy to increase oxygenation in both congestive heart failure and pulmonary edema. Position the patient in high Fowler's position to improve breathing. Administer blood pressure and cardiac medications, as ordered, to improve cardiac function. Administer antianxiety and/or pain medications, as ordered, to decrease patient anxiety and/or chest pain. In consultation with the physician, initiate

TABLE 15-5

Complications of Chronic Renal Disease by Body Systems (Continued)

ORGAN SYSTEM ASSESSMENT	SELECTED INTERVENTIONS
Peripheral Neuropathy	
Restless leg syndrome	Adequate dialysis treatment
Paresthesias	Exercise as tolerated
Motor weakness	Special foot care, etc., for diabetics, elderly
Paralysis	Nerve conduction studies for assessment
Endocrine	
Hyperparathyroidism	Adequate dialysis treatment
Hypothyroidism	Control of calcium/phosphorus
Amenorrhea/infertility	Sexual counseling/support
Impotence/low sperm count	
Psychologic/Social Environment	
Anxiety/depression	Ongoing support by professional staff
Denial	Psychiatric counseling/drug therapy if indicated
Psychosis	Assessment of family/significant other support
Level of compliance	Assessment of financial status/insurance coverage for illness
Support systems	Continuing education regarding disease, treatment, outcome
Adaptive responses	
Level of understanding	

hemofiltration procedures (discussed later in this chapter) or arrange for hemodialysis to remove the fluid overload to resolve this acute problem.

Before discharge, review the causes of the patient's fluid overload and provide appropriate patient teaching (if the patient is able to comprehend). For the patient with serious cardiac disease or renal failure due to intrinsic disease, avoid chastising the patient for increased fluid intake; instead, search for the source of the problem. For example, the diabetic patient with increased blood sugar levels develops thirst based on hyperosmolality; in this case, direct your teaching to causes of hyperglycemia and its correction rather than only to fluid intake problems.

High Risk for Injury: Electrolyte Imbalance Related to Multiple Causes The ESRD patient may require hospital care for life-threatening hyperkalemia, hyperglycemia or hypo- or hypercalcemia. These complications are reviewed in previous sections as well as in Chapter 16.

Direct your nursing interventions to the administration of drugs, as ordered, which will treat these electrolyte imbalances. As appropriate, make arrangements for dialytic therapy to protect the patient from further complications, such as seizures or cardiac arrest.

Hyperkalemia is usually a result of dietary indiscretion. Explore with the patient the possible sources of potassium in the diet and refer the patient to a dietitian for additional nutritional instruction and management. Assess for other sources of hyperkalemia, including bleeding, sites of infection (tissue breakdown), or use of medications or over-the-counter substances that are high in potassium.

Hyperglycemia in the patient with diabetes may result from dietary indiscretions, nonadministration or incorrect administration of insulin, or errors in blood glucose monitoring. In addition, sudden increases in blood sugar levels may indicate infection or other physiologic stressors. Perform frequent blood glucose monitoring and administration of insulin, as ordered. Assess the patient's insulin regimen and any changes that may have occurred in that regimen (blood glucose testing, changes in insulin preparation or storage, or changes in patient's routine activities). Observe for sites of infection which the patient may be unable to see (e.g., ulcers on the lower extremities). Consultation with the patient's dialysis staff may reveal further information regarding the patient's glucose control.

The patient's responses to your assessment may indicate specific follow-up needed for problems (e.g., lack of performance of blood sugars, broken glucose monitor, or lack of funds to buy testing strips).

Hypo/hypercalcemia may require acute hospitalization for patient observation and treatment. Observe the patient for the appropriate signs and symptoms of both of these conditions and protect the patient from life-threatening complications. Administer medications and fluids, as ordered, to treat these imbalances. Query the patient about dietary intake or the use of drugs or over-the-counter preparations which may have caused or contributed to hypo/hypercalcemia. As a complication of renal failure, hypocalcemia may be treated by the administration of vitamin D preparations to enhance calcium absorption. If the ESRD patient has undergone a parathyroidectomy to control bone disease and its complications, observe the patient frequently for signs of severe hypocalcemia. Twitching, seizures, development of a flap, or obtundation are critical findings requiring immediate intervention. Implementation of standing orders for reporting any changes to the physician and the IV administration of calcium, as ordered, are interventions which can correct these problems.

If acute electrolyte imbalances are treated successfully, the patient is discharged from the hospital without complications. If you have educated the patient about the prevention of these problems, the patient may not need to return to the hospital with similar problems. Establishing communication with the patient's dialysis staff and reporting your observations and findings can assist in long-term resolution or prevention of these complications.

High Risk for Injury: Access Failure Related to Knowledge Deficit The patient may be admitted to the hospital for revision or replacement of vascular or peritoneal access routes. Assess the patency of these routes following surgical implantation (discussed further in the next section). You may be able to determine that patients are performing procedures such as continuous ambulatory peritoneal dialysis incorrectly or caring for hemodialysis accesses in ways that contribute to their failure. Instructing patients regarding these procedures or referral to or consultation with other staff may prevent further access complications.

High Risk for Injury: Cardiac Complications Related to Uremia, Arteriosclerosis, or Hypertension The patient with ESRD is at increased risk of developing cardiac complications. Pericarditis has been associated with the uncontrolled uremic state. Adequate dialysis should resolve this complication and prevent its recurrence. If the patient is hospitalized with pericarditis, direct your care to the dysrhythmias or tamponade which can result. Closely observe the ECG tracings and interpret changes to prevent further insult. Provide symptomatic relief of pain associated with pericarditis, and prevent deterioration of cardiac function with appropriate medications, as ordered. Continued dialysis, often performed on a daily basis, will resolve uremic pericarditis. Your nursing care during this hospitalization is supportive. Attention to fluid volume, electrolyte balance, and nutritional status will enhance the patient's recovery from this complication.

Myocardial infarction (MI) may occur in the ESRD patient secondary to long-term complications of arteriosclerosis, hypertension, or both. Include in your care all of the assessments and interventions required for the MI patient, as described in Chapter 13. In addition, maintain the care required for the ESRD patient, including fluid control, medication administration, electrolyte balance, and continued dialysis.

High Risk for Fluid Volume Deficit Related to Bleeding Bleeding may result from anemia, platelet dysfunction from uremia, and heparin administration during hemodialysis. In your nursing assessment, include all the parameters of hematologic function. Also assess the patient's volume status related to blood loss. If your patient is hypovolemic, administer fluids, volume expanders, or transfusions, as ordered. Include the patient's responses to these interventions with stabilization of his or her volume status.

The patient who has suffered a cerebral hemorrhage will require interventions based on the site and extent of the hemorrhage (refer to Chapter 5 for further information). In addition, maintain blood pressure control via fluid control and drugs to prevent further insult. Direct your care to preventing complications, including pneumonia, contractions, or decubitus formation due to extended bedrest. Your support and education of the patient and family regarding rehabilitation possibilities and resources can provide the patient with hope and a positive attitude regarding recovery.

High Risk for Infection Related to Decreased Immunologic Function Because the ESRD patient has a blunted immunologic response to infections and routinely undergoes invasive procedures of hemodialysis or peritoneal dialysis, he or she is at high risk for infections. Such infections may range from localized infections (usually not requiring hospitalization) to septic events.

Assess access sites for signs of infection routinely. Also evaluate other data such as white blood cell counts and temperature elevations (even though they may be blunted). Early reporting of your findings will assist in verifying infection and initiating treatment.

During episodes of infection, administer appropriate antibiotics, as ordered, perform wound care if necessary, and maintain adequate nutrition for the patient. Conserving patient energy during your care prevents patient fatigue and catabolism. If the patient requires extended bedrest, provide appropriate pulmonary care to prevent pneumonia, skin care and positioning to prevent skin breakdown, and range of motion exercises to prevent muscle contraction.

Outcome Evaluation

ESRD patient outcomes following acute illness are variable. Morbidity and mortality risks for the ESRD patient remain high because of the multifactorial nature of the illness and its complications. Prevention or resolution of complications and maintenance of the patient's quality of life are the goals of the entire health care team. Evaluate the ESRD patient's progress using these desirable outcome criteria:

- Normal blood volume, as evidenced by blood pressure and heart rate within normal limits (WNL), and absence of peripheral edema and neck vein distention.
- Normal respirations.
- P_aO_2 WNL.
- Functional access route for continued dialysis.
- Patient able to state methods to prevent recurrence of complications requiring hospitalization.

Therapeutic Management of Renal Failure

Hemodialysis

Hemodialysis is a process of removing small molecules (end products of metabolism and electrolytes) from the vascular space by diffusion and filtration across a semipermeable membrane. The blood, on one side of the membrane, is referred to as the blood compartment. A fluid (dialysate) compartment on the opposite side of the membrane allows for equilibration of vital electrolytes in a normal concentration in the blood.

This semipermeable membrane also allows for the diffusion of particles into the vascular space from the dialysate to reestablish electrolyte balance. Fluid removal is achieved by creating a pressure gradient across the semipermeable membrane; water moves from an area of higher pressure in the blood compartment to an area of lower (negative) pressure in the dialysate compartment. Thus, the artificial kidney generally mimics the functions of the glomerulus of the healthy kidney.

Critical-care patients requiring hemodialysis are in varying states of illness, which influence their dialysis regimen. Specially trained dialysis nurses perform the actual hemodialysis. Depending on the organization of health care in your community, dialysis nurses may be from an outside agency or from the chronic dialysis facility. Some hospitals, however, provide hemodialysis training for critical-care nursing staff so that treatments will be performed by their own staff.

Because dialysis is readily available in nearly all critical-care units throughout the United States, it usually is initiated relatively early in the course of acute renal failure, thus avoiding the severe and life-threatening complications of uremia. The medical status of patients initiating treatment for ESRD may be so stable that they do not even require hospitalization to begin treatment. However, they may later require hospitalization for conditions related or unrelated to their renal failure and need continued dialysis treatment at that time.

NURSING TIP

Experienced Dialysis Patients

Patients who have been receiving hemodialysis may be very well informed about their treatment, including the procedure of hemodialysis, and they may be very vigilant of the treatment being performed. While patients rarely perform hemodialysis in their homes, many of them do participate in their own dialysis treatment in the outpatient facility. The knowledge and concerns that these patients express should be acknowledged and respected by you and your colleagues in the critical-care unit.

While the critical-care nurse may not be required to learn to perform hemodialysis, the nurse will perform or assist with other care the patient requires. You should understand the procedures involved in this life-supporting treatment so that you can understand and observe your patient for both the positive and negative effects of treatment. In addition, life-threatening complications which are directly related to these procedures may occur during or between the dialysis treatments. To respond appropriately to these complications, you need to understand how these treatments are performed, as the following examples show. You might be confronted by bleeding from a permanent fistula or graft in the chronic renal failure patient. You might observe blood pressure and weight changes in the patient who has just completed dialysis treatment; understanding and being able to interpret the fluid removal accomplished by dialysis allows you to integrate these hemodynamic changes into your patient care plan. You may be confronted by the more serious complication of seizure activity following a hemodialysis treatment; you need to understand that

this complication may be related to fluid shifts into cerebral tissues caused by the rapid removal of urea nitrogen from the vascular space, creating the "dialysis disequilibrium syndrome." This section therefore provides a description of the principles and technical performance aspects of dialysis treatment.

Equipment Required Three technical components are required for the performance of hemodialysis. These are the artificial kidney (the dialyzer), the delivery and monitoring system for the dialysate solution and the treatment parameters, and a vascular access system in the renal failure patient. The artificial kidney and dialysate delivery and monitoring system are contained in the hemodialysis machine, as shown in Figure 15–9.

The Artificial Kidney (Dialyzer) The dialyzer is a disposable unit which most commonly is designed as an enclosed bundle of hollow fibers (Figure 15–10).

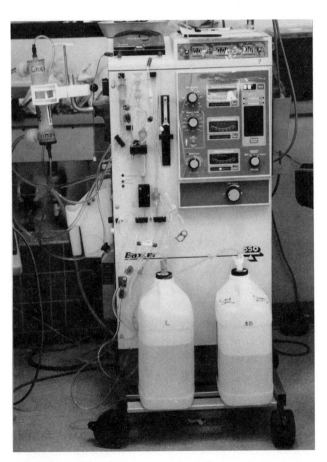

FIGURE 15–9

Hemodialysis machine with dialysate concentrate and artificial kidney in place (ready for use).

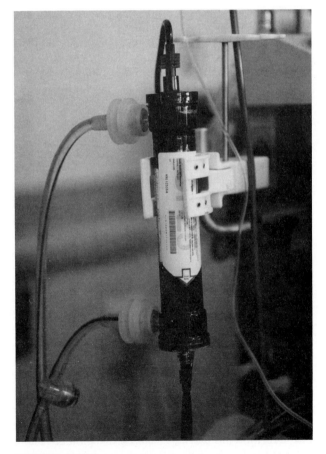

FIGURE 15–10

Hollow fiber dialyzer with blood lines and dialysate lines attached; dialyzer is filled with blood.

These hollow fibers serve as the semipermeable membrane, and the blood inside them constitutes the blood compartment. They usually are made of cellulose acetate, cuprophane, or other types of semipermeable materials. Blood flows into the hollow fibers from attached tubing at the top of the dialyzer and flows out from the bottom to be returned to the patient. Because of their configuration, the pressure within the blood compartment is relatively low. As blood flows from the top to bottom of the dialyzer, water, excess electrolytes, and end products of metabolism move by diffusion, filtration, and pressure gradients from the hollow fibers into the surrounding enclosed space, which is filled with dialysate solution. Depending on their concentrations, electrolytes may also move into the blood compartment from the dialysate. Acetate (a substance converted in the liver to bicarbonate) or bicarbonate diffuses from the dialysate into the blood compartment to correct the patient's metabolic acidosis. Disposable blood lines attached to either end of the dialyzer's blood compartment complete the extracorporeal circuit from the patient to the dialyzer and back to the patient.

In other technical designs of dialyzers, the semipermeable membrane may be designed as a parallel plate with flat bags containing the blood and dialysate flowing between these membranes. While the design may be different, the principles of dialysis remain the same.

The available surface area of the semipermeable membrane and its permeability to water, electrolytes, and waste products determine its efficiency in performing dialysis. The type of dialyzer is prescribed individually for the patient, according to the efficiency of dialysis required. You may observe the efficiency of dialysis by reviewing any changes in blood values that might be measured before and after dialysis.

Artificial kidneys hold blood volumes of 80–150 ml in their blood compartments. The blood lines going to and from each artificial kidney hold volumes of approximately 50 ml. Thus, the total volume of blood in the extracorporeal circuit (lines and dialyzer) during hemodialysis is approximately 200 ml. You will observe minimal hemodynamic changes with this loss of volume into the system. You may observe improvement in the cardiopulmonary function of patients initiating hemodialysis, due to this minor "phlebotomy" being performed. Blood flow through the artificial kidney is dynamic and rapid; a blood pump maintains this flow at 200–300 ml/min. During a dialysis treatment lasting several hours, the patient's total blood volume flows through the artificial kidney multiple times.

In your hypovolemic patient, the normal saline volume used to prime to dialyzer and blood lines can be infused into the patient, thus improving volume status. Fluid replacement or other IV infusions during dialysis (medications, blood or plasma expanders) can be administered through this extracorporeal circuit, thus eliminating the need for additional IV lines. Often, medical orders will specify administration of certain medications only during dialysis; you will need to ensure that these medications (or other infusions such as blood) will be available at the time of dialysis treatment.

Glucose may be added to the dialysate to remove additional fluid by creating an osmotic pressure gradient across the semipermeable membrane (in addition to the negative pressure gradient). Refer to the dialysis orders or confer with the dialysis nurse to determine the presence of glucose in the dialysate.

Potassium is the electrolyte (ion) most frequently altered in dialysate solutions. The concentration can range from 0 mg% to 4 mg% depending on the patient's current blood level of potassium. A relative hypokalemic state may be created by a hemodialysis treatment. If you review serum values between dialysis treatments, you will need to consider the patient's continuing intake of dietary potassium, as well as increased release of potassium from the intracellular space in catabolic patients or in patients who are resorbing red blood cells from bleeding or trauma sites. Because hypokalemia exacerbates digitalis toxicity, the patient who is receiving digitalis preparations will be dialyzed with solutions that have a higher K^+ concentration (4 mg/dl).

Dialysate Delivery and Monitoring Systems

In addition to mixing the dialysate solution that was described above, the dialysis machine also heats this solution and continuously monitors the correct mixture of dialysate by measuring its electrical conductivity. A vacuum pump generates negative pressure in the dialysate compartment to produce the pressure gradient required to remove excess fluid. Dialysate is generally maintained at 37°C; cooler dialysate is not harmful but may cause patient discomfort. However, overheated dialysate hemolyzes red blood cells and can be a life-threatening complication. The fail-safe systems on dialysis machines operate audible and visible alarms and initiate a by-pass flow of dialysate (diverting it from the dialyzer) when this and other harmful conditions occur.

A roller blood pump is integrated into this machine to maintain adequate blood flow through the dialyzer at the ordered rate. The pressure of blood flow through the dialyzer as measured through the arterial and venous blood lines (to and from the dialyzer) assures unobstructed blood flow. Should any change in pressure (decreased flow into the dialyzer or increased resistance to blood return to the patient) occur, audible and visible alarms are activated and blood flow stops. The dialysis nurse will assess and correct the cause of alarms before dialysis is reinitiated. You may need to assist in repositioning the patient to allow adequate blood flow through the access or in calming or restraining the patient as required to allow for maintenance of blood flow.

Because of the blood flow dynamics required for hemodialysis, the presence of air in the extracorporeal circuit is a life-threatening complication. An air embolus could occur easily and quickly in this system. A drip chamber and air leak detector are therefore present in the venous blood line to prevent such a complication. This detector system monitors the blood for increased clarity (air). When air is detected, the venous blood line automatically is clamped, the blood pump is stopped, and visible and audible alarms are activated.

Because all the monitors and alarms are integrated in the dialysis hardware, the hemodialysis procedure halts when an unsafe condition exists. These alarms can be cancelled only when the condition is corrected. You may observe that alarm conditions occur frequently during the dialysis of some patients and less frequently with others, usually due to differences in blood flow and pressure parameters within the system. The dialysis nurse is responsible for the interpretation and correction of these alarm conditions. As these alarms can be very frightening, direct your nursing intervention to reassuring the patient and family regarding these alarms. Also assist the dialysis nurse as required to minimize alarm situations.

The dialysis machine also contains a constant infusion pump for the delivery of heparin to the dialyzer at a set flow rate. Heparin usually is required to maintain anticoagulation in the extracorporeal circuit, depending on the hematologic status of the patient (refer to previous section). The amount of heparin that a patient receives during the dialysis treatment is recorded on the treatment record. The dialysis nurse may need to perform clotting studies at the bedside to adjust the rate of heparin infusion. Be aware of the heparin infusion requirements of the patient and his or her clotting or anticoagulation time at the end of the procedure to assess the patient's risk for bleeding following the hemodialysis treatment. Conferring with the dialysis nurse at the end of treatment will provide you with this information.

Advances in technology have been incorporated into dialysis hardware. Many systems now use computerized programs for monitoring and operation. Some machines also incorporate blood pressure monitoring devices.

Vascular Access for Hemodialysis While progress has been made in the placement of vascular access routes for hemodialysis, problems or complications with vascular access continue. Historically, arteriovenous (A-V) shunts were implanted surgically for the hemodialysis of both acute and chronic renal failure patients. While these external silastic arterial and venous tubes are no longer generally used in the United States, generic use of the term "shunt" continues in reference to any hemodialysis access method. More precise descriptions of vascular accesses are often needed to determine problems or complications. The critical-care nurse should be familiar with the various types of vascular accesses used for hemodialysis, assessment of their function, and assessment of complications which can occur. During the patient's stay in the hospital, you are the primary person who assesses access function and can prevent problems or complications that may occur with the patient's vascular access. This section reviews the various types of vascular accesses used for hemodialysis.

Subclavian Double-Lumen Catheters

Subclavian double-lumen catheters (Figure 15–11) frequently are placed for emergent initiation of hemodialysis in the patient with either acute or chronic renal failure. In addition, they are placed when a chronic renal failure patient experiences complications with a permanent vascular access. These catheters allow for blood to be withdrawn from the shorter outside lumen and returned via the longer internal lumen during hemodialysis. When hemodialysis is not being performed, these lumens are heparin-locked in the usual fashion. They generally are reserved only for hemodialysis use; do not use them for either intravenous fluid or medication administration or for blood specimen withdrawal without the explicit consent of the patient's physician.

Double-lumen catheters can be implanted into the subclavian vein, the femoral vein, or the jugular vein. Placement in the femoral vein prevents patient mobility, as the extremity needs to remain extended to prevent displacement, vascular injury, or kinking of the catheter. You may have to educate the patient about the need for immobility and to reinforce this need frequently. The placement of double-lumen catheters in a subclavian or jugular vein allows for more normal physical activity.

Care and complications associated with these catheters are similar to those required for single-lumen subclavian catheters. Double-lumen catheters are often left in place for several weeks as an access route for hemodialysis; thus, as the patient is discharged from the critical-care unit, you will need to

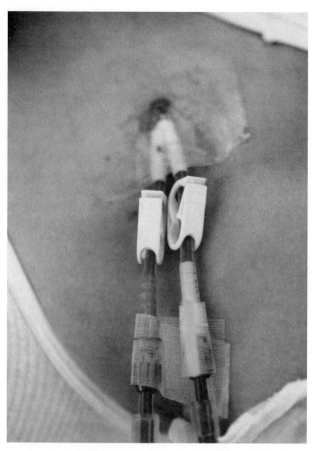

FIGURE 15–11

Subclavian double-lumen catheter in use for hemodialysis.

reinforce proper care to both other nurses and the patient and family.

A permanent surgically implanted double-lumen catheter also can be used as a hemodialysis access route; you should be aware of the presence of such a catheter when the patient is admitted to the critical-care unit. Some patients have had permanent catheters in place for months to years without complications.

Arteriovenous Fistula

The *arteriovenous* (AV) *fistula* (Figure 15–12) is intended to be a permanent access route. A fistula is created by the end-to-end, end-to-side, or side-to-side anastomosis of an artery and a vein. A fistula usually is created in the lower forearm; a single incision is made at the wrist for this anastomosis. Blood flow is directed from the artery directly into the vein (bypassing the capillary bed); the higher flow and pressure entering the venous system creates enlarged veins ("arterialization" of the venous system) above the anastomosis. These larger vessels with increased blood flow allow for the placement of large-gauge (15-gauge) needles

and the removal of blood at a flow rate adequate for the performance of dialysis (i.e., 300 cc). The "arterialization" process takes time to occur; this time is usually referred to as "development" or "maturing" of the fistula.

Care for the newly placed AV fistula following routine procedures for a postoperative incision. Elevate the extremity as necessary to prevent swelling from the operative procedure. Palpate or auscultate the pulse at the anastomosis site (if possible through the surgical dressing) to determine the continued presence of blood flow at the anastomosis. The presence of blood flow is described as a bruit (when auscultated) or a thrill (when palpated); you will hear a turbulence in the vessel as a "whooshing" sound or feel a vibratory, purring sensation. The increased blood flow can also be heard or felt in the venous system above the anastomosis.

When you admit the patient from surgery, inquire about the presence of this "bruit" or "thrill" in the operating and recovery room. Place a semipermanent mark (with a ballpoint pen or skin-marking pen) at the site of the bruit or thrill to make you and your colleagues' continued assessment of the fistula's patency relatively simple. In the immediate postoperative period, assess fistula patency frequently (every 30 minutes, then hourly and then every 2–4 hours). Observe not only for the presence of the bruit or thrill but also for the quality (increasing or decreasing strength or intensity) of the blood flow. Notify the physician when the quality of bruit decreases or when it becomes absent. Absence of a bruit indicates that flow has ceased through the fistula (clotting has occurred at the anastomosis or beyond it). Surgical intervention usually is required; a thrombectomy or revision of the fistula may be performed.

If your patient experiences hypotensive or hypovolemic episodes, assess the fistula's patency as soon as possible; the vascular anastomosis is subject to immediate flow changes when peripheral circulation is compromised. Direct your interventions to the prevention of such hypovolemic episodes.

In the immediate postoperative period, provide appropriate pain medications, as required. In addition to observing the presence of the bruit or thrill in the access, observe the extremity beyond the anastomosis site for continued vascular flow. The distal extremity should remain warm and pink without the presence of ischemic pain. Ask the patient to move the extremity to ensure mobility and integrity (if the fistula is in the forearm, have the patient move the fingers).

If you are caring for the patient after the immediate postoperative period, instruct and encourage the pa-

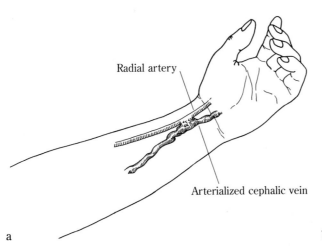

Radial artery

Arterialized cephalic vein

a

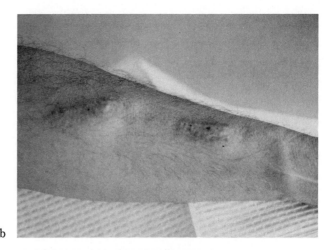

b

FIGURE 15–12

AV fistula. **a.** Schematic of vascular anastamosis, **b.** Photograph showing single incision at anastamosis (right) and typical multiple needle puncture sites.

tient to resume normal use and movement of the extremity to prevent neurologic or muscular damage as well as to enhance development of the fistula. Special exercises (e.g., squeezing a tennis ball) may be ordered or recommended by the physician and/or dialysis nurses to assist in fistula development.

Teach the patient to palpate the thrill as soon as appropriate, emphasizing that this should be performed at least daily or more frequently. If the patient finds palpation difficult, you may instruct him or her to listen to the bruit by placing the anastomosis (in the wrist) to the ear. If the patient has a stethoscope at home or is willing to obtain one, you may teach him or her to auscultate the bruit.

A steal syndrome may develop in a fistula, diverting blood flow from the distal extremity. This syndrome can result in loss of function of the hand or fingers and may require amputation due to the development of tissue necrosis. You may care for the patient in the critical-care setting who has experienced this complication. The loss of hand function can be devastating to the functioning patient. Ischemic and neurologic damage to the hand or fingers is a special risk for the diabetic patient, due to pre-existing disease. You will need to focus on providing supportive care, and referring the patient for psychologic support and functional retraining as needed.

Because the veins of the AV fistula are engorged and enlarged, the patient may perceive them as unsightly and try to hide them from sight. A more serious complication of this enlargement is the development of an aneurysm in the vein. Because the pressure within

the vein is actually arterial, the rupture of an aneurysm may be life-threatening; immediate swelling and pain in the fistula will occur. If this happens, place a tourniquet above the bleeding site as an emergent intervention to prevent hemorrhage. Also immediately notify the patient's physician.

Arteriovenous Grafts

Arteriovenous grafts are created by placing a graft between an artery and a vein, using end-to-side anastomoses (Figure 15–13). Several types of vessels may be used, including the patient's saphenous vein (removed and reimplanted), a bovine graft (the carotid artery of a cow which has been processed and sterilized), or an artificial substance such as expanded polyfluorotetraethylene (Gortex or Impra) which allows for tissue ingrowth into its surface. Other types of vascular grafts are inappropriate because they cannot reseal after needle puncture. AV grafts for hemodialysis can be placed in both the upper and lower portions of the arm as well as in the upper thigh. Rarely, grafts are placed in other areas of the body.

Assessing the patency of a graft is similar to assessing the patency of a fistula. The bruit or thrill may be present throughout the graft; in the immediate postoperative period, it can be felt or heard best at the site of venous anastomosis. If the graft is placed in the forearm, this anastomosis is most frequently just below the antecubital fossa at the incision site. Because grafts are tunneled through the subcutaneous tissue, more swelling and bruising may occur in the postoperative period. Keep the extremity elevated for several days following surgery. Creation of an AV graft is likely to

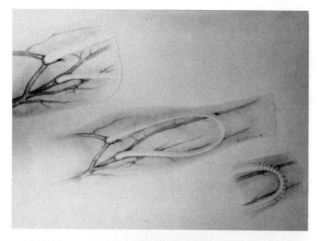

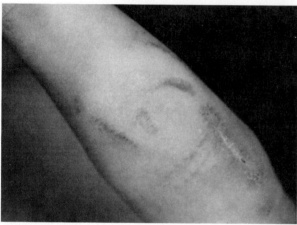

FIGURE 15–13

AV graft. **(top)** Schematic of AV graft implantation showing loop graft in lower arm. **(bottom)** Photograph of AV loop graft. Note previous site inside outer loop. (Top illustration: copyright Frederic Harwin.)

cause more pain than creation of a fistula; administer adequate pain medication to maintain patient comfort.

Complications associated with AV grafts may include clotting due to decreased blood flow, decreased volume, or external obstructions. Grafts also can develop false aneurysms in their surfaces which will need surgical repair. Finally, grafts may become stenotic, usually at their venous anastomosis. Observation of pressures in the extracorporeal circuit during dialysis allows the dialysis nurse to assess these complications.

Clotting in AV grafts often is corrected by balloon angioplasty, which restores blood flow. After any revision of a graft or fistula, assess frequently for patency (presence of bruit or thrill). After initial placement of fistulas or grafts, dressings may be applied which make it difficult to palpate or auscultate

blood flow. You may find that the use of a Doppler stethoscope will allow you to hear the bruit more easily.

Common Aspects of Care for Fistulas and Grafts

When auscultating or palpating to assess patency, also routinely observe for bleeding from the incisional sites and/or from old needle puncture sites in grafts and fistulas. Should bleeding occur, apply direct pressure over the site to control it. Bleeding after dialysis needle removal can be controlled in 5–10 minutes with direct pressure over the site. However, bleeding may be extended if the patient is suffering from other hematologic disorders.

Small dressings (2×2s) or band-aids should be applied for approximately 8 hours to a new needle puncture site. You should then remove the dressing to prevent infections from moisture that may accumulate in the dressing. Never place tape to encircle the arm when applying a dressing to a fistula or graft, because it may act as a tourniquet, restricting blood flow through the access and leading to clotting.

If bleeding occurs at the site of incision or anastomosis or possibly from a ruptured aneurysm, you will need to apply a tourniquet to control it. In this emergent situation, notify the physician immediately. Direct your care toward preventing blood loss and possible exsanguination rather than concern about the patency of the graft.

All vascular access routes are subject to infections, particularly at the needle puncture sites. Because of the high-flow, high-pressure nature of these accesses, the patient can quickly develop septicemia and bacterial endocarditis. Your assessment of the patient's vascular access (easily performed during bathing) should include inspection for areas of redness, swelling, or tenderness. Obtain a culture of any obvious drainage from any area of a fistula or graft.

In the hospital setting, you are the primary person to protect the patient's access from injury or complications: you will be performing the assessments to ensure that it is functioning properly and that it remains patent. Protect the access from blood drawing, blood pressure measuring, or other constrictions from clothing, positioning, bandages, or hospital identification bracelets. If the patient is cognizant and he or she has had the fistula or graft in place for some time, consult him or her about its care and function. Be aware that the patient has been taught to be very protective of the access and will refuse any treatment or care that might compromise its function. If you are caring for a patient who has had a newly placed permanent access, begin patient teaching regarding general observation and palpation or auscultation for patency. Finally, reassure the patient that the access

TABLE 15–6

Comparison of Hemodialysis and Peritoneal Dialysis

	HEMODIALYSIS	PERITONEAL DIALYSIS
Speed	Rapid—up to 8 hours per treatment	Slow—up to 72 hours initially, up to 12 hours per treatment thereafter. Can be advantage in patients who cannot tolerate rapid fluid and electrolyte changes.
Cost	Expensive	Manual—relatively inexpensive; automated—expensive
Equipment	Complex	Manual—simple and readily available; automated—complex
Vascular access	Required	Not necessary, so suitable for patients with vascular problems
Heparinization	Required: systemic or regional	Little or no heparin necessary, so suitable for patients with bleeding problems
Technical nursing skill necessary	High degree	Manual—moderate degree; automated—high degree
Complications (other than fluid and electrolyte imbalances common to all)	Dialysis disequilibrium syndrome (preventable) Mechanical dysfunctions of dialyzer	Peritonitis Protein loss (0.5 g/L of dialysate) Bowel or bladder perforation

will not interfere with his or her lifestyle or normal activities.

Peritoneal Dialysis

Employing the same general principles of osmosis, filtration, and diffusion as hemodialysis does, *peritoneal dialysis* uses the peritoneal membrane as the semipermeable membrane for dialysis. The peritoneum is rich in vasculature, from which end-products of metabolism, excess electrolytes, and water can move. An isotonic solution (dialysate) placed into the peritoneal cavity establishes a gradient for movement of both solutes and water. Peritoneal dialysis uses the principle of osmosis to promote fluid shifts out of the vasculature and into the dialysate solution.

Peritoneal dialysis usually is a continuous treatment. Except for the inflow and drainage periods, the dialysate solution is always present in the peritoneal cavity (this time is known as the dwell time). This procedure can be learned relatively easily by hospital nursing staff, with a minimal amount of special training. Thus, this is a procedure you may be performing in the critical-care unit.

Peritoneal dialysis has been used in acute uremia since the 1930s. Technologic advancements in peritoneal catheters, supplies, and techniques used for performance of the exchanges (draining dialysate out and replacing with new dialysate) make peritoneal dialysis a safe and effective treatment for both acute

and chronic renal failure. Peritoneal dialysis can be used to treat the uremic state of acute renal failure with success similar to that with hemodialysis (Table 15–6). It is especially useful for the patient who may not be able to receive heparin in an extracorporeal circuit due to the risk of hemorrhage. It may not be efficient enough for patients in severe catabolic states, and it may not be possible mechanically for patients with severe scarring or adhesions in the peritoneal cavity due to previous surgeries or infections.

Peritoneal Access Silastic catheters placed at the bedside using a trocar are frequently subject to leaking and infection. The development of permanently implanted silastic catheters has enhanced the long-term success of peritoneal dialysis. These catheters are implanted surgically using a small incision for entry into the peritoneal cavity; the catheter is tunneled through the subcutaneous tissue and exits from the skin at a distance from the peritoneal entry site (Figure 15–14). At the skin exit site, a cuff of Dacron material encircles the catheter; this cuff allows for tissue ingrowth and sealing of the tunnel that is created. The catheter exits from the skin via a snug puncture wound. A second cuff is often present on permanently implanted catheters at the point of exit from the peritoneal cavity. Tissue ingrowth at this site provides an additional barrier to fluid leakage and infection. An alternative method to surgical placement of these catheters uses a scope-type instrument which allows

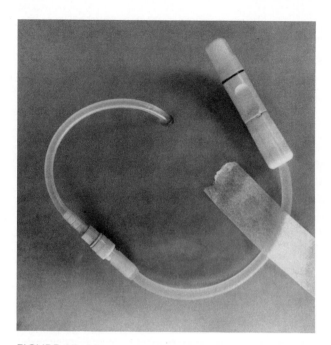

FIGURE 15–14

Peritoneal dialysis catheter with transfer set.

visualization and placement of the catheter through its lumen.

Silastic peritoneal catheters can remain in place for months to years without problems. There are multiple types of peritoneal catheters manufactured, with choice of a specific catheter determined by individual or institutional preference. All catheters have an end hole and multiple side holes to allow for efficient flow of dialysate fluid in and out of the peritoneal cavity.

After healing has occurred, routine care of these catheters includes daily washing in a shower, preferably using liquid soap. The patient should observe the exit site for redness, swelling, or drainage, which indicate an infection. Exit site infections usually are treated aggressively to prevent extension into the peritoneal cavity. The only restricted activity for patients with peritoneal catheters is swimming or soaking in untreated water, such as rivers, lakes, hot tubs, or Jacuzzis. Bandages may or may not be used to cover the exit site per patient preference. The presence of this catheter is often not noticeable to others, as it is covered by clothing.

Methods of Peritoneal Dialysis

Continuous Ambulatory Peritoneal Dialysis Continuous ambulatory peritoneal dialysis (CAPD) is a manual method of peritoneal dialysis which relies on multiple (usually four) daily exchanges of fluid. A prescribed volume of fluid (usually 2,000 ml for an adult) flows by gravity through a tubing set from a plastic bag or bottle. Before fluid is infused, the fluid that has been in the peritoneal cavity is drained by gravity into a plastic collection bag placed on the floor. This procedure is usually performed using aseptic, not sterile, technique. Spiking of the new dialysate solution bag and attachment of the tubing to the extension tubing on the catheter are performed in a way that prevents touching of the internal surfaces or ends of the tubing.

The average time required to complete a total exchange is approximately 30 minutes. Constant surveillance during the drain or fill periods is not required; however, valuable dialysis time should not be lost by allowing for extended drain periods. After the exchange procedure, disconnection of the tubing set, empty bags, and full bags of solution, with capping off of the catheter extension tubing, allows the patient to be quite mobile during the dwell time. CAPD exchanges are generally performed during the day at 4–6 hour intervals; fluid is left in the peritoneum overnight, providing the patient with uninterrupted sleep. More frequent exchanges of fluid increase the efficiency of dialysis for small solutes and fluid. Fluid removal is accomplished by the osmotic gradient that is created from the dextrose concentration of the dialysate solution. Three "strengths" of dextrose are currently available—1.5%, 2.5%, and 4.25%. Multiple individual patient variables influence the amount of fluid removed by each of these concentrations of dextrose. Use these different dextrose solutions in alternating or sequential patterns, as ordered, to remove fluid and maintain normal fluid balance. Determine fluid balance by changes in the patient's weight and blood pressure or the other complications of hypervolemia/hypovolemia discussed previously.

Because peritoneal dialysis is constant, there is no period of accumulation of fluid, end products of metabolism, or excess electrolytes between treatments.

CAPD is a self-care method of ESRD treatment. Patient training and education generally is accomplished on an outpatient basis. As the patient learns the ritual of exchanges, the need for aseptic technique is emphasized. Patients who have no health care knowledge, those who have minimal intelligence levels, and those who are illiterate often have been able to learn this treatment regimen successfully. Because all the supplies required for performance of a CAPD exchange are disposable, this technique of treatment is portable and can be performed in practically any setting. Nurses and patients have developed innovative techniques for performing CAPD while adhering to aseptic principles and practices. When the CAPD patient is hospitalized, he or she may wish and be able to continue performing these treatments. You may need to assist the patient or perform the exchanges if the patient is critically ill, has decreased energy, or seems to need a respite from this task.

Automated Peritoneal Dialysis Automated peritoneal dialysis is performed using equipment which cycles specific volumes of fluid in and out of the peritoneal cavity at set intervals of time. This equipment is computerized; the prescription for an entire treatment can be entered into the system. Flow problems that prevent inflow or outflow will activate audible and visible alarms. Outpatients generally use the cycler to perform multiple overnight exchanges; fluid is left in the peritoneal cavity for the entire day. This method allows the patient to be free of performing exchanges during the day. Cyclers are used in the hospital setting to provide peritoneal dialysis around the clock with a minimum of nursing time and intervention. If cyclers are used in your unit, dialysis staff may initiate or discontinue treatment. You should be trained to monitor this equipment.

The supplies required for the performance of peritoneal dialysis exchanges are not universal. Manufacturers have specific integrated systems for connections which are not interchangeable. Thus, the patient may have to bring his or her own supplies to the hospital to perform exchanges while the hospital is ordering these supplies. Hospitals should stock the supplies used by surrounding outpatient dialysis facilities to minimize this problem. Do not try to force any of the connections by using incompatible supplies because this can lead to contamination and infection.

Nursing Monitoring of Peritoneal Dialysis

High Risk for Fluid Volume Deficit Related to Excessive Fluid Removal Because the osmotic pressure gradient generated by the dextrose present in the dialysate removes excess fluid, you are able to control the fluid status of the patient. Assess the patient's volume status prior to initiating an exchange by evaluating patient weight, blood pressure, and presence of peripheral edema, congestive heart failure, or pulmonary edema.

Record the inflow and outflow volumes and types of solutions used for CAPD exchanges on a separate treatment record. This record will allow you to calculate the volume of fluid removed with this dialysis therapy. The volume of the outflow solution, should be equal to or greater than the inflow volume. The higher concentration of glucose removes more fluid (perhaps as much as 1,000 ml extra). If outflow volume is less than inflow, fluid has been retained. Reassess the patient carefully for signs of volume overload. If the patient is hypovolemic, however, and receiving no other sources of fluid intake, he or she may not be overloaded; the fluid absorbed from the peritoneum can correct the hypovolemia.

High Risk for Fluid Volume Excess Related to Catheter Malfunction Assess the patency of the peritoneal catheter by observing the flow of dialysate into the peritoneal cavity; 2 L of dialysate should flow into the peritoneum within 7–10 minutes. If flow is slower than that, record the time required for complete inflow and report this event to the physician. Inflow can be enhanced by increasing the height of the bag above the body. Normal height for adequate inflow is generally at arm's length above the body. Inflow problems usually are related to catheter displacement in the cavity, the omentum being wrapped around the catheter, or obstruction with fibrin. The catheter may require surgical manipulation or replacement. Attempts to disrupt fibrin formation have been made with the instillation of streptokinase or urokinase into the catheter. You may observe fibrin in the outflow as strands or flecks of white material; heparin is added to subsequent dialysate solution bags to prevent its formation.

Outflow should also be assessed by noting the time required for, and the briskness of, the flow. The outflow should begin immediately as a steady stream when the system is opened; it will slow to a drip at the end of the

---

NURSING DIAGNOSIS

Nursing diagnoses pertinent to the peritoneal dialysis patient include:

- high risks for fluid volume deficit
- fluid volume excess
- pain
- injury (hyperglycemia)
- impaired gas exchange
- altered nutrition
- infection

Your observations and interventions can prevent or provide successful resolutions to these complications.

outflow period (usually 20 minutes). The most frequent cause of outflow problems is constipation, which results in additional pressure against or occlusion of the catheter by the distended bowel. By assessing and maintaining the patient's normal bowel function through the use of medications or enemas if necessary, you can avoid or correct outflow problems. If outflow is reduced or absent, notify the physician.

High Risk for Pain Related to Peritoneal Distention or Infection Your patient may complain of pain at the initiation of peritoneal dialysis, due to the pressure generated by the increased volume of fluid within the peritoneal cavity. Distention or bloating discomfort is generally short-lived as the cavity adapts to this volume. Increased distention may occur at the end of the dwell time due to large volumes of fluid shifting into the cavity for removal. You may wish to give pain medication to relieve this discomfort at the beginning of the dialysis treatment. Also advise the patient that this discomfort will resolve.

NURSING TIP

Using Patient Twinges as a Time Clock

At the end of the dwell time, fluid distention and fluid shifts within the peritoneal cavity may cause sensations of discomfort. Patients accustomed to peritoneal dialysis may use these sensations, or "twinges," as a time clock for the drain segment of an exchange. Asking the patient to let you know when these twinges occur may individualize dwell time as well as convey respect for the patient.

Pain related to an episode of peritonitis (see below) has a sudden onset and is usually severe. Your patient may also exhibit rebound tenderness as well as generalized abdominal pain. Patients may be hospitalized with peritonitis and such severe pain that they are unable to continue their own treatment. Medicate them appropriately for relief of pain and assume responsibility for the performance of their dialysis exchanges.

High Risk for Injury (Hyperglycemia) Related to Absorption of Dextrose from the Dialysate You may need to perform glucose monitoring to verify that your patient's blood sugar is within normal limits. Assess and monitor the diabetic patient's blood sugar more carefully when he or she is undergoing peritoneal dialysis. You may be injecting regular insulin into the dialysate solution bag so that the patient can absorb it from the peritoneum. You will need to perform a blood glucose measurement to establish the insulin dose required. Nondiabetic patients also may absorb dextrose from the peritoneal cavity; while their blood sugars remain normal, they may gain unwanted weight secondary to its absorption.

High Risk for Impaired Gas Exchange Related to Increased Pressure of Fluid Within the Peritoneal Cavity Your care may include maintaining the patient in a Fowler's position and providing oxygen therapy to resolve the acute symptoms of dyspnea or atelectasis. Further assessment and intervention may be required for long-term resolution of this problem. You may also observe a decrease in these symptoms as the patient adapts to the volume of dialysate.

High Risk for Altered Nutrition: Less than Body Requirements Related to Protein Loss Assess the presence of a nutritional problem by reviewing the patient's serum albumin level, which reflects long-term protein intake. While the patient is in the hospital, encourage increased oral intake of protein. If the patient is unable to eat, administer total parenteral nutrition, as ordered, to enhance protein intake. If your patient is protein depleted, protect the patient from sources of infection which can be more severe or even life-threatening. Refer to Chapter 19 for further discussion of nutritional support.

High Risk for Infection Related to Contamination The peritoneal dialysis patient is at increased risk of developing peritonitis due to contamination of the cavity through multiple fluid exchanges. Use of aseptic procedures, employing good handwashing and masking during exchanges, minimizes the risk of peritonitis. If the catheter extension or other parts of the exchange system become contaminated, replace as ordered. Notify the physician of the contamination and initiate antibiotic therapy, as ordered.

Observe for cloudiness of the outflow, abdominal pain, and fever, which indicate peritonitis. Save the cloudy effluent and send it to the clinical laboratory for culture and sensitivity testing.

Exit site infections also may occur. Assess the exit site daily for signs of redness, swelling, and drainage. If drainage is present, obtain a culture for laboratory analysis. Do not apply ointments or other medications to the exit site if they are not specifically ordered. Finally, infections can occur in the tunnel through which the catheter is placed from the peritoneum to the skin. Report to the physician immediately any redness, pain or tenderness, and swelling beyond the exit site and along the catheter tunnel. Your early assessment of peritonitis and administration of antibiotics via the peritoneal dialysate solution and oral or IV routes can successfully resolve such infections without loss of effective dialysis.

Other more rare complications occur in patients undergoing peritoneal dialysis. Your general patient assessment may identify any of these other complications or problems.

Peritoneal dialysis is an effective method of treatment for both acute and chronic renal failure. Patients can perform peritoneal dialysis with minimal or no complications for years to sustain an acceptable quality of life. With better technology and decreased incidence of peritonitis and other complications, its use is increasing in the United States. When these patients require hospitalization, you may be able to continue their treatment of choice by performing their peritoneal dialysis exchanges. Patients and their families may be vigilant about the performance of this procedure by the staff because of their familiarity with and diligence in performing it at home. Your willingness to consult the patient and other staff, as needed, to maintain your skills in performing peritoneal dialysis, can ensure that your patient receives excellent nursing care during his or her hospitalization.

Continuous Ultrafiltration (Hemofiltration)

Continuous ultrafiltration is an extracorporeal treatment in which plasma water and nonprotein-bound solutes are removed from the blood primarily via the principle of convection. Indications for the use of continuous ultrafiltration include fluid overload in patients with acute or chronic renal failure, heart failure in patients who are diuretic-resistant or who become oliguric (develop acute renal failure), or chronic fluid overload without presence of renal failure (such as in ascites or nephrotic edema). The primary use of continuous ultrafiltration is in the fluid-overloaded, hemodynamically unstable patient in whom standard hemodialysis may cause further instability and hypotension, which prevents adequate fluid removal. The oliguric patient requiring large amounts of intravenous fluids may have extra fluid removed while electrolyte balance is maintained. Solute removal in acute or chronic renal failure can also be managed by continuous ultrafiltration. Removal of urea and creatinine may be inadequate, however, if a hypercat-

abolic state in the patient with acute or chronic renal failure generates these molecules. Finally, acid–base imbalance and/or specific electrolyte disturbances can be effectively treated with continuous ultrafiltration (Bosch and Ronco 1989).

This technology utilizes a specially developed extracorporeal filter, which is highly permeable to water and small to medium-sized molecules (Figure 15–15). The filter holds a small volume of blood and has a low resistance to blood flow through it. The ultrafiltrate produced in this treatment is a protein-free fluid whose electrolyte concentration is similar to that of plasma. Large amounts of water are also filtered due to pressure gradients maintained across the membrane. Access to blood flow is required both for flow to the filter and return of blood from the extracorporeal circuit. Specific methods of continuous ultrafiltration may require specific equipment and will be described in the following sections.

Continuous ultrafiltration employs the principle of a pressure gradient across a highly permeable membrane. The patient's arterial pressure usually maintains blood flow through the filter. This pressure generates

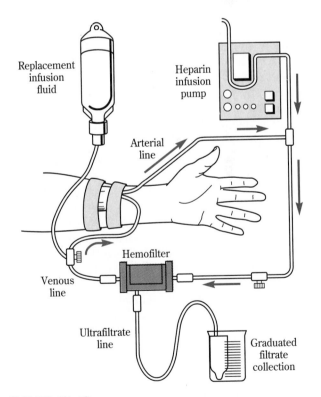

FIGURE 15–15

AV hemofiltration. (From Whittaker A et al.: Preventing complications in continuous arteriovenous hemofiltration. *Dimen Crit Care Nurs* 1986; 5:74.)

a hydraulic pressure in the filter; an opposing hydrostatic pressure, present on the outside of the membrane where the ultrafiltrate collects, is generated by the weight of the fluid column in the ultrafiltrate line. Finally, oncotic pressure, generated by plasma proteins, affects fluid removal via this membrane. A transmembrane pressure (the net pressure difference across the membrane) can be mathematically calculated (Bosch and Ronco 1989). This pressure gradient and the permeability of the membrane to water allows for the removal of as much as 10–15 L of water in a 24-hour period. Variations in pressure in the filter and height of the filter and ultrafiltrate bag will directly affect the transmembrane pressure across the filter and thus the amount of fluid removed.

Continuous Ultrafiltration Systems

As noted above, several variations of ultrafiltration are in use. These are described in the following paragraphs.

Continuous Arteriovenous Hemofiltration (CAVH) Continuous arteriovenous hemofiltration (CAVH) is the most commonly employed method of constant ultrafiltration. Large volumes of fluid can be removed during this treatment, along with large amounts of solutes and medium-sized waste products. Blood flows through the filter using the patient's mean arterial pressure and is returned into a vein. The filter should be placed at the level of the patient's right atrium to maximize outflow and minimize resistance to blood return. The ultrafiltration pressure gradient is established and maintained by the distance of the outflow chamber below the filter; increasing the distance between the filter and outflow chamber increases fluid removal, while decreasing the distance (raising the outflow bag) decreases the pressure gradient and fluid removal. Clamps placed at various places in the system also alter the pressure gradient and ultrafiltration achieved. Pumps may be employed in the system (e.g., ultrafiltrate line or collection chamber) to alter fluid removal. For the patient with fluid overload, electrolyte imbalance, and/or decreased renal function, this treatment may be adequate to control the azotemic or uremic state as well as the state of hydration. Because CAVH removes large amounts of fluid in short periods of time, fluid replacement via the extracorporeal circuit (into the venous line) may be necessary (Bosch and Ronco 1989). If only solute removal is necessary, all of the removed fluid can be replaced. In some patients, the administration of fluids (including hyperalimentation and crystalloids to treat the patient's primary condition or other complications) may provide adequate fluid replacement and eliminate the need for fluid

substitution via the extracorporeal circuit (Ludlow 1992).

Slow Continuous Ultrafiltration (SCUF) Slow continuous ultrafiltration is used to remove water rather than a solute load. The formation of ultrafiltrate is determined by changing the pressure gradient in the filter, which can be accomplished easily by increasing the height of the ultrafiltrate collection system or decreasing the blood flow through the filter. In addition, clamping the ultrafiltrate line can also alter the amount of fluid removed. Because smaller volumes of fluid are removed (150–300 ml/hour), this system can maintain or correct fluid balance in patients between hemodialysis treatments or in those who require less fluid removal.

Continuous Venous-Venous Hemofiltration (CVVH) The principles of hemofiltration remain unchanged in CVVH and the procedure utilizes the same membrane. Fluid and solute removal is similar to that obtained with CAVH, but arterial access is eliminated. A blood pump on the outflow line maintains blood flow through the filter.

Continuous Arteriovenous Hemofiltration Dialysis (CAVHD) Continuous arteriovenous hemofiltration dialysis (CAVHD) allows for the removal of large volumes of fluid and solutes using the same or a similar highly permeable filter. In addition, the use of dialysate in the fluid (ultrafiltrate) compartment allows for the diffusive transport of larger molecules at more efficient rates. CAVHD is indicated for the oliguric, fluid overloaded patient who is hypermetabolic and/or hypercatabolic and thus generating large amounts of urea and creatinine. CAVHD is usually indicated for the patient whose protein catabolic rate is greater than 1.5 g/kg per day (Sigler and Teehan 1990). While this patient usually would require hemodialysis to remove urea and creatinine, this procedure may be used in the hemodynamically unstable patient who may not tolerate the rapid fluid removal of dialysis. Fluid volume is maintained as for CAVH; fluid may be added to the extracorporeal circuit or replaced via other intravenous infusions. The dialysate flows in and out of the ultrafiltrate compartment of the filter. This dialysate must be sterile (due to the high permeability of the membrane) and should be solute-compatible with blood. The most frequently used solution is peritoneal dialysis fluid (refer to the earlier section on peritoneal dialysis). The dextrose concentration is usually 1.5%; dialysate flow is maintained at approximately 1 L per hour with the use of a constant infusion pump. Blood flow can be maintained via mean arterial pressure or by the use of a blood pump in a venous flow system.

Unlike in hemodialysis, the hemofilter membrane's high permeability allows for the removal of drugs in a manner similar to that of the human kidney. Thus, administration of drugs should be done in the usual fashion.

Vascular Access for Continuous Ultrafiltration Treatments This treatment requires access to the vascular system. Arteriovenous systems require catheterization of both an artery and a vein, usually central rather than peripheral vessels to ensure adequate blood flow with minimal resistance. Large-gauge catheters usually are placed in a femoral artery and vein. If the patient has a vascular access (graft or fistula) for chronic hemodialysis, arterial flow can be achieved from that vessel; however, return of blood flow should be performed through another peripheral vein (not the vascular access) to decrease venous resistance (Sigler and Teehan 1990). There have been reports of the surgical placement of AV shunts (silastic external tubes originally used for hemodialysis). These are placed peripherally, usually in the lower arm. Because external AV shunts are used infrequently today, consult older texts or references for further descriptions of their care. They do require special equipment for use which should be available in your hospital if they are to be used as access routes for this treatment.

Your nursing assessment and care of other vascular access routes for continuous ultrafiltration is the same as has been described earlier in this chapter. In particular, observe for redness or drainage associated with infection; obtain a swab culture of any drainage. Protect the catheter from displacement or kinking due to misalignment, while maintaining appropriate function of the extremity.

Anticoagulation and Continuous Ultrafiltration Because this treatment is performed in an extracorporeal circuit, blood can clot at any point in the system. Depending on the individual patient's medical condition, heparin anticoagulation is often required. Heparin can be infused into this system by the use of a constant infusion pump attached to the infusion line in the arterial tubing. Patient requirements for anticoagulation are determined by the patient's clotting parameters prior to treatment. The patient usually will receive approximately 2,000 units of heparin immediately prior to the initiation of treatment. Monitor adequate anticoagulation by performing whole blood partial thromboplastin times (PTTs) or activated clotting times (ACTs); these studies usually are not sent to the laboratory but instead are performed at the bedside by the nursing staff. Heparin infusion rates can be changed immediately based on the results. The physician's orders for treatment should include appropriate parameters for anticoagulation.

If clotting occurs in the extracorporeal circuit, the entire system must be replaced. In addition to abnormal clotting times, you may detect clotting by a decrease in the volume of ultrafiltrate formed in a given period of time.

Your patient is at increased risk of bleeding with this systemic anticoagulation, so you will need to assess the patient frequently for any signs or symptoms of acute bleeding. In addition, blood loss may occur across the filter membrane if it tears or ruptures. Observe the ultrafiltrate for the presence of blood.

Nursing Procedures for Continuous Ultrafiltration Critical-care units have adopted various procedures for continuous ultrafiltration. Some facilities may determine that the critical-care nurse has full responsibility for this treatment, including its initiation, monitoring, and discontinuation. Other units have utilized the resources of specialized staff, usually from the dialysis program, to initiate and discontinue treatment even if they are not continually present for monitoring. Because it is continuous, the critical-care nurse has some responsibility for this treatment and for the patient receiving it. While CAVH and its variations are often described as simpler than hemodialysis treatment, they are more labor intensive. A 1:1 staff/patient ratio is necessary due to the nursing interventions required. This treatment may be maintained for a relatively short period of time (less than 24 hours for simple fluid overload or electrolyte imbalances) or can continue for as long as a week without interruption.

The critical-care nurse should receive special instruction and skills training in the performance of continuous ultrafiltration. Review your own facility's procedures as needed. Maintain aseptic technique and universal guidelines for infection control during all aspects of this procedure.

Nursing Care During Continuous Ultrafiltration

High Risk for Fluid Volume Deficit Related to Filter Permeability The highly permeable filter used for ultrafiltration can remove massive amounts of fluid in a relatively short time. Monitor the patient's blood pressure and/or other volume parameters hourly or more frequently as indicated. Maintain blood pressure with intravenous fluid replacement and/or vasopressors. Measure ultrafiltrate volume hourly and replace,

NURSING DIAGNOSIS

Nursing diagnoses for the patient undergoing continuous ultrafiltration are:

- high risk for fluid volume deficit
- high risk for injury (bleeding)
- and high risk for fluid volume overload (inadequate treatment)

as ordered, with infusion fluid (via IV sites or into the hemofilter's venous line). Calculate total intake and output hourly to assess fluid balance. Assess and record other signs of improved fluid balance (improved respiratory function, lung sounds, and peripheral edema). Adjust the system as required for excessive fluid loss by increasing or decreasing the height of the collection bag, applying clamps, or adjusting pumps.

Obtain blood samples for chemistry studies, as ordered, and review results emergently. Adjust electrolyte intake via replacement fluids, as ordered.

High Risk for Injury: Bleeding Related to Heparinization and Other Factors Your careful monitoring of clotting parameters and accurate administration of heparin may prevent the complication of bleeding. However, your patient may be at greater risk of bleeding due to his or her primary illness or injury as well as other complications, such as disseminated intravascular coagulation. Frank hemorrhage from any site will result in signs and symptoms of hypotension and hypovolemia and should always be considered when assessing the patient's hemodynamic status. In addition, dislodgement of the arterial catheter may result in hemorrhage into the surrounding tissue and/or externally. Assess the catheter sites frequently and/or leave them exposed for continual observation.

High Risk for Fluid Volume Overload Related to Clotting Clotting in the blood lines or the filter decreases the surface area available for ultrafiltration and solute removal. Closely observe the system hourly for evidence of clotting, including darkening or separation of the blood in the filter, lines, or both. Prevent kinking or compression of the tubing to prevent decreased flow through the system and subsequent clotting. Observe for decreased ultrafiltrate formation without significant changes in the patient's volume status, which also indicates clotting. Because the volume of blood in this

extracorporeal circuit is quite small, the patient will likely not exhibit symptoms of significant blood loss. Repeated episodes of clotting will, however, produce loss of red cell mass and plasma proteins, which will require replacement via transfusion. Inadequate hemofiltration lengthens the period of fluid overload and electrolyte imbalance for your patient and can result in systemic complications described elsewhere in this text. If these occur due to clotting, your patient's stay in the critical-care unit may need to be extended. Your prevention of clotting by maintenance of appropriate anticoagulation ensures treatment success. If clotting occurs, your timely assessment and intervention of changing the hemofilter will ensure continued effective treatment.

Outcome Evaluation Outcome parameters should reflect the specific type of continuous ultrafiltration utilized. Correction of fluid overload can be assessed by:

- Patient weight WNL.
- Absence of peripheral edema.
- Blood pressure and other vascular volume measurements (CVP, etc.) WNL.
- Lungs clear and respiratory rate WNL.
- Skin warm and dry with normal turgor; moist mucous membranes.
- Serum osmolality WNL.

Electrolyte and acid–base balance can be assessed by:

- Serum electrolytes WNL for patient.
- Acid–base balance WNL as evidenced by normal CO_2 and blood pH.
- Patient has no signs or symptoms of electrolyte imbalance, e.g., absence of dysrhythmias, tetany, or altered level of consciousness.

Removal of waste products can be assessed by:

- BUN and creatinine WNL (or maintained in a steady state).
- Improving renal function in the oliguric patient, as evidenced by increased urine output, excretion of waste products and electrolytes, urine osmolality WNL, or improving signs or symptoms of uremia.

Methods of continuous ultrafiltration are increasingly employed in treating fluid and electrolyte imbalances in the hemodynamically unstable critical-care patient. When used with dialysate, continuous ultrafiltration also provides an alternative treatment to hemodialysis or peritoneal dialysis. The critical-care nurse needs to make expertise in this technology a part of his or her patient care activities.

Renal Transplantation

Renal transplantation is a treatment modality reserved for patients with ESRD. The critical-care nurse's role in renal transplantation varies according to the organization of patient care in acute care hospitals. Routine postoperative care of the transplant recipient may be provided in the critical-care unit, or the patient may be admitted to the critical-care unit only for management of complications.

In a more indirect fashion, the critical-care nurse's involvement with cadaver organ donation provides care for the renal transplant patient. It is often helpful for nurses to understand the end result of their care of organ donors.

All adult patients undergoing renal transplantation should have been educated fully about this treatment modality for their ESRD. The risks of the surgical procedure, risk of graft rejection, and the specific immunosuppressive regimen used by the transplant facility should be explained completely to the patient. The patient also should understand the potential side-effects and complications of the immunosuppressive drug regimen prior to receiving a kidney transplant.

Donor Sources   A functioning kidney may be obtained from either a cadaveric organ donor or a live donor. Usually, a live donor is a close genetic relative such as a sibling, parent, or adult child. Some renal transplant programs do use kidneys donated by a more distant relative or even a genetically unrelated individual who has a close emotional relationship with the recipient (e.g., spouse or close friend). The varying ethical issues and potential dilemmas created by these arrangements may or may not outweigh the benefit to both the donor and recipient. Organ donors routinely have reported that they derive much psychologic benefit from serving as donors (Simmons et al. 1987).

Cadaveric organ donors are individuals who have suffered total and irreversible cessation of brain function and whose cardiopulmonary functions and other organ viability are maintained by artificial interventions (ventilators, IVs, etc.). The vital organs and tissues donated by the patient or by the legal surrogate are removed during a sterile autopsy in the operating room setting and transported to the appropriate transplant facility. Each cadaveric organ donor provides two individuals with a renal transplant. An example in Chapter 3 briefly reviews the various aspects of the organ donation process. The staff of every hospital should have a local resource agency to provide ongoing education and assistance in the organ donation process.

It is currently against United States federal law for financial remuneration to be given to families of donors for cadaveric organ donation; organs and/or tissues may not be bought or sold. The disparity in numbers between cadaveric donors and organ recipients (too many potential recipients or too few donors) is a continuing problem in renal transplantation both in the United States and throughout the world.

Immunologic Compatibility of Donor and Recipient   Special immunologic testing between donor and recipient compatibility can minimize the possibility of immunologic destruction (rejection) of the transplanted kidney. This section briefly discusses immunology as it relates to renal transplantation. For further information on immunology, please refer to Chapter 18.

Human leukocyte antigens (HLA) are present on cell surfaces as identifiers of genetic identity. These antigens are inherited from our biologic parents, with half of the identifiable antigens coming from each parent. Thus, siblings have a one-in-four chance of receiving the same combination of HLA antigens. Children are always half-like their parents (unless their parents share genetic identity). Identical twins share the exact genetic identity (arising from the same ovum and sperm) and are thus considered immunologically privileged; renal transplants between identical twins have theoretically no possibility of immunologic rejection. HLA antigens can be identified from peripheral blood cells; after testing is completed, it should not need to be repeated—our genetic identity is not routinely subject to alterations. HLA compatibility of donor and recipient minimizes the recognition of the transplanted kidney as foreign tissue and thus decreases the possibility of transplant rejection.

Antibody typing and cross-matching also is performed prior to transplantation. Antibodies are directed against specific HLA types; because their presence at the time of transplantation would cause immediate graft rejection, antibody screening is performed at regular intervals for potential transplant recipients. These antibodies often are referred to as cytotoxic antibodies. Patients who have many antibodies (increased sensitization) may have difficulty receiving a transplant. Presence or absence of antibodies against a specific kidney donor (live or cadaveric) can be identified by performing cross-match testing between cells and sera (similar to blood transfusion cross-match testing). If the cross-match is negative, indicating absence of recipient antibodies directed against the donor, graft rejection is less likely. Antibodies against other identities may have been formed in response to blood transfusions, pregnancy, or prior transplants.

Final testing of potential donor and recipient thus includes both typing and cross-matching. The donor and recipient should share genetic HLA identity and have a negative cross-match prior to renal transplantation. If the donor and recipient are HLA identical, graft rejection is very unlikely; graft survival is reported as greater than 90% at 2 years after transplantation in this group.

Multiple manipulations of immune responsiveness between donor and recipient have been attempted by various transplant programs. These special protocols are employed either to better identify the possibility of immunologic response after transplantation or to alter the immune response to a specific genetic identity prior to transplantation. If you work in a hospital which performs transplants, you may wish to learn what procedures are used for transplant testing, donor selection, and recipient preparation.

Renal Transplant Surgical Technique A single kidney is implanted in the iliac fossa of the adult-size patient (Figure 15–16). The native kidneys rarely are surgically removed. The placement of the transplanted

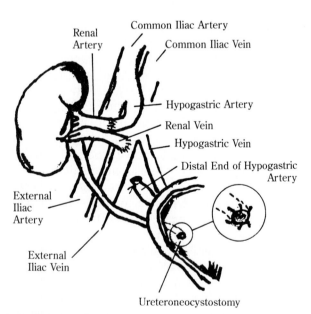

FIGURE 15–16

Schematic of a kidney transplant. (From Chatterjee S, *Manual of Renal Transplantation*, New York: Springer Verlag, 1979.)

kidney in this space allows for vascular anastomosis of the renal artery to the hypogastric artery; the renal vein is anastomosed to the iliac vein. The ureter of the donor kidney is implanted into the bladder using a ureteroneocystostomy technique. This extra-abdominal surgical technique provides for direct palpation of the kidney and allows for rapid recovery from the surgery. If removal of the transplanted kidney is necessary, the surgical procedure and patient recovery are similar.

The transplanted kidney can be visualized by various diagnostic studies. Blood flow to and from the kidney and excretory functions are most often measured through radionuclide scanning.

NURSING DIAGNOSIS

Nursing diagnoses for the renal transplant patient include:

- high risk for fluid volume deficit or excess
- pain
- high risk for infection
- high risk for altered urinary elimination

Nursing Care Following Renal Transplantation

High Risk for Fluid Volume Deficit or Excess Related to Function of New Kidney In the immediate postoperative period, the nurse caring for the renal transplant patient should frequently observe the patient's fluid balance. If the kidney functions immediately following transplantation, massive diuresis can occur, resulting in a dehydrated, hypovolemic patient. If the kidney does not function immediately, the patient is at risk of fluid overload resulting in cardiopulmonary complications.

Your careful measurements of the patient's intake and output after the return from surgery assist in assessment of fluid balance. Verify that the urethral catheter is patent and measure urine output via the urethral catheter hourly. Your interventions to maintain catheter patency will prevent increased pressure in the bladder which may disrupt the ureteral-bladder anastomosis (the ureteroneocystostomy).

Electrolyte imbalances may occur due to diuresis or fluid retention. Assess and observe the patient for sudden changes, particularly in sodium and potassium levels. Care of the diabetic patient receiving a renal transplant requires careful and frequent assessment of blood glucose levels as well as administration of insulin through either intravenous drips or subcutaneous injections.

Pain Related to Surgical Incision The patient who has undergone this surgery experiences pain. Administer medication, as ordered, for pain control. Your relief of pain will allow the patient to ambulate and to focus on learning about his or her continued care of the transplanted kidney. The patient may also experience pain during a rejection episode, due to swelling of the kidney. You will need to relieve this pain and address any anxiety about rejection that may accompany it.

High Risk for Infection Related to Immunosuppression Infection is a major risk to the immunosuppressed renal transplant patient. Use all precautions for prevention of infection described in this chapter and elsewhere. Assess catheters, IV lines, and wounds for possible infection. Because fever may be blunted due to corticosteroid use and/or continued renal failure, be aware of and report any alterations in temperature. Review white blood cell counts and use special precautions if the patient develops leukopenia. Reinforce health and hygiene practices that decrease the risk of infection, as needed.

High Risk for Altered Urinary Elimination Related to Graft Rejection The major risk following renal transplantation is loss of the graft due to an uncontrollable immunologic rejection response. Administer immunosuppressive medications, as ordered, both to prevent rejection and to treat a rejection episode. Multiple drugs in various combinations are currently used to suppress rejection responses. Observe the patient for the signs and symptoms of a rejection response, which may include pain over the kidney, decreased urine output, fluid retention with edema formation, elevated blood pressure, and elevated serum levels of urea nitrogen and creatinine. Assist in scheduling other studies, as ordered, such as a renal scan or a kidney biopsy. Provide emotional support to the patient during a rejection episode to minimize anxiety and/or depression.

Prevention of Transplant Graft Rejection Rejection episodes are mediated either by T cells, causing a cellular or acute rejection, or by B cells, mediating a chronic or humoral rejection. Immunosuppressive medications generally suppress acute (cellular) rejection responses by suppressing T cell formation. B cells or chronic rejection responses are not as specifically responsive to immunosuppressive medication.

The continued development and use of more effective immunosuppressive drugs provides hope that renal transplantation procedures will be more successful, with fewer rejection episodes causing loss of graft function and/or fewer side-effects or complications caused by the immunosuppressive therapy. The current clinically available immunosuppressive medications are reviewed briefly here. For more complete information, consult package inserts or drug reference texts, as well as current renal transplant literature.

1. Methylprednisolone (Solu-Medrol® or prednisone): Prednisone has been the mainstay of immunosuppressive therapy for renal transplantation, but it also causes a plethora of short- and long-term complications. Thus, current regimens attempt to minimize or eliminate its use. Prednisone causes all of the changes associated with Cushing's syndrome, with involvement of multiple organ systems. Patients who have been on prednisone for extended periods of time may have an Addisonian crisis after its discontinuation.

2. Azathioprine (Imuran®) is an immunosuppressive agent that specifically causes bone marrow (white blood cell) suppression. Monitoring the white blood cell count is essential to measuring the effectiveness of this drug. Use of Imuran specifically subjects the patient to the development of opportunistic infections. Hepatotoxicity is also a complication of this drug therapy.

3. Cyclophosphamide (Cytoxan®) is a chemotherapeutic/antimetabolite agent which acts as a bone marrow suppressant and thus decreases white blood cell formation. Cytoxan sometimes is used for patients who cannot tolerate Imuran due to hepatic disease (e.g., patients with hepatitis). The risk of opportunistic infection is equal to that with Imuran.

4. Cyclosporine is a fungal metabolite that acts as an immunosuppressive agent and is more specific to suppressing the response of helper T cells and possibly B cells which mediate the rejection response. Nephrotoxicity and hepatotoxicity are probably dose-related. The development of lymphomas and other solid tumors may be dose-related. Opportunistic infections are a continuing risk or complication. Fine tremors, hirsutism, and gum hypertrophy also may develop.

5. Monoclonal antibody (Orthoclone® OKT₃) is a specific antibody which prevents the rejection response by blocking the function of T cells. This drug can be administered only intravenously by bolus injection and is used only in

acute rejection episodes or as "rescue" therapy when all other immunosuppressive agents have failed. It is used in conjunction with other immunosuppressive agents.

6. Antilymphocyte/antithymocyte globulins (ALG/ATG) provide antibodies against lymphocytes or thymocytes that mediate rejection responses. This preventive therapy may be used in the early period following transplantation when the risk of rejection is the greatest. It is given via intravenous, intramuscular, or subcutaneous routes.

Both monoclonal antibody therapy and antilymphocyte or antithymocyte therapy are short-term treatments. Because of the sensitization to the globulin source that occurs, these agents cannot be repeated. A different animal source for the globulin production may allow additional courses of therapy.

Long-term Care and Survival Hospital stays following renal transplantation have been significantly shortened in recent years, with increased monitoring and surveillance performed on an outpatient basis. Patients should be aware that renal transplantation is not a cure for their ESRD but an effective alternative treatment. Patients must learn about and be responsible for their continued health care on an outpatient basis. They must assume responsibility for continued assessment of renal function by daily weights, early recognition of signs and symptoms of renal dysfunction or other complications, and continued necessary use of immunosuppressive drug therapy.

Summary

Renal function is a complex activity of human physiology. Alterations in or loss of renal function may cause both short-term and long-term effects on all organ systems. Expert understanding of renal function and the changes that occur with loss of function can guide the critical-care nurse's assessment and interventions with renal failure patients.

Care of the acute renal failure patient is directed toward maintaining as much renal function as possible, preventing complications, and replacing renal function through artificial means until it returns. All efforts are directed to saving the patient's life and ensuring a full recovery from the primary injury or illness and all of its complications.

For the patient with chronic renal disease, nursing efforts are directed to protecting remaining renal function and treating any systemic changes that may result from decreased renal function. The nursing interventions of care and education can assist the patient to understand the nature of the disease and the regimens necessary for management of real or potential complications. Such interventions can assist the patient in coping with his or her illness and maintaining a good quality of life.

The critical-care nurse's role in caring for the ESRD patient includes recognizing and managing complications which bring the patient into the hospital, preventing other complications from occurring during hospitalization, and maximizing rehabilitation.

Patients with chronic renal failure are living longer and healthier lives due to improvements in dialysis, transplantation, and various drug regimens and technologies. Decreased hospitalization for these patients is obviously a primary goal; when the need for hospitalization occurs, excellent nursing care is necessary to help them return to their pre-existing status.

REFERENCES

Anderson R et al.: Nonoliguric acute renal failure. *N Engl J Med* 1977; 216:1134–1138.

Crabtree A, Jorgenson M: Exploring the practical knowledge in expert critical-care nursing practice. Unpublished master's thesis, University of Wisconsin, Madison, 1986.

Cronin R et al.: Norepinephrine-induced acute renal failure. *Kidney Int* 1978; 14:115–125.

Bosch J, Ronco C: Continuous arteriovenous hemofiltration (CAVH) and other continuous replacement therapies: Operational characteristics and clinical use. In *Replacement of renal function by dialysis,* Maher J (ed). Boston: Kluwer Academic Publishers, 1989.

Gornick C, Kjillstrand C: Acute renal failure complicating aortic aneurysm surgery. *Nephron* 1983; 35:145–157.

Ludlow M, RN, MSN, Nephrology Clinical Specialist and Coordinator, Acute Dialysis, Stanford University Medical Center. Personal communication, 1992.

Myers B, Moran S: Hemodynamically mediated acute renal failure. *N Engl J Med* 1986; 314(2):97–105.

Paradiso C: Hemofiltration: An alternative to dialysis. *Heart Lung* 1989; 18(3):282–291.

Pfettscher S: Socioeconomic and Cultural Variables Influencing ESRD Treatment Decision-Making, 1991 (unpublished dissertation).

Reusch J, Anderson R: When acute renal failure complicates cardiac disease. *J Crit Illness* 1990; 5(2):108–114.

Schrier R: Acute renal failure. *Lifetime Medical Television,* 1986.

Sigler M, Teehan B: Continuous arteriovenous hemodialysis (CAVHD). In *Clinical Dialysis,* Nissenson A, Fine R, Gentile D (eds). Norwalk, CT: Appleton & Lange, 1990.

Simmons J et al.: *Gift of Life: The effect of organ transplantation on individual, family, and societal dynamics.* New Brunswick: Transaction Books, 1987.

Spurney R, Fulkerson W, Schwale S: Acute renal failure in critically ill patients: Prognosis for recovery of kidney function after prolonged dialysis support. *Crit Care Med* 1991; 19:8–11.

United States Renal Data System. National Institute of Diabetes and Digestive and Kidney Diseases. (1990). "United States renal data system: 1990 Annual data report." The National Institutes of Health, 1990.

Wilkes B, Mailloux L: Acute renal failure: Pathogenesis and prevention. *Am J Med* 1986; 80:1129–1136.

Wish J, Moritz C: Preventing radiocontrast-induced acute renal failure. *J Crit Illness* 1990; 5(1):16–31.

16

Fluid, Electrolyte, and Acid–Base Imbalances

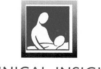

CLINICAL INSIGHT

Domain: The diagnostic and monitoring function

Competency: Detection and documentation of significant changes in a patient's condition

Becoming an expert critical-care nurse demands not only finely honing skills at detecting subtle physiologic changes but also developing the ability to present to the physician a convincing case for why this change is significant in this patient at this time. In the following example, from Crabtree and Jorgenson (1986, p. 133), Jill, a nurse, speaks eloquently of how she developed this skill. She describes an incident that occurred early in her career, while she was caring for a freshly postoperative patient who had undergone an abdominal aortic aneurysm repair.

My cardinal rule in nursing is, look at your patient. I don't care what any of the monitors say, what the papers say—look at your patient. . . . And, I looked

down, and the first thing I noticed was his Foley bag was totally full, and I said to this physician, I wonder what his K^+ is, and he said, don't worry about the potassium; don't worry about his I & O; you nurses get so hung up in this. And, he really verbally castrated me, and, well, I was worried about the potassium because I felt totally responsible. The surgeon would walk in and then would leave, and I had already learned that I really had to do my own thinking. So, I had a potassium drawn and, again—some people say this is very gutsy— who's going to pay for it? all these different things. I didn't worry about any of it. I worried about the patient. So, I had a potassium drawn, and it came back 2.8, and what I had never thought through was, now what am I going to do with this information? Because this surgeon that I had to call was, in my opinion, very difficult to deal with. So, now I'm in the position of, my God, Jill, you didn't *think this through. You've got to call him with this information. So, I called him at home. And I told him what the patient's potassium was, and we did rectify the situation. But, the point that I'm making is, how much energy, how much time I used up just taking care of one small detail. Where, now, today, I would never concern myself with this. I would follow through; none of my energy would be worrying about what the interaction was going to be with me. I would not hesitate to call him at home, and I wouldn't worry about it. But, it was I was so new in dealing with surgeons. I was the new kid on the block; what did I know? and I had to prove myself. And, I was very concerned with what the surgeons thought of me—their interactions with me—because to me the bottom line was, you had to get the order for the patient. And, there is a certain protocol that the nurse learns very early on: that she likes this relationship with the physician, or she's not going to get what the patient needs.*

Fluid, electrolyte, and acid–base disorders are common in the critically ill. The risk factors and signs and symptoms may be so subtle at times, however, that it takes special alertness to detect them and assertiveness to ensure appropriate treatment for them, as illustrated in the Clinical Insight. This chapter discusses the pathophysiology of each disorder and presents measures to assist you in nursing your patients more effectively.

FLUID AND ELECTROLYTE IMBALANCES

Assessment

As a critical-care nurse, you need to develop skill at effective assessment and intervention to protect the critically ill from the ravages of fluid and electrolyte imbalances. Such skill requires you to maintain a high index of suspicion in conditions that increase the patient's vulnerability to such imbalances. You should be able to anticipate and forestall the development of these disorders whenever possible. If they do occur, you should be able to recognize their signs and symptoms, alert the physician, and help him or her institute treatment early.

Table 16–1 presents a useful format for assessing the patient's fluid and electrolyte status. Assessment includes evaluation of serial body weights, fluid intake and output, serum and urine osmolalities, serum and urine electrolytes, and signs and symptoms.

TABLE 16–1

Fluid and Electrolyte Assessment Format

1. History_____

2. Physical_____

   Admission weight _____ date _____

   Yesterday's weight _____ date _____

   Today's weight _____ date _____

   Signs and symptoms (e.g., edema, skin turgor, character of sputum, pulse, blood pressure) _____

_____

3. Diagnostic procedures and laboratory tests

   Intake and output (24 hr) _____

   Osmolality: serum _____ urine _____

   Electrolytes: serum   Na$^+$ _____   K$^+$ _____   Cl$^-$ _____

                      Ca^{2+} _____   Mg^{2+} _____

             urine Na$^+$ _____   K$^+$ _____   Cl$^-$ _____

   Other _____

4. Other relevant data _____

Serial Body Weights

One of the most important interventions is to monitor body weights daily in patients susceptible to fluid imbalances.

The proportion of body weight that is fluid varies with the patient's sex and body fat content. In average-sized males, approximately 60% (40 L) of body weight is water. Women have more fat and less water than men: In average-sized females, water averages 50% (35 L) of body weight.

Fluid Compartments   Body fluid is divided into two main compartments: *intracellular* and *extracellular.* For a 70-kg man, about 25 L represents intracellular water, whereas about 15 L represents extracellular water. (Estimates of the volumes of fluid compartments vary considerably with the test substance used. Approximate percentages given here represent averages of those reported by various authors.) The extracellular compartment is subdivided into *functional* extracellular spaces, into and out of which fluid exchange can occur freely, and *nonfunctional* spaces, from which fluid is not readily accessible to the circulation. The functional spaces consist of fluid outside the cells in the vascular system *(plasma)* and that outside the cells in body tissues and cavities *(interstitial fluid).* Plasma equals about 3 L and interstitial fluid about 12 L. Dynamic fluid exchange occurs continuously among the intracellular, plasma, and interstitial compartments. Of these three, only the plasma can be influenced directly by fluid intake or elimination. For instance, when you drink water, the first fluid compartment that is affected is the plasma. The intracellular and interstitial compartments then respond to changes in the volume or concentration of the plasma.

Third-Spacing   Normally, the nonfunctional fluid space—fluid in peritoneal, pleural, cerebrospinal, bone, joint, and connective tissue—is small. *Third-spacing,* an abnormal alteration in physiologic function, occurs when fluid moves to spaces where it is functionally inaccessible, such as the interstitial space or peritoneal space. This can occur in conditions such as abdominal surgery, intestinal obstruction, liver disease (ascites), burns, peritoneal inflammation, decreased protein levels, and obstruction in lymph flow.

Intake and Output

For the internal environment to remain in a steady state from day to day, the intake and output of fluids must be equal (Table 16–2). The major routes of water intake

---

NURSING TIP

Estimating Fluid Gain or Loss

A rapid weight change (over 0.5 kg/day) suggests a fluid imbalance and often appears before other, more subtle signs and symptoms. One kilogram equals 2.2 lb and a liter of body fluid equals 2.2 lb. Accordingly, a general guideline is that a rapid weight gain of 1 kg reflects each liter of fluid retained and a loss of 1 kg reflects each liter lost. A patient's weight therefore can serve as a valuable guide to estimating fluid deficit or excess.

---

are ingestion of liquids (500–1,700 ml), the ingestion of water in foods (800–1,000 ml), and the oxidation of food and body tissues (200–300 ml). The primary normal routes of water output are urine (800–1,600 ml), water vapor excreted through the lungs and skin (600–1,200 ml), and feces (50–200 ml). There is an obligatory loss of approximately 600–800 ml daily of water vapor from the lungs and skin (insensible water loss). Vaporization from the lungs and skin occurs even when water intake is zero. It is important to note that the amount of water vapor lost from the lungs and skin may greatly increase with certain conditions such as fever and sepsis. In these conditions, as metabolism increases, so does production of water, which then is lost. Additionally, perspiration increases loss through the skin.

The osmolality of extracellular fluid is determined almost solely by sodium concentration. In turn, sodium concentration is controlled by two separate but closely associated systems: antidiuretic hormone (ADH) secretion and thirst (Guyton 1991). Oral intake is regulated by the thirst center, believed to be located in

---

TABLE 16–2

Average Intake and Output

INTAKE		OUTPUT	
Ingestion	500–1,700 ml	Wine	800–1,600 ml
Water in food	800–1,000 ml	Feces	50–200 ml
Oxidation of food and tissues	200–300 ml	Obligatory loss (skin, lungs)	600–800 ml
	1,500–3,000 ml		1,450–2,600 ml

the anterolateral hypothalamus. When plasma osmolality increases or blood volume decreases, intracellular dehydration stimulates the neurons in the thirst center and the person becomes thirsty and increases water intake.

Water output is under multiple controls, the most significant of which are antidiuretic hormone, aldosterone, and baroreceptors. *Antidiuretic hormone* is made in the supraoptic nuclei and stored in the posterior pituitary gland. Cells on the surface of the anterior hypothalamus, called *osmoreceptors,* sense changes in the sodium concentration of the extracellular fluid that bathes them. When osmotic pressure increases, the supraoptic neurons become dehydrated and discharge impulses to the posterior pituitary at a faster rate, so there is an increased release of ADH. (Conversely, when osmotic pressure decreases, ADH release falls.) ADH travels in the bloodstream to the kidneys. There it alters tubular permeability to water, increasing reabsorption of water (and therefore decreasing urinary output). The retained water dilutes the extracellular fluid, reducing its concentration toward normal. The restoration of normal osmotic pressure then feeds back to the osmoreceptors to inhibit their discharge. The thirst center and supraoptic nuclei are close together and appear to respond to the same stimuli.

Another substance that plays an important role in the control of extracellular volume is aldosterone. *Aldosterone* is a hormone secreted by the adrenal cortex in response to many stimuli. In probable order of decreasing importance, the three most potent stimuli are: (a) increased potassium concentration in extracellular fluid; (b) increased angiotensin II level (resulting from increased renin secretion by the juxtaglomerular apparatus in the kidneys); (c) decreased sodium concentration in extracellular fluid (Guyton 1991).

Aldosterone travels in the bloodstream to the kidneys, where it is believed to cause the formation of carrier proteins or enzymes necessary for active sodium transport through the tubular epithelium of the distal tubule and collecting duct (Guyton 1991). An increased level of aldosterone therefore causes increased sodium retention and an obligatory increase in water retention, thus reducing the urinary output. The retained sodium and water increase extracellular fluid volume and feed back to inhibit aldosterone secretion.

Baroreceptors that sense high-pressure (arterial) changes are located in the arch of the aorta and in each carotid sinus, just above the bifurcation of the internal and external carotid arteries. When arterial pressure drops, these receptors transmit fewer impulses from the carotid sinuses (via the Hering and glossopharyngeal nerves) and from the aortic arch (via the vagus nerves) to the vasomotor center. The decrease in impulses excites the sympathetic (cardioaccelerator and vasoconstrictor) center and inhibits the parasympathetic (cardioinhibitor) center. As a result, heart rate accelerates and the peripheral vasculature constricts, increasing the central blood volume. At the same time, sympathetic stimulation constricts the renal afferent and efferent arterioles. This constriction reduces glomerular filtration, so less water is excreted.

Serum Osmolality

When you consider the concentration of body fluids, it is important to realize that concentration may be expressed in several different ways. The term *concentration* in itself expresses the ratio between dissolved substances *(solutes)* and dissolving fluid *(solvent)*.

Concentration expressed as weight is equal to the grams of solute per 100 ml of fluid; an example is a serum albumin value of 5 g/100 ml, also reported sometimes as 5 g/dl or 5 g%. An *equivalent weight* equals the molecular weight of a substance divided by its valence. In clinical situations, this value is given as milliequivalents per liter of fluid (mEq/L). This method is often used for reporting serum electrolyte values, for example, a serum sodium level of 140 mEq/L.

Osmosis is the movement of water from a solution with fewer solute particles across a semipermeable membrane into a solution with more solute particles. An *osmol,* a unit for measuring osmotic pressure, is the gram molecular weight of a substance multiplied by the number of dissociating ions. Because of the small concentrations with which we work in clinical situations, values are expressed in thousandths of an osmol, that is, milliosmols (mOsm).

The *osmolarity* of a solution is the solute concentration per volume of solution, or mOsm/L. The *osmolality* is the solute concentration per weight of solvent, or mOsm/kg of solvent. In clinical practice, osmolarity and osmolality often are preferred to other measures of concentration, because they express the number of osmotically active particles without regard to their size, electrical charge, or molecular weight. In the body, the difference between osmolarity and osmolality normally is slight, and the terms often are used interchangeably. Normal serum osmolality consists primarily of sodium, its anions, glucose, and urea. The normal serum osmolality is 285–295 mOsm/kg.

Electrolytes

An *electrolyte* is a substance that will carry an electrical current when it is dissolved. The electrically charged particles into which it dissolves are called *ions.*

Negatively charged ions are *anions,* and positively charged ones are *cations.* For example, sodium chloride dissolves into a cation, sodium (Na^+), and an anion, chloride (Cl^-). Each ion has one ionic bond. The normal serum concentration for sodium is 135–144 mEq/L and for chloride 96–106 mEq/L. (The reason sodium concentration is higher than chloride concentration is that additional sodium exists in the serum in forms other than NaCl–for instance, as sodium bicarbonate ($NaHCO_3$).)

Often you will hear an electrolyte solution described in terms of its *tonicity,* that is, its osmotic pressure as compared to that of another solution, such as plasma. The tonicity of plasma is about 310 mEq/L. Tonicity is determined by adding the mEq of particles that cannot be ionized (such as urea), the mEq of those that can be but are not (such as undissolved sodium bicarbonate), and the mEq of ionized particles (anions plus cations). If the sum is within the range of 250–375 mEq/L, the solution is said to be *isotonic with plasma.* A *hypotonic* solution is less than 250 mEq/L, and a *hypertonic* one is over 375 mEq/L.

Electrolytes are taken into the body in food and fluids. They are lost normally through sweat and urine. They also may be lost through hemorrhage, vomiting, and diarrhea.

The distribution of electrolytes within fluid compartments and body fluids varies considerably. Intracellular fluid consists primarily of potassium, phosphate, proteins, and magnesium. Extracellular fluid consists primarily of sodium, chloride, and bicarbonate.

The signs and symptoms of fluid and electrolyte imbalances also vary considerably. They are discussed under individual disorders below.

Fluid Imbalances

The two primary fluid imbalances that occur are *fluid volume deficit* and *fluid volume excess.*

Fluid Volume Deficit

Information on fluid volume deficit is summarized in Table 16–3.

Signs and Symptoms Acute weight loss, dry skin and mucous membranes, poor skin turgor, hypotension, and oliguria indicate the patient has a fluid volume deficit. Infants and the elderly are particularly susceptible to this condition.

If the serum sodium concentration is normal (135–144 mEq/L), isotonic fluid must have been lost from the extracellular space *(hypovolemia).* An isotonic loss causes fluid and electrolytes to move out of the cell, so that both the extracellular and the intracellular compartments end up with volume deficits. When this occurs, the osmoreceptors in the hypothalamus stimulate ADH release and thirst to return body fluids to normal. If water intake remains inadequate, however, this mechanism is unable to restore normal fluid balance. Conditions that predispose to fluid volume deficit include decreased intake (anorexia, lethargy, unconsciousness); loss of electrolyte-rich secretions through blood loss, vomiting, diarrhea, fistulas, and nasogastric suction; and third-spacing. As with any fluid or electrolyte disorder, clues from the patient's history can be invaluable in identifying the imbalance present.

NURSING DIAGNOSIS

- Fluid volume deficit

Planning and Implementation of Care The treatment for fluid volume deficit requires replacement of both fluid and electrolytes with an isotonic solution, such as normal saline; plasma expanders; and replacement of specific losses, such as blood cells. (Of course, one must treat the cause, too. This point will not be belabored in the remaining discussions.)

Fluid Volume Excess

Information on this disorder is given in Table 16–4.

Signs and Symptoms Acute weight gain, bounding pulse, hypertension, edema, jugular venous distension, and pulmonary congestion suggest that the patient has a fluid volume excess. Combined intracellular and extracellular excesses can occur as a result of the intake of isotonic fluid.

Normal serum and urinary sodium concentrations confirm an isotonic imbalance. In this state, an increased volume of isotonic fluid in the extracellular space causes both fluid and electrolytes to move into the cell. The result is both extracellular and intracellular volume excesses. Pathologic conditions that can

TABLE 16–3

Fluid Volume Deficit

PREDISPOSING CONDITIONS	SIGNS AND SYMPTOMS	TREATMENT
Loss of Fluid and Electrolytes		
Gastrointestinal secretion loss:	Acute weight loss	Rehydration solutions
vomiting	Dry skin and mucous membrane	lactated Ringers
diarrhea	Skin turgor poor	normal saline
nasogastric suction	Hypotension	Plasma expanders
fistulas	Positive postural vital signs	albumin
Blood loss	Capillary filling time prolonged	plasmanate
Burns	Oliguria	Replacement of specific losses
Profuse diaphoresis	Thirst	blood cells
Diuretic abuse	Laboratory data:	
Decreased Intake	hemoglobin	
Anorexia	hematocrit } ↑ due to	
Lethargy	blood urea nitrogen } hemoconcentration	
Unconsciousness		
Unavailability	Serum osmolality ↑	
Third Spacing	Urine specific gravity and osmolality ↑	
Burns	Urinary sodium level ↓	
Intestinal obstruction		
Ascites		
Peritoneal inflammation:		
peritonitis		
pancreatitis		

produce this imbalance include increased ingestion or retention of isotonic fluid (for example, in steroid therapy, severe congestive heart failure, or hyperaldosteronism), and decreased renal excretion (for example, in chronic renal failure or severe stress).

NURSING DIAGNOSES

• Fluid volume excess

Planning and Implementation of Care The treatment of isotonic excess includes restricted intake of fluid and electrolytes, diuretics, dialysis, or continuous ultrafiltration.

Outcome Evaluation

Evaluate the patient's progress toward healthy fluid balance according to these outcome criteria:

• Weight within normal limits (WNL) for patient.
• Blood pressure and pulse volume normal for patient.
• Level of consciousness and respiratory rate normal for patient.
• Skin warm, dry, and with normal turgor.
• Moist mucous membranes.
• Urinary volume WNL for patient, ideal range 800–1,600 ml/24 hr.
• Serum sodium normal for patient, ideal range 135–145 mEq/L.
• Urinary sodium WNL for patient, ideal range 50–130 mEq/L.

TABLE 16–4

Fluid Volume Excess

PREDISPOSING CONDITIONS	SIGNS AND SYMPTOMS	TREATMENT
Increased Ingestion or Retention of Isotonic Fluid	Acute weight gain	Restricted intake of fluid and electrolytes
Excessive infusion of intravenous fluid, especially sodium chloride	Bounding pulse	Diuretics
Prolonged steroid therapy	Hypertension	furosemide
Hyperaldosteronism	Pitting edema	Dialysis
Severe congestive heart failure	Puffy face and eyelids	hemodialysis
Decreased Renal Excretion	Jugular venous distention	continuous arteriovenous ultrafiltration
Chronic renal failure	Pulmonary congestion:	
Severe stress (such as trauma, surgery)	shortness of breath	
	cough	
	crackles	
	pulmonary edema	
	Laboratory data:	
	hemoglobin and hematocrit ↓ due to hemodilution	
	serum osmolality ↓	
	urinary specific gravity and osmolality ↓	
	urinary sodium ↓	

- Serum osmolality WNL for patient, ideal range 285–295 mOsm/kg.
- Urinary osmolality WNL for patient, ideal range 500–800 mOsm/kg.

Sodium Imbalances

Roles of Sodium

Sodium, the major cation of the extracellular fluid, plays a crucial role in many body processes. Sodium has major responsibility for maintenance of normal osmolality (concentration) of body fluids. It is a part of many energy-dependent cell membrane transport mechanisms (e.g., the sodium-potassium pump). Because of its function in the maintenance of transmembrane cellular potential, it also plays a major role in the transmission of electrochemical impulses and in neuromuscular conduction. Finally, through its combination with anions during sodium reabsorption in the renal tubules and through its role in the sodium/potassium/hydrogen ion exchange mechanism in the kidney, it participates in consistency of acid–base balance in the body.

The normal serum sodium range is 135–145 mEq/L. Serum sodium concentration is controlled primarily by the renal system, under the major influence of the ADH–thirst mechanism. Aldosterone has a mild effect on sodium ion concentration (Guyton 1991). Although aldosterone is a potent stimulus for sodium reabsorption, the accompanying obligatory reabsorption of water means that extracellular volume increases but relatively little change in sodium concentration occurs.

The two primary imbalances of sodium are *hyponatremia* and *hypernatremia*. Differential diagnosis of sodium imbalances depends on the patient's history, the serum sodium concentration, and the urine sodium concentration. The serum sodium concentration expresses the relationship between the amount of sodium in the serum and the volume of plasma. If more water is lost than sodium, the sodium concentration rises. If more sodium is lost than water, the serum sodium concentration decreases.

TABLE 16–5

Hyponatremia

PREDISPOSING CONDITIONS	SIGNS AND SYMPTOMS	MECHANISM	TREATMENT
Water Intoxication (Dilutional hyponatremia)			
Excessive water ingestion	Fluid overload, *plus:*	Extracellular fluid excess, *plus:*	Fluid restriction
Excessive electrolyte-free IV solutions	Central nervous system:	Intracellular fluid excess	Diuretics
Excessive tap water enemas	Headache		Demeclocycline (for SIADH)
Irrigation of gastric tubes with water	Lethargy, confusion, delirium		
	Convulsions, coma		
Congestive heart failure	Gastrointestinal system:		
Inappropriate ADH secretion (SIADH)	Nausea, vomiting, diarrhea, cramps		
Hyperglycemia	Laboratory data:		
	Serum sodium ↓		
	Urine sodium ↓*		
	Urine specific gravity and osmolality ↓*		
Sodium Deficit			
Low-sodium diet	Dehydration, *plus:*	Extracellular fluid deficit, *plus:*	Replacement of sodium: normal saline solution; hypertonic (3%) sodium chloride solution
Diuretics	Central nervous and gastrointestinal systems: as above	Intracellular fluid excess	
Gastrointestinal losses:	Laboratory data: as above		
Severe vomiting			
Diarrhea			
Nasogastric suction			
Renal disease			
Adrenal insufficiency			

*except SIADH

Hyponatremia

Hyponatremia is defined as a serum sodium concentration of less than 135 mEq/L. A patient may become hyponatremic in two ways: ingestion or retention of excess water (water intoxication), and actual loss of sodium (Table 16–5). In *water intoxication,* also known as *dilutional hyponatremia,* an increased volume of water dilutes the serum sodium. The increased proportion of water causes water to move into the cell, so the patient develops both extracellular and intracellular fluid volume excesses. Situations that may produce this state are: (a) excessive water ingestion, through administration of electrolyte-poor intravenous (IV) fluids, tap water enemas, or irrigation of gastric tubes with water instead of saline; (b) congestive heart failure; and (c) the *syndrome of inappropriate secretion of antidiuretic hormone (SIADH).*

SIADH occurs when there is uncontrolled production of ADH; that is, ADH release is not triggered by decreases in blood volume but instead occurs ectopically. SIADH may occur in a number of disorders. The most common include neurologic conditions (head trauma, cranial surgery, and tumors) and pulmonary conditions (tumors, severe pneumonia, and mechanical ventilation). SIADH causes dilution of blood volume due to water retention by the kidneys; however, the feedback mechanism that normally would limit ADH production does not operate, and water retention continues. Urine volume usually is concentrated, due to water retention, and urine sodium is elevated, because the increased blood flow through the kidneys causes a sodium diuresis. SIADH is confirmed by comparison of serum and urine osmolalities; the serum osmolality will be considerably lower than the urine osmolality.

The other key mechanism by which hyponatremia can occur is true loss of sodium. A history of a low-sodium diet, diuretic use, gastrointestinal fluid losses, renal disease, or adrenal insufficiency usually is present. Because the patient loses sodium and water, an extracellular fluid volume deficit develops. However, since the extracellular sodium loss exceeds the water loss, water tends to move into the cells. True sodium deficit thus produces an extracellular fluid volume deficit and an intracellular fluid volume excess.

Signs and Symptoms The signs and symptoms of hyponatremia vary somewhat with the mechanism causing it. In both water intoxication and sodium loss, the patient has signs and symptoms of cerebral edema—for instance, headache, lethargy, and confusion—and gastrointestinal symptoms. In true sodium deficit, however, signs and symptoms of dehydration also may be present.

Laboratory values include a decreased serum sodium concentration, decreased urine sodium level (except in SIADH), and decreased urine specific gravity and osmolality (except in SIADH).

NURSING DIAGNOSES

Nursing diagnoses that may apply to the hyponatremic patient include:

- Pain
- Sensory-perceptual alteration
- Altered thought processes
- Diarrhea
- Fluid volume excess (with water intoxication) or deficit (with true sodium loss)

Planning and Implementation of Care Interventions for hyponatremia vary with its mechanism. Dilutional hyponatremia usually responds well to fluid restriction and diuretics. Demeclocycline (Declomycin) may be prescribed for the SIADH patient to block the action of ADH (Gotch 1991). In true sodium loss, the appropriate treatment is sodium replacement, with either normal saline or, in severe depletion, hypertonic sodium chloride. Implement the following nursing interventions in hyponatremia:

1. Assess for signs of fluid overload or dehydration.

2. In water intoxication, maintain fluid restriction and administer diuretics as ordered.

3. In true sodium deficit, administer sodium replacement, as ordered.

4. Weigh the patient daily.

5. Monitor vital signs every 2 hours and as needed.

Hypernatremia

Hypernatremia, a serum sodium concentration in excess of 145 mEq/L, can occur in two ways: a *disproportionate water loss,* or a sodium excess (Table 16–6). In the first situation, the patient loses more water than sodium; as a result, serum sodium concentration increases, and the increased concentration "pulls" fluid out of the cells. This type of hypernatremia is characterized by both extracellular and intracellular fluid volume deficits. Causes include actual water loss—for example, watery diarrhea, osmotic diuresis, and diabetes insipidus—and decreased water intake. In *sodium excess,* the patient ingests or retains more sodium than water. Examples are salt craving and excessive sodium bicarbonate administration. As the serum sodium concentration rises, water again is "pulled" out of the cells. This shift causes an extracellular volume excess in combination with an intracellular volume deficit.

Signs and Symptoms

Signs and symptoms again vary somewhat with the mechanism of the hypernatremia. In both types, central nervous system irritability is present, because the extra sodium concentration alters transmembrane electrical potential in such a way that cells become more easily excited. In addition, in water deficit, signs and symptoms of dehydration usually are present, whereas in sodium excess, signs and symptoms of fluid overload are observed.

Planning and Implementation of Care Hypernatremia due to water loss responds to isotonic or hypotonic fluid replacement. In contrast, hypernatremia due to sodium excess is managed with restricted sodium intake, hypotonic intravenous fluids, and diuretics. Implement the following nursing interventions:

1. Assess for symptoms of dehydration or fluid overload, depending on cause.

TABLE 16–6

Hypernatremia

PREDISPOSING CONDITIONS	SIGNS AND SYMPTOMS	MECHANISM	TREATMENT
Water Loss Exceeding Sodium Loss			
Watery diarrhea	Dehydration, *plus:*	Extracellular fluid deficit, *plus:*	Isotonic or hypotonic fluid replacement
Excessive osmotic diuresis	Central nervous system irritability:	Intracellular fluid deficit	
Diabetes insipidus	Restlessness, confusion,		
Fever	lethargy, stupor		
Excessive dialysis	Tremors		
	Seizures (if >160 mEq/L)		
	Coma (if >160 mEq/L)		
Decreased Water Intake			
Coma	Laboratory data:		
Unavailability of water	Serum sodium concentration ↑		
	Urine sodium concentration ↓		
	Urine specific gravity and osmolality ↑		
Sodium Excess			
Salt craving	Fluid overload, *plus:*	Extracellular fluid excess, *plus:*	Restricted sodium intake
Excessive sodium bicarbonate administration	Central nervous system irritability: as above	Intracellular fluid deficit	Diuretics
Excessive steroid administration	Laboratory data; as above		Hypotonic intravenous solutions
Hyperaldosteronism			
Renal failure			
Excessive sodium chloride administration			

NURSING DIAGNOSES

The nursing diagnoses that may apply to patients with hypernatremia include:

- Sensory-perceptual alteration
- Altered thought processes
- Fluid volume deficit (in disproportionate water loss) or fluid volume excess (in sodium excess)

2. Restrict sodium intake, if ordered.
3. Monitor intake and output.
4. Maintain IV therapy for replacement of fluid, if ordered.

5. Monitor vital signs every 2 hours and as needed.
6. Weigh the patient daily.

Outcome Evaluation

Outcome criteria appropriate for the patient with a sodium imbalance include the following:

- Level of consciousness WNL for patient.
- Skin warm, dry, and with normal turgor.
- Blood pressure, pulse volume, and pulse rate WNL for patient.
- Serum sodium concentration 135–145 mEq/L.
- Serum osmolality 285–295 mOsm/kg.
- Urine sodium WNL for patient, ideal range 50–130 mEq/L.

- Urine osmolality WNL for patient, ideal range 500–800 mOsm/kg.

Potassium Imbalances

Roles of Potassium

Potassium is the major intracellular cation; nearly 98% of total body potassium is found inside the cells. The extracellular concentration of potassium is 3.5–5.5 mEq/L, and it is important to remember that this small extracellular concentration is not an accurate reflection of the amount of total body potassium. Although large fluctuations in *intracellular* potassium can be tolerated by the body, even small fluctuations in *serum* potassium can be toxic.

Potassium plays a number of important roles in the body. It is one of the ions responsible for maintenance of cellular transmembrane electrical balance and therefore is instrumental in normal neuromuscular transmission. It participates in numerous intracellular processes, including enzyme systems involved in the production of energy, synthesis of protein and glycogen, and metabolism of carbohydrates. It also contributes to maintenance of normal cellular osmotic pressure and to normal acid–base balance. (The interrelationships between potassium balance and acid–base balance are explained in the section of this chapter on acid–base abnormalities.)

Potassium is absorbed from the gastrointestinal (GI) tract and freely filtered at the glomerulus. Most of it is reabsorbed in the proximal tubule, with the distal tubule primarily responsible for secretion of potassium. Potassium excretion is under multiple controls, the most important of which are the sodium load delivered to the tubules, acid–base status of the body, potassium intake, and aldosterone level. The kidney does not conserve potassium effectively, and urinary losses will continue even in the face of a potassium deficit.

Two imbalances of potassium exist: *hyperkalemia,* in which the serum potassium level exceeds 5.5 mEq/L, and *hypokalemia,* in which the serum potassium level is less than 3.5 mEq/L (Table 16–7).

Hypokalemia

Conditions that increase susceptibility to hypokalemia are numerous in the critically ill. As indicated in Table 16–7, general causes are: (a) inadequate dietary intake;

(b) loss of gastrointestinal secretions; (c) increased urinary loss; (d) aldosterone excess; and (e) intracellular potassium shift in alkalosis.

> ### ✎ NURSING TIP
>
> #### Preventing Hypokalemia
>
> An important responsibility of the critical-care nurse is preventing the development of hypokalemia. For example, consult the physician about adding potassium to the intravenous fluids of patients fasting postoperatively, particularly if they undergo GI suction or have diarrhea. Monitor serum potassium levels of patients on potassium-wasting diuretics, especially furosemide and ethacrynic acid. Be particularly alert with patients receiving both digitalis and diuretics, since hypokalemia potentiates digitalis toxicity.

Signs and Symptoms During hypokalemia, the serum deficit allows potassium to move out of the cell more easily than is normal. Since potassium has a positive charge, its loss results in increased negativity inside the cell, a condition known as *hyperpolarization.* Hyperpolarization reduces membrane excitability (responsiveness), making depolarization more difficult and prolonging repolarization.

On the ECG, the decreased responsiveness to stimuli may be seen as flattened T waves, prominent U waves, and depressed ST segments (Figure 16–1). However, these signs correlate poorly with the degree of hypokalemia. Because hypokalemia potentiates digitalis toxicity, you may see rhythms common in digitalis toxicity, such as ectopic beats and tachycardias. Ventricular asystole and fibrillation also may occur.

Skeletal muscle depression appears as progressive weakness, hypoactive reflexes, paresthesias, and paralysis. Smooth muscle hypoactivity causes the gastrointestinal symptoms of abdominal distention, paralytic ileus, anorexia, nausea, and vomiting. Central nervous system signs are uncommon but may appear as drowsiness or lethargy. The kidney's ability to concentrate urine is lost, so polyuria, nocturia, and thirst may be present. Hypotension, due to impaired vasoconstriction, and respiratory arrest may be late findings.

TABLE 16–7

Potassium Imbalances

PREDISPOSING CONDITIONS	SIGNS AND SYMPTOMS	TREATMENT
	Hypokalemia	
Inadequate dietary intake:	Flattened T waves	Treatment of cause
Lethargy, anorexia, coma, postoperative fasting	Prominent U waves	Increased potassium intake: foods, oral supplements, intravenous solutions
	ST depression	
Loss of gastrointestinal secretions:	Ventricular asystole or fibrillation	Correction of alkalosis
Persistent vomiting, diarrhea, gastrointestinal drainage, fistulas	Digitalis toxicity	Potassium-sparing diuretics
	Hypoactive reflexes	
Increased urine output:	Paresthesias	
Diuretics, diabetic acidosis, diuretic phase of renal failure, burn diuresis	Weakness, ascending flaccid paralysis	
	Hypotension	
Aldosterone excess:	Respiratory arrest	
Severe prolonged stress, corticosteroid therapy, adrenal tumor, Cushing's disease	Abdominal distention, ileus, anorexia, nausea, vomiting	
Intracellular shift:		
Alkalosis		
Hemodilution		
	Hyperkalemia	
Excessive intake:	Tall, peaked T waves	Treatment of cause
Rapid IV potassium administration	Prolonged PR interval	Limited potassium intake
Cellular breakdown:	Absent P waves	Emergency measures:
Crush injury, burns, stored bank blood transfusions	Prolonged QRS duration	Calcium chloride
	Bradycardia, escape rhythms	Sodium bicarbonate
Decreased urine output:	Ventricular asystole or fibrillation	Hypertonic glucose and insulin
Oliguric phase of renal failure	Weakness	Hemodialysis
Aldosterone deficiency:	Cramps	Nonemergency measures:
Addison's disease	Twitching	Ion exchange resins (e.g., Kayexalate/ sorbitol)
Extracellular shift:	Abdominal cramps, diarrhea	Peritoneal dialysis
Acidosis	Paresthesias, paralysis	Correction of acidosis
Hemoconcentration	Intestinal ileus	

Planning and Implementation of Care Minimize the effects of hypokalemia while you assist the physician to treat the disorder. Implement the following measures:

1. Conserve the patient's energy to lessen weakness and fatigue.

2. Relieve gastrointestinal discomfort symptomatically.

3. Be prepared for emergency defibrillation, cardiac massage, and artificial respiration if the person arrests.

4. Correct alkalosis if present. Treatment may include acetazolamide, which blocks the action of carbonic anhydrase. It thus increases excretion of bicarbonate and decreases the excretion of hydrogen ions. This action helps to correct the alkalosis.

5. Assess for signs and symptoms of decreased cardiac output, such as decreased blood pressure, increased pulse rate, decreased pulse amplitude, decreased urinary output, decreased peripheral pulses, and altered level of consciousness.

HYPOKALEMIA

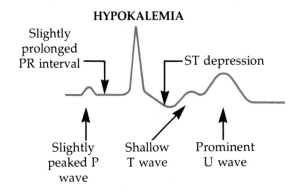

Slightly
prolonged
PR interval

ST depression

Slightly
peaked P
wave

Shallow
T wave

Prominent
U wave

NORMOKALEMIA

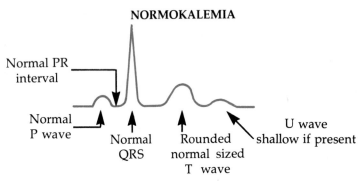

Normal PR
interval

Normal
P wave

Normal
QRS

Rounded
normal sized
T wave

U wave
shallow if present

HYPERKALEMIA

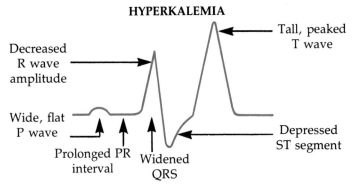

Decreased
R wave
amplitude

Tall, peaked
T wave

Wide, flat
P wave

Prolonged PR
interval

Widened
QRS

Depressed
ST segment

FIGURE 16–1

Effects of potassium levels on ECG.

NURSING DIAGNOSES

Depending on the degree and effects of hypokalemia, a number of nursing diagnoses may apply. These include:

- Decreased cardiac output (CO)
- Activity intolerance
- Self-care deficits
- Sensory-perceptual alteration
- Altered urinary elimination
- Altered tissue perfusion: peripheral

6. Increase the oral intake of potassium by giving potassium-rich foods, such as oranges, bananas, dried figs, and peaches, or oral potassium supplements if ordered. Oral potassium can produce small-bowel lesions, so alert the physician if the patient develops abdominal distention, pain, or gastrointestinal bleeding.

7. Administer intravenous potassium as ordered by the physician. Do not exceed a rate of 20 mEq/hr unless the patient is on a cardiac monitor and the physician specifically orders a faster rate.

8. Teach patients, especially those to be discharged on digitalis or diuretics, the importance of eating potassium-rich foods at home,

the signs and symptoms of hypokalemia, and the necessity of prompt medical attention if they appear.

Hyperkalemia

Conditions predisposing to hyperkalemia include excessive potassium intake, cellular breakdown, decreased renal excretion, aldosterone deficiency, and extracellular shift in acidosis (refer to Table 16–7). Preventive measures that can help protect patients from hyperkalemia include (a) ensuring that urinary output is adequate prior to administration of supplemental potassium and (b) treating acidosis promptly. For patients with renal failure, transfusions should be performed with fresh blood; as stored blood ages, its cells break down and release potassium.

Signs and Symptoms   In hyperkalemia, the excess serum potassium opposes the normal potassium leak from the cell in its resting state. As a result, the inside of the cell becomes less negative (more positive) than usual, a condition known as *hypopolarization*. Because fewer positive ions must flow in to initiate depolarization, the cell fires more easily. Action potential amplitude decreases, and repolarization is shortened. As the degree of hyperkalemia increases, however, the cell eventually has too many positive charges inside it to respond to stimuli. Impulse formation and transmission slow and eventually cease.

Progression of hyperkalemia often is associated with specific electrocardiographic signs that correlate with serum potassium levels (Marriott 1987). The earliest sign, which appears at a serum potassium level of about 6.5 mEq/L, is shortened repolarization, seen as tall, symmetric, peaked T waves. R wave amplitude decreases and ST depression develops. Above 7 mEq/L, atrial conduction slows, producing flattened P waves and prolonged PR intervals. As hyperkalemia worsens, atrial excitability ceases and P waves disappear, although QRS complexes remain. At 10 mEq/L, the QRS complexes widen. Eventually, at 11 mEq/L, they widen so much that they merge with T waves to form sine wave configurations. This abnormality occurs because some areas of the myocardium still are undergoing depolarization while others are being repolarized. Among the dysrhythmias that may appear are blocks, bradycardia, escape rhythms, and sinus arrest. Ventricular fibrillation or asystole may occur as terminal events.

In the earlier stages of hyperkalemia, skeletal muscle excitability is manifested by weakness, cramps, and twitching. During the later stages, when cellular excitability diminishes, skeletal muscle depression produces paresthesias and ascending flaccid paralysis, and smooth muscle hypotonicity causes intestinal ileus.

Planning and Implementation of Care   Severe hyperkalemia is present when the serum potassium level exceeds 7.0 mEq/L or the electrocardiogram (ECG) shows absent P waves, widened QRS complexes, or ventricular dysrhythmias. To relieve cardiac toxicity, potassium can be antagonized by IV administration of calcium chloride. This treatment does not lower serum potassium, and its effects are transient, so it must be followed by sodium bicarbonate and hypertonic glucose and insulin therapy. The bicarbonate helps to correct acidosis, encouraging the return of potassium to the intracellular space. The hypertonic glucose and insulin infusion also helps move potassium intracellularly. Insulin facilitates the movement of glucose into the cell, which carries potassium along with it. Details of the measures used in emergency treatment of hyperkalemia are summarized in Table 16–8.

TABLE 16–8

Emergency Treatment of Severe Hyperkalemia
(Serum K⁺ Above 7.0 mEq/L and/or ECG Signs)

AGENT	ONSET	DURATION	DOSE	MECHANISM	PROBLEMS AND IMPLICATIONS
Calcium chloride	1–5 min	1–2 hr	2.5–5.0 ml of 10% solution	Antagonizes effects on heart by raising threshold potential	Cardiac arrest in patients with digitalis toxicity No change in serum or total body potassium
Sodium bicarbonate	5 min	1–2 hr	1–2 amps	Promotes intracellular shift of K⁺	Sodium intake ↑ Metabolic alkalosis Serum K⁺↓ but not total body K⁺↓
Hypertonic glucose and insulin infusion	15 min	4–6 hr	250–500 ml of 10% dextrose with 10–15 units of regular insulin, over 30–60 min	Promotes intracellular shift of K⁺	Rebound hypoglycemia Serum K⁺↓ but not total body K⁺↓ Rebound hyperkalemia

Lesser degrees of hyperkalemia may be treated by administration of diuretics, dialysis, or cation-exchange resins. The most commonly used resin is sodium polystyrene sulfonate (Kayexalate) given orally or by retention enema.

Implement the following nursing interventions:

1. Monitor vital signs every 2 hours and as needed.
2. Monitor ECG and report significant changes in patterns to the physician.
3. Administer diuretics and cation-exchange resins as ordered.
4. Administer glucose and insulin, as ordered.

Outcome Evaluation

Use the following outcome criteria to gauge the patient's progress toward a healthy potassium balance:

- Serum potassium WNL for patient, ideally 3.5–5.3 mEq/L.
- Arterial blood gases WNL for patient, ideally pH 7.35–7.45, Po₂ 80–100 mm Hg, Pco₂ 35–45 mm Hg, and HCO₃ 23–28 mEq/L.
- ECG WNL for patient, ideally with normal sinus rhythm, rounded P waves, PR interval 0.12–0.20 second, QRS duration of 0.06–0.10 second, isoelectric ST segments, and rounded T waves.

- Deep tendon reflexes, neuromuscular irritability, and muscular strength WNL for patient.
- Gastrointestinal function WNL for patient.

Calcium Imbalances

Roles of Calcium

Calcium (Ca⁺⁺) is important in cellular excitability, excitation–contraction coupling, smooth muscle contractility, bone and tooth formation, blood clotting, and intracellular energy storage and use. Calcium is believed to bind with the protein linings of the sodium channels in the cell membrane. Its positive charges theoretically block the entrance of sodium. It thus helps to establish the normal resting membrane potential, in which the cell is more negative on the inside than on the outside of the membrane. In addition, calcium participates in slow-channel depolarization of cells (refer to the discussion of cardiac action potentials and calcium channel blockade in Chapter 12).

Calcium plays an important role in muscle contractility. Skeletal, cardiac, and smooth muscle all contain myofibrils of protein called actin and myosin. When a stimulus causes depolarization, calcium ions are released from their storage sites (cisternae, or sacs abutting the longitudinal tubules of the sarcoplasmic reticulum). Large amounts also diffuse from the transverse tubules into the sarcoplasm. The calcium allows actin and myosin to link up in cross-bridges. The subsequent breaking and reforming of the cross-bridges pulls the actin and myosin filaments closer together, producing the muscle contraction.

In blood coagulation, calcium is thought to be essential in the formation of prothrombin activator by the intrinsic and extrinsic pathways, the conversion of prothrombin to thrombin, and the stabilization of fibrin threads. Calcium also is important for activation of the complement system, circulating proteins that augment the clotting process.

Calcium exists in several forms in the body. Most calcium (approximately 99%) is found in the bone. Because of this large reservoir, it is usually unnecessary to add calcium to routine IV solutions. The other 1% is located in tissue spaces and extracellular fluid.

Extracellular calcium exists in three forms. About 45% of the total calcium is ionized. Ionized calcium is the form that is important physiologically because it can leave the capillaries and enter the cells. Approximately 50% of total calcium is nonionized and bound to plasma proteins. The remaining 5%, also nonionized, is combined with substances such as citrate, phosphate, and sulfate. Calcium can be released from the bound form and converted to the ionized form. This occurs during acidosis and can cause hypercalcemia. Conversely, during alkalosis the binding of calcium increases, reducing ionization and causing hypocalcemia. The ionized portion also varies with the level of plasma proteins. That is, as plasma protein levels decrease, the serum calcium level usually decreases. For every 1 g/dl change in serum albumin, there is a 0.8 mg/dl change in serum calcium. Therefore, when assessing calcium status, it is important to assess acid–base balance and protein levels also.

Calcium is absorbed from foods in the presence of normal gastric acidity and vitamin D. About 87% of calcium excretion is via the feces and the remainder is in the urine. The serum calcium level is controlled by two feedback loops, one involving parathyroid hormone and the other involving calcitonin. (The parathyroid glands also control the serum phosphorous level inversely with calcium.) When ionized serum calcium drops, the glands secrete increased parathyroid hormone. This hormone increases calcium absorption from the gastrointestinal tract, calcium reabsorption from the renal tubule, and calcium resorption (release) from bone. The resulting rise in calcium ion concentration feeds back to lower parathyroid hormone secretion. This control mechanism is slow, taking hours to days to function. When ionized calcium rises

excessively, the thyroid gland secretes calcitonin. This substance acts quickly and briefly to inhibit calcium reabsorption from bone. Acute changes in serum calcium also are buffered by the easily exchangeable calcium in the bones and some mitochondria.

The normal total serum calcium level is 8.5–10.8 mg%. Two imbalances of calcium exist: *hypocalcemia* (calcium deficit) and *hypercalcemia* (calcium excess). Table 16–9 summarizes information on these disorders.

Hypocalcemia

Conditions characterized by decreased calcium absorption, decreased calcium ionization, or increased calcium losses may lead to hypocalcemia.

Signs and Symptoms As with potassium imbalances, signs and symptoms of hypocalcemia are easier to remember if you understand the roles calcium plays in the body.

Hypocalcemia increases neuronal membrane permeability and allows sodium to enter the cell more easily than usual, facilitating spontaneous depolarization. Although this effect occurs in both the central and peripheral nervous systems, most manifestations appear peripherally. Central nervous system manifestations include irritability and convulsions. Early peripheral nervous system signs are numbness and tingling of the extremities, circumoral tingling, hyperactive reflexes, twitching, and muscular cramps. Smooth muscle hyperactivity may cause diarrhea, nausea, and vomiting.

Spasmodic muscular contractions (tetany) also may occur. At first, tetany may be latent unless you add another stimulus to depolarization, such as tapping the nerve or causing ischemia, or unless hyperventilation-induced alkalosis reduces calcium ionization and worsens the hypocalcemia. If you tap the facial nerve just below the temporal bone anterior to the ear, the facial muscles on that side of the head may twitch. This result is called a *positive Chvostek's sign*. Similarly, you can apply a blood pressure cuff to the arm and raise its pressure slightly above the patient's systolic level. If the hand folds in, *carpal spasm* (tetany of the hand) is present. This spasm following pressure on the nerves and vessels of the upper arm is known as a *positive Trousseau's sign*. As hypocalcemia progresses to approximately 6 mg%, tetany will appear even without added stimuli. Tetany usually is fatal at about 4 mg% (Guyton 1991).

Prolonged ventricular systole is seen on the ECG as a prolonged QT interval. Hypocalcemia theoretically

TABLE 16–9

Calcium Imbalances

PREDISPOSING CONDITIONS	SIGNS AND SYMPTOMS	TREATMENT
	Hypocalcemia	
Decreased calcium absorption:	Irritability	Treatment of cause
Vitamin D deficit, hypoparathyroidism	Convulsions	Seizure precautions
Immobilization of calcium in inflamed tissues:	Numbness and tingling of the extremities	CO_2 rebreathing
Massive subcutaneous infection, generalized peritonitis	Circumoral tingling	Possible emergency tracheotomy
	Hyperactive deep tendon reflexes	Calcium administration: intravenous, oral, dietary
Increased gastrointestinal loss:	Twitching	
Diarrhea, acute pancreatitis	Muscular cramps	
Increased urinary loss:	Diarrhea, nausea, vomiting	
Diuretic phase of renal failure	Positive Chvostek's sign	
Loop diuretics	Positive Trousseau's sign	
Increased calcium binding:	Carpopedal spasms	
Massive transfusions of citrated blood	Generalized tetany	
Alkalosis	Prolonged QT interval	
	Bronchospasm	
	Hypercalcemia	
Increased calcium intake:	Lethargy	Treatment of cause
Vitamin D excess, hyperparathyroidism	Coma	Saline solutions
Decreased urinary loss:	Constipation, nausea, vomiting	Diuretics
Oliguric phase of renal failure	Hypoactive deep tendon reflexes	Sodium bicarbonate
Increased ionization:	Weakness	Phosphate administration
Acidosis	Shortened QT interval	Mithramycin
	Bradycardia, heart blocks	Dialysis
Increased reabsorption from bone:	Digitalis toxicity	Reduced digitalis doses
Prolonged immobilization	Polyuria, thirst, dehydration	Acidification of urine
Malignant tumors (with or without metastasis to bone)	Renal calculi, flank pain	
	Deep bone pain, pathologic fractures	

causes dysrhythmias, diminished cardiac contractility, and bleeding due to inadequate clotting. In reality, however, death from tetany usually occurs first.

Planning and Implementation of Care Prevent complications of hypocalcemia while you assist the physician in treating it. Implement these measures:

1. Minimize the likelihood and effects of seizures by reducing environmental stimuli and placing the patient on seizure precautions.

2. Be prepared to assist with an emergency tracheotomy if laryngospasm occurs.

3. Administer calcium gluconate, chloride, or gluceptate as ordered by the physician. Do not

NURSING DIAGNOSES

Nursing diagnoses that may apply to the patient with hypocalcemia include:

- Pain
- Altered thought processes
- Sensory-perceptual alterations
- Diarrhea

add calcium to intravenous solutions containing bicarbonate or phosphate; it will precipitate. Five percent dextrose in water is a better diluent than normal saline, because saline can further calcium loss (Terry 1991).

4. Implement medical orders aimed at removing the cause of the calcium deficit.

5. IV infusions of calcium can cause cellulitis and/or tissue sloughing, so ensure that the IV is patent prior to infusion. Do not infuse at a rate >1 ml/min (usually 1 g = 10 ml).

6. Assess calcium levels during replacement therapy.

Hypercalcemia

A calcium excess is called *hypercalcemia*. Conditions that predispose to hypercalcemia include increased calcium intake, acidosis, increased bone reabsorption, malignant tumors, and hyperthyroidism.

Signs and Symptoms A calcium excess diminishes neuromuscular excitability theoretically because the extra calcium in the cellular pores repels sodium. Decreased excitability of the central nervous system is seen as lethargy or coma. Gastrointestinal signs include constipation, nausea, and vomiting. The skeletal muscles display hypoactive deep tendon reflexes and weakness. The ECG shows a shortened QT interval, indicative of a shortened ventricular systole. Decreased impulse formation and conduction may appear as bradycardia or heart blocks. Since hypercalcemia potentiates the effects of digitalis, rhythms of digitalis toxicity may occur. Because hypercalcemia impairs glomerular filtration and the kidneys' ability to concentrate urine, polyuria occurs and leads to thirst and dehydration. Renal calculi and flank pain also may appear. In hyperparathyroidism, increased parathyroid hormone causes excessive calcium resorption from the bones, and deep bone pain and pathologic fractures may occur. The effects of hypercalcemia begin at approximately 12 mg% and worsen as the level rises. Near 17 mg%, calcium precipitates throughout the body (Guyton 1991).

Planning and Implementation of Care For hypercalcemia, include these interventions:

1. Maintain ambulation or active or passive exercises to minimize bone cavitation. Avoid rough handling or trauma, which increase bone pain and can induce pathologic fractures.

NURSING DIAGNOSES

Among the diagnoses that may apply to the patient with hypercalcemia are:

- Sensory-perceptual alterations
- Decreased CO
- Activity intolerance
- Altered urinary elimination
- Pain

2. Record intake and output. Be sure intake is at least 1,000 ml over output to prevent dehydration.

3. Encourage a fluid intake of at least 4,000 ml daily to minimize possible precipitation of calcium as renal calculi. Maintain an acid urine by encouraging the intake of foods that acidify urine (such as cranberry juice) and by preventing urinary infections, which alkalinize the urine.

4. Strain all urine for renal calculi.

5. For patients on digitalis preparations, observe closely for signs of digitalis intoxication. Ask the physician about reducing digitalis doses.

6. Restrict dietary calcium.

7. Administer pharmacologic agents as ordered. These may include calcitonin and mithramycin if the cause is bone resorption.

8. Administer intravenous or oral phosphate, if ordered by the physician, to increase calcium excretion.

9. Administer sodium chloride and furosemide as ordered to cause diuresis and calciuresis.

Outcome Evaluation

Evaluate the patient's progress toward restoration of normal calcium balance according to the following outcome criteria.

- Serum calcium level 8.5–10.8 mg%.
- Normal deep tendon reflexes, muscular strength, and irritability (for example, negative Chvostek's sign and Trousseau's sign; no carpopedal spasms or other signs of tetany).

- Gastrointestinal function and urinary output normal for patient.
- Signs or symptoms of deep bone pain, renal calculi, or pathologic fractures absent or controlled by therapy.

Magnesium Imbalances

Roles of Magnesium

Magnesium is an essential catalyst for many important enzyme systems, especially those involved with carbohydrate metabolism and protein synthesis. It also is instrumental in the maintenance of normal ionic balance, osmotic pressure, neuromuscular transmission, and bone metabolism.

Magnesium is primarily an intracellular cation; a small amount (1.5–2 mEq/L) is found extracellularly. About half of the body's total is found in bones, with the remainder in muscles, soft tissues, and body fluids. Magnesium must be ingested daily. The body's requirement usually is met through eating chlorophyll-containing vegetables, meat, milk, and fruits. Extracellular magnesium concentration is regulated by the kidneys, though the mechanism is unclear.

Hypomagnesemia and Hypermagnesemia

Information on magnesium imbalances is summarized in Table 16–10. Conditions disposing to magnesium depletion are characterized by decreased intake or absorption or increased urinary excretion. States predisposing to magnesium intoxication are less frequent: excessive parenteral nutrition administration and oliguric renal failure.

Take measures to prevent magnesium imbalances. To avoid hypomagnesemia, encourage patients on oral intake to eat magnesium-containing foods. Ask the physician about magnesium supplements for alcoholic or malnourished patients, those suffering from excessive diarrhea or diuresis, and those receiving total parenteral nutrition.

To forestall hypermagnesemia, do not give drugs containing magnesium (such as antacids containing magnesium hydroxide) to patients in oliguric renal failure. When administering magnesium sulfate intravenously, do not exceed the rate recommended by the physician and watch for the signs of magnesium intoxication.

Signs and Symptoms Recognize the signs of magnesium disorders. Magnesium depletion causes increased neuronal excitability and neuromuscular conduction and produces signs and symptoms similar to those of hypocalcemia. At a serum concentration of 1 mEq/L or less, you may see twitches, muscle cramps, convulsions, or tetany.

Magnesium intoxication is rare and usually related to decreased renal function or abuse of magnesium sulfate as a cathartic. Magnesium excess depresses neuronal excitability and neuromuscular transmission. During hypermagnesemia, peripheral vasodilatation produces flushing. Tachycardia appears initially, due to hypotension, and later changes to bradycardia. Although ECG signs are not diagnostic of this disorder, you may observe certain changes including prolonged PR intervals and longer QRS durations. Drowsiness, loss of deep tendon reflexes, and weakness occur at between 5 and 10 mEq/L; above 10 mEq/L, coma and finally cardiorespiratory arrest ensue (Porth 1990).

Planning and Implementation of Care If signs of magnesium imbalances appear, notify the physician. Magnesium depletion is treated by correcting the underlying disorder and/or administering magnesium supplements. Magnesium intoxication is treated by slowing or discontinuing the administration of magnesium-containing drugs, by diuretics, and by dialysis. When appropriate to the patient's condition, teach ways to prevent the recurrence of magnesium depletion or intoxication. For instance, provide the renal failure patient with the names of antacids that do not contain magnesium.

Outcome Evaluation

- Use these outcome criteria to evaluate the patient's progress.
- Serum magnesium level 1.5–2 mEq/L.
- Normal neuromuscular excitability and deep tendon reflexes.
- Spontaneous respirations at rate normal for patient.
- ECG within patient's normal limits.
- Magnesium-depleted patient verbalizes knowledge of foods containing magnesium, awareness of importance of eating such, and ability to purchase them at home.
- Magnesium-intoxicated (oliguric renal failure) patient states intention to avoid magnesium hydroxide and names acceptable alternative antacids.

TABLE 16–10

Magnesium Imbalances

PREDISPOSING CONDITIONS	SIGNS AND SYMPTOMS	TREATMENT
	Hypomagnesemia	
Decreased intake or absorption: malnutrition, severe diarrhea, alcoholism	Mood alterations	Increased intake of magnesium-rich foods (chlorophyll-containing vegetables, meat, milk, fruits)
Increased urinary loss: diuretic phase of renal failure, diuretics, alcoholism	Twitches, paresthesias	Magnesium supplementation (oral or intravenous)
	Muscle cramps	Treatment of cause
Hyperaldosteronism	Positive Chvostek's and Trousseau's signs	
Hyperparathyroidism	Convulsions	
	Hypermagnesemia	
Decreased urinary excretion: oliguric phase of renal failure	Nausea, vomiting	Decreased intake of magnesium-rich foods
Excessive parenteral administration	Flushing	Use of nonmagnesium antacids
	Tachycardia leading to bradycardia	Slowing or discontinuation of parenteral magnesium
	Prolonged PR interval	Intravenous calcium to counteract Mg^{++}
	Prolonged QRS	Diuretics
	Drowsiness, weakness	Dialysis
	Loss of deep tendon reflexes	
	Weakness	
	Coma	
	Cardiorespiratory arrest	

ACID–BASE IMBALANCES

Assessment

Acid–base imbalances are ubiquitous in the critically ill. Their causes, signs, and symptoms can be subtle and confusing. A hasty or simplistic interpretation of arterial blood gas values can cause you to identify acid–base disorders incorrectly. It is essential that you develop a systematic method to detect these imbalances and that you interpret blood gas values only in the context of the clinical situation. This chapter recommends a clinically useful approach consisting of the following steps:

1. Consider the patient's history, noting conditions that predispose to imbalances.

2. Next, note signs and symptoms suggesting acid–base imbalances.

3. Then, interpret the blood gases.

In order to utilize this approach, you must have a sound understanding of normal acid–base physiology

as well as acid–base pathophysiology. Accordingly, the first portion of this assessment section is devoted to a review of key concepts in acid–base physiology.

Key Physiologic Concepts

Acids, Bases, and pH An *acid* is a substance that can release a hydrogen ion (H^+) when it dissociates; a *base* is a substance that can accept a hydrogen ion. Clinically, the H^+ concentration is expressed as pH. Since pH is the negative logarithm of the H^+ concentration, pH and H^+ concentration are related inversely. In other words, as H^+ concentration rises, pH falls; a low pH thus indicates the blood is more acid than normal. Similarly, a high pH indicates the blood is less acid (more alkaline) than normal.

Human metabolic processes produce several acids. The Krebs cycle, the major source of cellular energy, forms carbon dioxide and water as end products. Carbon dioxide and water combine to form carbonic acid (H_2CO_3), which is the most plentiful body acid. Because carbon dioxide can be excreted as a gas, it is sometimes referred to as a *volatile,* or respiratory, acid. Other less plentiful body acids, such as sulfuric acid and phosphoric acid, are breakdown products released by the metabolism of proteins or fats for energy or by other body processes. Because they cannot be excreted as a gas but instead must be excreted in water, they are called *nonvolatile, fixed,* or *metabolic* acids. Other metabolic acids are lactic acid, formed by anaerobic metabolism when tissues are hypoxic, and keto acids, commonly the result of metabolic pathways used when insulin is lacking.

The primary base in the body is bicarbonate. Lesser bases include forms of hemoglobin, protein, and phosphate.

To maintain the various life processes, human cells can tolerate only minor deviations in the concentration of hydrogen ions. Three primary systems interact to maintain the pH range most suitable for cellular processes. These systems are the chemical buffers in body fluids; the lungs; and the kidneys.

Chemical Buffers A chemical buffer consists of a weak acid and its salt. Chemical buffers are important because they are the body's first line of defense against an acid–base imbalance. When excessive acid or base is present, the chemical buffer system combines with it immediately, thus preventing pronounced changes in H^+ concentration.

There are four major chemical buffers in the body fluids, of which the most important are the bicarbonate/carbonic acid system in plasma and red blood cells. Other important buffers include the oxyhemoglobin/reduced oxyhemoglobin system (in red blood cells), the plasma protein system, and the phosphate system.

A variety of bicarbonate salts participates in the carbonic acid/bicarbonate system. Extracellularly, sodium bicarbonate is most important. Lesser salts in the extracellular fluid and those present in the intracellular fluid are potassium bicarbonate, calcium bicarbonate, and magnesium bicarbonate.

Carbonic Acid/Bicarbonate Buffer System As mentioned previously, carbonic acid is formed from carbon dioxide and water. It tends to dissociate into its ions: hydrogen and bicarbonate. This system can be expressed as follows:

$$H^+ + HCO_3^- \rightleftharpoons H_2CO_3 \rightleftharpoons CO_2 + H_2O$$

An important expression of this balance is the Henderson-Hasselbach equation. This equation states that the pH equals the sum of a constant value (pK) plus the logarithm of the ratio of bicarbonate to carbonic acid:

$$pH = pK + \log HCO_3^- \text{ (mEq/L)}/H_2CO_3 \text{ (mEq/L)}$$

Carbonic acid is a weak acid and dissociates readily. Since carbonic acid exists in the body mostly as CO_2 gas, one can substitute a P_{CO_2} value in the denominator of the equation. Clinically, P_{CO_2} is measured in mm Hg; to convert that value to mEq/L, multiply by 0.03.

$$pH = pK + \log HCO_3^- \text{ (mEq/L)}/P_{CO_2} \text{ (mm Hg)} \times 0.03$$

The normal ratio between bicarbonate and carbonic acid is 20:1. Since the log of this value is 1.3 and the pK equals 6.1, their sum gives the normal pH a value of 7.4. The normal range is considered to be 7.35–7.45. It is essential to remember that the pH is determined by the *ratio* between the two values rather than the absolute amount of HCO_3^- or carbonic acid. This fact has clinical importance, as will be demonstrated.

Respiratory Buffer System When the chemical buffers are unable to maintain balance, the respiratory and renal buffer systems come into play to control the concentrations of CO_2 and HCO_3^-, respectively.

The respiratory buffer system responds to an imbalance within minutes to hours. This system controls the level of CO_2, and therefore the level of carbonic acid, in the blood. When carbonic acid increases, the lungs increase their excretion of CO_2 gas by increasing the rate and depth of ventilation. If the body needs more acid, the lungs decrease ventilation, thereby retaining CO_2 and increasing the amount of carbonic acid.

Renal Buffer System The renal buffer system responds powerfully within hours to days to an acid–base imbalance. It affects pH primarily by controlling the concentration of bicarbonate ion in the extracellular fluid. It also excretes fixed acids (which the lungs cannot eliminate).

Bicarbonate is filtered freely at the glomerulus and "reabsorbed" in the proximal and distal tubules, collecting ducts, and thick part of the loops of Henle. In addition, the kidney has two important systems for creating new bicarbonate and excreting hydrogen ions: the ammonia buffer system and the phosphate buffer system.

Classification of Acid–Base Imbalances

Acidosis and Alkalosis The classification of acid–base abnormalities can be confusing, so the basic terms will be reviewed. Two general processes can cause the pH to deviate from normal: an acidosis or alkalosis. An *acidosis* is a process that causes *acidemia,* a state in which the blood is more acid than normal. An *alkalosis* is a process that causes *alkalemia,* a state in which the blood is more alkaline (less acidic) than normal. Information about acidoses and alkaloses is shown in Tables 16–11 and 16–12 and discussed in the remainder of the chapter.

Overview of Imbalances

The patient's history can provide valuable information in identifying acid–base disorders. Tables 16–11 and 16–12 give examples of significant conditions to note when reviewing the patient's history. The following paragraphs relate the types of acid–base disorders to predisposing conditions.

Single Disorders   An *acidosis* is present when there is an *acid excess or a base deficit* in the body, causing the blood's pH to be below 7.35. The acid excess can be a carbonic acid excess (in which case the condition is called *respiratory acidosis*) or a metabolic acid excess *(metabolic acidosis)*. A base deficit can occur only from metabolic causes, such as the loss of alkaline fluids via a fistula of the lower gastrointestinal tract.

TABLE 16–11

Respiratory and Metabolic Acidosis

PREDISPOSING CONDITIONS	SIGNS AND SYMPTOMS	TREATMENT
	Respiratory Acidosis	
Carbon Dioxide Retention		
Bronchial obstruction, chronic obstructive pulmonary disease	Hypoventilation (primary)	None (if compensated in chronic pulmonary disease)
Inadequate mechanical ventilation	Headache	Treatment of cause
Central nervous system depression (example: narcotic poisoning)	Restlessness, apprehension	Increased CO_2 elimination (by suctioning, aggressive pulmonary hygiene, or mechanical ventilation [cautiously to avoid alkalosis])
	Drowsiness, confusion, coma	
Neuromuscular disorders affecting respiration (example: poliomyelitis)	Acute respiratory failure	
	Hyperkalemia (peaked T waves, twitching, etc.)	Bicarbonate replacement
	Hypercalcemia (weakness, lethargy, flapping tremors, etc.)	Treatment of electrolyte imbalances
	Blood gas changes:	
	pH ↓	
	P_{CO_2} ↑	
	HCO_3^- normal or ↑	
	Metabolic Acidosis	
Excessive Metabolic Acids		
Starvation	Hyperventilation (compensatory)	Treatment of cause
Diabetic ketoacidosis	Headache	Bicarbonate replacement
Lactic acidosis	Drowsiness, confusion, coma	Treatment of electrolyte imbalances
Renal failure	Nausea, vomiting	
Hyperkalemia	Hyperkalemia	
	Hypercalcemia	
	Blood gas changes:	
	pH ↓	
	HCO_3^- ↓	
	P_{CO_2} normal or ↓	
Loss of Alkali		
Diarrhea		
Fistulas of lower gastrointestinal tract		
Chloride excess		

TABLE 16–12

Respiratory and Metabolic Alkalosis

PREDISPOSING CONDITIONS	SIGNS AND SYMPTOMS	TREATMENT
	Respiratory Alkalosis	
Increased CO$_2$ Excretion		
Hypoxia	Hyperventilation (primary)	Treatment of cause
Excessive mechanical ventilation	Giddiness, dizziness, syncope, convulsions, coma	Increased CO$_2$ retention (by decreased mechanical ventilation, breathing into paper bag, sedation, or 3–5% CO$_2$ administration)
Central nervous system stimulation (examples: pain, anxiety, hysteria, brainstem damage)	Hypokalemia (weakness, paresthesias, etc.)	
	Hypocalcemia (tingling, numbness, twitching, carpopedal spasms, tetany, convulsions, etc.)	Treatment of electrolyte imbalances
	Cardiac dysrhythmias	
	Blood gas changes: pH ↑ Pco$_2$ ↓ HCO$_3^-$ normal or ↓	
	Metabolic Alkalosis	
Loss of Metabolic Acids		
Nasogastric drainage	Hypoventilation (compensatory)	Treatment of cause
Vomiting	Hypokalemia	Increased H$^+$ retention (by administration of KCl)
Hypokalemia	Hypocalcemia	
Steroid administration	Cardiac dysrhythmias	Increased bicarbonate excretion (by administration of acetazolamide (Diamox) or ammonium chloride)
	Blood gas changes: pH ↑ HCO$_3^-$ ↑ Pco$_2$ normal or ↑	Treatment of electrolyte imbalances
Excessive Intake or Retention of Alkali		
Excessive sodium bicarbonate administration		
Chloride depletion: Diuretics		
Low-salt diet without chloride supplementation		

An *alkalosis* is present when there is either an *acid deficit or a base excess* in the body, causing the pH to be above 7.45. The acid deficit can be a carbonic acid deficit *(respiratory alkalosis)* or a metabolic acid deficit *(metabolic alkalosis)*. A base excess can occur only from metabolic causes (such as increased bicarbonate retention because of a chloride deficit) or from an exogenous source—for example, excessive infusion of sodium bicarbonate.

Respiratory acidosis, metabolic acidosis, respiratory alkalosis, and metabolic alkalosis are the four primary acid–base disorders.

Compensation When a primary disorder first occurs, it causes an abnormal pH and an abnormal value for the parameter associated with the system causing the imbalance. For instance, a respiratory acidosis causes an abnormal increase in Pco$_2$ and a resultant decrease in pH. The other value (in this case, HCO$_3^-$) is normal initially. At this point, the disorder is called *acute* or *uncompensated*. As time goes on, the system not causing the problem tries to compensate for it by altering its parameter to return the ratio of bicarbonate/carbonic acid to the normal 20:1; in this example, the kidney retains bicarbonate. If the alter-

TABLE 16–13

Mixed Disorders

COMBINATION	EXAMPLES	MECHANISMS
Mixed acidoses	Cardiac arrest Severe hypoventilation	Absent ventilation or hypoventilation→respiratory acidosis Hypoxemia→anaerobic metabolism→metabolic (lactic) acidosis
Mixed alkaloses	Patient with compensated respiratory acidosis rapidly and excessively mechanically ventilated	Elevated bicarbonate level→metabolic alkalosis Hyperventilation→respiratory alkalosis
Respiratory acidosis and metabolic alkalosis	Chronic obstructive pulmonary disease plus diuretics or low-salt diet without chloride replacement	Chronic obstructive pulmonary disease→respiratory acidosis Chloride depletion→obligatory bicarbonate retention→metabolic alkalosis
Respiratory alkalosis and metabolic acidosis	Hepatic and renal failure	Liver failure→toxic metabolites→hyperventilation →respiratory alkalosis Kidney failure→ ↓ H^+ excretion and ↓ bicarbonate production→metabolic acidosis

ation *is not* sufficient to return the pH to normal, the disorder is *partially compensated*. At this point, the pH, Pco_2 and HCO^-_3 all are abnormal. If the alteration *is* sufficient to restore a more normal ratio and hence a normal pH, the condition is called *chronic* or *fully compensated*. In this stage, the pH is normal but both the Pco_2 and HCO^-_3 values still are abnormal. Although their ratio causes the pH to be within the normal range, the pH usually tends more toward the acidic or alkaline end of the range, depending on the primary process.

In general, the pulmonary and renal systems compensate for each other. The renal system compensates for respiratory disorders by altering bicarbonate retention and hydrogen ion secretion. In respiratory acidosis, the kidneys compensate by increasing bicarbonate retention and accelerating hydrogen secretion. In respiratory alkalosis, the kidneys decrease bicarbonate retention and hydrogen secretion.

The lungs compensate for metabolic acid–base imbalances by varying CO_2 excretion. In metabolic acidosis, stimulation of the respiratory center increases the rate and depth of ventilation, so increased CO_2 is blown off. This compensation is limited, however: a falling Pco_2 eventually causes respiratory depression, returning Pco_2 toward normal. In metabolic alkalosis, the lungs decrease ventilation and therefore retain CO_2. Respiratory compensation for metabolic alkalosis also is limited, however. At a Pco_2

of about 60 mm Hg in most people, the hypoxic stimulus to respiration becomes dominant. This stimulus increases ventilation toward normal.

As mentioned earlier, the lungs respond to acid–base imbalances within minutes, while the kidneys take hours. As a result, compensation for metabolic imbalances occurs faster than compensation for respiratory imbalances.

Mixed Disorders   If two disorders occur simultaneously, the patient suffers from a *mixed disorder (mixed disturbance)*. There are four mixed disturbances (Table 16–13). Mixed disturbances result from either two processes with similar effects on the pH (such as respiratory and metabolic acidosis in cardiac arrest) or two processes with opposite effects on the pH (such as respiratory acidosis and metabolic alkalosis in the patient with chronic lung disease who is on diuretics).

Signs and Symptoms

Assess the patient for the clinical signs and symptoms of acid–base imbalances as described in the following sections.

Altered Level of Consciousness   Cerebral status changes result from alterations in cerebrospinal fluid pH. Confusion and coma often are present in acidosis, while dizziness and giddiness are more characteristic of alkalosis. Because CO_2 crosses the blood–brain barrier more quickly than HCO_3^- ions, these symptoms occur sooner in respiratory disorders than in metabolic ones.

Assess cerebral status by checking orientation to day, time, and location; ability to follow simple commands; and presence of dizziness or lightheadedness.

Ineffective Breathing Pattern Evaluation of ventilatory changes can be confusing, since they may either cause or compensate for acid–base imbalances. Hyperventilation can cause respiratory alkalosis or compensate for metabolic acidosis, in each case by increasing CO_2 elimination. Hypoventilation can cause respiratory acidosis or compensate for metabolic alkalosis, in each case by increasing CO_2 retention. Acid–base imbalances affect the respiratory center by altering the pH of arterial blood and cerebrospinal fluid. Acidosis lowers the pH, stimulates the respiratory center, and produces hyperventilation. Alkalosis raises cerebrospinal fluid pH and produces hypoventilation. To detect hypoventilation or hyperventilation, evaluate the rate and depth of respiration.

Respiratory failure may occur in acute respiratory acidosis when the P_{CO_2} reaches 60 mm Hg. A patient with chronic hypercapnia, however, may tolerate a P_{CO_2} above 60 mm Hg without developing acute respiratory failure. Because the slow development of hypercapnia has allowed time for the kidneys to increase the serum bicarbonate level in compensation, the chronic patient can maintain a more normal pH than an acutely afflicted person.

Impaired Gas Exchange or Tissue Perfusion Dysrhythmias, angina, or shock may result from hypoxia or from the electrolyte imbalances discussed later. Both acidosis and alkalosis cause shifts of the oxyhemoglobin dissociation curve. In alkalosis, the curve shifts to the left, decreasing dissociation of oxygen from hemoglobin. This effect contributes to tissue hypoxia. Acidosis shifts the curve to the right, so that hemoglobin releases oxygen more readily. However, acidosis also decreases responsiveness to catecholamines, which in turn can decrease myocardial contractility and dilate arterioles. As a result, less efficient circulation of the blood may counterbalance the increased availability of oxygen in the blood.

To detect dysrhythmias, angina, or shock, implement the following measures. Auscultate the apical pulse for irregularities and the presence of gallops or murmurs. Monitor the ECG for signs of new or increasing atrial or ventricular dysrhythmias. Also

monitor perfusion to the brain, heart, kidneys, and extremities.

Arterial Blood Gas Analysis

Definitive diagnosis of acid–base imbalances depends on arterial blood gas values. The values important in acid–base interpretation are the pH, P_{CO_2}, and a measure of base (HCO_3^- or base excess). Base excess, the preferred measure of metabolic activity, includes both bicarbonate and other buffer anions of whole blood, such as those of hemoglobin and plasma proteins. (It is reported as base mEq/L above or below the normal range of buffer base. Thus, a negative base excess actually means a base deficit.) When evaluating a patient's blood gases, always compare the reported values to the normals for your institution. Also compare them to the actual or expected normal values for your patient, as indicated by previous measurements or pre-existing conditions such as chronic obstructive pulmonary disease.

pH First evaluate the general acid–base status by examining the pH. The normal range is 7.35–7.45. If the value is lower than normal (below 7.35), an acidosis is present. If the value is elevated (above 7.45), an alkalosis is present. If the value is within the normal range, there are two possibilities: The patient could have a normal balance or a compensated abnormality. Since you cannot tell which situation exists from examining the pH alone, just note at this point whether the value is normal and, if so, whether it falls more toward the acid side of the normal range or more toward the alkaline side.

P_{CO_2} Evaluate the respiratory parameter by examining the P_{CO_2}. The normal range is 35–45 mm Hg. Decide whether the value is normal, elevated above 45 and therefore tending to make the blood acidic, or decreased below 35 and therefore tending to make the blood alkaline.

HCO_3^- or Base Excess Evaluate the metabolic parameter by examining the HCO_3^- or base excess. Normal ranges are 23–28 mEq/L for HCO_3^- and +2.5 to −2.5 for base excess. Decide whether the value is normal, elevated and therefore tending to make blood alkaline, or decreased and therefore tending to make the blood acidic. (For the sake of simplicity, only one measure of base is given in the following examples.)

Next, compare the pH, P_{CO_2}, and base value to each other. Since blood gas values can indicate a variety of disorders and stages of compensation, a given set of numbers may be compatible with more than one interpretation. Explain *each* value, considering *all* the possible interpretations.

After considering the possible interpretations of the values, choose the most probable one for your patient, based on the clues from the other patient data and the likelihood of a given disorder.

Following are principles and examples illustrating interpretation of acid–base values.

Abnormal pH and Abnormal Pco_2 or HCO_3^- If only the pH and one other value are abnormal, the blood gases indicate an acute primary disorder. You can identify the disorder by deciding which process the pH represents and which other value (the Pco_2 or HCO_3^-) is abnormal. For example:

pH 7.32
Pco_2 50 mm Hg
HCO_3^- 24 mEq/L

The pH is decreased, telling you that an acidosis is present. The HCO_3^- is normal, so a metabolic problem cannot be the cause. The Pco_2 is elevated, making the blood more acidic. The values thus indicate an acute respiratory acidosis.

Note that in this example the pH and the Pco_2 are changing in *opposite* directions. This example thus illustrates one of two *rules of thumb* that can help you to identify quickly the type of disturbance present:

1. *If the pH and Pco_2 are changing in opposite directions, a respiratory disorder is present.*

2. *If the pH and HCO_3^- are changing in the same direction, a metabolic disorder is present.*

Abnormal pH, Abnormal Pco_2, and Abnormal HCO_3^- If all three values are abnormal, they often indicate a primary disorder with incomplete compensation. For example:

pH 7.30
Pco_2 25 mm Hg
HCO_3^- 12 mEq/L

The pH is decreased, again telling you that an acidosis is present. The Pco_2 is decreased, tending to make the blood alkaline. The HCO_3^- is decreased, tending to make the blood acidic. As the pH and HCO_3^- are changing in the *same* direction, a metabolic disorder is present (second *rule of thumb*). The Pco_2 is decreased because the body is attempting to compensate for the disorder, but as the pH is still abnormal only partial compensation is present. The values thus indicate partially compensated metabolic acidosis.

Note that in this example, the Pco_2 and the HCO_3^- are changing in the *same* direction. This example illustrates a third *rule of thumb:*

3. *If the Pco_2 and the HCO_3^- are changing in the same direction, the body is compensating for an imbalance.*

(In this example, as the pH still is abnormal, the imbalance is only partially compensated.)

Normal pH, Abnormal Pco_2, and Abnormal HCO_3^- If the pH is normal but both the Pco_2 and the HCO_3^- are not, the values usually indicate a fully compensated primary disturbance. Determining whether the pH lies more toward the acid or the alkaline end of the normal range will help you decide whether the imbalance is an acidosis or alkalosis. For example:

pH 7.42
Pco_2 50 mm Hg
HCO_3^- 32 mEq/L

The pH is normal but more toward the alkaline end of the range. The Pco_2 is elevated, tending to make the blood acidic. The HCO_3^- is elevated, tending to make the blood alkaline. The values represent a metabolic alkalosis compensated by increased CO_2 retention.

This example also illustrates the third rule of thumb: If the Pco_2 and the HCO_3^- are changing in the same direction, the body is compensating for an imbalance. In this case, however, as the pH is normal, the imbalance is fully compensated.

Mixed Disorders At times, a patient will have both a respiratory and a metabolic imbalance present. Depending on the clinical circumstances, a combined or mixed disorder may consist of two acidoses, two alkaloses, or an acidosis plus an alkalosis. For example:

pH 7.20
Pco_2 55 mm Hg
HCO_3^- 20 mEq/L

The pH identifies the presence of a severe acidosis. The *pH* and *Pco_2* are changing in *opposite* directions, so a respiratory disorder is present (first rule). However, the *pH* and the *HCO_3^-* are changing in the *same* direction, so a metabolic disorder also is present (second rule). The values therefore indicate a mixed respiratory and metabolic acidosis. Such a combination may be seen in cardiac arrest, where respiratory acidosis may be present due to inadequate ventilation and metabolic acidosis may be present due to inadequate tissue oxygenation. This example illustrates a fourth *rule of thumb:*

4. *If the* Pco$_2$ *and the* HCO$_3^-$ *are changing in opposite directions, a mixed imbalance is present.*

Venous Acid–Base Values Thus far, we have been discussing arterial values. In some cases, an arterial blood sample may be unavailable and values may be determined instead on a mixed venous sample. Normally, the venous Pco$_2$ is slightly higher (40–50 venous versus 35–45 arterial), and the pH slightly lower (7.31–7.41 versus 7.35–7.45) than arterial blood. Venous bicarbonate and base excess values are about the same as arterial values.

Electrolyte Imbalances

Accurate diagnosis of acid–base imbalances requires arterial blood gas values, as already explained. However, a certain amount of information about acid–base imbalances can be gleaned from signs and symptoms of electrolyte imbalances and from the serum electrolyte panel routinely obtained on patients. This panel typically includes values for serum sodium, potassium, chloride, and CO$_2$ content. The following sections describe the complex interrelationships between acid–base balance and electrolyte balance.

Sodium (Na$^+$) Because there is so much sodium in the extracellular space, shifts in acid–base balance do not affect sodium balance significantly. An increased serum sodium level also does not affect acid–base balance much. A decreased serum sodium level, however, can be associated with great derangements in acid–base balance. The sodium deficit does not cause the derangements directly; the culprit is the accompanying chloride deficit. You may remember that the kidney can reabsorb sodium in three ways: with the negative chloride ion, with the negative bicarbonate ion, or in exchange for the positive potassium or hydrogen ion. In the presence of a depletion of both sodium chloride and water (such as in hypovolemic shock), the kidney will have a potent stimulus for sodium reabsorption. As relatively little chloride will be available in this situation, the kidney will reabsorb an increased percentage of the sodium with bicarbonate and an increased percentage in exchange for H$^+$ or potassium. Thus, hyponatremia, through its relationship to hypochloremia, may be associated with alkalosis and hypokalemia.

Potassium (K$^+$) Acid–base and potassium balance profoundly affect each other. Acidosis often is accom-

panied by hyperkalemia and alkalosis by hypokalemia. These associations are due to two mechanisms: exchange of potassium and hydrogen ions across the cell membrane, and altered renal excretion of potassium and hydrogen.

The body's cells contain buffer systems that can either accept or donate H$^+$ ions. H$^+$ ions and K$^+$ ions freely exchange across the cell membrane. Because the amount of extracellular K$^+$ is quite small compared to the intracellular amount, even small shifts of K$^+$ across the cell membrane cause significant changes in the serum level. In acidosis, excess H$^+$ ions in the serum migrate into the cell, where their buffering displaces K$^+$ ions. To maintain intracellular electrical balance, the K$^+$ ions diffuse out into the serum. As a result, acidosis can cause hyperkalemia. The Na$^+$/K$^+$/H$^+$ ion exchange mechanism in the kidney also plays a role in the interrelationships of K$^+$ imbalances and acid–base imbalances. In the kidney, Na$^+$ ions normally are retained in exchange for K$^+$ or H$^+$ ions. In acidosis, because H$^+$ ions are more abundant, the kidney tends to excrete H$^+$ ions rather than K$^+$ ions in exchange for sodium. As the excess H$^+$ ions block the secretion of K$^+$, hyperkalemia develops.

In alkalosis, the opposite situation exists. The intracellular buffers dissociate to release H$^+$ ions. As they move out of the cell, K$^+$ ions move in. Thus, alkalosis can cause hypokalemia. In addition, the kidney tends to retain H$^+$ ions, instead excreting K$^+$ in exchange for Na$^+$. This preferential retention of H$^+$ ions helps to compensate for the alkalosis, but it does so at the expense of further contributing to hypokalemia.

In contrast to the above situations, in which acid–base imbalances cause K$^+$ imbalances, the converse can also exist; that is, K$^+$ imbalances can cause acid–base imbalances. Hyperkalemia causes more K$^+$ ions to move intracellularly, displacing H$^+$ ions into the serum and producing acidosis. In the kidney, more K$^+$ ions are exchanged for Na$^+$, and the retention of H$^+$ ions increases the acidosis. Hypokalemia favors the transmembrane shift of K$^+$ ions in the opposite direction from hyperkalemia—that is, from the cell into the serum. To maintain intracellular electrical balance, more H$^+$ ions then move into the cell, leaving the serum alkalotic. In the kidney, fewer K$^+$ ions are available for exchange, so more H$^+$ ions are excreted, and the alkalosis deepens.

The signs, symptoms, and treatment of potassium imbalances are discussed in detail earlier in this chapter.

Calcium (Ca^{++}) Serum calcium exists in both ionized and nonionized forms. The ionized form is physiologically active. Calcium ionization increases in acidosis and decreases in alkalosis. As a result, an acidotic patient may have signs of hypercalcemia, while an alkalotic person often shows signs of hypocalcemia. Acidosis can mask hypocalcemia because of its ability to increase calcium ionization. When the acidosis is treated and pH returns to normal, twitching, convulsions, paresthesias, carpopedal spasms, tetany, and other signs of hypocalcemia may become evident.

For a complete discussion of signs, symptoms, and treatment of calcium imbalances, refer to this chapter's section on electrolyte imbalances.

Chloride (Cl⁻) Chloride is primarily an extracellular anion. Its serum concentration varies inversely with bicarbonate for two reasons: (a) it shifts across the cell membrane during buffering in exchange for bicarbonate (the chloride shift); and (b) renal absorption of chloride varies inversely with reabsorption of bicarbonate. For these reasons, hypochloremia can cause metabolic alkalosis, and vice versa; hyperchloremia can cause metabolic acidosis, and vice versa. The interrelationship of hypochloremia and metabolic alkalosis is particularly important clinically. As mentioned in the section on sodium, if insufficient chloride is present in the renal tubules, the kidney will reabsorb an increased proportion of sodium with bicarbonate, causing a metabolic alkalosis.

If the hypochloremic, alkalotic patient also has a stimulus for avid sodium retention, a vicious cycle may develop in which the electrolyte and acid–base imbalances reinforce each other. A clinical example is the person with chronic congestive heart failure who is on a low-salt diet without adequate chloride replacement. The abnormal volume regulation causes an intense stimulus for sodium reabsorption. Because of chloride depletion, an increased percentage of sodium will be reabsorbed with bicarbonate; the stimulus for sodium retention overrides the body's need to reduce alkali, and alkalemia worsens. As there also may be an increased renal exchange of potassium for sodium, hypokalemia may worsen also.

Serum Electrolyte Summary Because the changes in electrolyte balance are difficult to remember, they are summarized here.

The normal serum sodium level is 135–145 mEq/L. Hyponatremia, through its relation to hypochloremia, often is associated with alkalosis.

The usual serum potassium concentration is 3.5–5.5 mEq/L. Hyperkalemia often is present in acidosis or recovery from alkalosis. Hypokalemia may be associated with alkalosis or recovery from acidosis. A normal serum potassium may be present in the previously hypokalemic patient who becomes acidotic.

The normal serum calcium level is 8.5–10.8 mg/100

ml. Hypercalcemia may be present in acidosis and hypocalcemia in alkalosis.

The normal serum chloride concentration is 96–106 mEq/L. Hyperchloremia may be present in acidosis; hypochloremia frequently is associated with alkalosis.

CO₂ Content As mentioned earlier, the serum electrolyte panel usually includes a measurement of CO_2 content. CO_2 content consists of about 95% bicarbonate and 5% carbonic acid. It thus can reflect metabolic and/or respiratory activity. The normal CO_2 content is 24–30 mEq/L. CO_2 content is increased in respiratory acidosis and metabolic alkalosis. It is decreased in metabolic acidosis and respiratory alkalosis. Because of its relatively nonspecific nature, the CO_2 content value can indicate only that an acid–base abnormality is present. It cannot indicate whether that abnormality is an acidosis or alkalosis, nor can it pinpoint whether respiratory or metabolic dysfunction is at fault. To identify the type of imbalance, arterial blood gas values should be analyzed.

Anion Gap The serum electrolyte report can provide you with another useful clue to acid–base imbalance— called the *anion gap*, or delta—which helps differentiate the mechanisms of metabolic acidosis.

The anion gap is an expression of the excess unmeasurable anions in the body (the phosphate, sulfate, and other organic anions). To derive the value, add the bicarbonate and the chloride values (to get a sum of the measured anions) and subtract this sum from the Na⁺ level (the measured cation). The normal difference is 8–16 mEq/L. For example, if Na is 140, HCO_3^- 20, and chloride 100:

$$20 + 100 = 120$$

$$140 - 120 = 20 \text{ mEq of unmeasurable anions}$$

This value indicates there is an elevation of the unmeasurable anions in this patient.

The anion gap increases in metabolic acidosis resulting from an abnormal increase in organic acids. Examples are starvation, diabetic ketoacidosis, and lactic acidosis. The anion gap remains normal in metabolic acidosis owing to bicarbonate loss (for example, in diarrhea or lower gastrointestinal fistulas) or administration of chloride-containing acids, such as ammonium chloride.

Other Laboratory Data

Other laboratory data also may provide clues to causes of acid–base disturbances. For instance, an elevated blood urea nitrogen would suggest renal failure and possible metabolic acidosis, while abnormal pulmonary function tests would suggest potential respiratory acid–base imbalances.

NURSING DIAGNOSES

As is apparent from the earlier discussion of signs and symptoms, the most frequent nursing diagnoses for a patient with an acid–base imbalance are:

- Sensory-perceptual alteration
- Ineffective breathing pattern
- Altered tissue perfusion

Nursing measures for these diagnoses are discussed in detail in Chapters 3, 9, and 13.

Planning and Implementation of Care

Collaborate with the physician to relieve both the causes and the effects of acid–base disturbances.

Respiratory Acidosis

If the patient has a compensated respiratory acidosis from chronic pulmonary disease and is asymptomatic, no treatment is necessary.

Should the acidosis be acute and/or symptomatic, treatment is directed toward removing the cause. The nurse plays a major role in judicious use of a vigorous regimen of pulmonary hygiene to clear secretions and promote optimal ventilation. Mechanical ventilation may be necessary to lower the P_{CO_2} and maintain ventilation. If so, it must be provided cautiously. Excessive lowering of the P_{CO_2} can precipitate respiratory alkalosis. Also, if renal compensation is underway, a too-rapid lowering of the P_{CO_2} (before the elevated HCO_3^- level has time to decrease) can precipitate metabolic alkalosis.

Bicarbonate administration may be indicated if the acidosis is severe. Any electrolyte imbalances present also may require treatment. For example, significant hyperkalemia may necessitate insulin and dextrose infusions, ion exchange resins, or dialysis.

Metabolic Acidosis Treatment of metabolic acidosis involves both therapy of the underlying disorder and bicarbonate replacement. Treating the underlying disorder involves such activities as insulin and glucose administration in diabetic ketoacidosis, improvement of oxygenation in lactic acidosis so that aerobic metabolism can resume, and so on.

Respiratory Alkalosis

Respiratory alkalosis is treated by reducing the patient's need to hyperventilate. For example, correction of an underlying hypoxia often will restore the respiratory pattern, and therefore the P_{CO_2}, to normal. If the patient is being mechanically ventilated, decreasing the rate or tidal volume or adding extra tubing (to increase deadspace) will cause the P_{CO_2} to rise. Should the hyperventilation result from emotional excitement, having the person breathe into a paper bag is a convenient way to restore normal P_{CO_2} and eliminate the frightening symptoms of numbness, tingling, lightheadedness, and so on. This intervention must be followed by counseling to help the person become aware of the role he or she plays in inducing symptoms and to relieve emotional stress.

Metabolic Alkalosis

Metabolic alkalosis is treated by removing the underlying cause, promoting hydrogen retention, and by enhancing bicarbonate excretion. Examples of treating the underlying problem are relieving prolonged vomiting and replacing fluid and electrolytes lost through nasogastric suction. Depending on the patient's electrolyte status, hydrogen retention and bicarbonate excretion may be promoted by the administration of potassium chloride, acetazolamide, or ammonium chloride. If symptoms of calcium deficiency are present due to the decrease in ionized calcium, calcium gluconate may be given intravenously.

Mixed Disorders

Treatment of mixed disorders combines the principles governing the treatment of each individual disorder. For instance, to relieve a combined respiratory and metabolic acidosis due to severe hypoventilation, you must improve both ventilation (to relieve the respiratory acidosis) and oxygenation and circulation (to relieve the lactic acidosis). The combination of two acidoses or two alkaloses must be treated promptly and vigorously. They tend to block compensation for each other and thus produce severe acid–base and electrolyte disturbances. The combination of an acidosis and an alkalosis is tolerated better by the body. They tend to have opposite effects on the bicarbonate/carbonic acid ratio and thus produce a nearly normal pH.

General Nursing Care Measures

In addition to the measures specific to the acid–base disturbance(s), the nurse should provide the more general nursing care related to cerebral status changes; respiratory changes; and dysrhythmias, angina, or shock. For instance, for the confused patient, provide a safe environment, orient him or her to reality, and reassure him or her that the confusion probably will disappear as the condition is treated. Place the hyperventilating patient in a position that does not compromise diaphragmatic excursion. Decrease angina by assisting the person with activities of daily living to reduce myocardial workload. For more ideas on how to help these patients, review other chapters related to these symptoms.

Outcome Evaluation

Evaluate the patient's progress toward a healthy acid–base status. Judge the effectiveness of care by the following outcome criteria:

- Level of consciousness restored to preimbalance state.
- Respiratory rate and tidal volume WNL for patient.
- Cardiac rate and rhythm WNL for patient.
- Extremities warm and dry (and pink if the patient is Caucasian).
- Serum electrolytes WNL for patient.
- Arterial blood gases WNL for patient.

REFERENCES

Crabtree A, Jorgenson M: Exploring the practical knowledge in expert critical-care nursing practice. Unpublished master's thesis, University of Wisconsin, Madison, 1986.

Gotch P: The endocrine system. In *Core curriculum for critical care nursing,* 4th ed. Alspach J (ed). Philadelphia: Saunders, 1991.

Guyton A: *Textbook of medical physiology,* 8th ed. Philadelphia: Saunders, 1991.

Marriott H: *ECG/PDQ.* Maryland: Williams & Wilkins, 1987.

Porth CM: *Pathophysiology, concepts of altered health states,* 3d ed. Philadelphia: Lippincott, 1990.

Terry J: The other electrolytes: Magnesium, calcium, and phosphorus. *J Intravenous Nurs* 1991; 3(14):167–176.

17

Endocrine/Metabolic Disorders

CLINICAL INSIGHT

Domain: Effective management of rapidly changing situations

Competency: Identifying and managing a patient crisis until physician assistance is available

Because of the swiftness with which crises occur and the physician's inability to be continually at the bedside, critical-care nurses often must manage patient crises until physician assistance is available. Functioning with aplomb in these situations requires an amalgam of nursing and medical knowledge, gleaned during on-the-job training and polished by practice. Because delay or misjudgments can have severe repercussions, the nurse who can function with poise in the face of an ongoing crisis is a special nurse, as this exemplar from Benner (1984, pp. 116–117) shows.

I came on duty at 3 P.M. and was assigned to a fresh postop open heart surgery. The patient had returned to the ICU around 11 A.M. that day and had all the usual paraphernalia for postops—IVs, respirator, chest tubes, Foley catheters, etc. The patient had had a lot of IV fluid and blood replacement on days—this is the usual procedure for open heart surgery—give lots of fluid at first (usually have had mannitol), then level off. Blood pressure will drop as the patient begins to warm up and dilate peripherally, but will usually level off soon. However, this patient continued to be hypovolemic—low blood pressure, low central venous pressure—and was diuresing in enormous amounts. We were pouring fluids in, in an attempt to catch up, but were managing, barely, to stay even with output. Clearly something was amiss here. I telephoned the surgeon's exchange but was not able to locate him. I tried also to contact the assistant, but he was off call to another doctor who was not terribly familiar with open heart surgery. Meanwhile, we were pouring in fluids, blood and packed cells, without orders, just to stay even, for the patient was continuing this diuresis. I began reviewing the possible causes for this and decided a likely one was hyperglycemia. I then ordered a blood glucose level and the results came back—more than 600 mg percent. About this time the assistant surgeon had come back on call and I was finally able to contact him. He prescribed on the basis of the blood glucose level and we were then able to stabilize the patient.

The *endocrine system* regulates the secretion of hormones that alter metabolic function. *Metabolism* refers to the cellular processes that support the functions of the human body. Endocrine and metabolic disorders are common in critical-care units and are often secondary to other disorders. The nurse must be intimately familiar with this system and alert to its possible dysfunction, as illustrated in the Clinical Insight.

Overview

The endocrine system exerts its effect through hormones, or chemical messengers, transported through body fluids. Most hormones are synthesized by endocrine glands, secreted into the bloodstream, and subsequently transported to target organs or cells where they exert their action. However, some hormones reach the target organ through neurotransmission.

Hormones act by affecting the rate of cellular and organ responses; they do not initiate reactions. Most hormones circulate in the body in greater or lesser amounts depending on body need.

Control of hormone secretion varies. Some hormones are controlled by negative feedback, that is, as body levels increase, the stimulus for secretion decreases. Some hormones, like insulin, are secreted in response to the presence of metabolic substrates.

Although it is beyond the scope of this text to discuss the entire endocrine system, Figure 17–1 presents a graphic overview of its major components. It can be seen that the hypothalamus and pituitary are central to a majority of hormones. The hypothalamus regulates the system by secreting "releasing or inhibiting" hormones which then stimulate the pituitary. Notice also that the adrenal medulla (site of formation and release of epinephrine and norepinephrine) has a direct connection to the central nervous system (CNS). And finally, notice that the parathyroids and the pancreas are endocrine glands that have locally controlled hormone release mechanisms and do not have nervous system connections.

This chapter provides the critical-care nurse with an understanding of seven common endocrine/metabolic disorders, associated nursing care, and therapeutic techniques affecting endocrine/metabolic function.

DIABETIC KETOACIDOSIS

Assessment

Pathophysiology

Diabetic ketoacidosis (DKA) is an emergency condition resulting from inadequate amounts of insulin. Insulin, secreted by the pancreatic islet cells, is an anabolic hormone that facilitates the transport of glucose into cells for metabolic processes and inhibits the breakdown of glycogen stores, fats, and proteins (Yeates and Blaufuss 1990).

Diabetic ketoacidosis is one of three emergencies that may affect diabetic patients; the other two, hyperglycemic, hyperosmolar nonketotic coma and hypoglycemia, are discussed in later sections. It is important for the critical-care nurse to understand in detail the major pathophysiologic mechanisms that occur in these disorders. Table 17–1 compares the pathophysiologic mechanisms, serum glucose levels, and ketone levels in these three conditions. Insulin lack causes complex physiologic derangements, the most important of which follow.

Hyperglycemia and Hyperosmolarity Decreased cellular uptake of glucose results in increased serum glucose concentration (hyperglycemia), which in turn increases overall serum concentration (hyperosmolarity).

Dehydration The increased osmolarity provokes a fluid shift from the intracellular to the extracellular space as a compensatory mechanism to dilute the excess glucose. This fluid shift, which causes intracellular dehydration, is ineffective because it is counter-

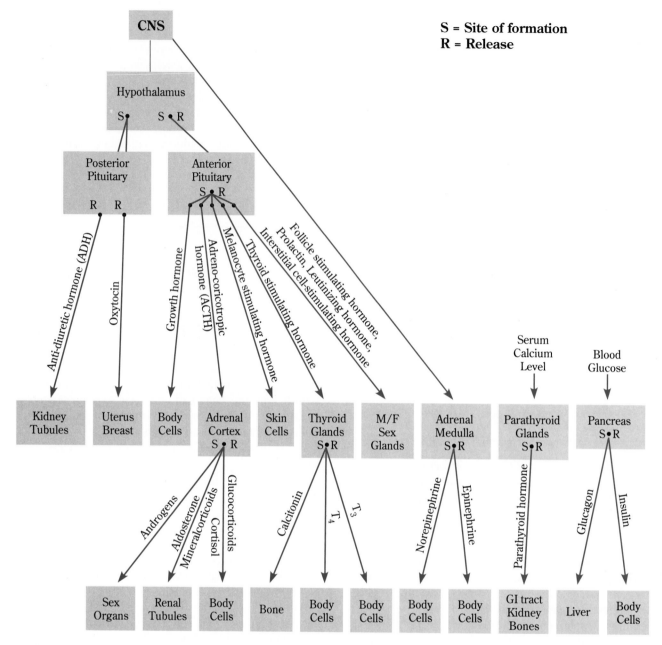

FIGURE 17–1

Endocrine hormones. *S,* Site of formation. *R,* Release. (Developed by Edward Glowgowski, RN, MS.)

acted by another compensatory mechanism, increased renal excretion of glucose. When glomerular filtration of glucose exceeds the transport maximum, glucose is spilled into the urine. This event usually occurs when the serum glucose level is greater than 180 mg/dl. The increased renal filtration of glucose is an important protective mechanism, but the glucose in the renal tubular filtrate increases osmotic pressure and pro-

vokes osmotic diuresis. The resulting extracellular volume depletion worsens dehydration and can result in hypovolemic shock.

Ketoacidosis Acidosis occurs as lipids used for metabolism yield keto acids. Because no carbohydrates are being metabolized, lipolysis (breakdown of fats) occurs as an alternate source of energy. In

TABLE 17–1

Pathophysiologic Mechanisms and Effects of DKA, HHNK, and Hypoglycemia

DKA	HHNK	HYPOGLYCEMIA
Physiologic Mechanisms		
↓ Insulin	↓ Insulin (relative)	↓ Serum glucose (possible ↑ insulin)
↑ Blood glucose	↑ Glucose	↓ Glucose production
Osmotic diuresis	No keto acid production	↓ Glycogen storage breakdown
Dehydration	Hyperosmolarity	
Lipolysis	Osmotic diuresis	
Fatty acids released	Dehydration	
Metabolic acidosis	Hypernatremia	
Hyperkalemia	Neurologic abnormalities	
↑ Protein catabolism		
Serum Glucose Level		
300–1,500 mg/100 ml	600–3,000 mg/100 ml	50 mg/100 ml or less
Ketones		
Elevated	Normal	Normal

addition, insulin normally inhibits lipase (an enzyme that stimulates lipolysis), so insulin lack accelerates lipolysis.

This breakdown results in free fatty acids, which are oxidized and cause accumulation of ketone bodies. Increased numbers of hydrogen ions (from the ketones) consume bicarbonate ions and result in metabolic acidosis (Porth 1990). In addition to the obvious effects of ketoacidosis, a decrease of extracellular sodium can occur. Keto acids have a low tubular reabsorption threshold in the kidneys. Thus, when the serum level of keto acids rises, a large amount is lost in the urine. The keto acids are mostly excreted along with extracellular sodium ions. The lost sodium ions are replaced in the extracellular fluid by hydrogen ions, worsening the acidosis (Guyton 1991). In addition, lactic acid accumulates secondary to anaerobic metabolism during decreased cellular oxygenation, further worsening the metabolic acidosis.

Other Pathophysiologic Effects DKA has many other effects. These include increased protein catabolism, overproduction of glucose by the liver, and decreased level of consciousness. Additionally, hyperkalemia occurs as potassium (normally an intracellular electrolyte) is displaced from cells into the serum during acidosis. Subsequently, hypokalemia occurs as potassium is lost if diuresis continues.

Risk Conditions

Diabetic ketoacidosis can occur in undiagnosed insulin-dependent diabetics with inadequate secretion of endogenous insulin. It also can occur in known diabetics who reduce the amount of insulin per dose or miss insulin doses entirely. Also at risk are people with an increased insulin need due to physical or emotional stress such as trauma, surgery, infection, or psychosocial stress disorders. The hormonal responses to stress responsible for the increased insulin need include release of glucagon from the liver, secretion of adrenal glucocorticoids, and adrenal secretion of catecholamines. Infection is the most common cause of DKA in these patients (Swearingen et al. 1991).

Signs and Symptoms

The client with DKA is acutely ill. Signs of dehydration from the osmotic diuresis include flushed dry skin, poor skin turgor, and dry mucous membranes. The patient, if conscious, will complain of the "three Ps": thirst (polydipsia), hunger (polyphagia), and large amounts of urine (polyuria) due again to osmotic diuresis. However, these characteristic early signs of

CRITICAL CARE GERONTOLOGY

Hyperglycemic Risk in the Elderly

As people age, glucose tolerance decreases. The average serum glucose 2 hours following a glucose load is 30% higher at 75 years of age than at 25 years. The decrease in glucose tolerance may be due to a decrease in insulin secretion or an inability to utilize insulin.

It is important for the critical-care nurse to be aware of glucose tolerance changes with aging and the risk for elderly patients in critical care. The stress of illness or injury can often precipitate hyperglycemia, and the elderly are particularly at risk (Carnevali and Patrick 1986).

Patients who have non-insulin-dependent diabetes are also much more at risk for HHNK, and this population usually includes the elderly. They may be able to secrete enough insulin to prevent ketone formation but not enough to prevent high serum glucose levels, hyperosmolality, and cellular dehydration.

lack of insulin may not always be associated with onset of DKA.

Respiratory symptoms include tachypnea, Kussmaul's breathing (deep respiration), and acetone odor to the breath, all compensatory mechanisms for metabolic acidosis. Acetoacetic acid is converted to acetone, which is volatile and can be exhaled through breathing. Acetone normally has a "fruity" odor and acetone breath is characteristic of diabetes mellitus and DKA. The presence of Kussmaul's respiration indicates severe acidosis.

Neurologic changes range from confusion to coma, related to dehydration and decreased cellular oxygenation. Deep tendon reflexes may be decreased or absent.

Cardiovascular signs include tachycardia related to sympathetic nervous system discharge, hypotension related to dehydration, and flushed skin related to increasing amounts of carbonic acid. The nurse may also observe electrocardiographic signs of hyperkalemia, such as peaked T waves, prolonged PR intervals and widened QRS complexes. Other presenting symptoms may include nausea, vomiting, and abdominal pain.

Laboratory Tests

Laboratory assessment will reveal an elevated serum glucose level. The serum glucose level typically is elevated to no more than 300–500 mg/dl because of the osmotic diuresis; however, serum glucose may soar to 1,000 mg/dl or higher in the severely volume-depleted patient or in one with impaired renal function. A widening anion gap $(Na - (Cl + HCO_3))$ reflects acid accumulation (normal is between 12 and 14 mEq/L). Also important are urine studies, to ascertain the presence of glucose and ketones. When the serum glucose level is above 300 mg, 100 g of glucose may be lost in the urine in 24 hours. Additionally 100–200 g of ketoacids may be lost in the urine in 24 hours. Arterial blood gases usually show a pH less than 7.30 and decreased bicarbonate levels. Increased plasma creatinine and blood urea nitrogen indicate decreased renal perfusion. Plasma osmolality will be above 300 mOsm/L. Electrolytes will demonstrate hyperkalemia due to displaced intracellular potassium (K^+) with acidosis, although a low total body potassium may be present with osmotic diuresis. Additionally, the serum sodium will be low because of urinary losses of sodium secondary to keto acid excretion; however, if the

NURSING DIAGNOSES

A variety of nursing diagnoses may apply to the patient with DKA.

- Fluid volume deficit
- Sensory-perceptual alteration
- Ineffective breathing pattern
- Knowledge deficit

patient is severely dehydrated, serum sodium will reflect normal or high levels (see Chapter 16 for detailed discussion of sodium). Finally, to differentiate and confirm DKA it is important to rule out other disorders. To this end, electrocardiogram (ECG) and cardiac enzymes are measured to rule out myocardial infarction; serum amylase is measured to rule out pancreatitis; and chest x-ray and urine and blood cultures are done to rule out possible infection.

Planning and Implementation of Care

DKA is a medical emergency. Early assessment, diagnosis, and intervention are vital to the patient's recovery from this life-threatening condition. A nursing care plan for the DKA patient appears nearby and selected aspects of it are discussed in the following section.

Fluid Volume Deficit Related to Osmotic Diuresis

Assess for signs of decreasing cardiac output, such as hypotension, and cool extremities related to sympathetic nervous system compensatory mechanisms. Insert an indwelling catheter to facilitate accurate hourly intake and output measurement, and monitor the fluid loss closely.

Fluid Replacement Rapid replacement of fluid is very important, because dehydration is the most immediate life-threatening aspect of the condition. As soon as intravenous access is established, administer the IV fluid ordered by the physician, usually 0.9% sodium chloride ("normal" saline, NS). The average fluid deficit in an adult is 3.5 L, and the usual initial replacement is 1–2 L in the first 2 hours (Yeates and Blaufuss 1990). Serum osmolality often is used as a guide for fluid replacement.

Although rapid fluid replacement is of utmost importance, continue to assess carefully for complications. The rapid fluid replacement can cause hemodilution, hypotonicity, and subsequent interstitial edema, which may account for the pulmonary and cerebral edema that has been occasionally observed with DKA.

When glucose levels reach 200–300 mg/dl, change the solution as ordered, most likely to 0.45% normal

---

NURSING TIP

Plasma Expanders

Plasma expanders such as albumin and plasma concentrates may be necessary to forestall impending vascular collapse. However, their administration should follow 2–3 L of normal saline, because the hypertonicity of plasma expanders can further cellular dehydration in a patient with a fluid deficit.

---

saline or dextrose in water. There are three reasons for doing so. First, more water than sodium is lost during an osmotic diuresis, so free water (hypotonic solution) will need to be replaced. Second, reducing the amount of chloride in the solution will reduce the possibility of hyperchloremia. Finally, a 5% glucose solution should be given before hypoglycemia is likely to occur, as discussed in more detail under the next nursing diagnosis (Yeates and Blaufuss 1990).

During fluid replacement therapy it is important to continually assess the patient for signs of circulatory overload, which may include the following: neck vein distention, crackles in lungs, increasing central venous pressure (CVP) and pulmonary artery pressures, tachycardia, and tachypnea.

Insulin Replacement Insulin deficiency is the primary cause of all of the problems of DKA, so it follows that replacement is an important part of the therapy, although insulin alone will not correct all of the changes with DKA. Insulin has four main effects. First, insulin facilitates *transport of glucose across the cellular membrane.* It allows uptake and use of glucose by almost all cells and tissues of the body. Second, insulin facilitates *storage of glucose,* in the form of glycogen, in the liver. The glycogen is broken down to glucose at different periods during the day to maintain an adequate blood glucose level. Third, insulin promotes *fatty acid synthesis.* Fatty acids are then transported to adipose cells to be stored. Additionally, fatty acids are utilized by the liver to synthesize triglycerides. Insulin also inhibits the pancreatic enzyme lipase that causes breakdown of fat cells into fatty acids. Finally, insulin stimulates *active transport of amino acids into cells,* inhibits protein catabolism, and inhibits liver glyconeogenesis (Guyton 1991).

NURSING CARE PLAN

Diabetic Ketoacidosis

Nursing Diagnosis	Signs and Symptoms	Nursing Actions	Desired Outcomes
Fluid volume deficit related to osmotic diuresis	Polyuria Polydipsia Weakness If severe: ↓ BP, ↑ HR, ↓ CVP, ↓ PCWP ↓ LOC	1. Assess vital signs frequently. Be alert for changes in HR, BP, CVP, and PCWP. 2. Measure I & O carefully. Report all output < 30 ml/hr. 3. Administer IV fluid as ordered. Assess for signs and symptoms of fluid overload, which may include dyspnea, jugular venous distention, and ↑ CVP and PCWP. 4. Monitor for lab results indicating imbalances caused by lack of insulin such as: 　↑ potassium 　↓ potassium 　↓ sodium 　↓ phosphate 5. Administer insulin as ordered. 6. Monitor blood sugar as ordered.	Patient is normovolemic: BP, HR, PCW, CVP WNL Urine output > 30 ml/hr. Skin turgor good. Awake and alert.
Sensory-perceptual alteration (decreased level of consciousness) related to cellular dehydration	Decreased LOC Unresponsiveness Confusion Disorientation	1. Assess patient's orientation and LOC frequently. 2. Maintain the bed in low position with side rails up. 3. Initiate seizure precautions.	Oriented to person, place and time.

The most common methods (routes) of insulin administration are intravenous (IV) or subcutaneous (SQ). In DKA, the IV route is preferred as it allows more reliable absorption and rapid onset of action. The amount administered should be guided by blood glucose levels assessed every hour. As stated previously, at approximately 250–300 mg/dl, the IV solution is changed to dextrose and water and/or the insulin dose is reduced. Generally, approximately 5–10 units per hour or 0.1 u/kg of body weight are given, and the blood glucose level decreases approximately 75–100 mg/dl per hour. Although some patients with DKA are insulin-resistant and require larger doses of insulin, most often low doses are effective.

Electrolyte Repletion Loss of electrolytes, including sodium, potassium, chloride, magnesium, phosphate, and calcium, is an important consideration in patients with DKA. Electrolytes are usually replaced via the IV route and monitored by serum electrolyte levels.

Potassium (K^+) repletion is a bit more complex. Potassium is primarily an intracellular ion, with only a very small amount in the serum, so serum levels do not reflect total body potassium (see Chapter 16 for detailed discussion of potassium). In acidosis, K^+ shifts out of the cells (secondary to large amounts of hydrogen ions), so the serum level will be high. As acidosis is corrected, however, K^+ will move back into the cells and K^+ deficit may become evident due to

NURSING CARE PLAN

Diabetic Ketoacidosis (Continued)

Nursing Diagnosis	Signs and Symptoms	Nursing Actions	Desired Outcomes
Ineffective breathing related to acidosis and decreased level of consciousness	Dyspnea Tachycardia ↓ Air exchange Skin color changes	1. Assess respiratory patterns frequently for (1) Kussmaul's breathing (rapid, deep breathing associated with acidosis); (2) signs of inadequate gas exchange, such as tachycardia, dyspnea, skin color changes (pallor or cyanosis), or decreased respiratory excursion. 2. Keep patient in semi-Fowler's position to minimize risk of aspiration. 3. Insert nasogastric tube if ordered to decrease likelihood of aspiration. Attach to low intermittent suction. 4. Assess ABGs for evidence of hypoxemia and acidosis.	Clear breath sounds throughout lung fields. ABGs within normal limits.
Knowledge deficit related to mechanisms of DKA	Patient and/or family ask questions and are ready to learn.	1. Give patient and/or family written and oral information on (1) causes, prevention, and signs and symptoms of DKA; (2) interventions such as frequent glucose testing; (3) importance of diet and fluid intake; (4) medical information bracelets; (5) support groups.	Patient and/or family understand disease process and treatment.

K^+ loss during osmotic diuresis. To prevent hypokalemia, potassium should be added to the IV when the serum potassium level reaches 4.5 mEq/L. Potassium phosphate salts may be given, which also will correct phosphate depletion. *Caution:* If the patient is oliguric, addition of potassium can cause hyperkalemia.

Other electrolytes to monitor are magnesium and phosphate. They usually will be low in patients with DKA. Phosphorus deficiency in DKA may be caused by tissue catabolism, decreased glucose and phosphorus uptake, and increased excretion with diuresis. Magnesium losses occur with diuresis. Both usually will self-correct to normal levels with fluid replacement and nutrition.

Acid–Base Balance   A significant number of patients with DKA do not require exogenous alkaline administration to correct acidosis. With prompt administration of fluid, electrolytes, and insulin, the kidney can begin to conserve bicarbonate and correct acidosis. However, the patient who is severely acidotic (pH less than 7.10) may require bicarbonate (Gotch 1991). The acidosis is corrected by administering either sodium bicarbonate or sodium lactate solution; correction should be guided by arterial blood gases and care should be taken not to overcorrect.

As discussed previously, acidosis causes an efflux of K^+ out of cells. As acidosis is corrected and K^+ is driven back into cells, an actual K^+ deficit secondary to osmotic diuresis may appear. Monitor electrolytes carefully and report changes and/or abnormal levels.

Carbon dioxide (CO_2) diffuses into cerebrospinal fluid (CSF) much faster than bicarbonate. As bicarbonate (HCO_3) is administered, part of it dissociates into CO_2 and diffuses into the CSF, causing a transient but potentially serious further drop in CSF pH. In the patient whose pH is moving more toward a normal range, this may manifest as a deepening coma.

Sensory-Perceptual Alteration (Decreased Level of Consciousness) Related to Cellular Dehydration

The changes in sensation and perception that occur with DKA range from mental confusion to coma. The causes of the neurologic problems are multifactorial. First, the osmotic diuresis causes severe cellular dehydration and altered metabolism, which may precipitate sensory-perceptual alterations. Second, the anerobic metabolism that occurs as a result of hypoxemia and acidosis also alters cerebral cellular metabolism and neuronal function. Finally, while insulin is being administered, there is risk of hypoglycemia, which will further impair cerebral and neuronal function.

Nursing care for the change in cerebral function should include decreasing the risk of vomiting and aspiration by positioning the patient on his or her side and having suction readily available. A nasogastric tube to low-intermittent suction may be ordered. If the patient is unconscious, it is important to have a cuffed endotracheal tube in place *prior* to gastric intubation to reduce the risk of aspiration.

Ineffective Breathing Pattern Related to Acidosis and Decreased Level of Consciousness

The patient with DKA will demonstrate changes in breathing patterns related to the acidosis and also may demonstrate changes related to the altered level of consciousness. Continually assess respiratory status for hyperpnea (Kussmaul's breathing), associated with acidosis, and decreased respiratory movements, which may be associated with cerebral cell dehydration.

Be alert for signs of inadequate gas exchange, which may include: decreased respiratory muscle excursion, tachycardia, dyspnea, and skin color changes (pallor or cyanosis). Report any changes in respiratory status, and administer oxygen as ordered. Be prepared for the possibility of endotracheal intubation. Assess arterial blood gases as ordered.

Knowledge Deficit Related to Mechanisms of DKA

DKA is a largely preventable disorder. When the patient and family are ready, institute a teaching program. An important function of the critical-care nurse is to initiate a program of self-care education, including signs and symptoms, appropriate interventions, and preventive measures. The teaching plan also needs to include information regarding medical identification bracelets or cards and available support groups.

Outcome Evaluation

Evaluation is based on the following outcome criteria:

- Plasma glucose less than 250 mg/dl.
- Electrolytes within normal limits (WNL).
- Serum osmolality WNL.
- Arterial blood gases WNL.
- Patient alert and oriented.
- Urine output WNL.
- Vital signs WNL.
- Skin turgor good.
- Mucous membranes moist.
- Patient and significant others understand treatment plan.

HYPERGLYCEMIC HYPEROSMOLAR NONKETOTIC COMA

Hyperglycemic hyperosmolar nonketotic coma (HHNK), a DKA-like syndrome with the absence of ketosis, is a medical and nursing emergency. It often is misdiagnosed because of a clinical presentation similar to cerebral vascular accidents and DKA. However, it does not occur as frequently as DKA. If not treated promptly and correctly, it is fatal.

HHNK is a disorder of insulin deficiency that results in hyperglycemia and hyperosmolarity but no ketoacidosis (refer to Table 17–1). The hyperglycemia occurs because of decreased peripheral glucose uptake related to a relative insulin deficiency. An osmotic diuresis with glycosuria follows, depleting electrolytes and precipitating extracellular and eventually intracellular dehydration. The dehydration and hyperglycemia increase serum osmolality. Cerebral impairment is the other major factor in HHNK, due in large part to dehydration of brain cells.

What causes HHNK rather than DKA? One theory holds that, with HHNK, lipolysis from adipose tissue is inhibited. Patients with HHNK have lower levels of circulating fatty acids and lypolytic hormones, growth hormone, and cortisol. The limited cortisol and stress response may contribute to the lack of maximal response and lack of ketogenesis (Leske 1985).

Assessment

Risk Conditions

It is important to be able to identify the patient at risk. Certain patients with recent onset of non-insulin-dependent (type II) diabetes may be able to secrete enough insulin to prevent ketosis but not enough to prevent high serum blood glucose levels, hyperosmolarity, and severe cellular dehydration. HHNK may also occur in previously stable patients whose insulin requirements increase, as with stress of surgery, trauma, or infection. HHNK also may be precipitated by pharmacologic therapy; for example, thiazide diuretics may decrease insulin release from the pancreas, as may diazoxide and phenytoin. Patients receiving high-calorie feedings, such as hyperalimentation and enteral feedings, also are at risk because of increased glucose load. Last, although it may occur in patients with type I or type II diabetes, HHNK is much less common in type I. Glucose processing dysfunction in type I is more likely to be associated with ketone formation and precipitation of DKA.

Signs and Symptoms

The signs and symptoms of HHNK all result primarily from the effects of the high serum glucose level, which generally is greater than 600 mg/dl and may be as high as 1,400–3,000 mg/dl. Symptoms often develop slowly and many are nonspecific. Serum osmolality usually is greater than 350 mOsm/L due to osmotic diuresis. Remember that serum ketones will be negative. Arterial blood gases usually are normal, because, without lipolysis, acidosis does not occur. It is important to note, however, that a slight acidosis may be present, related to either lactic acid production or decreased renal function, because of extracellular

(intravenous) dehydration and decreased perfusion. Electrolyte levels will vary. Electrolytes are lost with the osmotic diuresis, however; depending on the state of hydration, sodium levels may be high, normal, or low. Similarly, potassium is drawn out of the cells with dehydration, so serum potassium may be initially high; then, when volume depletion is corrected, a total body K^+ deficit may be unmasked. Also contributing to the K^+ deficit is the dehydration-stimulated aldosterone response, which results in the renal tubular reabsorption of Na^+ and secretion of K^+.

Laboratory signs of decreasing kidney function may be present. An elevated blood urea nitrogen and serum creatinine indicate decreased glomerular filtration.

Examination of the urine reveals glycosuria, because the renal reabsorption transport maximum has been exceeded. Urine will be negative for ketones.

Early in this syndrome, the alert patient may complain of feeling drowsy and thirsty and may appear confused. Detection of accompanying physical changes is very important to early diagnosis and intervention.

Physical assessment reveals clinical signs of dehydration, which may include dry mucous membranes, flushed dry skin, poor skin turgor, and postural hypotension. Sympathetic nervous system compensatory responses for the contracted intravascular volume include tachycardia, tachypnea, and constriction of peripheral blood vessels to shunt blood to more central organs. Of utmost importance and characteristic of this disorder are neurologic changes. These may be manifested by confusion, stupor or coma, or seizures. There is a direct relationship between plasma osmolality and degree of depressed cerebral functioning. Because of the severe neurologic abnormalities, this disorder has the risk of being misdiagnosed as cerebrovascular accident. Finally, although Kussmaul's respiration is not present, the tachypnea and shallow respirations that do occur are related to a disturbance in respiratory-center functioning.

NURSING DIAGNOSES

The following nursing diagnoses may apply to the patient with HHNK:

- Fluid volume deficit
- Sensory-perceptual alteration
- Altered tissue perfusion
- Knowledge deficit

Planning and Implementation of Care

Fluid Volume Deficit Related to Osmotic Diuresis

The problem of extracellular and intracellular dehydration needs to be treated promptly. The type and volume of fluid replacement generally is determined by the physician, based on cardiovascular and renal status. The following medical guidelines may be used when replacing fluids.

1. Administer isotonic saline (0.9% normal saline [NS]) if serum sodium is less than 130 mEq/L and plasma osmolality is less than 330 mOsm/L.

2. Administer hypotonic saline (0.45% NS) if serum sodium is greater than 145 mEq/L.

3. Usually, replace half the estimated loss in the first 12 hours and the rest in the subsequent 24 hours. This may be as much as 6–8 L in the first 12 hours.

4. When blood glucose reaches approximately 250 mg/dl, switch to 5% dextrose in water to prevent hypoglycemia, and/or switch from 0.9% NS to 0.45% NS to prevent lowering serum osmolality too rapidly, which can precipitate cerebral edema secondary to fluid shifts (Leske 1985).

Generally, patients with HHNK have a greater fluid deficit than patients with DKA because of a more prolonged and severe osmotic diuresis. Thus, they may require more fluid replacement. But remember, these patients often are elderly; may have renal, cardiac, or pulmonary disease; and are at risk for pulmonary edema and circulatory overload. Therefore, it is important to assess for signs of circulatory overload, such as crackles in lung fields, distended neck veins, shortness of breath, dyspnea, bounding pulses, increased pulmonary artery pressures, increased pulmonary capillary wedge pressure, and tachycardia. During correction of the fluid volume deficit, it is important for the critical-care nurse continually to assess the patient for signs of decreasing cardiac output, which may accompany circulatory overload. These may include decreasing urinary output, tachycardia, and decreasing blood pressure.

In addition to treating the fluid deficit, an important part of care is to reduce the blood glucose level below 300 mg/dl. The requirements for insulin usually are less than for patients with DKA, and some physicians treat HHNK with saline alone.

The goal of insulin therapy in HHNK is to gradually reduce the serum glucose level while preventing hypoglycemia and cerebral edema, as mentioned previously. (Cerebral edema is a complication that occurs from reducing serum osmolality too rapidly. If osmolality decreases rapidly, there is a substantial difference between brain cell osmolality and serum osmolality, causing a subsequent fluid shift to the intracellular space in the brain—hence, cerebral edema.) Usually, short-acting regular insulin is administered. It is best to use the IV route, because subcutaneous administration does not provide adequate absorption secondary to dehydration.

Restoring electrolyte balance is the next intervention. As discussed previously, electrolyte levels often are low, and electrolytes need to be replaced. Assess for symptoms of electrolyte imbalances and administer repletion therapy, as ordered. (See Chapter 16 for a detailed discussion of electrolyte imbalances.)

Sensory-Perceptual Alteration (Decreased Level of Consciousness) Related to Cellular Dehydration

Alterations in level of consciousness occur due to cellular dehydration in the central nervous system from the high plasma osmolality. It is important to assess level of consciousness and neurologic status frequently and to report any seizure activity. Remember, phenytoin reduces endogenous release of insulin, so it probably would not be indicated for HHNK-induced seizures.

Neurologic changes also may be due to cerebral edema secondary to decreasing osmolality too quickly and/or impaired electrolyte balance and ideally will be reversed as the imbalance is corrected.

Altered Tissue Perfusion Related to Osmotic Diuresis

Osmotic diuresis decreases plasma volume, and decreased tissue perfusion is mainly due to dehydration and hyperviscosity of the blood. These factors cause decreased preload, decreased cardiac output, decreased renal perfusion and function, decreased tissue perfusion and subsequent tissue hypoxia. Vascular thrombosis due to hemoconcentration also can occur (Swearingen and Keen 1991).

This problem will be relieved with fluid replacement. Assess for adequate renal output (½–1 cc/kg/hr), adequate tissue perfusion, and improving skin turgor. Additionally, observe for a decrease in sympathetic compensatory responses as evidenced by a return to sinus rhythm (from tachycardia), normal blood pressure, palpable peripheral pulses, and increasing skin temperature.

The respiratory center in the brainstem may be affected by the severe cellular dehydration that occurs with HHNK. It is important to continually assess respiratory function and report any changes. Assess for respiratory excursion, air movement on auscultation, skin color, shortness of breath, dyspnea, and sympathetic compensatory responses for hypoxemia.

Administer oxygen as ordered, monitor blood gas values, and prepare for endotracheal intubation if alterations in respiratory function are observed.

Knowledge Deficit Related to Insufficient Information Regarding Mechanisms of HHNK and Prevention

Although critical-care patients sometimes are not ready for teaching programs, after the acute episode assess the patient's readiness to learn and level of understanding and develop a teaching plan. This plan should include dietary restrictions and signs and symptoms of hyperglycemia and impending HHNK. It is always important to include family and/or significant others in teaching.

Outcome Evaluation

Evaluate the patient's progress according to these outcome criteria:

- Plasma glucose less than 300 mg/dl.
- Serum osmolality WNL.
- Patient alert and oriented.
- Vital signs WNL.
- Skin turgor good.
- Serum electrolytes WNL.
- Urine output WNL.
- Serum creatinine and blood urea nitrogen (BUN) WNL.

HYPOGLYCEMIA

Hypoglycemia is an emergency in which plasma glucose levels decrease to 50 mg/dl or lower.

Assessment

Risk Conditions

There are many potential causes of and contributing factors to hypoglycemia. The episode may be related to excessive insulin therapy or to change in absorption of insulin. It may be the result of insufficient nutritional intake or to decreased need for exogenous insulin (for example, from removal of stress, such as infection).

Medications and drugs also may precipitate a hypoglycemic episode—for example, excessive oral hypoglycemic agents (sulfonylureas) and alcohol, which inhibits gluconeogenesis by the liver. Finally, other health problems, such as liver disease (depleted glycogen stores) and adrenal insufficiency (insufficient glucocorticoids), may be contributing factors.

Signs and Symptoms

Signs and symptoms usually are apparent when the blood glucose level is less than 50 mg/dl (Gotch 1991). The onset of symptoms usually is more rapid than with DKA. The physiologic symptoms patients demonstrate generally are related to nervous system function—more specifically, cerebral function. The cerebral changes result from insufficient supply of glucose to the brain cells (the brain does not utilize alternative energy sources as well as other tissues do).

Patients usually first experience an inability to concentrate, apprehension, or light-headedness. Patients often are aware of these symptoms yet unable to verbalize their need for help. They often may present with slurred speech, trembling, and/or staggering gait, which may be mistaken for alcohol-induced signs. The central nervous system signs will progress to coma within minutes to an hour without treatment. It is important to recognize these signs and be aware of the possibility of hypoglycemia, because ignoring the signs may have a deleterious, even fatal, outcome.

The other signs involve the autonomic nervous system. Hypoglycemia stimulates release of catecholamines (epinephrine and norepinephrine). These hormones cause tachycardia, pallor, diaphoresis, cool skin, and tremors with potential seizure activity. This response is supported by glucocorticoid release from the adrenal glands, and liver glycogenolysis.

Diagnosis of hypoglycemia is based on low plasma glucose levels and on response when glucose is administered. Patients generally respond rapidly and dramatically to glucose administration.

NURSING DIAGNOSES

The following nursing diagnoses may apply to the patient with a hypoglycemic episode:

- Sensory-perceptual alteration
- Knowledge deficit

Planning and Implementation of Care

Sensory-Perceptual Alteration Related to Decreased Cerebral Cellular Metabolism

As discussed previously, the patient with hypoglycemia has central neurologic changes due to deficient glucose available to brain cells. These symptoms will promptly disappear with glucose administration. The key roles of the critical-care nurse in this situation are assessment and prompt intervention. Monitor the level of consciousness and neurologic status frequently.

If the patient is conscious, administer a simple carbohydrate, such as glucose gel, followed by a protein and carbohydrate snack, such as milk and crackers. If the patient is unconscious, start an intravenous line and be prepared to administer 50 ml of 50% dextrose IV push as ordered. Prior to administering 50% dextrose, check with the physician and draw blood for a chemistry panel. This action provides a way to assess blood sugar prior to glucose administration. When glucose is administered to an unconscious patient in the presence of uncomplicated hypoglycemia, consciousness will be promptly restored. An alternative

therapy (but not as effective) is to administer exogenous glucagon IV to stimulate liver glycogenolysis. Be aware of the possibility of recurrence of the episode. Consult with the physician about continued nutrient/glucose support, and monitor blood glucose level.

If these measures do not reverse the symptoms, the patient may not have uncomplicated hypoglycemia or may need more glucose.

Knowledge Deficit Related to Insufficient Information About Mechanisms of Hypoglycemia

Even though hypoglycemic episodes occur in stable, knowledgeable patients, they may be largely preventable. Patients need to know as much as possible about the causes and effects of hypoglycemic episodes. Using capillary blood glucose monitoring devices rather than urine glucose measurements provides for reliable control of blood glucose levels. Review diet and insulin doses with physician and patient. Discuss the importance of carrying simple carbohydrates, such as glucose gel. Finally, an episode of hypoglycemia usually is very frightening for the patient. Reassurance, explanations, and appropriate intervention by the nurse are vital. Also inform the patient about medical information (alert) bracelets and support groups available.

Outcome Evaluation

Evaluate the patient with a hypoglycemic episode based on the following criteria:

- Serum glucose level between 80 and 120 mg/dl.
- Patient awake and alert.
- Vital signs WNL.
- Patient and significant others understand treatment plan.

ACUTE ADRENAL INSUFFICIENCY

Acute adrenal insufficiency, sometimes known as Addisonian Crisis, is a life-threatening emergency characterized by deficiency of adrenal cortical hormones (specifically mineralocorticoids and glucocorticoids).

Assessment

Risk Conditions

Adrenal insufficiency may result from autoimmune disease, atrophy of the pituitary or adrenal gland, or acute deficiencies of aldosterone or cortisol. It sometimes is associated with abrupt withdrawal of steroids in a steroid-dependent patient or a period of stress in a steroid-dependent patient. This emergency may also occur in critically ill patients enduring tremendous physiologic stressors, such as infection, surgery, trauma, or acquired immune deficiency syndrome (AIDS).

Signs and Symptoms

The signs and symptoms all relate directly to lack of mineralocorticoids (aldosterone) and glucocorticoids (cortisol). The assessment usually will reveal hypotension, tachycardia, confusion, dry skin, and muscle weakness. The ECG may reveal signs of hyperkalemia, including peaked T waves, widened QRS complexes, and lengthened PR intervals.

Laboratory tests reveal decreased serum cortisol, decreased aldosterone level, decreased serum sodium, and increased serum potassium.

NURSING DIAGNOSES

The following nursing diagnoses may apply to the patient with adrenal insufficiency:

- Fluid volume deficit
- Knowledge deficit

Planning and Implementation of Care

Fluid Volume Deficit Related to Impaired Secretion of Aldosterone

Fluid volume deficit needs to be treated promptly to prevent severe hypovolemia and hypovolemic shock. Usually, 5% dextrose in normal saline is administered rapidly: 1 L in 1 hour, then 1–2 L over the next 6 hours. If the insufficiency is severe and the patient's condition critical, a pulmonary artery catheter may be placed for monitoring fluid replacement.

Monitoring the patient is critical. Observe for manifestations of hyperkalemia (lethargy, muscle weakness, or nausea) and hyponatremia (weakness or headache). Also monitor vital signs and hemodynamics. Report a blood pressure lower than 90/60 or a pulmonary capillary wedge pressure (PCWP) less than 6 mm Hg. If hypoglycemia is present, monitor serum glucose closely and administer glucose as ordered.

Knowledge Deficit Related to Long-Term Corticosteroid Replacement

The patient may need education about glucocorticoid (and possibly mineralocorticoid) replacement. Provide the patient, family, and significant others with information about long-term steroid replacement. Guidelines may include: take steroids with food, report weight gain of greater than 2 lb/week, notify the physician of periods of stress (which may require an increased dose), do not stop taking or miss doses, and avoid exposure to infectious diseases.

Outcome Evaluation

Evaluate the patient with adrenal crisis based on the following criteria:

- Blood pressure WNL.
- PCWP 4–12 mm Hg.
- Serum sodium WNL.
- Serum cortisol WNL.
- Patient awake and alert.

THYROID CRISIS

Assessment

Risk Conditions

Thyroid crisis, also known as *hyperthyroid crisis, thyroid storm,* and *thyrotoxicosis,* refers to the body's response to excessive amounts of circulating thyroid hormone. *Thyrotoxicosis* is simply a hyperthyroid state, whereas *thyroid crisis* and *thyroid storm* are emergency situations requiring critical care. The cause or precipitating factor in a crisis varies. A stressful situation may cause decompensation in a previously stable patient. Other possible causes include excessive exogenous thyroid hormone, withdrawal of antithyroid drugs, and palpation of the thyroid gland.

Signs and Symptoms

One of the main effects of thyroid hormone is to maintain the body's cellular metabolism. In a thyroid crisis, one of the presenting signs is an increase in body temperature related to accelerated metabolism. The increase in metabolic activity also uses a lot of body fluid, so the patient may be diaphoretic and dehydrated. Increased adrenergic activity causes tachycardia, increased blood pressure, and a hyperdynamic heart. Respiratory function eventually may deteriorate, and there may be skeletal muscle weakening because of muscle mass catabolism. The patient with thyroid crisis usually has an increased appetite, because of metabolic needs, and may have increased gastrointestinal (GI) motility. Skin is thin and friable. Red blood cell volume may be increased because of increased O_2 requirements; however, about 3% of patients have pernicious anemia. Nervous system changes such as nervousness, emotional lability, delirium, and tremors are common.

Laboratory Tests

Laboratory assessment of a thyroid crisis is based primarily on serum levels of triiodothyronine (T_3) and thyroxine (T_4), the thyroid hormones that regulate metabolic activity. The synthesis of these hormones depends on the presence of iodine in the gland. When T_3 and T_4 enter the bloodstream, they are bound by plasma proteins. In the periphery, thyroid hormone is freed and then active and available to the tissues and cells. Levels of T_3 and T_4 will increase during a thyroid crisis. Radionuclear scanning may demonstrate an enlarged or nodular thyroid. Radioactive iodine uptake may be measured to indicate the functional state of the thyroid gland. Radioimmunoassay studies demonstrate decreased plasma thyroid-stimulating hormone (TSH) concentrations in most patients (Guyton 1991). TSH is released by the anterior pituitary gland by a negative feedback mechanism stimulated by low circulating levels of thyroid hormone. Low TSH concentrations

rule out inappropriate pituitary secretion as the cause of the thyroid crisis.

NURSING DIAGNOSES

The following nursing diagnoses may apply to the patient with thyroid crisis:

- Fluid volume deficit
- High risk for altered body temperature
- High risk for decreased cardiac output
- High risk for impaired gas exchange
- Altered nutrition: less than body requirements
- Impaired tissue integrity
- Sensory-perceptual alteration

Planning and Implementation of Care

Fluid Volume Deficit Related to Increased Metabolic Activity

As discussed previously, patients may become dehydrated because of increased metabolism and diaphoresis. Therefore, fluid replacement is an important part of therapy. Assess for signs of dehydration, such as decreased urine output, poor skin turgor, and dry mucous membranes, and consult with the physician. Use caution when replacing fluids, however, and observe for any signs of congestive heart failure, such as increasing dyspnea, crackles in the chest, and increasing pulmonary vascular pressures. The patient may require large amounts of fluid to replace metabolic losses and maintain a state of hydration. At the same time, however, the patient is in a very hyperdynamic cardiovascular state secondary to increased adrenergic activity, so be alert for the risk of heart failure related to increased cardiac workload.

High Risk for Altered Body Temperature Related to Increased Metabolic Activity

Patients in thyroid crisis often present with hyperthermia related to the heat produced by exaggerated metabolic processes. Body temperature can increase to as much as 104°F. Assess rectal temperature, degree of peripheral vasodilatation, and diaphoresis. A hypothermia blanket may be used (see the section on therapeutic hypothermia). Also, institute general supportive measures that may help decrease metabolic rate, such as maintaining a quiet environment, reducing stimulation, and providing periods of undisturbed rest. It is important not to administer acetylsalicylic acid, because one of its actions is displacement of thyroxine from thyroid-binding hormones, making it available to tissues. Insulin may be required to prevent hyperglycemia from glycogenolysis.

High Risk for Decreased Cardiac Output Related to Increased Cardiac Workload Secondary to Increased Adrenergic Activity

The stress of thyroid crisis on the cardiovascular system is usually quite obvious as tachycardia, hypertension, and other signs of the hyperdynamic state. The increased inotropic state of the myocardium may be observed as bounding peripheral pulses, a systolic murmur on auscultation, and a precordial heave palpated at the apex. It is important to continually assess for dysrhythmias, most commonly tachycardias. Also assess for clinical indicators of adequate cardiac output, such as urine output, sensorium, vital signs, and tissue perfusion. Beta-adrenergic blocking drugs such as propranolol may be ordered to block the effect of catecholamines on the heart. Beta blockade also blocks the conversion of T_4 to T_3, the more metabolically active form of thyroid hormone. Vasodilators such as hydralazine and sodium nitroprusside may be used to reduce workload on the heart by decreasing afterload and systemic vascular resistance. An arterial line may be placed to facilitate accurate titration of the vasoactive drugs and measurement of systemic vascular resistance.

High Risk for Impaired Gas Exchange Related to Decreased Muscle Strength

During thyroid storm, the amount of protein in muscles decreases. Since thyroid hormone inhibits synthesis of protein, protein catabolism exceeds anabolism, and respiratory muscles weaken. In addition, if heart failure develops as a result of increased cardiac workload, pulmonary congestion ensues. Assess respiratory function frequently, auscultate the lungs, and administer oxygen as ordered.

Altered Nutrition: Less Than Body Requirements Related to Increased Nutrient Requirements

The patient in thyroid crisis cannot keep up with nutrient requirements for the increased metabolic activity. Supplemental feeding and vitamins are an important part of care. The patient should be weighed daily; if a state of adequate nutrition cannot be maintained, hyperalimentation should be administered.

Pharmacologic Therapy

Administer pharmacologic therapy to decrease the deleterious effects of thyroid crisis, as ordered by the physician. This therapy may include the following drugs.

- Propylthiouracil (PTU), administered orally, blocks the synthesis of thyroid hormones by interfering with conversion of T_4 to T_3.
- Methimazole (Tapazole) also works to inhibit thyroid hormone synthesis.
- Iodide inhibits the release of thyroid hormone from the gland. It should be given approximately 1–2 hours after PTU. This delay is important, because if administered earlier, PTU may cause the gland to accumulate iodide, which would be used for further synthesis.
- Glucocorticoids may be given to replace the rapidly metabolized cortisol. Dexamethasone, if used, also suppresses the conversion of T_4 to T_3.

Outcome Evaluation

Evaluate the recovery of a patient from thyroid crisis by the following criteria:

- Vital signs WNL.
- Body temperature normal.
- Patient awake and oriented.
- Skin warm and dry.
- State of hydration normal.
- Lung sounds clear bilaterally.
- Weight stable.
- Patient calm and steady.

THERAPEUTIC HYPOTHERMIA

Assessment

Candidates

Therapeutic hypothermia is the deliberate lowering of body temperature. Patients who may benefit from therapeutic hypothermia fall into two main categories. The first includes those who have a temperature above normal due to heat stroke, thyroid crisis, or infection, and who remain febrile in spite of antipyretics and conservative measures such as tepid baths, cooling fans, and ice packs. These patients are candidates for hypothermia because each degree centigrade of temperature elevation above normal raises metabolism approximately 7%; this elevation increases physiologic stress in a patient whose resources may be nearing depletion due to the critical nature of the illness.

The second group of patients includes those who are normothermic and who suffer an insult whose effects can be minimized by reducing the normal metabolic demand. Examples are patients undergoing cardiovascular surgery or neurosurgery and patients with acute cerebral ischemia or edema, severe gastrointestinal bleeding, or persistent coma following cardiac arrest. Both groups may be helped by moderate hypothermia, which can reduce the total metabolic demand by 50%. The effect on the function of individual organs varies, with some, such as the brain, being affected profoundly and others, such as the kidney, being affected minimally.

Signs and Symptoms

To comprehend the signs and symptoms seen in hypothermic patients, it is helpful to understand the major physiologic principles of thermoregulation. Body temperature is controlled by the *thermoregulatory center* in the anterior hypothalamus (Guyton 1991). Two types of sensory receptors supply information to the thermoregulatory center: the peripheral receptors, which sense surrounding or ambient temperature, and the central receptors, located near the center itself, which sense the temperature of blood. The thermoregulatory center uses a number of mechanisms to preserve body temperature, among which are shunting of blood and shivering.

The body's thermoregulatory zones can be conceptualized as three concentric rings. The outermost zone is the *shell,* which consists of the skin and subcutaneous adipose tissue. The skeletal muscles form the middle zone. The innermost zone, the *core,* consists of the viscera, which the body tries to protect at all costs, whether body temperature falls precipitously or gradually.

The physiologic effects and signs and symptoms of hypothermia correlate roughly with the degree of temperature drop. They are summarized in Tables 17–2 and 17–3.

NURSING DIAGNOSES

Nursing diagnoses applicable to the hypothermic patient may include:

- Altered tissue perfusion
- Sensory-perceptual alteration
- Impaired gas exchange
- High risk for impaired skin integrity
- High risk for decreased cardiac output
- High risk for injury

Planning and Implementation of Care

Induction of Therapeutic Hypothermia

The range of therapeutic hypothermia associated with the greatest physiologic benefit and least hazard is the moderate range, 28–32°C. Since this is the range used most commonly at the bedside, this chapter will focus on effects of moderate hypothermia and *not* those of deep hypothermia (below 28°C).

To initiate hypothermia, place a hypothermia blanket on the bed, provide a light sheet on top of the blanket if indicated to maintain skin integrity, and precool the blanket if possible. Place the patient on the blanket. Prepare the skin and extremities if needed, depending on the equipment used. Monitor core temperature with the thermistor of a pulmonary artery catheter or with a rectal probe. If a rectal probe is used,

TABLE 17–2

Physiologic Effects of Hypothermia

Mild 32–37°C	Neurologic: autonomic stimulation
	Metabolic: basal metabolic rate (BMR) increased 3 × normal
Moderate 28–32°C	Neurologic: cerebral metabolism 66% of normal, cerebral blood flow 70% of normal, CSF pressure 64% of normal
	Metabolic: BMR 50% of normal, depressed hypothalamic thermoregulation
	Cardiac: HR 50% of normal, prolonged diastole
	Respiratory: decreased CO_2 production, leftward shift of O_2/hemoglobin dissociation curve, total O_2 demand 50% of normal
	Liver: depressed function
	Kidney: moderately decreased glomerular filtration rate
Severe 20–28°C	Metabolic: BMR < 25% of normal, paralyzed thermoregulation, mixed metabolic and respiratory acidosis
	Cardiac: prolonged systole, prolonged conduction time, depressed pacemaker activity, hemoconcentration, hypovolemia
Profound below 20°C	Absent thermogenesis

TABLE 17–3

Signs and Symptoms of Hypothermia

Mild 32–37°C	Level of consciousness: agitation→confusion→apathy
	Heart: HR increased→decreased; BP increased→decreased
	Peripheral vasoconstriction: intense→decreased
	Respiration: respiratory rate increased→decreased
	Musculoskeletal: shivering moderate→intense→decreased
	Muscular coordination: poor→staggering
Moderate 28–32°C	Level of consciousness: stupor→coma
	Heart: dysrhythmias
	Respiration: decreased RR, decreased gag and cough reflexes
	Musculoskeletal: shivering alternating with rigor
Severe 20–28°C	Respiration: severe depression, absent gag reflex
	Musculoskeletal: absent reflexes, rigor
	Heart: high risk of ventricular fibrillation
Profound below 20°C	Level of consciousness: coma→isoelectric electroencephalogram
	Heart: ventricular fibrillation→asystole
	Respiration: apnea
	Musculoskeletal: rigidity

insert it at least 2 inches, making sure it is not embedded in feces. Tape the probe in position. Because probes and machines may be inaccurate, it is a wise precaution to periodically check the patient's temperature with a rectal thermometer during hypo-thermia induction and maintenance. If desired, a second hypothermia blanket may be placed on top of the patient to enhance cooling.

During induction, monitor the patient closely for the phenomena of drift and after-fall.

Drift *Drift* is defined as a sudden change in body temperature greater than 1°C in 15 minutes. Many nurses have observed that drift precedes frank shivering, shock, and dysrhythmias.

After-Fall *After-fall* is the phenomenon of continuing drop in core temperature after the hypothermia machine is turned off and the blanket remains in contact with the body. During hypothermia the periphery cools more than the core, so even after hypothermia is discontinued, the warmer core continues to lose heat to the superficial tissues; in addition, temperature may drop as chilled blood is returned from the periphery. Therefore, the cooling device should be reset and the top cooling blanket (if used) removed when the rectal temperature is a few degrees centigrade above the desired temperature. The patient usually shows an after-fall of 2–5°C. Drift and after-fall are intensified when the patient is obese.

Effects

Altered Tissue Perfusion Related to Normal Thermoregulatory Responses Monitor vital signs, neurologic status, and peripheral perfusion every 15 minutes until stable, and then every 1–2 hours. During the first 20 minutes of hypothermia, the heart rate (HR) rises, blood pressure (BP) increases, and respiratory rate accelerates due to sympathetic and metabolic responses to the drop in temperature. The body initially responds to the cold stimulus by conserving body heat and increasing heat production. Peripheral vasoconstriction minimizes surface heat loss, and skin coldness and pallor occur. Vasoconstriction increases venous return, which causes the blood pressure to rise. Increased heat production is achieved by shivering, a potent response which occurs in nearly all people exposed to intense cold.

After about 20 minutes, vasoconstriction ceases and superficial blood flow returns. Reactive hyperemia causes reddened skin. As body heat continues to be lost, all vital signs decrease. They stabilize at lower levels when the desired degree of hypothermia is maintained. At moderate hypothermia, the cardiac refractory period and ventricular relaxation are prolonged. The heart rate slows, coronary arterial filling is proportionally enhanced, and ventricular contractility improves.

Urinary output does not change significantly. Although a moderate decrease in glomerular filtration occurs, secretion of antidiuretic hormone is inhibited. Thus, the urinary output will increase and

the urine osmolality and specific gravity may decrease; however, electrolyte excretion by the kidney is unchanged.

It is crucial that you interpret the patient's vital signs and urinary output in light of the expected changes. For example, a heart rate of 90 beats per minute at 30°C is an abnormal finding that requires prompt investigation. Similarly, a progressive drop in urinary output may signal the onset of hypovolemia or renal failure.

During hypothermia, fluid shifts from the intravascular space into the intracellular and interstitial spaces. This shift leaves the blood more concentrated, and thrombosis and embolization may occur. Use support stockings, frequent turning, and range of motion exercises. See Chapter 8 for further suggestions on avoiding this complication.

Shivering, a normal physiologic response to cold, is produced by stimulation of the temperature control center in the posterior hypothalamus. This center appears to respond to superficial temperature receptors in the skin, which detect changes in skin temperature, and deep thermoreceptors in or near the hypothalamus (Guyton 1991).

It is important to prevent or minimize shivering in the hypothermic patient for several reasons. Shivering increases the patient's discomfort. It also accelerates the metabolic rate, heart rate, arterial pressure, venous pressure, cerebrospinal fluid pressure, oxygen consumption, carbon dioxide production, depletion of glycogen stores, and production and accumulation of lactic acid. These effects occur at a time when perfusion to the core organs already is reduced. Since blood flow to the muscles is increased during shivering, the temperature gradient between the core and periphery steepens, and core heat loss worsens. Shivering therefore is only a short-term mechanism for coping with hypothermia, with numerous undesirable effects.

To minimize shivering (without pharmacologic therapy) implement the following:

1. Prevent rapid cooling of the distal limbs. Slowing their rate of heat loss appears to slow the change in core temperature. Wrap the upper extremities from fingertips to elbows and the lower extremities from toes to knees, until the patient has stabilized at the desired temperature.

2. During induction of hypothermia, initially set the blanket temperature to provide a steep gradient between it and the patient (15°C is a common initial setting). If core temperature drops more than 1°C per 15 minutes, reduce the

gradient between the patient and blanket by increasing the blanket temperature.

3. Observe the patient for shivering. Premonitory signs of frank shivering are muscle tremor artifact on the ECG, and tensing or clenching of the masseter muscles, which close the jaw. Actual shivering begins in the masseters as a twitch and moves to the neck or pectoral areas. Frank shivering in the extremities and chattering teeth are later signs that usually necessitate pharmacologic intervention.

4. If shivering occurs, try reducing the rate of temperature decline by removing the top blanket or increasing the blanket temperature. If this action is contraindicated by the gravity of the patient's condition, the physician may prescribe chlorpromazine (Thorazine) in doses of 10–25 mg. The effect of chlorpromazine on shivering is unpredictable. In addition, it causes vasodilatation, which produces hypotension, tachycardia, and increased core heat loss.

The physician may also order diazepam (Valium) or midazolam (Versed). Another drug used to treat hyperthermia is IV dantrolene (Dantrium). It acts on peripheral skeletal muscles to inhibit calcium release from the sarcoplasmic reticulum (Thomas 1989).

Sensory-Perceptual Alteration (Altered Level of Consciousness) Related to Decreased Cerebral Metabolism Cerebral metabolism drops more than the rest of the body, approximately 6.7% per degree centigrade. Cerebral blood flow decreases about one-third, while cerebral metabolic demand diminishes about 54%. Since the decrease in cerebral metabolism is greater than the decrease in cerebral blood flow, cerebral perfusion is relatively improved. Cerebrospinal fluid pressure drops 5.5% per degree centigrade with moderate hypothermia.

At normal temperatures, the brain is slightly colder than the rest of the body. With surface cooling, it becomes 1–2°C warmer than the body core. Highly integrated centers are depressed first by hypothermia, providing a valuable cerebral protective mechanism even at moderately hypothermic levels. The sensorium, including hearing, fades at a body temperature of 33–34°C.

Nursing implications related to the decreased sensorium include applying artificial tears and taping the eyelids shut if blinking becomes infrequent. To evaluate changes in the level of consciousness, assess the more primitive responses, such as those elicited by noxious stimuli, rather than higher integrative responses.

Impaired Gas Exchange Related to Decreased Temperature and Decreased Tissue Perfusion
The respiratory system undergoes several significant changes during hypothermia. Carbon dioxide production decreases, but ventilation decreases more rapidly. This imbalance between carbon dioxide production and excretion can lead to respiratory acidosis. Oxygen uptake increases, but cold shifts the oxyhemoglobin dissociation curve to the left, reducing the dissociation of O_2 from the red blood cells. This effect contributes to tissue hypoxia, which can precipitate ventricular irritability. If the hypoxic patient shivers, the cells must rely more heavily on anaerobic metabolism for energy production, which produces lactic acid and ketone bodies as by-products. Because circulation is reduced, these by-products accumulate and metabolic acidosis can occur.

Minimize the risk of acidosis by monitoring arterial blood gases (ABGs) closely. Prevent shivering. If shivering occurs, consideration must be given to increased oxygen consumption, so administer oxygen as ordered. Promote ventilation through elevating the head of the bed, turning the patient frequently, and implementing a program of chest physiotherapy to enhance CO_2 elimination and removal of secretions. The physician may prescribe the addition of 2–5% CO_2 to the patient's ventilation. This treatment induces respiratory acidosis, which shifts the oxyhemoglobin dissociation curve back toward normal (the Bohr effect), thus promoting the release of oxygen to the tissues. It also dilates the cerebral vasculature, thus enhancing cerebral perfusion.

High Risk for Impaired Skin Integrity Related to Decreased Perfusion and Decreased Level of Consciousness Skin breakdown and frostbite can result from both diminished perfusion to the skin and the patient's decreased awareness of skin damage. Take the following steps to avoid these problems.

Keep the face, hands, and feet off the blanket. Place lamb's wool between the fingers and toes. Cover the hands and feet loosely with cotton and wrap them with stretch gauze. When bathing the patient, use tepid water and massage the skin gently to avoid producing heat. Turn the patient at least every 2 hours to relieve pressure points and massage the skin gently. To maintain the hypothermia, turn the blanket with the patient.

High Risk for Decreased Cardiac Output Related to Dysrhythmias Be alert for dysrhythmias. Dysrhythmias (other than sinus bradycardia, which is an expected response) are unlikely to occur with moderate hypothermia if precautions are taken to ensure slow cooling and to avoid unintended deep hypothermia. During hypothermia, the total cardiac refractory period lengthens and the vulnerable period is prolonged. An ectopic ventricular beat falling during the vulnerable period may initiate ventricular tachycardia or fibrillation. The likelihood of ectopic beats producing ventricular tachycardia or fibrillation does not increase dangerously during hypothermia until the temperature drops below 28°C. To minimize ventricular irritability, limit the temperature drop to 1°C per 15 minutes and (preferably) do not allow the core temperature to go below 28°C.

Hypothermia prolongs all intervals on the ECG. In addition, it often causes a slowly inscribed terminal portion of the QRS, called a J wave or Osborn wave. This wave is an incidental finding. It is most pronounced in leads V_3–V_6.

Other electrocardiographic findings may include a fine muscle tremor and, at lower hypothermic levels, atrial fibrillation with a slow ventricular response.

High Risk for Injury Related to Altered Drug Absorption Because decreased perfusion alters the absorption of drugs, avoid subcutaneous and intramuscular injections; give medications intravenously instead. If a medication must be given intramuscularly, use a deep injection technique.

Although few liver functions are decreased by moderate hypothermia, the ability to detoxify morphine and some barbiturates is reduced. The physician may prescribe reduced doses or substitutes for these drugs.

Rewarming

When hypothermia is no longer needed, rewarm the patient gradually. Although active (artificial) surface rewarming can be used, it carries the danger of warming the periphery before the core. The still-cold heart then may be unable to produce a cardiac output (CO) adequate for the metabolic demands of the warmer areas. Dilatation of the surface vessels causes blood pooling, a diminished venous return, and a further decrease in cardiac output. These conditions may lead to "rewarming shock."

When therapeutic hypothermia has been used, natural rewarming is preferred. Simply remove the cooling blanket and place a bed blanket over the patient. The temperature should return to normal at the rate of approximately 1.0°C per hour.

Possible Complications

Shock and Acidosis During the rewarming period, which may take several hours, observe for shock and acidosis. Shock may result from too rapid warming, as explained earlier; this can occur even if the rewarming is achieved naturally. Acidosis may result from inadequate perfusion of the warmer areas or a release of the lactic acid that accumulated during shivering. During rewarming, the level of consciousness, pulse, blood pressure, and respiratory rate should increase proportionately to the core temperature. When any decrease or disproportionate increase occurs, alert the physician, who may want to investigate other possible causes (such as a bleeding ulcer), prescribe vasopressors, or initiate recooling.

Cumulative Drug Effects During the rewarming phase, remember to observe for the cumulative effects of previously administered drugs, particularly those given intramuscularly. Also, remember that hearing will return at about 34°C; you can use this knowledge to gradually reorient the patient to the surroundings.

Ulcers Another problem that may appear during rewarming is gastritis or peptic ulceration. During hypothermia, pepsin production continues, although the secretion of gastric juice diminishes. When rewarming occurs and gastric juice flow increases, it contains an increased concentration of pepsin. Notify the physician if signs of gastritis or ulceration appear. These signs may include abdominal pain, rigid abdomen, dark stools (guaiac positive), hematemesis, or changes in vital signs (tachycardia and hypotension) if bleeding is significant.

Overhydration Rewarming causes fluid to shift from the intracellular and interstitial spaces back into the intravascular compartment. If fluids were not given cautiously during hypothermia, signs of overhydration may appear during rewarming. Recognition and management of fluid volume excess is discussed in detail in Chapter 16.

Outcome Evaluation

Evaluate the patient according to the following outcome criteria:

- Temperature WNL.
- BP and pulse WNL.

RESEARCH NOTE

Oliver S, Fuessel E
Control of postoperative hypothermia in cardiovascular surgery patients.
Crit Care Nurs Quart 1990; 12(4):63–68.

CLINICAL APPLICATION

Safe and effective rewarming of postoperative cardiac patients is the responsibility of the critical-care nurse. The nurse, the physician, and hospital policy usually determine whether mechanical heating blankets, warmed thermal blankets, or room temperature blankets are used. However, prior to this study, there was no research supporting any method of rewarming as best for the patient.

Twenty-one postoperative patients were studied after the protocol had received the full support of the cardiovascular surgeons. Prior to surgery, informed consent was obtained from the patient or from the patient's legal guardian. All patients had postoperative temperatures of less than 35°C (95°F). The differences in temperatures (rang- ing from 33.9°C–34.3°C) were not significant.

Subjects were assigned randomly to one of three study groups. Their torsos and extremities were covered with:

1. Thermal blankets, or
2. Heated thermal blankets, warmed for 2 hours at 110°F (43°C) and changed hourly, or
3. Heated blankets, warmed to 105°F (40.5°C) and covered with one thermal blanket

Core temperature, monitored with a Swan-Ganz thermal sensor, was recorded every 30 minutes. Nurses assigned to the patients monitored their hemodynamics and ABGs, as well as checking them frequently for shivering, changes in vital signs, and dysrhythmias.

Results demonstrated no significant baseline temperature differ- ences between blanket type and time to rewarm. The only variable that reached statistical significance (0.04) was body type. Overweight patients took longer to rewarm. However, blanket type did not influence this result significantly.

CRITICAL THINKING

Weaknesses: The sample size was small. Before practice decisions can be made with a sound research base, the study needs to be duplicated with a larger sample size.

Strengths: This study addresses a common nursing intervention and suggests that using heated blankets is unnecessary. This finding may result in cost savings as well as saving nursing time.

- ABGs WNL.
- Level of consciousness (LOC) WNL.
- Urinary output 60–100 ml/hr.

DIABETES INSIPIDUS

Diabetes insipidus (DI) is a disorder in which there is a deficiency of antidiuretic hormone (ADH). It can be primary (from hypothalamic dysfunction), secondary (from destruction to the hypothalamus from surgery, tumor, or trauma), or nephrogenic (from decreased kidney responsiveness to ADH). Whatever the cause, a deficiency of ADH results in the body's inability to conserve water and subsequent uncontrolled diuresis.

DI is frequently temporary and is often observed in patients following cranial trauma, infection, or surgery. Transient DI usually resolves in 5–7 days.

Assessment

Risk Conditions

Patients in critical care with head injury, cranial infections such as encephalitis, brain tumors, or cranial surgery are all at risk because of potential damage to the hypothalamus. Any conditions that increase intra-cranial pressure may cause DI which may be transient until intracranial pressure normalizes.

Signs and Symptoms

If the patient is awake, he or she may complain of severe thirst and increased urine output. Often, the critically ill patient is not responsive and thus will not be able to increase fluid intake. The patient with DI will have increased urine output (4–16 L/24 hours), decreased skin turgor, dry skin, dry mucous membranes, and tachycardia (nervous system response to dehydration).

Laboratory Tests

Sodium levels will be high. Urine specific gravity will be low (1.001–1.005). If plasma osmolality is tested, it will be high (normal is 295 mOsm/kg).

NURSING DIAGNOSES

The following nursing diagnoses may apply to the patient with DI:

- Fluid volume deficit
- High risk for altered tissue perfusion (cerebral)
- Knowledge deficit

Fluid Volume Deficit Related to Uncontrolled Diuresis

One of the most important aspects of care for the patient with DI is fluid replacement. Usually, hypotonic IV fluids are used to replace loss in unconscious patients who cannot take fluid orally. Fluids will be given rapidly to restore hemodynamic stability (if dehydration is severe) and then replaced based on urine output. Monitor hemodynamic measurements and intake and output.

ADH replacement therapy may be administered on a physician's order. Many different forms of synthetic ADH are available. Common preparations used in critical care include:

1. Aqueous vasopressin (Pitressin), given nasally or subcutaneously. Onset is quick (within ½ hr), and the drug is short-acting.
2. Desmopressin acetate (DDAVP), IV, SQ, or intranasally. Onset is within 1 hour, and the effects last 4–8 hr.
3. Vasopressin tannate in oil (Pitressin tannate in oil). This preparation is given deep intramuscularly (IM) and may only need to be administered once every 2–3 days because it is absorbed slowly.

NURSING TIP

Vasopressin Administration

After giving intramuscular injections of vasopressin tannate in oil, administering 1–2 glasses of water may help reduce gastrointestinal cramping and discomfort.

Any of these preparations may cause increased GI activity and cramping. The nasal preparations may cause nasal irritation. Because the preparations cause fluid retention, carefully monitor the patient for fluid overload. Signs may include headache, increased BP, signs of congestive heart failure, distended neck veins, and shortness of breath.

Altered Cerebral Tissue Perfusion Related to Severe Dehydration

Alterations in level of consciousness (LOC) may be observed for several reasons. First, the same disorder that is causing DI also may be causing changes in LOC; an example is increased intracranial pressure. Another cause of decreased LOC may be severe dehydration; providing adequate hydration will help improve LOC.

If you are caring for a patient with head injury, nursing measures to decrease intracranial pressure are appropriate. See Chapter 5 for details on such interventions.

Knowledge Deficit Related to Unfamiliar Disorder

Although critical-care patients often are not ready for extensive teaching programs, it is important for you to plan for patient, family, and significant other education. The plan should include effects of synthetic ADH preparations, accurate measurement of intake and output, importance of daily weights, and signs and symptoms of dehydration and fluid overload.

Outcome Evaluation

Evaluate the patient's progress according to the following outcome criteria:

- Normovolemia, as evidenced by BP, CVP, PCWP, and HR WNL.
- Stable weight.
- Serum and urine osmolality WNL.
- Patient alert and oriented.
- Skin turgor good.
- Urine output WNL.

SYNDROME OF INAPPROPRIATE ANTIDIURETIC HORMONE

Syndrome of inappropriate antidiuretic hormone (SIADH) is characterized by an excessive release of and response to ADH that causes increased fluid volume, low plasma osmolality, and hyponatremia. Because the high ADH levels impair normal regulatory mechanisms, SIADH eventually results in water intoxication if not treated. It is often caused by central nervous system disorders or by an injury causing hypothalamic or pituitary dysfunction; however, it also has been associated with positive pressure ventilation, which decreases venous return and stimulates ADH release.

Assessment

Risk Conditions

Many patients in critical care are at risk because there are many causes of SIADH. These include head injury, neoplasms, infections, vascular disorders, cancer chemotherapy, pulmonary infections, and positive pressure ventilation.

Signs and Symptoms

Initially, an alert patient may complain of headache, lethargy, anorexia, nausea, restlessness, and/or weakness. Nursing assessment will reveal decreased urine output, with concentrated urine. Changes in LOC become apparent as water intoxication occurs. Edema is usually *not* present.

Diagnostic studies will reveal low serum sodium, low plasma osmolality, elevated urine osmolality and

NURSING TIP

Assessing Edema with SIADH

The patient with SIADH is hyponatremic, and the fluid retention is hypotonic. Because of the low sodium content, edema will often NOT be present.

specific gravity, and high urine sodium. The diagnosis of SIADH is often based on a "water load" test. A dehydrated patient is given water and overhydrated. The urine output and serum osmolality then are monitored. A normal patient will respond to the water load by increasing output of dilute urine, to maintain normal serum osmolality. In contrast, patients with SIADH demonstrate decreased serum osmolality and no change in urine output or concentration because they retain the extra fluid.

NURSING DIAGNOSES

The following nursing diagnoses may apply to the patient with SIADH:

- Fluid volume excess
- Sensory-perceptual alteration

Fluid Volume Excess Related to Impaired Regulatory Mechanisms

Assess the patient carefully for changes indicating water intoxication, including changes in LOC, headache, fatigue, and weakness. It is vital that you monitor intake and output and IV fluid therapy. Based on urine output, the patient will be on fluid restriction—usually less than 1,000 ml/day.

Patients with severe hyponatremia may be given isotonic or hypertonic sodium chloride solutions. Fluid administration will be accompanied by IV furosemide (Lasix) or an osmotic diuretic to promote diuresis and prevent worsening of water intoxication.

Sensory-Perceptual Alteration Related to Altered Cellular Function

As stated, the patient with SIADH may experience changes in LOC, because water intoxication and hyponatremia alter cerebral cellular function. Institute seizure precautions and keep the bed in a low position. Always maintain an open airway. If the patient is confused, reorient him or her frequently. Remember also that changes in LOC may be due to the primary disorder and not solely to water intoxication and hyponatremia.

Outcome Evaluation

Evaluate the patient's progress according to the following outcome criteria:

- Balanced intake and output.
- Plasma and urine osmolality and serum sodium WNL.
- Patient alert and oriented.
- Normovolemia, as evidenced by BP, CVP, PCWP, and HR WNL.

REFERENCES

Bacchus H: Heading off a diabetic crisis. *Emerg Med* 1989; 21(20):20–24, 26, 31–32.

Benner P: *From novice to expert: Excellence and power in clinical nursing practice.* Menlo Park, CA: Addison-Wesley, 1984.

Cagno J: Diabetes insipidus. *Crit Care Nurse* 1989; 9(6):86–93.

Carnevali D, Patrick M: *Nursing management for the elderly,* 2d ed. Philadelphia: Lippincott, 1986.

Epstein C: Fluid volume deficit for the adrenal crisis patient. *Dimen Crit Care Nurs* 1991; 10(4):210–217.

Germon K: Fluid and electrolyte problems associated with diabetes insipidus and syndrome of inappropriate ADH. *Nurs Clin North Am* 1987; 22(4):785–96.

Gotch P: The endocrine system. In *Core curriculum for critical care nursing.* Alspach J (ed). Philadelphia: Saunders, 1991.

Guyton A: *Textbook of medical physiology,* 8th ed. Philadelphia: Saunders, 1991.

Johnson D: Metabolic and endocrine alterations in the multiple injured patient. *Crit Care Nurs Quart* 1988; 11(2):35–42.

Kim M, McFarland G, McLane A: *Pocket guide to nursing diagnoses,* 3d ed. St. Louis: Mosby, 1989.

Lee K, Stotts N: Support of the growth hormone–somatomedin system to facilitate healing. *Heart Lung* 1990; 19(2):157–163.

Leske J: Hyperglycemic hyperosmolar nonketotic coma: A nursing care plan. *Crit Care Nurse* 1985; 5:49–56.

Lumley W: Recognizing and reversing insulin shock. *Nursing 89* 1989; 19(9):34–41.

Mathewson M: Antidiuretic hormone. *Crit Care Nurse* 1986; 5(5):88–92.

Michael S, Sabo C: Nursing management of the diabetic patient receiving nutritional support. *Focus Crit Care* 1990; 17(4):331–338.

Oliver S, Fuessel E: Control of postoperative hypothermia in cardiovascular surgery patients. *Crit Care Nurs Quart* 1990; 12(4):63–68.

Poe C, Taylor L: Syndrome of inappropriate ADH: Assessment and nursing implications. *Oncol Nurs Forum* 1989; 16(3):373–381.

Porth C: *Pathophysiology: Concepts of altered health states,* 3d ed. Philadelphia: Lippincott, 1990.

Price S, Wilson L: *Pathophysiology: Clinical concepts of disease processes,* 3d ed. New York: McGraw-Hill, 1986.

Swearingen P, Keen J: *Manual of critical care,* 2d ed. St. Louis: Mosby, 1991.

Thomas S: Malignant hyperthermia. *Crit Care Nurse* 1989; 9(6):58–68.

Yeates S, Blaufuss J: Managing the patient in diabetic ketoacidosis. *Focus Crit Care* 1990; 17(3):240–248.

18

Immunologic Disorders

CLINICAL INSIGHT

Domain: The helping role

Competency: Being with a patient

When words no longer comfort a patient, expert nurses provide solace through their very presence. The exquisite comfort provided by deeply felt, unspoken communication elegantly exemplifies the primacy of caring in expert nursing practice. In this extract, from Crabtree and Jorgenson (1986, p. 107), Kelly, the nurse, talks about Jon, an AIDS patient. Jon is struggling with whether to request resuscitative measures if he "blue carts" (has a cardiac arrest)—knowing that he would thereby expose others to the disease. Kelly describes how Jon, surrounded by people who love him, wrestles with his poignant dilemma:

> *Then we decided that we needed to talk to him about what he wanted done . . . did he want to be a blue cart? We needed to explain to him totally*

what a blue cart was. His sister was in the room, and he had a very close friend, who was also a nurse—a public health nurse—and she had come in. We sat down with him and said, this is what a blue cart is. . . . You will have to be bagged; there will be a lot of people in the room; more than likely you will have central lines placed because everything was peripheral at this time. Then I told him that blood will be everywhere, and there will be a lot of people exposed to it. And, there's probably not a whole lot we could do because of the cancer; your lungs are just not responding to treatment, and we're not oxygenating you, and I just flat out told him, somebody's going to be pushing on your chest; you may have to be shocked a couple times; I stressed the facts of everything.

Armed with this explicit information, Jon reaches the decision Kelly already knew he would—and she remains to comfort him with her very presence.

> *He was very aware of his disease and how it affected other people, and he said, no, I don't want to be coded because I don't want to expose people to that, to me, not knowing what's going to happen, getting blood all over, tracking blood everywhere, and I respected his opinion, and he seemed to deal real well with knowing that. But, after we were all done talking about it, he just, like, held on to my hand and just, you know. And then, afterwards, he wrote me a note saying, thank you for being so honest and thanks for being here, and he said he just wanted time, he said, just to be with me for a few minutes even though we were so busy in the unit; it's like I can't just walk out on him, so I stayed in there with him for a while.*

One may take issue with Kelly's choice of words in describing for Jon what "resuscitative measures" would entail. Nevertheless, her actions illustrate two important aspects of excellent nursing care: being honest with the patient in presenting the information he needed to come to a decision, and not abandoning him after the decision was made. Even though some patients in the critical-care setting will choose to forgo "high-tech" medical interventions, the nurse continues to care for, and "be there" for, the patient.

The number of patients in critical-care units with immunologic disorders has been increasing over the past few years. This chapter provides the nurse with knowledge about immunity and an understanding of the interventions currently used in the care of the patient with immunologic dysfunction. Even more challenging than meeting these patients' physical needs is remaining sensitive to their emotional needs, as illustrated in the Clinical Insight.

After a review of immunity, this chapter focuses on four immunologic disorders challenging the critical-care nurse: anaphylaxis; acquired immune deficiency syndrome (AIDS); immunosuppression and/or graft rejection in the recipient of an organ transplant; and sepsis or septic syndrome. These disorders illustrate the spectrum of immune response. Anaphylaxis results from an excessive or inappropriate response of the immune system to a foreign substance. Both AIDS and the therapeutic immunosuppression needed for successful organ transplantation are at the other end of the immune response continuum—lack of function by the immune system. In sepsis the immune system, whether initially normal or already compromised, is taxed to its limit.

Related Anatomy and Physiology

Immunity is the body's ability to resist infectious organisms that otherwise would damage tissues and organs. The body's first line of defense against invasion by pathogenic microorganisms is the barrier provided by intact, normal skin and mucous membranes. A second source of resistance is the microbicidal nature of gastric acid and of many of the digestive enzymes. These defense mechanisms usually are not considered immunologic because they do not involve leukocytes (white blood cells). However, the barrier function of the skin is enhanced by the antigen-presenting activity of the Langerhans cells found at the dermal-epidermal junction. Similarly, the passive barrier function of the mucous membranes is augmented by the presence of antibodies (class IgA) on the membranes. Antigen presentation and antibody secretion are two key components of the immune response. Both will be discussed further below.

Innate and Adaptive Immune Responses

Most immunity is provided by the immune system, a complex system of organs, tissues, and cells throughout the body. The primary organs of the immune system include the thymus, bone marrow, lymph nodes, and spleen. The primary cells are the lymphocytes, macrophages, and neutrophils. Two processes underlie the function of the immune system: general processes, which produce the *innate immune response,* and specific processes, directed at particular invading agents, which produce the *adaptive immune response.* The innate immune response (usually called "inflammation"), is rather stereotyped; it varies only slightly with the nature of the initiating event. The purposes of inflammation are to remove the debris produced by tissue injury, to control any microorganisms that may be present, and to initiate healing. The adaptive immune response is what is usually thought of as "immunity" or "acquired immunity." It involves recognition of foreign elements (either cells or acellular agents such as viruses) as "non-self," marking of these elements to facilitate their destruction, destruction of the foreign elements, and induction of immunologic memory so that the body's response upon re-exposure to the same agent will be much more prompt and effective.

Types of Leukocytes

Understanding the events which make up the innate and adaptive immune responses will be facilitated by a summary of the classes and functions of leukocytes, which are the body's mobile units of protection. All leukocytes are descendants of the bone marrow stem cells (Figure 18–1), which also give rise to erythrocytes and platelets. Leukocytes are subdivided into *lymphocytes* and nonlymphocytes. Lymphocytes, which are the most distinctive leukocytes, themselves constitute a varied group. Lymphocytes are involved primarily in the adaptive immune response; their subclasses and functions are discussed below.

The *non*lymphocytic leukocytes are classified as either *granulocytes* or nongranulocytes. Granulocytes (so called because they contain numerous granules) are also termed *polymorphonuclear* leukocytes (sometimes abbreviated to *PMNs* or *polys*) because of the varied shapes of their nucleus. Granulocytes are divided further, on the basis of their staining characteristics, into *neutrophils, eosinophils,* and *basophils.*

In the healthy adult, neutrophils are by far the most numerous granulocytes in the blood (Fischbach 1992), and they are the first leukocytes to enter damaged tissue during the innate immune response. Neutrophils phagocytose both microorganisms and damaged components of host tissue. Eosinophils are weakly phagocytic cells, but their functions are poorly understood. They are believed to detoxify inflammatory mediators released by basophils and mast cells, but eosinophils can also release substances which are toxic to host tissue, especially epithelia (Barnes 1989). Eosinophils also secrete cysteinyl leukotrienes, toxic substances which are derivatives of arachidonic acid (Austen 1992; Lewis et al. 1990).

Basophils participate in hypersensitivity reactions. When activated, they release stored compounds, including histamine and heparin. Basophils constitute a very small percentage of circulating granulocytes (Fischbach 1992). In allergic reactions they may enter tissues other than blood. *Mast cells,* descendants of the bone marrow stem cells, migrate to and take up residence in other tissues. Large numbers are found in skin, the respiratory tract, and the intestine. Mast cells,

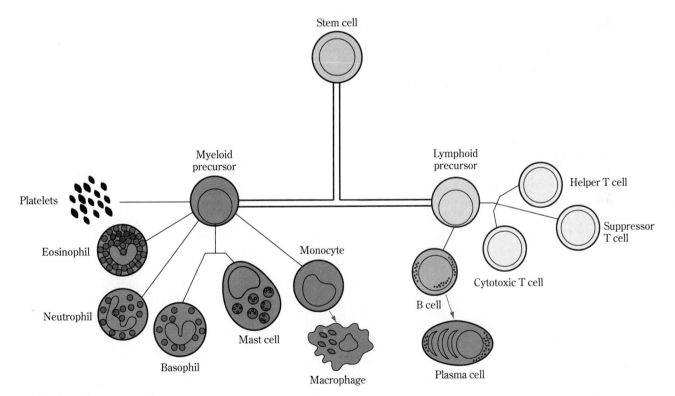

FIGURE 18–1

Cells of the immune system. (From Schindler, Lydia: *Understanding the Immune System.* U.S. Department of Health and Human Services, Public Health Service, National Institutes of Health, 1988.)

like basophils, contain and release histamine, but mast cells also secrete several compounds which basophils (whether in blood or in solid tissues) do not (Austen 1992).

Monocytes are nongranulocytic, nonlymphocytic leukocytes which circulate in small numbers in the blood of healthy persons. When tissue damage occurs, monocytes enter the damaged area and differentiate into *macrophages*. Macrophages are powerfully phagocytic and secrete many substances that help to initiate the adaptive immune response (see below). Many tissues also contain resident macrophages, whose varied names were assigned before their common nature as macrophages was recognized. Examples include alveolar macrophages, mesangial cells of the kidney, osteoclasts in bone, microglia in the central nervous system, Kupffer cells in the liver and Langerhans cells in the skin.

The Innate Immune Response

Inflammation is initiated by any injury to cells; the presence of pathogenic microorganisms is not required. The innate immune response consists of three phases: the vascular phase, phagocytosis, and resolution.

Vascular Phase Cellular injury causes the production or release of chemicals that diffuse to surrounding blood vessels, inducing arteriolar dilatation and increasing the permeability of the microcirculation (especially the venules) to proteins (Garrison 1990). These chemicals, called "mediators of inflammation," include cellular secretory products such as *histamine* and the *prostaglandins*. Enzymes in plasma and interstitial fluid act on substrates present in those same fluids to produce *kinins,* which also function as inflammatory mediators.

The result of this initial vascular phase of inflammation is the delivery into the injured tissue of proteins, such as clotting factors and antibodies, as well as smaller molecules which function as metabolic fuel for the cells and building blocks for tissue repair. In addition, the mediators attract leukocytes from blood into the damaged area. The vascular phase of inflammation is responsible for the classic local physical signs of redness, swelling, warmth, and pain. The pain is due to the actions of the chemical mediators on the endings of small-diameter nerve fibers.

Phagocytosis The next phase of inflammation involves the actions of leukocytes that enter the damaged tissue from blood. Neutrophils enter early; monocytes enter more slowly, then differentiate into macrophages. Both neutrophils and macrophages phagocytose damaged tissue elements and microorganisms. Phagocytosis of a living cell proceeds in two steps, which use different compounds.

In the first step of phagocytosis, the phagocyte surrounds the microbe and creates a membranous chamber inside the cell with the phagocytosed particle inside. Following the phagocyte's engulfment of the microbe, the phagocyte produces *reactive oxygen metabolites* (ROMs), which kill the microbe. Reactive oxygen metabolites include hydrogen peroxide, superoxide, oxygen free radicals, and several other compounds. ROMs kill by attacking lipids in the microbe's membranes (Burton 1990). Since this action is not specific for microbial lipids, ROMs are potentially dangerous to host tissue should they be released from the phagocyte into extracellular fluid. Such release does occur when phagocytic cells are very highly activated or die "in action." ROMs are increasingly being recognized as a cause of tissue damage in many instances of trauma or obstructive ischemia, such as a heart attack (Odeh 1991).

In the second step in phagocytosis, enzymes break down the engulfed material, whether it is tissue debris or a dead microbe. Phagocytes synthesize numerous enzymes which collectively can break down virtually any constituent of a cell. Important examples of enzymes that can destroy host tissue if they are released into extracellular fluid include lipases and such proteases as elastase and collagenase. As with ROMs, enzymes released from phagocytes are being recognized as a significant cause of pathology (MacNee et al. 1989; McGowan and Hunninghake 1989). Stabilizing neutrophil and macrophage cell membranes, thereby minimizing release of ROMs and enzymes, is one rationale for the administration of glucocorticosteroids to certain patients with severe infections (see section on PCP later in this chapter).

The combination of digested tissue debris and leukocytes is the liquid called pus. Since pus may contain traces of enzymes and other active compounds, it is important to minimize its accumulation and its contact with healthy tissue.

Resolution Activated neutrophils and macrophages secrete a variety of "signal molecules" (Table 18–1). Initially called either *monokines* or *lymphokines,* these molecules (all peptides) are now labeled *cytokines* because they have been found to be secreted by several types of cells. Cytokines whose amino acid sequence has been determined are identified as *interleukins* and are numbered according to the order in which they

TABLE 18–1

Functions of Cells and Molecules Involved in Immunity

ELEMENT	FUNCTION IN THE IMMUNE RESPONSE
Cells	
B-cell	Lymphocyte that resides in the lymph nodes or spleen, where it is induced to replicate by antigen-binding and macrophage and helper T cell interactions; its progeny (clone members) form memory cells or plasma cells
Plasma cell	Antibody-producing "machine"; produces huge numbers of the same antibody (immunoglobulin); represents further specialization of B cell descendants
Helper T-cell	A *regulatory* T cell that binds with a specific antigen presented by a macrophage; upon circulating into the spleen and lymph nodes, it stimulates the production of other cells (killer T cells and B cells) that help fight the invader; acts both directly and indirectly by releasing lymphokines
Killer T-cell	Also called a cytotoxic T cell; recruited and activated by helper T cells; its specialty is killing virus-invaded body cells, as well as body cells that have become cancerous
Suppressor T-cell	Slows or stops the activity of B and T cells once the infection (or onslaught by foreign cells) has been conquered
Memory cell	May be a descendant of an activated B or T cell; generated during the initial immune response (primary response); may exist in the body for years thereafter, enabling it to respond quickly and efficiently to subsequent infections or meetings with the same antigen
Macrophage	Engulfs and digests antigens that it encounters, and presents parts of them on its plasma membrane for recognition by T cells bearing receptors for the same antigen; this function, antigen presentation, is essential for normal helper T cell function; also releases chemicals that activate the T cells
Molecules	
Antibody (immunoglobulin)	Protein produced by a B cell or its plasma cell offspring, and released into the body fluids (blood, lymph, saliva, mucus, etc.), where it attaches to antigens and acts to neutralize them (by precipitation or agglutination), or "tags" them for destruction by phagocytes (neutrophils) or for lysis by chemicals (complement)
Lymphokines	Chemicals, including the following, released by sensitized T cells: • Migration inhibitory factor (MIF)—inhibits migration of macrophages, thus keeping them in the immediate area • Macrophage-activating factor (MAF)—"activates" macrophages to become killers • Interleukin II—stimulates T cells to proliferate • Helper factors—enhance antibody formation by plasma cells • Suppressor factors—suppress antibody formation or T cell-mediated immune responses • Chemotactic factors—attract leukocytes (neutrophils, eosinophils, and basophils) into the inflamed area • Lymphotoxin (LT)—a growth inhibitor and cell toxin; causes cell lysis • Gamma interferon—helps make tissue cells resistant to viral infection; also released by macrophages
Complement	Group of blood-borne proteins that are activated when they become bound to antibody-covered antigens; when activated, complement causes lysis of the microorganism and enhances the inflammatory response
Monokines	Chemicals, including the following, released by activated macrophages: • Interleukin I—stimulates T cells to proliferate and causes fever • Interferon—helps protect tissue cells from virus particles that have invaded them by preventing replication of the virus particles within them

From Marieb E: *Essentials of human anatomy and physiology,* 2d ed. Menlo Park: Benjamin/Cummings, 1988; 244–245

were sequenced (Herberman 1989). Prominent among the cytokines released during the inflammatory process are *interleukin-1* (IL-1) and *tumor necrosis factor* (TNF, also called *cachectin*). These molecules act synergistically to initiate the adaptive immune response, to intensify inflammation, and to generate the *acute phase response,* which is responsible for the systemic manifestations of inflammation—fever, somnolence, and malaise (Herberman 1989). IL-1 also stimulates the growth of endothelial cells (which form new blood vessels) and of fibroblasts, which secrete the collagen, elastin, and proteoglycans of extracellular matrix (Handschumacher 1990). Thus, the third phase of inflammation initiates the process of tissue repair.

Reactivation of Tuberculosis in the Elderly

Many of today's elderly were exposed to the tuberculosis bacillus when they were young. Some were able to "fight off" the organism without developing an active infection. Others developed active disease but were treated successfully. However, the bacillus is very hard to kill. In some cases, the person's macrophages were able to engulf the bacillus but weren't able to kill it. In such cases, the bacillus remains alive but confined to a phagocytic vesicle in the cytoplasm of the macrophage—unless the macrophage itself dies. When the macrophage dies, the bacillus is released and is once again able to cause disease. Thus, an elderly person who has no memory of having had TB, or who was successfully treated and has been noninfectious for decades, may develop the disease and transmit it. Not all elderly persons harbor the organism, and not all macrophages die as a person ages, but it is essential to be aware of these possibilities.

The Adaptive Immune Response

The innate immune response is relatively nonspecific; its course is similar whether the cause of tissue damage is heat, physical trauma, a toxic chemical, or a pathogenic microorganism. The immune system can also mount a defense against microorganisms which is exquisitely specific, but only on the second or later exposure to that particular organism. This specific response, developed as a result of events during the first exposure, constitutes the adaptive immune response. The adaptive immune response involves the actions of several types of lymphocytes as well as macrophages.

Types of Lymphocytes Lymphocytes are found primarily in lymph nodes and special lymphoid tissues, such as the spleen, bone marrow, and submucosal areas of the gastrointestinal tract (Guyton 1991). Lymphocytes are descendants of bone marrow stem cells (Figure 18–2). There are two major groups of lymphocytes: those that secrete antibodies, and those that do not. Some prolymphocytes—those that will not secrete antibodies—leave the marrow and travel by way of the bloodstream to the thymus, where they mature under its influence. These are the *T lymphocytes,* which generate a type of acquired immunity called *cell-mediated immunity,* because some activated T cells directly kill target cells (Figure 18–3). T lymphocytes include several subgroups: helper T cells, cytotoxic T cells, and suppressor T cells. It is possible that some T cells perform the functions of more than

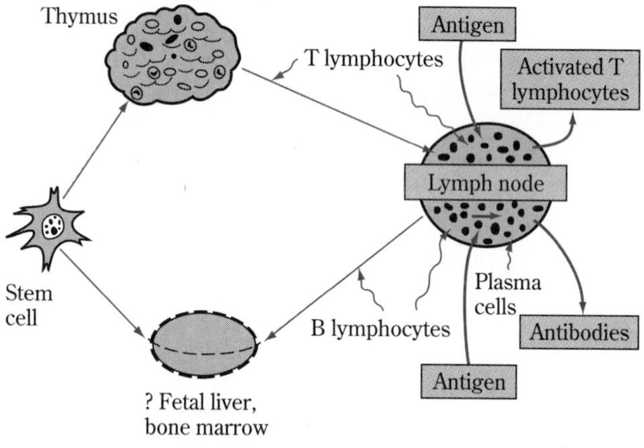

FIGURE 18–2

Formation of antibodies and sensitized lymphocytes by a lymph node in response to antigens. This figure also shows the origin of *thymic* (T) and *bursal* (B) lymphocytes that are responsible for the cell-mediated and humoral immune process of the lymph nodes. (From Guyton A: *Textbook of medical physiology,* 8th ed. Philadelphia: Saunders, 1991 p. 375.)

one of these types; the issue is still controversial (Miller 1990; Podack and Kupfer 1991). *Helper T cells* play a pivotal role in regulating almost all immune functions. They stimulate growth of cytotoxic and suppressor T cells and assist B lymphocytes (discussed below) in becoming specific and maturing to their antibody-secreting stage. *Cytotoxic T cells* directly kill

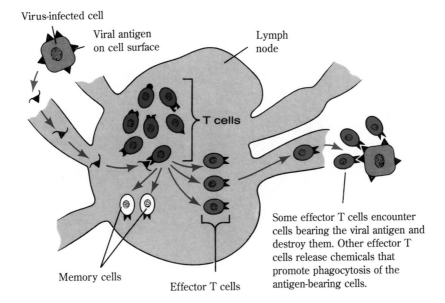

Virus-infected cell

Viral antigen
on cell surface

Lymph
node

T cells

Some effector T cells encounter
cells bearing the viral antigen and
destroy them. Other effector T
cells release chemicals that
promote phagocytosis of the
antigen-bearing cells.

Memory cells

Effector T cells

FIGURE 18–3

Diagrammatic representation of the events of a cell-mediated immune response. The
presence of an antigen stimulates some T lymphocytes to differentiate into
effector T cells, such as cytotoxic cells. Cytotoxic cells destroy the cells that bear
the antigen which stimulated their differentiation (see text for details). Other T cells
remain in the lymph node as memory cells. (From Spence A: *Basic human anatomy*, 3d ed. Redwood City, CA: Benjamin/Cummings, 1990 p. 345.)

target cells bearing a specific protein in their membrane. *Suppressor T cells* damp down the adaptive immune response to minimize damage to host tissue.

B lymphocytes secrete antibodies, thus generating the second type of acquired immunity, called *humoral immunity* (Figure 18–4). B lymphocytes do not require direct action by the thymus in order to mature, although they do need "help" from T lymphocytes.

A third class of lymphocytes are the "null cells," so named because they lack the proteins specific to either T or B lymphocytes. Among the null cells is a group called *natural killer* (NK) cells. These cells induce lysis (rupture) of host tissue cells infected by a variety of viruses. Several of the interleukins, including IL-1, stimulate activity of NK cells.

Antigens and Antigen-Presenting Cells An *antigen* is a chemical which can be recognized by a lymphocyte. What is recognized is a characteristic fragment of the antigenic molecule; the fragment is called an *epitope* (Cohen 1988). Many antigens are proteins, but some polysaccharides, single-strand nucleic acids, and even small molecules (if attached to a protein) can be antigenic. Each individual's immune system determines what molecules are antigenic for it. Thus, the immune system of a person who is allergic to penicillin recognizes the penicillin molecule (usually combined

with a protein) as an antigen, while the immune system of a person who is not allergic to penicillin does not. A given person's immune system can consider a particular molecule antigenic at one time in the person's life but not at another, which explains why allergies may be outgrown or may develop for the first time in mid-life.

Most lymphocytes do not recognize any antigens until the antigen has been engulfed, partially digested, and presented to the lymphocyte by an *antigen-presenting cell,* for example a macrophage. The macrophage selects the epitope and inserts it into its own cell membrane attached to endogenous glycoproteins which form the *human leukocyte antigen* (HLA) group. These glycoproteins are encoded by a complex of genes, located on the short arm of chromosome 6, called the *major histocompatibility complex* (MHC).

HLA glycoproteins form two classes. HLA Class I molecules are expressed by most cells in the body. They are labeled HLA-A, HLA-B, and HLA-C. Because these were recognized early in the course of work on tissue transplants, they are called the major histocompatibility antigens. HLA Class II molecules are usually expressed only by cells of the immune system, especially B lymphocytes, monocytes, and macrophages; they are coded by genes labeled HLA-DP, HLA-DQ, and HLA-DR (Krensky et al. 1990). Each gene in the MHC has many alleles (alternative forms of the same gene),

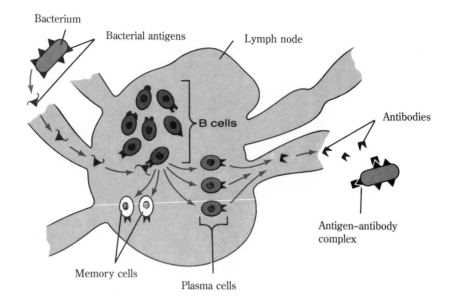

FIGURE 18–4

Diagrammatic representation of the events of a humoral immune response. In response to the presence of an antigen, antibodies are produced by plasma cells, which develop from B lymphocytes. The antibodies are released into the lymph and blood, where they facilitate the destruction of the antigen which stimulated their synthesis. Some B cells remain in the lymph nodes as memory cells. (From Spence A: *Basic human anatomy,* 3d ed. Redwood City, CA: Benjamin/Cummings, 1990 p. 345.)

so the "tissue type" (group of HLA glycoproteins expressed by the cells of one individual) is usually quite distinctive. Each gene occupies a specific position, or locus, on the chromosome. Most persons are heterozygous (have two different alleles) at all six loci, so complete matches between the tissue types of two individuals are unusual unless the persons are identical twins (Krensky et al. 1990).

HLA Class I proteins present antigens to cytotoxic T cells. The antigenic peptide (the epitope) presented by Class I molecules is usually derived from proteins secreted by host tissues, such as viral proteins produced during viral replication (Bjorkman and Parham 1990). Following such antigen presentation, the cytotoxic T cell is specific for that protein. It will recognize the viral protein on the surface of host cells as "foreign" and will lyse cells infected by that particular strain of virus.

HLA Class II proteins usually present epitopes derived from exogenous proteins, such as those made by bacteria or fungi, to helper T lymphocytes. Once a helper T cell has had antigen presented, it is thereafter specific for that antigen only. This activated helper T cell will proliferate, and members of the resulting *clone* (a group of identical cells derived from a common precursor) will activate B lympho-

cytes to make antibodies which react with that antigen.

To summarize: the adaptive immune response is initiated when antigen-presenting cells present epitopes derived from foreign proteins to T cells. If the activated T cell is a cytotoxic cell, the response, called *cell-mediated immunity,* consists of lysis by the cytotoxic T cell of cells displaying that epitope (Podack and Kupfer 1991). If the activated T cell is a helper T cell, the response is called *humoral immunity* because it results in the synthesis and release of antibodies by B lymphocytes. A B lymphocyte in its antibody-secreting mode is called a *plasma cell.* Most antigens simultaneously activate both T lymphocytes and B lymphocytes (Guyton 1991). The adaptive immune response renders the body better able to resist the infecting organism on later exposures because some of the activated T and B cells become *memory cells,* which can recognize the antigen immediately (without another round of antigen presentation) and respond to it at once.

Antigen-Antibody Complexes Antibodies react with their epitopes whether the epitope is part of a noncellular structure floating freely in body fluids (such as a virus particle) or part of a cell (an infected host cell in the case of viral epitopes or a microbial cell in the case of bacterial or fungal epitopes). These antibodies may render the agent harmless to the host by reacting with the sites the microbe or toxin uses to attach to host cells. With this active site occupied, the microbe or toxin cannot gain access to host cells and eventually is phagocytosed by a macrophage or a granulocyte. Since antibodies have at least two identical antigen-binding sites, they may also form *antigen-antibody complexes* with the antigens. Such a complex, containing one or more copies of the antibody and two or more copies of the antigen, is much more attractive as a target for phagocytosis than a single free copy of the antigen is. Antibodies may coat foreign cells if the epitope is part of the cell's membrane, thus rendering the cells very likely to be phagocytosed.

Complement Cascade Another very important method by which antibodies cause the destruction of the antigen is by activating the *complement cascade.* Complement is a term for a group of nine major plasma proteins plus additional regulatory proteins.

Formation of an antigen-antibody complex involving some (not all) immunoglobulins of the G and M classes activates the cascade. The complement cascade may also be activated by the external membranes of some bacteria and yeast (even without antibodies attached to them), by aggregations of immunoglobulins A or E, or by endotoxin, lysosomal enzymes (released from phagocytes), and plasmin. The final five proteins in the cascade cooperate to generate a membrane-spanning pore which allows extracellular fluid to enter the antigen-bearing cell, killing it (Herberman 1987; Podack and Kupfer 1991). Activation of complement proteins results in the production of several small peptides or fragments which attract leukocytes to the area, powerfully stimulate phagocytosis, and intensify or prolong the inflammatory response.

An important reciprocal excitatory relationship exists between the complement cascade and the coagulation and fibrinolysis systems. Strong activation of the complement system promotes activation of both blood coagulation and clot lysis. Strong activation of the coagulation cascade also promotes activation of complement. Such reciprocal stimulation makes sense when the body is reacting to trauma, since massive microbial invasion and severe bleeding are both possibilities. However, this reciprocal relationship also means that patients with multiple trauma, sepsis, or both, are at risk for massive and inappropriate activation of coagulation and clot lysis—that is, disseminated intravascular coagulation (DIC).

Assessment of Immune Function

Risk Conditions

Most patients admitted to critical-care units are at risk either for immunosuppression or for strong activation of the immune system. Immunosuppression reduces and may eliminate the ability to fight off infection. Even appropriate activation of the immune system carries risks, due to the inevitable production of reactive oxygen metabolites and lytic enzymes and to the potential for widespread activation of the blood coagulation and fibrinolytic systems. Inappropriate activation of the immune system may result in allergic reactions, including anaphylaxis, in response to either environmental allergens or substances administered for therapeutic or diagnostic purposes. It is appropriate to assess every critically ill patient for the presence of factors which *may* contribute to alteration in immune function. These factors include (but are not limited to): acute stress, chronic stress, advanced age, poor nutrition, surgical or traumatic disruption of tissue structure, certain therapeutic drugs and recreational drug abuse.

Acute Stress Acute stress generates a complex mixture of signals to the immune system. Some of these activate immune responses; others inhibit them. As stress becomes chronic, the balance shifts in favor of immunosuppression, due to prolonged secretion of endogenous glucocorticoids. Glucocorticoids inhibit secretion of interleukins during antigen processing and presentation. They also suppress the killing activity of cytotoxic T cells (Handschumacher 1990) and the synthesis of mediators of inflammation, including prostaglandins and leukotrienes (Haynes 1990). Glucocorticoids reduce the numbers of circulating lymphocytes (especially T cells), monocytes, eosinophils and basophils, while increasing the number of circulating neutrophils. The decrease in lymphocytes, monocytes, and eosinophils is due to their sequestration in the extravascular space, not to destruction of the cells (Haynes 1990). Glucocorticoids impair healing by favoring the breakdown of collagen. Note that glucocorticoid administration is likely to suppress both local and systemic signs of inflammation, making detection of an infection more difficult.

Advanced Age Advanced age may cause reduced immune function, although in any given individual it is often difficult to separate the effects of age from those of other factors such as poor nutrition, medications, or chronic disease(s). While age does not appear to alter the relative proportions of T and B lymphocytes or of helper to suppressor T cells, there is evidence that age reduces the ability of T lymphocytes to proliferate when stimulated (Miller 1990). Age also appears to reduce both the secretion of interleukin-2 (IL-2) by activated T cells and the ability of immune system cells to respond to IL-2 (Miller 1990). IL-2 normally stimulates the differentiation of helper, suppressor, and cytotoxic T cells and NK cells (Herberman 1989). The effects of age directly on B cell function, if any, are controversial (Miller 1990).

Additional Conditions Malnutrition reduces the availability of the amino acids, essential lipids, and vitamins necessary for mitosis, mediator synthesis, and formation of antibodies (Keusch and Farthing 1990). Many drugs are known to affect some aspect of either the innate or the adaptive immune responses. The administration of broad-spectrum antimicrobial drugs, for example, kills off much of the normal flora, allowing microbes usually controlled by the normal flora to proliferate and cause superinfections.

Laboratory Tests of Immune Function

White Blood Cell (WBC) Count and Differential Laboratory examination of a peripheral blood smear

can give useful information regarding the nature of antigens to which the patient has been exposed and the nature and adequacy of the body's response. The total *white blood cell count (WBC)* normally ranges between 5,000 and 10,000 per cubic millimeter (Fischbach 1992). An increased total white cell count is a relatively nonspecific finding, since it may indicate inflammation from any cause (an elevated total white cell count is part of the "acute phase response" described earlier). Less commonly, an elevated total white cell count may be the result of malignancy of the bone marrow. A decreased total white cell count usually indicates either generalized suppression of the bone marrow or diversion of large numbers of maturing marrow cells into the pathways for red blood cell or platelet synthesis. Just after a viral infection, suppression of the immune system is common and may be reflected in decreased production of leukocytes with consequent reduced white cell count.

The *differential count* involves determining what fraction of total circulating leukocytes are lymphocytes, granulocytes (neutrophils, eosinophils and basophils), or monocytes. As a routine part of the differential, the relative numbers of mature and immature granulocytes also are determined. Because of their highly segmented nucleus, mature granulocytes are called *"segs."* In the absence of severe allergies or parasitic infestation, neutrophils make up the vast majority of segs. Immature granulocytes are called both *bands* and *stabs.* (The name "band cell" was assigned because the originally bar-shaped nucleus appears to be constricted by an invisible band as it

CRITICAL-CARE GERONTOLOGY

Immune Function in the Elderly

Changes in immunocompetence occur in both very young and very old patients. A number of causes of age-related immune deficiency have been identified in the elderly, including thymic involution, altered antibody production, and decreased antibody response (Gurka 1989). Thymic involution causes deficiencies in number and quality of T cells in the system, predisposing the pa-

tient to infection with intracellular organisms and viruses, as well as to an increase in malignancies. Alterations in antibody production and antibody response, secondary to the natural decline in B-cell performance with increasing age, allow infections to become more easily established (Gurevich 1989).

Additionally, elderly patients who develop infections or septic pro-

cesses may not present with classic signs and symptoms. Many older individuals seek medical treatment because of vague complaints of anorexia, malaise, and weakness. Normal physiologic mechanisms are blunted, with a less conspicuous febrile response and a decreased urge to cough (Petrucci, Booth-Blaemire and Watson 1989).

begins to segment). For historical (rather than physiologic) reasons, an increased percentage of band forms among circulating granulocytes is called a *shift to the left,* while a deficit of band forms is labeled a *shift to the right.* In most instances the vast majority of band forms will be immature neutrophils. An increased percentage of neutrophils with a shift to the left (indicating that the bone marrow is forming new granulocytes) most often indicates a bacterial infection, although there are other causes. Such a report is "both good news and bad news," bad in that the person probably has an infection, good in that his immune system is responding appropriately. A shift to the right can be an ominous sign because the bone marrow is not forming or releasing new granulocytes, potentially leaving the individual with impaired defenses.

A decreased neutrophil count also can indicate that the bone marrow is favoring the formation of other types of leukocytes. For example, during a viral infection, the lymphocyte count will often rise while the neutrophil count falls. The monocyte count typically rises late in the course of an inflammatory response (recall that monocytes enter damaged tissue more slowly than neutrophils do; they are also released from bone marrow more slowly). Infection with microorganisms that are very difficult to kill, for example, in tuberculosis, Hansen's disease (leprosy), and malaria, also increases monocytes.

Determination of Lymphocyte Classes Because different classes of lymphocytes express different groups of proteins on their surfaces, it is possible to use monoclonal antibodies against these lymphocyte antigens to determine what percentage of lymphocytes in a sample belong to each class. All T lymphocytes express the CD3 antigen. Helper T cells also express the CD4 antigen, while suppressor T cells express CD8 along with CD3. The CD19 antigen is an early B-cell marker; CD20 is also a B-cell marker (Fischbach 1992). The helper/suppressor (T4/T8) ratio may be reported; in the healthy immune system it is greater than 1.0.

Culture and Sensitivity (C/S) Samples of blood and other body fluids often are obtained for culture of one or more pathogen(s) responsible for a suspected infection. This information is useful for decisions to institute or to discontinue isolation. Pathogen identification plus sensitivity studies allow medical selection of appropriate antimicrobial therapy. Table 18–2 lists precautions which can help to ensure that C/S specimens yield accurate information. Accuracy is particularly crucial in the critical-care setting, where the patient's condition may be changing rapidly and delayed or incorrect decisions may prove devastating (Warren, Danner and Munford 1992).

Measurement of Complement Components Recall that activation of the complement cascade results in attachment of some of the complement proteins to antigens. Thus, complement activation reduces the concentration of freely circulating inactive forms while fixing or consuming the activated proteins. Commonly measured components include C1q, C3, and C4. C3 depletion often precedes the onset of shock (Fischbach 1992).

TABLE 18–2

Methods for Ensuring Optimal Culture Results

1. **Notify the laboratory if the patient is on antibiotics.** In the ideal situation, cultures are obtained before antibiotic therapy is begun, but when this is not possible, notification of the laboratory that antibiotic therapy has already begun will enable laboratory personnel to make any changes necessary in culture technique.

2. **Communicate the identity of suspected organisms to the laboratory staff.** This will enable selection of appropriate culture media and incubation conditions.

3. **Transport specimens to the laboratory without delay.** Some significantly pathogenic organisms are sufficiently fragile that they will die if transit is delayed, or overgrowth of contaminants may occur.

4. **Obtain sufficient quantities of the material to be cultured, at appropriate times.** Blood cultures require three 10-mL specimens for 99% accuracy and are best obtained before the patient's temperature spikes. Sputum and urine cultures are best taken when the patient arises in the morning.

5. **Take wound, skin, and soft tissue cultures from freshly cleaned areas.** Old drainage should be removed with saline and a 4- by 4-inch gauze pad and fresh drainage collected with a swab.

Data from Gurevich I: *Infectious diseases in critical care nursing: prevention and precautions.* Rockville, MD: Aspen, 1989, pp. 15–34, 37–54.)

Anaphylaxis

Assessment

Pathophysiology *Anaphylaxis,* strictly defined, is a life-threatening immune response mediated by IgE and requiring a sensitizing exposure to the antigen before the exposure on which the anaphylactic episode occurs (Bochner and Lichtenstein 1991). *Anaphylactoid* reactions do not necessarily require a previous sensitizing exposure and/or are not mediated by IgE (Bochner and Lichtenstein 1991). Anaphylaxis and anaphylactoid reactions are indistinguishable during acute presentation and are treated similarly.

Anaphylaxis, the most extreme and dangerous form of immunologic *hypersensitivity,* results from a rapid massive release of mediators. In a hypersensitivity reaction, the immune response significantly injures the host. *Autoimmune diseases* result from attack by the immune system against antigens which are normal components of host tissue (endogenous antigens). In contrast, allergic reactions, including anaphylaxis, are a consequence of unusual activity of the immune system following exposure to an exogenous antigen (also called an *allergen*). A person who develops an allergic disease is said to exhibit *atopy* or an *atopic tendency.* (The term derives from the Greek, meaning "out of place.") Such an individual's immune system manufactures and secretes unusually large amounts of class E antibodies (IgE). In addition, an atopic person's immune system may treat as antigenic such intrinsically harmless substances as pollens, food proteins, or therapeutic drugs. Even in the case of an intrinsically damaging substance such as an insect venom, the harm done by the atopic host's immune response far exceeds the damage resulting from direct action of the venom on host tissue.

IgE is synthesized, as are all antibodies, by B lymphocytes. Upon its release from the lymphocyte, IgE is rapidly taken up by both basophils and mast cells, which attach it to their plasma membrane with the antigen-binding sites facing the extracellular fluid. When the antigen is reintroduced into the body on a later exposure it reacts with the IgE, triggering release of inflammatory mediators from the mast cells and basophils. Among the compounds released are histamine and leukotrienes C_4, D_4 and E_4 (Lewis, Austen and Soberman 1990). The histamine causes vasodilatation and increased microvascular permeability to proteins. The mixture of leukotrienes, formerly called "slow-reacting substance of anaphylaxis," exerts a potent constricting effect on the airways (Lewis, Austen and Soberman 1990).

Risk Conditions Several categories of substances can initiate anaphylaxis (Table 18–3). Note that these include both environmental antigens and substances administered for diagnostic or therapeutic purposes. Thus, a patient already in a critical-care setting could experience an anaphylactic reaction during the course of care.

Signs and Symptoms Upon examination, the patient experiencing an anaphylactic or anaphylactoid reaction demonstrates characteristic signs and symptoms, usually occurring within 20 minutes or less of exposure to the causative agent. There is generalized flushing and urticaria with pruritus, followed by extreme shortness of breath due to bronchospasm and fluid shifts into the alveoli. Often, angioedema (swelling of the hands, feet, lips, and tongue) is seen. The edema of the lips and tongue further compromises ventilation. Peripheral vasodilatation increases the volume of blood in capillary beds, thereby slowing venous return and lowering cardiac output. The intravascular volume is reduced due to the leakage of fluid into tissues across the highly permeable vessels of the microcirculation, producing a relative hypovolemia and further impairing venous return and cardiac output. The combination of reduced cardiac output with peripheral vasodilatation lowers both systolic and diastolic blood pressure, potentially compromising cerebral and coronary blood flow as well as glomerular filtration. The patient may feel a sense of impending doom (Summers 1990).

NURSING DIAGNOSES

The following nursing diagnoses may apply to the patient in anaphylaxis:

- Ineffective airway clearance
- Impaired gas exchange
- Decreased cardiac output
- High risk for injury
- Fear of suffocation
- High risk for altered health maintenance

Planning and Implementation of Care

Ineffective Airway Clearance Related to Angioedema and Bronchospasm As in any emergent situation, first priority must be given to maintenance of a patent airway. Independent measures for mainte-

TABLE 18–3

Substances Associated with Anaphylactic and Anaphylactoid Responses

1. **Foods**
   Eggs or egg whites
   Beans and nuts
   Milk
   Potatoes
   Citrus fruit
   Seafood, especially shellfish
   Corn
   Chocolate

2. **Insect Bites and Stings**
   Venomous snakes
   Bees
   Hornets
   Fire ants
   Wasps
   Yellow jackets
   Jellyfish

3. **Biologics**
   Antisera
   Vaccines
   Fresh frozen plasma
   Platelets
   Gamma globulin
   Adrenocorticotropic hormone (ACTH)
   Pituitary extract
   Albumin
   Insulin
   Cryoprecipitate
   Red blood cells
   White blood cells
   Acetylcysteine
   Thyroid stimulating hormone (TSH)
   Chymopapain
   Plasma protein fractions

4. **Diagnostic Compounds**
   Iodinated contrast agents
   Bromosulfophthalein
   Iopanoic acid (Telepaque)
   Dehydrocholic acid

5. **Anesthetics and Anesthetic Adjuncts**
   Procaine
   Cocaine
   Succinylcholine
   Ketamine
   d-Tubocurarine
   Lidocaine
   Thiopental
   Barbiturates
   Pancuronium
   Atracurium

6. **Antibiotics**
   Penicillins
   Vancomycin
   Tetracyclines
   Streptomycin
   Sulfonamides
   Cephalosporins
   Clindamycin
   Erythromycin
   Nitrofurantoin

7. **Nonsteroidal Anti-inflammatory Drugs**
   Salicylates
   Naproxen
   Ibuprofen

8. **Analgesics**
   Morphine
   Meperidine
   Codeine

9. **Miscellaneous Drugs**
   Dextran
   Mannitol
   Thiazides
   Parenteral iron compounds
   Hydroxyethyl starch
   Protamine
   Cyclosporine

10. **Miscellaneous Other Agents**
    Seminal fluid
    Sulfites
    Exercise
    Methylmethacrylate glue

Data from Dickerson M: Anaphylaxis and anaphylactic shock. *Crit Care Nurse Quart* 1988; 11(1):68–74 and Mathewson Kuhn M: Anaphylactic versus anaphylactoid reactions: Nursing interventions. *Crit Care Nurse* 1990; 10(5):121–136.

nance of airway patency include positioning the head and neck in hyperextension, insertion of oral or nasal airways, and orotracheal or nasotracheal suction (Kersten 1989). Collaborative measures to restore upper airway patency in the presence of edema include nasotracheal or orotracheal intubation. Treatment of lower airway obstruction due to bronchoconstriction requires the collaborative measure of epinephrine administration, subcutaneously or intravenously. For the subcutaneous route, use 0.2–0.5 ml of 1:1000 solution, as ordered; dilute the dose to 1:10,000 for the intravenous route. Repeat the dose every 5–15 minutes until the patient responds. Other possible collaborative pharmaceutical interventions include bronchodilators, such as aminophylline or metaproterenol. Monitor vital signs closely because, once the drugs are effective, the hypotension may be replaced by hypertension with extreme tachycardia, potentially inducing myocardial ischemia (Goldschlager 1988). In addition, collaborative administration of corticosteroids *may* help to shorten prolonged reactions, especially those involving bronchospasm (Bochner and Lichtenstein 1991). However, corticosteroids are not the first-line treatment for anaphylaxis.

Impaired Gas Exchange Related to Alveolar Flooding Fluid shifts from the capillary bed into the pulmonary alveoli and/or pulmonary interstitium impair exchange of gases across the waterlogged alveolar-capillary interface. The resulting hypoxemia usually responds to collaborative intervention with increased inspired oxygen concentration (Kersten 1989). Refer to Chapter 9 for further information on oxygen administration.

Decreased Cardiac Output Related to Fluid Shifts The genesis of the fluid shift and reduced cardiac output is explained under Signs and Symptoms (p. 520). Epinephrine administered to prevent lower airway occlusion also causes vasoconstriction. If intravascular volume is replaced by rapid fluid infusion (a collaborative intervention), the vasopressor effect of epinephrine can help to return the intravascular volume to normal (Burns 1990; Rice 1991).

High Risk for Injury Related to Continued Exposure to Antigen Once the patient's airway, breathing, and circulation are maintained or restored, the antigen must be removed to prevent development of further symptoms. If the causative agent has been administered intravenously, stop the infusion immediately, and change the bag and tubing down to the catheter hub. In the case of intravenous (IV), intramuscular (IM), or subcutaneous drug administration, place a tourniquet above the site to delay absorption and circulation of the offending substance until treatment is underway. If an insect sting is the culprit, remove the stinger by scraping, to prevent rupture of the venom sac and release of additional antigen into the patient's body fluids. If a food is the causative factor, absorption may be reduced or prevented by induction of emesis. If emesis is initiated, be sure to protect the already compromised airway (Dickerson 1988).

Fear of Suffocation Related to Dyspnea Shortness of breath, especially of sudden onset as in an anaphylactic episode, can elicit extreme fear of suffocation. This can become a vicious cycle, with fear causing hyperpnea which may worsen the respiratory status, exacerbating the sensation of dyspnea and making the patient even more fearful (Kersten 1989). To break this cycle, acknowledge the reality of the threat to the person's vital functions. Give the person permission to express the fear (Rossman Jillings 1990). To reassure the person and convey the belief that the situation is manageable, point out the definitive interventions being undertaken to correct the situation.

High Risk for Altered Health Maintenance Related to Lack of Knowledge of Safety Precautions Before the patient who has suffered an anaphylactic episode is released from care, provision must be made for identifying the antigen which provoked the episode and for teaching the patient or significant other(s) how to avoid re-exposure. For example, as a collaborative intervention for a person being discharged, instruct the person and significant other(s) in the self-administration of epinephrine, if appropriate (Bochner and Lichtenstein 1991).

Outcome Evaluation

Evaluate the patient's progress according to the following expected outcome criteria:

- A patent airway.
- Maintenance of patient's normal P_aO_2 on room air.
- Vital signs within normal limits for the patient.
- Urine output greater than 30 ml per hour.
- Adequate skin turgor, mucous membrane moisture and capillary refill.
- Absence of further exposure to the causative agent.
- Verbalization of a realistic understanding of the danger associated with future anaphylactic episodes and of measures to minimize the risk.

Acquired Immune Deficiency Syndrome

Acquired immune deficiency syndrome (AIDS) has rapidly become a major health problem in the United States and in the world, reaching epidemic proportions (Anderson and May 1992). The virus associated with AIDS has been identified as the *human immunodeficiency virus* (HIV). Two types of HIV have been identified; HIV-1 is the cause of almost all HIV infections in the United States, while HIV-2 is currently found mostly in Africa. Infection with HIV reduces the body's ability to mount an immune response, making the person vulnerable to certain malignancies and to the opportunistic infections which indicate that progression to AIDS has occurred (Vaishnav and Wong-Staal 1991). AIDS is the final stage in the continuum of HIV infection. Earlier stages may include an initial acute illness (see p. 524 under Signs and Symptoms); an asymptomatic period which may last for years; chronic lymphadenopathy; or symptomatic HIV disease (previously called the AIDS-related complex or ARC), a constellation of symptoms consisting of persistent fever, weight loss, diarrhea, peripheral neuropathy, dementia, or myelopathy (Lewis 1988).

The drugs available to treat HIV infection delay progression to AIDS, reduce the number and severity of opportunistic infections, and lengthen survival, but they do not cure the disease (Graham et al. 1992; Moore et al. 1991). Therefore, the person with AIDS who receives care in the critical-care setting is experiencing an acutely life-threatening episode superimposed on a chronic illness which must be regarded as ultimately fatal.

Assessment

Pathophysiology

Infectious Process HIV has been identified as a member of the retrovirus group. Retroviruses use the enzyme *reverse transcriptase* to convert their genomic RNA into DNA, which is then inserted into the host genome. (The genome is an organism's complete set of chromosomes.) HIV gains entry into helper T cells by reacting with the CD4 glycoprotein, after which the virus is taken into the cell by endocytosis or the virus initiates fusion of its own lipid membrane with that of the T cell (Vaishnav and Wong-Staal 1991). Following insertion of the DNA copy of the viral genome into the T cell's DNA, replication of the HIV is controlled by both host cell factors and viral factors. In T cells, HIV replication requires an antigen to activate the T cell (Vaishnav and Wong-Staal 1991). This explains why concurrent infection with several other viruses or parasites accelerates progression of HIV infection (Greene 1991). Furthermore, HIV infection reactivates many latent DNA viruses which had previously produced active infection, such as herpesviruses and hepatitis viruses (Vaishnav and Wong-Staal 1991).

Effect on Helper T Cells HIV infection of helper T cells first reduces their function, then kills them. Several mechanisms by which HIV kills T cells have been proposed, including induction of autoimmune attack by other elements of the immune system (Vaishnav and Wong-Staal 1991; Beardsley 1991).

Some killing probably occurs as huge numbers of new HIV particles bud off from an infected cell, since the virus incorporates some of the host cell's membrane into its own lipid membrane envelope. Depletion of helper T cells impairs those immune functions which depend on T-cell help, such as activation of B lymphocytes and cytotoxic T cells.

Effect on Macrophages Cells of the monocyte/macrophage group express CD4 molecules to a lesser extent than the helper T cells, so HIV gains access to them more slowly than to the T cells (Greene 1991). However, macrophages replicate HIV without having to be activated by exposure to an antigen. Furthermore, these cells convey HIV into other organs, particularly the central nervous system (CNS). DNA transcripts of HIV are integrated into the genomes of glia and endothelial cells in the CNS, which thus becomes a protected reservoir for HIV. None of the drugs currently available can excise the viral genome without killing the cell. In rodents, HIV induces increased calcium permeability in the cell membrane of neurons, which rapidly kills the nerve cells. It is not known whether the same mechanism accounts for the CNS symptoms of the *AIDS-dementia-complex* (Vaishnav and Wong-Staal 1991).

HIV-infected monocytes secrete abnormally large amounts of cytokines (Keusch and Farthing 1990), which may account for some of the wasting seen in AIDS. Cachectin, one of the cytokines present in excess, inhibits the storage of fat (Herberman 1989). HIV is also found in the wall of the intestine, where it may directly affect intestinal function (Keusch and Farthing 1990).

Rapid Mutation of Virus The genome of HIV is unusually complex, and its reverse transcriptase is unusually error-prone (Vaishnav and Wong-Staal 1990). This accounts for the rapid mutation of the virus, which greatly complicates efforts to create an effective vaccine. Each viral isolate represents "a mixture or 'swarm' of microvariants that are highly related but distinguishable" (Vaishnav and Wong-Staal 1990). The genome of HIV particles isolated from a given patient changes as the disease progresses, and even closely related HIV isolates can have different cytopathic effects.

Risk Conditions Transmission of the virus takes place from person to person through infected body fluids and depends on several factors. The virus must be: (a) present in the fluid, (b) alive and stable in the fluid, (c) transmitted in a viable state, in a sufficient quantity to a susceptible host, and (d) able to gain access to the host's tissues and invade host cells. HIV is transmitted most commonly by intimate sexual contact involving exchange of semen or vaginal fluid; by direct injection of blood or blood products containing the viral genome into tissue (as in a needle stick or injection of illicit drugs); or perinatally from mother to fetus (Table 18–4). Infection is dose related; for example, although small amounts of the virus have been identified in sweat and saliva, casual contact, sharing eating utensils, and hugging and kissing are not believed to transmit the virus (Quinn 1990).

Signs and Symptoms

Primary or Acute Infection   Primary or acute infection with HIV may be asymptomatic or may induce a mononucleosis-like syndrome (which often goes undiagnosed) (Clark et al. 1991). The acute illness includes fever, sweats, lethargy, malaise, myalgia, arthralgia, headache, photophobia, diarrhea, sore throat, lymphadenopathy, and sometimes a maculopapular rash distributed primarily on the torso (Tindall et al. 1990).

Viral Replication   Viral replication begins almost immediately; infectious cytopathic virus can be detected in plasma, peripheral-blood mononuclear cells, and cerebrospinal fluid during the most symptomatic period of the primary illness and *before* any antibodies to HIV are generated (Clark et al. 1991). The high

levels of replication decline (without pharmacologic intervention) in as little as 10 days, to as low as 1% of peak levels (Daar et al. 1991). In some patients, this fall in viremia coincides with the appearance of antibodies to HIV. The means by which the viremia is reduced may include activation of cytotoxic T cells (Baltimore and Feinberg 1989).

Viral isolates obtained following the reduction in viremia are often of "microvariants" that replicate slowly and are of low cytopathic potency (Vaishnav and Wong-Staal 1990). The immune system may have successfully dealt with rapidly replicating variants in the initial inoculum, but slowly replicating variants have nevertheless succeeded in becoming integrated into host DNA. Over a long period (up to a decade or more) these low-cytopathic variants erode the immune system, paving the way for eventual emergence of aggressive, strongly cytopathic variants generated by the continuing production of mutations during reverse transcription (Vaishnav and Wong-Staal 1990). The patient is usually asymptomatic during the long period of reduced viremia, but the virus is not truly latent (Baltimore and Feinberg 1989), and the person must still be considered capable of transmitting the virus.

Clinical AIDS   Severe erosion of immune function is heralded by the development of symptomatic disease,

TABLE 18–4

Guidelines for Preventing Transmission of HIV to Health Care Workers

Although HIV seroconversion in health care workers is very rare, there have been several reported cases. The following guidelines are recommended by the Centers for Disease Control to prevent transmission of HIV between all patients and all health care workers (Gerberding 1990).

1. All health care workers who perform or assist in invasive procedures must be educated regarding the epidemiology, modes of transmission, and prevention of HIV infection.

2. Wear gloves when touching mucous membranes or nonintact skin, and use other appropriate barrier precautions when indicated (e.g., masks, gowns, and eye coverings if aerosolization or splashes are likely to occur).

3. After delivery of an infant, use appropriate barrier precautions when handling the placenta or the infant until blood and amniotic fluid have been removed.

4. Use care to avoid injuring the hands with needles, scalpels, and other sharp instruments.

5. A health care worker who has exudative lesions or weeping dermatitis should not assist in invasive procedures or other direct patient care activities.

6. Routine serologic testing for evidence of HIV infection is *not* necessary for health care workers who perform invasive procedures or for patients undergoing invasive procedures.

7. All health care workers with evidence of any illness that may compromise their ability to adequately and safely perform invasive procedures should be evaluated medically.

8. If an incident occurs that results in exposure of a patient to the blood of a health care worker, the patient should be informed and recommendations for management of such exposures should be followed.

Data from Gerberding J: Occupational HIV transmission: Issues for health care providers. In: *The medical management of AIDS,* 2d ed. Sande M, Volberding P (eds). Philadelphia: Saunders, 1990, pp. 57–65.

such as Kaposi's sarcoma; one of many opportunistic infections (*Pneumocystis carinii* pneumonia, toxoplasmosis, cryptococcosis, cryptosporidiosis, or *Candida* esophagitis); or nonopportunistic infection by such pathogens as mycobacteria, cytomegalovirus (CMV), herpesvirus, *Salmonella,* and *Shigella* (Keusch and Farthing 1990).

Diagnosis of AIDS   Diagnosis of AIDS is based on criteria established by the Centers for Disease Control (CDC): (a) the presence of specific opportunistic infections in patients who are seronegative for HIV or whose serologic status is unknown, or (b) the existence of laboratory criteria including a positive HIV antibody test and a low helper T cell lymphocyte count.

Tuberculosis has emerged explosively as a health problem in HIV-positive persons (Snider and Roper 1992; Barnes et al. 1991). *Mycobacterium tuberculosis* is one of the first organisms to cause disease in an HIV-infected person, even before *Pneumocystis carinii.* The incidence of active tuberculosis (TB) in AIDS patients is about 500 times that in the general population. HIV infection increases both the risk of reactivation of latent tuberculosis and the rate of progression in those newly infected by the mycobacterium. In those with advanced HIV infection, tuberculosis usually involves other organs in addition to the lungs (Barnes et al. 1991). Roughly 8% of HIV-infected persons with positive skin tests to TB antigen will develop active infection *each year,* in marked contrast to the risk of only 10% in a *lifetime* among HIV-negative persons with positive TB skin tests (Barnes et al. 1991). A negative skin test in an HIV-positive patient is not reassuring, however, because many such persons do not react appropriately to intradermally administered antigens. (Langerhans cells of the skin, which are important in antigen presentation for intradermally administered antigens, are infected and destroyed by HIV.) Development of drug resistance among *M. tuberculosis* strains is occurring; almost 90% of cases of drug-resistant TB in the United States are in HIV-positive persons (Snider and Roper 1992). There have been several documented instances of spread of TB among HIV-positive patients in hospitals, possibly facilitated by cough-inducing procedures. Mortality in HIV-positive patients infected by drug-resistant strains of *M. tuberculosis* is between 70% and 90%, with a very fast course (Snider and Roper 1992).

Laboratory Studies   Laboratory studies in AIDS (as opposed to earlier stages of HIV-related disease) demonstrate *cutaneous anergy* (lack of response to intradermal or subcutaneous administration of antigenic stimuli) in many persons with AIDS. Lymphope-

nia is profound; CD4+ lymphocytes in particular are reduced, usually below 0.2×10^9/L (Corey and Fleming 1992), and the CD4+/CD8+ (helper/suppressor) ratio is less than 1.0. Antibodies to HIV may be demonstrable, but as AIDS progresses the antibody titer may fall due to accelerating destruction of the adaptive immune system (Lewis 1988; Tindall et al. 1990; Hollander 1990).

NURSING DIAGNOSES

Because of the complexity of AIDS, there will be multiple applicable nursing diagnoses in any one person with AIDS during any particular episode of critical illness. The appropriate diagnoses will differ from time to time in the life of an individual person with AIDS and will also vary among persons with AIDS. Physical needs will depend on the stage of illness and the particular opportunistic infection being experienced. Even more importantly, psychologic and spiritual needs are highly specific to the individual. Applicable nursing diagnoses may include but certainly are not limited to:

- High risk for infection
- Impaired gas exchange
- Sensory-perceptual alteration
- Altered nutrition: less than body requirements
- Altered oral mucous membrane
- Fluid volume deficit
- Pain
- Activity intolerance
- Anticipatory grieving
- Social isolation

Planning and Implementation of Care

High Risk for Infection Related to Immunosuppressed State   Septicemia can occur with any opportunistic infection. Persons with AIDS are at high risk for nosocomial infections as well as community-acquired opportunistic and nonopportunistic infections. Thoroughly wash your hands before and after caring for a person with AIDS, and maintain strict aseptic technique during invasive procedures. Instruct the patient and visitors about the importance of washing their hands. Assist bedfast patients to turn and deep breathe at least every 2 hours and to carry out any prescribed ventilatory exercises. Encourage oral intake as much as possible to help maintain adequate fluid balance. Assess frequently and thoroughly for newly developing signs and symptoms of infection; look for clouding of urine, visual disturbances, fever, episodes of chilling and diaphoresis, worsening of dyspnea, or signs of inflammation at previous IM or IV sites. Check laboratory reports for alterations in WBC count or differential.

Impaired Gas Exchange Related to Diffuse Alveolar Consolidation A frequent admitting diagnosis for a person with AIDS in a critical-care unit is *Pneumocystis carinii* pneumonia (PCP). The taxonomic classification of *P. carinii* is still in dispute. It is usually referred to as a protozoan, but its enzyme complement, RNA composition, and cyst wall composition resemble those of fungi more than those of protozoa (Walzer P., 1991). Transmission appears to be by airborne particles, but their exact nature is not known. Transmission is so efficient that by age 3 most children are seropositive and the organism is considered a normal resident of the respiratory tract. PCP is almost unknown except in immunosuppressed individuals, and infection in those who are HIV-positive is considered reactivation of a latent infection (Walzer P., 1991).

Because the organism is considered part of the normal flora, CDC guidelines have not recommended isolation of those with PCP. However, Walzer P. (1991) recommends that immunocompromised patients without PCP be isolated from those with known active PCP, based on epidemiologic evidence of person-to-person spread (i.e., a new infection rather than reactivation) among debilitated patients. There are probably multiple strains of the organism, which may explain how a "new" infection can arise in a person who already carries the organism. Incubation time is long: 1–2 months (Walzer P. 1991). It is therefore possible, if a new strain is acquired nosocomially, for the newly infected person to be dismissed from the hospital unaware of the infection.

The pathology of PCP is poorly understood. On autopsy, the lungs evidence a "mononuclear-cell infiltrate in the interstitium" and "proteinaceous fluid and organisms *[P. carinii]* in alveoli" (Consensus Statement 1990). The latter is reminiscent of the adult respiratory distress syndrome (ARDS). Granulocytes are found in bronchoalveolar lavage fluid. Lymphocytes and various cytokines are also believed to have a role in the inflammation. Hypoxemia at diagnosis is the best predictor of the severity of the episode. Five to thirty percent of persons with PCP will develop respiratory failure, and most of these patients will die from it (Consensus Statement 1990).

In addition to examining the laboratory report to ascertain the degree of hypoxemia, assess respiratory status frequently. Auscultate lung sounds. With PCP, the lungs may sound clear, or diffuse crackles may be present. Because PCP is a diffuse process, no particular lobe of the lung is affected (Rosen 1990). Observe respiratory excursion, check the color of skin and mucous membranes, and monitor heart rate (which may increase as a compensatory mechanism for hypoxemia). Note the presence of a cough. Place the individual in high Fowler's position, if this is comfortable. Collaborative treatment includes administration of increased fraction of inspired oxygen and of medications, as ordered, most commonly trimethoprim-sulfamethoxazole and pentamidine. These drugs are tolerated poorly, and side effects may include rash, neutropenia, and severe vomiting (Carr 1988). Mechanical ventilation may be necessary to maintain oxygenation while treatment takes effect. Initiation of chemotherapy for PCP is often accompanied, for 2–3 days, by worsening of symptoms, probably due to worsening of inflammation (Consensus Statement 1990). Control of inflammation to prevent tissue damage is achieved with corticosteroids (Montaner et al. 1990).

Most persons who are HIV-positive, whether or not their condition has progressed to clinical AIDS, will be on antiretroviral medication. They may be receiving zidovudine, didanosine, dideoxycytidine, foscarnet, or some combination of these, in addition to pentamidine or dapsone as prophylaxis against PCP. Review the interactions of these drugs with any new medications ordered.

Sensory-perceptual Alteration Related to Pathogen Invasion of the CNS HIV itself, as well as numerous opportunistic pathogens, can affect the central nervous system, causing abscesses, meningitis, or encephalopathy. Initially, persons with AIDS complain of decreased attention span, loss of memory, decreased mental acuity, or personality changes (Price and Brew 1990). Progression of disease or the onset of a new opportunistic infection may be heralded by headache, which can be followed by seizures, sensory or cognitive deficits, and coma. If the pathogen is *Cryptococcus neoformans,* pharmacologic therapy may include amphotericin B (IV) or fluconazole (oral). Monitor the patient carefully for side effects such as fever, neutropenia, anemia, and liver dysfunction. Toxoplasmosis encephalitis usually is treated with sulfadiazine or pyrimethamine, both given orally. Monitor for nephrotoxicity, gastrointestinal distress, and/or hypersensitivity (Carr 1988). If the patient is being treated with antitubercular drugs, be aware that rifampin and antifungal agents may impair each other's effectiveness (Corey and Fleming 1992). Independent nursing interventions include monitoring for neurologic signs such as headache and changes in mentation or level of consciousness. Reorient the patient frequently, and protect him or her from injury.

Altered Nutrition: Less Than Body Requirements Related to Oral Pain, Anorexia, Accelerated Metabolism, and/or Diarrhea This problem has been referred to as the wasting syndrome associated with AIDS. Numerous etiologic factors are involved, and the problem is usually worse than it appears from the data on height and weight because the person with AIDS often has increased extracellular fluid volume, which can mask a diminution in cellular mass (Keusch and Farthing 1990). The disease process itself induces increased use of protein from body stores, while reduced nutrient intake can be severe enough to justify the term "starvation" and result in depletion of fat stores. Anorexia may be related to fatigue, fear, anxiety, depression, or oral pain resulting from stomatitis. Malabsorption of ingested nutrients results from infections of the intestinal tract. While infections and inflammatory processes usually increase metabolic rate, there is evidence that in at least some AIDS patients the resting metabolic rate is reduced below normal, perhaps a compensatory response to diminished nutrient intake (Keusch and Farthing 1990).

Intervene with independent measures such as consultation with the patient and a clinical dietitian to plan a diet with adequate protein and calories, offering soft foods and foods that can be easily swallowed, serving small portions, and encouraging significant others to bring in favorite foods. If the individual is not tolerating oral feedings, consult the physician early for collaborative intervention, as malnutrition is more difficult to reverse once the deficit is significant. Refer to Chapter 19 for further information on nutrition.

Altered Oral Mucous Membrane Related to Oral Candidiasis, Malnutrition, or Chemotherapy Impairment of oral mucous membrane integrity is seen specifically as stomatitis, pharyngitis, or esophagitis from *Candida* infection related to the incompetent immune system, altered nutritional status, and/or a side effect of chemotherapy. Observe the individual for reddened or inflamed mucous membranes, ulcerations, and white opaque lesions on mucous membranes.

Independent nursing care measures include assisting with frequent oral hygiene and ensuring fluid intake of at least 2,500 cc/day. Consult the guidelines of the Taskforce on Nutritional Support in AIDS for suggestions on how to manipulate temperature, texture, acidity, and flavor of foods to achieve adequate nutrition in patients for whom eating is uncomfortable (Keusch and Farthing 1990). Collaborative interventions include administration of prescribed medications.

Fluid Volume Deficit Related to Poor Intake and Diarrhea Fluid deficit may be related to anorexia or to the severe unrelenting diarrhea that often occurs with infection during AIDS. The critical-care nurse can independently encourage fluid intake and monitor for signs of dehydration and electrolyte imbalance (see Chapter 16). Collaborative interventions include administration of prescribed antidiarrheal agents, such as Lomotil®.

Pain Related to Immobility, Neuropathy, or Pathologic Lesions Pain associated with AIDS may be related to immobility, neurologic involvement (peripheral neuropathy), dyspnea, swelling of Kaposi's sarcoma lesions, and herpes or *Candida* infections, to name only a few of the factors which may be involved. Often it is difficult to relieve the pain completely; rather, seek to decrease it to a tolerable level. Independent nursing interventions may involve positioning for comfort, using therapeutic touch, and instructing the patient in meditation techniques, use of guided imagery, and distraction. Narcotic analgesics may be given as a collaborative intervention, usually orally or IV since decreased muscle mass makes IM injections difficult. Achieve and maintain pain relief through optimal timing of analgesic administration; do not allow pain to reintensify before the next dose.

Activity Intolerance Related to Malnutrition and Fluid Deficit AIDS often afflicts young, independent people. Encourage independence as much as possible to maintain an optimal level of activity and self-care. It is important to be sensitive to the person's needs and desires for independence.

Anticipatory Grieving Related to Fatal Disease The diagnosis of AIDS, and the subsequent implications, usually will be a source of anxiety, fear, concern, anger, and depression. Everyone involved will go through a grieving process when the diagnosis is made. The nurse can have a positive effect with independent nursing interventions. Encourage verbalization of fear and help significant others to project a calm and concerned attitude. Involve all significant others in teaching, and explain all procedures to the patient. The use of relaxation exercises or guided imagery can relieve stress, and visualization exercises can facilitate utilization of inner strength. It is essential that the caretaker support the coping mechanisms used by the person and significant others.

Social Isolation Related to Stigma of Disease

Coping with a potentially terminal illness is difficult even with a large social support network, but being diagnosed with AIDS can cost a person income, living quarters, health insurance, dignity, and social support. The diagnosis of AIDS challenges an individual's coping mechanisms to their maximum; it is imperative to mobilize as much support as possible from significant others and community resources.

Early and deliberate assessment and intervention connecting persons with AIDS and support networks relieves the risk of social isolation and maladaptive coping associated with this stigmatized condition (Nyamathi and van Servellen 1989). You can help to reduce the patient's social isolation while he or she is in the critical-care setting by interacting with him or her every time you come into the room (i.e., make sure you nurse the patient, not just the tubes and monitors). Deliberately stop in the patient's room even when the call light isn't on; this lets the patient know that you care about him or her and aren't minimizing your contact because he or she has AIDS. Use touch to comfort and to enhance the patient's sense of your presence if your assessment of the patient's feelings about the use of touch indicate it is appropriate.

Outcome Evaluation

Evaluate the patient's progress according to these criteria:

- Arterial blood gases are within normal limits.
- Patient is alert and oriented in all domains.
- Patient is free of nosocomial infection.
- Nutritional status is optimal.
- Oral mucous membrane is intact, or alterations do not impair or restrict oral intake.
- Patient verbalizes optimum pain relief.
- Patient is physically active as tolerated.
- Urine output is optimum ($\geq$30 ml/hour) with adequate skin turgor.

- Patient and significant others verbalize a sense of hope accompanied by realistic planning for the future.
- Patient has adequate social services and support network.

Organ Transplantation Immunology

Since the first transplantation of kidneys between monozygotic twins in 1954, organ transplantation has become an important treatment modality for end-stage organ failure. Currently several organs are being transplanted successfully from living donors or from cadavers, including hearts, single lungs, pancreases, livers, kidneys, and bone marrow. This section presents immunologic aspects of caring for the patient undergoing transplantation. The legal and ethical aspects are presented in Chapter 3. Surgical aspects of renal transplantation are covered in Chapter 15.

Blood samples from potential donors are ABO-typed for blood group determination and cross-matched with the recipient's blood for compatibility. If the recipient has antibodies to the donor's antigens, transplantation may be contraindicated because of the risk of graft rejection. The blood samples also are HLA tissue-typed to identify antigens in donor and recipient tissues. HLA histocompatibility minimizes the risk that the recipient's body will reject the transplanted organ as foreign tissue. In addition, leukocytes from donor and recipient are incubated together in a mixed leukocyte culture (MLC). The degree of compatibility is most helpful in screening living related donors (Waltzer W. 1991).

Physiopharmacology of Immunosuppression

Acute rejection episodes are mediated by T cells, so immunosuppressive medications are used to suppress T cell response. Successful transplantation is a delicate balancing act. On the one hand, insufficient immune suppression causes rejection and allows the development of graft-versus-host disease if the transplanted organ contains lymphocytes. On the other hand, excessive immunosuppression leaves the patient open to opportunistic infections and to malignancies. Immunosuppression usually is begun shortly before transplantation takes place, to blunt the initial response of the immune system to the foreign cells. The choice of immunosuppressant drug depends on the organ to be transplanted, the recipient's health status (for example, the degree of kidney and liver functioning or the state of pregnancy) and the preference of the physician. Following transplantation, the dose of immunosuppressant gradually is reduced to maintenance level. Episodes of rejection are treated by briefly raising the dose of immunosuppressant.

Specific drugs used include prednisone, a glucocorticoid (see the earlier section on "Assessment of Immune Function," subsection on "Risk Conditions" for mechanisms of action); cyclosporine; azathioprine (Imuran) and various antibodies. Cyclosporine inhibits an early step in the response of helper T cells to stimulation by antigens or by regulatory molecules (Handschumacher 1990). Although it does not suppress bone marrow functioning, cyclosporine is significantly nephrotoxic. Azathioprine inhibits mitosis and therefore suppresses bone marrow functioning rather nonspecifically.

Other agents that have been used during rejection episodes include *antilymphocyte globulin* (ALG) and *antithymocyte globulin* (ATG). These drugs provide antibodies against the lymphocytes or thymocytes that mediate rejection. ATG induces lysis of thymus-derived lymphocytes and suppression of T-cell functioning (Handschumacher 1990). More specific antibodies, called *monoclonal antibodies,* are directed against

NURSING DIAGNOSIS

A nursing diagnosis pertinent to the patient who has undergone homograft transplantation, no matter what the specific type of transplantation, is:

- High risk for infection

either the antigen-receptor expressed by T cells or the CD3 glycoprotein complex. *OKT₃*, a monoclonal antibody against the CD3 complex, blocks the function of T cells (all of which express the CD3 glycoproprotein) but does not lyse them (Handschumacher 1990). Please refer to Chapter 15 for further information on immunosuppression in transplant recipients.

Signs and Symptoms of Rejection

Classic presenting signs and symptoms of rejection include fever, hypertension, tenderness over the transplanted organ, and a recurrence of the original signs and symptoms of organ failure. Most transplant

ADVANCES IN CRITICAL-CARE TECHNOLOGY

Monoclonal Antibodies

Monoclonal antibodies are antibodies produced by the members of a B-lymphocyte clone. Since the cells of a clone are identical and are descended from a single B lymphocyte, only a single type of antibody is produced by the clone (for example, only IgM directed against a single antigen). This is in marked contrast to the heterogeneous mixture of antibodies (of all classes and directed against an enormous variety of antigens) found in "gamma globulin."

To generate a monoclonal antibody, the gene for the desired antibody is inserted into cells derived from a myeloma—a tumor of B lymphocytes (Figure 18–5). Myeloma cells proliferate readily, so that adequate quantities of the desired antibody are produced. Antibodies against the Lipid A component of gram-negative bacterial endotoxin have been tested in septic patients (Ziegler et al. 1991; Wolff 1991). The results have sparked a controversy (Warren, Danner and

Munford 1992; Wenzel 1992), with some investigators concerned about the safety and the cost/benefit ratio. Antibodies to interleukin-1 and to tumor necrosis factor, two of the cytokines whose concentrations are elevated in the blood of septic patients, are also available (Wolff 1991). The development and testing of these antibodies offers new hope for septic patients, who otherwise have a poor prognosis.

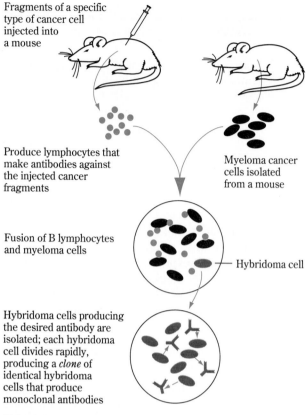

Fragments of a specific type of cancer cell injected into a mouse

Produce lymphocytes that make antibodies against the injected cancer fragments

Myeloma cancer cells isolated from a mouse

Fusion of B lymphocytes and myeloma cells

Hybridoma cell

Hybridoma cells producing the desired antibody are isolated; each hybridoma cell divides rapidly, producing a *clone* of identical hybridoma cells that produce monoclonal antibodies

FIGURE 18–5

Monoclonal antibodies. From Marieb E: *Essentials of human anatomy and physiology,* 2d ed. Redwood City, CA: Benjamin/Cummings, 1988.

recipients experience several rejection episodes and overcome them successfully. Rejection is, however, a medical emergency and should be identified and treated immediately (Waltzer W., 1991). In the case of renal transplantation, distinguishing rejection of the transplanted kidney from nephrotoxicity due to cyclosporine may require a biopsy of the transplanted kidney (Handschumacher 1990).

Planning and Implementation of Care

High Risk for Infection Related to Immunosuppression The patient who is therapeutically immunosuppressed is as much at risk of infection as is the individual with AIDS. Independent and collaborative nursing interventions for this person include surveillance for signs and symptoms of infection, strict handwashing, minimization of invasive procedures and indwelling lines, and limitation of exposure of the patient to individuals with known infections.

Outcome Evaluation

Compare the condition of your patient with the following outcome criterion:

- Patient remains afebrile and free of signs and symptoms of infection.

Sepsis/Septic Syndrome

Defining sepsis is a controversial issue in critical care. To eliminate confusion, the definitions to be used in this section are as follows:

Bacteremia is the asymptomatic presence of bacteria in the blood. *Sepsis* is the presence of suspected infection and systemic symptoms (specifically tachypnea, tachycardia, and hypo- or hyperthermia). The term *septic syndrome* describes the septic patient who demonstrates evidence of one or more organ systems in failure, such as oliguria, severe hypoxemia, changes in mental status, or lacticacidemia. *Septic shock* characterizes the patient with sepsis syndrome who exhibits hypotension. Estimates of the incidence of true sepsis range from 70,000 to 300,000 cases per year, with a mortality rate approaching 50%. If the illness progresses to septic shock, mortality has been estimated as high as 90% (Bone 1991).

Assessment

Pathophysiology The pathophysiologic mechanisms of sepsis result from activation of the innate immune response throughout the body. What differentiates sepsis from the "normal" inflammatory process in localized tissue damage is only the greater intensity of the response. Dispersion of microorganisms throughout the body results in massive activation of phagocytic cells, which release large quantities of lytic enzymes and reactive oxygen metabolites as well as numerous interleukins and cytokines. Reactive oxygen metabolites damage lipids indiscriminately. Lytic enzymes break down extracellular matrix as well as cellular structures. Both of these processes further stimulate phagocytosis, developing a vicious cycle that is intensified by the effects of interleukins and cytokines.

The chemical mediators of inflammation dilate virtually all systemic arterioles and induce an enormous increase in cardiac output, as the body seeks to maintain normal blood pressure and ward off distributive shock. Increased microvascular permeability in all tissues leads to hypovolemia, further stressing the cardiovascular system, which eventually reaches its limit and is unable to maintain normotension. Onset of hypotension signals the transition from septic syndrome to septic shock. The septic state also predisposes to the development of disseminated intravascular coagulation secondary to endothelial damage by microorganisms and strong activation of the immune system.

A fortunate few patients in septic shock respond to fluid infusion and pharmacologic intervention with vasopressor or cardiostimulant drugs. Failure to respond may result from the depressant effects on the heart of lactic acid and other toxic molecules produced by ischemic tissue (Table 18–5). Another possible explanation for the eventual fatal hypotension despite aggressive intervention is exhaustion of arteriolar smooth muscle cells from sustained contraction in the absence of adequate perfusion. Early detection of sepsis and aggressive intervention to identify and treat the responsible organisms while supporting the circulatory system provide the only hope for a successful outcome (Hoffman and Lefkowitz 1990).

Risk Conditions A number of risk factors for the development of sepsis have been identified. The most important is leukopenia with an absolute WBC count of less than 1,000/cubic mm. Lack of intact skin or mucous membranes exposes the patient to the normal flora of the body surfaces as well as to any pathogenic organisms present there. *Staphylococcus, Pseudomonas,* and *Candida* are present among the normal flora and can cause sepsis in a susceptible host. Surgical procedures or trauma that result in contamination of the peritoneal cavity by intestinal contents place the patient at high risk from the normal intestinal flora, including *Escherichia coli, Enterobacter,* and *Serratia.* Indwelling invasive lines provide a route for the cutaneous microflora to reach the circulation. Diabetes mellitus, uremia, and chronic administration of corticosteroids all result in decreased resistance to microbial invasion (Tolkoff-Rubin and Rubin 1990). Advanced age *may* diminish immune system functioning. Chronic illness and long-term malnutrition are additional immunocompromising states (Piper and Crawford 1990; Keusch and Farthing 1990).

Signs and Symptoms Just as the toxic effects of the mediators involved in sepsis are systemic, so are the signs and symptoms of sepsis. The classic presentation includes flushed skin, tachycardia, tachypnea, and fever. Some patients, especially those at the extremes of age, present with hypothermia. During the septic stage, before impaired tissue perfusion develops, urine

TABLE 18–5

Mediators of Sepsis

MEDIATOR	SYSTEMIC EFFECTS
Cytokines	
Tumor necrosis factor	Profound hypotension
	Pulmonary edema
	Thrombocytopenia
	Leukopenia
	Fever
	Endothelial disruption and fibrin formation
	Release of interleukin-1 and prostaglandins
	Platelet activation
	Anorexia
	Nausea
	Inhibition of fatty acid synthesis
Interleukin-1	Synergistic action with tumor necrosis factor, increasing the strength of its effects.
Free radicals of oxygen	Lung injury
	Cell death
Proteases	Destruction of interstitial architecture
Prostaglandins and thromboxanes	Profound systemic vasodilatation
	Bronchoconstriction
	Platelet aggregation
	Pulmonary vasoconstriction

Data from Stroud M, Swindell B, Bernard G: Cellular and humoral mediators of sepsis syndrome. *Crit Care Nurs Clin North Am* 1990; 2(2):151–159.

output may be inappropriately high for the fluid intake, and the urine concentration will be relatively low, similar to that of plasma. Once the septic syndrome develops, additional signs and symptoms arise from impaired perfusion of one or more organs. Reduced renal blood flow may cause oliguria and eventually azotemia. Disorientation, confusion, lethargy, agitation, or obtundation may be present if cerebral blood flow is insufficient. Jaundice, stress ulceration, and gastrointestinal (GI) bleeding may develop as a result of hypoperfusion of the GI tract.

Laboratory Data Laboratory values depend on the particular event that made the patient vulnerable to sepsis, as well as on the state of the immune system before sepsis set in and the duration of the septic state. Although an increased white cell count (with a leftward shift in the differential) is the most common alteration during sepsis, decreased numbers of leukocytes have also been reported. The latter result would be expected if the patient is immunosuppressed. Elevated blood urea nitrogen (BUN) and creatinine levels may be seen once renal blood flow declines or if it was low before the onset of sepsis. There may be thrombocytopenia, with or without lengthened prothrombin and partial thromboplastin times. A mixed acid–base abnormality is most common, comprised of metabolic acidosis, caused by poor tissue perfusion, combined with respiratory alkalosis, due to hyperventilation (Balk and Bone 1989).

Planning and Implementation of Care

The following interventions are designed to support the body as it attempts to fight the widespread infection. None of these interventions actually reverses the septic state; doing so requires the collaborative intervention of administration of appropriate antimicrobial drugs (Hoffman and Lefkowitz 1990). Unless the infection is eliminated, recovery will not occur.

Fluid Volume Deficit Related to Hyperventilation and Elevated Urine Output Increased insensible water loss through the respiratory tract accompanies hyperventilation. Renal vasodilatation due to the mediators of inflammation renders the kidney unable to conserve water. Keep careful records of intake and output and assess for skin turgor and moistness of mucous membranes. Since fluid absorption from the GI tract may be poor, consult the physician about

the collaborative intervention of intravenous fluid administration.

High Risk for Altered Body Temperature: Fever Related to Pyrogens or Hypothermia Related to Depressed Immune Response Fever is commonly experienced by patients suffering from sepsis or septic syndrome, and the possible benefit of this elevation in body temperature remains a matter of controversy. Systemic hyperthermia may assist in slowing the reproduction of or actually killing microorganisms with a narrow range of thermal tolerance. However, the elevation in metabolic rate associated with increased body temperature increases the demands on an already taxed circulatory system. Some authorities recommend not treating a temperature below 39°C and treating higher temperatures only in children with a history of febrile seizures. Most agree that using medication to reset the hypothalamic temperature regulatory center is preferable to using a cooling blanket or packing the patient in ice, since the latter may cause powerful vasoconstriction in the periphery while the core temperature remains elevated (Pierson 1988).

If the patient is hypothermic, provide additional blankets. Use heating pads only with great caution, since reduced peripheral perfusion renders the skin more susceptible to thermal damage.

Altered Nutrition: Less Than Body Requirements Related to Restricted Oral Intake or Elevated Metabolic Rate Oral intake, especially of foods, may be restricted due to poor absorption by the hypoperfused GI tract. If such restriction exists, consult the physician about the collaborative intervention of intravenous nutritional support. If oral intake is permitted, encourage and assist the patient to consume frequent small servings of easily absorbed foods.

Anxiety Related to Seriousness of Illness Anxiety is defined as "A state in which the individual experiences feelings of uneasiness (apprehension) and activation of the autonomic nervous system in response to a vague, nonspecific threat" (Carpenito 1992). The septic patient will probably be aware that "something is wrong" even if his or her condition has not been fully discussed with him or her. To help allay anxiety, answer questions honestly. Explain all interventions, unless doing so appears to increase the patient's anxiety. Be present for the patient by interacting with him or her whenever you are in the room to perform a technical procedure and by checking on the patient even when no alarms are sounding and the call light isn't on. Physical comfort measures such as freshening linens, giving a backrub, providing oral care, or applying a cool cloth to the face or forehead also allow you to reassure the patient emotionally. With some patients, touch is a very effective means of reducing anxiety. Evaluate the patient's response to your touch carefully, since some patients prefer that touch be minimized.

Decreased Cardiac Output Related to Relative Hypovolemia The mediators released as part of the inflammatory process cause movement of fluid from the intravascular to the interstitial space by opening the tight junctions between capillary endothelial cells, allowing leakage of proteins as well as smaller solutes and water out of the vasculature. In sepsis, this capillary leak can be sufficient to require significant amounts of fluid replacement. The choice of colloid versus crystalloid for fluid replacement is a matter of some dispute. Since the microvasculature of the septic patient is excessively permeable to solutes, including protein, colloids may not remain in the vascular space.

If they do cross into the interstitial space, their presence worsens edema by drawing additional water out of the vasculature. Independent nursing actions to facilitate replenishment of intravascular volume include encouraging oral intake as appropriate and possible, encouraging activity (even if only repositioning) to mobilize fluid pooled in dependent tissues, and positioning limbs higher than the heart so that the hydrostatic pressure gradient favors reabsorption of fluid into capillaries and flow of blood toward the heart. Collaborative interventions may also include judicious use of vasopressor drugs to facilitate venous return (Hoffman and Lefkowitz 1990). Keep in mind, however, that vasopressors work only as long as there is peripheral volume to return; increased intravascular volume must precede vasopressor therapy. Cardiostimulant drugs may also be used, especially those which increase cardiac output without constricting renal blood vessels (Hoffman and Lefkowitz 1990).

Altered Tissue Perfusion in One or More Organ Systems (Renal, Cerebral, Cardiopulmonary, Gastrointestinal, Peripheral) Related to Relative Hypovolemia Independent nursing interventions in this patient population include surveillance for signs of decreased perfusion, such as poor distal pulses and delayed capillary refill; nausea or vomiting from GI ischemia; and others mentioned in the section on Signs and Symptoms. Interventions for promoting perfusion are the same as those mentioned above for increasing cardiac output (Littleton 1988).

Impaired Gas Exchange Related to Alveolar Infiltration by Viscid Exudate The existence of sepsis or septic syndrome is the single biggest risk factor for the development of the adult respiratory distress syndrome (ARDS). In ARDS the alveolar-capillary membrane becomes extremely permeable to protein, allowing the accumulation of a viscid, proteinaceous exudate which may include red blood cells, both interstitially and in the alveoli. The increased permeability is probably due at least in part to damage to the membrane by reactive oxygen metabolites released by activated phagocytic cells.

Monitor the patient carefully for increasing tachypnea, increasingly difficult breathing, falling P_aO_2, and respiratory alkalosis. Declining P_aO_2 despite oxygen supplementation is an important sign of ARDS. Intubation should be instituted early if needed. Further information on ARDS can be found in Chapter 8 and nursing measures for impaired gas exchange in Chapter 9.

Outcome Evaluation

Evaluate the patient's progress using these outcome criteria:

- P_aO_2 is within normal limits.
- Vital signs are stable.
- Urine output is adequate (at least 30 ml/hour) with good skin turgor and moist mucous membranes.
- Peripheral pulses are palpable, and capillary refill takes less than 3 seconds.
- Core temperature is maintained within normal limits.
- Patient is free of infection.

REFERENCES

Anderson R, May R: Understanding the AIDS pandemic. *Sci Am* 1992; 266(5):58–66.

Austen K: Systemic mastocytosis. *N Engl J Med* 1992; 266(5):58–66.

Balk R, Bone R: The septic syndrome: Definition and clinical implications. *Crit Care Clin* 1989; 5(1):1–6.

Baltimore D, Feinberg M: HIV revealed: Toward a natural history of the infection. *N Engl J Med* 1989; 321(24):1673–1675.

Barnes P: A new approach to the treatment of asthma. *N Engl J Med* 1989; 321(22):1517–1527.

Barnes P et al.: Tuberculosis in patients with human immunodeficiency virus infection. *N Engl J Med* 1991; 324(23): 1644–1650.

Beardsley T: Cross reaction. *Sci Am* 1991; 265(6):56–57.

Bjorkman P, Parham P: Structure, function and diversity of class I major histocompatibility complex molecules. *Annu Rev Biochem* 1990; 59:253–288.

Bochner B, Lichtenstein L: Anaphylaxis. *N Engl J Med* 1991; 324(25):1785–1790.

Bone R: Let's agree on terminology: Definitions of sepsis. *Crit Care Med* 1991; 19(7):973–976.

Burns K: Vasoactive drug therapy in shock. *Crit Care Nurs Clin North Am* 1990; 2(2):167–178.

Burton G: Vitamin E: Antioxidant activity, biokinetics, and bioavailability. *Annu Rev Nutr* 1990; 10:357–382.

Carpenito L: *Nursing diagnosis: Application to clinical practice,* 4th ed. Philadelphia: Lippincott, 1992.

Carr G: Medical treatment of persons with AIDS/ARC. Pages 131–140 in *Nursing care of the person with AIDS/ARC,* Lewis A (ed). Rockville, MD: Aspen, 1988.

Clark S et al.: High titers of cytopathic virus in plasma of patients with symptomatic primary HIV-1 infection. *N Engl J Med* 1991; 324(14):954–960.

Cohen: The self, the world and autoimmunity. *Sci Am* 1988; 258(4):52–60.

Consensus statement on the use of corticosteroids as adjunctive therapy for Pneumocystis pneumonia in the acquired immunodeficiency syndrome. The National Institutes of Health–University of California Expert Panel for Corticosteroids as Adjunctive Therapy for Pneumocystis Pneumonia. *N Engl J Med* 1990; 323(21): 1500–1504.

Corey L, Fleming T: Treatment of HIV infection—Progress in perspective. *N Engl J Med* 1992; 326(7):484–486.

Crabtree A, Jorgenson M: Exploring the practical knowledge in expert critical-care nursing practice. Unpublished master's thesis, University of Wisconsin, Madison, 1986.

Daar E et al.: Transient high levels of viremia in patients with primary human immunodeficiency virus Type 1 infection. *N Engl J Med* 1991; 324(14):961–964.

Dickerson M: Anaphylaxis and anaphylactic shock. *Crit Care Nurs Quart* 1988; 11(1):68–74.

Fischbach F: *A manual of laboratory & diagnostic tests,* 4th ed. Philadelphia: Lippincott, 1992.

Garrison J: Histamine, bradykinin, 5-hydroxytryptamine, and their antagonists. Pages 575–599 in *The pharmacological basis of therapeutics,* 8th ed, Gilman A et al. (eds). New York: Pergamon Press, 1990.

Goldschlager N: Shock. Pages 62–66 in *Critical care medicine,* Luce J et al. (eds). Philadelphia: Saunders, 1988.

Graham N et al.: The effects on survival of early treatment of human immunodeficiency virus infection. *N Engl J Med* 1992; 326(16):1037–1042.

Greene W: The molecular biology of human immunodeficiency virus type 1 infection. *N Engl J Med* 1991; 324(5):308–317.

Gurevich I: *Infectious diseases in critical care nursing: Prevention and precautions.* Rockville, MD: Aspen, 1989.

Gurka A: The immune system: Implications for critical care nursing. *Crit Care Nurse* 1989; 9(7):24–35.

Guyton A: *Textbook of medical physiology,* 8th ed. Philadelphia: Saunders, 1991.

Handschumacher R: Immunosuppressive agents. Pages 1264–1276 in *The pharmacological basis of therapeutics,* 8th ed, Gilman A et al. (eds). New York: Pergamon Press, 1990.

Haynes R: Adrenocorticotropic hormone; adrenocortical steroids and their synthetic analogs; inhibitors of the synthesis and actions of adrenocortical hormones. Pages 1431–1462 in *The pharmacological basis of therapeutics,* 8th ed, Gilman A et al. (eds). New York: Pergamon Press, 1990.

Herberman R: Elements of the immune system. Part 1 of the *ImmunoPrimer Series,* Pittsburgh: Cetus, Inc., 1987.

Herberman R: Cytokines. Part 3 of the *ImmunoPrimer Series,* Pittsburgh: Cetus, Inc., 1989.

Hoffman B, Lefkowitz R: Catecholamines and sympathomimetic drugs. Pages 187–220 in *The pharmacological basis of therapeutics,* 8th ed, Gilman A et al. (eds). New York: Pergamon Press, 1990.

Hollander H: Care of the individual with early HIV infection: Unanswered questions, including the syphilis dilemma. Pages 93–101 in *The medical management of AIDS,* 2d ed, Sande M, Volberding P (eds). Philadelphia: Saunders, 1990.

Kersten L: *Comprehensive respiratory nursing: A decisionmaking approach.* Philadelphia: Saunders, 1989.

Keusch G, Farthing M: Nutritional aspects of AIDS. *Annu Rev Nutr,* 1990; 10:475–501.

Krensky A et al: T-Lymphocyte–antigen interactions in transplant rejection. *N Engl J Med* 1990; 322(8):510–517.

Lewis A: HIV: The basics. Pages 3–9 in *Nursing care of the person with AIDS/ARC,* Lewis A (ed). Rockville, MD: Aspen, 1988.

Lewis R, Austen K, Soberman R: Leukotrienes and other products of the 5-lipoxygenase pathway—Biochemistry and relation to pathobiology in human diseases. *N Engl J Med* 1990; 323(10):645–655.

Littleton M: Pathophysiology and assessment of sepsis and septic shock. *Crit Care Nurs Quart* 1988; 11(1):30–47.

MacNee W et al.: The effect of cigarette smoking on neutrophil kinetics in human lungs. *N Engl J Med* 1989; 321(14):924–928.

Mathewson Kuhn M: Anaphylactic versus anaphylactoid reactions: Nursing interventions. *Crit Care Nurse* 1990; 10(5):121–136.

McGowan S, Hunninghake G: Neutrophils and emphysema. *N Engl J Med* 1989; 321(14):968–970.

Miller R: Aging and the immune response. Pages 157–180 in *Handbook of the biology of aging,* 3d ed, Schneider E, Rowe J (eds). San Diego: Academic Press, 1990.

Montaner J et al.: Corticosteroids prevent early deterioration in patients with moderately severe *Pneumocystis carinii* pneumonia and the acquired immunodeficiency syndrome (AIDS). *Ann Intern Med* 1990; 113:14–20.

Moore R et al.: Zidovudine and the natural history of the acquired immunodeficiency syndrome. *N Engl J Med* 1991; 324(20):1412–1416.

Nyamathi A, van Servellen G: Maladaptive coping in the critically ill population with acquired immunodeficiency syndrome: Nursing assessment and treatment. *Heart Lung* 1989; 18:113–120.

Odeh M: The role of reperfusion-induced injury in the pathogenesis of the crush syndrome. *N Engl J Med* 1991; 324(20):1417–1422.

Petrucci K, Booth-Blaemire E, Watson K: Aging, immunity, and critical care nursing. *Crit Care Nurs Clin North Am* 1989; 1(4):787–794.

Pierson D: Hyperthermia. Pages 563–567 in *Critical care medicine,* Luce J, Pierson D (eds). Philadelphia: Saunders, 1988.

Piper J, Crawford G: Septic shock. *Prob Crit Care* 1990; 4(1):90–119.

Podack E, Kupfer A: T cell effector functions: Mechanisms for the delivery of cytotoxicity and help. *Annu Rev Cell Biol* 1991; 7:479–504.

Price R, Brew B: Management of the neurologic complications of HIV-1 infection and AIDS. Pages 161–177 in *The Medical Management of AIDS,* 2d ed., Sande M, Volberding P (eds). Philadelphia: Saunders, 1990.

Quinn T: Global epidemiology of HIV infection. Pages 9–16 in *The Medical Management of AIDS,* 2d ed., Sande M, Volberding P (eds). Philadelphia: Saunders, 1990.

Rice V: Shock, a clinical syndrome: An update. Part 3: Therapeutic management. *Crit Care Nurse* 1991; 11(6):34–39.

Rosen M: Intensive care of patients with AIDS. *Crit Care Report* 1990; 1:224–233.

Rossman Jillings C: Shock: Psychosocial needs of the patient and family. *Crit Care Nurs Clin North Am* 1990; 2(2):325–330.

Snider D, Roper W: The new tuberculosis. *N Engl J Med* 1992; 326(10):703–705.

Stroud M, Swindell B, Bernard G: Cellular and humoral mediators of sepsis syndrome. *Crit Care Nurs Clin North Am* 1990; 2(2):151–159.

Summers G: The clinical and hemodynamic presentation of the shock patient. *Crit Care Nurs Clin North Am* 1990; 2(2):161–166.

Tindall B et al.: Primary HIV infection: Clinical, immunologic and serologic aspects. Pages 68–81 in *The Medical Management of AIDS,* 2d ed., Sande M, Volberding P (eds). Philadelphia: Saunders, 1990.

Tolkoff-Rubin N, Rubin R: Uremia and host defenses. *N Engl J Med* 1990; 322(11):770–772.

Vaishnav Y, Wong-Staal F: The biochemistry of AIDS. *Annu Rev Biochem* 1991; 60:577–630.

Walzer P: Pneumocystis carinii—New clinical spectrum? *N Engl J Med* 1991; 324(4):263–265.

Waltzer W: Clinical application: Clinical organ transplantation. Pages 1204–1212 in *Critical care nursing: Clinical management through the nursing process,* Dolan J (ed). Philadelphia: Davis, 1991.

Warren H, Danner R, Munford R: Anti-endotoxin monoclonal antibodies. *N Engl J Med* 1992; 326(17):1153–1157.

Wenzel R: Anti-endotoxin monoclonal antibodies—A second look. *N Engl J Med* 1992; 326(17):1151–1153.

Wolff S: Monoclonal antibodies and the treatment of gram-negative bacteremia and shock. *N Engl J Med* 1991; 324(7):486–488.

Ziegler E et al.: Treatment of gram-negative bacteremia and septic shock with HA-1A human monoclonal antibody against endotoxin—A randomized, double-blind, placebo-controlled trial. *N Engl J Med* 1991; 324(7):429–436.

19

Gastrointestinal Disorders

CLINICAL INSIGHT

Domain: The helping role

Competency: Maximizing the patient's participation and control in his or her own recovery

Expert nurses know how critically important it is that a patient be emotionally available to participate in recovery. Maximizing such participation requires the patient to have faith that he or she will get through the ordeal and to recognize his or her own power to influence recovery. A patient's commitment to engage in healing activities can be a hard-won step in recovery. It is a particularly difficult one if the patient is demoralized by prolonged illness and the feeling of being treated like an object. In the following exemplar, from Benner (1984, pp. 60–61), an expert nurse achieves a patient turnaround by challenging the patient to choose recovery.

The patient was a 36-year-old man who had a history of multiple surgeries and complications. He had

a history of ulcers and came as a transfer from another hospital after having surgery for hemorrhagic pancreatitis. He ended up with another surgery from which he emerged minus most of his pancreas and with multiple tubes, a huge abdominal wound, several IVs, etc. He was a person who had always been independent and was having an extremely hard time coping with being ill and helpless. He finally reached a point where he was so angry and so depressed that he refused any further treatments, procedures, and blood work. He also refused to ambulate or do much of his self-care.

I went in to talk to him. He told me, "I'm so sick of being poked all the time, and not having any say in any of this. I'm so helpless. People are constantly doing things to me!" I told him that while the circumstances would be hard to change, he could shift his point of view. I told him that he did have a choice in all of this, and that instead of seeing him-

*self as having things being done to him, he could
view it as things being done for him to help him get
better. I told him that while he felt helpless about
what we were doing to him physically, he was
the only one who could help himself mentally by
keeping this whole thing in perspective . . . that he
needed to remember that he was a person . . . that
he was more than this sickness he was going
through. I couldn't really tell if I was getting
through.*

*The next morning when I came to work, I saw
him sitting out in the hall by the window laughing
and smiling. When I asked him what had changed
for him, he said, "You were right! I'm just going
to choose to be here and let all of you help me get
well as fast as I can!"*

*I really felt like I made a difference in this man's
life in helping him cope with circumstances he
thought were beyond his control, just by helping him
tap into inner strengths.*

As illustrated in the Clinical Insight, the nurse can be instrumental in helping patients maintain both faith in their recovery and awareness of their power to influence it. Such nursing support is particularly important with patients whose illness requires prolonged hospitalization, which is often true with gastrointestinal (GI) disorders.

Nutrition is defined as the intake, digestion, and absorption of nutrients and the removal of solid waste products. To meet nutritional needs normally, a person requires a functioning GI system. This chapter therefore begins with a review of abdominal assessment and the most common GI abnormalities seen in the critically ill: upper GI bleeding, acute pancreatitis, hepatitis, and liver failure. It then discusses nutrition in the critically ill patient.

GASTROINTESTINAL (GI) SYSTEM

GI Assessment

Gastrointestinal (GI) assessment provides essential data on the baseline status of GI functioning as well as dysfunctional states. The assessment consists of two key areas: the focused history and the physical exam. A suggested format is shown in Table 19–1.

History

In eliciting the GI history, assist the patient to focus on the current chief complaint and ask the patient about both general and specific signs and symptoms. *General symptoms* include changes in appetite or energy levels, and weight loss or weight gain. *Specific symptoms* about which to inquire include pain, nausea and vomiting, diarrhea or constipation, and heartburn or indigestion. The location of abdominal pain can be confusing, especially in the beginning stages of a disorder, as pain may be referred along transmission pathways to a site distant from its source. The pain arising from an organ *(visceral pain)* often is dull, poorly localized, and hard for the patient to describe. In contrast, pain from the skin, peritoneum, or muscle wall *(somatic pain)* is sharp and easier to localize.

The history should include information from the patient and family about recent past events, family history of GI problems, and previous treatments.

Physical Examination

The health assessment continues with a physical examination of the patient's general appearance, mouth, abdomen, anus, and rectum.

Mouth Examine the mouth for adequacy of dentition, tongue movement, and oral hygiene. Also note whether the gag and swallow reflexes are intact.

Abdomen Next, examine the patient's abdomen. As you do so, keep in mind the location of various abdominal organs (Figure 19–1). Instead of following the usual sequence of inspection, palpation, percussion, and auscultation, alter the order to inspection, auscultation, percussion, and palpation. Auscultation precedes percussion and palpation in the GI assessment because the latter two can change the frequency of bowel sounds. Percussion precedes palpation because it usually is easier to identify the location of abdominal organs through percussion than through palpation. As you examine specific organs, you may find it helpful to alternate percussion and palpation. The following is a procedure for abdominal examination.

Be particularly careful when examining the person experiencing abdominal pain. Ask her or him to point to the area of pain, and examine that area last.

1. Inspect the abdomen, looking especially at its contour and symmetry. Also look for pulsations,

TABLE 19–1

Abdominal Assessment Format

1. Chief current complaint _____
2. Related History _____
3. Physical Assessment

   Mouth: Dentition _____

       Tongue _____

       Oral hygiene/mucous membranes _____

       Gag reflex _____

       Swallow reflex _____

   Abdomen

       Inspection _____

       Auscultation _____

       _____

   Percussion and palpation:

       Liver _____

       _____

       Spleen _____

       _____

       Tenderness _____ Rigidity _____ Free fluid _____

   Anus and rectum _____
4. Laboratory tests and diagnostic procedures

   _____
5. Other _____

   _____

scars, and distended superficial veins (seen in portal obstruction and venous thrombosis).

2. Auscultate the abdomen in all four quadrants. Apply the stethoscope diaphragm lightly to listen for *bowel sounds*. Normal bowel sounds are soft intermittent noises that occur about every 2–10 seconds and vary in frequency, intensity, and pitch. Sounds that are intensified, weak, or absent are abnormal. Loud gurgling sounds signify either increased intestinal motility, as in diarrhea or nervous tension, or early intestinal obstruction. Occasional weak sounds suggest poor peristalsis. Absent sounds occur after handling of the bowel during surgery, during severe electrolyte disturbances, in peritonitis, and in advanced intestinal obstruction. Listen for 5 minutes in each quadrant before deciding whether bowel sounds are absent.

   Use the bell of the stethoscope to listen for vascular sounds and rubs. *Bruits* (audible turbulence of blood flow within an artery or vein caused by narrowing or partial obstruction of the vessel) may be audible in patients with arteriosclerosis, hypertension, aortic aneurysms, masses compressing the aorta, or renal artery stenosis. *Peritoneal friction rubs* (audible sounds due to contact of the peritoneum against an inflamed, enlarged organ and/or inflammation of the peritoneum itself) may be heard over the right lower costal margin, related to hepatic tumors or abscesses, or over the left lower costal area, related to splenic infarction.

3. Percuss the abdomen lightly. Normally, you will hear tympany over the stomach and intestine (that is, over most of the abdomen). *Tympany* is a long, very hollow sound that indicates gas in an enclosed chamber. It resembles the sound you can hear by puffing out your cheek and percussing it. Over solid organs, a short, high-pitched sound (called *dullness*) will be heard. (If you wish to review percussion technique and the characteristics of percussion notes, see Chapter 7.)

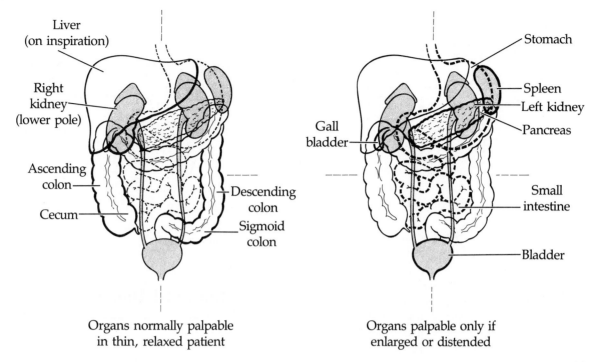

Liver
(on inspiration)

Right
kidney
(lower pole)

Ascending
colon

Cecum

Descending
colon

Sigmoid
colon

Stomach

Spleen

Left kidney

Pancreas

Gall
bladder

Small
intestine

Bladder

Organs normally palpable
in thin, relaxed patient

Organs palpable only if
enlarged or distended

FIGURE 19–1

Abdominal organs.

Estimate the size of the *liver* by percussing in the right midclavicular line, down from lung resonance to dullness, and up from abdominal tympany to dullness. It is important to note both the location of the borders and the distance between them. The liver can normally be palpated 4 cm below the right costal margin (Bates 1987). A normal-sized liver may be displaced downward, as in emphysema, or upward, as in ascites or abdominal tumors. As a result, a liver edge below the costal margin does not necessarily indicate liver enlargement.

4. Palpate the abdomen lightly. Use light touch to feel for tenderness and resistance. Resistance may be voluntary, due to patient discomfort, ticklishness, or apprehension, or involuntary, due to peritoneal irritation. If you encounter resistance, try to differentiate the type by ensuring that the patient is relaxed—make sure he or she is positioned comfortably and your hands are warm; try to distract the patient with conversation. You also can feel for the normal relaxation of the abdominal muscles on expiration. Rigidity that continues in spite of these maneuvers probably is involuntary.

Palpate areas of known tenderness last. If pain is present, check for rebound tenderness, a reliable sign of peritoneal inflammation. *Rebound tenderness* is pain that occurs after the release of pressure. To elicit this response, press firmly over a quadrant of abdomen other than the tender one and release the pressure suddenly. If the patient feels a sharp stab of pain over the suspected area (*not* over the site on which you pressed), rebound tenderness is present. This test can provoke severe pain and muscle spasm, which interfere with further examination. For this reason, it is wise to postpone it until the end of the examination.

5. To palpate the *liver,* stand on the patient's right side (Figure 19–2). Slide your left hand under and parallel to the eleventh and twelfth ribs. Place your right hand on the abdomen, below the lower border of liver dullness that you identified previously. Point your fingers toward the right costal border. Ask the patient to take a deep abdominal breath, blow it out, and take another deep breath. As the patient exhales, gently push your fingers inward and upward under the costal margin. You may be able to feel a firm ridge of pressure come down to meet your fingertips; this is the lower border of the liver. If you feel the edge, repeat the maneuver medially and laterally. An alternate technique is

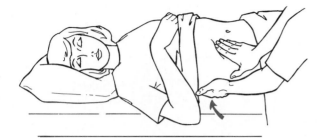

FIGURE 19–2

Palpation of liver.

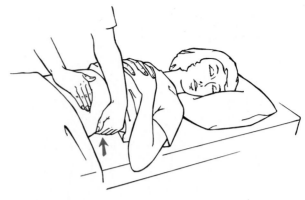

FIGURE 19–3

Palpation of spleen.

the *hooking* method: Stand at the patient's right shoulder. Hook the fingers of both hands over the right costal margin, and feel for the liver edge as the person inhales deeply. Note the smoothness of the edge and any tenderness. Since the liver normally is not palpable, *blunt percussion* over the liver is an alternate method of detecting tenderness. To perform blunt percussion, place your left hand on the lower right lateral rib cage. Make a fist with your right hand and lightly strike your left hand.

The *spleen* is not palpable unless it is enlarged about three times its normal size. To check for splenic enlargement, stand at the patient's right side (Figure 19–3). Reach over the patient and place your left hand under the left lower ribs. Place your right hand below the left costal margin on the anterior abdomen. Ask the patient to take a deep breath, lift with your left hand, and press inward with your right. As the normal spleen cannot be felt, be cautious if you do palpate the spleen. An enlarged spleen is friable and may rupture with aggressive palpation.

Anus and Rectum   Complete the physical examination of the gastrointestinal system by examining the anal area and rectum. Examine the anal area for hemorrhoids, fissures, rectal prolapse, or skin excoriation. If the date of the last bowel movement is not known, consult with the physician for contraindications to rectal examination (for example, vagal stimulation could result in bradydysrhythmias). Early detection of fecal matter in the rectum can avoid the development of a fecal impaction, but it may be necessary to delay this examination if the patient's condition is unstable or might be adversely affected by rectal stimulation. If a rectal examination provides stool on the gloved finger, check it for the presence of visible and occult blood.

Upper GI Hemorrhage

Assessment

Risk Conditions   Gastrointestinal hemorrhage may occur from upper or lower GI sources. There are four categories of bleeding sources:

- *Arterial,* common with bleeding ulcers which have eroded through an arterial wall
- *Venous,* commonly found with esophageal varices
- *Capillary,* demonstrated most commonly in erosive gastritis
- *Mixed arterial and venous,* as in Mallory-Weiss syndrome.

Upper GI bleeding sources include peptic ulcer of the stomach and duodenum, marginal ulcers resulting from ulcer formation at the anastomotic sites following GI reconstructive surgeries, acute hemorrhagic gastritis, esophageal varices, erosive tumors of the stomach and duodenum, and Mallory-Weiss syndrome. *Mallory-Weiss syndrome* is a linear, nonperforating tear of the gastric mucosa near the juncture between the esophagus and the stomach. It usually results from an episode of violent vomiting, most often in patients with a history of alcoholism, gastritis, or esophagitis. About 75% of upper GI bleeds result from duodenal, gastric, or esophageal ulcers; 20% from erosive gastritis; and 5% from esophageal varices.

Lower GI bleeding sources include erosive tumors of the rectum, colon, or distal ileum; diverticular disease of the colon; inflammatory bowel disease (colitis and Crohn's disease); and hemorrhoids (internal, external, or both).

Signs and Symptoms The patient's clinical presentation will vary with the amount and speed of blood loss. Factors to include in assessment are presenting signs and symptoms, focused history (note particularly previous episodes of hematemesis, hematochezia, or melena), vital signs, and rapid systems assessment for signs of decreased perfusion.

Vital signs correlate roughly with the degree of blood loss. When blood loss is less than 500 ml, supine vital signs are likely to be normal due to compensatory mechanisms. Blood loss of 500–1,000 ml causes sympathetic stimulation sufficient to cause tachycardia, and the patient may complain of being thirsty, dizzy, or nauseated. Blood loss in excess of 1,000 ml may cause frank hypovolemic shock, with cool, clammy skin, rapid, thready pulse, and decreased level of consciousness.

An important clue in assessing the patient with a history of blood loss or suggestive symptoms but normal or equivocal vital signs is the response to the *postural vital signs* (tilt) test. This test compares vital signs in the recumbent position with those in the upright standing or sitting position. Do not perform this test if syncope, marked tachycardia, hypotension, or shock are present. To assess postural vital signs, work with a colleague (or by yourself if a cardiac monitor is available) to simultaneously measure the blood pressure (BP) and pulse while the patient is recumbent. Then sit the patient up and immediately measure the BP and pulse again. (Be sure to observe the patient closely for fainting during the sitting up.) The comparison is considered *positive* for the presence of orthostatic hypotension if the systolic BP drops more than 10 mm Hg or if the pulse increases more

than 20 beats per minute. A pulse increase of 20 beats or more per minute with no change in BP indicates a blood loss of 500 ml or less; a pulse increase of 30 beats per minute and a 10 mm Hg fall in BP correlate with a loss of approximately 1,000 ml.

Additional physical signs of blood loss may be detectable. Pale conjunctiva suggest a hemoglobin value of less than 10 g%. Pale palmar skin folds suggest a hemoglobin value of less than 6 g%. Hemodynamic assessment should be followed by a rapid systems assessment, to include observation of peripheral blood flow (pulses, color and temperature of peripheral tissues); urinary output; and mentation status.

Hematemesis (vomiting of blood) is common and usually indicates that the patient is bleeding from a source above the ligament of Treitz at the duodenojejunal junction. The blood may be bright red if bleeding is so profuse that there has been little time for gastric juices to act on it. Conversely, the blood may look like coffee grounds if bleeding has been slower and gastric juices have converted hemoglobin to a brown breakdown product.

Blood also may be present in stools, but its presence is of equivocal diagnostic value. The stool may appear black and sticky (tarry), bright red, or maroon. As little as 60 ml of blood in the gastrointestinal tract can cause *melena* (tarry stool). A black stool usually indicates an upper GI bleed, but also may be present in a lower GI bleed. *Hematochezia* (the presence of bright red blood passed rectally) usually occurs with a rapid lower GI bleed, but it also may indicate massive upper GI bleeding with markedly increased GI motility. The color of the stool also is affected by the intake of food; for example, beets can produce a red stool, whereas iron can produce a dark one. Stools should be tested for occult bleeding if they appear normal.

Planning and Implementation of Care

Planning and implementation of care can be divided into two phases: *emergency care,* to control shock; and *definitive care,* to control bleeding. Nearby is presented a nursing care plan for acute upper GI hemorrhage. The following section expands on selected aspects of care.

Fluid Volume Deficit Related to Hemorrhage

Diagnostics and Patient Stabilization Early insertion of nasogastric (NG) tubes serves three important functions in active GI bleeding. First, the insertion of a large-bore NG tube will provide diagnostic information about the volume, color, and characteristics of blood in the stomach. Secondly, gastric aspiration of blood and clots will facilitate the body's own control of hemostasis, since the presence of clots and blood breakdown products may stimulate acid production and prolong or even abolish the clotting process in the stomach. Thirdly, evacuation of the stomach prior to endoscopy can reduce the risk of aspiration during the diagnostic intervention.

Gastric Cooling The efficacy of iced fluid lavage of the stomach to vasoconstrict vessels providing vascular flow to bleeding sites is controversial. Studies have demonstrated variable results using both iced and room-temperature tap water and saline (Dusek 1984). The addition of a topical adrenergic agent, norepinephrine (Levophed), two ampules per liter of fluid, may provide some additional vasoconstriction and "buy some time" while the patient is prepared for diagnostic endoscopy. The most significant variable in iced fluid lavage is effective technique (Table 19–2).

Laboratory Monitoring Following initial baseline laboratory tests (see care plan), patient status and

TABLE 19–2

Principles of Effective Iced Fluid Lavage

Use large volumes (2–3 L).

Tap water is less expensive than, and as effective as, saline.

Instill 200-cc volumes.

Allow to "dwell" in stomach for 1–2 min.

Hand aspirate total dwell volume each lavage with large syringe.

Stop after 30 minutes (if return not clear by then, it probably won't ever be).

Protect patient's airway during lavage (because of increased risk of aspiration and stimulation of vomiting).

response to therapy are evaluated by lab tests every 8–12 hours. Table 19–3 summarizes those tests usually monitored for the patient with GI bleeding.

Blood Transfusions Blood transfusions are crucial. Monitor the patient for a possible transfusion reaction, as well as for complications of massive transfusions, such as hypocalcemia related to binding of circulating calcium by blood preservative (citrate).

NURSING TIP

Blood Transfusions

The hematocrit should rise 3% with each 500 ml of blood administered; if you do not observe this response, the patient still may be bleeding actively.

Immediate surgery is indicated if more than 6–8 units of blood must be administered, if transfusions are ineffective in maintaining BP, or if bleeding persists more than 24 hours.

Anxiety Related to Self-Soiling and Precarious Health Status Patients often are acutely embarrassed about being unable to control their vomiting and diarrhea. The odors are unpleasant, and getting these excretions on one's body may activate memories of childhood struggles for mastery over one's body. It is helpful to reassure the patient that you understand it is impossible to control the vomiting and diarrhea. Keep the patient clean, and provide mouthwash to rinse blood out of the mouth after vomiting episodes. All caregivers should practice universal precautions when providing patient hygiene and/or assisting the patient with an episode of emesis or toileting. Wearing gloves usually should be adequate; however, consider protective eyewear and impermeable gowns for patients with projective vomiting and active, uncontrolled diarrhea.

The patient with an upper GI bleed is anxious and frightened. The sight of one's own blood is very upsetting, and patients often fear that they are bleeding to death. A calm, professional attitude as you institute emergency procedures can convey a sense of safety to the patient. In addition, it is helpful to indicate that you understand the patient's fright and that everything is being done to stabilize the condition.

NURSING CARE PLAN

Acute Upper Gastrointestinal Bleeding

NURSING DIAGNOSIS

Fluid volume deficit related to bleeding/hemorrhage and loss of volume

SIGNS AND SYMPTOMS

Red blood or coffee-grounds material in naso-gastric tube or emesis
Sticky black or dark red stools
If 30% or more of blood volume lost, shocklike symptoms:
  increased heart rate
  cold, clammy skin
  shallow respirations
  decreased blood pressure
If less than 30% of blood volume lost:
  pallor
  weakness
  positive orthostatic vital signs
Decrease in urine output
Increase in body temperature

NURSING ACTIONS

1. Maintain a large-caliber intravenous access.
2. Prepare for possible insertion of pulmonary artery line and arterial line for assessment of hemodynamic status.
3. Insert nasogastric tube.
4. Initiate intragastric lavage of iced saline or iced tap water.
   a. Keep accurate records of amount used for irrigation.
   b. Continue until return is clear or for total of 30 minutes.
5. Administer colloids and crystalloids as ordered to replace volume.
   a. Insert Foley catheter and maintain urine output of at least 30 cc/hr.
   b. Assess hemodynamic parameters (CVP/RAP, PCWP, PAP, BP, HR, CO).
   c. Whole blood or packed cells are best volume expander (due to O_2 carrying capacity).
   d. After multiple transfusions, consider replacement of clotting factors, calcium and platelets.
6. Administer vitamin K as ordered.
7. Monitor BUN, electrolytes, hemoglobin, and hematocrit.
8. Administer vasopressin/nitroglycerin infusions as ordered to control bleeding. Monitor for side effects such as hypertension, chest pain, abdominal pain, oliguria (see Definitive Care text).

DESIRED OUTCOMES

Normal circulating blood volume.
Hemorrhage controlled.
Hemodynamic stability.

(Continues)

NURSING CARE PLAN

Acute Upper Gastrointestinal Bleeding (Continued)

NURSING DIAGNOSIS	SIGNS AND SYMPTOMS	NURSING ACTIONS	DESIRED OUTCOMES

Impaired tissue integrity related to mucosal damage to GI tract and/or esophageal varices	Frank bloody emesis
	History of alcoholism
	Black, sticky, or dark red stools
		1. Administer histamine H_2-receptor antagonists such as cimetidine or ranitidine to aid in healing of mucosa via reduction of acid production and release
		2. Administer antacids as ordered (pH goal of ≥ 5.0)
		3. Assist with insertion of a tamponade tube, as ordered.
		  a. Check patency of each lumen prior to insertion.
		  b. Explain procedure to patient.
		  c. Assess vital signs during procedure.
		4. Once the tube is in place:
		  a. Ensure that x-ray is taken to confirm placement.
		  b. Inflate the gastric balloon with 200–500 cc of air. Watch for bradycardia during inflation of gastric balloon, due to vagal nerve stimulation.
		  c. Inflate the esophageal balloon with air to 25–45 mm Hg.
		  d. Secure tube using slight traction. (Football helmet or catcher's mask provides effective anchor.)
		  e. Keep scissors at bedside for emergency deflation of balloons in case of esophageal rupture and tracheal occlusion by the balloon, as evidenced by sudden onset of respiratory distress and/or back pain.
			Absent or decreased bleeding from GI mucosa or esophageal varices

NURSING CARE PLAN

Acute Upper Gastrointestinal Bleeding (Continued)

NURSING DIAGNOSIS	SIGNS AND SYMPTOMS	NURSING ACTIONS	DESIRED OUTCOMES

		f. Ensure patency of gastric aspiration port and oropharyngeal port. Tubes are not vented, so apply to intermittent suction source.
		g. Deflate esophageal balloon and reinflate as ordered.
		h. Keep the head of the bed elevated to increase ventilation.
		i. Check nostrils, mouth, and lips at least every 2 hours to prevent pressure sores.
		j. Monitor for continued bleeding.
		5. Assist with removal of tube.
		   a. Usually removed after 24 hours of no bleeding.
		   b. Balloons usually are deflated for several hours prior to removal. Always release traction first, then deflate esophageal balloon next and gastric balloon last.
		6. Assist with injection sclerotherapy as a possible therapy for continued bleeding.
		7. Assist with bedside endoscopy for diagnosis of tissue damage.	

Altered tissue perfusion (decreased renal) related to decreased volume and compensatory vasoconstriction	Decreased urine output (30 cc/hr or less) Serial increased potassium level Serial increases in BUN and creatinine High specific gravity of urine Presence of protein in urine	1. Assess hemodynamic parameters for indications of adequate vascular volume. 2. Assess urine output and specific gravity hourly. 3. Monitor serum levels of electrolytes, urea nitrogen, and creatinine. 4. Administer crystalloids and colloids as ordered to maintain vascular volume.	Urine output equal to or greater than 30 cc/hr. Serum electrolytes within normal limits BUN and creatinine normal Specific gravity normal

(Continues)

NURSING CARE PLAN

Acute Upper Gastrointestinal Bleeding (Continued)

NURSING DIAGNOSIS	SIGNS AND SYMPTOMS	NURSING ACTIONS	DESIRED OUTCOMES
High risk for impaired gas exchange related to hemoglobin deficit or to pulmonary edema from fluid overload	Dyspnea Shortness of breath Crackles and/or wheezing heard on auscultation of chest Increased PCWP and RAP Increased HR, decreased BP Pink, frothy sputum Abnormal arterial blood gases	1. Monitor ABGs. 2. Administer supplemental oxygen, as ordered. 3. Monitor hemodynamic status carefully during crystalloid and colloid replacement. Avoid "overfilling" vascular tank until definitive intervention (may precipitate rebleeding). 4. Assess frequently for: congestion in chest as evidenced by crackles, and wheezes, dyspnea, shortness of breath, orthopnea, cough with pink, frothy sputum. 5. If signs or symptoms occur, notify physician promptly and prepare to assist in treatment of pulmonary edema.	ABGs within normal limits. Chest clear to auscultation. Hemodynamic stability. CVP 6–8 SBP ≥100 MAP ≥60
Sensory-perceptual alteration related to increased blood ammonia levels (secondary to increased protein load from GI bleeding)	The following signs and symptoms may vary and/or appear in combination: Irritability Changes in level of consciousness Euphoria Increased drowsiness Confusion Slowed response Neuromuscular irritability	1. Administer antacids or histamine H_2-receptor antagonists as ordered to reduce bleeding. 2. Assess and monitor: BUN level, ammonia level, level of consciousness, neuromuscular function. response, alertness. 3. Avoid therapies that may increase blood ammmonia levels, such as: antacids with ammonium chloride, excessive diuresis. 4. Initiate actions to prevent encephalopathy as ordered: lactulose to promote excretion of ammonia, antibiotics to decrease formation of nitrogen-forming intestinal bacteria, volume replacement.	Patient is alert and oriented. Absence of encephalopathy.

NURSING CARE PLAN

Acute Upper Gastrointestinal Bleeding (Continued)

NURSING DIAGNOSIS	SIGNS AND SYMPTOMS	NURSING ACTIONS	DESIRED OUTCOMES
		5. If symptoms occur: 　a. Reorient patient frequently. 　b. Provide a safe environment. 　c. Administer sorbitol or magnesium citrate as ordered to decrease intestinal flora. 　d. Administer low-protein nutritional support. 　e. Administer lactulose as ordered to promote excretion of ammonia.	
Anxiety related to hospitalization, critical illness, or fear of death	Patient and family appear anxious, showing signs of fear: increased heart rate rapid, shallow breathing irritability asking numerous questions verbalizations of anxiety	1. Reassure patient. 2. Explain all procedures. 3. Maintain a calm, unhurried atmosphere. 4. Encourage verbalization of anxiety and fears. 5. Allow rest periods between treatments. 6. Keep patient warm and as comfortable as possible. 7. Demonstrate competency and efficiency.	Absence of anxiety, or tolerable level of anxiety.

An upper GI hemorrhage often is acutely frightening to the family as well. For guidelines on nursing interventions with family members, please consult Chapter 3.

Definitive Care The bleeding vessel often can be located with *fiberoptic endoscopy,* usually performed within 24 hours of admission. A local anesthetic is used, and the patient is sedated. *Electrocautery* or *sclerotherapy* may be used to treat sites of bleeding. If the patient continues to bleed or is bleeding very rapidly (more than 0.5 ml per minute), *arteriography* is performed to visualize the arterial systems. Selective arteriography allows direct intra-arterial infusion of vasopressin to control bleeding. Upper GI series and barium studies have limited value in an active GI bleed, since disruptions in intestinal mucosa cannot definitively

identify if that particular site is bleeding actively or is scar tissue from a previous bleed.

Medical approaches to control bleeding include antacid administration, cimetidine or ranitidine administration, and tamponade of bleeding vessels. *Antacids* are used to promote healing and usually are titrated to achieve a gastric pH of 5.0 or more; therefore, the pH of the nasogastric aspirate is checked prior to administration.

Cimetidine (Tagamet) is a specific histamine antagonist at a histamine$_2$ (H$_2$) receptor site in gastric parietal cells. Although its use in prophylaxis of duodenal ulcers and treatment of hypersecretory disorders is accepted, its use in preventing and treating acute ulceration is controversial. Cimetidine can cause central nervous system side effects; hematologic disorders; slowed metabolism of warfarin-type

TABLE 19–3

Laboratory Monitoring Following GI Bleeding

TEST/FREQUENCY	RESULTS EXPECTED	RATIONALE
Hemoglobin, hematocrit (q8–12hr)	Within normal limits initially—lag time of 4–6 hours postbleed for decreased values	Re-equilibration takes 4–6 hr. Equal volumes of serum and cells are lost. Body compensates for lost volume by hemodilution, and crystalloid fluids given also dilute blood.
WBC (q12hr)	Increased counts postbleed (15,000–40,000)	Body responds to insult; hypovolemia exacerbates elevation of WBC.
Platelet counts (q12hr)	Initially normal; decreased after volume restored	Hemostasis consumes platelets. As clotting factors are used, coagulopathy may ensue.
Prothrombin time, partial thromboplastin time, and thrombin time (q12hr)	Decreased times to half normal times	Body attempts hemostasis.
Serum sodium (q8–12hr)	Initially normal; decreased following volume restoration transiently; elevated over time postbleed	Initially hemoconcentration followed by hemodilution; over time, body responds to conserve sodium and water to maintain volume.
Serum potassium (q8–12hr)	Initially normal; decreased following volume restoration transiently; elevates over time	As above, with sodium; elevation over time as transfusions liberate potassium to serum and breakdown of red blood cells (RBCs) in intestine liberates additional potassium; hypovolemia may induce renal impairment.
Serum calcium (q12hr)	Normal to decreased levels; markedly decreased circulating levels following massive transfusions of stored blood	Preservative (citrate) in stored blood binds circulating calcium.
Serum lactate (q12hr)	Elevated levels	Shock/hypovolemia, citrate in blood transfusions, and anaerobic metabolism all elevate levels.
Serum ammonia (q12hr)	Possible elevated levels	Liver dysfunction impairs clearance of blood breakdown products in intestines, resulting in elevated blood levels with encephalopathy.
Serum glucose (q8–12hr)	Mild elevation (hyperglycemia)	Stress causes release of epinephrine, inducing glycogenolysis.
Blood urea nitrogen (q12–24hr)	Increased levels 24–48 postbleed	Blood breakdown in intestinal products overwhelm kidneys' ability to clear.
Serum creatinine (q12–24hr)	Elevated levels	Hypovolemia/shock leads to decreased glomerular filtration.
Serum enzymes (q24hr; q8 hours x3 for CPK)	Elevated levels	Hypovolemia/shock decreases perfusion to organs, damaging tissues of kidney, liver, lung, and heart.
Arterial blood gases (as necessary per status)	Early respiratory alkalosis; late metabolic acidosis	Decreased perfusion to lung during shock stimulates hyperventilation; later lactic acid build-up leads to acidosis.

anticoagulants, aminophylline, and diazepam; and false-positive tests for occult blood. When both oral cimetidine and antacids are being used, they should be administered at separate times, as antacids decrease cimetidine absorption.

Ranitidine (Zantac), another histamine H$_2$-receptor antagonist, has fewer side effects. Side effects may include nausea, constipation, and GI pain; blood dyscrasias; and central nervous system (CNS) effects. Current histamine antagonist therapy includes admin-

NURSING TIP

Administering Antacids

One method of antacid administration that is both effective and efficient is the every-two-hour administration dwell and release schedule. Just prior to administration of the antacid, evaluate the stomach pH. Administer the antacid, clamp the tube for one hour, and then open it to suction for one hour.

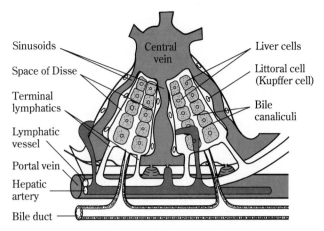

FIGURE 19–4

Basic structure of a liver lobule, showing the hepatic cellular plates, the blood vessels, the bile-collecting system, and the lymph flow system composed of the spaces of Disse and the interlobular lymphatics. (Reprinted from Guyton, Taylor, and Granger [as modified from Elias]: *Circulatory physiology two: Dynamics and control of the body fluids.* Philadelphia: Saunders, 1975.)

istration orally and by intermittent and continuous intravenous infusions.

Cytoprotection of gastric mucosa may be accomplished by the administration of *sucralfate* (Carafate). This medication forms an ulcer-adherent complex which then "protects" the disrupted gastric mucosa from the action of acid and digestive enzymes. Sucralfate should not be administered concomitantly with antacids, and if given via NG tube, the tube should be well irrigated after the dose.

Aqueous pitressin (vasopressin) and nitroglycerin infusions are used as a temporary measure to reduce blood supply to bleeding sites in acute upper GI bleeding. Vasopressin works on smooth muscle of the GI tract and on all parts of the vascular bed. Vasopressin has a very short half-life (20 minutes) and therefore must be administered by intravenous (IV) infusion. Because of significant dose-related side effects, a standardized dilution is recommended for close monitoring and control. Initial therapy is begun at 0.3–0.4 units per minute for 12–24 hours, and then the drug is tapered gradually until discontinued. Significant side effects include: decreased arterial oxygenation (decreased cardiac output, mixed venous O_2 and tissue oxygenation); coronary artery spasms; a possible direct toxicity on the myocardium and reflex vagal activity; peripheral vascular spasms; decreased renal perfusion; and severe tissue necrosis if the drug extravasates into tissues at the IV site.

Vasopressin is used in conjunction with a nitroglycerin infusion because effective high-range doses of vasopressin alone lead to the significant side effects mentioned above. Concomitant administration of a nitroglycerin infusion maintains coronary perfusion and cardiac output (Burns and Martin 1990). Table 19–4 provides suggested dilutions and administration schedules. Vasopressin/nitroglycerin infusions are most commonly used in the management of bleeding esophageal varices. Transdermal application of vasopressin also has been used; however, its therapeutic effect may be of limited value in an acute bleed. Transdermal vasopressin may be utilized best in the management of chronic portal hypertension to prevent bleeds (Toyonaga et al. 1991).

As liver disease progresses, chronic inflammation and fibrosis within the sinusoids and channels of the liver lobule produces intrahepatic obstruction of the portal blood flow. Figure 19–4 illustrates the basic structure of the liver lobule. Blood flow through the portal circulation is normally a low-flow system, with average pressures of 7–11 mm Hg. With congestion of the liver sinusoid network due to fibrotic changes (commonly seen in alcoholic cirrhosis), the portal pressures rise to as high as 40–45 mm Hg. This elevation in pressure produces backup of blood and congestion of those organs normally drained by the portal system, principally the spleen and the GI tract (Figure 19–5). The vessels of the upper stomach and distal esophagus are unable to tolerate these pressure elevations, and the usual sequela is rupture of these distended and now fragile vessels. Rupture of these vessels may occur in response to a sudden increase in abdominal pressure due to physical exertion, vomiting, forceful coughing and sneezing, straining at stool, or mechanical trauma (blind insertion of an NG tube, endoscopic procedures, or ingestion of excessive roughage or incompletely chewed food).

TABLE 19–4

Vasopressin/Nitroglycerin Therapy Protocol*

VASOPRESSIN (VP)

250 U/250 cc 5% dextrose in water (D$_5$W) (1 U/ml)

1. Start with 15 U vasopressin (VP) in 50 ml D$_5$W over 15 min.
2. Begin VP drip between 0.4 U/min and 0.6 U/min.

NITROGLYCERIN (NTG)

100 mg/250 cc D$_5$W (400 mcg/ml)

1. Initiate nitroglycerin (NTG) drip.
2. Increase NTG drip in increments of 10 to 40 mcg/min maintaining systolic BP > 100 mm Hg (to a maximum of 400 mcg/min).
3. May substitute with NTG paste or sublingual form once patient stabilizes.

DESIRED RATE (U/MIN)	ML/MIN	DROPS/MIN OR ML/H	DESIRED RATE (MCG/MIN)	ML/MIN	DROPS/MIN OR ML/H
0.1	0.1	6	10	0.1	2
0.2	0.2	12	20	0.1	3
0.3	0.3	18	30	0.1	5
0.4	0.4	24	40	0.1	6
0.5	0.5	30	50	0.1	8
0.6	0.6	36	60	0.2	9
0.7	0.7	42	70	0.2	11
0.8	0.8	48	80	0.2	12
0.9	0.9	54	90	0.2	14
1.0	1.0	60	100	0.3	15
1.1	1.1	66	110	0.3	17
1.2	1.2	72	120	0.3	18
1.3	1.3	78	130	0.3	20
1.4	1.4	84	140	0.4	21
1.5	1.5	90	150	0.4	23
			160	0.4	24
			170	0.4	26
			180	0.5	27
			190	0.5	29
			200	0.5	30
			210	0.6	32
			220	0.6	33
			230	0.6	35
			240	0.6	36
			250	0.6	38
			260	0.7	39
			270	0.7	41
			280	0.7	42
			290	0.7	44
			300	0.8	45
			310	0.8	47
			320	0.8	48
			330	0.8	50
			340	0.9	51

TABLE 19–4

Vasopressin/Nitroglycerin Therapy Protocol* (Continued)

DESIRED RATE (U/MIN)	ML/MIN	DROPS/MIN OR ML/H	DESIRED RATE (MCG/MIN)	ML/MIN	DROPS/MIN OR ML/H
			350	0.9	53
			360	0.9	54
			370	0.9	56
			380	1.0	57
			390	1.0	59
			400	1.0	60

*For use in variceal bleed.

Excerpted from Burns S, Martin M: VP/NTG therapy in the patient with variceal bleeding. *Crit Care Nurs* 1990; 10(9):42–49. © 1991 Cahners Publishing Company.

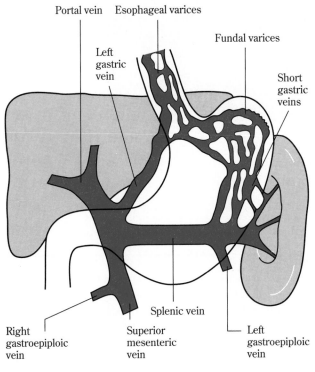

FIGURE 19–5

Congested portal blood circuit with back-up to gastric and esophageal vessels. (From: Misiewicz J, Pounder R, Venables C (eds): *Diseases of the gut and pancreas.* Oxford, England: Blackwell Scientific Publications, 1987.)

Bleeding esophageal varices occur in 60% of patients with cirrhosis. They are a medical emergency with a mortality rate of 50% in first-time bleeds (Navab, Schiller and Slaton 1984; Grew et al. 1984).

This condition requires prompt intervention with hemodynamic stabilization, vasopressin/nitroglycerin infusions, and most often the insertion of a tamponade tube for direct compression of the bleeding sites. (Figure 19–6 illustrates one such tamponade tube in its therapeutic position.) The nursing care plan highlights nursing considerations during insertion and ongoing therapy with esophageal-gastric tamponade tubes.

Injection sclerotherapy is utilized as a definitive treatment for bleeding esophageal varices as well as bleeding rectal varices. Sclerotherapy consists of the injection, via endoscope, of a coagulating substance directly into each varix. An intense inflammatory response ensues, which then scars over the weakened and ruptured vessel, thereby providing definitive hemostasis and control of bleeding. Injection sclerotherapy is 80% effective and may be done emergently if the patient is stable; however, it most often is performed 3–4 days after patient stabilization. The treatments are repeated at weekly intervals for a few weeks, then monthly and quarterly until all the varices are obliterated. Side effects from injection sclerotherapy include: esophageal ulceration; stricture; perforation; retrosternal burning pain; bacteremia/sepsis; aspiration pneumonia; bradycardia; allergic response to medications used; and possible long-term dysphagia motility disorder.

Surgical intervention for bleeding esophageal varices requires abdominal and thoracic incisions for access, transection of the gastroesophageal junction, oversewing, and reanastomosis. In a patient who already is compromised by hepatic dysfunction and often by malnutrition, prognosis with this surgery is very poor.

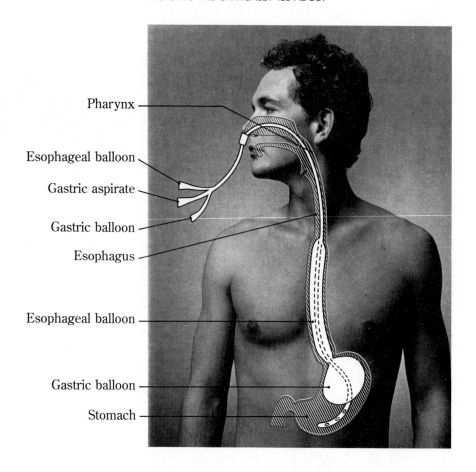

FIGURE 19-6

Triple-lumen esophageal-nasogastric (Sengstaken-Blakemore) tube. (From Swearingen P: *The Addison-Wesley photo atlas of nursing procedures,* 2d ed. Redwood City, CA: Addison-Wesley, 1991, p. 249.)

Outcome Evaluation

Evaluate the patient's progress according to these desirable outcome criteria:

- Vital signs within normal limits (WNL).
- No complaints of dizziness, thirst, or syncope.
- Postural vital signs negative; that is, systolic BP change of less than 10 mm Hg and pulse change of less than 20 beats per minute.
- No hematemesis or hematochezia.
- Hemoglobin, hematocrit, and red blood cell count WNL.
- Arterial blood gas values WNL.
- Relaxed appearance.

Acute Pancreatitis

The pancreas is a soft, lobulated accessory organ of digestion. It measures approximately 4–6 inches and is located in the epigastric region of the abdomen behind the duodenum and spleen. The pancreas is divided physically into three sections—the head, which lies in the curve of the duodenum, the body, and the tail, which contacts the spleen. The duct of Wirsung (main pancreatic duct) runs the length of the organ and joins the common bile duct to drain the exocrine secretions of the pancreas into the duodenum for the digestion of fats, proteins, and carbohydrates. An accessory duct (duct of Santorini) is present in about 15–20% of the population.

Pancreatic enzymes normally are released via the duct of Wirsung into the entrance to the duodenum (ampulla of Vater) in a controlled manner following the stimulus of ingested food and fluids. Pancreatic secretions normally are colorless, are produced in a volume

TIPS: TRANSJUGULAR INTRAHEPATIC PORTOSYSTEMIC SHUNT

A transjugular intrahepatic portosystemic shunt is an intervention to reduce portal hypertension in patients with variceal hemorrhage.

The Technology The management of patients with portal hypertension and subsequent variceal hemorrhage remains a challenging and complex task. Current interventions include attempts at reduction of portal pressures with oral doses of propranolol (Inderal); management of acute variceal hemorrhage with tamponade tubes and infusions of vasopressin and nitroglycerin; injection sclerotherapy, both prophylactically and emergently following actual variceal bleed; and surgically created portosystemic shunting procedures. Although surgical shunting procedures have been associated with the lowest frequency of rebleeding, surgical shunting is associated with a significant morbidity and mortality (Cello et al. 1987; Rikkers et al. 1987). Shunting operations usually are limited for the 10–15% of patients who do not respond to endoscopic sclerotherapy. Surgical shunting has not been demonstrated to impact long-term survival for patients with advanced liver disease. Less than 50% of patients who bleed from varices survive 30 days, whether or not they have had portosystemic shunting-surgery or sclerotherapy (Ring et al. 1992).

Attempts to identify alternatives to surgical shunting for portal decompression were begun as early as 1969 (Rosch et al. 1969). A percutaneous technique was employed to create a parenchymal liver tract between the inferior vena cava and portal vein, thereby diverting blood flow from the diseased liver to the general circulation. Further research in animal models (Palmaz et al. 1986) resulted in use of expandable stents (devices employed to maintain patency of an operative area and support structures during healing) to keep the parenchymal tracts, created by percutaneous needle insertion, patent in blood flow.

Percutaneous intrahepatic shunts in humans, using angioplasty balloons to establish transparenchymal channels, were reported in 1982 (Colapinto et al. 1982). A transjugular intrahepatic portosystemic shunt (TIPS) procedure in humans, utilizing a balloon expandable stent, was performed on a patient in 1988 (Richter 1990). The patient, with alcoholic cirrhosis and portal hypertension, had multiple admissions for massive esophageal bleeding that was refractory to endoscopic sclerotherapy. The procedure successfully created an intrahepatic shunt and significantly reduced portal pressures. Further refinement of the TIPS procedure resulted in a technique that successfully reduces portosystemic pressures (average portosystemic pressures were reduced from 36 to 11 mm Hg) with decompression of gastroesophageal varices. No mortality has been associated with the procedure and reported morbidity is limited to one incident of stent migration to the left lower-lobe pulmonary artery (Zemel et al. 1991).

The procedure is indicated in cirrhosis with portal hypertension, in refractory documented or symptomatic (bleeding) varices (gastroesophageal and/or rectal), and in end-stage liver disease to minimize or eliminate the threat of variceal bleed in patients who are awaiting liver transplantation.

The procedure is usually performed in the interventional radiology or imaging department and takes about 2 hours. The patient receives mild intravenous sedation and local anesthetic to the right neck. The right internal jugular vein is accessed percutaneously with ultrasonographic guidance. A long sheath is advanced through the right atrium to the inferior vena cava. An angiographic catheter then is manipulated into either the right or middle hepatic vein and the sheath advanced. The catheter then is exchanged for a biopsy needle, which is advanced from the hepatic vein into a portal vein branch, connecting a hepatic vein with the right or left portal vein across the liver parenchyma. Portal pressure and a portal venogram are obtained. An angioplasty balloon catheter is placed and inflated across the hepatic parenchymal tract. A self-expanding metallic stent (Wallstent) is placed into position in the parenchymal tract. The stent will become incorporated into the liver tissue as the healing process is completed. Upper gastrointestinal endoscopy is performed following the procedure to verify that variceal decompression has been achieved. Sonographic Doppler is used to verify shunt patency at 3–6 month intervals thereafter.

Patient Care Considerations Because the procedure is done using a jugular venipuncture and fluoroscopic and transabdominal ultrasound guidance, there is little risk for hemorrhage, even for those patients with coagulopathies. Other potential risks and discomforts include jugular or portal vein thrombosis, peritoneal bleeding and/or infection, stent thrombosis, pulmonary embolism, and hepatic encephalopathy.

Following the procedure, patients are returned to the nursing unit for routine postangioplasty observation. A small sterile dressing is applied to the puncture site, and the patient is monitored additionally for signs of hemodynamic instability and intra-abdominal hemorrhage (a drop in blood pressure with elevation in pulse, narrowing pulse pressure, and increasing abdominal girth).

of approximately 1,500–2,000 ml per day, and have a pH of 8.0–8.3. In addition to digestive enzymes, pancreatic fluids contain a high concentration of sodium, bicarbonate, water, and potassium. The beta cells of the pancreas (islands of Langerhans) produce and secrete the hormone insulin into the blood stream for regulation of blood glucose.

Pancreatitis is the acute or chronic inflammation of the tissues of the pancreas due to the premature activation and release of proteolytic enzymes, which then autodigest the organ itself. The inflammatory and autodigestive process leads to tissue necrosis; precipitation of calcium with resultant hypocalcemia; release of necrotic toxins, precursors to sepsis; leakage into the peritoneum of large volumes of pancreatic exudates rich in albumin; shock and death.

The Marseille-Rome classifications (Sales, Bernard and Gullo 1990; Sarles et al. 1989) describe pancreatitis as a spectrum of inflammatory lesions in the pancreas and in the pancreatic tissues leading to edema, hemorrhagic and fat necrosis, and destruction of exocrine parenchyma and fibrosis. The classifications of pancreatitis include: class 1) acute pancreatitis; class 2) chronic pancreatitis; class 3) infected cysts or necrotic abscesses, called pseudocysts; and class 4) perilobar fibrosis without evident loss of exocrine parenchyma.

Assessment

Risk Conditions The etiologies and precipitating factors of pancreatitis include: heredity, infections, metabolic, traumatic (accidental and surgical), drug ingestion, and mechanical. Table 19–5 summarizes these factors. By far the most common etiology of pancreatitis is chronic alcohol ingestion.

It is unclear exactly how alcohol abuse overcomes the natural safeguards of the pancreas and initiates premature pancreatic enzyme activation. Several mechanisms have been hypothesized; they are summarized as follows. First, alcohol stimulates and increases gastric and pancreatic secretions, which may induce duodenal inflammation and spasm of the ampulla of Vater. Alcohol also decreases gastric pH, which is another stimulus for secretion of alkaline pancreatic fluid. In the presence of ampulla obstruction, stimulation of the pancreas can precipitate pancreatitis. Second, prolonged alcohol intake produces histologic changes in pancreatic tissue and the ducts, which may cause obstruction and cell membrane changes. It is important to note that not all people who abuse alcohol develop pancreatitis, indicating that other factors possibly are involved.

TABLE 19–5

Etiologies and Precipitating Factors in Pancreatitis

Heredity

Special protein (PSP) prevents calcium precipitation. Dominant hereditary trait observed in children of both sexes; biochemical modification is decrease of PSP in pancreatic juice (Multigner et al. 1985).

Metabolic

Chronic alcohol ingestion results in changes in pancreatic exocrine secretion, protein precipitation within ducts, obstruction, inflammation, autodigestion (over 60% cases after 6–8 years of chronic heavy alcohol ingestion).

Hypercalcemia

Hyperlipidemia—abnormally high- or low-lipid diets

High-protein, high-fat diets

Protein/fat malnutrition (observed in some tropical countries)

Hyperparathyroidism

Drugs

Corticosteroids, thiazide diuretics, sulfonamides, oral contraceptives, tetracycline, excessive doses of acetaminophen

Mechanical

Trauma

Cholecystitis, cholelithiasis (obstruction of gall stones 20% of cases)

Bile/duodenal reflux into pancreatic duct

Postoperative complication of gastric, biliary, duodenal surgery

Ischemia following shock states

Pancreatic tumor

Infection

Vital hepatitis, mumps, coxsackievirus

Signs and Symptoms The most common clinical feature of acute pancreatitis is severe abdominal pain. It may begin gradually or suddenly, but once present it is unrelenting. It usually is located in the epigastrium, and often radiates to the back, chest, and flank areas. It is relieved by sitting forward. Nausea, vomiting, and abdominal distention, which may accompany the pain, usually are caused by hypomotility and peritonitis. Peritonitis occurs with cell and tissue destruction. If the condition is severe, shock may be present due to loss of large amounts of plasma into pancreatic and parapancreatic tissue. This hemorrhage may cause retroperitoneal bruising *(Grey-Turner's sign)* and discoloration around the umbilicus *(Cullen's sign)*. Pleural effusion may be present. Additionally, low-grade fever and tachycardia are common.

Diagnostic Studies In addition to the severe and often incapacitating abdominal pain experienced by patients with acute episodes of pancreatitis, a marked elevation in the total serum amylase level is the hallmark sign.

Total serum amylase measures all three forms of amylase—salivary amylase, macroamylase (released by intestinal walls), and pancreatic amylase. Total serum amylase levels in acute pancreatitis may rise to 2½ times normal values within 6 hours of the onset of an attack, peaking at about 24 hours, and may remain elevated for several days. Values about 1,000 IU are characteristic. Total serum amylase may rise dramatically in several other intra-abdominal events, including small bowel obstructions, mesenteric infarctions, and perforated ulcers. Isoamylase determinations differentiate acute pancreatitis from other abdominal events. The isoamylase ratio reflects a comparison of salivary amylase to pancreatic amylase. The normal ratio is about 50%, and a ratio exceeding 80% indicates acute pancreatitis.

Urine amylase and serum lipase levels also elevate for about 5–7 days following an acute episode of pancreatitis. An amylase/creatinine clearance ratio of >5% indicates pancreatitis. Other abnormal laboratory values expected are leukocytosis; marked variances in hemoglobin and hematocrit depending on fluid volume status, degree of compensation and hemorrhage; elevation of serum and urine bilirubin levels; decreased serum albumin values, frequently less than 3.2 g/dl; elevated serum triglyceride levels; and variances in serum electrolyte values (commonly hypocalcemia and, with NG suction, hypokalemia and hyponatremia).

Arterial pH is frequently decreased, related to shock states, toxic peritoneum, and sepsis. Decreased arterial Po_2 results from a variety of physical and physiologic impairments, and respiratory dysfunction may progress to the adult respiratory distress syndrome. In

NURSING DIAGNOSES

The nursing diagnoses that may apply to the patient with acute pancreatitis include the following:

- Fluid volume deficit
- Pain
- High risk for altered nutrition: less than body requirements
- High risk for infection

TABLE 19–6

Diagnostic Imaging in Findings or Rationales Diagnosis of Pancreatitis

Abdominal Films

Demonstrate hollow viscera close to pancreas, denoting ileus of stomach, duodenum, proximal ileum calcifications, adhesions.

Chest Films

Pleural effusions in 5–17% of patients, left side greater than right.

Bilateral diffuse alveolar consolidation, atelectasis.

Diaphragmatic elevation due to peritonitis.

Upper GI Studies

Delayed gastric emptying, enlarged duodenum related to edema of head of pancreas.

Stomach displacement due to pseudocyst formation.

IV Cholangiography

To rule out acute cholecystitis of biliary tree as cause of symptomatology.

Abdominal Ultrasound

Reflects organ/structural edema, inflammatory processes, gallstones, calcifications of pancreatic ducts, abscesses, hematoma, organ enlargement, pseudocysts.

Computerized Tomography (CT) Scan

Identifies tumors, pseudocysts, dilated/calcified pancreatic ducts.

Paracentesis

Diagnostic use for assay of elevated pancreatic amylase, blood; therapeutic use for reduction of peritoneal fluid impairing respiratory dynamics.

adequate respiratory dynamics result from accumulations of peritoneal fluid under the diaphragm and from pleural effusions, which are present in 5–17% of patients with acute pancreatitis.

Serum glucose and urine glucose levels may be elevated as the inflammatory process affects endocrine (beta cell) function of the pancreas. Additionally, increased glucagon release and increased secretion of adrenal glucocorticoids may contribute to hyperglycemia. Table 19–6 highlights other diagnostic studies that assist in the diagnosis of pancreatitis.

Planning and Implementation of Care

This section organizes nursing care by nursing diagnosis. An alternate way to remember care using a mnemonic is presented in Table 19–7.

Fluid Volume Deficit Related to Hemorrhage
Monitor the patient carefully for signs of hemorrhage

TABLE 19–7

Intervention for Acute Pancreatitis

Intervention for acute pancreatitis can best be summarized and remembered using the mnemonic PANCREAS.

P = PAIN: The pain experienced during acute attack can be severe; meperidine (Demerol) is the drug of choice to minimize potential for spasm of sphincter of Oddi that morphine may cause.

A = ANTISPASMODIC DRUGS: These may be helpful to decrease motility and stimulation of the GI tract during acute attack.

N = NASOGASTRIC SUCTION: Patient's oral intake should be restricted to put the pancreas at rest and remove stimulation of enzyme release; nasogastric suction can assist in managing abdominal distention, ileus, and pancreatic stimulation by hydrochloric acid that is released by stomach and enters duodenum. Histamine blockers may also be used to decrease acid production and release.

C = CALCIUM: Transient hypocalcemia develops in ⅓ of patients; clinical tetany is rare; calcium sequestration in areas of fat necrosis occurs; if clinical signs of hypocalcemia occur, replace calcium.

R = REPLACEMENT OF FLUIDS AND ELECTROLYTES: With large volumes of NG losses and fluid shifts into peritoneum, replacement of effective circulating volume is essential to maintain hemodynamics; albumin loss is significant and replacement may be indicated to minimize capillary leak syndrome, especially in pulmonary bed.

E = ENDOCRINES: Control of hyperglycemia is achieved with insulin; glucagon, calcitonin, and somatostatin are sometimes used.

A = ANTIBIOTICS: Antibiotics are given in all cases with fever and frequently with all cases of acute pancreatitis, since it is difficult to differentiate signs and symptoms of infection from those of aseptic pancreatic necrosis; usual drugs are cefotaxime, mezlocillin, cefalothin, and cephamandole.

S = STEROIDS: Corticosteroids may be administered during acute attacks.

Other interventions may include: heparin, administered if disseminated intravascular coagulation occurs or in low doses to prevent thromboembolic complications; peritoneal dialysis to remove toxic substances; and peritoneal tap when collection of fluid in the peritoneal space impairs respiratory dynamics, resulting in atelectasis.

and decreased fluid volume such as: decreased blood pressure, increased heart rate, peripheral vasoconstriction, and decreased urine output (30–40 cc/hr). In addition, Grey-Turner's sign and Cullen's sign may indicate retroperitoneal and/or parapancreatic bleeding. Hemodynamic monitoring with a pulmonary artery line may be used to guide and evaluate fluid replacement. A right atrial pressure less than 2 mm Hg and a pulmonary capillary wedge pressure (PCWP) less than 4 mm Hg may indicate hypovolemia.

Administer fluid, blood replacement, and plasma expanders as ordered by the physician. Care must be taken when administering hyperosmotic solutions, such as albumin, because rapid fluid shifts may precipitate fluid overload.

Hypovolemia may contribute to renal failure with decreased renal perfusion, so monitor urine output hourly.

Pain Related to Inflammation Meperidine is the analgesic usually used for relief of the pain associated with pancreatitis. It is less likely to cause spasm of the sphincter of Oddi than an opiate such as morphine sulfate. Assist the patient to a position of comfort, usually Fowler's with knees flexed, as this relaxes abdominal muscles. Maintain bedrest to minimize pain and facilitate rest. Additionally, restrict the patient's oral intake to decrease stimulation of pancreatic secretions.

The critical-care nurse may also intervene with nonpharmacologic techniques such as relaxation, massage, distraction, and guided imagery to enhance analgesic effect.

Altered Nutrition: Less than Body Requirements Related to Restricted Oral Intake, Nasogastric Suction, Anorexia, and Vomiting The patient with pancreatitis is at risk for nutritional deficiency for several reasons. First, the patient's oral intake is restricted in order to decrease pancreatic secretions. Second, nasogastric suction is used to decrease abdominal distention and flow of acid into the small intestine, which stimulates pancreatic secretion. Finally, prior to hospitalization and implementation of suction, the patient has most likely been anorexic and nauseated and has experienced vomiting.

When nutritional support is needed, total parenteral nutrition often is administered and continued for approximately 2–3 weeks. The administration of lipids or amino acids intravenously does not stimulate the pancreas.

When symptoms improve, patients begin refeeding very gradually on clear liquids. Resumption of oral intake within the first 2 weeks may cause exacerbation and a return to restricted oral intake with IV hydration may be necessary.

High Risk for Infection Related to Leakage of Enzymes The patient with pancreatitis is at risk for infection from peritonitis, pancreatic abscess, or pancreatic pseudocyst. These complications usually occur in the second or third week after the onset of pancreatitis. Monitor the patient for signs of infection, such as increased white blood cells (WBC), increased polymorphonuclear cells (PMNs), increased temperature, and abdominal pain and rigidity.

Because of the toxicity of pancreatic secretions, peritoneal lavage may be done to remove the exudate and help prevent sepsis. However, lavage has not been shown to prevent pancreatic necrosis.

A treatment sometimes used for infected pseudocysts is aspiration by introducing a catheter into the cyst for drainage. If this is not possible, surgical removal is required. Another indication for surgery is necrotizing pancreatitis, as the necrotic tissue and abscess areas must be completely removed.

Surgical Management of Pancreatitis Generally, surgical intervention is contraindicated in uncomplicated episodes of pancreatitis. If the diagnosis is uncertain, diagnostic laparoscopy may be used. Placement of drains and irrigation catheters in the peritoneal space, and possibly t-tube placement in the biliary tree, may be of some use in the management of fulminant pancreatitis. Mortality rates from acute pancreatitis average about 10%, and for hemorrhagic pancreatitis, rates approach 50% (Way 1990). Respiratory insufficiency and significant hypocalcemia are indicators of a poor prognosis. Surgical options include debridement of necrotic pancreatic tissues, total pancreatectomy (resulting in insulin-dependent diabetes), pancreatectomy with islet cell autotransplantation (patient's own healthy cells injected into portal vein and into the liver), and segmental pancreatic autotransplantation (healthy segments of pancreas reimplanted and anastomosed to femoral vessels).

Outcome Evaluation

Evaluate the patient's progress according to the following outcome criteria:

- Fluid balance normal.
- Urine output 30 cc/hr or greater.
- Vital signs within normal limits.
- Relief of pain.
- No evidence of infection.
- No evidence of hemorrhage.
- Electrolytes within normal limits.
- No manifestations of electrolyte imbalance (e.g., tetany).

Liver Failure

The liver is the body's largest parenchymal organ. This pear-shaped organ, weighing about 1,400–1,600 g (2% of body weight), lies under the diaphragm and is strategically placed between the intestinal and general circulatory systems. The liver's complicated structure supports its critical metabolic, vascular, excretory, and secretory functions (Table 19–8). Liver cells, once chronically damaged and replaced with fibrotic tissues, do not continue to function; however, the liver is able to generate new cells if the precipitating factors originally causing damage have been eliminated. The Kupffer cells, located within the liver's parenchymal network, are the body's most important part of the reticuloendothelial system. These cells break down hemoglobin to bilirubin, form globulins and immune bodies, and act as scavengers to clear bacteria,

TABLE 19–8

Summary of Liver Functions

Vascular Functions

Stores blood volume and can release up to 400 cc as needed to maintain effective circulating volume.

Kupffer cells filter bacteria from the blood.

Secretory Functions

Hepatocytes produce bile to aid in absorption of fats.

Conjugates bilirubin so it is water-soluble for excretion.

Removes unused cholesterol.

Metabolic Functions

Stores sugar in the form of glycogen.

Reconverts glycogen to glucose as needed for energy.

Converts amino acids and fatty acids into new glucose (gluconeogenesis).

Stores fat as triglycerides.

Converts fatty acids to acetyl CoA (by a process called *beta oxidation*) for use in energy production.

Converts excess acetyl CoA to ketones.

Synthesizes serum proteins (albumin, globulins, and fibrinogen).

Deaminates amino acids (removes an amino group so proteins can be used for energy production).

Converts ammonia to urea.

Produces vitamin-K-dependent clotting factors.

Detoxifies hormones and drugs.

Storage Functions

Stores large quantities of vitamins A, D, and B_{12} and iron.

Stores vitamins E and K.

corpuscular, and macromolecular elements from the blood.

Four major vessels supply and drain the liver. The *hepatic artery* provides oxygenated blood to liver tissues, the *hepatic vein* drains the liver, the *bile duct* drains bile produced in the liver to the gall bladder, and the *portal vein* delivers blood from the intestines to the liver for filtration and detoxification of nutrients and ingested medications. The bile duct, portal vein, and hepatic artery all travel together in what is termed the portal triad. This triad of vessels is juxtaposed among the liver cells, Kupffer cells, bile capillaries, and lymphatics in the dense sinusoid cavities and duct systems that support the complex function of the liver (refer to Figure 19-4).

Liver failure may result from several different pathophysiologic states that destroy or disrupt the structural elements of liver tissue. When significant amounts of parenchymal cells are progressively damaged and replaced with fibrotic tissue, the complex functions of the liver are impaired, leading to life-threatening failure of the organ. Liver dysfunction may occur with a sudden onset or may develop insidiously over a period of years, depending on its etiology.

The process of destruction of liver cells and decreasing liver function is called *cirrhosis*. Cirrhosis has three main types, all of which eventually lead to liver failure. *Postnecrotic cirrhosis* is characterized by massive necrosis of liver cells and formation of fibrous nodules. *Portal,* or *alcoholic (Laennec's), cirrhosis* is characterized by fatty deposits and inflammation progressing to necrosis. Laennec's cirrhosis occurs because of alcohol's direct toxic effect on the liver. The by-product of alcohol oxidation, acetaldehyde, causes mitochondrial membrane damage and necrosis of hepatocytes. Alcohol also inhibits release of triglycerides from the liver (by increasing storage) and increases synthesis of fatty acids, thereby producing fatty infiltration and obstruction in the liver. *Biliary cirrhosis* begins in the bile ducts and is characterized by inflammation and scar formation in the ducts, eventually causing obstruction and destruction.

Assessment

Risk Conditions There are three main precipitating conditions for hepatic failure: Laennec's (alcoholic) cirrhosis, postnecrotic cirrhosis, and biliary or obstructive processes. In *Laennec's cirrhosis,* the patient's history usually reflects alcohol abuse plus another stressor, such as a recent drinking binge, infection, GI bleeding, surgery, or sedative use. *Postnecrotic cirrho-*

sis is usually associated with viral hepatitis or hepatic destruction from toxic industrial chemicals. Ingested drugs in prescribed dosages, as well as self-overdosages, can exert direct toxic effects on liver cells. *Obstructive processes* can occur with chronic biliary infections or ductal obstruction. In critically ill patients, liver failure also may be associated with circulatory failure and/or shock.

Signs and Symptoms The symptoms associated with the clinical presentation of liver failure vary with the severity and the extent of hepatic destruction. With early liver dysfunction, the patient may present with weakness, anorexia, weight loss, abdominal discomfort or pressure, and lack of energy. As the dysfunction progresses and the liver deteriorates, virtually every bodily system is affected.

Cardiovascular Symptoms Initially, the patient has a hyperdynamic cardiovascular system with flushed skin, hypertension, bounding pulses, and an enhanced precordial impulse. Blood pressure eventually decreases due to fluid transudation and release of vasoactive substances from the damaged liver. (Fluid transudation occurs because decreased albumin synthesis decreases plasma oncotic pressure, leading to ascites formation and decreased effective circulating volumes.) Dysrhythmias may occur because of electrolyte changes.

Respiratory Symptoms Ascites may cause pressure on the diaphragm and prevent normal lung expansion. Additionally, a pleural effusion may compress lung tissue as ascitic fluid leaks into the pleural space. The patient may become hypoxemic.

Renal Symptoms Urine output decreases because of decreased renal perfusion.

Neurologic Symptoms Clinical manifestations range from minor personality changes to coma. Most neurologic changes result from accumulation of ammonia in the blood due to the liver's inability to convert it to urea. The excess ammonia then enters the central nervous system. Additionally, the decreased storage of B vitamins may cause peripheral nerve degeneration and sensory alterations. Clinical symptoms vary greatly and may manifest very quickly (hours to days) or may appear gradually over the course of a week or more. Table 19–9 highlights the stages of hepatic coma and clinical manifestations.

Hematologic Symptoms Coagulation problems occur because of deficient clotting factors. Bruising, nosebleeds, and gingival bleeding are common. The pa-

TABLE 19–9

Stages of Hepatic Coma

STAGE	CLINICAL MANIFESTATIONS
One	
Prodromal	Apathy, confusion
	Impaired mentation
	Mild tremor
	Diminished intellectual function
	Behavior alterations
	Mild ECG abnormality
	Elevated blood ammonia levels
	Normal psychomotor skills
Two	
Impending Coma	Inappropriate behavior
	Drowsiness
	Lack of awareness, lethargy
	Tremor present with asterixis
	Moderate ECG abnormalities
	Increased blood ammonia levels
	Some abnormal psychomotor skills
Three	
Stupor	Confusion
	Somnolence but arousable
	Tremors
	Disorientation
	Severe ECG abnormalities
	Abnormal psychomotor skills
Four	
Coma	Unconsciousness, possible response to deep stimuli
	Vital sign alterations
	Loss of reflexes
	Seizures
	Severe ECG changes

tient also may have petechiae associated with thrombocytopenia.

Fluid/Electrolyte Symptoms Electrolyte levels vary with fluid balance. Initially, sodium and water retention occur in the intravascular spaces due to decreased metabolism of antidiuretic hormone (ADH) (prolonged half-life). As the liver becomes congested and portal vein pressure increases, fluid eventually seeps into the peritoneal cavity (ascites) and plasma volume decreases. This decrease results in compensatory

mechanisms: release of ADH, release of aldosterone, and activation of the renin-angiotensin system. These mechanisms also result in sodium and water retention and eventually may cause dilutional hyponatremia. Other electrolyte disturbances include:

- Hypokalemia due to diarrhea, aldosterone, or diuretics.
- Hypocalcemia due to decreased dietary intake and decreased absorption of vitamin D.
- Hypomagnesemia due to inability of the liver to store magnesium.

Gastrointestinal Symptoms Fetor hepaticus, a sweetish, almost fecal odor to the breath, is thought to be due to accumulation of methyl-mercaptan. Because of the increased portal vein pressure, varices may develop, most frequently in rectal and esophageal vessels. These may be an additional source of gastrointestinal bleeding in hepatic failure.

Immunologic Symptoms Patients with hepatic failure have increased susceptibility to infection due to dysfunction of the filtering Kupffer cells.

Dermatologic Symptoms Jaundice occurs because of accumulation of bilirubin. Palmar erythema and erythema of the soles of the feet occur due to arteriovenous anastomoses.

Diagnostic Procedures Diagnostic procedures in liver failure include laboratory screens, diagnostic imaging, biopsies, and endoscopies. Table 19–10 presents diagnostic findings in liver failure.

NURSING DIAGNOSES

Nursing diagnoses that may apply to the patient with hepatic failure include:

- High risk for fluid volume alteration*
- High risk for electrolyte imbalance*
- Sensory-perceptual alteration
- Altered nutrition: less than body requirements
- High risk for infection
- High risk for impaired gas exchange
- Impaired skin integrity
- High risk for altered urinary elimination

*non-NANDA diagnosis

TABLE 19–10

Diagnostic Findings in Liver Failure

DIAGNOSTIC TEST LABORATORY TESTS	FINDING OR RATIONALE
CBC	Decreased hemoglobin and hematocrit, demonstrating recent GI bleeding and the liver's inability to store the hematopoietic factors of iron, folic acid, and vitamin B_{12}. Decreased white blood cell counts and platelets associated with splenomegaly and/or elevated WBC, indicating current infection.
Prothrombin time	Prolonged, reflecting decreased synthesis of prothrombin and impaired absorption of vitamin K.
Serum albumin and total proteins	Decreased, reflecting impaired protein synthesis.
BUN and creatinine	BUN may elevate with hypovolemia/GI bleeding. Elevated creatinine level reflects impaired renal perfusion.
Serum ammonia levels	Elevated, reflecting impaired hepatic synthesis of urea.
Serum glucose levels	Decreased due to liver's inability to store glycogen; decrease also may reflect malnutrition.
Cholesterol levels	Either decreased, reflecting liver's inability to synthesize cholesterol, or elevated due to obstruction.
Bilirubin levels (total and direct)	Elevated, reflecting liver's dysfunction.
Enzyme tests	Elevated, reflecting hepatocellular or biliary tissue damage/necrosis. Specific enzymes tested are AST (aspartate aminotransferase, formerly known as SGOT, serum glutamicoxaloacetic transaminase); ALT (alanine aminotransferase, formerly known as SGPT, serum glutamic-pyruvic transaminase); alkaline phosphatase, and lactic dehydrogenase.
Hepatitis antibodies test	To assess for active hepatitis as etiology.
Urine and stool tests	May indicate increased urine urobilinogen and reduced fecal urobilinogen, which is observed with jaundice.
IMAGING STUDIES	
Abdominal ultrasound	May demonstrate biliary obstruction.
Abdominal x-rays	Denote liver enlargement, peritoneal involvement, possibly tumor.
Liver scan	Hepatic structure abnormalities.
Liver biopsy	Extent of liver tissue involvement/damage.
Angiography of liver and mesenteric vessels	Detail liver circulation and evaluate for portal hypertension.
Electroencephalogram	To evaluate for generalized slowing of frequency of brain waves, confirming encephalopathy.
Endoscopies	Sources of upper and lower GI bleeding may be demonstrated.

Planning and Implementation of Care

High Risk for Fluid Volume Deficit Related to Hemorrhage The risk of hemorrhage is present for several reasons. First, there are decreased amounts of vitamin-K-dependent clotting factors. Second, thrombocytopenia related to splenomegaly usually is present. Finally, the increased portal venous pressure causes (a) development of collateral channels in systems with lower pressure, and (b) congestion in the venous systems, which results in engorged varicose veins. This engorgement can manifest as hemorrhoids and dilated abdominal veins *(caput medusae)*.

Another manifestation of collateral circulation is varices of esophageal submucosa and the upper stomach. Bleeding varices are a life-threatening med-

ical emergency. (See the section of this chapter on Upper GI hemorrhage.)

High Risk for Fluid Volume Alteration Related to Ascites The ascites that occurs with liver failure is the result of several complicating factors. It can be understood by looking at Figure 19–7. Management of ascites may include the following:

- Dietary sodium limited to 200–500 mg/day.

- Fluids restricted to approximately 1,500 cc/day.

- Weight, intake and output (I & O), and abdominal girth calculated daily.

- Diuretics given with an aldosterone antagonist such as spironolactone.

- Intravenous albumin given to increase plasma oncotic pressure.

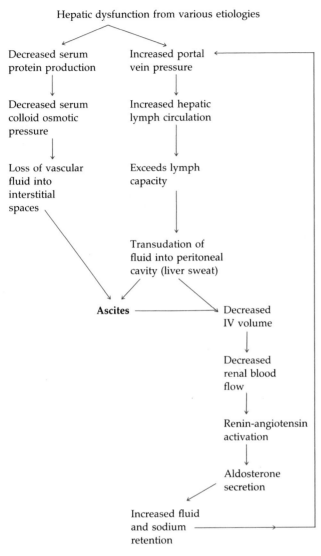

Hepatic dysfunction from various etiologies

Decreased serum protein production

Decreased serum colloid osmotic pressure

Loss of vascular fluid into interstitial spaces

Increased portal vein pressure

Increased hepatic lymph circulation

Exceeds lymph capacity

Transudation of fluid into peritoneal cavity (liver sweat)

Ascites

Decreased IV volume

Decreased renal blood flow

Renin-angiotensin activation

Aldosterone secretion

Increased fluid and sodium retention

FIGURE 19–7

Formation of ascites. (Adapted from Dodd RP: Ascites: When the liver can't cope. *RN* (October) 1984; 26–30. Copyright © 1984 Medical Economics Company, Inc., Oradell, N.J. Reprinted by permission.)

- Therapeutic paracentesis, using a small indwelling catheter for temporary relief, if respiratory function is impaired.

If ascites is refractory to medical management, peritoneovenous shunt procedures may be done. The collecting cannula lies in the peritoneal cavity, and the outflow tubing is tunneled through subcutaneous tissue to the internal jugular vein. Important nursing actions for a patient with a shunt include the following:

1. Maintain the patient in a supine position to facilitate flow.

2. Assist the patient with deep breathing to encourage flow.

3. Check the patency of the shunt with a Doppler flow meter.

4. Observe for central fluid overload from drainage of fluid into the jugular vein.

5. If fluid overload occurs, treatment will include:
   a. Positioning the patient upright
   b. Combination of digoxin and furosemide
   c. Shunt ligation by the physician

High Risk for Electrolyte Imbalance Related to Fluid Shifts The risk of electrolyte imbalance is present due to fluid shifts related to the development of ascites and from sodium and water retention. As the diseased liver is unable to synthesize albumin and the colloid osmotic pressure falls, fluid shifts into the peritoneum. The body senses a decreased effective circulating plasma volume, and hormonal response is initiated. Excessive amounts of ADH are secreted by the posterior pituitary to signal sodium and water retention. The diseased liver is unable to inactivate this hormone. Increased levels of aldosterone, renin, and angiotensin also are initiated in order to conserve sodium and water to counteract the lowered effective circulating volumes.

Potassium deficiency is also seen in liver dysfunction. Chronic diuretic therapy—used to manage ascites, secondary hyperaldosteronism, and renal tubular acidosis—and intravenous administration of glucose solutions contribute to hypokalemia. Zinc deficiencies, particularly common in alcoholic cirrhosis, impair wound healing and the immune response. Monitoring serum and urinary electrolytes is critical in patients with liver dysfunction. Replacement of electrolytes (especially sodium, potassium, and magnesium), fluids, and deficient minerals may be indicated at regular 8–24 hour intervals.

Sensory-Perceptual Alteration Related to Ammonia Retention Elevated plasma ammonia is a common occurrence in patients with hepatic failure. This problem is manifested as changes in neuromuscular and mental status. In early stages, patients show irritability, confusion, and clouding of the sensorium. As it progresses, the patient may proceed into coma and demonstrate asterixis (a characteristic hand-flapping tremor demonstrated with elevated blood ammonia levels).

Treatment is aimed at decreasing the amount of toxic protein metabolites that are absorbed into the blood. Initially, treatment includes excluding protein from the diet. Since bacterial breakdown of protein in the large intestine is the main source of ammonia, this exclusion lessens ammonia production. Another treatment involves introducing lactulose into the GI tract. Lactulose passes unchanged into the large intestine, where it is metabolized by bacteria, producing lactic acids and carbon dioxide. This decreases the pH to about 5.5, which favors conversion of ammonia to ammonium ions and subsequent excretion in the stool. The laxative action of lactulose further enhances evacuation of ammonia-rich stools.

Neomycin may also be used as a common treatment for hepatic encephalopathy. It is a nonabsorbable antibiotic that decreases the amount of urease-containing bacteria in the bowel, thereby decreasing ammonia production. For this purpose, it is given orally or by enema.

Altered Nutrition: Less than Body Requirements Related to Altered Hepatic Metabolism Liver dysfunction produces changes in carbohydrate, fat, and protein metabolism and alterations in storage and metabolism of vitamins and minerals. During liver dysfunction, catabolism creates a nutritional deficit that must be supplemented with high caloric intake. The calorie sources during encephalopathic states must not include protein sources, since the diseased liver is unable to metabolize proteins. Energy needs are met by intravenous or oral ingestion of high-calorie (1,600 calories/day) carbohydrate nutrients. Fat sources are used to supply essential fatty acids and energy but are contraindicated if jaundice is present, since the appearance of jaundice indicates decreased levels of bile salts, which are important in the absorption of fat. Supplements of vitamins and minerals are added to calorie sources since liver storage is impaired. Once encephalopathy has subsided, the gradual introduction of protein sources may begin at 20 g/day, with close monitoring for recurrence of the symptoms of encephalopathy. Protein intolerance may become chronic, depending on the severity and chronicity of liver dysfunction.

High Risk for Infection Related to Decreased Detoxification of Bacteria by Liver With hepatic dysfunction, the liver Kupffer cells do not adequately filter and detoxify bacteria. Additionally, splenomegaly may contribute to leukopenia. These two conditions predispose the patient to infection. An increase in circulating corticosteroids due to the stress response may further decrease the immune response.

High Risk for Impaired Gas Exchange Related to Ascites and Possible Pleural Effusion As the patient with hepatic failure is predisposed to respiratory problems, frequently assess for adequate gas exchange. The patient is usually more comfortable and able to expand the chest in a semi-Fowler's position.

Listen for adequate and clear lung sounds at least every 2 hours, and administer oxygen as indicated.

Impaired Skin Integrity Related to Impaired Circulation and Nutritional Deficit Skin care is of utmost importance for the patient with hepatic dysfunction, because of jaundice, dry skin, and decreased peripheral circulation. Turn frequently, massage bony prominences, and keep the skin clean and dry. See "Altered Skin Integrity" in the Hepatitis section for additional concerns, observations, and interventions.

High Risk for Altered Urinary Elimination Related to Decreased Renal Perfusion A serious complication of hepatic failure is decreased renal blood flow, decreased glomerular filtration, and subsequent renal failure. Renal failure in the presence of hepatic failure, termed *hepatorenal syndrome,* has a high mortality rate. Treatment is directed toward improving hepatic function and supporting renal function and includes:

- Fluid and electrolytes to maintain hemodynamic stability.
- Dextran or albumin to increase intravascular volume and increase glomerular filtration.
- Discontinuation of potentially nephrotoxic drugs such as neomycin.
- Monitoring of lab values indicative of renal function, such as blood urea nitrogen (BUN) and creatinine.

Outcome Evaluation

Evaluate the patient's progress according to the following criteria:

- Patient is alert and oriented.
- Patient exhibits no signs of infection.
- Nutritional status is adequate.
- Gas exchange is adequate.
- No signs of hemorrhage.
- Abdominal girth is not increasing.
- Liver function tests within normal limits.
- Hemodynamics stable.

Hepatitis

The term hepatitis refers to a range of inflammatory processes within the tissue of the liver. As hepatocytes are damaged, the cells become necrotic, and accumulation of necrotic debris in the liver parenchyma, portal ducts, and lobules alters the structural and functional capacity of the liver. The liver's critical metabolic, vascular, excretory, and secretory functions are impaired or may fail.

Assessment

Risk Conditions   Hepatitis can have many etiologies. The differential diagnosis must consider pathologies of hepatitislike disorders such as Wilson's disease, Budd-Chiari syndrome, sickle cell crisis, or veno-occlusive disease (Mandell et al. 1990). Anoxic liver injury and alcoholic and cholestatic liver diseases must also be considered because their syndromes resemble acute viral hepatitis. Drug-related acute hepatitis (see Table 19–11 listing common causes of drug-related injury) is not as common as viral hepatitis but is a serious pathology and a major cause of fulminant hepatic failure.

Acute viral hepatitis is a common disease, affecting 1–2 of every 1,000 people in the United States. The incidence rates of acute viral hepatitis have been rising slowly over the past 20 years according to the U.S. Centers for Disease Control (Mandell et al. 1990). Infection may be acute, chronic active, chronic persistent, autoimmune chronic, or drug-related chronic.

The primary etiology of hepatitis remains viral infection. Table 19–12 summarizes the five major known categories of agents that may lead to acute viral hepatitis. Historically, hepatitis was divided into the two types of hepatitis, type A and type B. It has been demonstrated that there are many viral agents that can cause hepatitis (Mandell et al. 1990). Non-A, non-B hepatitis includes several clinical entities, but the virus for only one type (hepatitis C) can be isolated at present. Laboratory tests to isolate other types of non-A, non-B hepatitis will be available in the future. Additional types of hepatitis are hepatitis D (delta hepatitis) and hepatitis E, enterically transmitted. Table 19–13 provides a viral hepatitis summary for hepatitis classifications A, B, C, D and E, indicating occurrence, etiologies, transmission, and periods of communicability.

Other viral agents that can affect the liver secondarily and result in a hepatitislike syndrome include cytomegalovirus (CMV), the Epstein-Barr virus (EBV), herpes simplex, varicella-zoster, measles, rubella, rubeola, and the coxsackie B viruses.

Hepatitis B is of particular concern, for the reasons presented in Table 19–14. High-risk conditions for this type of hepatitis are presented in Table 19–15.

Signs and Symptoms   In general, the clinical manifestations of hepatitis are divided into four stages: an incubation period; a preicteric phase; an icteric phase; and the convalescent period (Figure 19–8). The incubation period of viral hepatitis may be as short as 2 weeks to as long as 6 months. Averages are as follows:

Hepatitis A:	30 days (range 15–45 days)
Hepatitis B & C:	70 days (range 30–180 days)
Hepatitis non-A, non-B:	50 days (range 15–150 days)
Epidemic non-A, non-B:	40 days (range 15–60 days)

Delta hepatitis (hepatitis D) has no well documented incubation periods available (Mandell et al. 1990).

The initial symptoms of acute hepatitis are usually nonspecific and vague. Frequently the first symptoms patients report are general malaise and overall weakness. Headaches, fatigue, low-grade fevers and flu-like symptoms are also reported by patients during the preicteric phase. Anorexia, nausea and vomiting, and dull right upper quadrant pain may be reported as the preicteric phase develops, typically lasting for about 3–10 days. The icteric phase of hepatitis is indicated by the appearance of varying degrees of jaundice, dark urine, and light, clay-colored stools. The icteric phase lasts from 1–3 weeks. Approximately 40% of patients with jaundice experience pruritus (Mandell et al. 1990). Most patients report some subjective improvement in symptoms once the icteric phase begins, with appetite returning gradually and nausea and vomiting subsiding. Weight loss and liver and spleen enlargement may also be demonstrated during the icteric phase. Variability in reported and observed symptoms is one of the most characteristic features of acute hepatitis.

Diagnostic Tests   In addition to the signs and symptoms presented by the patient and observed by the caregiver, laboratory findings are characteristic and assist in making the diagnosis of acute hepatitis. The most distinctive changes are demonstrated in the dramatic elevations in the aminotransferases—aspartate aminotransferase (AST, SGOT) and alanine aminotransferase (ALT, SGPT). These values rise to over eight times normal, peaking at onset of jaundice and falling with recovery (Mandell et al. 1990). The ALT level is the specific enzyme that denotes actual liver damage. The other enzyme assays reflect biliary obstruction and/or cholestasis. Table 19–16 summarizes the laboratory studies and findings that assist in the diagnosis and management of hepatitis.

TABLE 19–11

Causes of Drug-Related Liver Injury

AGENT CLASS	AGENT	FREQUENCY OF OCCURRENCE*	TYPE OF INJURY
Analgesic	Acetaminophen	Dose-related	Hepatitis
	Aspirin	Dose-related	Hepatitis
Anesthetic	Halothane	Rare (0.01–0.1%)	Hepatitis
	Methoxyflurane	Rare	Hepatitis
Antiarthritic	Allopurinol	Rare	Granuloma/hepatitis
	Indomethacin	Very rare	Hepatitis
	Phenylbutazone	Rare	Granuloma/mixed
Antibacterial	Carbenicillin	Low†	Hepatitis
	Erythromycin estolate	Low	Cholestasis
	Nitrofurantoin	Rare	Mixed
	Oxacillin	Rare	Hepatitis
	Sulfonamides/sulfones	Rare	Hepatitis
	Tetracycline	Dose-related	Steatosis/necrosis
Antifungal	Ketoconazole	Rare	Hepatitis
Antineoplastic	Azathioprine	Rare†	Cholestasis
	6-Mercaptopurine	Common (10–35%)†	Hepatitis
	Methotrexate	Dose-related	Fibrosis
	Mithromycin	Rare†	Necrosis
Antituberculosis	Isoniazid	Low (1%)	Hepatitis
	Para-aminosalicylic acid	Low (0.1–1%)	Hepatitis
	Rifampin	Low	Hepatitis
Cardiovascular	Methyldopa	Low	Hepatitis
	Quinidine	Rare	Granuloma/hepatitis
	Thiazides	Very rare	Mixed
	Amiodarone	Low (1–3%)	Steatosis/necrosis
Endocrinologic	17-Alkylated androgens	Dose-related	Cholestasis
	Chlorprompamide	Rare	Cholestasis
	Oral contraceptives	Rare	Cholestasis
	Propylthiouracil	Rare	Hepatitis
	Tolbutamide	Very rare	Cholestasis
Neuro- and psychopharmacologic	Dantrolene	Low (1–2%)	Hepatitis
	Monoamine oxidase inhibitors	Low	Hepatitis
	Phenothiazines	Low (1–2%)	Cholestasis
	Phenytoin	Rare	Hepatitis
	Valproic acid	Low (1–2%)	Steatosis/necrosis

*The frequency of occurrence is an estimate from the literature: common ≃ > 2%, low ≃ 0.1–2%, rare <0.1%, very rare ≃ isolated case reports only.
†Dose-related to some degree.

Reprinted from Mandell G, Douglas R, Bennett J: *Principles and Practice of Infectious Diseases,* 3d ed. New York: Churchill-Livingstone, 1990.

TABLE 19–12

Hepatitis Nomenclature

	ABBREVIATION	TERM	DEFINITION/COMMENTS
Hepatitis A	HAV	Hepatitis A virus	Etiologic agent of "infectious" hepatititis; a picornavirus; single serotype.
	Anti-HAV	Antibody to HAV	Detectable at onset of symptoms; lifetime persistence.
	IgM anti-HAV	IgM class antibody to HAV	Indicates recent infection with hepatitis A; detectable for 4–6 months after infection.
Hepatitis B	HBV	Hepatitis B virus	Etiologic agent of "serum" hepatitis; also known as Dane particle.
	HBsAg	Hepatitis B surface antigen	Surface antigen(s) of HBV detectable in large quantity in serum; several subtypes identified.
	HBeAg	Hepatitis B e antigen	Soluble antigen; correlates with HBV replication, high titer HBV in serum, and infectivity of serum.
	HBcAg	Hepatitis B core antigen	No commercial test available.
	Anti-HBs	Antibody to HBsAg	Indicates past infection with and immunity to HBV, passive antibody from HBIG, or immune response from HB vaccine.
	Anti-HBe	Antibody to HBeAg	Presence in serum of HBsAg carrier indicates lower titer of HBV.
	Anti-HBc	Antibody to HBcAg	Indicates prior infection with HBV at some undefined time.
	IgM anti-HBc	IgM class antibody to HBcAg	Indicates recent infection with HBV; detectable for 4–6 months after infection.
Non-A, non-B hepatitis (including hepatitis C)	PT-NANB	Parenterally transmitted	Diagnosis by exclusion. At least two candidate viruses, one of which has been named hepatitis C virus; shares epidemiologic features with hepatitis B.
Hepatitis D	HDV	Hepatitis D virus	Etiologic agent of delta hepatitis; can cause infection only in presence of HBV.
	HDAg	Delta antigen	Detectable in early acute delta infection.
	Anti-HDV	Antibody to delta antigen	Indicates present or past infection with delta virus.
Hepatitis E	ET-NANB	Enterically transmitted	Diagnosis by exclusion. Causes large epidemics in Asia, Africa, and Mexico; fecal-oral or waterborne.

Modified from U.S. Department of Health and Human Services, Centers for Disease Control: Protection against viral hepatitis, *MMWR*, February 9, 1990; 39(RR-2):6.

Planning and Implementation of Care

Medical management of hepatitis consists of supportive care during the course of illness. No chemotherapeutic agent has proven effective, nor have corticosteroids (Grimes, Grimes and Hamelink 1991).

Activity Intolerance Related to Low Energy Level
During the acute and convalescent phases of hepatitis, patients demonstrate activity intolerance. Because of the liver's critical role in metabolism, energy storage and liberation of those stores are impaired. Nutritional deficits also contribute to activity intolerance. Nursing staff must assist the patient, other members of the health care team, and the family to honor the patient's rest requirements. Frequent periods of undisturbed rest and grouping of activities are beneficial. Severity of symptoms will determine the patterns of activity that are best tolerated by each patient.

TABLE 19–13

Viral Hepatitis Summary

	HEPATITIS A	HEPATITIS B	HEPATITIS C	HEPATITIS D	HEPATITIS E
Occurrence	Worldwide; sporadic and epidemic, with a tendency toward cyclic recurrence; outbreaks in institutions	Worldwide; endemic; highest in young adults, homosexual men, heterosexuals with multiple sex partners, parenteral drug users, and health care and public safety workers	Worldwide; accounts for 90% of posttransfusion hepatitis in the United States	Worldwide; occurs epidemically and endemically in populations at risk for HBV infection	Epidemic and sporadic cases, particularly in developing countries; highest in young adults; rare in children or elderly
Etiologic agent	Hepatitis A virus (HAV)	Hepatitis B virus (HBV) Delta agent may coinfect with HBV	Hepatitis C virus (HCV)	A viruslike particle (HDV, or the delta agent); coinfects with HBV	Viruslike particle (HEV)
Reservoir	Humans and captive primates	Humans and possibly captive primates	Humans, chimpanzees	Humans, chimpanzees	Humans, chimpanzees
Transmission	Person to person by fecal-oral route; contaminated food, water, shellfish	Direct and indirect contact with blood, saliva, and semen; sexual contact; perinatal	Percutaneous exposure to blood; person-to-person and sexual transmission have not been defined	Similar to HBV, including sexual contact	Contaminated water; person to person by fecal-oral route
Period of communicability	Latter half of incubation period to 1 wk after onset of jaundice	During incubation period and throughout clinical course of disease; carrier state may persist for years	From 1 or more wks before symptom onset, indefinitely during chronic and carrier states	Throughout acute and chronic disease	Not known; probably similar to HA
Susceptibility and resistance	Usually affects children and young adults; immunity after infection probably lasts for life; 45% of population has hepatitis A antibodies	All age groups; disease is mild in children; lifetime immunity follows infection if antibody to HBsAg develops and HBsAg is negative	All age groups; degree of immunity following infection is unknown	All persons susceptible to HB, HBV carriers; disease is severe in children	Unknown; no explanation for epidemics among young adults; pregnant women have highest fatality

Modified and reprinted from: Grimes D, Grimes R, Hamelink M: *Infectious diseases.* St. Louis: Mosby Yearbook, 1991, p. 106.

Altered Nutrition: Less than Body Requirements Related to Anorexia, Nausea, Vomiting, and Digestive Dysfunction Nutritional deficits are related to the anorexia, nausea, vomiting, and alterations in the digestive processes that accompany hepatitis. As highlighted in the previous section on hepatic dysfunction, calorie sources should be primarily carbohydrates in frequent, small feedings, supplemented with small amounts of fat sources *after* jaundice has subsided. Alcohol abstention is advised for a minimum of 6 months following acute hepatitis. Patients should be counseled to consult with their physician before ingesting any medications, since the liver's ability to detoxify drugs is impaired.

Altered Skin Integrity Related to Irritation from Bile Salts During an episode of hepatitis, hepatic cellular function is impaired. The enterohepatic circulation of bilirubin and the excretion and reabsorption of bile salts is disrupted, leading to jaundice and pruritus. Bile pigments have an affinity for the skin and mucous membranes. As bile pigments and salts build up in the blood, the skin is unable to eliminate all of them. The retained bile salts irritate cutaneous sensory nerves,

NURSING DIAGNOSES

Nursing diagnoses that may apply to the patient with hepatitis include:

- Activity intolerance
- Altered nutrition: less than body requirements
- Altered skin integrity
- High risk for infection
- High risk for fluid volume deficit
- High risk for altered health maintenance

producing itching or pruritus. Approximately 40% of hepatitis patients with jaundice report significant pruritus at the peak of the icteric phase (Mandell et al. 1990). Patients attempt to gain relief from the aggravating and relentless itching by frequent, often violent scratching, which may disrupt skin integrity. Bathing may bring some symptomatic relief; however, avoid using soaps, since they may exacerbate drying of the skin and itching. Frequent baths with clear, cool water or with nonirritating soaps, such as Aveeno oatmeal soap, may provide some relief. Apply oil-based lotion after bathing.

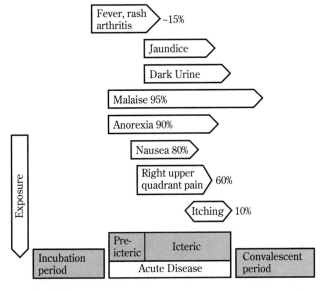

FIGURE 19–8

Timing, frequency, and major symptoms of viral hepatitis. (Reprinted from: Mandell G, Douglas R, Bennett J: *Principles and practice of infectious diseases.* New York: Churchill-Livingstone, 1990, p. 1002.)

TABLE 19–14

Hepatitis B Virus Infection in the United States

- 300,000 persons infected each year.
- Primarily young adults infected with HBV.
- Over 10,000 patients with HBV require hospitalization annually.
- An average of 250 die annually of fulminant disease following infection with HBV.
- Infectious carrier pool in U.S. is estimated at 750,000–1,000,000.
- 25% of carriers develop chronic active hepatitis, which often progresses to cirrhosis.
- Risk of developing primary liver cancer 12–300 times greater in HBV carriers.
- Annual death rate estimated at 4,000 persons from HBV-related cirrhosis and more than 800 deaths from HBV-related liver cancer.

Source: Centers for Disease Control: Protection against viral hepatitis. *MMWR* February 9, 1990; 39(RR-2):20.

Pharmacologic interventions for symptomatic relief of pruritus include use of topical anesthetics (Lanacaine) and oral medications such as cyproheptadine (Periactin), diphenhydramine (Benadryl), and hydroxyzine (Atarax). Phenothiazides and antihistamines are contraindicated for patients in advanced encephalopathic states. Use of the binding resin, cholestyramine

---

TABLE 19–15

Hepatitis B: High-Risk Conditions and Behaviors

Hepatitis B is found in all body fluids and is transmitted through blood and body-fluid contact. High-risk behaviors include the following:

- Contact with contaminated needles (intravenous drug users, accidental needle and sharps injuries by health care providers)
- Tattooing, piercing, acupuncture, dental and medical invasive procedures where properly cleaned instruments are not used
- Body fluids in contact with infected nail files, razor blades, eating utensils, and toothbrushes (HBV can live in saliva)
- Unsafe sex practices—multiple sexual partners
- Unprotected sexual activities with contact and/or exchange of bodily fluids
- Transfusions with blood or blood products infected with Hepatitis B (now rare due to routine screening of blood for HBsAg and current donor selection procedures)

From Colbruno, Michael. Hepatitis A & B. . . HIV news in S.F. Sentinel 2/6/92 and Grimes, Grimes, Hamelink *Infectious Diseases.*

TABLE 19–16

Laboratory Studies and Findings in Acute Hepatitis

DIAGNOSTIC TEST	FINDINGS
Serum enzymes	
Aspartate aminotransferase (AST, SGOT) and alanine aminotransferase (ALT, SGPT)	At least eight times normal during clinical disease; indicators of liver damage; peak at onset of jaundice and fall during recovery; may be 20–50 times normal for hepatitis B and 10–20 times normal for non-A, non-B hepatitis, persisting at 2–5 times normal for months
Alkaline phosphatase	1 to 3 times normal
Lactic dehydrogenase (LDH)	1 to 3 times normal
Creatine phosphokinase (CPK)	Normal
Serum bilirubin	Elevated: measures extent of liver dysfunction; ratio of direct to indirect fraction—1:1
Prothrombin time	Normal; elevated only in severe fulminating hepatitis
Venereal disease research laboratory test (VDRL)	False positive
Hepatitis A	
Stool specimen: immune electron microscopy, radioimmunoassay, or enzyme immunoassay	Positive for HAV 2–4 wks after exposure, remains until onset of clinical disease, then is negative
	HAV may be absent from stool by time patient is hospitalized
Serology: radioimmunoassay (RIA) or ELISA test	Fourfold rise in anti-HAV antibodies between early disease and convalescence
	Identification of IgM antibodies during early disease indicates present infection; peaks at 3 months and then drops
	IgG peaks after clinical disease and persists for life; high levels indicate past infection and present immunity
Hepatitis B	
Serum antigen tests: radioimmunoassay, enzyme immunoassay	HBeAg and HBsAg in serum 1–2 wks after exposure and 2–7 wks before onset of clinical disease; peaks and begins to drop during clinical disease
	HBsAg remains in serum of chronic carriers for life; positive tests indicate present infection or carrier state
	Positive test in carrier with disease symptoms may misdiagnose infection with HAV or NANB
Serum antibody tests: radioimmunoassay	Anti-HBe increases during clinical disease and peaks during convalescence; anti-HBe begins rising during convalescence; both persist and gradually decrease over time; anti-HBs rises rapidly during late convalescence and persists
	Carriers are always HBeAg-positive and/or HBsAg-positive and anti-HBs-negative
	For screening purposes: anti-HBs >10 RIA sample ratio units indicates immunity
Non-A, non-B hepatitis	
If above tests are negative in patient with clinical symptoms of viral hepatitis, non-A, non-B is suspected	
Hepatitis C	
One serologic test for parenterally transmitted hepatitis C is recently available	

Reprinted from: Grimes D, Grimes R, Hamelink M: *Infectious diseases.* St. Louis: Mosby Yearbook, 1991, p. 109.

(Questran), may be helpful to bind the bile salts for excretion in the stool rather than via the skin. The drug, given in powdered form at a dose of 12–16 g/day, should be mixed in milk or juice and swallowed quickly, as it has a gritty consistency and a nitrogenous odor.

Impaired skin integrity may also result from nutritional deficits. Malnutrition and vitamin and mineral deficiencies place patients at increased risk for skin breakdown and significantly delay wound repair.

Liver failure also impairs the synthesis of clotting factors. A prolonged prothrombin time increases the risk of skin bruising and breakdown as well. Indicators of bleeding tendencies include purpura on forearms, axilla, and other skin surfaces, bleeding gums following oral hygiene, and bruising following injections and/or phlebotomy, even when small-gauge needles are used.

Monitor skin condition and integrity closely (every 8–12 hours). Alter patient position every 2 hours during periods of immobility and decreased levels of consciousness. Employ pressure relief devices *before* skin breakdown occurs. Provide nutritional supplements based on need as identified by initial and ongoing assessments.

High Risk for Infection Related to Communicability of Virus   Patients infected with the hepatitis virus may infect others and should be educated about transmission routes and high-risk behaviors (refer back to Table 19-15 for specific information).

The Occupational Safety and Health Administration requires health care workers to practice universal precautions to protect themselves from blood-borne infections. Universal precautions apply to all patients to prevent the spread of hepatitis and other infectious diseases. Wear gloves when you anticipate direct contact with moist body substances (blood, urine, pus, feces, saliva, or drainage of any kind). Wash hands and other skin surfaces immediately and thoroughly if contaminated with body substances, and immediately after gloves are removed. Wear an impervious gown when you anticipate soilage of clothing with any body substances. Wear a mask and protective eyewear when you anticipate splashing or aerosolization of body substances into your mouth, nose, or eyes during the rendering of critical-care services. These universal precautions provide protection from the hepatitis viruses.

High Risk for Fluid Volume Deficit Related to Nausea, Vomiting, and Diarrhea   The risk of volume depletion exists because of the episodic nausea, vomiting, and diarrhea experienced by patients infected with hepatitis. Hydration should be maintained by frequent, small volumes of nutritious fluids around the clock, with intravenous supplementation whenever oral intake is inadequate to maintain hydration.

High Risk of Altered Health Maintenance Related to Knowledge Deficit   Patients and families will require simple but thorough information about the pathophysiology of hepatitis, transmission risks, prevention of spread, and potential chronicity. Nurses must assess and reinforce the patient and family's understanding of the importance of follow-up liver function tests, maintenance of dietary regimen, and avoidance of all drugs and alcohol. Hepatitis B carriers must be educated that their blood and secretions are infectious and that they should not donate blood. Close contacts should be evaluated for hepatitis B vaccine.

The following guidelines to prophylaxis are taken from Mandell et al. (1990).

Acute Hepatitis A   All family members and close personal contacts of patients with acute hepatitis A should be advised to receive immune serum globulin (ISG) as soon as possible following exposure. The immune globulin may be given up to 4 weeks after exposure but is most effective if given within 7–14 days.

Acute Hepatitis B   Prophylaxis is appropriate only for persons with sexual or blood-borne contact with patients with hepatitis B. The most common prophylactic recommendation is administration of hepatitis B immune globulin (HBIG) as soon as possible following exposure and repeated one month later. Postexposure immunization with hepatitis B vaccine may attenuate or even prevent a clinical course of hepatitis B. Most often recommended following exposure to hepatitis B is an injection of HBIG and hepatitis B vaccine, followed by subsequent injection of the vaccine at 1 and 6 months following exposure. Table 19–17 summarizes the Centers for Disease Control's recommendations for Hepatitis B prophylaxis following percutaneous or permucosal exposure. These recommendations are a model for all parenterally transmitted forms.

Acute Hepatitis C and D   Recommendations for hepatitis C and D are the same as for hepatitis B.

Acute Hepatitis Non-A, Non-B   There is no current proven efficacy in any mode of prevention of non-A,

TABLE 19–17

Recommendations for Hepatitis B Prophylaxis Following Percutaneous or Permucosal Exposure

	TREATMENT WHEN SOURCE IS FOUND TO BE:		
Exposed person	HBsAg-positive	HBsAg-negative	Source not tested or unknown
Unvaccinated	HBIG × 1* and initiate HB vaccine[†]	Initiate HB vaccine[†]	Initiate HB vaccine[†]
Previously vaccinated Known responder	Test exposed for anti-HBs 1. If adequate,[§] no treatment	No treatment	No treatment
	2. If inadequate, HB vaccine booster dose		
Known nonresponder	HBIG × 2 or HBIG × 1 plus 1 dose HB vaccine	No treatment	If known high-risk source, may treat as if source were HBsAg-positive
Response unknown	Test exposed for anti-HBs 1. If inadequate,[§] HBIG × 1 plus HB vaccine booster dose	No treatment	Test exposed for anti-HBs 1. If inadequate,[§] HB vaccine booster dose
	2. If adequate, no treatment		2. If adequate, no treatment

*HBIG dose 0.06 ml/kg IM.
[†]HB vaccine dose
[§]Adequate anti-HBs is ≥ sample ratio units by RIA or positive by EIA.

Reprinted from U.S. Department of Health and Human Services, Centers for Disease Control: Protection against viral hepatitis. *MMWR* February 9, 1990; 39 (RR-2): 20.

non-B hepatitis. Regular sexual contacts with patients with non-A, non-B hepatitis are recommended to receive immune serum globulin (ISG) following exposure, since it may have some effect in attenuating the course of the disease.

Because of the delay in presentation of symptoms, and therefore diagnosis, of acute hepatitis, standard recommended procedure includes injection of ISG immediately, with vaccination programs for sexual contacts or blood exposures if serology proves type B or delta hepatitis.

Outcome Criteria

Evaluate the patient's progress according to the following criteria:

- Alert and oriented
- No fever, headache, anorexia, nausea or vomiting
- No dark urine, clay-colored stools or jaundice
- Liver function tests within normal limits
- Ability to participate in usual physical activities

- Nutritional status adequate to maintain stable weight and skin integrity
- Fluid volume status adequate to maintain effective hemodynamics
- No signs or symptoms of infection
- Ability to verbalize knowledge of communicability of hepatitis virus, including modes of transmission and high risk behaviors

Liver Transplantation

When hepatitis or other etiologic agents lead to fulminant hepatic failure, the most promising therapy is liver transplantation. With the refinement of immunosuppressive agents such as cyclosporin A, liver transplantation is now an accepted approach to the management of severe hepatic failure. Approximately 1,200–1,500 liver transplants are done annually in the United States in over 50 medical centers. The 2-year survival rates range from 60–90% (Mandell et al. 1990). As with all transplantation interventions, access to viable organs remains the greatest challenge to transplant programs.

NOURISHMENT OF THE CRITICALLY ILL

Nutritional Assessment

As the key provider of care to the critically ill patient, it is essential that you be aware of common risk factors for and signs and symptoms of nutritional deficit so that you can promptly alert the appropriate member of the critical-care team. In most cases, a registered dietitian is available to thoroughly assess a patient's nutritional status.

The nutritional assessment can be divided conveniently into three major parts: diet history, physical examination, and laboratory data. A suggested screening assessment format is shown in Table 19–18.

History

Patterns of Eating and Elimination Include in your assessment the person's usual eating and elimination patterns. A knowledge of preferred foods, portion sizes, and meal frequency can be quite helpful in encouraging food intake in the anorexic patient. An awareness of normal bowel elimination patterns is essential in preventing constipation, fecal impaction, or unnecessary use of laxatives, enemas, or suppositories.

Conditions That Limit Nutrient Intake or Absorption Patients may become malnourished through two general mechanisms: limited nutrient intake or absorption, and increased nutrient demand. Be alert for conditions that limit the patient's intake and absorption of nutrients.

High-risk conditions for malnourishment include the following (Weinsier, Heimburger and Butterworth 1989):

- Pre-existing depletion
  - Alcoholism
  - Gross underweight
  - Gross overweight
  - Recent weight loss of 10% or more of usual body weight
- No oral intake for more than 5 days on simple IV solutions
- Drugs with catabolic or antinutrient properties: steroids, immunosuppressants, antitumor agents
- Prolonged nutrient losses: renal dialysis, draining abscesses or wounds, fistulas or short-gut syndromes, malabsorption syndromes

Conditions That Increase Needs Injury or stress can increase resting metabolic expenditure significantly. The Harris-Benedict equation and multiples by Long et al. (1979) provide one way of estimating caloric needs. However, the best means of estimating caloric needs in critically ill patients is measurement of the resting energy expenditure (REE), multiplied by an

TABLE 19–18

Nutritional Assessment

1. History
   Eating and elimination patterns _____

   Conditions limiting nutrient intake _____

   Conditions increasing needs _____

2. Physical examination
   General appearance _____
   Height _____
   Weight: Current _____ Usual _____ Ideal _____ Loss _____
3. Laboratory tests _____

activity factor (Van Way 1991; Schlichtig and Ayres 1988). Please see the nearby box, Indirect Calorimetry, for more information about this technique. Although 2,000–3,000 calories will meet daily maintenance needs for most hospitalized adults, certain patients—such as those with acute head injury or burns—may require up to 4,000 kcal/day. Protein intake for an average, healthy adult is 0.8 g/kg body weight per day based on the Recommended Dietary Allowances (1989).

Numerous conditions can increase protein/caloric needs. High-risk patients include those with the following conditions:

- Massive burns
- Severe infection
- Extensive trauma
- Prolonged fever

The most dramatic demand occurs in major burns, where requirements can increase up to four to six times normal.

Physical Examination

Physical examination can provide important indicators of malnourishment. The usual parameters evaluated by the nurse in a screening examination are general appearance, height, and weight.

General Appearance Many signs of nutritional deficiency are apparent on assessment of the general appearance of the patient. Among the signs of possible nutritional deficiencies are the following:

- Thin, frail appearance
- Hair loss
- Scaly skin
- Stomatitis

The most important anthropometric parameter evaluated by the nurse is weight. Ideally, when evaluating weight, compare the current and usual weights to the ideal weight for the patient's height, using standardized height/weight tables. Also compare present weight to usual weight, noting particularly the approximate change in weight and the time period in which it has occurred. Finally, compare the amount and rapidity of recent weight loss with values indicating protein-calorie malnourishment: 2% weight loss in the last week, 5% in last month, or 10% in last 6 months (Williams 1986). Weight trends may be hard to assess in patients with unstable volume status.

Another useful measure of nutritional deficiency is a recent absolute weight loss of 10 or more pounds. Although crude, this measure is statistically meaningful: Seltzer (1982) found that a recent loss of more than 10 pounds correlated with increased mortality. This measure has the advantage of immediate availability without need to resort to mathematical calculation or reference tables. It can alert you to the increased risk of mortality and the need for prompt consultation with a nutrition expert.

Protein stores can be clustered in two categories: muscle protein and visceral protein (Keithley 1983). In the critically ill patient, muscle protein is assessed through anthropometric measures such as height, weight, and muscle measurements (for example, mid-upper-arm muscle circumference) (Keithley 1983; Schlichtig and Ayres 1988). Anthropometrics may be difficult to evaluate when the patient has edema or cannot sit.

Laboratory Data

Among laboratory findings suggesting malnutrition are decreased hemoglobin and hematocrit levels. Measurement of serum albumin, prealbumin, total lymphocyte count, transferrin, and total iron-binding capacity are important because they reflect the status of visceral protein—primarily of the liver and immune tissues (Schlichtig and Ayres 1988). However, in critically ill patients lab values such as serum albumin may be low for nonnutritional reasons (e.g., liver disease or dilutional factors).

Low serum albumin (less than 2.5 g/dl) may affect the critically ill patient's tolerance of enteral feedings (Brinson et al. 1987). Providing albumin is postulated to enhance feeding tolerance by decreasing bowel wall edema (Moss 1982).

In the critically ill patient who becomes stressed or septic and/or requires ventilatory support, the key assessment factors are weight, sodium, potassium, phosphorus, magnesium, and nitrogen balance. In the nutritionally depleted patient, potassium and phosphorus ions move out of the cells to maintain normal serum levels. With the provision of glucose, which stimulates endogenous insulin release, these ions are shifted back into the cells, producing symptoms related to hypokalemia and hypophosphatemia. Hypophosphatemia has a significant effect on respiratory functioning, and the patient with compromised respiratory function may require ventilatory support.

Nitrogen balance is one of the most objective measurements for monitoring adequacy of nutritional therapy in the critically ill patient (Wilmore 1980). The

ADVANCES IN CRITICAL-CARE TECHNOLOGY

INDIRECT CALORIMETRY

"Is this patient getting enough nutrition?" "What's the calorie goal?"

Do these questions sound familiar? They are commonly asked by physicians and nurses in the critical-care setting when their patients are on specialized nutritional support.

What is the best way to determine calorie requirements? Although formulas such as the Long formula (see Table 19-20) have been used to estimate needs, studies suggest that these methods may not always be valid for hospitalized patients. Results may lead to under- or overfeeding of the patient, which may lead to complications such as malnutrition (in the case of underfeeding) or hepatic steatosis, increased CO_2 production, and fluid overload when patients are overfed, especially with TPN.

The Technology Indirect calorimetry represents the state of the art in terms of measuring energy expenditure in the critically ill. The development of portable metabolic carts which measure gas exchange has moved this technique from the research setting to the bedside. These carts contain a gas analyzer, connected to a tube into which the patient breathes, and a computer which uses the gas analysis data to calculate the person's energy expenditure.

How does indirect calorimetry measure energy expenditure? Total daily energy expenditure (daily calorie requirement) is the sum of the basal metabolic rate (BMR), specific dynamic action (SDA), and the energy used during activity. *Note:* SDA represents the incremental increase in energy expenditure associated with eating.

Components of Total Energy Expenditure:

Total kcals/day =
$$BMR + SDA + Activity$$

The source of the energy (kcals) expended is a combination of food and/or stored body fuel which combines with oxygen to produce carbon dioxide, water and energy. (The following equation shows how one body fuel source, glucose, is oxidized in this manner.)

Oxidation of Glucose to Produce Energy:

$$C_6H_{12}O_6 + 6\,O_2 \rightarrow 6\,CO_2 + 6\,H_2O + 678\,\text{Calories}$$

Indirect calorimetry measures the volume of O_2 consumed (VO_2) and the amount of CO_2 expired (VCO_2).

The data obtained by the metabolic cart measurement (VO_2 and VCO_2) are plugged into the cart's computer, which then calculates the individual's energy expenditure using a formula similar to the following one. Urinary nitrogen results may also be used, if available, but are not strictly necessary.

Weir formula for Calculating Energy Expenditure:

Calories = [3.941 (VO_2) + 1.106 (VCO_2)] 1.44 − 2.17 (UN)*

*UN = urinary nitrogen

Patient Care Considerations During an indirect calorimetry study, the patient is instructed to lie quietly so that activity is not a factor being measured. Thus, the study usually measures two of the three components of energy expenditure. (The two components are BMR and SDA, also known as resting energy expenditure, REE). If the patient is relatively inactive (e.g., a sedated or comatose ICU patient), the activity component may be quite low, so that resting energy expenditure is approximately the same as total energy expenditure.

---

general formula for nitrogen (N) balance is: N balance = N intake − N output. Nitrogen balance usually is calculated by the dietitian. Measurement of urinary urea nitrogen losses requires a 24-hour urine collection. The urine is kept on ice to avoid excretion of nitrogen from bacteria, thus altering the measurement. Negative nitrogen balance in patients receiving 0.8–1.5 g protein/kg/day suggests that the patient is receiving either inadequate calories or inadequate protein to spare protein and achieve an anabolic state. During severe stress and sepsis, zero nitrogen balance may be the maximal response that can be achieved (Wilmore 1980).

Malnutrition

Physiology of Starvation

In their classic article on nutrition in the critically ill, Stotts and Friesen (1982) delineated the metabolic characteristics of malnutrition. Early starvation begins within several hours of absent food intake; when the glucose from ingested food has been utilized, blood sugar decreases to 10–15% below its baseline value. This drop initiates two compensatory mechanisms: *alteration in insulin–glucagon balance* and *gluconeogenesis.*

Alteration in Insulin–Glucagon Balance When serum glucose falls, the level of circulating insulin decreases. This decrease in turn stimulates *glycolysis,* the breakdown of liver glycogen stores. Unfortunately, the glycogen stores are exhausted within a few hours, so the rise in blood glucose is only temporary. The altered insulin–glucagon balance also initiates *lipolysis,* the breakdown of fat into free fatty acids and glycerol, both of which can be used by the heart and other body parts for energy production. Finally, the insulin–glucagon change also initiates *proteolysis,* the breakdown of muscle tissue, which releases amino acids that the liver subsequently converts into glucose. Thus, proteolysis is an important energy source for glucose-dependent organs, especially the brain.

Gluconeogenesis The other compensatory mechanism initiated by a drop in serum glucose is *gluconeogenesis,* the formation of glucose from breakdown products of incomplete metabolism (lactate and pyruvate), amino acids, and glycerol. During this period of rapid catabolism, muscle mass decreases; urinary nitrogen loss accelerates; and rapid weight loss occurs, due to protein loss and an associated osmotic diuresis. This stage lasts up to 5 days if the patient ingests nutrients soon after injury (Moore and Brennan 1975) and up to 10 days if no nutrients are ingested (Saudek and Felig 1976).

Late Starvation If nutritional supplementation is not resumed, the patient enters the stage of late starvation after several days (Stotts and Friesen 1982). In this stage, the metabolic rate slows and the body's major energy source becomes fat, with the brain in particular adapting to the use of ketone bodies as its major energy source. The ketones also affect protein catabolism, so that muscle releases less of one amino acid, *alanine,* and more of another, *glutamine.* Alanine, the primary amino acid released during protein breakdown in the nonstarvation state, produces urea; thus in late starvation, when alanine release slows, urinary urea levels drop. Glutamine metabolism produces ammonia as a by-product, so urinary ammonia levels increase. Weight loss continues, but at a slower rate.

If starvation continues for several months and fat stores are exhausted, the body turns to protein as its only remaining source of energy. Protein in muscles, organs, and cells is metabolized for energy, until death ensues.

The Injured or Infected Patient It is important to realize that fuel mobilization and utilization differ in patients with injury or infection as compared to patients who merely are nutritionally depleted. The nutritionally depleted patient follows the pattern of starvation and hypometabolism described above. In contrast, the injured or infected patient develops a hypermetabolic state and greater glucose mobilization in the immediate posttrauma period (Stotts and Friesen 1982). These differences are believed to be mediated by the release of catecholamines, epinephrine, and norepinephrine, triggered by sympathetic nervous system stimulation. The metabolic response of the injured or infected patient also is affected by the stress-provoked release of pituitary hormones, particularly adrenocorticotropic hormone (ACTH). ACTH in turn stimulates the release of glucocorticoids, which promote glucose mobilization, and mineralocorticoids, which promote retention of sodium and water. The mineralocorticoid activity delays the onset of osmotic diuresis and rapid weight loss for up to 24–48 hours posttrauma.

NURSING DIAGNOSES

The nursing diagnoses appropriate for the malnourished person vary, depending on the cause and stage of starvation as well as on individual responses. Examples of single diagnoses are:

- Fatigue
- High risk for infection

A more global or general diagnosis is "altered nutrition: less than body requirements" or, more simply stated, "nutritional deficit."

Planning and Implementation of Care

Nutritional Supplementation Patients maintained solely on routine intravenous solutions receive highly inadequate nutrition. For example, a liter of 5% dextrose in water contains only approximately 170 calories of hydrated glucose. For the patient able to meet nutritional needs through *oral feeding,* ways to enhance the intake of adequate nutrients include such well-known nursing measures as small, frequent feedings, selection of foods the patient enjoys, provision of a pleasant eating environment, and social interaction during meals. Dietary supplements may be prescribed for patients whose calorie needs cannot be met with the usual oral diet. A calorie count may be ordered to evaluate whether or not the patient is meeting his or her needs.

For the patient unable to meet physiologic needs through oral intake, nutritional support via *enteral* or *parenteral* routes may be prescribed. If the patient has relatively normal GI function, *enteral feeding* is preferable.

Enteral Feeding Tube feeding is less expensive than parenteral nutrition and also provides nutrients in a more physiologic manner. More importantly, enteral feeding appears to prevent the gut atrophy and decreased mucosal digestive enzyme activity that occur with parenteral nutrition, thereby maintaining the integrity of the gut (Levine et al. 1974; Feldman et al. 1976). Enteral feeding also is hypothesized to reduce the incidence of sepsis and even multiple organ system failure by maintaining the gut barrier and thereby preventing the translocation of gut bacteria across the gut mucosa and into the systemic circulation (Rolandelli et al. 1990).

Indications Tube feeding is generally indicated for patients with functional GI tracts who are unable to consume adequate amounts of energy (kcals) and/or nutrients by mouth. More specifically, tube feeding is suggested as part of routine care for these conditions: protein-calorie malnutrition with inadequate oral intake for the previous 5 days, normal nutritional status with less than 50% of required oral intake for the previous 7–10 days, severe dysphagia, major full-thickness burn, massive small-bowel resection in combination with administration of total parenteral nutrition (TPN), or low output (<500 cc/day) enterocutaneous fistulas (ASPEN 1987). Tube feeding may also be appropriate for patients who have undergone major trauma, radiation therapy, mild chemotherapy, and liver or kidney failure.

Choosing an Appropriate Formula A nutritional consultation by a registered dietitian can be helpful in deciding which of the available formulas is the best choice in a given situation. Choosing an appropriate formula from among the more than 50 that are available for adults can be a difficult task, but the dietitian can make the decision more easily by using one of the many formula classification systems that group formulas by similar characteristics (Table 19–19).

To use the formula classification system, the clinician first asks whether the patient has a disorder causing malabsorption or maldigestion. If so, an elemental (or "pre-digested") formula is often indicated. If the patient has no absorption or digestion problems and simply needs routine tube feeding, a polymeric formula will usually be appropriate. Once the decision is made to use formulas in this group,

TABLE 19–19

Tube Feeding Formula Classification

Elemental

For patients with minimal absorptive/digestive capability; protein is in the form of amino acids and/or short peptides.

Polymeric

For routine use either short-term (nonblenderized polymeric) or long-term (blenderized polymeric); protein is in the intact form.

Disease-specific

For patients with a special need or a disease which might benefit from the *unique feature(s)* of a formula in this class; protein may be in any form, i.e., amino acids, peptides, or intact.

Modular Components

For patients who would benefit from having a "custom-made" formula or from having their formula supplemented with a nutrient or nutrients from one or more modular components.

Adapted with permission from DeBourgh G, Wapensky T, Guthrie S: Guidelines for Tube Feeding at California Pacific Medical Center-Pacific Campus, San Francisco, 1989.

other factors must also be considered, because polymeric formulas vary in many respects, for example, in the extent to which they contain lactose, fiber, and certain types of nutrients. If the patient has a specific disease state that may benefit from nutritional manipulation, a disease-specific or a specially designed formula made from modular components is probably the best choice.

Tube Placement Feeding tubes may be placed either into the stomach (e.g., nasogastric or gastrostomy) or into the small intestine (e.g., nasointestinal or jejunostomy). Gastrostomy and jejunostomy placement are usually indicated for long-term feeding. Both types of placement are contraindicated when the patient has ascites, peritonitis, severe immunosuppression, or an esophageal obstruction (Bockus 1991).

The literature suggests that small-bowel feeding may offer the patient some protection against aspiration (Metheney et al. 1986). However, a study which compared aspiration rates in patients fed via either nasogastric or nasoduodenal tubes concluded that intragastric delivery of tube feeding is equally as safe as delivery into the duodenum (Strong et al. 1992).

Once the tube is placed, an x-ray should be obtained to verify tube placement. Infusion of formula into a misplaced tube can cause serious problems, including aspiration pneumonia or hydrothorax. An x-ray is the most reliable method of checking placement. Once radiographic confirmation of correct placement is obtained, other methods are used to check tube placement. They include: 1) aspiration of recognizable gastric contents, 2) auscultation of insufflated air, 3) checking the pH of fluid aspirated by a syringe, and 4) ruling out inadvertent respiratory placement by checking for coughing, choking, or cyanosis, asking the patient to speak, and observing for bubbles when the proximal end of the tube is held underwater (Metheney 1988). All of these methods are potentially fallible. Case reports show that on occasion, fluid aspirated via the tube and assumed to be gastric contents was, in fact, fluid obtained from the respiratory tract (Metheney 1988). In addition, a study of the effectiveness of the auscultatory method in predicting tube location in acutely ill patients concluded this method was ineffective in determining the location of the tube in the GI tract (Metheney et al. 1990). According to this study, checking the pH of aspirates may be useful in verifying tube placement; however, more research is needed in this area.

Initiating Tube Feeding Feedings may be administered by either continuous drip or bolus (intermittent) schedules. The continuous drip method is recommended for critically ill patients (Schlichtig and Ayres 1988). This method is associated with less risk of gastric distention and aspiration, and fewer metabolic problems (Guenter et al. 1990).

Continuous Drip Feedings Generally patients can be given full-strength isotonic, or even mildly hypertonic (e.g., 430 mOsm/kg), polymeric formulas by continuous drip if they have relatively normal GI function (Keohane et al. 1984). Very hypertonic formulas may be diluted to half strength or started at a lower rate to help achieve tolerance. To help prevent the risk of aspiration, be sure to elevate the head of the bed (HOB) to at least 30° during the feedings.

Initiate tube feeding in critically ill patients at a low rate. Advancement schedules vary; however, tube feedings (using isotonic formula) often are started at 25 cc/hr. The rate may be advanced every 8–12 hours, as long as the feeding is tolerated, until the goal rate is reached. If dilute tube feeding is started, it is very important to avoid increasing both the rate and the strength simultaneously, since if intolerance develops, it would be impossible to determine which change caused the problem.

Checking gastric residuals is a common practice thought to help alert the nurse to the risk of aspiration. Residuals are only checked when the patient has a feeding tube in the stomach, not in the small bowel. They are usually checked every 4 hours for continuous drip feedings. A large residual may indicate gastric atony. (Clinicians vary on the definition of "large residual," i.e., 10–20% greater than or even up to twice

the hourly rate). If the residual is large the tube feeding should be stopped and the residual refed. The residual should be rechecked in one hour. If it is still high, the physician should be notified (Bockus 1991). Sometimes the use of metaclopramide (Reglan) can be helpful in resolving the problem, as it increases gastric motility (Perkel et al. 1979).

NURSING TIP

Using Dye to Detect Tube Feeding Aspiration

Blue food coloring (1 ml dye per 500 ml formula) may be added to the formula to help detect whether aspiration has occurred. Blue is a non-physiologic color. If aspiration is suspected and suctioning produces blue secretions, it may be assumed that aspiration has occurred.

To keep the tubing patent, it is important to flush warm water (20–30 cc q 4 hr) through it. In addition, flush the tubing before and after giving medications via the tube. For example, flush the tube with 20 cc warm water prior to administering medications, then follow each medication with a 5-cc flush, then flush again with 20 cc warm water after the last medication is given (Bockus 1991). Cranberry juice should not be used as a flushing solution as it is associated with a higher incidence of obstruction of feeding tubes (Wilson and Haynes-Johnson 1987; Metheney et al. 1988).

Whenever medications are ordered by tube, liquid medications are the preferred form. If a liquid medication is not available, pills or tablets may be crushed and administered through the tube in some cases; however, this is not true for all medications, such as enteric coated capsules. The pharmacist can be helpful in providing guidance regarding how medications can best be administered to the tube-fed patient.

To minimize the risk of infection, several measures may be taken. First, hang formula for no longer than 8–12 hours (Kohn and Keithley 1989). Open formula may be kept covered in the refrigerator for 24 hours. Secondly, change the bag and delivery tubing (but not the feeding tube itself) every 24 hours (Schlichtig and Ayres 1988). Rinse the bag prior to adding new formula. Finally, the use of sterile, canned, undiluted formulas is recommended.

Complications of Tube Feeding Several types of complications can occur when patients are tube-fed. These complications may be classified as 1) mechanical, 2) gastrointestinal, or 3) metabolic. Of these types, gastrointestinal complications are the most common, and diarrhea is the major type of GI complication, especially in critically ill patients. One study found a 41% overall incidence of diarrhea related to tube feeding in critically ill patients studied over a 1-year period (Kelly et al. 1983).

Many factors have been associated with the development of diarrhea in tube-fed patients, including antibiotics, lactose intolerance, hyperosmolar formulas, bacterial contamination of the formula, low serum albumin levels, and use of medications. As with all complications related to tube feeding, investigation to determine the cause is recommended so that appropriate intervention may be identified. For more information, the reader is referred to the excellent review of complications of enteral feeding and suggested interventions by Kohn and Keithley (1989).

Total Parenteral Nutrition (TPN) Parenteral nutrition is prescribed for patients unable to meet nutritional needs through the GI system. Two routes are available: peripheral venous nutrition and central venous nutrition. *Peripheral venous nutrition* is appropriate for the patient with relatively lower caloric needs. Patients who need large amounts of calories and protein, however, usually require central venous nutrition, as the solutions used have greater caloric and protein density than do peripheral venous nutrition solutions.

The technique of *central venous nutrition* is referred to by several names, including *total parenteral nutrition* (TPN) and *hyperalimentation*. Among the patients who can benefit from this technique are those with high-output (>500 cc/day) gastrointestinal fistulas, bowel obstructions or resections, severe burns, or inflammatory bowel disorders. The nursing care of the person receiving TPN is complex. Because of the degree of nursing skill required, the remainder of this chapter is devoted to this nutritional technique.

Total parenteral nutrition (TPN) is the delivery of total nutrition into the superior vena cava by means of a solution containing hypertonic glucose, crystalline amino acids, minerals, and vitamins. Indications for TPN are the following: 1) conditions that interfere with nutrient absorption (for example, bowel obstruction, short bowel syndrome, or radiation enteritis), 2) the need for complete bowel rest (e.g., pancreatitis or chylous fistula), 3) persistent vomiting or diarrhea (e.g., GI side effects of chemotherapy or radiation or hyperemesis gravidarum) and 4) inability to tolerate tube feedings (e.g., inability to maintain safe access for enteral feedings or inability to achieve nutrient requirements in 7–10 days) (Worthington and Wagner 1989; ASPEN 1986). TPN is initiated on a physician's order.

Initiating TPN Therapy

Baseline Laboratory Values Before starting the infusion, ensure that baseline laboratory values are obtained. Because of the complexity of TPN therapy, numerous baseline studies should be done. Authors differ somewhat on which studies to do and how frequently. The following studies usually are obtained before TPN is instituted: serum electrolytes, serum osmolality, fasting blood sugar, complete blood count, blood urea nitrogen, and serum albumin and lipid levels. In addition, weigh the patient and obtain a chest x-ray, electrocardiogram (ECG), and urinalysis.

Adequate Hydration Ensure adequate hydration. If the above studies or clinical evaluation indicate suboptimal hydration, consult with the physician and administer whatever fluids he or she recommends. Adequate hydration prior to the institution of TPN is essential. Not only is it technically difficult to insert the catheter in a constricted vein, but inadequate hydration also increases the risk of hyperglycemic hyperosmolar nonketotic coma.

Catheter Insertion The catheter is inserted under local anesthesia, usually into the subclavian vein. This vein has a greater blood volume than other veins, so the hypertonic TPN solution is diluted more rapidly. This approach also allows the patient to move the neck and arms freely after insertion and simplifies the application of an occlusive dressing. The internal jugular vein, which may be used instead, is less desirable because it has a lesser volume, use of this site limits neck movement, and nearby hair makes it difficult to apply an occlusive dressing. The brachial and axillary veins are avoided. Their smallness limits blood flow between the catheter and the vessel wall. The concentrated solution and limited arm movement that occur with use of brachial or axillary veins both predispose to phlebitis.

Potential Complications The numerous potential complications of catheter insertion include injury to the vein, thrombosis, pneumothorax, arterial puncture, air embolism, dysrhythmias, and cardiac tamponade. Since these are the same as with any central venous catheter, see Chapter 11 if you wish to review signs, symptoms, and treatments. To help avoid these complications, maximize venous distention immediately prior to catheter insertion by positioning the patient as follows: Place a towel roll along the spine so the shoulders drop posteriorly, turn the head to the side opposite the insertion site, and place the patient in Trendelenburg position if tolerated.

Catheter Placement The physician will use a 2-inch 14-gauge needle and a 3-ml syringe to locate the vein by passing the needle through the skin, toward the suprasternal notch, and behind and below the clavicle. Once blood is obtained, the physician will have the patient hold a breath and bear down (Valsalva maneuver) while the physician holds the needle hub, disconnects the syringe, and passes an 8-inch 16-gauge catheter its full length into the vein. When blood appears, attach the catheter hub to an isotonic intravenous solution. Tell the patient to breathe again, and flush the catheter. The physician will withdraw the needle and cover it with the needle guard to minimize the chance of shearing the catheter. The physician then will place a single suture to keep the catheter in place and apply an antiseptic ointment. Finally, the physician will paint the skin with benzoin, apply a dressing, secure a loop of the tubing over the dressing to decrease traction on the catheter, and apply an occlusive dressing.

Starting the TPN Solution Obtain a stat chest x-ray to confirm proper placement of the catheter tip. It is important to verify catheter placement by x-ray because the catheter can curl up or travel up the internal jugular vein instead of going down the innominate vein into the superior vena cava. Once catheter placement is verified, discontinue the isotonic solution and begin the TPN solution.

Nutrients Supplied via TPN Table 19–20 shows how nutrient requirements are calculated. As mentioned earlier, when protein undergoes proteolysis, tissue nitrogen is excreted. The negative nitrogen balance will continue even if exogenous nitrogen is supplied, unless adequate calories also are supplied. When both adequate calories and nitrogen are provided, the calories will be used for energy and the nitrogen for protein synthesis.

Calories Calories in IV nutrition are supplied primarily by carbohydrate and fat, although protein also can be used for energy. Although fat contains more calories per gram than carbohydrate or protein, fat emulsions cannot be used for total caloric intake because the rate of utilization of fat is limited and because the body requires the intake of some carbohydrate and amino acids as well as fat. Hypertonic glucose is used most frequently because it is inexpensive, available in several concentrations, and relatively safe.

Nitrogen Nitrogen (N) can be supplied as protein or amino acids. Although the body can use protein

supplied in plasma, whole blood, or albumin, time and energy are required to convert it to forms suitable for protein synthesis. Although protein hydrolysates used to be the main source of N, synthetic crystalline amino acids now are used exclusively because they provide N in a form more easily and completely used by the body. Most amino acid solutions contain both essential and nonessential amino acids. However, some specialized amino acid formulations developed for patients with renal disease contain only (or primarily) essential amino acids (e.g., Aminosyn RF). Other specialized amino acid formulations (containing higher proportions of branch chain amino acids than standard formulations) have been developed for use in liver disease (e.g., Hepatamine) and stressed states (e.g., Aminosyn-HBC).

Ratio of Calories to Nitrogen As mentioned previously, calories must be supplied so that the nitrogen will be used for protein synthesis. The ratio of calories to nitrogen necessary for protein synthesis is approximately 150–250 cal to 1 g N. In stressed, critically ill patients, lower calorie/nitrogen ratios (e.g., 100:1) are used. Usually, amino acids are added to a 70% stock of dextrose solution to obtain the proper calorie/nitrogen ratio. Depending on its composition, the TPN solution's osmolality will be approximately 1,200–2,000 mOsm/kg. As normal serum osmolality is about 290 mOsm/kg, these solutions are extremely hypertonic.

Electrolytes A variety of electrolytes may be added to the solution. In the absence of definitive data on daily needs for some electrolytes, their supplementation must be determined empirically. In addition, supplementation is influenced by the multiplicity of factors affecting electrolyte needs in a given patient. Furthermore, minimal and optimal amounts of electrolyte intake may differ. For these reasons, the prescribed electrolyte supplementation may vary considerably from patient to patient and institution to institution. As electrolyte compositions of the different commercial solutions also vary, the physician should specify the desired total concentration of each electrolyte per liter. The pharmacist will add to the commercial solution the amounts necessary to provide the desired concentration.

Sodium chloride usually is added for maintenance and potassium for protein synthesis. Because potassium is excreted when muscle breaks down, patients in negative nitrogen balance often have a potassium deficit. If protein is supplied without potassium, these patients will be unable to synthesize protein. Calcium often must be provided; although intestinal loss ceases with hyperalimentation, urinary loss is exaggerated by immobilization. Magnesium deficit is common in

TABLE 19–20

Calculation of Nutrient Requirements for the TPN Patient

Use the actual body weight to compute nutritional requirements. Optimal weight gain with nutritional support is 0.5–1.0 kg per week. If weight gain is the goal, this can be achieved by giving 500 kcal per day *in addition to* calculated caloric requirements.

Caloric Requirements

Consider the Harris-Benedict equation, with multiples developed by Long et al. (1979), to calculate caloric requirements:
Men: $(66 + 13.7W + 5H - 6.8A) \times AF \times IF$
Women: $(655 + 9.6W + 1.8H - 4.7A) \times AF \times IF$
where W = weight (in kg), H = height (in cm), A = age (in years), AF = activity factor, and IF = injury factor.

ACTIVITY FACTOR:		INJURY FACTOR:	
Confined to bed	1.2	Minor operation	1.20
Out of bed	1.3	Skeletal trauma	1.35
		Major sepsis	1.60
		Severe thermal burn	2.10

Protein Requirements

The range is 0.8–2.0 g/kg body weight:

Normal	0.8–1.0 g/kg body weight
Moderate stress	1.0–1.5
Severe stress	1.5–2.0

Consider using 0.8 g protein/kg initially until nitrogen balance data can be obtained.

Fat Requirements

Approximately 30% of the nonprotein calories should be given via a fat emulsion. A minimum of 4% of nonprotein calories must be given as fat to meet linoleic acid requirements and to avoid essential fatty acid deficiency. Patients with increased CO_2 production may require 50% of their calories from the fat emulsion.

Trace Elements and Vitamin Requirements

Trace elements and vitamins are added to TPN solution in accordance with current AMA group guidelines.

Trace Elements

Daily recommended intakes (established by the Nutrition Advisory Group AMA Dept. of Foods and Nutrition) are:

Zinc	2.5–4.0 mg	Manganese	0.15–0.8 mg
Copper	0.5–1.5 mg	Chromium	10–15 mcg

This requirement can be met by adding an appropriate amount of the trace element formula (TEF) to the patient's TPN per day.

Vitamins

Daily recommended intakes (established by the Nutrition Advisory Group AMA Dept. of Foods and Nutrition) are:

Ascorbic acid	100 mg	Pyridoxine	4 mg
Vitamin A	3300 IU	Niacinamide	40 mg
Vitamin D	200 IU	Dexpanthenol	15 mg
Thiamine	3 mg	Vitamin E	10 IU
Riboflavin	3.6 mg	Biotin	60 mcg
Folic acid	400 mcg	Vitamin B_{12}	5 mcg

These requirements can be met by adding 10 ml *per day* of MVI-12® or its equivalent to the patient's TPN. Trace element formula and vitamins are ordered on a daily basis. The pharmacy staff should place the appropriate amount in each bottle to accumulate the daily dose.

starvation. Although magnesium is necessary for optimal functioning of enzyme systems, the amount that should be supplied has not been established definitely. Iron is supplied only if the patient is deficient; if so, it must be given intramuscularly rather than in the TPN solution.

Vitamins and Trace Elements Detailed discussion on the need for vitamins and trace elements (such as zinc and cobalt) is beyond the scope of this text. The patient usually is given 10 ml of fat- and water-soluble vitamins daily. Trace elements must be added to the solution. For a more complete discussion, consult the Review Article (1980), cited in the reference list.

Prospects for the Future Although conventional parenteral nutrition is based on the delivery of hypercaloric solutions, investigators have called into question the usefulness of delivering more calories than the patient can use (Robin et al. 1981). Injured and infected patients have a different pattern of fuel mobilization and utilization than do patients who are just nutritionally depleted. Similarly, the former also have a different pattern of response to substrate administration (Elwyn 1980; Kinney and Felig 1979). Excessive glucose administration (when all nonprotein calories are provided as glucose) may result in increased CO_2 production and increased O_2 consumption (Robin et al. 1981). The increased CO_2 production and O_2 consumption produce significant increases in ventilation, and may precipitate respiratory distress in the patient with poor pulmonary function (Askanazi et al. 1980). Burke et al. (1979) demonstrated that, in severely burned patients, there are maximal infusion rates beyond which no manifestations of additional increases in glucose oxidation or protein synthesis are observed. Moreover, they noted large fat deposits in the livers of their patients who had received TPN for 3 weeks or more preceding death from massive burns. They therefore suggested there may be a limit to the "physiological cost-effectiveness" of hypercaloric solutions. Robin et al. (1981) recommended that each patient requiring TPN be treated with an individualized approach that limits energy intake to approximate energy expenditure and utilizes fat as a significant energy source. Optimal nutritional support for the critically ill patient requires further research to define increased caloric needs and further assessment of optimal amino acid profiles and types of fat emulsion, particularly in stressed or septic patients.

Importance of Physical Activity Promote optimal utilization of the calories and protein TPN provides by maintaining the patient's physical activity. If the patient can tolerate ambulation, encourage it. If not, provide activity through active or passive exercises. Exercise minimizes protein breakdown, helps to ensure that weight is gained as lean muscle rather than adipose tissue, and lifts your patient's spirit as he or she sees bodily strength increasing. Explain the exercise's importance, and together set short-term goals by which the patient can judge improvement.

Potential Complications Prevent and/or respond promptly to complications of TPN. As you would expect with so complex a therapy, the potential problems are numerous. They include allergy, infection, hyper- or hypoglycemia, fluid overload, protein overload, bleeding, metabolic acidosis, fatty acid deficiency, and electrolyte imbalances.

Allergy Observe for allergic reactions to IV lipid solutions. An initial "test dose" of IV lipid (at 1 ml per minute for 15–30 minutes) is usually infused. If adverse effects such as headache, dyspnea, flushing, sweating, skin rash, temperature elevations of 3–4°C, chills, nausea and vomiting, back pain, muscle aches, dizziness, diplopia, or blurred vision occur, the infusion should be stopped. Fat emulsions contain egg phosphatides and may contain either soybean or safflower oil; therefore, patients should be asked if they are allergic to these foods prior to administration of IV lipid.

Infection Guard against infection by following these guidelines:

1. Prevent infection through meticulous aseptic technique.

2. Use as few connections in the line as possible. Avoid "piggybacks" and stopcocks, and tape all connections securely. (These measures will prevent both infection and air embolism.) Some physicians advocate the use of filters in the line. Others avoid them, because they may clog, or release a bolus of bacteria if they break; furthermore, they may stop bacteria but not their toxins.

3. Refrigerate solutions until 30 minutes before use, when you may allow them to warm naturally. Solutions usually are ordered daily from the pharmacy, which prepares them under a laminar-flow hood.

4. Do not hang solution that appears cloudy or has a precipitate. Do not save a discontinued bottle and rehang it later.

5. Minimize fibrin deposition along the catheter. Fibrin deposition is believed to provide a focus for infection and thrombosis. Do not administer

blood through the line, nor withdraw blood samples (unless checking for contamination of the catheter itself). Also, avoid using the line to measure central venous pressure.

6. Avoid administering drugs routinely via the line, as they may precipitate. (Most physicians do not add antibiotics routinely to the TPN solution, either. Routine use can promote superinfections, and some antibiotics may interact with chemicals in the fluid.)

7. Change the bottle, intravenous tubing, and filter (if you are using one) at least every 12–24 hours, following unit protocol. Place the patient flat and have the patient perform a Valsalva maneuver while you change the tubing to avoid a possible air embolism.

8. Change the dressing when soiled, and according to protocol (typically every other day). As you do, examine the skin for erythema and any drainage. Examine the catheter to be sure it still is sutured in place, and make sure the needle guard still is closed. (You may find it helpful to grasp the catheter *hub* with a hemostat while you change the extension tubing. Do *not* clamp the catheter itself; although you may prevent an air embolus, you may produce a catheter embolus!) Redress the site occlusively. Chart the procedure and your observations, and alert the physician to any troublesome signs, such as a loose suture.

9. Observe the patient closely for indications of bacterial or fungal infection. The most common bacterial contaminant is *Streptococcus.* The catheter also may become contaminated with *Candida.* Because *Candida* sepsis may be asymptomatic in its early stages, routine weekly blood and urine cultures for both bacteria and fungi should be performed. Redness, swelling, heat, or tenderness at the insertion site or along the catheter course; fever; or chills are signs of infection. If you suspect infection, alert the physician. Change and culture the bottle, tubing, and filter. Blood cultures will be drawn from both the catheter and a peripheral vein to identify possible foci of infection other than the catheter itself, such as a urinary tract, respiratory, or wound infection. If one is identified, the physician will treat that infection and leave the catheter in place. If no other source can be located, the doctor will remove and culture the catheter. TPN may be resumed at another site. Note that only the development of a new infection warrants catheter removal. The pa-

tient with an established infection may be started on TPN precisely to reverse the nutritional depletion that contributed to that infection.

Hyperglycemia Be alert for hyperglycemia. The development of hyperglycemia is undesirable for a number of reasons. Excess glucose increases serum osmolality, causing fluid to shift out of the cells. It also causes an osmotic diuresis, resulting in both extracellular and intracellular dehydration. The increased volume of plasma dilutes the serum sodium—producing hyponatremia—and dilutes the serum bicarbonate—creating a hypertonic metabolic acidosis.

Hyperglycemia can result from an excessive total load of glucose, too rapid an infusion rate, or diminished glucose tolerance. Prevent hyperglycemia by incorporating these measures into the patient's care:

1. During the initial stabilization period (4–7 days), increase the TPN rate gradually according to the physician's orders and the patient's tolerance. TPN increases the glucose, protein, osmolar, and volume loads on the patient. Most patients can increase their ability to cope with these loads if they are introduced slowly. One example of administration follows. On the first day, the physician may order administration of 1,000 ml of TPN solution over 24 hours and the rest of the patient's fluid requirements as routine intravenous fluid. Each day, one liter of TPN solution may be added and one liter of other fluid deleted, until the total desired TPN solution is being administered, typically 1–2 liters a day.

2. Maintain the flow rate ordered by the physician. Most physicians specify that a constant flow rate be maintained over 24 hours to prevent deleterious swings in blood glucose and serum osmolality. Use an infusion pump to maintain the flow of solution within 10% of the rate ordered by the physician. Check the accuracy of the flow rate periodically. Time-tape the bottle to indicate how much solution should be infused over a given period. This will provide a double check on pump accuracy. Do *not* increase flow rate to "catch up" an infusion that is behind schedule.

3. Monitor blood glucose levels with indicator reagent strips (BG chemstix) every 6 hours, as ordered. Anticipate that the blood glucose will rise. It should stabilize under 200 mg%.

4. Check urine glucose and ketones every 6 hours, using a freshly voided specimen, to

detect renal glucose spillage and ketone production. Urinary glucose and ketones should be negative. Due to variations in renal threshold for glucose, urine glucose determinations do not indicate accurately blood glucose levels.

5. Expect that diabetic patients or those with relative pancreatic insufficiency will need exogenous insulin. Administer supplementary insulin as ordered.

6. Exogenous insulin also often is needed due to the critically ill patient's altered glucose metabolism. Anticipate that patients who are on high-dose steroids or undergoing increased stress (such as during surgery, the early postoperative period, or sepsis) will have a relative glucose intolerance. These patients will need insulin coverage when TPN is used.

7. Anticipate that patients with cardiac, renal, or hepatic disease will require adjustments in TPN volume or composition.

8. Monitor the patient for signs of hyperglycemia. Signs of hyperglycemia are: an increased urinary output, a urinary glucose level of 3–4$^+$, and/or a ketone level greater than small; confusion, headache, lethargy, convulsions, or coma; nausea, vomiting, or diarrhea; dehydration; and a blood glucose level over 200 mg%. Notify the physician, who will order the infusion rate slowed or supplemental insulin administered.

9. If a decreased level of consciousness is accompanied by profound dehydration, a blood sugar over 600 mg%, and a serum osmolality over 350 mOsm/L, the patient has developed a *hyperglycemic hyperosmolar nonketotic state* (HHNK). This disorder is discussed in Chapter 17.

Hypoglycemia   Hypoglycemia also is a constant threat to patients on TPN. Signs and symptoms of hypoglycemia include profuse sweating, palpitations, convulsions, and/or coma, accompanied by a normal urine volume and negative urinary glucose level. Hypoglycemia can occur as a rebound phenomenon if the TPN solution is stopped suddenly, especially in patients receiving exogenous insulin. In this situation, the pancreas continues to produce high levels of insulin, causing blood glucose to drop precipitously. Prevent rebound hypoglycemia with these measures:

1. Use an infusion pump to maintain a constant flow rate.

2. Prevent kinking, clotting, and displacement of the catheter. If the flow slows, check for these causes. If they are absent, try changing the filter, if one is in use.

3. Avoid giving blood or other solutions through the catheter, which will interrupt the flow of TPN solution.

4. If the patient is receiving insulin, give it intravenously rather than subcutaneously. By doing so, any accidental interruption in solution flow will be accompanied by an appropriate interruption in insulin administration.

5. If the patient is receiving exogenous insulin, keep urine glucose at 0, to prevent chronic water loss. Monitor BG chemstix readings to prevent hypoglycemia.

6. If you are unable to use an infusion pump and there is an unplanned interruption in administration, restart the infusion promptly; doing so may prevent a hypoglycemic reaction.

7. If abrupt changes in flow occur, notify the physician promptly so he or she can order appropriate changes in therapy.

8. When the physician orders the solution discontinued, taper it off gradually. Guidelines are presented later in this chapter.

Fluid Overload   Observe for fluid overload. Weigh the patient daily under the same conditions, and maintain strict intake and output records. Also consult with the physician about the expected rate of weight gain from tissue synthesis; the goal usually ranges up to 2 pounds per week. More may be desirable, especially if the patient's hydration is very poor. A gain in excess of the amount for a specific patient may represent fluid overload rather than increased lean body mass. Patients without cardiac, renal, or hepatic disease usually can tolerate 3,000–4,000 ml of fluid per day.

Protein Overload   Watch for signs of protein overload. Monitor the BUN and creatinine daily until stable and then weekly. If signs of prerenal azotemia appear, the physician may change from the previous TPN solution to solutions containing a lower amount of amino acids and/or a higher proportion of essential amino acids to lower the protein load on the kidneys.

Bleeding   Be alert for bleeding. Monitor the complete blood count (CBC), prothrombin time, and platelet count weekly. Malnourished patients often have anemia and/or hypoproteinemia. Alert the physician if you suspect either condition, as administration of whole blood, plasma, or albumin may be needed. Patients on TPN as their sole source of nutrition will generally require weekly vitamin K administration to maintain a normal prothrombin time, since this vitamin is not found in standard adult vitamin formulations.

Metabolic Acidosis Be alert for the signs of metabolic acidosis. They include restlessness, disorientation, coma, hyperventilation, hyperkalemia, arterial pH below 7.35, and serum bicarbonate below 23 mEq/L. Possible causes of metabolic acidosis in TPN patients include hyperglycemia, excessive additions of sodium chloride or potassium chloride to TPN solutions, or administration of crystalline amino acid solutions that contain cationic amino acids or that are derived from chloride or hydrochloride salts. If the problem results from excessive sodium or potassium chloride administration, the physician can substitute sodium or potassium bicarbonate, acetate, or phosphate for electrolyte replacement.

Fatty Acid Deficiency Watch for signs of fatty acid deficiency. Scaly skin, skin eruptions around the nose and mouth, mouth or tongue tenderness, hair loss, poor skin turgor, poor wound healing, and decreased resistance to infections result from fatty acid deficiency. Such deficiency occurs because hypertonic dextrose provokes hyperinsulinemia, which in turn inhibits lipolysis, and because the TPN solution may not contain fatty acids. Alert the physician if you note these signs, and administer fat emulsions as ordered.

Commercially available fat emulsions contain safflower or soybean oil, egg yolk phospholipids, and glycerin in water (Gever 1981). Two to three 500-ml bottles may be administered weekly through a Y-site or piggyback into a peripheral venous line. Daily administration of smaller volumes of lipid is also common. If a filter is used in the peripheral line, the fatty acid (lipid) emulsion should be connected below it because the fat particles can be trapped in the filter. Inspect the bottle before administration to detect separation of the emulsion. Avoid shaking the bottle, because shaking can cause aggregation of fat particles and separation of the emulsion. You may give fat emulsion safely via a peripheral vein because it is isotonic. Do not add any drugs, electrolytes, or other nutrients to the bottle because you may disturb the emulsion's stability. For the first 15 minutes, give the solution at the rate of 1 ml/min while you observe for dyspnea, allergic reactions, vomiting, or chest pain. If no untoward reactions occur, you may increase the rate to the limit specified by the physician, typically 500 ml over a 6–12 hour period or even over 24 hours.

Some hospitals use "3 in 1" TPN solution in which all 3 solutions (dextrose, amino acids, and lipid) are mixed together in one bag. This eliminates the need to give IV lipid separately.

Electrolyte Imbalances Maintain electrolyte balance. Monitor serum electrolytes daily until stabilized and weekly thereafter. Watch for signs and symptoms of developing imbalances. Potential electrolyte imbalances during TPN include hypo/hypernatremia, hypokalemia, and hypophosphatemia.

Changes in weight, blood pressure, pulse volume, skin turgor, level of consciousness, and respiratory rate may indicate sodium imbalances, which are discussed in detail in Chapter 16. Hyponatremia is fairly common and may be due to true sodium loss or dilution of serum sodium by fluid shift from the intracellular to extracellular compartment. As mentioned above, sodium is added routinely to the solution to meet maintenance needs.

Hypernatremia may occur secondary to excessive osmotic diuresis. If the elevation in serum sodium is accompanied by lethargy, hyperventilation, or coma, suspect the occurrence of hyperglycemic hyperosmolar nonketotic state, mentioned earlier.

Weakness, cramps, nausea or vomiting, paresthesias, and ECG changes suggest hypokalemia, also discussed in Chapter 16. Potassium needs are increased during TPN, due to stress, osmotic diuresis, and increased protein synthesis.

Weakness, confusion, respiratory failure, paresthesias, seizures, coma, and dysarthria may be signs of hypophosphatemia. This condition can develop from the increased demand for phosphate for glycolysis and production of proteins, membrane phospholipids, deoxyribonucleic acid, and adenosine triphosphate (ATP), and from the increased need for buffering of acidic wastes produced by the accelerated metabolic rate. A diminished phosphate level can cause decreased levels of ATP and 2,3 diphosphoglycerate in red cells (Janson et al. 1983). Since these compounds bind to hemoglobin, their deficiencies are associated with a leftward shift of the oxyhemoglobin dissociation curve; that is, the red cells' affinity for oxygen is increased, so less oxygen is available to the tissues. Hypophosphatemia also may produce a decreased ATP level in leukocytes, leading to a theoretical decrease in ability to combat infection (Janson et al. 1982). To prevent these problems, the physician often will order 10–15 mEq/L of phosphate added to the TPN solution. Since supplemental phosphate can cause a drop in serum calcium, calcium must be provided also. Calcium and phosphate may be added to separate bottles, because they can precipitate when mixed together at certain concentrations.

Vitamin–Mineral Abnormalities Be alert for signs of vitamin and mineral deficiencies. For example, monitor the patient for signs and symptoms of poor wound healing, impaired immunity, and mental abnormality (Review Article 1980).

Discontinuation of TPN The physician will discontinue TPN when the condition necessitating its use is alleviated and the patient shows progress toward adequate nutrition. The rate of solution usually is tapered to avoid insulin rebound and hypoglycemia.

While returning to oral intake, the patient may have little appetite because of all the glucose being supplied intravenously. Slowing the infusion rate and providing appetizing meals, perhaps with some pleasant social interaction, will help to stimulate appetite. A cyclic TPN regimen, which condenses the TPN infusion into a shorter period of time (e.g., 12 hours), may be tried to allow the patient to eat when the infusion is off.

REFERENCES

Gastrointestinal Disorders

Bates B: *A guide to physical examination,* 4th ed. Philadelphia: Lippincott, 1987.

Benner P: *From novice to expert: Excellence and power in clinical nursing practice.* Menlo Park, CA: Addison-Wesley, 1984.

Burns S, Martin M: VP/NTG therapy in the patient with variceal bleeding. *Crit Care Nurse* (October) 1990; 10(9):42–49.

Cello J et al.: Endoscopic sclerotherapy versus portacaval shunt in patients with severe cirrhosis and acute variceal hemorrhage. *N Engl J Med* 1987; 316:11–15.

Colapinto R et al.: Creation of an intrahepatic portosystemic shunt with a Grantzig balloon catheter. *Canad Med Assoc J* 1982; 126:267–268.

Dusek J: Nursing rules—Fact or myth?: Iced gastric lavage slows bleeding in gastric hemorrhage. *Crit Care Nurse* (July/Aug) 1984; 8.

Grew W et al. Endoscopic variceal sclerotherapy: Experience with 30 patients. *Southern Med J* 1984; 77:1091–1094.

Grimes D, Grimes R, Hamelink M. *Infectious diseases.* St. Louis: Mosby Year Book, 1991.

The Lippincott Manual of Nursing Practice, 5th ed. Philadelphia: Lippincott, 1991.

Mandell G, Douglas R, Bennett J (eds): *Principles and practice of infectious diseases,* 3d ed. Chapters 102–103. New York: Churchill Livingstone, 1990.

Multigner L et al.: Pancreatic stone protein. II. Implication in stone formation during the course of chronic calcifying pancreatitis. *Gastroenterol* 1985; 89:387–391.

Navab F, Schiller T, Slaton D. Management of variceal hemorrhage. *Southern Med J* 1984; 77:1302–1307.

Palmaz J et al.: Expandable intrahepatic portacaval shunt in dogs with chronic portal hypertension. *Am J Roentgenol* 1986; 147:1251–1254.

Richter G et al.: Transjugular intrahepatic portacaval stent shunt: Preliminary clinical results. *Radiology* 1990; 174:1027–1030.

Rikkers L et al.: Shunt surgery versus endoscopic sclerotherapy for long-term treatment of variceal bleeding. *Ann Surg* 1987; 206:261–271.

Ring E et al.: Using transjugular intrahepatic portosystemic shunts to control variceal bleeding before liver transplantation. *Ann Intern Med* 1992; 116:304–309.

Rosch J, Hanafee W, Snow H: Transjugular portal venography and radiologic portocaval shunt: An experimental study. *Radiology* 1969; 92:1112–1114.

Sales H, Bernard J, Gullo L. Pathogenesis of chronic pancreatitis. *GUT* 1990; 31:629–632.

Sarles H et al.: Classifications of pancreatitis and definition of pancreatic diseases. Letter to the editor in *Digestion* 1989; 43:234–236.

Sarles H: Classification et definition des pancreatitis. Marseille-Rome 1988. *Gastroenterol Clin Biol* 1989; 13:857–859.

Toyonaga A et al.: Selected summaries: Nitroglycerin in the treatment of portal hypertension. *Gastroenterol* 1991; 101(2):552.

U.S. Department of Health and Human Services, Public Health Service, Centers for Disease Control: Protection Against Viral Hepatitis. *MMWR* February 9, 1990; 39(RR-2):6.

Way L (ed). *Current surgical diagnosis and treatment,* 9th ed. San Mateo, CA:, Appleton & Lange, 1990.

Zemel G et al.: Percutaneous transjugular portosystemic shunt. *JAMA* 1991; 266(3):390–393.

Nutrition

American Society of Parenteral and Enteral Nutrition (ASPEN). Guidelines for the use of enteral nutrition in the adult patient. *JPEN* 1987; 11: 435–439.

American Society of Parenteral and Enteral Nutrition (ASPEN): Guidelines for use of total parenteral nutrition in the hospitalized adult patient. *JPEN* 1986; 10:441–445.

Askanazi J et al.: Respiratory distress secondary to a high carbohydrate load: A case report. *Surgery* 1980; 87:596.

Bockus S: Troubleshooting your tube feedings. *Am J Nurs* 1991; 91:24–29.

Brinson R, Anderson W, Singh H: Hypoalbuminemia-associated diarrhea in critically ill patients. *J Crit Illness* 1987; 2:72–78.

Burke J et al.: Glucose requirements following burn injury. *Ann Surg* 1979; 190:274–278.

DeBourgh G, Wapensky T, Guthrie G: Guidelines for tube feeding at California Pacific/Medical Center—Pacific Campus, San Francisco, 1989.

Elwyn D: Nutritional requirements of adult surgical patients. *Crit Care Med* 1980; 8:10–36.

Feldman E et al.: Effects of oral versus intravenous nutrition on intestinal adaption after small bowel resection in the dog. *Gastroenterol* 1976; 70:712–719.

Gever L: Intravenous lipids. *Nurs 81* (Nov) 1981; 160–161.

Guenter P et al.: Administration and delivery of enteral nutrition. In *Clinical nutrition—Enteral and tube feeding,* 2d ed. Rombeau J, Caldwell M (eds). Philadelphia: Saunders, 1990.

Janson C et al.: Hypophosphatemia. *Ann Emerg Med* 1983; 12:107–116.

Keithley J: Infection and the malnourished patient. *Heart Lung* 1983; 12:23–27.

Kelly T, Patrick M, Hillman K: Study of diarrhea in critically ill patients. *Crit Care Med* 1983; 11:7–9.

Keohane P et al.: Relation between osmolality of diet and gastrointestinal side effects in enteral nutrition. *Brit Med J* 1984; 288:678–680.

Kinney J, Felig P: The metabolic response to injury and infection. *Endocrinol* 1979; 3:1963–1968.

Kohn C, Keithley J: Enteral nutrition—Potential complications and patient monitoring. *Nurs Clin North Am* 1989; 24:339–353.

Levine G et al.: Role of oral intake in maintenance of gut mass and disaccharidase activity. *Gastroenterol* 1974; 67:975–982.

Long CL et al.: Metabolic response to injury and illness: Estimation of energy and protein needs from indirect calorimetry and nitrogen balance. *JPEN* 1979; 3:452–456.

Metheney N: Measures to test placement of nasogastric and nasointestinal feeding tubes: A review. *Nurs Res* 1988; 37:324–329.

Metheney N, Eisenberg P, McSweeney M: Effect of feeding tube properties and three irrigants on clogging rates. *Nurs Res* 1988; 37:165–169.

Metheney N, Eisenberg P, Spies M: Aspiration pneumonia in patients fed through nasoenteral tubes. *Heart Lung* 1986; 15:256–261.

Metheney N et al.: Effectiveness of the auscultatory method in predicting feeding tube location. *Nurs Res* 1990; 39:262–267.

Moore F, Brennan M: Surgical injury: Body composition, protein metabolism, and neuroendocrinology. Pages 169–224 in *Manual of surgical nutrition,* Ballinger W (ed). Philadelphia: Saunders, 1975.

Moss G: Malabsorption associated with extreme malnutrition: Importance of replacing plasma albumin. *J Am Coll Nutr* 1982; 1:89–92.

Perkel M, Moore C, Hersh T: Metaclopramide therapy in patients with delayed gastric emptying. *Dig Dis Sci* 1979; 24:662–666.

Recommended Dietary Allowances, 10th edition. Subcommittee on the Tenth Edition of the RDA's, Food and Nutrition Board, Commission on Life Sciences, National Research Council. Washington D.C.: National Academy Press, 1989.

Review Article: Trace metal abnormalities in adults during hyperalimentation. *JPEN* 1980; 5:424–429.

Robin A et al.: Influence of hypercaloric glucose infusions on fuel economy in surgical patients: A review. *Crit Care Med* 1981; 9:680–686.

Rolandelli R et al.: Critical illness and sepsis. In *Clinical nutrition—Enteral and tube feeding,* 2d ed. Rombeau J, Caldwell M (eds). Philadelphia: Saunders, 1990.

Saudek C, Felig P: The metabolic events of starvation. *Am J Med* 1976; 60:118–125.

Schlichtig R, Ayres S: *Nutritional support of the critically ill.* Chicago: Year Book Medical, 1988.

Seltzer MH: Instant nutrition assessment: Absolute weight loss and surgical mortality. *JPEN* 1982; 6:218–221.

Stotts N, Friesen J: Understanding starvation in the critically ill patient. *Heart Lung* 1982; 11:469–478.

Strong R et al.: Equal aspiration rates from postpylorus and intragastric-placed small-bore nasoenteric feeding tubes; a randomized, prospective study. *JPEN Nutrition* 1992; 16:59–63.

Van Way C: Nutritional support in the injured patient. *Surg Clin North Am* 1991; 71:537–541.

Weinser R, Heimburger D, Butterworth C: Hospital-associated malnutrition. In *Handbook of clinical nutrition,* 2d ed. St Louis: Mosby, 1989, p. 132.

Williams S: *Essentials of nutrition and diet therapy,* 4th ed. St Louis: Times Mirror/Mosby College Publishing, 1986.

Wilmore DW: *The metabolic management of the critically ill.* New York: Plenum, 1980.

Wilson M, Haynes-Johnson V: Cranberry juice or water? A comparison of feeding tube irrigants. *Nutr Support Serv* 1987; 7:23–24.

Worthington P, Wagner B: Total parenteral nutrition. *Nurs Clin North Am* 1989; 24.

20

Multisystem Disorders

CLINICAL INSIGHT

Domain: Effective management of rapidly changing situations

Competency: Contingency management: rapid matching of demands and resources in emergency situations

Labile situations are the norm in critical-care nursing, and coping with them can be exhilarating and exhausting. These situations demand an immediate response, and often it is the expert who steps forward to take charge. Acting with confidence in the midst of disaster requires extensive clinical experience. Maintaining credibility during catastrophes requires a track record; precious minutes can be lost if others challenge leadership. In the crucible of a crisis, however, role distinctions often fall away when others recognize and respect the authority conferred by expertise. Managing life-threatening crises successfully also requires an intimate knowledge of how the health

care system works, as illustrated in the following paradigm (Benner 1984, pp. 115–116). Here, a nurse talks about fighting for the life of a patient with a carotid bleed while coping with the news that the patient has no blood in the blood bank and directing a panicked ICU resident.

By this time the problem is blood, we need blood, and so I said "OK, someone call the blood bank and get us some blood." And the nurse said, "We just called and there's none down there." No one had caught that the patient was sitting up there with no blood in the blood bank. So we took off a blood (sample) from the arterial line and sent it down for a type and cross-match. Meanwhile, I started plasmanate and lactated Ringer's, because the mean pressure was dropping to about 30 and the blood was just pumping out of his mouth. About this time the ICU resident came in. He said, "What shall I do?" And I said, "You need to go down to the blood bank and get some type-specific blood for this patient, because a nurse can't get that. You're the only person who can get type-specific blood." It was the best thing he could do under the circumstances. I said, "Bring two units, they will only give you two at a time, no matter how bad. But bring two and get back here as soon as you can." So he took off.

(Fluid resuscitation was successful and the patient's bleeding was controlled in time for surgical repair of the artery.)

Introduction

Multisystem problems are usually complex and difficult to comprehend; however, all of the disorders presented in this chapter share common concepts. First, the chapter analyzes shock as the result of cellular hypoxia, and malignant inflammation as the result of prolonged hypoperfusion. Then it examines the sequelae of shock and inflammation organ system by organ system, and discusses appropriate nursing care measures.

Shock

Cardiovascular health depends on the successful interaction of three elements: the heart pump, the blood vessels, and the blood volume. Shock—an acute process of hemodynamic and metabolic derangements leading to decreased delivery of oxygen to the cell—results from disruption of one or more elements in this triad. It is an ever-present specter in the care of the critically ill.

Assessment

Risk Conditions You can determine which patients are at risk for shock by conceptualizing three major types of shock based on the three components of the cardiovascular system.

Hypovolemic Shock Rice (1991) defines hypovolemic shock as decreased tissue perfusion due to decreased effective intravascular volume resulting from internal fluid shifts or external losses of fluid. For purposes of this discussion, we will define hypovolemic shock as

inadequate tissue perfusion due to loss or sequestration of body fluid that is then unavailable for restoration to the circulating volume. This definition differentiates hypovolemic shock from distributive shock (discussed below).

Fluid volume deficit following profound hemorrhage, excessive diuresis, or severe dehydration may lead to hypovolemic shock. Internal or external hemorrhage can result in blood loss, and thermal injuries or large exudative lesions may cause plasma loss. Fluid can be lost from the gastrointestinal tract by vomiting, diarrhea, fistulas, ostomies, or suction. Diuretic administration, diabetes insipidus, or hyperglycemia may cause excessive loss of fluid through the kidneys. Any of these fluid losses can result in dehydration and hypovolemic shock, especially when fluid volume replacement is inadequate.

Cardiogenic Shock Cardiogenic shock results from failure of the heart to pump adequately. During *coronary cardiogenic shock,* pump failure results from ischemia or infarction due to compromised coronary arterial circulation, whereas during *noncoronary cardiogenic shock,* pump failure results from abnormalities of the cardiac muscle or heart valves. For more information on cardiogenic shock, please consult Chapter 13.

Distributive Shock Distributive shock, which includes neurogenic shock and vasogenic shock, is caused by abnormal distribution of blood volume due to altered vessel resistance. *Neurogenic shock* results from loss of normal sympathetic vasoconstrictor stimuli, which leads to vasodilatation. The blood vessels expand beyond normal blood volume capacity, causing a relative hypovolemia. Possible causes are spinal cord injury, severe pain, and vasomotor center depression due to drug overdose. *Vasogenic shock* results from diminished arterial resistance and increased venous capacitance due to the release of vasodilating substances. Clinical examples include anaphylactic shock and septic shock.

Pathophysiologic Changes

Hypovolemic Shock Hypovolemic shock primarily results from a defect in the microcirculation. In the compensated stage of hypovolemic shock, sympathetic stimulation constricts both the precapillary sphincter and the venule. As a result, fluid flow through the capillary decreases and pressure inside the capillary drops. The disparity in pressure between the outside and inside of the capillary promotes the movement of fluid from the interstitium into the blood vessels, thus increasing circulating blood volume.

If shock persists and there is a prolonged decrease in capillary flow, decompensation occurs and a self-perpetuating cycle of events develops. The long period of diminished flow results in microcirculatory hypoxia and acidosis, which increase capillary permeability. The acidosis also promotes relaxation of the capillary sphincters, allowing more blood to enter the capillary. As venule constriction continues, capillary pressure increases. The increased pressure, combined with the increased capillary permeability, causes fluid to flow out of the capillaries into the tissues, worsening the drop in circulating blood volume and creating the self-perpetuating cycle.

On the cellular level, shock disrupts vital cellular activities. Sodium/potassium transport mechanisms falter with the accumulation of excess sodium inside and excess potassium outside the cell. Altered cellular permeability allows proteins and water to enter the cell, causing intracellular swelling. Mitochondria become depressed, and oxygen metabolism suffers.

Normally cells receive energy from a highly complex series of chemical reactions (Guyton 1991), diagrammed in Figure 20–1. During glycolysis, glucose is split to form pyruvic acid. This step does not require oxygen. In addition to the pyruvic acid, the cell produces a small number of hydrogen atoms and a small amount of energy, which is used in the synthesis of the high-energy bonds of *adenosine triphosphate* (ATP). These phosphate bonds store energy until the cell needs it. The pyruvic acid is converted to acetyl coenzyme A (CoA) and enters the Krebs (citric acid) cycle, during which the acetyl portion is broken down into carbon dioxide and hydrogen atoms. These hydrogen atoms, along with those released during glycolysis, undergo oxidative phosphorylation, during which huge amounts of energy are released and again stored as ATP.

Cellular hypoxia has drastic effects on energy availability. It is unknown whether this energy deficit results from decreased energy production or whether adequate energy production accompanied by insufficient formation of ATP causes energy to be lost as heat rather than stored as ATP.

Because glycolysis does not require oxygen, it continues to provide a small amount of energy, as well as pyruvic acid and hydrogen atoms. These elements cannot be metabolized in the Krebs cycle or undergo oxidative phosphorylation in the absence of oxygen. Instead, the excessive amounts of pyruvic acid and hydrogen atoms combine to produce lactic acid. The lactic acid diffuses out of the cell into the extracellular fluid, thus allowing glycolysis to continue providing energy for a few minutes. This shift from aerobic to anaerobic metabolism has three important consequences: (a) cellular activities are hampered severely due to lack of available energy; (b) the increased demand for glucose causes rapid depletion of glycogen stores; and (c) lactic acidosis deranges the body's acid–base and electrolyte balances. By the time metabolic acidosis is detectable in arterial blood gas values, significant physiologic derangement has occurred. Refer to Chapter 17 for further detail.

If the patient resumes adequate oxygenation, the lactic acid can be reconverted to pyruvic acid and utilized in the Krebs cycle. If not, the worsening

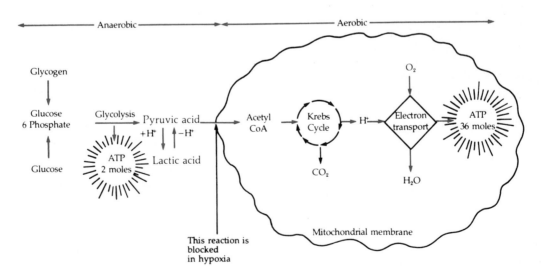

FIGURE 20–1

Cellular aerobic and anaerobic energy production.

metabolic acidosis and loss of energy will result in cellular destruction.

As cells are damaged, disruption of their lysosomes frees proteases and other enzymes, which may hasten cellular destruction. These enzymes also are believed to provoke the release or activation of bradykinin, histamine, and other substances that cause severe vasodilatation and depress the heart. These mediators also increase vascular and cellular permeability leading to fluid loss from the intravascular and intracellular compartments.

Septic (Endotoxin) Shock The pathophysiology of septic shock deserves special recognition because of the increasing importance of sepsis in mortality among the critically ill. The major pathogens responsible for septic shock are the aerobic, Gram-negative organisms, particularly *Escherichia coli,* the *Klebsiella-Enterobacter-Serratia* group, *Proteus,* and *Pseudomonas aeruginosa* (Roach 1990).

The cell walls of Gram-negative bacilli contain lipopolysaccharides, which are released as endotoxin when the bacteria die. This endotoxin is a principal cause of the pathogenicity of these organisms, which produce a type of septic shock called *endotoxin shock.*

The release of endotoxin stimulates the immunologic system, causing complement activation. The complement cascade produces these important effects:

1. Attraction of leukocytes to the injured area. These leukocytes increase bacterial destruction, causing further release of endotoxin.

2. Production of inflammatory chemical mediators. Cells damaged by infection release powerful chemical substances. The most important of these substances are histamine and lysosomal enzymes, which cause severe inflammatory injury.

3. Release of histamine from mast cells. This release causes vasodilatation, increased capillary permeability, and decreased peripheral resistance.

Lysosomal enzyme release damages surrounding tissue, and, in conjunction with endotoxin, activates vasoactive polypeptides. One of the most significant vasoactive polypeptides is bradykinin, a powerful vasodilator that significantly increases capillary permeability.

Sepsis stimulates the sympathetic nervous system, resulting in greatly increased catecholamine release. Beta stimulation causes an increase in heart rate and cardiac contractility. The metabolic rate also increases, generating more body heat. The resulting increase in cardiac output causes a hyperdynamic state during which the patient feels warm because of vasodilatation and increased heat production—hence the term "warm shock." Because vasodilatation increases the capacity of the vascular bed, blood pressure is low despite the increased cardiac output. The increased capillary permeability causes marked extravasation of fluid from the vascular space, further contributing to the disparity between the capacity of the vascular bed and the available blood volume.

As septic shock evolves, the hemodynamics change from vasodilatation to vasoconstriction, provoked by the marked constrictive effects of the catecholamines and prostaglandins released from damaged tissue. Perfusion of organs slows because of hypotension and vasoconstriction. Ischemia of the splanchnic bed triggers the release of myocardial depressant factor (MDF). As venous return decreases and MDF depresses contractility, cardiac output drops. In this hypodynamic state, the patient is in "cold shock." From this point on, the pathophysiologic events are similar to those of hypovolemic shock.

Blood gas values may vary, depending on the progression of septic shock. Initially, there is respiratory alkalosis due to hyperventilation induced by endotoxin. As septic shock progresses, metabolic alkalosis may develop. The cause of this alkalosis is unclear and may be related to impaired anaerobic metabolism that results in a reduction in lactate production relative to the degree of hypoxemia. Metabolic (lactic) acidosis is a late development attributed to profoundly disrupted cellular metabolism. It may occur in combination with respiratory acidosis if pulmonary deterioration becomes so severe that carbon dioxide elimination is impaired.

The septic shock patient is at particular risk for developing adult respiratory distress syndrome (ARDS) and disseminated intravascular coagulation (DIC). Endotoxin directly damages pulmonary vascular endothelium (Vaughan and Brooks 1990). Disruption of capillary endothelium and increased permeability result in platelet aggregation, pulmonary vasoconstriction, pulmonary interstitial edema, leakage of fluid and protein into alveoli, and surfactant reduction. Because of alveolar collapse, diminished pulmonary perfusion, and impaired oxygenation, the patient develops the hallmarks of ARDS—widespread atelectasis, profound ventilation/perfusion imbalances, severe hypoxemia, pulmonary edema, and finally respiratory failure.

In addition to the effects of complement activation mentioned earlier, the complement sequence also triggers both the intrinsic and extrinsic coagulation pathways. The accelerated coagulation in turn triggers

TABLE 20–1

Hemodynamic Responses in Different Types of Shock

TYPE	HYPOVOLEMIC	CARDIOGENIC	SEPTIC		NEUROGENIC
			Early	Late	
Cause	Decreased Circulating Blood Volume	Depressed Cardiac Contractility	Vasodilatation Due to Endotoxins		Peripheral Vasodilatation Due to Loss of Nervous Stimulation
Filling pressures	↓	↑	↓	↑	↓
Cardiac output	↓	↓	↑	↓	normal or ↑
Systemic vascular resistance	↑	↑	↓	↑	↓
Pulmonary vascular resistance	normal	normal	↑	normal	normal

From Bodai B, Holcroft J: Use of the pulmonary artery catheter in the critically ill patient. *Heart Lung* 1982; 11:406–416. Reprinted by permission of the C.V. Mosby Company.

accelerated fibrinolysis—the classic "setup" for disseminated intravascular coagulation.

Signs and Symptoms The traditional criteria for shock are a systolic blood pressure (BP) below 70 mm Hg; confusion or other signs of diminished cerebral perfusion; pale, cool, clammy skin; a urinary output below 30 ml per hour; and metabolic acidosis. If you rely on these classic signs, however, you may deprive many of your patients of prompt assistance in the early stages of shock. These signs are late; they may not occur in some shock states (especially early septic shock); and/or they may be inappropriate for a given patient—such as the hypertensive patient—in whom shock can occur within the range of seemingly normal systolic pressures.

Early detection and aggressive management of shock are important, so it is vital that you watch for early signs. Hemodynamic responses in the different types of shock are presented in Table 20–1.

Hypovolemic Shock In early hypovolemic shock, powerful compensatory mechanisms activate when the blood pressure starts to drop. Baroreceptor stimulation excites the vasomotor center in the medulla, leading to tachycardia; arteriolar constriction, which increases systemic vascular resistance; and venoconstriction, which increases circulating blood volume. The kidneys also attempt to restore blood volume via ADH- and aldosterone-mediated sodium and water retention. As a result, cardiac output (CO) increases to near-normal

levels. The blood flow is redistributed away from the skin and kidneys to preserve the vital heart and brain.

The signs and symptoms of this compensated stage of shock correlate with its pathophysiology. Pulse rate is slightly increased, and BP is normal or slightly decreased. However, positive postural vital signs may be present at this stage of hypovolemic shock; that is, compared to supine vital signs, sitting vital signs reveal a systolic BP drop of 10 mm Hg or more and a pulse increase of 20 beats per minute or more. Positive postural vital signs indicate the presence of orthostatic hypotension due to the body's inability to compensate for the challenge of a sudden change in position while also compensating for the developing shock. The skin of the periphery is cool and pale, with poor capillary filling evident in the nail beds. Urinary output is slightly decreased. The patient is alert and oriented.

As shock deepens to approximately 25% loss of circulating blood volume, the pulse is rapid and thready, and frank hypotension is evident. The skin of the trunk is cool. Oliguria (urinary output below 30 cc per hour) is present and the patient is markedly thirsty. Restlessness, confusion, or agitation develop. The respiratory rate increases in response to the continuing biochemical abnormalities.

In late shock, with loss of 40% or more of circulating blood volume, the pulse is very rapid and weak. BP drops below 80 mm Hg systolic. The skin appears mottled or cyanotic and feels cold. Urinary output drops below 20 cc per hour, and the patient is disoriented. Finally, when just a few minutes of life remain, the skin becomes deeply pale or cyanotic, sensation decreases, and unconsciousness ensues.

Cardiogenic Shock Similar events occur in cardiogenic shock, with one area of exception. In hypovolemic shock, cardiac filling pressures are normal or slightly low in the compensated stage, and definitely low in the decompensated stage, because of the actual loss of blood volume. In cardiogenic shock, filling pressures are elevated because of the vascular congestion that results from the heart's inability to pump effectively.

Septic Shock Hemodynamic parameters in septic shock are significantly different from those in other types of shock. In *early sepsis,* beta stimulation results in increased CO, but vasodilatation causes a drop in filling pressures and systemic vascular resistance. Pulmonary vascular resistance increases due to the release of prostaglandins from injured vascular endothelium and platelets (Houston 1990). In *late septic shock,* when the heart is failing, cardiac output falls and filling pressures rise. Catecholamine and prostaglandin releases result in generalized vasoconstriction, so systemic vascular resistance increases.

NURSING TIP

Hypotension

A "normal" blood pressure can be deceptive. Keep in mind that a drop in blood pressure is one of the last symptoms of shock, and watch the patient's respiratory rate and heart rate for signs of acceleration. Early intervention means an improved chance of recovery.

The signs and symptoms of septic shock correlate with its pathophysiology; however, the signs of sepsis prior to the onset of shock are subtle. They include restlessness, confusion, tachycardia, and increased respiratory rate. In the *hyperdynamic, "warm shock"* state, the patient becomes hypotensive but the skin is warm and dry or flushed. Confusion, restlessness, and hyperventilation increase. In the *hypodynamic, "cold shock"* state, the patient resembles one in late hypovolemic shock, with cold and clammy skin and severe oliguria. Because of the copious interstitial fluid accumulation, the patient shows signs of fluid overload and pulmonary congestion. This appearance is deceptive, however, inasmuch as the effective circulating fluid volume is severely reduced.

Endotoxin's effect on the temperature-regulating center of the hypothalamus may lead to confusing temperature changes. Initially, the patient may be hypothermic due to depression of the center. Later, the patient may become hyperthermic as a result of the temperature-stimulating effects of the endotoxin and of pyrogen release from leukocytosis.

Laboratory Data Laboratory data can provide valuable assistance in assessing the degree and type of shock. The most common laboratory parameters in shock, their normal values, changes during shock, and the mechanisms of abnormalities are presented in Table 20–2.

Prevention The nurse plays a critical role in prevention of shock. For example, to prevent hypovolemic shock, the nurse can: (a) closely monitor the intake and output of traumatized patients, patients on diuretics, and patients unable to satisfy their thirst, e.g., unconscious patients; (b) promptly control frank bleeding; and (c) securely fasten arterial line connections to avoid accidental disconnection and hemorrhage. Septic shock may be prevented by removing sources of infection, such as contaminated IV lines and infected or necrotic tissue, and enhancing host defenses.

NURSING DIAGNOSES

Because of the rich complexity and diverse causality of shock, there are many applicable nursing diagnoses for patients in shock, including:

- Altered tissue perfusion: global*
- Impaired gas exchange
- Altered urinary elimination
- Altered nutrition: less than body requirements

*non-NANDA diagnosis

Planning and Implementation of Care

Altered Tissue Perfusion Related to Loss of Circulating Blood Volume If you detect signs of rapidly

TABLE 20–2

Common Laboratory Data in Shock*

TEST	NORMAL	IN SHOCK	MECHANISM
Blood Chemistries			
NUTRITIONAL SUBSTANCES			
Glucose	70–100 mg/100 ml	↑ Early ↓ Late	Sympathetic stimulation Depletion of body glycogen stores; decreased liver function
Serum proteins			
Total	6.0–7.8g/100 ml	↓	Leakage from capillary and decreased synthesis in liver cells
Albumin	3.2–4.5g/100 ml	↓	
Globulin	2.3–3.5g/100 ml	Normal or ↓	Larger particle size, less leaks from capillary
EXCRETORY SUBSTANCES			
Urea nitrogen	5.0–20.0 mg/100 ml	↑	Decreased renal excretion
Creatinine	0.6–1.2/mg 100 ml	↑	Decreased renal excretion
Bilirubin			
Total	0.5–1.2 mg/100 ml	↑	
Direct (conjugated)	up to 0.2 mg/100 ml	↑	Liver cell damage
Indirect (unconjugated)	0.1–1.0 mg/100 ml	↑	
FUNCTIONAL SUBSTANCES			
Sodium	136–142 mEq/L	↑ Early	↑ aldosterone causing renal retention of sodium
Potassium	3.8–5.0 mEq/L	↑ or ↓ Late ↓ Early ↑ Late	Altered renal function (ATN) ↑ aldosterone causing renal excretion of potassium Acidosis, cell necrosis, and decreased renal function
Chloride	95–103 mEq/L	↓ Early ↑ Late	Alkalotic state and bicarbonate excess Acidotic state and bicarbonate deficiency
Carbon dioxide (carbonate)	21–28 mEq/L	↑ Early ↓↓ Late	Alkalotic state Severe metabolic and respiratory acidosis
SERUM ENZYMES			
Creatine phosphokinase (CPK)	5–35 U/ml	↑	Necrosis of muscle cells and/or heart cells
Aspartate aminotransferase (AST, SGOT)	15–40 U/ml	↑	Necrosis of heart cells and/or liver cells
Alanine aminotransferase (ALT, SGPT)	15–35 U/ml	↑	Necrosis of liver cells
Lactic dehydrogenase (LDH)	150–450 Wroblewski U/ml	↑	Necrosis of liver and/or heart cells
Amylase	60–160 somogyl U/100 ml	↑	Necrosis of pancreatic cells
Lipase	0–1.5 Cherry-Crandall U/ml	↑	Necrosis of pancreatic cells

developing shock, promptly identify the type of shock and take appropriate emergency measures:

1. Mentally review the patient's history, and quickly look for clues to the cause of shock, such as a site of active bleeding.

2. Perform these emergency measures according to unit protocol:

A. For hemorrhagic shock, control bleeding if possible. For frank bleeding from hemodynamic lines, reconnect the line or shut it off between the break and the patient. For blood vessel ruptures, apply direct pressure and elevate the site.

B. For hypovolemic shock, elevate the patient's legs. This increases circulating

TABLE 20–2

Common Laboratory Data in Shock* (Continued)

TEST	NORMAL	IN SHOCK	MECHANISM
BLOOD CULTURES	No growth	Positive	Variety of causative microbes
Hematology			
Hemoglobin	male 14.0–16.5 g/100 ml female 12.6–14.2 g/100 ml	↓	Hemorrhage (if present)
Hematocrit (packed cell volume = PCV)	male 42–52% female 37–47%	↑ or ↓	Fluid leakage from the capillary Loss of blood (Note: does not occur until 6 hrs after blood loss)
Red blood cell count	male 4.6–6.2 million/ml female 4.5–5.4 million/ml	↓	Hemorrhage (if present)
White blood cell count	4,500–11,000/ml	↑	Body's response to infection (if present)
Platelet count	150,000–400,000/ml	↓	Platelet aggregation and microemboli
Coagulation test:			
Prothrombin time (PT)	12–14 sec	Prolonged	Hypercoagulable state (if present)
Partial thromboplastin time (PTT)	45–65 sec	Prolonged	Hypercoagulable state (if present)
Arterial Blood Gases			
pH	7.38–7.42	↑ Early ↓ Late	Hyperventilation and carbon dioxide exhalation Carbon dioxide retention and lactic acid production
P_{CO_2}	35–45 mm Hg	↓ Early ↑ Late	Hyperventilation Hypoventilation
P_{O_2}	80–100 mm Hg	↓	Hypoventilation and hypoperfusion (ventilation/perfusion imbalances)
Bicarbonate	22–28 mEq/L	↓ Late	Severe acidotic state
Urine Measurements			
Creatinine clearance	male 1.0–2.0 g/24 hr female 0.8–1.8 g/24 hr	↓	Impaired renal excretion
Osmolality	500–800 mOsm/L	↑ Early ↓ Late	Water retention, secondary to ADH Inability of the kidney to concentrate urine
Specific gravity	1.001–1.035	↑ Early ↓ Late	Same as for osmolality (influenced by administration of Dextran)
Sodium	80–180 mEq/24 hr	↓ Early ↓ or ↑ Late	Sodium reabsorption secondary to aldosterone Abnormal renal function
Potassium	40–80 mEq/24 hr	↑ Early ↓ or ↑ Late	Potassium excretion secondary to aldosterone Abnormal renal function

*Normal values cited from: Halsted JA: *The laboratory in clinical medicine*, Philadelphia: WB Saunders, 1976.

Excerpted from: Rice V: Shock, a clinical syndrome. Part 3: The nursing care: Prevention and patient assessment. *Crit Care Nurse* (July/Aug) 1981; 38–39. © 1991 by Cahners Publishing Company.

blood volume 400–800 ml by promoting venous drainage from the legs. Do not use this measure for patients with cardiogenic shock, increased intracranial pressure, or active bleeding from the head and neck; increasing the circulating blood volume can worsen these conditions. Trendelenburg's position, popular in the past treatment of shock, is used less often because of its detrimental effects on diaphragmatic excursion—and therefore ventilation—as well as its tendency to further lower BP by reflex depression of baroreceptor activity (Gotshall, Wood, and Miles 1989).

C. Administer supplemental oxygen so that the blood that reaches the tissues is optimally oxygenated.

D. If there are no IV lines in place, establish two large-bore IV lines to facilitate rapid administration of fluid.

3. Consult with the patient's physician about further interventions.

4. Establish baseline values and initial diagnostic data by recording a 12-lead electrocardiogram (ECG) and obtaining routine laboratory studies, such as a complete blood count; type and cross-match; serum electrolytes; arterial blood gases; and urinalysis. Obtain additional specimens, such as blood cultures, as indicated.

5. Assist the physician in inserting an arterial line and a central venous or pulmonary artery (PA) catheter to monitor hemodynamic pressures. Insert a Foley catheter with urimeter to monitor urinary output. Monitor these parameters every 15 minutes to 1 hour, depending on the severity of shock and the rapidity of its progression.

6. Administer a fluid challenge as appropriate. Evaluation of the preceding data frequently identifies the type(s) of shock present, however, in many cases the data are equivocal. For example, low blood pressure and decreased urinary output may be present in any type of shock, so the physician may ask you to administer a fluid challenge to evaluate the patient's hemodynamic response to an increased blood volume. The appropriate amount of fluid challenge can be titrated by judicious use of hemodynamic data. Although the details vary among physicians, one common protocol is presented in Table 20–3.

Depending on the patient's condition and the physician's preference, crystalloids, colloids, and/or blood may be given to restore fluid volume. The characteristics of the most commonly used solutions are presented in Table 20–4. The amount of solution used depends on the fluid volume lost and on the degree of vascular capacitance.

Whatever fluids are used, remember to closely monitor intake and output, follow the trend of vascular pressures, and watch for the signs of fluid overload discussed in Chapter 16.

Altered Tissue Perfusion Related to Excessive Vasoconstriction A wide variety of inotropes, vasoconstrictors, and vasodilators can be used to treat patients with hemodynamically significant hypotension. They include dopamine, dobutamine, amrinone, norepinephrine, sodium nitroprusside, and intravenous nitroglycerin. The rationale for use, actions, and side effects are presented in Chapter 13 and the Appendix. Keep in mind, however, that these drugs will not maintain peripheral perfusion if fluid volume is inadequate; in fact, their use in hypovolemic patients can cause further tissue death and worsen shock, so hypovolemia must be corrected before or concomitantly with their use.

Impaired Gas Exchange Related to Ventilation-Perfusion Imbalance Impaired gas exchange resulting from microatelectasis, microemboli, increased

TABLE 20–3

Fluid Challenge Protocol According to Weil and Rackow

1. Obtain baseline measurements of either the pulmonary capillary wedge pressure (PCWP) or central venous pressure (CVP) for an initial 10-minute observation period prior to beginning fluid administration.

2. Determine the infusion rate based on the filling pressure:

PCWP	Fluid Infusion Rate
<12 mm Hg	20 cc/min
12–18 mm Hg	10 cc/min
>18 mm Hg	5 cc/min

CVP	Fluid Infusion Rate
<12 cm H_2O	20 cc/min
12–18 cm H_2O	10 cc/min
>18 cm H_2O	5 cc/min

3. Infuse the appropriate amount of fluid for 10 minutes via an infusion pump. If at any time during the infusion, the PCWP increases by more than 7 mm Hg (or if the CVP increases by more than 5 cm H_2O), *discontinue the infusion.*

4. At the end of the 10-minute infusion period, measure the PCWP or CVP. If the PCWP has increased by 3 mm Hg or less (or if the CVP has increased by 2 cm H_2O or less), repeat the fluid challenge.

   If the PCWP has increased more than 3 mm Hg but less than 7 mm Hg (or if the CVP has increased more than 2 cm H_2O but less than 5 cm H_2O):
   a. Discontinue the infusion, and observe the patient for 10 minutes
   b. During this 10-minute observation period, if the PCWP falls to within 3 mm Hg of the initial PCWP (or if the CVP falls to within 2 cm H_2O of the initial CVP), administer another fluid challenge over another 10-minute period.
   c. During this 10-minute observation period, if the PCWP does not fall to within 3 mm Hg of the initial PCWP (or if the CVP does not fall to within 2 cm H_2O of the initial CVP), discontinue the fluid challenge.

Excerpted from Rice V: Shock management. Part I: Fluid volume replacement. *Crit Care Nurse* 1984; 4:80–81. Based on data from Weil MH, Rackow EC: A guide to volume repletion. *Emerg Med* 1984; 16:101–110. © 1991 by Cahners Publishing Company.

shunting, increased pulmonary congestion, and worsening acidosis is particularly dangerous because it superimposes respiratory acidosis on metabolic acidosis, and the combination can be lethal.

Independent nursing interventions include maintenance of a patent airway (by using the head-tilt maneuver, inserting a pharyngeal airway or assisting with endotracheal intubation) and keeping the airway clear of secretions by suctioning as necessary. Assessment of respiratory rate and rhythm, chest excursion, and lung sounds should take place at least every hour. Arterial blood gas values need to be checked at least every 4 hours for trends, especially hypoxemia, hypercapnia, and acidosis. The nurse may also provide aggressive pulmonary hygiene measures to prevent the development of atelectasis and pneumonia in this patient population.

Collaborative nursing interventions include administration of supplemental oxygen appropriate for the patient's needs. Initially, the patient in a relatively light degree of shock may be managed with a nasal cannula, oxygen mask, or Venturi mask. As shock becomes more profound and the patient is intubated, oxygen may be administered via a mechanical ventilator.

Altered Urinary Elimination Related to Decreased Renal Perfusion To prevent acute renal failure, monitor urinary volume and maintain output above 30 ml/hr, and monitor blood urea nitrogen (BUN), creatinine, and urine electrolytes as ordered. In addition to fluid administration, the physician may prescribe diuretics, usually mannitol or furosemide (Lasix). Monitor patients carefully during diuresis; fluid overload and congestive heart failure may occur with osmotic diuretics, rapid diuresis may provoke cardiovascular collapse, and a variety of electrolyte imbalances may develop during diuresis. Acute renal failure is discussed in detail in Chapter 15.

Altered Nutrition (Less Than Body Requirements) Related to Diminished GI Perfusion Paralytic ileus may result from autonomic hyperactivity, but even if it does not, it is unwise to create an increased need for blood flow to the digestive organs while blood is shunted preferentially away from them. For the duration of the shock episode, it is appropriate to give the patient nothing by mouth and to insert a nasogastric catheter to drain the stomach. Collaboratively, provide nutritional supplementation as ordered, but be sure bowel sounds are present before resuming oral feedings.

Definitive Care Specific correction of the cause of shock is also necessary, although at times it may be appropriate to wait until the patient's hemodynamic status is stabilized. Collaborate with the physician in treating the underlying cause of shock, for example by sending the patient in hemorrhagic shock to surgery to ligate bleeding vessels or starting intravenous antibiotics on a patient in septic shock.

Complications of shock may include myocardial infarction (MI), ARDS, acute renal failure, DIC, and

TABLE 20–4

Guide to Parenteral Fluid Replacement

TYPE	DESCRIPTION	USES	SPECIAL CONSIDERATIONS
Whole Blood and Blood Products			
Whole blood	Complete blood	To replace volume and maintain Hgb at 12–14 g/100 ml. Given in slow or rapid hemorrhage and hypovolemic shock	Best replacement for loss of whole blood is whole blood.
Red blood cells (packed, fresh or frozen)	Whole blood with 80% of plasma removed	To correct RBC deficiency and improve oxygen-carrying capacity of the blood. Given in anemia, slow hemorrhage, with PCV ↓ 25–30% Frozen (thawed) RBCs given to organ transplant patients (because freezing destroys leukocytes) Used in cardiogenic shock (avoids fluid overload)	Frozen (thawed) RBCs—very expensive. Washed RBCs (suspended in saline) may be given in progressive shock to ↓ red cell adhesiveness (↓ fibrinogen coating).
Plasma (fresh or frozen)	Uncoagulated plasma separated from whole blood	To restore plasma volume in hypovolemic shock without ↑ PCV To restore clotting factors (except platelets)	Used effectively for immediate volume replacement.
Plasma protein fraction (Plasmanate) (Plasma-plex)	5% solution of selected proteins from pooled plasma in buffered stabilized saline diluent (0.9% NaCl). Contains albumin, alpha and beta globulins	To expand plasma volume (while cross-matching is being completed) in hypovolemic shock. To correct hypoproteinemia and increase serum colloid osmotic pressure	Use cautiously in patients with CHF (due to added fluid) and in patients with renal failure (due to added proteins). Is osmotically equivalent to plasma. Does not carry danger of hepatitis (heat-treated).
Albumin 5% or 25% (Albuminate)	Aqueous fraction of pooled plasma	To increase serum colloid osmotic pressure and expand plasma volume in shock (while cross-matching is being completed)	Does not carry danger of hepatitis (heat-treated). Use cautiously in patients with CHF. In shock, leaky capillaries may ↑ tissue proteins and augment interstitial and intracellular edema (may remain in circulation longer than crystalloid solutions). 5% albumin is osmotically equivalent to plasma.
Platelets	Platelet sediment from platelet-rich plasma, resuspended in 30–50 cc of plasma	To restore platelets (in thrombocytopenia) and to maintain normal blood coagulability	

cardiopulmonary arrest. MI, ARDS, acute renal failure, and cardiopulmonary arrest are discussed in previous chapters; DIC will be addressed later in this chapter.

Outcome Evaluation

Without vasopressor or vasodilator support, the patient should ideally maintain these outcome criteria:

- Arterial blood pressure within 10 mm Hg of preshock levels.
- Adequate perfusion of vital organs, as manifested by a return to preshock level of consciousness, cardiac status, and renal function.
- Adequate peripheral perfusion, as manifested by warm, dry skin, and by peripheral pulse volume within normal limits (WNL) for patient.
- Arterial blood gases and serum electrolytes WNL for patient.

TABLE 20–4

Guide to Parenteral Fluid Replacement (Continued)

TYPE	DESCRIPTION	USES	SPECIAL CONSIDERATIONS
Plasma Substitutes (pharmaceutical plasma expanders)-Hypertonic Solutions			
Dextran	Large polysaccharide polymer of glucose		
LMWD (Dextran 40) (Rheomacrodex) (Gentran 40)	Solution that contains 10% dextran (average molecular weight = 40,000) in 0.9% NaCl or in 5% dextrose in water	To rapidly expand plasma volume	Used if PCV ↑ 30%. Lasts about 12 hours. ↓ platelet adhesiveness, so may ↑ bleeding from raw surfaces (avoid in hemorrhage). May ↓ capillary sludging in progressive shock. Alters urine specific gravity.
HMWD (Dextran 70) (Macrodex) (Gentran 70)	Solution that contains 6% dextran (average molecular weight = 70,000) in 0.9% NaCl or 5% dextrose in water	To effectively expand plasma volume for up to 24 hours	May leak from capillary less readily than LMWD. ↑ platelet adhesiveness. Alters urine specific gravity. Same molecular weight as human plasma albumin.
Hetastarch (Hespan) (Volex)	500 ml unit of a 6% solution containing a synthetic polymer of hydroxethyl starch in normal saline	To expand plasma volume	Potential dilution of clotting factors with resultant coagulation changes. Potential circulatory overload in patients with severe CHF and compromised renal function. Increased serum amylase level, peaking within one hour of IV administration and persisting for 3–4 days. Do not use if solution is cloudy or deep brown. Monitor clotting studies and platelet counts. Compatibility with other substances is not established: infuse through separate line. Maximum infusion rate in hemorrhagic shock is 20 ml/kg/hr. Monitor serum albumin.
Crystalloid Solutions (contain electrolytes and water)			
Isotonic Solutions:			
Normal Saline	0.9% NaCl in water	To ↑ plasma volume when RBC mass is adequate	Contains 154 mEq/L sodium. Replaces losses without altering normal fluid concentrations.
Lactated Ringer's (Hartmann's)	Normal saline to which K⁺ and Ca⁺ have been added; also contains buffers	To replace fluid and to buffer pH (contains lactate, which is quickly converted to bicarbonate to buffer acidosis)	Contains 130 mEq/L sodium, 3 mEq/L calcium, 4 mEq/L potassium 28 mEq/L lactate, 109 mEq/L chloride.
Ringer's	Normal saline to which K⁺ and Ca⁺ have been added	To replace fluid and to give additional K⁺ and Ca⁺. Contains high concentration of chloride and may increase plasma chloride level	Contains 147 mEq/L sodium, 4 mEq/L potassium, 5 mEq/L calcium, 156 mEq/L chloride.
Hypotonic Solutions:			
½ normal saline	0.45% NaCl in water	To raise total fluid volume	Contains 77 mEq/L sodium and 77 mEq/L chloride. Rapidly leaves vascular space; may potentiate interstitial and intracellular edema. Dilutes plasma proteins and electrolytes.
D₅W (physiologically hypotonic)	5% dextrose in water	To raise total fluid volume and to provide calories for energy (200 calories/1,000 cc)	Glucose is metabolized rapidly so that water remains in vascular space (hypotonic). Dilutes plasma proteins and electrolytes.

Excerpted from Rice V: Shock management: Part I. Fluid volume replacement. *Crit Care Nurse* 1984; 4:71–73. © 1991 by Cahners Publishing Company.

Multiple Organ Systems Failure (MOSF)

Prevention and Early Detection

Multiple organ system failure can be characterized as "a failure of host defense homeostasis in which the products of this defense are injurious to the host as well as to the invading organisms" (Macho and Luce 1989). The most frequent initial clinical presentation of MOSF is septic, and the respiratory and cardiovascular systems are frequently affected early in the course of the syndrome. The key to treatment of the syndrome, from both a nursing and a medical perspective, is early detection of a septic clinical picture. In addition, tissue oxygenation must be maintained by manipulation of hemoglobin, oxygen saturation, and cardiac index (Harper 1992). Such surveillance and early maximization of oxygen transport indices are the most effective prevention of the cascade of organ failures that characterize MOSF.

Pathophysiology

Malignant Inflammation Inadequate tissue oxygen delivery quickly leads to cellular dysfunction and shock. Key to this cellular dysfunction is the development of lactic acidosis and subsequent cellular destruction. The body's natural defenses deteriorate, and endogenous bacteria can initiate an inflammatory response; if cellular destruction continues, the ensuing inflammatory response can become systemic and generalized. This malignant inflammatory response causes metabolic and circulatory derangements in every body system (Pinsky and Matuschak 1989).

One of the causes of systemic inflammatory processes is the release of proinflammatory mediator substances by a variety of cells—including tissue macrophages and circulating monocytes—when stimulated by the invading normal flora. Some of these mediators are discussed in Chapter 18. A pivotal mediator was initially isolated in patients with neoplastic disease who either had radical decrease in tumor mass or suffered from severe weight loss. Thus, the same chemical was variously called *tumor necrosis factor* (TNF) and *cachectin* (Beutler 1989). This chemical has been the center of investigation for some years and is suspected of causing (directly or indirectly) many of the metabolic and cellular changes associated with both the septic syndrome and multiple organ

systems failure (Pinsky and Matuschak 1989). These changes will be described relative to each organ system.

Oxygen Utilization in Multiple Organ Systems Failure On the cellular level, the primary effect of malignant inflammation is a change in the ability of the cell to utilize oxygen. Because of this change in oxygen utilization, the maintenance of aerobic cellular metabolism depends on *supranormal* oxygen delivery by the cardiopulmonary system. If sufficient oxygen is not delivered—if oxygen delivery is not persistently *higher than normal*—the cell falls into anaerobic metabolism, accumulates lactic acid, and dies. It may therefore be incumbent upon experienced critical-care nurses and physicians to monitor oxygen delivery and consumption in patients whose clinical presentation results in a high index of suspicion for malignant inflammatory processes. This surveillance includes intermittent or continuous monitoring of cardiac index, arterial blood gases, mixed venous oxygen saturation ($S\bar{v}O_2$), and hemoglobin level. Oxygen *delivery* can then be calculated using the following formula:

$$\dot{D}O_2 = C.I. \times [(S_aO_2 \times 1.36 \times Hgb) + (P_aO_2 \times 0.003)] \times 10$$

where $\dot{D}O_2$ = oxygen delivery, C.I. = cardiac index, S_aO_2 = arterial oxygen saturation, Hgb = hemoglobin, and P_aO_2 = arterial partial pressure of oxygen. The P_aO_2 component is often neglected because its contribution to the total delivered amount of oxygen is so small. Eliminating this component, oxygen *consumption* can then be calculated using the following formula:

$$\dot{V}O_2 = [(S_aO_2 - S\bar{v}O_2) \times 1.36 \times Hgb] \times C.I. \times 10$$

The same abbreviations apply, with the addition of $\dot{V}O_2$ = oxygen consumption and $S\bar{v}O_2$ = mixed venous (pulmonary artery) oxygen saturation. Normal values for $\dot{D}O_2$ are 520–720 ml/min/m^2 and for $\dot{V}O_2$ are

---

NURSING TIP

Mixed Venous Blood Gases

When drawing mixed venous blood samples from the distal port of a pulmonary artery line, the balloon must be deflated and the sample drawn slowly, with a 5-ml or larger syringe, to avoid contaminating it with arterialized blood from flow distal to the catheter tip.

CRITICAL-CARE GERONTOLOGY

Many changes occur during aging that impact recovery from shock and multiple organ systems failure. Every physiologic process functions less efficiently with increasing age, and the hallmark of aging is a progressive stiffness or rigidity in many systems, including the arterial, pulmonary, and musculoskeletal systems. With increasing age, pulmonary changes include a decrease in diffusion capacity across the alveolar-capillary interface, leading to less efficient pulmonary function. Changes in the stomach include both decreased secretion of hydrochloric acid and slowed emptying

time. These changes make the elderly patient more susceptible to translocation of bacteria from the gut into the bloodstream. Loss of cellular function, including alteration of nutrient pathways, cellular secretion, and neuroendocrine control mechanisms, depletes the ability of the aging client to recover from multiple organ systems failure. Finally, all these changes combine to make the elderly critically ill patient especially subject to multisystem complications. (McCance 1990)

Careful assessment of the elderly critical-care patient should include the following:

1. Strength of the neuromuscular mechanism of ventilation
2. Thirst, dehydration, and adequacy of intravascular volume
3. Nutritional status, along with presence or absence of impaired appetite, chewing, or swallowing
4. Alterations in sensory processing, making the elderly critical-care patient more susceptible to delirium and confusion
5. Mobility limitations
6. Pain, especially of musculoskeletal origin

110–140 ml/min/m^2. The supranormal values commonly found in survivors of multiple organ systems failure are a $\dot{D}o_2$ greater than 550 ml/min/m^2 and a $\dot{V}o_2$ greater than 167 ml/min/m^2 (Shoemaker 1989).

Circulatory Effects of Multiple Organ Systems Failure

Under normal circumstances, it is the function of the circulatory system to prevent tissue hypoxia by maximizing tissue oxygen delivery during periods of increased oxygen demand. This maximization occurs in three ways: through a decrease in precapillary sphincter tone, which increases the number of perfused capillaries; a decrease in arteriolar tone, which decreases systemic vascular resistance and increases regional blood flow; and an increase in cardiac output. In addition, the tissues increase the percentage of available oxygen that they extract from the blood stream *(oxygen extraction ratio)* [Bersten and Sibbald 1989]. In malignant systemic inflammation—multiple organ systems failure (MOSF)—oxygen demand skyrockets due to an increase in metabolism secondary to the effects of inflammatory mediators. Additionally, oxygen extraction is blunted, which causes a phenomenon known as *flow-dependent oxygen consumption;* the more oxygen presented to the tissues, the more they consume. If oxygen delivery is inadequate, as in

hypotension, pump failure, hypovolemia, or hypoxemia, oxygen consumption drops and cellular acidosis ensues. Oxygen demand exceeds oxygen supply, causing an *oxygen debt.*

On the supply side, a compound called *myocardial depressant factor* has been isolated from patients with MOSF. This compound decreases ventricular contractility, ejection fraction, and cardiac output. Myocardial ischemia may also contribute to pump failure (Bersten and Sibbald 1989).

Assessment The flow-directed pulmonary artery catheter is used to access mixed venous circulation in the pulmonary artery and thereby calculate and assess oxygen consumption. In addition, right atrial and pulmonary wedge pressures may assist in determining appropriate preload, which can be altered by the peripheral vasodilatation characteristic of this syndrome. Other indices of circulatory adequacy include level of consciousness, urine output, capillary refill time, and arterial blood pressure (preferably directly measured by intra-arterial catheterization).

Planning and Implementation of Care

Altered Tissue Perfusion (Global) Related to Systemic Vasodilatation and Myocardial Depression Independent nursing interventions related to this nursing diagnosis include surveillance of patient status (as in

NURSING DIAGNOSES

Nursing diagnoses for the patient with circulatory effects of MOSF are partially addressed in the section on shock, p. 599. The primary nursing diagnoses relating to circulatory factors include:

- Altered tissue perfusion (global)
- Decreased cardiac output

Assessment, p. 599) and maintenance of the patient at rest in order to decrease metabolic and circulatory demand. Collaborative interventions include administering vasoconstrictors and fluid, and providing inotropic support to restore effective ventricular contractility.

Decreased Cardiac Output Related to the Presence of Circulating Myocardial Depressant Factors Independent nursing interventions for this nursing diagnosis are virtually identical to those above.

Outcome Evaluation   At discharge from the critical-care unit, the patient with circulatory effects of MOSF should optimally demonstrate these criteria:

- Return to baseline level of consciousness.
- Vital signs stable.
- Capillary refill time less than 2 seconds.
- Freedom from dependence on vasopressors or inotropic drugs.
- Urine output greater than 30 ml/hour.

Pulmonary Effects of Multiple Organ Systems Failure

Neutrophil activation and inflammatory mediator secretion (see Chapter 18) have been implicated in the pathophysiology of adult respiratory distress syndrome (ARDS). Please refer to Chapter 8 for nursing care related to ARDS.

Metabolic Effects of Multiple Organ Systems Failure

The inflammatory mediators released during MOSF cause multiple changes in cellular metabolism. The release often culminates in a phenomenon called *hypermetabolism,* which is well characterized in the

literature. This phase usually begins 3–4 days after the patient's initial resuscitation and can occur concomitantly with ARDS. Liver and renal involvement are common, as reflected by elevated serum creatinine and bilirubin levels. The increase in tissue oxygen demand due to systemic effects of inflammatory mediators causes a flow-dependent state, and if oxygen delivery is marginal or inadequate, cellular damage results. A fall in systemic vascular resistance occurs, and vasoactive amines (epinephrine and norepinephrine) are released. Cardiac output and index increase, and the cells begin to metabolize more amino acids and fewer carbohydrates as the preferred substrate to fuel the increased energy expenditure (Cerra 1989).

In addition, organs of the gastrointestinal system can suffer tissue ischemia related to the systemic hypoperfusion caused by the inflammatory process. The reperfusion of these highly vascular organs after resuscitation allows systemic release of the toxic mediators that were produced by the normal flora of the gut during this hypoxic interval; this effect may contribute significantly to the systemic inflammatory process. As a result, stress ulcers may occur, along with central lobular necrosis of the liver and ischemic pancreatitis (Collins 1990).

Assessment

Signs and Symptoms Each organ may be assessed individually. Stomach ulceration surveillance involves intraluminal pH measurement, using pH paper or, optimally, an indwelling nasogastric tube with an electrical pH sensor. Diagnosis of stomach ulceration is typically confirmed by positive guaiac findings in the stomach secretions or stool. Pancreatic dysfunction is often heralded by pain, restlessness, agitation, diaphoresis, and/or nausea and vomiting. Intestinal ischemia and ileus are demonstrated by abdominal distention, hyper- or hypoactive bowel sounds, and abdominal pain. Vomiting and diarrhea are also typical (Collins 1990).

Nutritional assessment, pivotal to the care of the patient with gastrointestinal failure, is discussed in Chapter 19.

Laboratory Data The transition to the hypermetabolic state has several laboratory hallmarks. Urine nitrogen excretion is greatly increased. Serum glucose is elevated due to high hepatic glucose release and a relative insulin resistance. Plasma ketones are negligible. Serum albumin and transferrin are decreased secondary to lowered levels of synthesis (Cerra 1989).

Measurement of serum calcium, magnesium, lipase, and amylase levels assists in assessment of pancreatic function. Glucagon release from the ischemic pancreas causes calcitonin release from the thyroid, which reduces serum calcium and magnesium levels. Lipase and amylase elevate, and lipase remains increased for a longer period of time. Definitive diagnosis of pancreatic abscess or pseudocyst is confirmed by computed tomography of the abdomen, which reveals a fluid-filled cavity. Bleeding may occur in the retroperitoneal space, revealed by a decrease in the hemoglobin and hematocrit levels. Assessment of hepatic function is accomplished using laboratory tests, including direct and indirect bilirubin, serum ammonia, aspartate aminotransferase (AST [SGOT]) and alanine aminotransferase (ALT [SGPT]) levels. All of these values are elevated in hepatic failure, discussed in Chapter 19 (Collins 1990).

NURSING DIAGNOSES

Nursing diagnoses for patients with metabolic effects of MOSF are partially addressed in the section on shock, p. 591. The primary nursing diagnosis relating to metabolic factors is:

- Altered nutrition (less than body requirements) related to impaired absorption and metabolism of presented nutrients

Planning and Implementation of Care   Independent nursing interventions relating to this diagnosis are primarily limited to surveillance, and collaborative nursing interventions are centered around supplementing the patient's nutritional intake. As with any patient, use of the gut for feeding preserves the integrity of the mucosal barrier and can provide adequate nutritional supplementation if no ileus or ischemia are present. However, most patients in multiple organ systems failure have been taking nothing by mouth (NPO) for some time and will demonstrate lactose intolerance due to the loss of lactase from the brush border of the intestinal lumen (Mathewson Kuhn 1990). This loss is temporary but can cause an interval of diarrhea, bloating, and increased production of intestinal gas.

The results of the nutritional assessment performed by nursing, dietary, or medical personnel are used to plan caloric and nutrient dosages using current guidelines. Suggested therapies include: 30–35 nonprotein calories/kg/day, with 3–5 g/kg/day as glucose, and fat emulsions restricted to less than 1 g/kg/day; achievement of nitrogen equilibrium without concern for exact caloric balance; and use of modified (high branched-

chain) amino acid formulas to achieve positive protein synthesis as measured by plasma prealbumin and/or transferrin levels (Lekander and Cerra 1990).

Outcome Evaluation   At discharge from the critical-care unit, the patient with metabolic effects of MOSF should optimally demonstrate:

- Independence from hyperalimentation with positive nitrogen balance.
- Active bowel sounds with formed stools.
- Maintenance of adequate serum glucose levels without ketonemia or hyperosmolarity.
- Absence of abdominal pain, tenderness, or anorexia.

Hematologic Effects of Multiple Organ Systems Failure (Disseminated Intravascular Coagulation [DIC])

Bleeding diatheses in critical care are most frequently a consequence of multiple organ systems failure. With hepatic function impairment, clotting factors manufactured in the liver are depleted; in addition, venous stasis secondary to hypoperfusion can activate the clotting cascade in small vessels, further depleting stores of clotting factors. This phenomenon can lead to the syndrome known as *disseminated intravascular coagulation* (DIC).

Assessment   The assessment of the patient at risk for hematologic failure centers on awareness of risk factors and the detection of bleeding.

Risk Conditions   Numerous conditions place patients at risk for development of DIC, including:

- *Tissue injury.* Trauma, burns, crush syndrome, snake bite
- *Antigen/antibody reactions.* Anaphylactic reactions, incompatible blood transfusions, transplant rejections
- *Obstetric emergencies.* Abruptio placentae, amniotic fluid embolism, incomplete abortion, retained dead fetus
- *Neoplasms.* Leukemia, solid tumors
- *Infections.* Septic shock
- *Prolonged hypotension.*
- *Acidosis.*

In a patient with DIC, procoagulant release initiates uncontrolled microcirculatory clotting. Several procoagulants have been implicated, including bacterial

RESEARCH NOTE

Baggs J et al.: The association between interdisciplinary collaboration and patient outcomes in a medical intensive care unit. *Heart Lung* 1992; 21(1):18–24.

CLINICAL APPLICATION

Nurses who work in critical-care units are aware that the relationship between physicians and nurses in their unit has an influence on patient care. When the landmark study by Knaus et al. (1986) demonstrated a relationship between interdisciplinary collaboration in critical care and patient mortality, many nurses saluted the empirical validation of what their experience already told them. Since that time, however, the nursing and medical literature has discussed but not validated or duplicated Knaus' group's findings.

The study carried out by Baggs and her colleagues (both physicians and nurses) examines the relationship between the amount of interdisciplinary collaboration involved in the decision to transfer a patient from critical care and the eventual fate of the patient. Both staff nurses and ICU residents completed a battery of instruments including the Collaborative Practice Scales, a Decision About Transfer scale, and a measurement of the number of alternatives available in a given patient transfer decision. In addition, the 286 consecutive patients whose transfer was examined were evaluated using the Acute Physiology and Chronic Health Evaluation (APACHE II) severity of illness scale. Correlations between the amount of collaboration reported separately by nurses and physicians, the individual patient's severity of illness, and the eventual patient outcomes were calculated.

A statistically significant correlation was demonstrated between the amount of collaboration the nurses perceived in the transfer decision and the risk of negative patient outcome ($p = 0.02$). Residents' report of the level of collaboration was not so related ($p = 0.859$). APACHE II scores were used to control for the severity of patient illness during the multiple linear regression analysis. Interestingly, the correlation between nurses' and physicians' perception of collaboration was quite low, as calculated by the Pearson product-moment statistic ($r = 0.10$, $p = 0.10$).

What all these statistics mean is that when nurses perceived the decision to transfer a patient as a collaborative one, the transfer's risk to the patient decreased from 16% to 5%, a threefold reduction.

CRITICAL THINKING

Limitations: The study is limited, having been conducted at a single site with a single group of physicians and nurses. Physicians and nurses may not define collaboration in the same way. In addition, collaboration itself may not really be the variable causing the difference, but only a perception of the staff actually related to another, unknown variable.

Strengths: Both this study and the work by Knaus and associates emphasize that critical-care nurses have a duty to convey to physician colleagues all the information that may be pertinent when treatment decisions are made and the physicians have a duty to listen.

---

toxins, free hemoglobin, and fragments of cancer or placental tissue. If the procoagulants damage the endothelial wall, they can activate the intrinsic clotting pathway, the complement system, or the plasmin/kinin system. If they injure tissue, the procoagulants can activate the extrinsic clotting pathway. In many instances, the triggering event activates more than one pathway (Bell 1990).

Whatever the triggering mechanism, explosive thrombin production occurs, causing three major problems: *diffuse fibrin deposition in the microcirculation, avid consumption of clotting factors,* and *provocation of the fibrinolytic system.*

Almost all patients with DIC have suffered an episode of prolonged hypotension. In hypotension, arterial vasoconstriction combined with capillary dilatation and the opening of preferential arteriovenous shunts leads to stagnation of blood in many capillaries. The blood pooled in the capillaries rapidly becomes acidotic, which exacerbates the situation, as acidemia is itself a procoagulant. As the abnormal procoagulants accumulate in the acidotic blood, widespread clotting occurs in the microcirculation, and in turn causes pervasive organ ischemia and necrosis. As the capillaries of an average adult represent a total length of approximately 100,000 miles, clotting factors are consumed faster than they can be replaced, hence the term *consumption coagulopathy* sometimes used to describe DIC.

The presence of thrombin also activates the fibrinolytic system, which acts as a homeostatic mechanism to maintain patency of the microcirculation in compensation for the widespread obstruction to blood flow caused by the diffuse clotting. The fibrinolytic system limits clotting and in so doing produces *fibrin degradation products* (FDPs, also known as FSPs [fibrin split products]). The FDPs also act as anticoagulants, interfering with the activity of thrombin, fibrin, and platelets (Guyton 1991).

Following the initial clotting and fibrinolysis, a web of fibrin and FDPs is left in the microcirculation. This web mechanically damages red blood cells trying to pass through it, producing fragmented red blood cells, schistocytes, and hemolytic anemia. As a result of the decreased availability of coagulation factors and the increased presence of anticoagulants, the patient's blood is unable to form stable clots where they are needed, and bleeding occurs into the skin, from body orifices, and at sites of catheters and incisions.

Signs and Symptoms   DIC can occur in chronic, subacute, and acute forms. The *chronic* form is seen in patients with chronic DIC-provoking disorders, such as leukemia. With the *subacute* form, the typical laboratory indications of DIC are present but the patient does not yet show clinical signs. In the *acute* form, the earliest sign is slow venous bleeding, appearing as blood oozing from multiple sites, such as sites of indwelling vascular catheters and blood sample punctures, or around nasotracheal or nasogastric tubes. The integumentary system displays subcutaneous ecchymoses, petechiae, and purpura. Symptoms may progress to acrocyanosis (patchy cyanosis of the fingers and toes) or necrosis of extremities. Signs of organ ischemia and necrosis, such as seizure activity, angina or acute tubular necrosis, may be present. Finally, frank gastrointestinal bleeding or other life-threatening bleeding episodes may occur.

Laboratory Data   Laboratory measures of hematopoiesis and coagulation can provide helpful assessment clues when used as adjuncts to the patient's history and physical examination.

Complete Blood Count (CBC) and Reticulocyte Count

The complete blood count (CBC) is a series of tests that provides a comprehensive evaluation of the blood's formed elements. This common group of laboratory tests measures red blood cells *(erythrocytes),* white blood cells *(leukocytes),* and *platelets* (Figure 20–2). Red blood cells (RBCs) have three major functions: oxygen transport, carbon dioxide transport, and acid–base buffering. In the normal adult, RBC production occurs in the marrow of membranous bones; for example, the vertebrae, sternum, ribs, and pelvis. Production is stimulated by *erythropoietin,* a glycoprotein formed primarily in the kidneys in response to hypoxia. Normal red blood cell formation requires the presence of amino acids, iron, vitamin B_{12}, folic acid, and other nutrients (Guyton 1991).

Red blood cell measures contained in the CBC are the red cell count, hemoglobin level, and hematocrit. The normal *red cell count* varies with sex, age, altitude, and exercise. It usually falls within 5.1–5.8 million per ml for males and 4.3–5.2 million per ml for females. *Hemoglobin* is an iron–protein complex, formed and carried inside RBCs, that functions in O_2 and Co_2 transport and in acid–base buffering. Males usually have a hemoglobin level between 14 and 18 g per 100 ml and females between 12 and 16 g per 100 ml. The *hematocrit* expresses the volume percentage of red blood cells in whole blood and normally ranges between 40% and 54% for males and between 37% and 47% for females. The red cell count, hemoglobin level, and hematocrit usually follow the same trend. Elevated values, for instance, occur with hemoconcentration due to blood loss, dehydration, and polycythemia. Decreased values are seen in fluid overload, recent hemorrhage, and anemia.

Additional information on red cell production is available from a separately ordered reticulocyte count. *Reticulocytes* are immature RBCs, which usually represent 0.5–2.0% of the RBC count. An increased reticulocyte count indicates an accelerated rate of RBC production, as would be seen in hemolysis or hemorrhage. A decreased count indicates depressed bone marrow production of red cells, as in aplastic anemia, or acute blood loss.

The CBC contains a total white cell count and a differential white cell count (see Chapter 18 for further discussion of white blood cells).

Platelets (thrombocytes) are also formed in the bone marrow. The normal platelet count is 250,000–400,000/ ml. Platelets initiate blood clotting, as explained in detail in the next section on blood coagulation. The platelet count is decreased in most leukemias and idiopathic thrombocytopenic purpura, and elevated in some anemias, severe hemorrhage, and thrombocytosis (Guyton 1991).

Blood Coagulation

Blood coagulation involves an intricate sequence of chemical reactions that remains only partly understood despite years of investigation. The following simplified explanation is based on Guyton (1991).

When a blood vessel ruptures, hemostasis occurs in several steps. First, vessel spasm limits the amount of blood loss. Second, a platelet plug forms when platelets adhere in layers to the roughened endothelial surface. Third, a blood clot forms. Fourth, fibroblasts invade

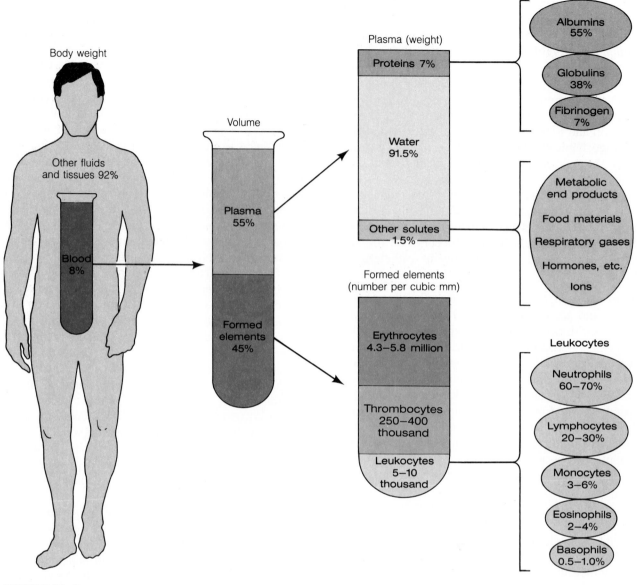

FIGURE 20–2

Components of blood. (From: Spence A: *Basic human anatomy,* 2d ed. Redwood City, CA: Benjamin/Cummings, 1986.)

the clot and organize it into fibrous tissue within 8–10 days, or, less commonly, the clot dissolves.

Prothrombin and fibrinogen, two plasma proteins formed by the liver, are instrumental in clotting. Coagulation occurs in three major steps: the *formation of prothrombin activator* (Stage I), the *conversion of prothrombin to thrombin* (Stage II), and the *conversion of fibrinogen to fibrin* (Stage III).

Prothrombin can be activated by two systems, both of which are difficult to describe, as steps in the coagulation process cascade, and several steps occur simultaneously (Figure 20–3). Vascular injury initiates

an intrinsic activator system, whereas tissue damage initiates an extrinsic system. Although separated for analytic purposes, these systems interact in the patient.

Trauma to the blood or blood contact with subendothelial collagen appears to initiate the *intrinsic pathway.* The initiating event causes platelets to release platelet phospholipids, and it activates Factor XII, which in turn activates Factor XI, which subsequently activates Factor IX. Activated Factor IX next activates Factor VIII, which in the presence of platelet phospholipids and calcium activates Factor X.

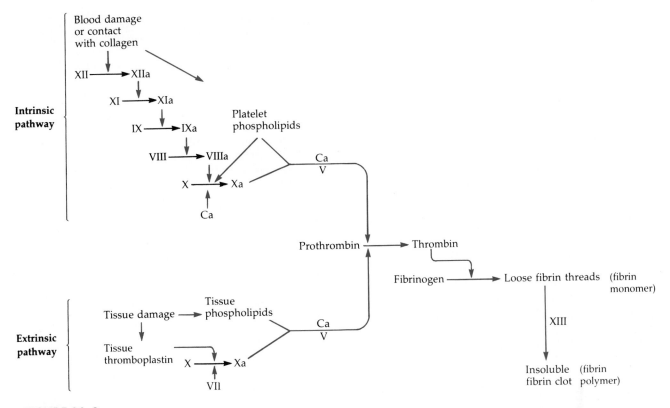

FIGURE 20–3

Coagulation process.

In the *extrinsic system,* damaged tissue releases thromboplastin and tissue phospholipids. Thromboplastin interacts with Factor VII in the presence of calcium and tissue phospholipids to activate Factor X.

From the activation of Factor X, clotting proceeds almost identically for both pathways. Activated Factor X interacts with Factor V, calcium, and platelet or tissue phospholipids to convert prothrombin to thrombin. Thrombin is a proteolytic enzyme that in turn converts fibrinogen to fibrin.

Loose fibrin threads adhere to the vessel wall, forming a network that traps platelets, RBCs, and plasma. Factor XIII forms the loose threads into an insoluble fibrin clot, which then retracts, squeezing out the plasma and further binding the margins of the vessel rupture. Large numbers of platelets, which apparently bond the fibrin threads together, are needed for the retraction.

The formation of fibrin activates a fibrinolytic system that limits clotting to the area of injury. When a clot is formed, it incorporates a plasma protein called *plasminogen* (profibrinolysin). Although the mechanisms are unclear, plasminogen can be activated by several substances. Activated plasminogen becomes plasmin (fibrinolysin), a proteolytic enzyme that di-gests the fibrin threads and destroys the surrounding clotting factors.

Endogenous anticoagulants normally prevent spontaneous blood clotting and clot extension. Among the most important anticoagulant determinants are the smoothness of vascular endothelium and a negatively charged inner layer of endothelium that repels platelets and clotting factors. Also, the rapidity of blood flow tends to carry clotting factors away from a developing clot, thereby limiting clot size. In addition, the clot's fibrin threads trap most of the thrombin, and antithrombin-heparin cofactor and fibrin degradation products released during fibrinolysis inactivate the remainder.

Finally, the blood contains heparin, a strong anticoagulant produced primarily by the mast cells located around the capillaries in the lungs and liver. Heparin interrupts both coagulation and fibrinolysis by inhibiting the action of thrombin (thereby inhibiting platelet aggregation and the conversion of fibrinogen to fibrin), inhibiting the activation of Factor X (thereby blocking both the intrinsic and extrinsic pathways contributing to thrombin formation), and preventing further extension of already developed clots.

Coagulation Profile

A coagulation profile is used as a preoperative screening measure or as an aid in diagnosing a bleeding disorder. Although numerous tests may be ordered, the most common are the clotting time, activated partial thromboplastin time, prothrombin time, and fibrinogen level. As with other laboratory tests, normal values vary among laboratories.

The clotting or coagulation time is a general indicator of the blood's clotting ability and is used to evaluate the intrinsic pathway. It is determined on a venous sample by a number of methods, most commonly either the *activated clotting time (ACT)* or the Lee-White procedure. For the *Lee-White procedure,* blood is mixed gently at 30-second intervals, and the time required for it to clot is noted. Because numerous factors participate in the clotting process, this test is nonspecific for clotting abnormalities. For the ACT, a substance that activates Factor XII is added to the blood. A prolonged clotting time may indicate anticoagulant therapy, liver disease, or a deficiency of any factor except VII. Results are influenced by extraneous factors such as tube size and room temperature.

Because standardized results for the clotting time are so difficult to obtain, some physicians prefer the *activated partial thromboplastin time (APTT),* which tests both the intrinsic and common pathways. The range of normal values is 30–40 seconds. It, too, reflects the general clotting ability of the blood but is faster, more sensitive, and more easily standardized.

The clotting time and activated partial thromboplastin time are used primarily to monitor patients on heparin, but they also are used to detect bleeding tendencies and evaluate hemorrhagic disorders.

Blood used for the *prothrombin time* is a nonfasting, venous sample that is oxalated after drawing to prevent the conversion of prothrombin to thrombin. In the laboratory, calcium is added to neutralize the oxalate, thromboplastin is added to provoke the conversion of prothrombin to thrombin, and the time necessary for fibrin threads to appear is noted. The test thus bypasses the intrinsic clotting process and evaluates the extrinsic system as well as Stages II and III. A control value is also reported, based on the concurrent reactivity of reagents used in the test. The normal prothrombin time is 12–15 seconds. A prolonged prothrombin time may indicate coumarin therapy, liver disease, vitamin K deficiency, or obstructive jaundice due to the deficiency of bile salts blocking intestinal absorption of vitamin K. The prothrombin time is the preferred test for monitoring oral anticoagulant therapy.

The *fibrinogen level* is determined on plasma extracted from a venous blood sample. The normal level

---

NURSING TIP

Drawing Coagulation Studies

If agency protocol allows you to draw blood for coagulation studies from an indwelling arterial line, be sure that other samples are drawn first and that at least 5 ml of fluid has been pulled back before any blood is taken for testing (Harper 1988).

---

is 200–400 mg/100 ml, which decreases in fibrinolytic disorders and in DIC.

A test for the presence of *fibrin degradation products* (FDP) or *fibrin split products* (FSP) may be ordered with hematologic disorders. The levels of these products increase when clot lysis is occurring, whether the lysis is provoked endogenously, such as during DIC, or exogenously, such as during treatment with tissue plasminogen activator or streptokinase.

When a platelet disorder is suspected, the bleeding time and the platelet count are evaluated. The bleeding time measures the platelets' ability to adhere and aggregate, and the platelet count determines the actual number of circulating platelets. Both tests are important for diagnosis. For example, a patient on large doses of aspirin may have adequate numbers of platelets; however, because aspirin prevents platelet aggregation and adhesion, bleeding time will increase.

Although the patient's clinical history is important in diagnosis, DIC is primarily a laboratory, rather than clinical, diagnosis. A panel of tests is evaluated to detect the presence and progress of DIC. The most common laboratory tests used to diagnose DIC are (a) prothrombin time, (b) partial thromboplastin time (PTT), (c) fibrinogen level, (d) platelet count, and (e) fibrin degradation products. In DIC, the prothrombin time and PTT are prolonged due to the depletion of prothrombin and Factor V. The fibrinogen level decreases due to fibrinogen depletion, and the platelet count diminishes due to platelet consumption. In contrast to the decrease in the fibrinogen level and the platelet count, fibrin degradation products increase.

Planning and Implementation of Care

Fluid Volume Deficit Related to Hemorrhage Independent nursing interventions for this diagnosis are primarily related to surveillance. Observe for the subtle signs that signal the onset of DIC. In addition to

NURSING DIAGNOSES

Because of the complexity of the hematologic effects of multiple organ systems failure, multiple nursing diagnoses may apply, including:

- Fluid volume deficit
- Pain
- Altered tissue perfusion
- Impaired gas exchange
- Altered level of consciousness*
- Fear

*non-NANDA diagnosis

TABLE 20–5

Treatment for Massive Blood Loss

1. Ensure a stable and adequate airway and determine baseline vital signs.
2. Obtain two large-bore intravenous accesses, and draw baseline laboratory studies, including CBC, coagulation studies, and electrolytes.
3. Give crystalloid rapidly until vital signs stabilize.
4. Place direct pressure on any accessible hemorrhage sites.
5. Determine the extent of blood loss, using patient symptoms.
   < 1,000 ml: anxiety
   1,000–1,500 ml: tachycardia, tachypnea, capillary refill > 2 sec
   > 1,500 ml: hypotension, oliguria
6. Order appropriate amounts of crossmatched packed RBCs.
7. Heat the room, warm all solutions, and use a warming blanket to maintain body temperature.
8. If more than 6–8 units of packed RBCs are administered, give fresh frozen plasma with every other unit of RBCs.
9. Give platelets, one unit for every unit of RBCs administered, after at least 8 units of RBCs have been infused.
10. Measure coagulation studies, platelets, and calcium periodically during resuscitation and after.
11. If hypocalcemia is discovered, monitor QT intervals thereafter and administer calcium by slow IV push.

Based on Yeston N, Niehoff J, Dennis R: Transfusion therapy. In *Critical care*, Civetta J, Taylor R, Kirby R (eds). Philadelphia: Lippincott, 1988.

---

observing for the persistent oozing and integumentary signs mentioned earlier, test all secretions and drainage for the presence of occult blood. Observe the degree of bleeding from wound sites, and check for the onset of vaginal bleeding in women. In addition, monitor the blood pressure, and try to prevent surges by keeping the patient calm, using anxiolytics as necessary. Sudden increases in mean arterial pressure can disturb unstable clots and initiate new bleeding episodes. Use judicious fluid administration to prevent hypotensive episodes that can contribute to the self-perpetuating clotting cycle in DIC.

During collaborative interventions, monitor laboratory values, and evaluate the risk of bleeding episodes and the effectiveness of treatment measures. In conjunction with physician caregivers, administer medical and pharmacologic therapy as ordered, treating hypotension and acidosis when present, and monitoring any heparin therapy. Heparin usually is given as a continuous IV infusion with the rate titrated to coagulation values. Use an infusion control device and monitor it closely to ensure its accuracy. Also monitor the clotting time—the therapeutic level usually is 2–3 times normal. Finally, remember to double-check heparin's compatibility with other drugs to avoid accidental over-anticoagulation. Blood products may be administered to the patient with a falling hematocrit instead of, or in addition to, heparinization. Replacement of clotting factors by fresh frozen plasma, cryoprecipitate, and platelet transfusion are the most common methods (Bell 1990).

Many institutions have a transfusion protocol for any patient who shows signs of severe hemorrhage. Table 20–5 describes a sample protocol. It is important to replenish serum calcium, which can be bound by the anticoagulants in banked blood. Also, replenishing platelets is important because fresh frozen plasma dilutes the available platelets in the blood.

Pain Related to Tissue Ischemia   Obstruction of the microvasculature causes ischemic pain. It is important, therefore, to use independent nursing interventions, including distraction and imagery, for analgesia. If these measures fail, assess the patient's need for pain medications. Give pain medications intravenously whenever possible, to provide maximum effectiveness and to avoid creating another potential bleeding site.

Altered Tissue Perfusion Related to Peripheral Microthrombi   Clots in the microcirculation can cause large perfusion deficits. Monitor peripheral perfusion by checking peripheral arterial pulses, skin temperature and color, and capillary filling time.

Impaired Gas Exchange Related to Intrapulmonary Hemorrhage   Intraparenchymal hemorrhage can occur with DIC and obstruct gas exchange at the alveolar-capillary interface. Observe for early signs of hypoxemia, particularly tachycardia, increased respiratory rate, and restlessness. Monitor arterial blood gas values for the development of hypoxemia and hypercapnia.

Altered Level of Consciousness Related to Intracerebral Hemorrhage Intraparenchymal hemorrhage may also occur in the brain, so evaluate the patient's neurologic status frequently. When assessing level of consciousness in patients who do not respond to verbal stimuli, avoid or minimize the use of painful stimuli such as pinching or pressure, which can result in ecchymoses.

Fear Related to Uncertainty of Prognosis The sight of blood produces an emotional response, especially in those patients who are not used to such occurrences. Provision of emotional support is an integral part of independent nursing care of the multisystem organ failure patient. To promote the development of rapport, consistently assign the same nurse to care for the patient. To relieve the patient's and family's anxiety, provide brief explanations of procedures and encourage short, frequent family visits.

You can also use relaxation exercises or guided imagery to relieve patient or family stress. Center visualization exercises on assisting the patient and family to capitalize on inner strengths and mobilize energy for recovery. Support the coping mechanisms used by the patient and family unless they are pathologic. If they are, teach and encourage substitution of healthier coping mechanisms. See Chapters 2 and 3 for suggestions.

ADVANCES IN CRITICAL-CARE TECHNOLOGY

Experimental Therapies of Shock and Multiple Organ Systems Failure

The following discussion is based on information from Baue (1990) and Reines and Cook (1992).

THE TECHNOLOGY

Clinical research on the treatment of shock (especially endotoxin-in-mediated septic shock) and of multiple organ systems failure has produced a number of experimental therapies that show promise in decreasing the morbidity and mortality associated with these clinical crises. A number of experimental therapies focus on chemical inflammatory mediators and on immune modulation.

Inflammatory Mediators An overwhelming response to injury with systemic activation of inflammatory mediators, such as those discussed in Chapter 18, is a major factor in producing multiple organ systems failure. A number of therapies in development focus on blocking these cytokines with monoclonal antibodies that attach and inactivate them. One mediator to which monoclonal antibodies have been developed is tumor necrosis factor (TNF), which is capable of inducing shock even in isolation.

Immune Modulation In addition, monoclonal antibodies have been developed against the lipids found in endotoxin manufactured by Gram-negative bacteria. This endotoxin acts as a major activator of the immune response in both sepsis and MOSF.

Superoxide Scavengers Phagocytosis by granulocytes is accompanied by the release of a number of toxic forms of oxygen, including superoxide anion (O_2^-), hydrogen peroxide, and hydroxyl radicals (OH^-). The hydrogen peroxide forms other toxic chemicals within the cell, notably hypochlorous acid and halogens. Substances have been developed that protect the body from these toxic oxygen radicals; the best experimental documentation exists for *superoxide dismutase*. These treatments remain experimental, however.

PATIENT CARE CONSIDERATIONS

As with all experimental treatments, good nursing care demands that patients and/or surrogates be aware of the nature of such therapies and give informed consent for their use. In addition, the high cost of many of the new immunotherapeutic agents—sometimes thousands of dollars per dose—is a consideration in settings where the likelihood of reimbursement is limited or where a large proportion of patients are un- or underinsured. Critical-care nurses must keep abreast of the frequent changes in types of assistance for patients for whom the cost of medical care can be a limiting factor; often, social service personnel can be helpful in advocacy for such patients and should be consulted early.

Outcome Evaluation   At discharge from the critical-care unit, the patient with hematologic effects of MOSF ideally will demonstrate these outcome criteria:

- Absence of signs and symptoms of spontaneous hemorrhage.
- Absence of detectable blood in urine, stool, and gastric drainage.
- Normal skin turgor, capillary refill time, skin color, and peripheral pulses.
- Absence or control of pain.

Renal Effects of Multiple Organ Systems Failure

Hypoperfusion has dramatic effects on renal function; in fact, urine output is frequently used as an index of circulatory adequacy. Renal autoregulatory ability is lost below a mean arterial pressure of approximately 75 mm Hg, and poor perfusion of renal tissues for more than 25 minutes results in some degree of renal function impairment (Lancaster 1990). Assessment, diagnosis, and treatment of acute renal failure is discussed in detail in Chapter 15.

Prognosis: Effect of Number of Organ Systems in Failure

A number of studies in the past decade correlating the number of organ systems in failure with the probability of survival show two organ systems in failure associated with a mortality rate from 64–83%, and three systems in failure leading to a fatal outcome in 82–98% of those studied (Knaus and Wagner 1989). These studies, however, use very liberal definitions of organ failure; for example, pulmonary failure was defined as three days of ventilator dependence. Multiple organ systems failure is a serious complication of any critical illness, but precise mortality estimates are not available and are of questionable use in evaluating an individual case.

Ethical Issues in Multiple Organ Systems Failure

Given the dismal prognostic statistics cited above, patients in multiple organ systems failure are often candidates for life support removal. These discussions often occur in the context of utilization review, a shortage of critical-care beds and nurses, and increasing levels of professional burnout. A complete discussion of ethical issues in these cases is beyond the scope of this volume; consult Chapter 2 for a discussion of general ethical issues.

Multisystem disorders include a spectrum of syndromes that are a result of our ability to prolong the lives of those who, without technologic intervention, would have died from their initial pathophysiologic processes. As technology advances, the prevalence of these syndromes may increase. Critical-care nurses must prepare to face the challenges presented by these patients and their families.

REFERENCES

Baue A: *Multiple organ failure: Patient care and prevention.* St. Louis: Mosby-Year Book, 1990.

Bell T: Disseminated intravascular coagulation and shock: Multisystem crisis in the critically ill. *Crit Care Nurs Clin North Am* 1990; 2(2):255–268.

Benner, P: *From novice to expert: excellence and power in clinical nursing practice.* Menlo Park, CA: Addison-Wesley, 1984.

Bersten A, Sibbald W: Circulatory disturbances in multiple systems organ failure. *Crit Care Clin* 1989; 5(2): 233–254.

Beutler B: Cachectin in tissue injury, shock, and related states. *Crit Care Clin* 1989; 5(2):353–367.

Cerra F: Hypermetabolism–organ failure syndrome: A metabolic response to injury. *Crit Care Clin* 1989; 5(2):289–300.

Collins A: Gastrointestinal complications in shock. *Crit Care Nurs Clin North Am* 1990; 2(2):269–278.

Gotshall R, Wood V, Miles D: Modified head-up tilt test for orthostatic challenge of critically ill patients. *Crit Care Med* 1989; 17(11):1156–1158.

Guyton A: *Textbook of medical physiology,* 8th ed. Philadelphia: Saunders, 1991.

Harper J: The use of heparinized intra-arterial lines to obtain coagulation samples. *Focus Crit Care* 1988; 15(5):51–55.

Harper J: Third level hemodynamics. *Dimen Crit Care Nurs* 1992; 11(3):130–143.

Houston M: Pathophysiology of shock. *Crit Care Nurs Clin North Am* 1990; 2(2):143–150.

Knaus W et al.: An evaluation of outcome from intensive care in major medical centers. *Ann Intern Med* 1986; 104:410–418.

Knaus W, Wagner D: Multiple systems organ failure: Epidemiology and prognosis. *Crit Care Clin* 1989; 5(2):221–232.

Lancaster L: Renal response to shock. *Crit Care Nurs Clin North Am* 1990; 2(2):221–233.

Lekander B, Cerra F: The syndrome of multiple organ failure. *Crit Care Nurs Clin North Am* 1990; 2(2):331–342.

Macho J, Luce J: Rational approach to the management of multiple systems organ failure. *Crit Care Clin* 1989; 5(2):379–392.

Mathewson Kuhn M: Nutritional support for the shock patient. *Crit Care Nurs Clin North Am* 1990; 2(2):201–220.

McCance K: Altered cellular and tissue biology. In *Pathophysiology: The biologic basis for disease in adults and children,* McCance K, Huether S (eds). St. Louis: Mosby, 1990.

Pinsky M, Matuschak G: Multiple systems organ failure: Failure of host defense homeostasis. *Crit Care Clin* 1989; 5(2):199–220.

Reines HD, Cook JA: Prostaglandins. Pages 123–141 in *Multiple system organ failure,* Fry, DE (ed). St. Louis: Mosby-Year Book, 1992.

Rice V: Shock, a clinical syndrome: An update. Part 1. An overview of shock. *Crit Care Nurs* 1991; 11(4):20–27.

Roach A: Antibiotic therapy in septic shock. *Crit Care Nurs Clin North Am* 1990; 2(2):201–220.

Shoemaker W: Shock states: Pathophysiology, monitoring, outcome prediction, and therapy. In *Textbook of critical care,* 2d ed, Shoemaker W et al (eds). Philadelphia: Saunders, 1989.

Shoemaker W: Therapy of shock based on pathophysiology, monitoring, and outcome prediction. *Crit Care Med* 1990; 18(1):S19–S25.

Vaughan P, Brooks C: Adult respiratory distress syndrome: A complication of shock. *Crit Care Nurs Clin North Am* 1990; 2(2):235–253.

Yeston N, Niehoff J, Dennis R: Transfusion therapy. In *Critical care,* Civetta J, Taylor R, Kirby R (eds). Philadelphia: Lippincott, 1988.

21

Trauma

CLINICAL INSIGHT

Domain: The helping role

Competency: The healing relationship: creating a climate for and establishing a commitment to healing

Trauma nursing involves a great deal of caring about, as well as caring for, a critically ill patient. In the Trauma Intensive Care Unit (TICU), the patient requires sensitive, healing touch and support from nursing staff who care intensely about life and about the quality of the patient's experience in the unit. Trauma nursing staff are strong, intelligent, decisive people with an overwhelming need to do things right the first time. Trauma care is team work, and collaborative practice facilitates a positive outcome for the patient. You, the nurse, are in a unique position to provide support and reassurance as well as physical care to further enhance a positive outcome.

Here, a nurse demonstrates expertise in identifying a critically ill 19-year-old patient's needs and in following through using feedback from the patient, excellent patient education, and reassuring touch in the face of extreme circumstances. The patient has undergone a limb-saving procedure—surgical repair of a bullet laceration of the right femoral artery and vein—sustained when he was shot while committing a felony. He has returned from the postanesthesia care unit on a ventilator, with an arterial line, Foley catheter, and right chest tube in place. This exemplar demonstrates the essential nature of the team concept and collaborative practice in planning and coordinating care, as Nancy, an expert nurse, describes how she works with Dan, a recent graduate of the critical-care residency program, and with the patient.

Dan says, "Come look at this foot. I can't get a pulse, and it's blue. Looks like he's developed a

*compartment syndrome." "OK, Dan," I reply, "call
the orthopedic surgeon on tonight." Dan says,
"Ortho is on the way. He wants us to set up for pressure monitoring and check with O.R. (operating
room) for a room if we need to do fasciotomies, but
he says he will do them in the room here if we
don't have an O.R. available." I approach the bedside and speak to Jeff, the patient. "Hi, I'm Nancy.
I am a nurse. I will be helping Dan. The pain in
your leg is from a lack of blood to your lower leg
and foot. It's so swollen that the blood can't get
down to your toes. We are going to give you something for the pain. We're going to check the pressure
in your leg (compartment). When you are all
numb, your doctor will make some cuts so that the
pressure on the artery will be relieved. It hurts now,
but the blood will be able to go through the artery,
and then most of the pain will go away." Jeff signals
consent after being informed that if he does not
have the fasciotomies he could lose his foot. I say to
him, "We are going to give you some medicine in
the tubing, three kinds. The first (morphine sulfate)
will make the pain go away and make you really
sleepy. The second (midazolam, Versed) will relax you—you may go to sleep—and help you forget
how scary this feels right now. Before I give the
last one (vecuronium, Norcuron, a neuromuscular
blocking agent), you may be asleep. You may still be
able to hear us. When I give you this medicine you
will not be able to open your eyes; you won't be
able to breathe by yourself, but this machine that is
breathing with you now will do it all; you'll be
fine. Dan and I will be right here the whole
time. . . . We know that you won't be able to move.
You won't hurt either, because I am going to give
you lots of medicine to help you relax and feel
no pain. What questions do you have?" Jeff responds
with a shoulder shrug, looking scared. "Remember,
we'll be right here with you until you wake up."
Jeff dozes off, the vent takes over with full, regular
respirations, vital signs stay stable, and heart rate
is unchanged during the procedure (one nice objective measure that he is feeling no pain or anxiety,
which would cause a catecholamine release and
increase heart rate). The next day, I see Jeff again.
"Hi, Jeff." I read Jeff's lips around the endotracheal tube: "Thanks. I remember your voice. You
stayed with me and talked to me. I felt scared, but
I could hear your voice."*

Trauma is defined as injury resulting from an
external force. It may be accidental, self-inflicted, or the
result of an act of violent aggression. By its very nature,
trauma is thrust upon an individual suddenly and

dramatically; there is no time for psychologic preparation. The nurse plays a pivotal role not only in caring for
the patient physically after a traumatic experience but
also in helping the person cope psychologically with
the aftermath of trauma. The importance of caring in
trauma practice cannot be overestimated. Without
benefit of caring, the patient's body may survive, but
the patient may be so traumatized by the event and by
the treatment that normal function is no longer
possible.

This chapter describes the physiologic and psychologic manifestations of traumatic injury and its treatment in the critical-care setting, not in the prehospital
or resuscitative area. It presents concepts related to the
initial phases of treatment only when they are essential
to the *critical-care management* of this complex patient.
The discussion assumes mastery of assessment skills
and the foundation presented in other chapters within
this text. Additional material includes an overview of
trauma care systems and their development and a
discussion of geriatric considerations and research
challenges.

Scope of Trauma

Traumatic injury is a major public health problem. It is
the leading cause of death in persons up to 44 years old
and the fourth most prevalent cause of death in persons
of all ages. Motor vehicle crashes are the most frequent
cause of death for people 1–34 years old.

Deliberate or accidental injury kills about 150,000
Americans annually and permanently disables an
additional 400,000 people. Approximately $58 billion
are spent annually on auto crashes alone (Zador 1991).
In its report on trauma, "Injury in America: A Continuing Public Health Problem," the 1991 Committee on
Trauma Research for the National Research Council
reports that 15 years after its first publication the
problems have not changed very much (Champion et
al. 1990).

Nearly 55% of patients die as a result of inadequate
availability of services (Trunkey and Lewis 1991).
Hypoxia and hypovolemia are major causes of death in
15–35% of all victims of head injury (Trunkey and
Lewis 1991). With a well-implemented trauma system,
endotracheal intubation can be carried out in the field
and could result in the survival of 40% of those
head-injury patients.

Trauma may be categorized into minor or major
injuries. *Minor trauma* is a single-system injury that
does not pose a threat to life or limb. Appropriate
treatment can be provided in hospital emergency

departments. On the other hand, victims of *major or multiple trauma*—serious single- or multiple-system injuries—require immediate and specialized intervention to prevent loss of life or limb. For victims of major trauma, the first hour after injury is a critical period in which definitive care predicts survival. Regionalization of trauma care and the designation of trauma centers helps to ensure that such patients receive optimum care.

The Trauma System Concept

A systems approach to trauma care requires a coordinated system of triage and treatment in the field, an organized communication network, air and ground transportation, trauma centers (tertiary centers designated within a population area), public and professional education programs, and a scientific plan for the evaluation of care. The Committee on Trauma of the American College of Surgeons has published documents describing four patient components and five societal components of a trauma system (Trunkey and Lewis 1991). The four patient components of the trauma system are: (1) access to care through an organized emergency medical services system; (2) prehospital care and transportation during the first critical hour after injury; (3) hospital care, including a skilled, caring staff of specialists available 24 hours a day; and (4) rehabilitation to promote return to the community and minimize disability. The five societal components of the trauma system are: (1) prevention, (2) disaster medical care, (3) education, (4) research, and (5) the economics of trauma care or resource allocation. Selected aspects of these patient and societal components are discussed in the sections that follow.

Trauma Prevention

Prevention is a major goal of responsible trauma care, for most injuries can be avoided; trauma is rarely an accident. The American College of Surgeons, in its 1986 guidelines entitled, "Hospital and Prehospital Resources for Optimal Care of the Injured Patient," has challenged our society to institute active prevention programs, because prevention is the most cost-effective method for reducing death and disability from trauma. Prevention is very difficult, however, because it requires that we confront societal problems such as alcohol consumption (as it relates to driving), handgun control, mandatory restraints, helmet laws, and violent

crimes associated with drugs. As critical-care nurses, responsible adults, and caring human beings, we must meet the challenge, because we are in an ideal position to facilitate change and make prevention a reality.

Alcohol Abuse "Alcoholism" refers to the repeated ingestion of alcohol, resulting in dependence, physical disease, and other types of harm including psychologic and social problems (Grupp, Perlanski and Stewart 1991). Alcohol abuse is a major contributor to trauma; approximately 80% of drivers involved in fatal vehicular crashes have blood alcohol concentrations (BAC) over the legal limit, which varies by state. Alcoholic trauma patients, who may have chronic debility, pre-existent organ failure, and/or withdrawal symptoms, are at high risk for complications during the critical-care phase.

The prevention and treatment of alcohol abuse is beyond the scope of this chapter; however, several programs bear mentioning. Community programs such as Mothers Against Drunk Driving have been instrumental in raising social awareness of the consequences of drinking and driving and toughening the laws against violators of drunk driving statutes. School programs such as Students Against Drunk Driving have been helpful in educating school-age children about the consequences of drinking and driving.

Management of chronic alcoholism remains a serious problem for our society, despite the existence of Alcoholics Anonymous and other intervention and recovery programs. Research on physiologic factors that control alcohol intake suggests a possible new approach. This work indicates that the renin-angiotensin system, which is a potent mediator of fluid and electrolyte balance, modulates alcohol intake (Grupp et al. 1991). This discovery may result in new and more effective pharmacologic treatments for reducing alcohol intake, such as the administration of angiotensin-converting enzyme (ACE) inhibitors. A collaborative consultation service of pharmacologic intervention and behavior modification for chronic alcohol abusers would be one prevention program in which critical-care nurses could participate.

Head and Spinal Cord Injuries Prevention of head and spinal cord injuries has been addressed by several school programs that encourage students to "think first" before diving into shallow water. Other programs have been successful in passing motorcycle helmet laws. Data collected in every state that adopted a helmet law, rescinded it, and then reinstated the law indicated that the cost savings and the number of lives saved were substantial when helmets were worn (McSwain and Belles 1990). Without mandatory helmet laws, use of protective helmets drops 50%. The

CRITICAL-CARE GERONTOLOGY

Geriatric Patients Require Special Care

Preventing geriatric accidents will result in improved quality of life and decreased cost of hospitalization. One recommendation to older adults might include a safe driving course; these courses are offered in many states through the American Association of Retired Persons. Seniors should be reminded to avoid the use of alcohol or to use great care and limit the amount consumed, because their balance, posture, and gait, as well as their fluid and electrolyte levels, are affected. Consistent use of the "buddy system," in which seniors call each other daily, go shopping together, and walk in pairs can help prevent assaults. Careful environmental assessment can ensure that seniors avoid common hazards in the home such as electric cords, throw rugs, small tables, and other objects. The American Trauma Society or your local trauma center can assist you in finding or supporting a prevention program.

Elder abuse remains a major source of geriatric trauma. Laws regarding reporting elder abuse and neglect may vary from state to state. Family coping programs to prevent caregiver burnout have been very helpful in supporting significant others in caring for patients after discharge (Hogstel 1991).

average hospital stay for a helmeted rider is 5.8 days and for nonhelmeted riders 11.8 days.

Violent Assaults   Violence is endemic in our society. Neighborhood Watch programs, which decrease burglary, use of guns, and other violent activity, can help prevent penetrating trauma. As critical-care nurses, we must commit some of our professional activity to injury prevention in our homes, schools, and communities.

Research

"The Major Trauma Outcome Study: Establishing National Norms for Trauma Care" (Champion et al. 1990) is a retrospective descriptive study of injury severity and outcome. One hundred thirty-nine centers nationwide contributed data to the study, which established consistent, systematic reporting and analysis systems for trauma populations. Information from the study forms the largest database in the United States. The study reported an average length of stay of 9.2 days—which is longer than the 7 day figure previously reported by Trunkey and Lewis (1991)—and a 9% mortality rate. These data may be biased, because the study does not include all populations triaged commonly as "trauma." Definitions for terms such as "severely," "critically," or "fatally" injured were unclear, and "severely" injured patients may or may not have been included by all centers. Early trauma center triage patterns in community settings employed strict trans-portation criteria, and many critically injured patients died en route or were never admitted to trauma centers. Systematic nationwide trauma data collection is in its infancy and will continue to grow and provide meaningful statistics on evaluation and outcome for patients, hospitals, and prehospital care systems.

Nursing Roles in Trauma Care

Currently, critical-care nurses specially trained in trauma patient care find challenging responsibilities in independent and interdependent environments. Practice roles in multiple areas of trauma nursing practice are listed below:

- Prehospital care includes direct field care, surface transportation, fixed-wing aircraft and helicopter transportation, and advanced practice roles in rural areas.
- Hospital roles and responsibilities differ depending upon the organization. Clear, exact position descriptions are essential for effective team interaction. Staff are often cross-trained to practice in resuscitation as well as in intensive care areas. Critical-care skills are needed in trauma resuscitation areas and Emergency Department settings, Surgical Intensive Care or Trauma Intensive Care Units, Surgery, and Postanesthesia Care Units. Experienced education and research teams are

critical to improving patient care, increasing positive outcomes, developing specific techniques, and facilitating staff education.

- Trauma Nurse Clinician roles are emerging as a case management approach to decreasing hospitalization costs (Shaver et al. 1991; Songne and Holmquist 1991). Models of care and position descriptions vary. In one model in centers that receive patients inconsistently throughout a 24-hour period, the role may include full-time resuscitation responsibility: the primary nurse follows the patient from resuscitation through surgery and recovery to critical-care admission. Another model may follow a discharge planning style, and some centers employ Clinical Nurse Specialists to support and augment primary professional care.

- Nurses are taking on the role of forensic examiner, especially in rural areas. Trauma experience is invaluable in such a position.

Nursing Process in Trauma

This chapter, which is oriented to the bedside staff nurse caring for the trauma patient, presents general nursing care in trauma first, followed by care related to specific injuries. (An aspect of care pertinent only to chest trauma patients, for example, will be covered in the section on chest trauma rather than in the general nursing process section.)

Assessment

A prioritized, systematic approach to assessing the multiple trauma patient is the key to planning and implementing effective care. The trauma patient arriving in the critical-care unit from the Emergency Department, Trauma Resuscitation Area, Surgery, or Postanesthesia Unit *ideally* has been resuscitated fully. "Resuscitated fully" means the airway has been stabilized, adequate blood and fluids have been administered to reverse hypovolemic shock, and initial injuries have been identified and treated to the point where the patient is considered "stable." Realistically, critically injured trauma patients often are still unstable on admission to the critical-care unit. On admission, therefore, it is essential to ensure that the patient meets these criteria:

- Airway is patent and/or isolated with endotracheal intubation.

- Ventilation is controlled with adequate tidal volume.

- Arterial blood gases are within normal limits for the patient's age and usual state of health, if known.

- Arterial blood pressure is normal for the patient's age and usual state of health.

- Heart rate is within normal range (indicating that volume resuscitation is adequate).

- Pulmonary artery line pressures, if available, are central venous pressure (CVP) 3–8 cm H_2O (2–6 mm Hg), pulmonary capillary wedge pressure (PCWP) 4–12 mm Hg, cardiac index (CI) 4–5.5 L/m^2, systemic vascular resistance (SVR) 800–1,200 dynes (or slightly higher in the presence of stress).

- Capillary refill is present in all extremities and takes less than 3 seconds.

- Temperature is 96–99°F (35.5–37.5°C).

- Intracranial pressure (ICP) and cerebral perfusion pressure (CPP) are at acceptable levels, or measures are in place to decrease them to optimal levels.

- No obvious external bleeding or signs of shock are present.

- Foley catheter is in place and draining at least 30 ml per hour.

- Bladder or pulmonary artery (PA) temperature, if measured, correlates with less accurate measures, such as oral, tympanic, rectal, or axillary temperature.

- Abdomen is soft and is not distended.

- Abdominal drains, if present, are draining but drainage is within expected limits. Irrigant, if used, is infusing and being removed continuously.

- Traction to cervical spine or extremities, if present, is intact and functional.

- All intravenous (IV) sites inserted in the field have been discontinued and replaced.

Older patients may have pre-existent chest and bony chest wall disease, which must be considered when interpreting "normal values." Normal tidal volume for a person with chronic obstructive pulmonary disease (COPD), for example, may be 400–600 ml and oxygen saturation levels may be between 60% and 75%. This patient normally may have a lower hematocrit (Hct) level than a healthy patient and may have a depleted fluid volume status due to chronic diuretic intake. The patient's serum potassium level may be low, with concomitant magnesium depletion. The nurse's awareness of such expected findings enables him or her to individualize assessment and intervention for the patient.

Mechanism of Injury Identification of the *mechanism of injury* (MOI) involves defining the *who, what, where, when,* and *why* of the injuring event. The prehospital report sheet or the emergency resuscitation record can help identify these factors, and if the patient is alert and oriented, he or she may be able to help. Table 21–1 lists some factors that may be used to ascertain necessary details. The key point in identifying the mechanism of injury is to personalize it for each individual patient, that is, to determine the amount of

force that was directed at *that* patient's body tissue at the moment of impact. Knowledge of the mechanism of injury and the transfer of energy to organs is vital in predicting and managing the injuries of the trauma patient in critical care.

Importance of Index of Suspicion Not all injuries are initially apparent; for example, blunt injuries are particularly difficult to diagnose because surface trauma may not be present. The complete history of the mechanism of injury may reveal information that will heighten your index of suspicion regarding actual and potential injuries. Subsequently, the physical examination will become more individualized as areas of the

TABLE 21–1

Factors to Assess to Determine Traumatic Force and Body Areas Most Susceptible to Injury

MOTOR VEHICLE ACCIDENTS	FALLS	PENETRATING TRAUMA
Estimated speed of accident:	Height of fall	*Gunshot Wounds*
Freeway vs surface street	Any evidence of stopping distance	Location of wounds
Direction of vehicle impact:	Surface onto which victim fell	Caliber/velocity of weapon
Frontal	Position which victim was found after fall	Distance from which patient was shot:
Lateral	Evidence of any other injury prior to fall (gunshot wounds, stab wounds, physical assault)	Close range
Rear		Long range
Damage to vehicle:		Character of wounds:
Front end		Size
Rear end		Extent of external tissue destruction
Side doors caved into passenger space		Powder burns surrounding wounds (indicates victim was shot at close range)
Steering wheel bent		Number of "shots" heard by bystanders or victim
Windshield broken		
Position of victim in vehicle:		*Stab Wounds*
Front seat—driver/passenger		Location of wounds
Back seat		Type of weapon
Victim ejected from vehicle		Length of blade
Seat belt/no seat belt		Depth of penetration
Extrication of victim required		
Another passenger (in same or other vehicle) dead at scene		
Motorcycle:		
Helmet/no helmet		
Protective clothing		
Distance victim found from motorcycle		
Pedestrian:		
Type of vehicle that struck victim		
Traveling speed of vehicle		
Estimated distance victim was thrown and body points of impact		

body are preidentified for risk and in-depth assessment. This focus leads to earlier identification and treatment of all injuries and greatly affects mortality and morbidity following multiple trauma. The knowledgeable critical-care nurse maintains a high index of suspicion in assessing the trauma patient, determining appropriate diagnoses, and implementing specialized nursing care.

The critical-care nurse frequently has more interaction with, and longer direct care responsibility for, the major trauma victim than any other health care professional. Therefore, it is essential that the critical-care nurse acquire and maintain advanced knowledge and skills specific to the needs of critically injured patients.

The following case study illustrates the importance of maintaining a high index of suspicion for other injuries while assessing trauma patients, to avoid overlooking occult internal injuries that can lead to preventable deaths.

A 56-year-old, unrestrained male patient with a history of previous upper left arm amputation was in a head-on crash with an 18-wheel dual trailer truck going 45 mph. On admission, his cervical spine x-ray was reviewed and cervical vertebrae C_1 through C_5 were viewed. The standard review requires a "swimmer's view," to see C_6 and C_7. This view was impossible due to a fracture of the patient's right humerus. His level of consciousness (LOC) was altered in the field. Diagnostic peritoneal lavage (DPL) was negative, no other injuries were identified, and the patient was admitted to the TICU for observation. Within 24 hours, he was quadriplegic as the result of undiagnosed cervical spinal fracture at C6–7. Another 72 hours passed with an unstable clinical course and the patient died from mediastinitis. Mediastinitis is a common complication of unrecognized or undiagnosed tracheal and bronchial tears resulting from blunt chest trauma.

This rare, dramatic case illustrates the critical need for understanding mechanisms of injury and maintaining a high index of suspicion even when diagnostic tests do not reveal injuries.

NURSING TIP

Discovery of Hidden Injury

Knowing the mechanism of injury can help you predict potential injuries and identify hidden injuries early.

Principles of Mechanism of Injury Critical-care nurses who understand the concepts of kinetic energy and the body's response to blunt and penetrating forces will be better equipped to assess and manage these challenging trauma injuries. Blunt or penetrating injury occurs when an energy load applied to the body exceeds the body's ability to withstand that energy. This energy load, defined as *kinetic energy* or the energy of motion, is represented by the following equation:

$$\text{Kinetic energy} = \text{Mass} \times \text{Velocity}^2/2$$

The extent of the injury depends on the amount of energy absorbed by the tissues, organs, or structures at the time of impact. In an auto crash, for example, kinetic energy is dissipated in two impacts: the primary impact as the auto hits another object and the secondary impact as the body collides with parts of the car. When an auto hits a tree at high speed and suddenly stops, the primary impact stops the car, but any objects in the vehicle continue forward until they, too, hit stationary objects.

The extent and severity of the injury are influenced by both the kinetic energy and the stopping distance of the body. The amount of energy that is directed at body tissues is called *force*.

$$\text{Force} = \text{Kinetic energy}/\text{Stopping distance}$$

The greater the stopping distance, the greater the dissipation of kinetic energy and the smaller the extent of injury (May 1984). People may be spared extensive injury if the stopping distance is great. For example, a fall from 15 feet onto a 3-foot steel plate may be fatal, whereas a fall from 55 feet into a soft cushion designed to break the fall may result in no injury at all.

Tension, compression, and shear are three basic forces that affect a given mass. *Tension* tends to pull tissues apart, *compression* tends to push them together, and *shear* causes tissues to override one another (May 1984). Injury results from one or more of these forces, which may be either direct or indirect. A *direct* force causes injury by direct impact or forced compression. An *indirect* force causes injury during rapid acceleration or deceleration as body tissues and vessels are stretched, rotated, and torn from points of attachment. The torso is especially rich in structures subject to potential disruption by indirect forces. The "little stalks" of the bladder (urethra), lungs (bronchi), duodenum (ligament of Treitz), aorta (ductus arteriosus), heart (aorta at the valve), and head (spinal cord) may be damaged simply from falling or jumping (vertical loading) or from sudden stops (deceleration injuries).

The severity of the body's response to an injuring force depends upon:

- The area over which the force is concentrated (the smaller the area, the stronger the force). Maxillofacial trauma, for example, increases the index of suspicion for cervical spinal injuries. Blunt forces of great magnitude applied to broad surfaces cause multiple injuries.

NURSING TIP

Nursing Intervention with Spinal Cord Injury

Assume the patient has a cervical spine injury until it is ruled out. Failure to do so may result in quadriplegia or death. Cervical spine injury is ruled out by radiologic examination of all seven cervical vertebrae and by physical examination.

- The location of the impact. Bony structures such as the ribs may protect the lungs and heart from direct injury, although these organs can be injured indirectly through contusion. There are no bony structures protecting the abdominal organs anteriorly, so if the pelvis is fractured, there is a greater likelihood that the underlying structures will be damaged as well. Upper abdominal contents are easily displaced, frequently limiting the extent of injury.
- The quality and quantity of the safety equipment in use. Leather clothing and helmets protect the motorcycle rider; seat belts, shoulder restraints, air bags, and child restraint systems protect the auto user from the dashboard, steering wheel, and windshield and from ejection from the vehicle.
- The injuring object in penetrating trauma (knife and bullet wounds). Knives are low-velocity impact weapons, and damage is usually limited to a relatively small area along the wounding tract. Morbidity and mortality depend upon the structures involved, the general health of the victim, and the development of complications from the wound. Bullet wounds, however, are quite different (Trunkey and Lewis 1991). The transmission of kinetic energy from the bullet may form a temporary cavity in the surrounding tissue, and this water-vapor-filled cavity may be 30 times larger than the bullet that entered. Additionally, bullets develop "yaw and tumble," meaning they enter and then begin to turn "head over heels" within the soft tissue, enlarging the cavitation even further. This cavitation enlargement is related to striking velocity and size of the bullet; however, this information is not needed for treatment decisions or for surgical exploration or debridement, which is required to remove debris and necrotic tissue. The patient with a gunshot wound is at great risk for infection and sepsis; in addition to local tissue ischemia and necrosis, there will be contamination with debris as the bullet travels through clothing and through bone and other bodily tissues.

Possible Precipitating Factors In single-person accidents, it is important to consider acute myocardial infarction, stroke, seizure, hypoglycemia, and attempted suicide as possible precipitating events. Frequently, older individuals have diabetes, or underlying cardiac or cardiovascular disease for which they are being treated with beta blockade, calcium channel blockers, cardiac glycosides, or other pharmacologic agents and/or a pacemaker or an automatic internal cardiac defibrillator (AICD). Consider the following case study:

An 89-year-old man with a history of well-controlled hypertension was admitted to the TICU from trauma resuscitation after crashing into a signal-light standard on the corner of two busy streets near his home. Vital signs on admission were blood pressure (BP) 100/60, heart rate (HR) 70, respiration rate (RR) 24, and temperature 36°C. He was unconscious and pallid, with surgically treated fractures of the right fibula, tibia, and femur. This patient had an excellent identification system—a Medic-Alert bracelet and a wallet card with a detailed medical history. Although he had no history of stroke or acute myocardial infarction (MI), the staff had a high index of suspicion about acute MI because of its incidence in the elderly. Nursing staff instituted routine electrocardiographic monitoring and saw 4-mm ST segment depression in leads II and V_1, an indicator of myocardial injury. The physician was alerted, and the 12-lead electrocardiogram (ECG) demonstrated anterior changes indicating acute MI in progress. Angioplasty was performed and the process of acute MI was reversed.

Planning and Implementation of Care

Once the emergent phase has passed and the condition of the patient stabilizes, the critical-care nurse determines which aspects of care have priority. Infection, sepsis, and multiple organ failure are the major

NURSING DIAGNOSES

Among the most common nursing diagnoses in trauma patients are the following:

- Ineffective airway clearance
- Ineffective breathing patterns
- Impaired gas exchange
- Decreased cardiac output
- Hypothermia
- High risk for infection
- Impaired physical mobility
- Altered nutrition: Less than body requirements
- High risk for multiple organ systems failure*
- Pain
- Post-trauma response
- Sleep disturbance

*non-NANDA diagnosis

physical complications that are commonly seen in the multiple trauma patient, and the psychosocial problems associated with multiple trauma are numerous. This section discusses selected aspects of these nursing diagnoses pertinent to trauma patients. More general aspects of the nursing diagnoses are discussed in detail in other sections of this text, and the interventions identified there apply to the multiple trauma patient.

Ineffective Airway Clearance Related to Airway Obstruction Airway obstruction in the multiple trauma patient may be due to one or more of the following conditions:

- Tongue displacement or swelling
- Presence of blood or vomitus
- Soft tissue facial or neck trauma
- Instability of maxillary or mandibular structures

Airway management is critical because of the oxygen debt that is inevitable in tissue injury. Basic concepts of airway management are presented in Chapter 9. Suction the patient as needed, and be prepared to assist with intubation or a surgical airway procedure as needed. The compromised airway is managed most effectively with endotracheal intubation; however, several available mask and nasal appliances—such as non-rebreather oxygen masks—

may assist patients who do not have facial or neck fractures. In an experimental, double-blind study, Helfman et al. (1991) found that during emergent intubation, esmolol consistently protected against vasomotor instability. Although further investigation is required, it appears that this agent, coupled with neuromuscular blocking agents, may be important during intubation and subsequent management in the critical-care setting.

Nursing research in the area of suctioning is abundant and should be reviewed for current recommendations pertaining to trauma patients. For example, hyperventilation and hyperoxygenation prior to suction have become the standard of practice in critical-care nursing. A study by Stone et al. (1991), however, indicates that hyperventilation and hyperoxygenation may increase mean arterial pressure (MAP), cardiac output (CO), pulmonary artery pressure (PAP) and peak airway pressure. These increases may in turn increase ICP and therefore be deleterious for patients with increased ICP (Stone et al. 1991). ST segment depression has been documented during suctioning (Bell 1992), so careful monitoring of ST segment changes during suctioning is also important.

Hemodynamic and oxygen transport changes following endotracheal suctioning were evaluated by Lookinland (1991) in a study of 24 adult trauma patients. Several protocols, all using hyperinflation and hyperoxygenation, yielded no statistical differences among techniques. Schmitz (1991) found in a very small study of five patients with adult respiratory distress syndrome (ARDS) that placing patients in a semiprone position increased gas exchange as measured by arterial blood gas samples. Although these studies used small populations, the results are specific to trauma patient populations and therefore are important in the care of trauma patients.

Most studies of trauma patient populations report very high rates of nosocomial pneumonia. Rodriguez, Gibbons and Bitzer (1991) studied trauma patients undergoing emergent intubation, and reported that 44.2% of mechanically ventilated patients acquired pneumonia. They found Gram-negative pathogens in 72% of the group, resulting in increased morbidity; however, there was no increase in mortality. Blunt trauma, head injury, and hypotension remained significant predictors for the development of nosocomial pneumonias. The experience within one author's institution is similar; however, the nosocomial pneumonia rate has been reduced to below 25% with the use of specialty beds, competency-based suctioning demonstrations, and closed suctioning systems (Bell 1991). Adequate fluid resuscitation on admission, nutritional support within 24 hours, and mobilization within 48 hours are critical to preventing pneumonia in trauma patients (Rodriguez, Gibbons and Bitzer 1991).

Ineffective Breathing Patterns Ineffective breathing patterns in the multiple trauma victim may be related to the following situations:

- Decreased level of consciousness (head injury, drugs, alcohol)
- Tension pneumothorax
- Flail chest
- Pulmonary vessel injury with large hemothorax
- Penetrating chest trauma
- Pulmonary contusion
- Tracheal-bronchial tear
- Spinal cord injury
- Pain from any combination of injuries

Observe the patient with any of the above identified injuries for the following signs and symptoms of ineffective breathing: dyspnea, tachypnea, tachycardia, hypotension, asymmetric chest wall expansion, paradoxical chest wall movement, use of accessory or abdominal muscles for breathing, distended neck veins, tracheal shift, decreased lung sounds, bloody secretions from the airway, and reduced arterial Po_2. Measures to alleviate the ineffective breathing patterns are directed toward the specific cause and include chest tube insertion for hemo/pneumothorax, use of high-flow oxygen, and intubation and mechanical ventilation.

Hunter (1989) found neuromuscular blocking agent use essential in the management of pulmonary function in trauma care; however, nurses must be knowledgeable about the specific agent in use. Many agents designed for use in the intraoperative period have half-lives that are too long for use over a period of 24 or more hours. Some are fat-soluble and will have effects long after the agent is discontinued (Davidson 1991). Institutional standards should require periods in which the drugs are discontinued for patient assessment. When therapeutic levels of neuromuscular blockade are used, patients are completely paralyzed. Because trauma patients are likely to have skeletal and soft tissue pain, they must also receive adequate sedation and narcotic analgesia for pain relief. (Consider the likely levels of fear and anxiety if a patient were to have a fractured neck and pelvis, be fully aware and in pain but unable to speak due to pharmacologic paralysis.) Anti-inflammatory drugs and benzodiazepines are also helpful.

Impaired Gas Exchange This problem may result from injury to the central nervous system, the chest, or the abdomen, or it may be caused by major hemorrhage. Chapters 8 and 9 discuss recognition and management of conditions that can impair gas exchange in trauma patients, such as pulmonary edema and shunting. Monitor the patient's respiratory and cardiovascular status continuously, and optimize oxygen delivery to all severely injured trauma patients, who may require increased oxygen delivery to offset the tremendous increase in oxygen consumption. Administer humidified high-flow oxygen (6–8 L) to all multiple trauma patients. Monitor arterial blood gas values and ventilatory parameters.

Decreased Cardiac Output Common causes of decreased cardiac output in the multiple trauma patient are:

- Acute, major blood loss
- Cardiac tamponade
- Aortic or other major vessel dissection
- Tension pneumothorax
- Multiple organ systems failure

The following section focuses on decreased cardiac output due to acute blood loss (hypovolemic shock). The remaining causes are discussed later in the chapter. Chapter 20 discusses assessment and management of hypovolemic shock in detail.

NURSING TIP

Nursing Assessment of Arterial Blood Pressure without Equipment

A "rule of thumb" from the prehospital care field may help you estimate systolic blood pressure: A palpable carotid pulse correlates with a blood pressure of at least 60 mm Hg, a femoral pulse correlates with at least 70 mm Hg, and a radial pulse correlates with at least 80 mm Hg.

Resuscitation Solutions Major blood loss in the trauma patient is replaced with crystalloid, colloid, hypertonic solutions, packed red blood cells, or a blood substitute. Large-bore (14–16-gauge) peripheral intravenous catheters are used for rapid volume replacement, which is essential for survival. Crystalloids, such as normal saline or Ringer's lactate, are infused as indicated by patient status and estimation of blood loss. Blood products should be available for immediate use as indicated.

Careful monitoring for transfusion reactions is imperative in the multiple trauma patient. When it is essential to initiate blood replacement with noncross-matched type O-negative blood, there is minimal risk of a major transfusion reaction (Unkle, Smejkal and Snyder 1991). In about 4% of the population, however, delayed development of antigen-antibody complexes can occur, making subsequent cross-matching more difficult after administration of multiple units. There is great controversy over when or if to administer platelets in trauma care, but many studies suggest platelet administration concurrent with or after the tenth unit of packed cells (Trunkey and Lewis 1991).

The use of hypertonic saline (HS) has been studied over several years, and recent studies indicate that it appears to exacerbate bleeding in uncontrolled hemorrhage (Reed, Johnson and Chen 1991). Research indicates that at least one contributing mechanism may be the ability of hypertonic saline to dilate blood vessels (Halvorsen, Gunther and Dubick 1991). If hypertonic saline is able to override the normal vasoconstrictive response to injury, this mechanism could explain the increased bleeding. Reed, Johnson and Chen (1991) found that administering HS to less than 10% of normal circulating volume produced no significant effect on prothrombin time (PT), activated partial thromboplastin times (APTT), or platelet aggregation activity; however, larger volumes had a significant impact on these variables.

Hypertonic saline and dextran solutions used in resuscitation demonstrate highly reproducible results: plasma volume is expanded rapidly and myocardial contractility is increased, dependent upon preload increase and afterload reduction. When administered as 250 ml of 2,400 mOsm/L solution, hypertonic saline/dextran represents a 600-mOsm load of sodium chloride. Interstitial fluid depletion yields up to 1 L of circulating volume. Hematocrit levels drop rapidly, indicating dilution. Mean arterial pressures rapidly return to normal, and shock-induced oxygen debt is rapidly corrected. The solution also causes a cutaneous flushing and sensation of warmth and a profound diuresis (Trunkey and Lewis 1991). Halvorsen, Gunther and Dubick (1991) found that a 4-ml/kg bolus of 7.5% sodium chloride in a 12% dextran 70 solution may be more effective in increasing the hemodynamic response than other solutions previously recommended.

Human resuscitation without using blood is an area of intense research interest. Multiple liquid perfluorochemical compounds that have high solubilities for oxygen and carbon dioxide when emulsified in a suitable aqueous medium have been used as blood substitutes, and they provide adequate gas transport.

Absence of adverse effects and rapid clearance from the liver are essential in any compound used. Mukherji and Sloviter (1991) describe perfluorodecalin, an emulsion that shows great promise as a superior resuscitation fluid compatible with dextran, other plasma substitutes, and human blood. However, studies involving large-scale critical-care utilization of such solutions are not yet available.

Military Anti-Shock Trouser (MAST) Suit The military anti-shock trouser (MAST) suit, also known as the pneumatic anti-shock garment (PASG) (Figure 21–1), may be used along with fluid resuscitation to raise the systolic blood pressure to an acceptable level (100 mm Hg). Use of the suit has been controversial since its introduction into civilian prehospital use. When used with a backboard, the suit currently is considered useful for splinting the lower extremities and pelvis, applying pressure to decrease bleeding, and increasing fluid volumes to the chest. Ideally, a patient will not arrive in the critical-care unit with the MAST suit in

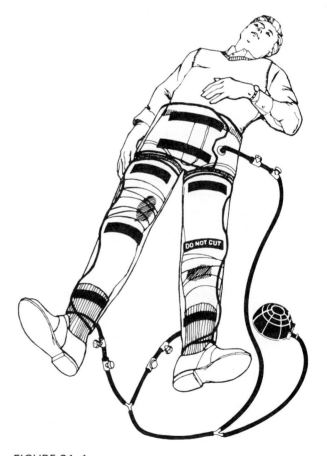

FIGURE 21–1

Pneumatic antishock garment (PASG). (Reprinted from Hammond B, Lee G: *Emergency Nursing,* 1984. By permission of David Clark Co., Inc. Worcester, MA.)

place; however, if he or she does, there are several cautions related to its use. Always monitor suit pressures and peripheral pulses; pressures greater than 30 mm Hg for more than 2 hours may result in significant ischemia to the lower extremities. Monitor the patient's fluid volume status carefully. When the patient is stable enough for a suit removal trial, deflate the suit beginning with the abdomen first. Never cut or open the garment when it is inflated, and never open a leg compartment first.

Hypothermia Hypothermia can contribute to difficulty in resuscitating the acute trauma patient and can increase the number and severity of postoperative complications. Obtaining accurate vital signs becomes a challenge in the hypothermic—and therefore maximally vasoconstricted—patient. In the relatively stable trauma patient, there is no difference between direct and indirect methods of monitoring arterial blood pressure (Norman, Gadaleta and Griffin 1991); however, when vital signs vary significantly, direct monitoring is more accurate, especially in the patient with hypothermia or shock (Gregory, Flancbaum and Townsend 1991). To detect hypothermia early, monitoring either urinary bladder temperature or pulmonary artery temperature is valuable (Earp and Finlayson 1991). In the patient in frank shock or hypothermia, correlate the urinary bladder temperature (if available) and the pulmonary artery temperature to determine the most accurate body temperature. Capillary blood glucose measurement is oxygen dependent; peripheral stasis and diminished blood flow decrease oxygen content and may alter results. Therefore, measure blood glucose with venous blood samples rather than capillary blood samples.

Shivering associated with hypothermia (35.5°C) will increase oxygen consumption up to 500% (Feroe and Augustine 1991). This effect is particularly important in the very old and the very young, because their oxygen and metabolic reserves are more quickly depleted. If your patient is shivering, collaborate with the physician to identify the cause, if possible. Sources of shivering include hypothermia, administration of cold fluids and blood, altered thermoregulatory function in fever, exposure in general care, chemical mediators, and neural factors (Holtzclaw 1990). Generally, trauma patients become hypothermic from exposure. In a study by Gregory, Flancbaum and Townsend (1991), 92% of patients lost heat while in the emergency department. Convective warming is particularly useful in rewarming patients, as are warmed fluids, warm blankets to decrease exposure and radiation of heat to the environment, and infrared sources.

High Risk for Infection Related to Wound Contamination Traumatic wounds are considered dirty injuries. Often the trauma occurred in an unclean environment, or wounding instruments were thrust through dirty clothing, so the wounds frequently contain foreign debris. Despite surgical intervention, they remain contaminated and place the patient at great risk for infection. Surgical repair in the immunosuppressed trauma patient likewise exposes the patient to the risks of infection.

Adequate ventilation; oxygenation; fluid resuscitation; debridement and repair of wounds; the use of universal precautions; and the changing of lines, dressings, and tube insertion sites are the first priority interventions against infection. Wound management is a collaborative problem, frequently involving the wound, skin, or enterostomal specialist. The following guidelines apply in sound wound management:

- Use meticulous universal precautions. Conscientious use of universal precautions is essential to protect both the staff and the multiple trauma patient (Jackson and Lynch 1990).
- Use strict aseptic technique when applying and changing dressings.
- Because catheter insertion sites are considered wounds, change catheters and dressings based on Centers for Disease Control guidelines.
- Regularly evaluate wounds for signs of inflammation, purulent drainage, and ischemia. Observing the wound location, size, and depth, the presence of any exudate, infection, or necrosis, and the condition of the surrounding skin, is essential to positive outcome (Cruzzel and Stotts 1990).
- Regularly evaluate the appropriateness of the dressing. No single wound dressing can be used for all wounds or all stages of healing. Avoid circumferential dressings, which can restrict circulation.
- Avoid tape; use fishnet mesh tubes or "stretch gauze" to hold dressings, if appropriate.
- Avoid wound cross-contamination when several wounds are present.
- Collect drainage in "ostomy" type collection devices. These are available in "large wound" size for wounds 12–30 cm in length. Abdominal wounds and draining incisions often require this appliance.
- Establish and maintain adequate nutrition and hydration as soon as possible.
- Ensure adequate tetanus prophylaxis: tetanus toxoid 0.5 ml intramuscularly (IM) if previous

immunization is current; human immune globulin 250 units IM if immunization status is unknown.

- Assess concealed wounds, such as those under plaster, bulky dressings, or restraint devices. Anywhere there is pressure or a concealed wound, there is high risk for skin breakdown, and purulence can go unnoticed.

- Where appropriate, include family members when changing dressings. Many patients will be discharged from the hospital with family members who will be responsible for complex dressing changes. Experience has shown that the earlier family members are included in procedures, the more successful they are in performing them at home (Johanson et al. 1988).

Impaired Physical Mobility Related to Activity Restrictions Research has shown that positioning the trauma patient for optimum comfort, oxygenation, and prevention of skin ischemia decreases complications. External fixators and specialty beds have dramatically increased mobility and decreased complications such as skin breakdown and pulmonary stasis. Patients would benefit from further research on positioning and other therapies that reduce the hazards of immobility and the devastating effects of pulmonary or infectious complications.

If the team is unable to mobilize the multiple trauma patient, serious consideration should be given to the use of specialty beds. One type, the kinetic continuous rotation bed (Roto Rest Trauma Bed) (Figure 21–2), allows continuous turning of the patient with cervical or other spinal cord injury, femoral fractures requiring traction, or massive soft tissue damage. This motion promotes removal of pulmonary secretions, decreases pulmonary complications such as pneumonia and atelectasis, and decreases development of pressure sores, venous stasis, pulmonary emboli, postural hypotension, urinary stasis, muscle wasting, and bone demineralization. This bed does not adversely affect ICP dynamics (Gentilello et al. 1988). Airbag beds are another type of specialty bed. One type of airbag bed turns the patient side to side and the other inflates and

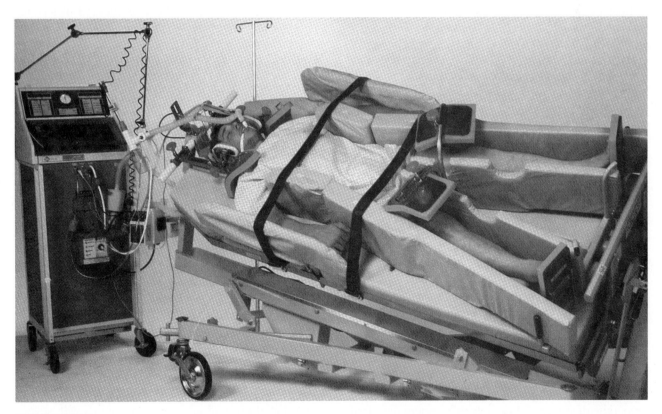

FIGURE 21–2

Roto Rest® Kinetic Treatment Table. May be used with cervical traction using Gardner-Wells tongs or Halo ring, as well as with orthopedic injuries requiring traction. (Photo courtesy of Kinetic Concepts, Inc., San Antonio, Texas. Used with permission. Roto Rest®—KCI's registered trademark for its oscillating support surfaces.)

deflates from head to foot. Choose a bed that best meets the patient's needs, but avoid airbag beds for patients in traction or those with spinal cord injury.

Oxygenation, as measured by arterial blood gas determination, is increased by placing the trauma patient in the prone position offered by the Stryker frame or Circ-O-Lectric bed. Turning the patient with the "good lung" or nondiseased lung in the dependent position increases oxygenation and decreases shunting when compared to the supine position (Fontaine and McQuillan 1989).

Altered Nutrition: Less than Body Requirements Related to Iatrogenic Starvation Chapter 19 discusses concepts of nutrition in the critically ill. Hypermetabolism in the trauma patient usually prevents the body's normal response to starvation. The catabolic trauma patient risks losing one pound, or more, of lean muscle mass and fat per day. Once the patient resumes eating, he or she actually may develop a nutritional deficit because of a simple inability to consume adequate numbers of calories to meet metabolic demands.

Inadequate nutrition is a collaborative problem that requires a team approach. Initial nutritional management may begin with enteral nutrition or total parenteral nutrition. Intestinal feeding is preferable for a variety of reasons. Early enteral feeding results in fewer, less severe infections, a reduction in hypermetabolism, and a reduction in neurologic complications (Trunkey and Lewis 1991). In addition, early enteral feeding may decrease the potential for bacterial translocation (movement of bacteria across the mucosal barrier), a well-described phenomenon associated with multiple organ systems failure (Trunkey and Lewis 1991). Small intestinal feeding tubes permit day-one feeding in all patients except those with severe abdominal trauma or those in barbiturate coma. It is always advisable to add color to enteral feedings to identify them should they enter the trachea or leave the alimentary canal via fistulae or perforations. Use green or blue dye, never red (because it looks like blood) or yellow (because a large amount is needed to color tan feeding solution, and the liquid may be confused with *Pseudomonas*-containing sputum).

Considerations for the geriatric patient may include a reduction of calories and an increase in vitamins C, D, and folic acid, calcium, zinc, and iron. These changes reflect the decreased basal metabolic expenditure that occurs with age and an increased need for vitamins and minerals commonly lacking in adequate amounts in the geriatric diet but essential in increased amounts for wound healing (Dowe 1989; Foreman 1989; Hogstel 1991).

NURSING TIP

Feeding the Patient with a Wired Jaw

Once healing is adequate to permit the introduction of food, patients with extensive maxillofacial injury who do not have jejunostomies may prefer blenderized feedings that they can push through a tube into their mouths. Milk shakes are often a good start and a tasty change from enteral liquid feedings.

Special considerations apply to the patient with head, facial, or chest trauma, or abdominal trauma with reconstruction to the upper gastrointestinal tract. Percutaneous gastrostomy—placement of a feeding tube through the abdominal wall by endoscopy, often during initial surgical management of injuries—is preferred for these patients. This method of feeding into the duodenum can be implemented on the first or second day of hospitalization and assists in decreasing intestinal flora in the pulmonary system, minimizing aspiration into the airways, and allowing earlier initiation of nutritional supplements (Kirby, Clifton and Turner 1991). *Because of the risk of entering the brain, never attempt to insert a nasogastric tube in a patient with known or suspected facial or posterior pharyngeal injury.*

High Risk for Multiple Organ Systems Failure Following injury, intubation with mechanical support, malnutrition, or large-scale exposure to pathogenic organisms, the body immediately begins to mobilize a sophisticated series of neurohumoral and cellular responses to repair the damage and increase the potential for survival. Prolonged periods of hypoxia and inadequate tissue perfusion are the major factors leading to alterations in cellular activity that increase the risk of organ failure. Multiple organ system failure is discussed in Chapter 20.

Pain Related to Traumatic Injury Pain from traumatic injury can be severe. Epidural analgesia is superior to systemic analgesics in patients with severe blunt chest trauma (Mackersie, Karagianes and Hoyt 1991). Continuous epidural infusion of opiates is the preferred treatment for these patients. This method of pain control decreases the frequency of complications, increases the patient's sense of well-being, and decreases hospital stay. Frequently, these patients report nausea, which is controlled with prochlorperazine. Adequate pain management, as well as turning, coughing, and deep breathing, are the keys to decreasing the necessity for intubation and the frequency of pneumonia or atelectasis. A combination of continuous infusion and patient-controlled dosing is very helpful in pain management in the multiply injured individual. Intravenous narcotics, especially morphine, generally are tolerated well; meperidine has active metabolites, which may not be desirable in the head-injured patient.

Post-Trauma Response Related To Traumatic Experience One of the most challenging aspects of nursing care for the trauma patient is the provision of psychosocial support for the patient, family, and friends as they attempt to cope with the injury. Because a traumatic event is sudden, unexpected, and disruptive, the psychologic and sociologic results can be devastating if not recognized and included in the treatment regimen. During the initial resuscitation, life-saving procedures will be implemented simultaneously, sometimes without prior explanation to the patient. The invasive procedures, in combination with memories of the incident resulting in injury, are often overwhelming to the trauma patient.

Post-trauma response is a well-defined, sustained, emotionally painful response to a traumatic event. The patient may re-experience the traumatic event in flashbacks, intrusive thoughts, dreams, or nightmares and may feel survival guilt, self-blame, shame, and/or fear of repetition, death, or loss of bodily control. The patient may have other feelings, including confusion, numbness, or restlessness.

The first nursing intervention that may be helpful is reassuring the patient that he or she is in a safe place. Assist the patient and the family to begin to process the event by talking and expressing feelings of anger, fear, or guilt. You may also help them make connections with support people and evaluate the support they are given. Consultation with and referral to mental health professionals may be helpful in managing the patient's and family's emotional reactions.

Establishing early rapport facilitates coping. To ensure that families get information and to establish trust in a timely manner, assign one volunteer from a family support group to the family in crisis. In one model, in use at Eden Hospital Medical Center, Castro Valley, California, specially educated volunteers are recruited from the community to assist families during the resuscitation and early admission phase of the crisis. A volunteer assists the nurses and social worker with delegated activities and remains with the family until the patient is admitted to the clinical unit. The volunteer helps orient the family to the unit and collaborates with professional nursing staff throughout the patient's stay, including attendance at patient care conferences. This volunteer communicates basic information, assists with the decision-making process, and remains a consistent source of support and comfort to the family.

Multidisciplinary conferences that include family members help them perceive themselves as members of a team of people focused on reducing morbidity and mortality and promoting recovery and wellness. These conferences also help the team evaluate the coping strategies of the patient and family.

Sleep-Pattern Disturbance Related to Multiple Factors Drugs, environmental stimuli (such as constant lighting), pain, fear, anxiety, immobility, and temperature variations all contribute to the trauma patient's sleep deprivation. Sleep deprivation can lead to physical and psychologic symptoms such as memory loss, disorientation, agitation, decreased motivation, delusions, and paranoid or psychotic behavior. These manifestations are disturbing to the patient, family, and visitors, as well as to the nursing staff. The geriatric patient is most susceptible to sleep disruption due to the length of time required to fall asleep, the loss of stage 4 deep sleep, frequent awakenings, and altered sensory input (sight and hearing may already be impaired). Being in a strange environment without his or her usual support system also may increase the patient's anxiety, thereby decreasing sleep ability (Foreman 1989).

Maintain sensitivity to sleep pattern disturbances, and intervene before the patient experiences a personality change. Maintaining a night-day pattern is essential. After the first 48 hours, few patients are so unstable that they cannot be permitted to rest during the night with regular monitoring. Even providing 90-minute undisturbed periods may be helpful. Ideally, care can be safely clustered in 2- to 4-hour periods. Post-trauma stress often interrupts sleep with nightmares. Support, reassurance, and psychiatric, social service, and/or trauma clinical nurse specialist consultation, coupled with relaxation, touch, and chemical or other therapy, may be helpful.

Outcome Evaluation

The overall goal for the acute period is to transfer the patient from the critical-care unit to the general medical-surgical unit or rehabilitation facility with intact and functional respiratory, cardiovascular, neurologic, genitourinary, and gastrointestinal systems.

Evaluate the patient's progress and the effects of interventions based on these criteria:

- Level of consciousness stable.
- Airway patent.
- Blood gas values within expected limits for this patient.
- Vital signs within normal limits for this patient.
- Capillary refill in less than 3 seconds.
- Evidence of progressive wound healing.
- Mobility optimal within obvious limitations and physician's orders for range of motion.
- Previously uninjured skin intact, with no evidence of redness or breakdown.
- Skin on the occiput of the head and sacrum intact, especially in the patient on the Roto Rest or Stryker bed.
- Weight maintained within appropriate range for this patient.
- Nutrition optimal, as shown by pre-albumin and transferrin levels within normal limits.
- Infection, purulence, and erythema absent around external fixators or pin sites.
- Bowel and bladder function within normal limits for this patient.
- Pain statements and behaviors indicating an adequate comfort level.
- Periods of undisturbed sleep.
- Patient and significant others utilizing appropriate coping mechanisms.

Specific Traumatic Injuries

Traumatic injuries, which are classified as blunt, penetrating, chemical, and burn injuries, may occur in isolation or combination. *Penetrating trauma* (gunshot wounds and stabbings) frequently occurs in urban inner-city areas; *blunt trauma,* often associated with motor vehicle accidents, falls, assaults, and other similar mechanisms of injury, is seen more frequently in rural and suburban areas. Burns resulting from thermal, chemical, and electrical accidents are often included in discussions of trauma. Some counties, however, may not include burns in their trauma triage protocols, depending upon tertiary referral center availability. Burns are discussed in a separate section later in this chapter.

Head Injury

Each year approximately 500,000 people in the United States sustain head injuries, and another 10,000 suffer spinal cord injuries (Davis 1990). The most common cause is motor vehicle accidents; other causes include falls, violence, and sports-related accidents. About 60% of victims have positive blood alcohol levels, making assessment very difficult until the levels have dropped. The simplest head injury can result in a loss of memory so severe that patients are unable to balance a checkbook or go to the grocery store for more than three items.

NURSING TIP

Assessing Memory in the Head-Injured Patient

The Galviston Orientation Amnesia Test (GOAT) is a ten-item test of orientation to time, place, person, and present and past events. This assessment can be very helpful in predicting memory loss prior to discharge (Foreman 1989). Some patients who have sustained minor head injury feel that they are "going crazy" because they have memory deficits. Referral to a neuropsychologist or head injury support group may be very helpful. Patient and family education related to potential memory problems can assist in earlier identification and treatment of this very disturbing problem.

Mechanism of Injury Several mechanisms operating individually or simultaneously produce the injuries associated with head trauma. An *acceleration* injury occurs when a moving object, such as a lead pipe, strikes the head. A *deceleration* injury results when the head hits a stationary object, such as a cement sidewalk. The brain is often injured at the site of the impact *(coup)* and on its opposite side, where the force of the injury makes the brain rebound against the rigid skull *(contrecoup).*

Types of Head Injury There are three common classes of head injuries: skull fractures, focal brain injuries, and diffuse brain injuries.

Skull Fractures The skull may fracture in the vault or the base. The following types of fractures all occur in the vault. A *linear* fracture is a single crack. A *comminuted* fracture describes a fragmented bone. In a *depressed* fracture, bone is displaced downward into the brain. A basilar fracture involves bone at the base of the skull. Any of these fractures may be closed (the scalp is intact) or compound (there is an external opening through the scalp). Compound fractures communicate directly with intracranial contents, providing a direct route for bacterial invasion of the brain (Figure 21–3).

Basilar skull fractures warrant special attention because of the risk of infection. The base of the skull is divided into the anterior, middle, and posterior fossae. Because the dura closely adheres to the bone, a fracture results in a dural tear and leakage of cerebrospinal fluid. Organisms can enter via the dural tear, putting the patient in danger of an intracranial infection. Rhinorrhea, periorbital ecchymosis (raccoon's eyes), and subconjunctival hemorrhage are clinical signs of anterior fossa fracture. Otorrhea (drainage from the ear), ecchymosis over the mastoid bone (Battle's sign), hemotympanum, and (sometimes) facial nerve palsy result from a middle fossa fracture.

Focal Brain Injuries: Intracranial Hematomas Brain injuries can be grouped into two categories: focal and diffuse. Focal injuries constitute about 50% of head injuries and account for about 66% of deaths due to brain injury (Trunkey and Lewis 1991). These injuries result from intracranial hemorrhage associated with compound or closed head injury. When a single vessel or many small bridging vessels are torn, the blood collects and forms an expanding mass lesion, a hematoma. Hematomas are classified as: (1) epidural, (2) subdural, or (3) intracerebral (Figure 21–4).

In an *epidural hematoma,* arterial bleeding occurs between the skull and the dura, most commonly because of fracture of the temporal bone and tearing of the middle meningeal artery. Because the bleeding has

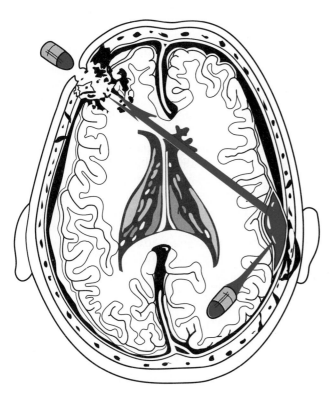

FIGURE 21–3

Gunshot wound to the head with entry wound, fracture with bone fragments, hemorrhage, fracture and lodgement in the occiput. (Reprinted with permission of New York Regional Transplant Program, Inc., and Biocom, Ltd., New York.)

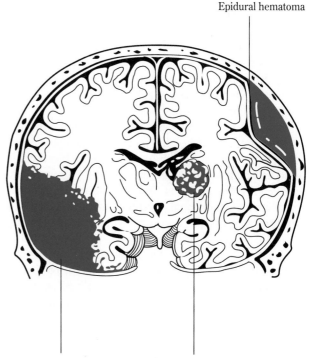

Epidural hematoma

Subdural hematoma   Intracerebral hematoma

FIGURE 21–4

Epidural hematoma, subdural hematoma and intracerebral hematoma. (Reprinted with permission of New York Regional Transplant Program, Inc., and Biocom, Ltd., New York.)

NURSING TIP

Planning Life-Saving Interventions

An intracranial bleed results in only a very small blood loss into the closed skull. When the skull is closed, there is no obvious external bleeding, and the patient is still in shock, you must consider the chest, abdomen, retroperitoneum, and pelvis as sources of blood loss.

to strip the dura away from the skull, which is difficult to do, the bleeding tends to be confined. Because the bleeding is under great pressure, however, it quickly can become life-threatening, so an epidural hematoma is a neurosurgical emergency. In its classic presentation, the patient typically loses consciousness at the scene, regains consciousness and is oriented, and then progressively and rapidly deteriorates.

With a *subdural hematoma,* bleeding occurs in the space between the dura and the arachnoid, usually due to tearing of small cerebral arteries or bridging veins. The bleeding can spread over the hemispheres and exert direct pressure on the brain, generally producing a progressive degeneration culminating in coma due to brainstem compression.

Subdural hematomas are categorized based on the amount of time between the injury and the appearance of signs and symptoms. *Acute* subdural bleeding is often associated with significant primary impact damage, such as contusions and lacerations. Signs and symptoms of neuronal dysfunction and increased intracranial pressure present within 24–48 hours. *Subacute* subdural hematomas yield symptoms within 2 days to 2 weeks. Clinical presentation, which may include localizing signs such as a dilated pupil and abnormal motor response or generalized signs of increased intracranial pressure, depends on the area of the brain involved. *Chronic* subdural hematomas may not cause symptoms for over 2 weeks or until months later. Due to the time lag and the seeming insignificance of the blow to the head, patients may not remember the initial injury. Headache, mental confusion, drowsiness, and/or seizure activity may occur.

An *intracerebral hematoma* frequently accompanies contusions or lacerations, especially if there has been a penetrating head injury. Clinical presentation of intracerebral hematoma combines neuronal dysfunction due to cerebral contusion or laceration with intracerebral bleeding. The patient is generally unconscious from the time of the injury. Localizing signs include hemiplegia on the contralateral side and a dilated pupil on the side of the clot. As intracranial pressure increases, signs of transtentorial herniation with accompanying changes in respirations, pupils, and motor response occur.

The diagnosis of focal injury is made by computerized tomography (CT) scanning. Epidural hematomas may require immediate surgical intervention to evacuate clots and ligate bleeding vessels, optimizing the patient's chances of a more favorable outcome. Acute, subacute, and chronic subdural hematomas that are large enough to produce significant symptoms require surgical evacuation. Small subdural hematomas may be followed medically if symptoms are receding. With intracerebral bleeding, parenchymal involvement means that neurologic deficit generally is permanent, regardless of whether medical or surgical management is used.

Diffuse Brain Injuries Diffuse brain injuries include mild concussion, classic cerebral concussion, and prolonged coma (Trunkey and Lewis 1991). Diffuse axonal injury (DAI) is classified as mild, moderate, or severe. It may produce a prolonged coma (longer than 6 hours) that results from diffuse axonal damage rather than from a mass lesion, that is, bleeding or brainstem compression. If coma is present, both hemispheres, the reticular activating system, and/or the brainstem are involved.

Mild DAI results in coma lasting 6–24 hours (Trunkey and Lewis 1991). Although this injury may produce permanent damage, it more commonly causes temporary cognitive or memory deficits. Moderate DAI results in coma lasting more than 24 hours and is associated with little or no brainstem compression. Significant morbidity and a 20% mortality rate can be expected (Trunkey and Lewis 1991). Severe DAI results in coma for more than 24 hours, when there is no mass lesion. There is usually extensive damage to axons of the cerebrum and brainstem, and mortality is as high as 57% (Trunkey and Lewis 1991).

Nursing Considerations in Head Trauma

Risk of Brain Herniation Both intracranial hematomas and diffuse brain injuries result in increased intracranial pressure and may lead to brain herniation. Astute nursing assessment and prompt intervention at the earliest signs of increased intracranial pressure and impending herniation are critical to patient survival. Chapter 4 presents neurologic assessment techniques, and Chapter 5 covers increased intracranial pressure and brain herniation syndromes in detail.

Trendelenburg Position   The safety of Trendelenburg positioning during chest physiotherapy (CPT) in the head-injury patient is a concern, because conventional flat CPT may not clear secretions adequately but the head-down position may raise ICP. Fontaine and McQuillan (1989) state that the Trendelenburg position does not compromise the head-injury patient during chest physiotherapy when duration does not exceed 10 minutes; however, ICP, MAP and cerebral perfusion pressure (CPP) should be closely monitored. A study by Lee (1989), however, suggests that the head-down position is hazardous even for short periods of time because it produces intracranial hypertension in most instances. A study by the Maryland Institute for Emergency Medical Services Systems (Walleck 1992) examined this question further. Trendelenburg positioning during CPT was ordered on head injury trauma patients undergoing ICP monitoring. Sedation and neck alignment supports were utilized to prevent intracranial hypertension. These authors conclude that Trendelenburg position could be used for the head-injury patient population if ICP, MAP, and CPP are monitored closely. All authors conclude that positioning varies from individual to individual and that further study is necessary.

Controlled Hyperventilation   Continuous hyperventilation is advocated in a number of texts on traumatic coma, but there is still considerable debate about its usefulness (Hind 1987; Beckler and Gardner 1985). (See Chapter 5 for further discussion of controlled hyperventilation.) Although benefits of controlled hyperventilation on cerebral hemodynamics have been documented in the normal brain, recent evidence suggests that these effects are not uniform throughout the injured brain (Muizelaar et al. 1988; Walleck 1989). A study by Muizelaar et al. (1991) suggests that prophylactic use of sustained hyperventilation for periods of 5 days retards recovery from severe head injury, and outcomes are statistically worse at 3 and 6 months but not at 12 months. Further clinical research is necessary to determine the benefit of hyperventilation in patients with severe brain injury.

Family Support and Organ Donation   Families of head-injury patients may be asked to make difficult decisions, including whether to donate organs and tissues if the injury is fatal, whether or not to begin nutrition in a patient for whom additional care would be futile, deciding placement for chronically noninteractive patients, and choosing rehabilitation facilities for those with potential for recovery. Mirr (1991) identified six factors that affect the decision-making of families of patients with severe head injury: personal functioning, relationships, information, uncertain outcomes, the

environment, and emotions. Decisions fell into five categories: medical treatment, personal, financial, ethical, and legal decisions. This study supports providing families with as much time as possible in which to make decisions.

Patients with traumatic head injuries frequently are pronounced brain dead. When the patient has a fatal injury, the act of organ donation may help families grieve with a more positive outcome. Some families will discuss the decision and will volunteer the information without assistance. Others need time to realize that death has occurred and that disposition of the body is inevitable. Death is a very difficult concept to grasp when the patient appears alive because the body is warm and pink and the ventilator is making the patient breathe.

Research has demonstrated the importance of sensitive timing in approaching the family about organ donation (Vernale and Packard 1990). Delay asking the family if they would like information about organ donation until the patient has been declared brain dead. After brain death is declared, the patient is dead, and the removal of a ventilator does not require a family decision. If organ donation is not going to occur, the ventilator is disconnected from the body just as if cardiopulmonary death had occurred. Sensitivity to the family's need to be with the body during this time is important. Helping the family understand death with continuing cardiac function is at times challenging. Explain that there may be spinal cord reflex activity during the cardiopulmonary death. This is energy that is expended similar to a light bulb which is about to fail; it may light for an instant and then be dead. Children may have specific questions which should be answered at their level.

Rarely will a patient have the opportunity to donate organs when facing non-neurologic death; often, organ systems have been too stressed to permit retrieval. Constant contact with the organ procurement organization is essential to the retrieval of any organs which can be salvaged. For example, in a fatal liver injury, death may be certain without a liver transplant; if none is found the patient will die, but the patient's kidneys, lungs and pancreas may still be viable.

The rapport you have established with the family will be essential for the family and nursing staff dealing with brain death. Collaboration with the social worker on the team, with the family support system, or with volunteers from previous patient populations may be very helpful. A case example illustrates the support that families with previous experience can offer.

A 12-year-old male was admitted to the TICU after being hit by an "out-of-control" motorcycle. Although there were

RESEARCH NOTE

Rosner M, Daughton S
Cerebral perfusion pressure management in head injury.
J Trauma 1990; 30(8):933–941

CLINICAL APPLICATION

The accepted treatment of increased intracranial pressure includes a reduction in intravenous fluid volume, hyperventilation to decrease carbon dioxide levels, elevation of the head of the bed, and frequently administration of an osmotic diuretic such as mannitol. Maintenance of a particular ICP range often is used as an end point, with measurement of cerebral perfusion pressure (CPP) frequently overlooked.

Cerebral perfusion pressure (equal to the mean arterial pressure minus the intracranial pressure) provides a tool for evaluating the blood flow to the brain. Normally 80–90 mm Hg, the CPP begins to fail at approximately 40 mm Hg, with irreversible brain damage occurring at approximately 30 mm Hg. This study evaluated whether trauma patients with a Glasgow Coma Scale (GCS) score of less than 7 could be safely managed based on CPP.

A convenience sample of 34 consecutive patients admitted to the Neurosurgical Intensive Care Unit at the University of Alabama, Birmingham, was studied. The treatment protocol was enacted on all 34 patients with a GCS of less than 7. ICP was monitored by frontal ventriculostomy. Fluid orders were written so that hourly intake equaled output plus 30 ml. Cerebrospinal fluid (CSF) drainage was the first method of regulating ICP increases. When CSF drainage alone was inadequate to maintain adequate CPP, systemic pressors were used routinely to titrate MAP. Negative sodium balance was maintained, monitored by serum and urine sodium levels. Mannitol was used, but furosemide (Lasix) was not used in combination unless the patient was considered to be overhydrated. All patients were nursed in the supine position. Oxygen saturation was 90% or more, and CO_2 levels were maintained at 35 torr. Neuromuscular blocking agents were used to control ventilation, and morphine sulfate also was used for pain control as patients began to wake up.

The investigators performed careful assessments of neurologic function and found an optimal CPP for each patient. Overall, CPP was maintained at 84 ± 11 mm Hg. ICP was 23 ± 9.8 mm Hg, MAP averaged 106 ± 11 mm Hg, and CVP was 8.0 ± 3.7 mm Hg. Average fluid intake was 5.3 ± 3.9 L/day, and urinary output averaged 5.0 ± 4.0 L/day. Albumin and packed red blood cells were used for volume expansion. Hemoglobin was maintained at 11.4 ± 1.4 gm/dl.

Overall mortality was 21%. Three patients (8%) died from uncontrolled ICP, all due to protocol errors. Four patients died from avoidable complications. More than 50% of the patients who normally would have died or had poor outcomes have had excellent or good recovery.

CRITICAL THINKING

Limitations: The sample size was small. There were a substantial number of avoidable errors in conducting the study. The results cannot be generalized to patients with a GCS above 7.

Strengths: This study addressed an important method of patient care management: basing management on CPP. The authors found that the outcome was very positive when patients (1) were maintained in a flat position, rather than with the head of bed elevated; (2) had adequate volume expansion; (3) had normal sodium balance; and (4) occasionally received mannitol, but not to the point of causing a negative fluid balance. Most important, they found that maintaining the optimal CPP for each patient improved outcome.

very few external, soft tissue injuries, the child was areflexic and soon pronounced dead. The parents, previously separated, were alone. The mother of a patient who had died two years before came to the TICU to offer her support. Her intervention assisted the overwhelmed health care team and nursing staff and provided continuous support for the parents through the funeral and beyond.

Not all volunteers are acceptable support personnel; care should be taken to assure the expertise and availability of these potentially invaluable people.

When brain death is probable, notify the organ procurement organization (OPO) in your area for possible organ and tissue donation. OPO staff can help decide whether a patient is a candidate for major organ donation, as shown in the following example.

A 16-year-old male was admitted with meningococcal meningitis. Without consultation with the OPO, many staff would not consider a patient with this history as an organ donor. In this case, however, antibiotics had been started on admission, so he was considered a potential donor. Within 72 hours after admission, he was declared brain dead, and seven organs were transplanted.

In addition to assisting with identifying potential donors, the OPO staff can help manage the donor and guide family and nursing staff through the donation process. In an effort to increase the number of organs available for transplantation, many OPOs are involved in studying organizational and family response to donation opportunities. For further discussion of issues related to organ donation, see Chapter 3.

Spinal Cord Injury

Surviving a spinal cord injury (SCI) presents great challenges for patients and their families. The injured person suddenly finds the world turned upside down and inside out: a frightened mind held captive by a body that won't move. Complete independence is abruptly replaced with total dependence on others for all activities of daily living.

Mechanisms of Injury Traumatic injury more commonly affects the cervical area of the spine. Flexion, extension, rotation, and/or compression forces cause vertebral fractures and dislocations, disruption of longitudinal ligaments, and spinal cord damage. Maximum mobility and force of movement make C_7 the most common site of cervical fractures.

Cervical Spinal Cord Injury This section addresses the cervical-cord-injury, or quadriplegic, patient. Challenges to the health care team begin immediately after the injury occurs and continue into rehabilitation.

Nursing Considerations in Spinal Cord Injury

Spinal Precautions When a patient is brought to the hospital by the prehospital providers in "full spinal immobilization," he or she is immobilized on a long backboard with a hard cervical collar, sandbags to the neck, and adhesive tape or body straps across the forehead, shoulders, and pelvis. The patient must remain immobilized until the spinal cord injury is ruled out (usually by radiographic determination) or definitive stabilization is achieved, for example, by application of cervical traction tongs, a Halo device, or open-reduction and internal fixation.

All patients suspected of head and neck injuries will have cervical spine films taken. Anteroposterior films assess alignment, and the lateral view assesses stability. Odontoid and oblique views may be ordered based on organizational protocols and physician preference. Computerized tomography (CT scan) or myelography may be employed to visualize the problem if plain films are not conclusive. Throughout the diagnostic workup, the head and neck must be immobilized to prevent further injury.

Spinal Decompression and Stabilization Early management of the patient with an injured spinal cord centers on decompression and stabilization. Indications for surgical intervention include open, penetrating injuries, an unstable spine, and progressive neurologic deficit.

Nonsurgical reduction and stabilization of the cervical spine is accomplished using skeletal traction, including Gardner-Wells skull tongs and a Halo ring (Figure 21–5). Gardner-Wells tongs have two spring-loaded pins that are seated into the temporal bone just above and in front of the ears. After the tongs are inserted, weights are applied to restore the normal alignment of the spinal column. The physician determines the amount of weight used. The nurse ensures that weights hang freely at all times, so that traction is not interrupted. To assess alignment, x-rays may be taken after weights are applied and with each increase. If the neurosurgeon knows that the patient will eventually be fitted for a Halo brace, the ring may be placed and traction applied as needed, so that a change from the tongs to a Halo device will not be necessary. The SCI patient should be placed on a Roto Rest, Stryker, or other trauma bed that allows the patient to be turned without disruption of the traction. Studies demonstrate preference for the Roto Rest bed, concluding that this bed improves reduction and stabilization and reduces complications (McGuire, Green and Eismont 1988; Brackett and Condon 1984).

Investigational trials of drug agents that enhance recovery after spinal cord injury are currently underway. Halpern (1991) found methylprednisolone contributed to significant neurologic recovery in patients with spinal cord injury. The National Institute of Neurologic Disorders and Stroke of the National Institute of Health recommend onset of therapy within 8 hours and completion within 24 hours (Halpern 1991). Administration should include an intravenous loading dose of 30 mg/Kg over 15 minutes, and, after a 45-minute waiting period, the infusion of 5.4 mg/Kg for 23 hours (Halpern 1991).

Nursing assessment includes frequent neurologic checks, including recording of sensory dermatome

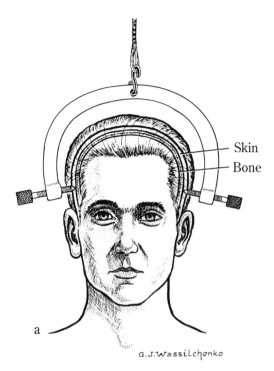

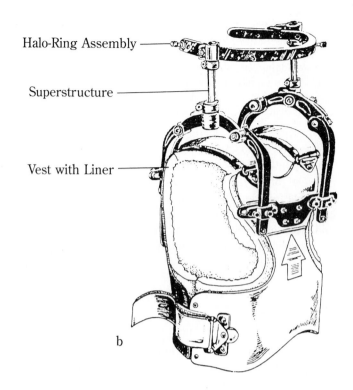

Skin
Bone

Halo-Ring Assembly
Superstructure
Vest with Liner

a

b

G.J.Wassilchenko

FIGURE 21–5

a. Gardner-Wells tongs **b.** Halo vest structure (Reproduced by permission from:
a: Rudy E: *Advanced neurological and neurosurgical nursing,* 1984, St Louis: Mosby,
p. 404; b: Illustration courtesy of Durr-Fillauer.)

patterns. The rating scale for documentation of sensation described by Trunkey and Lewis (1991) ranges from S0, the absence of sensation, to S4, complete recovery. A motor scale ranges from M0, no motor activity at all, to M5, contraction against resistance and normal power. Patients may demonstrate a motor skill on admission and yet, within a few minutes to an hour, be unable to demonstrate the same skill.

Spinal Shock Spinal cord injury directly interferes with the cord's ability to transmit impulses descending from the brain. *Spinal shock,* the complete suppression of all reflex activity below the level of the injury, occurs immediately after injury and lasts from days to months. Flaccid paralysis is a hallmark of spinal shock. Tendon reflexes diminish or disappear, and temperature regulation is lost. Loss of vasomotor tone due to loss of sympathetic activity causes arterial vasodilatation and venous pooling, leading to hypotension. Because the parasympathetic nervous system is unopposed, marked bradycardia can occur. Management of these two acute complications consists of administration of IV fluids, a vasopressor, and/or atropine. If the bradycardia does not respond to atropine, a temporary transvenous pacer must be placed to maintain good

perfusion. Frequent monitoring of vital signs and the ECG for cardiac dysrhythmias is imperative.

The combination of vasodilatation and the inability to shiver causes heat loss, so an additional problem related to the loss of sympathetic tone is difficulty maintaining a normal body temperature. Take the patient's temperature every 4 hours and minimize body exposure to the environment. It may be necessary to employ additional warming methods to maintain normal body temperature.

The reappearance of involuntary reflexes signifies that spinal cord shock is abating. The anal reflex may be tested, as it frequently is one of the earliest to return. With the return of reflex activity, the development of spasticity poses a problem for the quadriplegic.

Altered Urinary Elimination Pattern In the acute phase of spinal cord shock, the patient has an atonic bladder because impulses from the brain are unable to reach it, and a urinary catheter must be inserted to prevent urinary retention. In the acutely unstable patient, an indwelling catheter may be used for a few days to monitor output closely, after which intermittent catheterization is employed to maintain bladder capacity. Because an overdistended bladder can cause ischemia, which predisposes tissue to bacterial invasion and infection, strict aseptic technique should be used when catheterizing patients. When spinal shock abates, the bladder becomes spastic and reflex emptying may occur.

Altered Bowel Elimination Bowel dysfunction results in ileus and fecal retention. The abdomen should be assessed for the presence of bowel sounds, after which the stomach may need to be decompressed with a nasogastric tube.

Spinal-cord-injury patients with neurogenic bowels often develop diarrhea or impaction related to immobility, ingestion of foods or fluids, or infection. Team collaboration with the patient and especially with dietitians skilled in problem solving may yield solutions. For example, adding yogurt or buttermilk to the diet may decrease diarrhea during antibiotic therapy.

It is essential that the patient maintain a daily bowel program to decrease the incidence of impaction. Bowel control can be regained in most cord-injury patients with an appropriate program. Bowel evacuation should begin as soon as the patient is over the critical period. Constipation should be prevented, as it may trigger autonomic dysreflexia or aggravate spasticity. A high-roughage diet, plenty of fluids, and the use of stool softeners, mild cathartics, suppositories, or digital stimulation are all part of a bowel retraining program.

Altered Nutrition: Less than Body Requirements Depending on associated gastrointestinal injuries and bowel function, the patient's nutritional requirements are met via parenteral or enteral feeding. Recent research demonstrates that the spinal-cord-injury patient may have an obligatory negative nitrogen balance, although the reason for this phenomenon remains unclear (Rodriguez, Clevenger and Osler 1991). Chronic paraplegia and quadriplegia are marked by a reduction in energy of up to 67% and progressive loss of lean body mass (Rodriguez, Clevenger and Osler 1991). The exact mechanism for the phenomena is unknown, but immobilization and denervation atrophy may be contributing factors. Decreased thyroid function, as well as tumor necrosis factor and interleukin-1, appear to be mediators of altered protein metabolism following injury. The spinal-cord-injury patient develops a virtually irreversible negative nitrogen balance in the acute injury period, therefore efforts to achieve a positive nitrogen balance will result in overfeeding (Rodriguez, Clevenger and Osler 1991).

High Risk for Infection Infection is both an acute and chronic threat to the spinal-cord injury patient. Potential sources of infection are the lungs, skin, and bladder.

The loss of intercostal and abdominal muscles to assist in effective airway clearance leaves the quadriplegic prone to atelectasis and pneumonia. Good pulmonary hygiene, along with early mobilization, may help decrease pulmonary infections.

The patient's skin is another potential site for infection. The insertion sites of the skull tongs should be inspected daily for signs of redness or excess drainage. Pin care should include cleansing with hydrogen peroxide and betadine, followed with a sterile split 2×2 dressing.

The development of a decubitus ulcer poses an infection risk, delays the rehabilitation process, and can aggravate spasticity or precipitate an episode of autonomic dysreflexia. The key is prevention. Be sure to scrutinize the skin for reddened areas, and straighten the linen so there are no bumps or wrinkles that put pressure on the patient's skin. Pay special attention to pressure points, and establish a turning schedule.

Intermittent catheterization or use of condom catheters is preferred to use of indwelling Foley catheters for the prevention of bladder distention and urine pooling (stasis).

Altered Tissue Perfusion Related to Autonomic Dysreflexia Autonomic dysreflexia, a massive sympathetic discharge stimulated by sensory input that cannot traverse the spinal cord to communicate with the brain, is a potentially life-threatening situation seen in patients with cord lesions above the T_6 level. This phenomenon does not occur until spinal cord shock is over (Mitchell et al. 1988). Signs and symptoms include throbbing headache, flushing of the face and neck, nasal congestion, sweating above the lesion, hypertension, and bradycardia. A distended bladder, full rectum, decubitus ulcer, ingrown toenail, bladder spasm, or other stimuli may trigger this autonomic dysreflexia. The primary danger to the patient is that uncontrolled hypertension will precipitate a stroke. Management focuses on eliminating the cause; however, if the cause is not easily ascertained, then blood pressure control is instituted.

Identify patients at risk for developing autonomic dysreflexia by tagging their chart to alert hospital personnel to the condition. In-depth patient/family education is vital, because this condition will be a problem for the patient for the rest of his or her life.

High Risk for Ineffective Individual Coping Most patients notice the loss of sensation and motor function and transient pain for an unidentified period. Paresthesias (burning or tingling) or hyperesthesias (increased sensitivity) may also be a source of discomfort. The patient's greatest suffering, however, is psychologic.

The spinal-cord-injury patient experiences many areas in which his or her self-concept is disrupted, including body image, self-esteem, role performance, personal identity, and sexual function. The quality of life issue is dealt with differently by every patient and family. Each SCI patient must find a reason for participating in rehabilitation and in independent living after discharge. Some patients may value life to the extent that even profound physiologic and functional dependency requires nothing more than adaptation and altered goal setting. Other patients may be so devastated that they judge their lives as meaningless and they become intent on self-destruction.

Usually, patients and families are capable of making informed choices and the health care provider acts as advocate, giving information upon which to base decisions (Sullivan 1990). The health care team should not project personal feelings about the patient's anticipated quality of life. It is very important that patients know that the level of their functioning will not be stable for some time, so it is often very difficult to judge rehabilitation potential accurately in the hospital.

Patient education should include information about sexual function. Many male patients continue to produce active sperm and could participate in artificial insemination. Penile implants may permit the patient to return to a normal pattern of sexual activity. Women may become pregnant and deliver babies while paraplegic.

High Risk for Ineffective Family Coping Acute spinal cord injury occurs about 10,000 times each year, and patients can expect to return to the community to live within 10% of a normal lifespan (Sullivan 1990). This devastating injury affects between 120,000 and 150,000 people in the United States (Sullivan 1990). The families and friends of these individuals assume a tremendous task in assisting the injured person to rebuild a life and return to optimal functioning. Generally, family members' psychologic adaptation to sudden, unexpected injury is similar to the adaptation process for death and grief.

Chapter 3 discusses communication with the patient and family. The following humanistic principles are particularly important in caring for spinal-cord-injury patients and their families.

- Know what the physician has told the patient and family so you can reinforce what they have been told.
- Communicate openly and honestly with the patient and family.
- Provide reassurance by touching. (Be sure to touch areas that the patient can feel.)

- Stand in the patient's visual field so the patient knows to whom he or she is talking.
- Avoid talking "about," "over," or "for" the patient.
- Always explain what is being done and why.
- Allow the patient some control over daily activities.
- Provide for privacy.
- Pay special attention to personal care that maintains the patient's sexual self-image (e.g., encourage the use of after-shave cologne, make-up, nail polish).
- Acknowledge the family's feelings, and include family members in daily care activities as soon as possible.

Chest Trauma

Chest injuries account for 25% of all sudden trauma deaths in the United States (Del Rossi 1990). Head trauma is the only fatal injury surpassing chest trauma in incidence. Trauma to the chest is life-threatening and requires accurate diagnosis and immediate intervention. Concomitant injury to abdominal organs is also a common cause of death in these patients.

Mechanism of Injury Injuries to the chest and upper abdomen are commonly referred to as torso trauma. Chest trauma can involve the heart, lungs, esophagus, diaphragm, and/or great vessels. Because the ribs extend over the liver, spleen and other structures, forces applied to the rib cage may be transmitted to lower "chest" or abdominal structures. In blunt trauma, hydraulic forces (fluids forced under tremendous pressure) also may injure structures.

The critical-care nurse needs to be vigilant for the signs and symptoms suggesting the presence of chest trauma (Table 21–2). Fractured chest bones indicate that underlying structures may be injured, and these underlying injuries (such as pulmonary contusion and cardiac contusion) are not always apparent initially. Stab or gunshot wounds to the midpectoralis muscle may result in laceration of the pectoral branch of the thoracoacromial artery, causing bleeding that may be very difficult to control.

Diagnostic studies include chest x-ray, CT scanning, angiography, electrocardiography, and pulse oximetry (Table 21–3). Laboratory tests include electrolyte panels, particularly calcium levels. The myocardium, which is highly dependent upon calcium, may be calcium depleted as a result of the resuscitation. The presence of catecholamine, calcium overload, and

TABLE 21–2

Anatomic and Physiologic Signs and Symptoms Associated with Chest Trauma

ANATOMIC

Paradoxical chest wall movement

Chest wall abrasions, contusions, ecchymosis

Open wounds (penetrating and perforating)

Tracheal deviation

Distended neck veins

Chest wall crepitus

PHYSIOLOGIC

Dyspnea, shortness of breath

Tachypnea

Respiratory distress, mild to severe

Cyanosis

Decreased or absent breath sounds

Hyperresonance or dullness to percussion

Signs of hypovolemic shock

Chest pain, especially on inspiration

Muffled heart sounds

Pulsus paradoxus

Widened mediastinum

Cardiac dysrhythmias

NURSING TIP

Assess the Polytrauma Patient Carefully and Completely

When trauma is sustained to the torso above the diaphragm, carefully assess below the diaphragm for additional injury. Bullets can change direction, and blunt trauma can cause "hydraulic injury" to other structures. (Hydraulic injury results from structures moving into and against each other due to pressure on the fluid within them.)

---

energy interruption, and the generation of oxygen-free radicals during reperfusion after prolonged resuscitation or in cardiac contusion, may contribute to alterations in cardiac output (Chisholm 1990).

Types of Chest Trauma   Types of chest trauma include tension pneumothorax, open pneumothorax

TABLE 21–3

Diagnostic Studies Commonly Used to Assess Chest Trauma

STUDY	DIAGNOSTICALLY SIGNIFICANT DATA
Laboratory:	
Complete blood count (CBC)	Hemoglobin/hematocrit
Electrolytes	Baseline data
Arterial blood gas	$\uparrow$ Pco_2; $\downarrow$ Po_2; $\downarrow$ pH
Urinalysis	Positive for blood
Radiography: chest x-ray	Collapsed lung; widened mediastinum
Electrocardiogram	Elevated ST segment; dysrhythmias
CT scan	Fluid, thoracic bony deformity
Arteriogram	Intact vascular supply
Echocardiogram	Pericardial effusion, valve function, ejection fraction
Doppler echo	Valvular integrity

(sucking chest wound), massive hemothorax, flail chest with underlying pulmonary contusion, cardiac tamponade, and cardiac contusion and concussion (Table 21–4). Although these conditions are stabilized in the field or emergency department, they continue to pose risks for the patient in the ICU because they may recur or worsen.

Tension Pneumothorax   Mechanical ventilation, especially with the addition of positive end-expiratory pressure and underlying, undetected tracheal or bronchial injuries, may lead to the development of tension pneumothorax. Classic signs and symptoms include:

• Severe dyspnea and slightly-to-significantly decreased arterial oxygen saturation levels, usually measured continuously by pulse oximetry

• Absent lung sounds on the affected side

• Tracheal deviation away from the affected side

• Decreased systolic blood pressure

• Increased central venous pressure, as demonstrated by pressures of 15–20 cm H_2O or distended neck veins 3–4 cm above the clavicle at 45° in a semi-Fowler's position.

The measure for immediately relieving the tension pneumothorax is decompressive thoracostomy with a large-bore (14–16-gauge) needle in the second intercostal space, midclavicular line, followed by chest tube

TABLE 21–4

Specific Chest Injuries, with Pathophysiology, Classic Signs and Symptoms, and Nursing and Medical Interventions

INJURY	PATHOPHYSIOLOGY	SIGNS AND SYMPTOMS	NURSING/MEDICAL INTERVENTIONS
Tension pneumo- thorax	Air enters the pleural space on inspiration without any mechanism for release. Intrathoracic pressure increases on affected side, resulting in complete collapse of the lung. Occurs more frequently than cardiac tamponade.	Severe shortness of breath Respiratory distress Tracheal deviation to unaffected side Distended neck veins (may be flat if severe hypovolemia) Decreased or absent breath sounds, affected side Hyperresonance on percussion, affected side	1. Prepare for insertion of 14–16–gauge needle into 2nd intercostal space in midclavicular line of affected side. 2. Prepare for insertion of chest tube into 5th/6th intercostal space, anterior to midaxillary line.
Open pneu- mothorax (sucking chest wound)	Defect in chest wall allows passage of air from atmosphere into pleural space and out of the pleurae.	Respiratory distress Tachypnea, grunting Penetrating chest wound Sucking sound as air enters pleural space Unilateral decrease or absence of breath sounds, affected side	1. Cover wound with sterile, occlusive dressing. 2. Monitor for development of tension pneumothorax. 3. Remove dressing if tension pneumo- thorax develops. 4. Prepare for insertion of chest tube into 5th/6th intercostal space, anterior to midaxillary line. 5. Definitive care usually is surgical care of chest wall defect.
Massive hemothorax	Accumulation of 1,500 ml or more of blood in pleural space. May cause severe hemodynamic compromise due to major blood loss, mediastinal shift, and compression of unaffected lung.	Signs of shock Dyspnea Unilateral decrease or absence of breath sounds, affected side Dullness to percussion, affected side Distended or flat neck veins	1. Restore blood volume with crystal- loid, blood, and/or colloids before chest tube insertion. 2. Consider PASG. 3. Consider autotransfusion. 4. Prepare for insertion of large-bore chest tube 5th/6th intercostal space, anterior to midaxillary line. 5. Continuous monitoring of chest tube drainage. 6. Emergency thoracotomy if severe hy- povolemia or unable to control blood loss.
Flail chest	Usually occurs in relation to blunt trauma with the flail segment resulting in paradoxical movement of the chest wall. Occurs when two or more ribs are fractured in at least two sites, or when the sternum is separated from the rib cage due to multiple fractures. Results in impaired ventilation and gas exchange due to pain and associated lung injury.	Shortness of breath, respiratory distress Flail segment, paradoxical chest wall movement Severe chest pain, affected side Crepitus and abnormal chest wall movement may be palpable	1. Stabilization of flail segment by inter- nal fixation with endotracheal intuba- tion and mechanical ventilation .2. Control of pain with intercostal nerve blocks and/or systemic intravenous analgesics. 3. Aggressive respiratory care. 4. If severe respiratory distress, endo- tracheal intubation and ventilatory support.

TABLE 21–4

Specific Chest Injuries, with Pathophysiology, Classic Signs and Symptoms, and Nursing and Medical Interventions (Continued)

INJURY	PATHOPHYSIOLOGY	SIGNS AND SYMPTOMS	NURSING/MEDICAL INTERVENTIONS
Cardiac tamponade	Most often occurs from a penetrating injury to the myocardium, which results in an acute accumulation of blood in the pericardial sac. May less frequently result from blunt cardiac trauma. Results in alterations in diastolic filling of ventricles and mechanical function of the heart. Venous hypertension often occurs due to the backup of blood resulting from the decreased diastolic filling.	Signs of shock Beck's triad (increased venous pressure with jugular venous distention—may be absent in severe hypovolemia; decreased blood pressure, muffled heart sounds) Pulsus paradoxus (fall in systolic BP >15 mm Hg during inspiration) Possible inability to palpate apical pulse Dyspnea, possibly Kussmaul's respirations	1. Pericardiocentesis by the subxyphoid route (pericardial blood has Hct lower than venous blood and will not clot). 2. Placement of central line to assess central venous pressure. 3. Emergency thoracotomy if unable to aspirate pericardial blood. 4. Definitive care requires thoracotomy for surgical repair of cardiac injuries.

insertion. Tension pneumothorax is discussed further in Chapter 8.

Flail Chest and Underlying Pulmonary Contusion Flail segments (chest wall segments that move paradoxically with ventilation) with subcutaneous emphysema are common in chest trauma patients. The usual treatment is internal fixation with endotracheal intubation and mechanical ventilation, and neuromuscular blocking agents may be very helpful in initially controlling the flail segments.

Pulmonary contusion may underlie flail segments or may occur due to blunt trauma without flail chest. Intrapulmonary shunting and reduced compliance increase the difficulty in maintaining adequate ventilation. Restlessness, tachycardia, tachypnea, and/or wheezes may indicate hypoventilation. Assessment includes the color and quantity of sputum (bloody sputum is unusual) and levels of arterial oxygen saturation as measured by pulse oximetry and arterial blood gases. Adequate supplemental oxygen, pain relief, and chest physiotherapy are important measures for maintaining adequate oxygenation. Intubation and meticulous endotracheal care help prevent complications related to prolonged hypoxemia. Infection also is very common in the patient with pulmonary contusion (Trunkey and Lewis 1991).

Cardiac Tamponade Cardiac tamponade, which results from the accumulation of blood in the pericardial sac, is accompanied by a significant reduction in cardiac output. Patients usually demonstrate Beck's

triad as long as fluid volume status has been adequately restored: increased venous pressure (as evidenced by jugular venous distention and increased CVP and right atrial pressures), muffled heart tones, and hypotension. Pulse pressure narrows and pulsus paradoxus appears.

Successful resolution may require various treatments. In a pericardiocentesis—a short-term, emergency measure to relieve cardiac tamponade—an 18-gauge needle or over-the-needle catheter is inserted into the pericardium and fluid is aspirated. Frequently, a catheter is capped and left in place to provide further aspiration, if needed, before definitive surgical exploration and repair can occur. The aspirate will not clot unless there is a massive fresh bleed into the pericardium; in that case, aspiration—even with a large-bore (19-gauge) spinal needle—will be inadequate to remove the obstruction. Thoracotomy, sternotomy, or creation of a pericardial window may be necessary to diagnose and treat the source of bleeding. If the cause of the tamponade is a penetrating injury to the heart, an emergency thoracotomy will be necessary to repair the injury and relieve the tamponade. Especially in the event of sudden cardiovascular collapse with electromechanical dissociation, cardiac tamponade must be ruled out. Cardiac tamponade is discussed further in Chapter 13.

Cardiac Contusion and Concussion When trauma occurs to the heart, cardiac contusion or concussion may result. Histopathologically, cardiac contusion resembles acute myocardial infarction, in that erythrocytes leak into myofibril interspaces resulting in edema and myocardial necrosis. After the area infiltrates with leukocytes, the well-demarcated hemorrhage is absorbed and a scar of variable size is formed. Small subepicardial areas likely will have no sequelae; however, full-thickness contusions of the wall may result in ventricular aneurysm formation and/or rupture of the myocardium. Contusion and concussion differ only in that contusion results in tissue necrosis, whereas concussion has no necrosis but often presents with fatal dysrhythmia (Bartlett 1991). Monitoring is critical and may demonstrate a number of nonspecific ST–T wave changes to full-blown ST segment ischemic changes with activity, suctioning, or any increase in oxygen demand (Bell 1992). Continued surveillance for signs or symptoms of decreased cardiac output, oxygenation deficit, or dysrhythmia is also critical.

The use of continuous, multiple-lead ST analysis can assist in identification of cardiac ischemia related to blunt chest trauma. Effective nursing response to clinically significant changes may also minimize expensive invasive or noninvasive diagnostic follow-up. This is especially true when the nurse effectively treats cardiac ischemia or ventricular dysrhythmia at the bedside. Additional research is needed to establish the clinical and prognostic significance of ST segment changes in the immediate post chest trauma patient (Bell 1992). In many centers, routine cardiac workup for suspected cardiac contusion includes a 12-lead ECG, measurement of a creatine phosphokinase myocardial band (CPK-MB) isoenzyme level, echocardiogram, and invasive diagnostics. This patient requires symptomatic, prompt treatment of ventricular dysrhythmia and identification of the cause of tachydysrhythmias and congestive heart failure (Trunkey and Lewis 1991). Regular auscultation for valvular or septal disruption may be life saving.

When cardiac injury is suspected, emergent two-dimensional echocardiography is a valuable tool in the triage of stable penetrating trauma patients. Small effusions can be monitored and followed, thus preventing unnecessary thoracotomy. Large effusions must be treated surgically.

Nursing Considerations in Chest Trauma There are two additional general considerations in caring for patients with chest trauma: pain related to chest tube removal, and complications of chest trauma.

Gift, Bolgiano and Cunningham (1991) published the results of a study in which 36 patients described sensations of burning, pain, pressure, pulling, and soreness on chest tube removal. Interestingly, the reported intensities of sensation did not differ between patients who received analgesia before the procedure and those who did not, between mediastinal and pleural tube removal, or between sexes or ages. (This study did not, however, indicate the time between drug administration and chest tube removal, an important variable.) Although chest tube removal happens rapidly, it may upset the patient if it is performed unexpectedly, so patient education is very important. Prior to the procedure, advise the patient that the chest tube will be removed and offer premedication for reduction of anxiety and pain. Distraction and relaxation techniques may be helpful as well.

Complications of chest trauma include adult respiratory distress syndrome, discussed in Chapter 8, and multiple organ system failure, presented in Chapter 20.

Abdominal Trauma

Mechanism of Injury and Types of Abdominal Trauma The abdominal wall offers minimal protection from injury of the underlying organs. Blunt trauma, most common, frequently results from motor vehicle accidents and physical assault. Penetrating abdominal trauma frequently results from stabbing and gunshot wounds. The liver and spleen are the most frequently injured abdominal organs.

Aggressive surgical management of abdominal injuries has been the standard. Recently, however, conservative management has been effective in children, and this approach has produced a positive outcome in adult patients as well (Kimura and Otsuka 1991).

Several diagnostic studies, including diagnostic peritoneal lavage, CT scanning, and magnetic resonance imaging (MRI), may be performed in an effort to spare the patient from undergoing surgical laparotomy. Diagnosis by diagnostic peritoneal lavage (DPL) or CT scanning alone often does not provide sufficient information.

DPL is an internationally recognized method of assessing intraperitoneal bleeding. A catheter is placed into the peritoneum through a very small incision just below the umbilicus. One liter of warmed saline solution is instilled and then allowed to drain. A gross estimate of the amount of red blood cells (for example, as shown by the ability to read newsprint through the fluid) or laboratory analysis determines the requirement for further diagnostic evaluation and surgery. This very safe procedure may replace the need for full laparotomy in the patient with altered level of consciousness, lower thoracic injury, pelvic fracture, abdominal wall contusion, or multiple system injury (Trunkey and Lewis 1991). Henneman, Marx and Moore (1990) report that DPL has a 93% accuracy with a complication rate of 0.3%. DPL detects some self-limited solid visceral injuries but misses a significant percentage of hollow visceral injuries. DPL does not, however, replace physical examination and good surgical judgment (Henneman, Marx and Moore 1990).

CT scanning is notoriously inadequate for diagnosing ruptured viscus. Harris (1991) reports that the use of CT for diagnosis of hepatic and intra-abdominal injury is insufficient and may delay surgical intervention. In cases of major hepatic injury, delaying treatment may delay the diagnosis of significant associated injury and thereby increase mortality (Harris 1991). However, utilization of multiple diagnostic procedures and assessment of potential or actual shock may be helpful in successfully eliminating unnecessary surgical intervention for minor hepatic injury. Kimura and Otsuka (1991) report the reliability of ultrasonography in detecting hemoperitoneum in blunt abdominal trauma. Ultrasonography is a rapid, safe, noninvasive method of assessing the abdomen and may replace DPL.

Nursing Considerations in Abdominal Trauma

Chest wall contusions, and/or chest wall ecchymosis are common in blunt trauma to the torso. If you observe these hematomas, be alert for the possibility of injury to the underlying structures, especially the liver, spleen, abdomen, or uterus. Retroperitoneal hematoma frequently is present after blunt trauma to the anterior or posterior surface of the torso. Surgical intervention varies according to the individual and with concomitant injury.

In motor vehicle accidents, the seat belt can produce major structural injury. Because the belt crosses the body diagonally, injuries may include fracture of the clavicle, scapula, and/or ribs; contusion of the heart or lung; and disruption of the small bowel (especially at the ligament of Treitz), kidney, spleen, and liver. You may observe Grey Turner's sign (hematoma along the flanks), or Cullen's sign (periumbilical hematoma), which may signal retroperitoneal bleeding or pancreatitis.

Major concerns for the abdominal trauma patient are establishing hemodynamic stability, recognizing and identifying occult injuries, determining the risk of sepsis, and instituting nutritional and psychosocial support for the patient and significant others. The

ADVANCES IN CRITICAL-CARE TECHNOLOGY

Abdominal Pressure Monitoring

THE TECHNOLOGY

Abdominal pressure monitoring is a relatively simple procedure that may help determine increased intra–abdominal pressures. The procedure is similar to compartment pressure monitoring done when orthopedic, crush or peripheral vascular injury occurs.

A catheter is placed into the abdomen and attached to a transducer, but fluid is not infused through this catheter. Size and location of this catheter differ based on the surgeon or center. Laparoscopic assessment with insertion of the catheter may replace diagnostic peritoneal lavage and perhaps initial CAT scan in some centers.

A trend plot must be established for a specific position because gravitational or respiratory forces in a sitting position may not be the same as supine. Side-lying positions need to be trended as well.

PATIENT CARE CONSIDERATIONS

Usual pressures are 0 mm Hg or subatmospheric. Pressures above 20 mm Hg are considered elevated and may result in ischemia and necrosis of the surrounding tissues if not treated promptly. Postoperative abdominal pressures usually measure 3–15 mm Hg.

The reference point for transducer placement is the symphysis pubis. The patient must be either supine or in a semi-Fowler's position. Careful documentation of position is required.

major early life-threatening concern in abdominal injuries is severe blood loss and resulting hemorrhagic shock (see Chapter 20).

Peritonitis and sepsis are life-threatening concerns that cause increased mortality and morbidity in the later stages of care. Injury that results in bowel perforation is likely to cause virulent bacterial bowel contents to leak into the peritoneum, with subsequent peritonitis and septic shock. The gut plays a central role in sepsis, shock response, and trauma pathophysiology, because it acts as a barrier that may be impaired by microbial translocation resulting from ischemia, malnutrition, stress, chemical alteration, and/or antibiotics. (See Chapter 20 for further discussion.)

The critical-care nurse has a particularly important assessment challenge with the medically managed patient during the first 72 hours after injury. Abnormal vital signs, increasing abdominal tenderness, guarding, and changed pain pattern are all important observations that must be communicated to the surgeon, as iatrogenic trauma (from DPL or from insertion of lines and tubes) and delayed response to trauma may not appear until several hours later. Pain radiating to the left shoulder, referred to as *Kehr's sign,* is a classic finding in patients with splenic rupture and is caused by blood below the diaphragm irritating the phrenic nerve.

Abdominal trauma rarely results in injury to the kidneys that is severe enough to require surgical removal of both kidneys. Frequently, however, abdominal trauma does lead to acute renal failure or multiple organ failure. The trauma patient in acute renal failure may require continuous hemofiltration, because cardiovascular instability and hypotension often accompany intermittent hemodialysis in the critically ill or unstable patient. (See Chapter 16 for further details.)

Orthopedic Trauma

Orthopedic trauma, often the most visibly dramatic injury, must be managed only after life-threatening situations have been assessed and appropriately treated. In the initial resuscitation period, the team must focus on the primary survey and ensure a patent airway, effective ventilation, and adequate circulation. Amputation, neurovascular compromise (loss of pulse or sensation), and uncontrolled hemorrhage do require immediate attention during resuscitation; however, without an airway there is no reason to continue resuscitation.

Types of Orthopedic Trauma Orthopedic injuries include fractures, sprains, strains, ligament tears,

tendon lacerations, arterial disruption, and joint dislocations. Definitive care for these injuries includes accurate diagnosis, reduction of dislocations, application of splints and casts, traction, or surgical procedures. Detailed attention to medical management is beyond the scope of this chapter; however, the brief discussion below will provide a framework for planning nursing care.

Orthopedic injuries may result in an obvious deformity or they may be obscured because there are no visual signs of injury and the patient does not complain of pain. As with other forms of trauma, a history of the accident and information about the mechanism of injury provide data to guide the assessment process. Typical signs of orthopedic injury include obvious deformity of the injured extremity, pain, swelling, muscle spasm, crepitus, limited movement, and possible neurovascular compromise. Signs of shock may appear due to a substantial blood loss from either external hemorrhage or internal bleeding resulting from disruption of tissue and vessels.

Open reduction and internal fixation or external fixation are best performed within 6 hours of the injury, because after the first 24 hours, the hazards of immobility and deconditioning increase. Frequently, these patients will be restored to weight bearing within 48 hours in the absence of pelvic ring or acetabular fractures.

Pelvic and Acetabular Fractures Although very painful, pelvic and acetabular fractures are frequently stable and they usually do not require surgery. When surgery is indicated, there are very few reasons for delaying internal or external fixation of extremity or compound pelvic fractures. External fixation may hasten mobilization of the patient with open-book pelvic fracture and therefore decrease the complications related to immobility.

Fibular and Tibial Fractures and Dislocations Patients with distal fibular and tibial fractures may have longer recovery times than those with complex femoral fractures, due to the limited vascular supply to these areas. *Dislocations* result when joints exceed the normal range of motion and the joint surfaces are no longer intact. Unrecognized or irreducible dislocations increase the risk of nerve or vascular damage and osteonecrosis.

Open Fractures Open fractures involving skin disruption require surgery for debridement to minimize the risks of clostridial and pyogenic infections. They are classified as grade I, which includes small wounds caused by low-velocity trauma and little soft tissue trauma; grades II and IIIA, which include wounds of

2–6 cm that require stabilization with rods, pins, or plates; grade IIIB, which involves extensive soil/manure contamination and requires extensive plastic repair; or grade IIIC, which includes a vascular injury requiring repair followed by stabilization of the orthopedic injury. Immediate administration of antibiotics is vital in limiting infections. Hyperbaric oxygen treatment, although controversial, may be instituted for major soft tissue injury with clostridial invasion. Cultures are not usually useful at admission because colonization and growth patterns generally change over the next 48–72 hours (Trunkey and Lewis 1991).

Nursing Considerations in Orthopedic Trauma
Nursing care requires careful assessment. The "five Ps" (pain, pallor, pulselessness, paresthesias, and paralysis) often are used to assess orthopedic injuries. Additional assessment must include comparison of the injured extremity with the uninjured extremity. Assessment of blood loss should take into consideration actual external loss and estimated blood loss into the closed space. Blood losses may be substantial: 1,000–1,500 ml per femur and 2,000 ml or more for the pelvis (Trunkey and Lewis 1991). This blood loss frequently requires transfusion replacement for 4–7 days. Special attention to occult injuries or frequently missed injuries is important during the assessment phase of care. Assessment of respiratory status is essential due to the high potential for embolization. Immobilized patients are at great risk for deep-vein thrombosis preventable by early mobilization. Early physical and occupational therapy consultations minimize disability and encourage early mobilization.

Compartment Syndrome Compartment syndrome is a complication of orthopedic injury that occurs as pressure increases inside the fascial compartment enveloping the injury site. This condition compresses nerves, vessels, and muscle, and must be identified immediately to prevent permanent damage. The increasing pressure may result from internal bleeding and swelling or from external sources such as a cast or pneumatic antishock garment. Compartment syndrome occurs predominantly in relation to injuries involving the lower leg and forearm.

Signs and symptoms associated with compartment syndrome include progressive, severe pain that is frequently unrelieved by narcotic analgesics; paresthesia (a loss of sensation or numbness); absent or decreasing distal pulse; cyanosis or pallor of a distal extremity; delayed capillary refill; and loss of motor function. An increased compartment pressure becomes evident with measurement.

Immediate intervention is based on early recognition of signs and symptoms. Elevation of the affected extremity to the level of the heart will help prevent further swelling. The critical-care nurse prepares for a fasciotomy if compartment pressure is greater than 40 mm Hg. The fasciotomy will immediately relieve ele-

ADVANCES IN CRITICAL-CARE TECHNOLOGY

Compartment Pressure Monitoring

THE TECHNOLOGY

Compartment pressure monitoring is used to measure the compartment pressure in an extremity that has sustained either crush or ischemic injury. To measure compartment pressure you need an over-the-needle catheter, a transducer, and a monitor that is equipped to measure pressures from 1 mm Hg to 300 mm Hg. The transducer and catheter are flushed and filled with fluid, the catheter is inserted into the compartment, and the transducer is attached and then opened to the compartment for a pressure reading.

PATIENT CARE CONSIDERATIONS

It is critical that a flush device *not* be attached, because infiltration of fluid into an already distended compartment could be responsible for significant damage to muscles, blood vessels, and nerves. Normal compartment pressure is 20 mm Hg or less, with 21–40 mm Hg indicating decreased tissue perfusion and 41 mm Hg or above signaling ischemia.

vated compartment pressure and may prevent permanent neurovascular damage and possible loss of limb.

External Fixator Care External fixator care remains controversial, and a review of the literature shows that no one procedure is superior. There is general consensus that until there is evidence of erythema or purulence, no care is required (Goldberger, Kruse and Stender 1987). Nevertheless, some advocate a variety of cleaning and dressing techniques.

Burns

After a major thermal insult—one of the most devastating traumas—the patient has to cope not only with its complex physiologic sequelae but also with its psychologic effects and long-term implications for the quality of life. Nursing care of the burned patient is one of the most demanding—and yet most satisfying—challenges faced by the critical-care nurse.

SPECIAL FEATURE

Pregnancy: A Collaborative Problem in Trauma Nursing Care

The detailed management of the pregnant trauma patient is beyond the scope of this chapter; once the patient has reached the critical-care unit, consultation with labor, delivery, and postpartum colleagues is strongly advised. Fetal monitoring may be instituted if the fetus is yet undelivered. (Normal heart rate for the fetus is 120–160 beats per minute.)

Maternal cardiac output increases to 6–7 L/min by the end of the first trimester and remains elevated throughout pregnancy. Although fluid volume increases, preload may be compromised by placing the patient in a flat supine position, as the gravid uterus may compress the vena cava. Turning the patient slightly will permit the normal compensatory mechanisms for hemorrhage (increased peripheral resistance, increased cardiac index, and increased respiratory rate) to occur. Compression of the vascular structures in the pelvis may increase the pressure distally and increase retroperitoneal hemorrhage or blood loss from pelvic fractures. Keep the patient in a left lateral recumbent position if at all possible.

Due to the increase in plasma circulating volume, normal hematocrit for the pregnant trauma patient is about 36%, and the hemoglobin is about 12 g/dl. Signs of shock may not become evident until 30–35% of circulating volume is lost. Placental fetal perfusion depends upon maternal blood pressure. With acute hemorrhage, uterine blood flow may be reduced 10–20% before changes in maternal blood pressure are noted, due to compensatory vasoconstriction (Trunkey and Lewis 1991). If the patient is delivered by Cesarean section, pitocin is commonly administered to facilitate uterine contraction. This drug may impact resuscitation drug and fluid effects.

Because the gravid uterus alters the normal configuration and location of the abdominal structures, knowledge of the gravid anatomy is very important. The larger the uterus and fetus, the greater the risk of placental separation (abruptio placentae). Generally, when placental separation occurs, the uterus becomes tender and irritable, and labor is common. The stretching of the rectus muscles can result in little or no guarding or rigidity despite significant injury.

The decision to attempt Cesarean section will depend on the condition of the mother and fetus. Some surgeons may opt for the infant in the face of certain maternal death, others for the mother if fetal death is clear, and others for maintaining the maternal-fetal unit if there is a risk of both maternal and fetal death. Each case is different, and each team needs to make such decisions based upon the data available.

It is important that pictures be taken if the fetus dies. If possible, obtain footprints, a lock of hair, and a photograph, as these may be the only evidence the parents have of their baby. These items may facilitate the grieving process by helping the parents to see the reality of the baby's birth and death. Support for the mother and her family is essential as soon as her condition and ability to interact allow it.

Once survival is predicted, consideration is given to postpartum lactation and its impact on the mother's fluid, electrolyte, and breast tissue status. The care plan is developed in collaboration with the patient, her family, and the health care team. A review of the literature was not helpful in guiding bonding, visiting, or breast-feeding guidelines for trauma populations. To assist you in decision-making, integrate your assessment of the patient, team collaboration, and institutional policies.

Key Concepts

The skin is composed of three layers: the epidermis, the dermis, and the hypodermis, or subcutaneous fat (Figure 21–6). The *epidermis,* the outermost layer, is thin and nonvascular. It consists primarily of epithelial cells, which form a protective coating and are shed constantly. The epidermis contains *keratin,* which limits fluid loss, and *melanin,* which contributes to the basic color of the skin. The complex structure of the *dermis,* the middle layer, consists of blood vessels, sensory receptors for temperature, pain, touch, and pressure, portions of hair follicles, sebaceous glands, and ducts of sweat glands. The deepest layer is the *hypodermis,* the subcutaneous fat (containing the roots of sweat glands and hair follicles), under which lie the fascia, muscles, and organs.

The skin has important physiologic functions. It protects the interior of the body, and plays major roles in perception, temperature regulation, and fluid and electrolyte balance. In addition, its outward appearance forms an essential defining feature of a person's self-identity and self-concept.

Assessment

Burn agents are usually classified as *thermal, electrical, chemical,* and *radiation.* Thermal agents, the most common, include flames, scalding substances, and hot tar.

Signs and Symptoms The signs and symptoms of a burn vary with the extent of skin damage (Table 21–5).

Burn Depth The degree of burn varies with the intensity and duration of exposure to the burning agent. In addition, areas may have different degrees of burn, i.e., areas of severe burn may be surrounded by areas of lesser burn. The full extent of a burn may not be apparent for several hours or days. A lesser-degree burn can convert to a greater-degree burn if the burning process continues or if the blood supply to the area is impaired due to edema, hypotension, infection, or pressure.

Superficial Partial-Thickness Burns (First-Degree Burns) Superficial partial-thickness burns involve only the epidermis; a sunburn is a common example. The signs and symptoms are similar to those of epidermal inflammation: redness and pain, with little edema. The skin remains dry and intact at the time of the burn. It desquamates within 3–7 days, and spontaneous healing occurs within a few days.

Deep Partial-Thickness Burns (Second-Degree Burns) Deep partial-thickness burns involve both the epidermis and dermis, and often are the result of exposure to flames, scalding substances, or hot tar. Because the epidermis is involved, the sensory receptors, the capillaries, the hair follicles, and the sebaceous and sweat glands are damaged. The burn is characterized by a red or mottled appearance, blanching on pressure, intense pain, and moderate edema. The skin has blisters or vesicles that increase in size, with apparent oozing and weeping of fluid. Hair is still present. Healing usually occurs spontaneously within about 3–5 weeks but the burned area sometimes requires skin grafting.

Full-Thickness Burns (Third-Degree Burns) Full thickness burns result from thermal, chemical, or electrical agents and they involve all three layers of the skin. (An extremely deep burn may also involve muscle and bone.) Because all the structures in the dermal layer

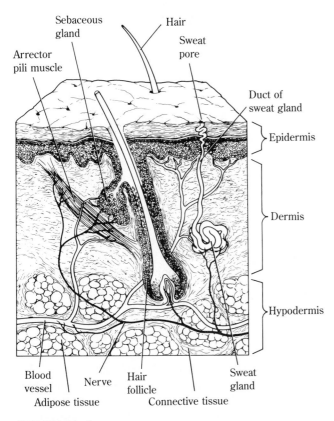

Sebaceous gland

Hair

Sweat pore

Arrector pili muscle

Duct of sweat gland

Epidermis

Dermis

Hypodermis

Blood vessel

Nerve

Hair follicle

Sweat gland

Adipose tissue

Connective tissue

FIGURE 21–6

Structure of the epidermis, dermis, and hypodermis layers. (From: Spence A, Mason E: *Human anatomy and physiology,* 3d ed. Menlo Park, CA: Benjamin/Cummings, 1987, Fig. 5.2a.)

TABLE 21–5

Classification of Burns

BURN TYPE	AREA DAMAGED	CHARACTERISTICS
Partial Thickness		
Superficial	Epidermis	Erythema
		Pain
		Little or no edema
		Dry, intact skin
Deep	Epidermis	Erythema
	Dermis	Blanching on pressure
		Hair still present
		Blisters that increase in size
		Intense pain
		Minimal to moderate edema
		Oozing/weeping
Full Thickness	Epidermis	Dry
	Dermis	Blisters absent or do not increase in size
	Hypodermis	Red, white, or charred (blackened and depressed)
		Leathery texture
		No pain
		No blanching on pressure
		Blood vessels may be visible

are destroyed, the burn, which may appear red, white, or charred, does not blanch on pressure, and the area of full-thickness burn is painless. It may have a dry, leathery texture, and either no hair is present or the hair pulls out easily. Blisters are absent or, if present, do not increase in size. Blood vessels may be visible in the exposed tissue. These extensive burns cannot heal spontaneously and always require skin grafting.

Burn Area   There are several methods for determining the amount of burned area. A quick, convenient method used in the prehospital or emergency department setting is the classic *rule of nines,* which assigns percentages to various areas of the body (Figure 21–7). For small or peculiarly shaped burns, the size of the burn may be compared to the size of the patient's palm as the palmar surface approximates 1% of the total body surface area (TBSA). The rule of nines is relatively inaccurate for determining specific therapies, as it does not account for differences in body proportions among age groups. The Lund and Browder chart, which correlates body surface area percentages with age (Figure 21–8), is the most precise determinate of burn extent.

Burn Severity   The severity of a burn can be categorized as *minor, moderate,* or *major* according to the classic guidelines developed by the American Burn Association (ABA) (1976). The categories are determined by the *depth* of burn, *area* of burn, and *high-risk factors.* According to the ABA guidelines, patients with major burns should be cared for in a regional burn center.

A major burn presents with any of the following characteristics: (a) a full-thickness burn greater than 10% TBSA; (b) a partial-thickness burn greater than 25% TBSA; (c) a burn in a critical area: the face, eyes, ears, hands, perineum/genitalia, or feet; or (d) a high-risk burn. A high-risk burn is complicated by inhalation injuries, electrical burning, fractures or other major trauma, pre-existing serious medical disease (such as diabetes or heart failure), or age below 2 years or above 60 years. Social circumstances indicating abuse (such as child abuse or spouse abuse) or possible poor compliance with follow-up care also constitute high-risk situations.

Nursing Diagnoses

Burn care may be conceptualized as a continuum with three overlapping periods: the emergent (resuscitation) period, the acute period, and the rehabilitative period. The *emergent period* lasts from the onset of injury to 2 days–2 weeks posttrauma, depending on the severity of injury (Dyer and Roberts 1990). The *acute period* lasts from the end of the emergent period until all of the full-thickness burns are covered with autografts (grafts from elsewhere on the patient). The *rehabilitation period* may last up to 5 years except with a severely burned infant or small child, in which case the social and physical rehabilitation may last until the child is fully grown.

These three periods are distinguished by the emphasis placed on different aspects of the burn patient's recovery. In the emergent period, the major concerns are maintenance of pulmonary functioning and cardiovascular integrity. In the acute period, the primary concerns are protection against infection and enhancement of wound healing. In the rehabilitation period, the chief concern is the patient's restoration to useful participation in society.

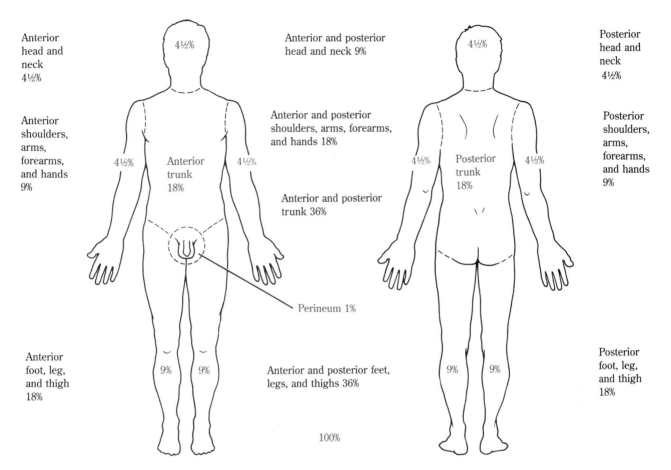

Anterior head and neck 4½%

4½%

Anterior and posterior head and neck 9%

4½%

Posterior head and neck 4½%

Anterior shoulders, arms, forearms, and hands 9%

4½%   Anterior trunk 18%   4½%

Anterior and posterior shoulders, arms, forearms, and hands 18%

4½%   Posterior trunk 18%   4½%

Posterior shoulders, arms, forearms, and hands 9%

Anterior and posterior trunk 36%

Perineum 1%

Anterior foot, leg, and thigh 18%

9%   9%

Anterior and posterior feet, legs, and thighs 36%

9%   9%

Posterior foot, leg, and thigh 18%

100%

FIGURE 21–7

Estimating the extent of burns on the body surface area using the rule of nines.
(From: Spence A, Mason E: *Human anatomy and physiology,* 3d ed. Menlo Park, CA: Benjamin/Cummings, 1987, Fig. 5.7.)

This section focuses on nursing care during the emergent and acute periods. For further information on rehabilitation, the reader is referred to the burn literature, particularly Dyer and Roberts (1990).

Planning and Implementation of Care

Pain Related to Exposure of Sensory Receptors Initially, the patient with a major burn is alert and oriented, although intensely anxious. If the patient's level of consciousness is decreased, alternative causes should be investigated—for example, associated head trauma, decreased cardiac output (shock), inhalation of toxic materials, carbon monoxide poisoning, or drug or alcohol overdose.

The patient with a full-thickness burn may not need much immediate pain control, because the skin's pain receptors have been destroyed and the full-thickness burn area is anesthetized. Deep partial-thickness burns, however, are extremely painful. Patients rarely have only full-thickness burns and will experience pain from other burn sites. Analgesia can be provided with intravenous morphine titrated to achieve pain control.

Impaired Gas Exchange Related to Upper or Lower Airway Injury Burned patients can develop upper airway obstruction, manifested by laryngeal edema, laryngospasm, or profuse airway secretions due to mucosal trauma in the naso- and oropharynx. This damage can occur with or without actual smoke inhalation. Observe for the signs of stridor, dyspnea, and intense hoarseness; if these signs are present, the patient requires intubation for airway protection until the swelling subsides in a few days.

Ineffective gas exchange also can result from lower

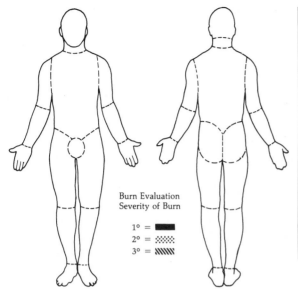

Lund and Browder Chart								
	AGE-YEARS					%	%	%
AREA	0-1	1-4	5-9	10-15	ADULT	2°	3°	TOTAL
Head	19	17	13	10	7			
Neck	2	2	2	2	2			
Ant. Trunk	13	17	13	13	13			
Post. Trunk	13	13	13	13	13			
R. Buttock	2½	2½	2½	2½	2½			
L. Buttock	2½	2½	2½	2½	2½			
Genitalia	1	1	1	1	1			
R.U. Arm	4	4	4	4	4			
L.U. Arm	4	4	4	4	4			
R.L. Arm	3	3	3	3	3			
L.L. Arm	3	3	3	3	3			
R. Hand	2½	2½	2½	2½	2½			
L. Hand	2½	2½	2½	2½	2½			
R. Thigh	5½	6½	8½	8½	9½			
L. Thigh	5½	6½	8½	8½	9½			
R. Leg	5	5	5½	6	7			
R. Foot	3½	3½	3½	3½	3½			
L. Foot	3½	3½	3½	3½	3½			
					Total			

Burn Evaluation
Severity of Burn

1° = ▬
2° = ▨
3° = ▧

FIGURE 21–8

Lund and Browder chart for precise determination of burn extent. (Adapted from
Lund C, Browder N: The estimation of areas of burns. *Surg Gynecol Obstet* (Oct.)
1944; 79:352–358.) By permission of *Surgery, Gynecology & Obstetrics.*

NURSING DIAGNOSES

The following nursing diagnoses may apply
during the emergent and acute periods.

- Pain
- Impaired gas exchange
- Decreased cardiac output
- Altered tissue perfusion
- Altered urinary elimination
- Altered bowel elimination
- Impaired thermoregulation
- Altered nutrition: less than body
  requirements
- High risk for infection
- High risk for disuse syndrome
- High risk for poor wound healing*
- High risk for ineffective individual coping
- High risk for ineffective family coping

*non-NANDA diagnosis

airway damage related to inhalation injury. With the
exception of steam burns, the lower airway usually is
not directly burned, as heat is dispersed on inhalation.
Usually, lower airway damage is related to inhalation of
the toxic products of combustion, which cause a
chemical pneumonitis.

Be alert for dyspnea, tachypnea, cough, crackles,
and gurgles, as well as decreasing Po_2. On admission,
the patient should receive a chest x-ray, have blood
drawn for baseline arterial blood gases, and a sputum
specimen sent for culture and sensitivity. The critical-
care nurse should be especially alert for lower airway
damage with smoke inhalation. Clues to smoke inhalation include a history of being burned in an enclosed
space, singed nasal hairs, burns around the nose and
mouth, and carbonaceous particles in the sputum. If
smoke inhalation is suspected, the physician may elect
to perform a laryngoscopy or bronchoscopy on admission to the critical-care unit. Positive findings include
carbon particles and mucosal erythema, swelling,
blistering, and sloughing.

Carbon monoxide poisoning may result in poor gas
exchange. Because carbon monoxide has a greater
affinity for hemoglobin, oxygen saturation is significantly impaired. Symptoms associated with increased
levels of carbon monoxide are confusion, headache,
dyspnea, nausea, vomiting, hallucinations, ataxia,
coma, and, finally, cardiopulmonary arrest. A carboxy-
hemoglobin level should be drawn on any patient with

a history suggesting smoke inhalation. The normal value is less than 5%.

Another factor that may cause impaired gas exchange in the initial postburn period is a circumferential burn of the chest, which limits thoracic expansion necessary for respiration and commonly leads to alveolar hypoventilation. A circumferential chest burn is relieved via escharotomy. In this procedure, the physician uses a scalpel or electrocautery to make linear incisions through the burn eschar down to the layer of superficial fat. Two incisions extend bilaterally from the clavicle to the bottom of the rib cage and another incision extends across the mid-chest to form an "H," thus alleviating the restriction caused by the tightening eschar.

Initial airway care should include intubation if there is upper airway damage; administration of humidified oxygen; frequent auscultation of breath sounds; monitoring of arterial blood gases; measurements of tidal volume, vital capacity, and inspiratory force every 4 hours; suctioning as necessary; and encouraging the patient to turn, cough, and breathe deeply every hour. Carbon monoxide poisoning is treated with 100% oxygen, or, if available, hyperbaric oxygenation.

The importance of pulmonary care continues during the acute period, but emphasis shifts from management of early complications, such as airway obstruction, to later complications, primarily ARDS and pneumonia. For principles of care related to these disorders, please consult Chapter 8.

Decreased Cardiac Output Related to Burn Shock and Other Factors *Burn shock* is the term used to describe the hypovolemic shock suffered by patients with major thermal insults. In the first 24–36 hours postburn, capillary permeability increases significantly. This increase is most marked at the site of injury, but also occurs throughout the rest of the body. The leaky capillaries allow fluid, electrolytes, and proteins to translocate into a nonfunctional interstitial space, nicknamed "the third space." This fluid movement and the accumulation of cellular debris exceed the ability of the venous ends of the capillaries and the lymphatics to absorb the excess fluid. The degree of fluid shift can be difficult to comprehend; a patient with a 40% TBSA burn may have up to 75% of his or her plasma volume in the third space (Davies 1982). In addition, fluid is lost via the exposed surface of the burn. Other factors that contribute to decreased cardiac output include hypothermia, acidosis, decreased coronary artery perfusion, and—in extensive burns—the possible release of a myocardial depressant factor.

Nursing measures to combat burn shock include the prompt establishment of IV lines and management of the fluid replacement prescribed by the physician. Fluid resuscitation must be aggressive to combat the deleterious effects of burn shock.

The content of the fluid used in the initial 24-hour resuscitation period is controversial. Some experts argue that it should consist partially of crystalloids and partially of colloids, as both crystalloids and colloids are lost in burn shock. Others believe that colloids are contraindicated because they can leak into the interstitial space, pulling fluid along with them, thus increasing the likelihood of pulmonary edema. According to Demling (1987), the most popular resuscitation fluid in the United States is crystalloid, particularly lactated Ringer's solution. Fluid resuscitation in the burn patient is dynamic; no single formula can be considered correct. An understanding of the pathophysiology of burn shock will result in the best choice for the individual patient.

A number of different formulas may be used to guide fluid resuscitation (Table 21–6). When replacement of both crystalloids and colloids is preferred, the Brooke formula is usually the formula of choice. If crystalloid therapy alone is preferred, the most commonly used formula is the Baxter (Parkland) formula. One-half the amount of fluid is given in the first 8 hours postburn (*not* postadmission), when the capillary leak is greatest; one-quarter in the next 8 hours; and the final quarter in the next 8 hours. This calculation is only a guideline; the least amount of fluid necessary to produce adequate tissue perfusion should be used. Fluid replacement after the initial 24 hours involves colloids, crystalloids, and electrolyte-free solutions in varying amounts according to the patient's needs.

The adequacy of fluid resuscitation must be carefully monitored by the physician and nurse according to vital signs, peripheral perfusion, urinary output, and hemodynamic parameters. Hematocrit values also are used to monitor fluid resuscitation. In the immediate postinjury period, the hematocrit rises due to hemoconcentration. As fluid volume is restored, the hematocrit drops, reflecting adequate fluid resuscitation.

Given the massive amounts of fluid that may be administered, meticulous monitoring of infusions and precise intake and output records are essential. If the burn exceeds 25% of TBSA, a central line should be inserted for fluid resuscitation, blood samples, and administration of intravenous narcotics and other medications.

The end of burn shock is signalled by the onset of spontaneous diuresis about 48 hours postburn, due to the mobilization of burn edema and reestablishment of normal capillary permeability. Monitor the patient carefully for signs of excess fluid volume, congestive

TABLE 21–6

Fluid Resuscitation Formulas, First 24 Hours*

FORMULA	URINE OUTPUT	RATE OF INFUSION	BASIS FOR CALCULATED VOLUME
Brooke			
Colloid: 0.5 ml/kg/% burn (plasma protein solutions, e.g., albumin)	Adult: 0.5–1.0 ml/kg/hr Child: 1.0 ml/kg/hr	One-half the total in the first 8 hours; one-quarter the total in the next 8 hours; one-quarter the total in the next 8 hours	Burn surface area to a maximum of 50% of TBSA. Burns greater than 50% are calculated the same as 50% of TBSA
Crystalloid: 1.5 ml/kg/% burn (lactated Ringer's), 5% dextrose in water: 2,000 ml/meter^2			
Parkland			
Crystalloid: 4 ml/kg/% burn (lactated Ringer's)	Same as for Brooke	Same as for Brooke	Total burn area for all sizes of burns
Monafo			
Hypertonic saline (Na 250 mEq/L, lactate 150 mEq/L, Cl 100 mEq/L)	Same as for Brooke	Rate and volume titrated to urine production	

*It must be remembered that the "first 24 hours" means from the time of the burn injury, not from the beginning of treatment.

Sources: Demling R: Fluid replacement in burned patients. *Surg Clin North Am* (Feb) 1987; 67(2):15–30; Trofino R (ed): *Nursing care of the burn injured patient.* Philadelphia: Davis, 1991, pp. 154–155.

heart failure (CHF), and pulmonary edema. During this diuretic phase, fluid infusion rates can be titrated based on urinary output and tissue perfusion.

Weigh the patient on admission (to establish a baseline weight prior to the peak of edema), and weigh daily thereafter. Edema development gradually increases over the first 3 days, and the patient can be expected to gain approximately 15% of baseline weight during the initial few days. Burn edema has a gel-like consistency due to its high protein content. It is slowly mobilized over a period of about 2 weeks.

During the first 24–36 hours, cellular destruction and impairment of the sodium-potassium pump cause hyperkalemia. During this period, avoid adding potassium to intravenous solutions and monitor the patient for ECG signs necessitating treatment of the hyperkalemia. After 72 hours, hypokalemia may develop during burn diuresis. During this time, add potassium to intravenous solutions to replace urinary losses, as ordered, and monitor for signs of hypokalemia. Hyperkalemia and hypokalemia are discussed in detail in Chapter 16.

Altered Tissue Perfusion Related to Progressive Thrombosis Several interrelated factors cause progressive ischemia in major burn trauma patients. Aggregation of platelets and leukocytes and intravas-

cular hemolysis cause sludging of cellular debris in the microcirculation. In conjunction with decreased perfusion due to decreased CO, this sludging causes thrombosis of both the micro- and macrocirculation. Monitor peripheral pulses, skin temperature, and capillary filling closely. If pulses are not palpable, check flow with an arterial Doppler. Watch perfusion of the fingers especially closely, because fingers have poor peripheral perfusion. Elevating the extremities helps to reduce edema formation, thereby improving capillary flow. Medications must be given intravenously due to the unreliability of tissue perfusion.

Perfusion is particularly likely to become compromised in a circumferential burn of an extremity; the constriction of the eschar, combined with the tissue pressure from edema formation, can severely impair blood flow. An escharotomy (surgical incision of the eschar) is indicated if (a) distal pulses become weak or absent; (b) distal unburned skin becomes cyanotic; (c) capillary filling weakens; or (d) progressive paresthesias or motor impairment develop. A fasciotomy (surgical incision through the fascia to expose underlying tissue) may be necessary with electrical burns, to release the pressure caused by major edema and to assess tissue viability.

Patients with massive burns develop a profound anemia, characterized by abnormal red blood cell

(RBC) morphology and decreased RBC half-life. Hemolysis begins when red blood cells are destroyed by heat as they pass through the burned areas or become trapped in swollen capillaries. Hemolysis contributes to capillary thrombosis, and the resulting anemia may significantly reduce oxygen-carrying capacity.

The initial injury may destroy up to 10–15% of the RBC mass. The initial destruction is followed by a progressive anemia whose exact etiology is unknown but may be an extrinsic mechanism unrelated to initial heat or mechanical damage (Davies 1982). In addition, the patient loses blood during debridement. Most patients require transfusions of packed red cells to maintain acceptable serum hematocrits.

Altered Urinary Elimination Related to Volume Changes

If the burn exceeds 20% of TBSA, a Foley catheter is inserted and the urinary output is monitored hourly. Urine flow from an indwelling catheter should be maintained at 30–50 ml per hour. Send a urinary specimen to the laboratory for routine examination and culture and sensitivity on admission. Dark, concentrated urine may be present due to sludging of hemoglobin or myoglobin from damaged cells, indicating massive hemolysis or tissue destruction and possible renal damage. The abnormal concentration usually clears with adequate fluid administration, although mannitol may be indicated if the concentration is pronounced.

Altered Bowel Elimination Related to Paralytic Ileus and Gastric Hemorrhage

Development of gastric dilatation and paralytic ileus is a normal response to the stress of a major burn. The patient should not be allowed oral food or fluids until bowel sounds return. A nasogastric tube usually is placed because of the danger of vomiting and aspiration. The intense thirst present for the first 2 days, which is a compensatory mechanism for the fluid volume deficit, may be relieved with ice chips and mouth swabs.

Gastrointestinal (GI) hemorrhage can occur due to hemorrhagic gastritis, which develops secondary to capillary congestion and rupture, or Curling's ulcer. Nursing measures to prevent GI bleeding include checks of nasogastric fluid aspirate pH and occult blood every 2 hours, administration of antacids through the nasogastric tube every 2 hours, and administration of ranitidine or cimetidine, as ordered.

Impaired Thermoregulation Related to Heat Loss

A significant amount of body heat is lost through a major burn. Beginning in the emergent period, the patient should be kept warm by using a heat cradle and maintaining a warm environmental temperature.

Altered Nutrition: Less Than Body Requirements, Related to Stress Response

As part of the normal physiologic response to an overwhelming stress, the burned patient becomes hypermetabolic, developing increased catecholamine release, increased glucose production from the breakdown of glycogen (glycogenolysis) and formation of glucose from fats and proteins (gluconeogenesis), and protein catabolism leading to negative nitrogen balance. The increased metabolic rate peaks at about 1 week postburn. Because of these factors, the patient needs to be protected from additional environmental stressors, provided with as much uninterrupted rest as possible, and given a high-calorie diet of approximately 5,000–6,000 calories per day. Once bowel sounds have returned, oral feedings are preferred. If nutritional needs cannot be met through oral feedings, enteral feedings and/or total parenteral nutrition may be necessary. Weigh patients daily to monitor the effectiveness of the program.

High Risk for Infection Related to Broken Skin, Traumatized Tissue, and Suppressed Inflammatory Response

Infection presents a major problem for seriously burned patients, in whom sepsis is a leading cause of death. The skin is the body's first line of defense against infection, so loss of the skin barrier is a significant risk factor, and the burn wound itself is a frequent source of infection. In addition, the injured tissue is a superb culture medium. Finally, the inflammatory response is impaired following a major burn. In full-thickness burns, blood vessels undergo coagulation necrosis, so white blood cells cannot reach burned tissue. Even areas without complete arterial occlusion suffer impaired defenses; although phagocytic cells may be able to reach them, the neutrophils' ability to kill ingested bacteria is depressed (Hunt and Eriksson 1986).

Because of these factors, burn patients are at high risk for infection, from both themselves and their environment. Burn wounds often are colonized by the patient's endogenous GI, respiratory, and skin flora (autocontamination). Exogenous sources of infection include invasive procedures, such as IV catheterization, hemodynamic monitoring line insertion, Foley catheterization, hyperalimentation, and endotracheal intubation. Manipulation of the burn wound during hydrotherapy, debridement, and surgery also can seed the bloodstream with infectious organisms.

Wound infections occur with a variety of organisms, especially Staphylococcus aureus, Pseudomonas aeruginosa, beta-hemolytic Streptococcus, and Candida albicans (Pruitt 1984). Tetanus prophylaxis is provided on admission. Meticulous attention to wound assessment

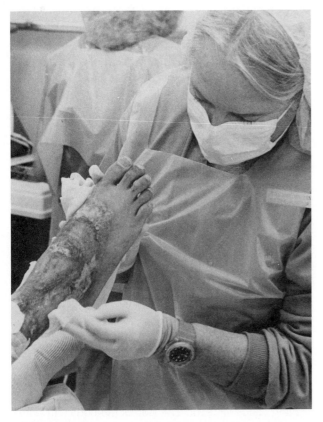

FIGURE 21–9

A burn nurse inspects the wounds of a patient while preparing him for hydrotherapy. (Photo courtesy of Claire Dyer, Bothin Burn Center, St. Francis Memorial Hospital, San Francisco.)

is critical (Figure 21–9). Measures to reduce infection include conscientious use of aseptic technique when providing wound care, and decontamination of equipment such as the hydrotherapy tanks.

If wound infection is not controlled, bacteria will seed the bloodstream, resulting in bacteremia that may lead to septicemia. Bacteremia is the colonization of microorganisms greater than 10^5 per gram of viable tissue (Salisbury et al. 1983). In major burns, bacteremia is a constant threat to the patient until the burn wound is completely covered by autografts. It is not uncommon for the patient to have recurrent episodes of bacteremia following hydrotherapy treatment and/or major debridement procedures because of the overwhelming shower of bacteria from the infected burn wound during these procedures. Be alert for signs of impending septicemia, such as fever, chills, malaise, elevated white blood cell (WBC) count, increased pulse or respiratory rate, gradual hypotension, and altered mental status. Treatment includes aggressive wound cleansing, daily wound and blood cultures, administration of appropriate antimicrobials and antipyretics as ordered by the physician, and promotion of adequate rest and nutrition.

Overwhelming septicemia can provoke the development of septic shock, which carries a high mortality. Its development in the burn patient is an ominous prognostic sign.

High Risk for Disuse Syndrome Related to Contractures Hypertrophic scarring and contractures of scar tissue can cause severe functional impairment of burned areas. Because contractures tend to form in positions of comfort, it is important to begin splinting burned areas in functional positions early, and to explain to the patient why you are doing so. Turn the patient at least every 2 hours, and consult a physical therapist to design a program of range-of-motion exercises and appropriate splinting. Encourage the patient to exercise in bed and to ambulate as soon as possible.

High Risk for Poor Wound Healing Related to Inadequate Wound Care Wound healing may be conceptualized as a triad of interrelated factors: wound damage, endogenous host defense mechanisms, and exogenous support for healing. As the manager of the healing support mechanisms prescribed by the physician, the critical-care nurse plays a crucial role in the healing process.

Therapeutic approaches can be broadly subdivided into conventional and aggressive therapies. *Conventional therapy* consists of hydrotherapy with debridement of necrotic tissue, application of topical antimicrobials and dressings, and skin grafting. *Hydrotherapy* is used to soften eschar, wash away topical agents, and aid in debridement. Unfortunately, hydrotherapy may increase the risk of wound contamination, is very painful, and causes heat loss. *Debridement*—a procedure dreaded by burn patients because it causes severe pain—involves removal of eschar, either with forceps and scissors or scalpel, or with wet-to-dry dressings that are peeled away from the burn wound surface.

A variety of methods of wound care is appropriate for burn patients. In the open (exposure) method, wounds are left exposed to air. This method allows easy visibility of the site and it enhances dryness, but it may require reverse isolation and use of a warm room to minimize heat loss. Dry occlusive dressings, consisting of thick bandages, are used less frequently because they limit observation and mobility and may promote infection. They are used primarily to stabilize grafts. The most commonly used method of wound care is partial exposure. A thin layer of antimicrobial cream, which may be covered by a thin layer of gauze, is

TABLE 21–7

Topical Preparations Used in Burn Care

PREPARATION	ADVANTAGES	DISADVANTAGES	NURSING ACTIONS
Silver sulfadiazine	Wide-spectrum antimicrobial Antifungal Nonstaining Relatively painless Usable without dressings No systemic metabolic abnormalities	Less eschar penetration than Sulfamylon Decreased granulocyte formation	Check for allergy to sulfa; sometimes causes rash.
Mafenide acetate (Sulfamylon)	Eschar penetration Effective with *Pseudomonas* Topical of choice for electrical burns Suitable for open method of treatment Used for gram-negative organisms	Severe pain and burning sensation (lasts 30 min) Acidic breakdown product Carbonic anhydrase inhibitor Ineffective against fungi May cause hypersensitivity rash	Administer pretreatment analgesic. Monitor for metabolic acidosis and hyperventilation. Check for allergy to sulfa; observe for rash.
Povidone-iodine (Betadine)	Antifungal Wide-spectrum microbicidal	Iodine absorption Staining of clothing Dressing necessary Metabolic acidosis	Assess for allergy to iodine. Check serum iodine levels.
Bismuth tribromphenate (Xeroform)	Petroleum-based gauze, so conforms to wound	Painful removal	Alert patient to discomfort before removing.
Silver nitrate	Low cost	Continuous wet soaks Superficial penetration Black staining Stinging Electrolyte imbalances (low sodium, low chloride, low calcium), alkalosis	Keep dressings wet. Perform active debridement. Check serum electrolytes daily.
Sutilains (Travase)	Enzymatic debriding agent (digestion of necrotic material)	Refrigeration necessary Irritation of wound and skin Can cause some bleeding Can cause fluid loss Painful on partial-thickness burn	Limit use to 10–15% of burn surface at one time. Observe for infection. Cross-hatch eschar if necessary to allow optimal penetration. Monitor fluid balance. Assess need for analgesic.

applied. Various antimicrobial agents are available; the advantages and disadvantages of different agents are summarized in Table 21–7.

Aggressive therapies consist of *tangential or staged removal of eschar* down to a bleeding base (granulating tissue), followed with dressings and grafting. Compared to conventional therapy, early aggressive surgical therapy shortens hospitalization, reduces the de-velopment of sepsis, and decreases scar formation; however, it increases blood loss. Eschar excisions can begin during the first week postburn. In the past, they have been limited to removal of no more than 15% of TBSA at one procedure, although some centers are experimenting with more liberal guidelines.

Grafts are used to cover or close an open wound. *Synthetic grafts* are used as temporary biologic dress-

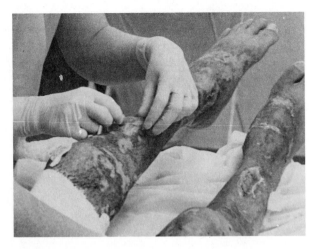

FIGURE 21–10

Burn nurses work in teams, assessing the wounds for signs of infection and for areas of healing and graft "take." In this photograph, the nurse carefully removes the dressing protecting the new grafts and debrides the burn eschar by removing the non-viable tissue. (Photo courtesy of Claire Dyer, Bothin Burn Center, St. Francis Memorial Hospital, San Francisco.)

ings to minimize infection, prevent fluid and heat loss, and protect nerve endings. The terms *heterografts, homografts,* and *skin grafts* refer to tissue. Biologic skin can be obtained from animals such as pigs *(heterografts or xenografts)* or human cadavers *(homografts or allografts);* both are temporary. Homografts and heterografts are used to prepare the granulating wound bed for grafts of the patient's own skin *(autografts),* the only permanent coverage.

The wound in Figure 21–10, for example, is covered in cultured epithelial autografts (CEA). Skin excised from an unburned area the size of a postage stamp (2 cm^2) was cultured over 21 days to produce epithelial sheets sufficient to cover 60% of this patient's body surface. Extremely fragile, the CEA grafts require gentle handling, for the slightest amount of pressure can destroy them.

Autografts are used to provide permanent coverage for full-thickness burns. *Split-thickness skin grafts,* which include the epidermis and part of the dermis, are used more commonly than full-thickness grafts, because they "take" more easily and require less time to heal. Split-thickness grafts can be taken from anywhere there is intact skin; preferred donor sites are those that match the skin texture of the area to be grafted and that will be covered by clothing, such as the thigh. Skin layers are removed with a dermatome.

Sheet grafts, which are used to cover the face, hands, fingers, and jointed areas, are left exposed to the air and are carefully rolled with sterile cotton-tipped applicators to remove trapped fluid or air that accumulates. *Mesh grafts* are put through the Tanner dermatome, which meshes them and allows expansion to three or more times their original size. These grafts, which are used to cover large surface areas such as the chest, back, arms, and legs, are dressed and kept moist for the first 48–72 hours postgrafting. The graft sites are immobilized by splints to ensure the grafts will "take." Although mesh grafts have the advantage of numerous openings through which fluid can drain, they have the disadvantages of additional portals for infection and an unattractive appearance, which cosmetically limits their use to areas that will be covered by clothing.

For a graft to take, it must be placed on a healthy recipient bed that can generate granulation tissue and a capillary network. The graft must be immobilized for up to 10 days until a fibrin network and granulation tissue are firmly established (Tompkins and Burke 1992). Blood flow usually is established by the third day. Nursing responsibilities during the early postgraft period include: (a) prevention of shearing between the graft and site by appropriate positioning, dressings, and sedation; (b) removal of serous accumulations or hematomas under the graft, if approved by the surgeon; and (c) observation of the graft site for infection. More conservatively, dressings may be left in place for up to 10 days. When they are removed, range-of-motion exercises may be resumed.

Donor sites must be cared for and observed carefully for signs of infection. They usually are covered with a light gauze dressing and left exposed to air, with drying encouraged by use of a heat lamp. Analgesics may be necessary for the first day or two.

High Risk for Ineffective Individual and/or Family Coping Related to Psychotraumatic Experience
Among the most challenging aspects of caring for the burned patient is the provision of psychologic support for the patient, family, and friends as they cope with the devastating impact of the burn (Figure 21–11). Psychologic reactions may include: (a) anxiety or fear about prognosis and treatment; (b) anger at self or others for contributing to the burn accident; (c) guilt for not being "more careful" to avoid dangerous circumstances; (d) resentment (if the person views the burn as undeserved punishment); and (e) increased awareness of vulnerability, especially if the burn results from an act of senseless violence. Patients often go through a grieving process for loss of their body image; loved ones may undergo a parallel grief process for loss of the patient's appearance or other valued characteristics.

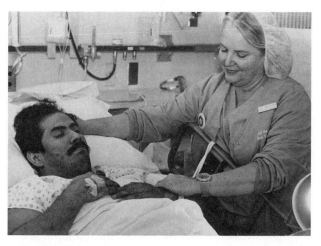

FIGURE 21–11

When the patient is back in bed, the nurse reassesses him for alterations in comfort. The pain, anxiety, and knowledge of scarring and disfigurement add to the problems and concerns the burn patient faces. The nurse's caring is an important aspect of psychologic support for the burned patient. (Photo courtesy of Claire Dyer, Bothin Burn Center, St. Francis Memorial Hospital, San Francisco.)

Depending on the individual, applicable nursing diagnoses may include post-trauma response, anxiety, altered family dynamics, fear, grieving, rational anger state, social isolation, disturbed self-concept, and spiritual distress. Among the most effective nursing measures for helping burned patients and their families are: (a) projecting a calm, confident attitude as procedures are performed; (b) being as honest and hopeful as reality allows; (c) giving "bad news" in small doses appropriate to current coping levels; (d) focusing on the achievement of small goals; (e) willingly repeating explanations, which often are not heard initially through the screen of fear, pain, and anxiety; (f) preparing family and friends for bedside visits; (g) seeking assistance and consultation with psychologists and other burn team members skilled at dealing with psychotrauma; and, after the initial life threat has passed, (h) putting the patient and loved ones in contact with successfully rehabilitated burn survivors. See Chapters 2 and 3 for further information on helping the patient and family cope with the experience.

Outcome Evaluation

The following criteria may be used to judge the patient's progress:

- Vital signs within normal limits (WNL).
- CVP and pulmonary artery (PA) readings normal.
- Alert and oriented level of consciousness.
- Urinary output 30–50 ml per hour during resuscitation phase.
- Bowel sounds present.
- Ventilation and oxygenation adequate as manifested by lung sounds and arterial blood gases WNL.
- Wounds free of infection, as demonstrated by wound cultures <10^5 organisms/g of viable tissue; negative blood, urine, and sputum cultures; no discoloration of wounds; decreased drainage; and absent odor.

Conclusion

Trauma nursing is an exciting, challenging, dynamic, and growing aspect of critical-care nursing practice. In order to deliver effective nursing care, the critical-care nurse must understand and integrate the variety of data representing multiple organ systems. Based on these data, the critical-care nurse develops a plan of care that addresses life-threatening problems in order of priority and prevents delays in intervention and treatment. This approach enables the critical-care nurse to have the greatest impact on the patient with traumatic injury. The care of the multiple trauma patient is often multidisciplinary, involving all hospital departments. The critical-care nurse, in conjunction with the primary surgeon, coordinates these efforts to provide optimal care and to minimize the physiologic and psychologic impacts of the injury.

The American Association of Critical Care Nurses (AACN) has announced research priorities that will help the critical-care nurse refine his or her practice based on sound nursing research. These research priorities include techniques to optimize pulmonary function and prevent complications, wean mechanically ventilated patients, and provide nutritional support. Research also will focus on strategies for preventing infection and determining the accuracy of noninvasive monitoring devices, as well as other topics. The Emergency Nurses Association, in collaboration with the American College of Surgeons and the Committee on Trauma, provides numerous educational programs to build skills in prehospital and resuscitative phases of trauma patient care; the Trauma Nurse Core Course offered throughout the United States is a good example. The greater the knowledge of the prehospital, resuscitative, and intraoperative phases, the better the foundation for the critical-care nurse's practice.

REFERENCES

Multiple Trauma

American College of Surgeons: Hospital and Prehospital Resources for Optimal Care of the Injured Prehospital Patient. 1986.

Bartlett R: Myocardial contusion: Using the index of suspicion for assessing blunt chest trauma. *Dimen Crit Care Nurs* 1991; 10(3):133–139.

Becker D, Gardner S: Intensive management of head injury. Pages 1593–1599 in *Neurosurgery,* Vol. 2, Wilkins R, Rengachary S (eds). New York: McGraw-Hill, 1985.

Bell N: Nosocomial pneumonia [unpublished quality assurance study]. Eden Hospital Medical Center, Castro Valley, California 1991.

Bell N: The clinical significance of continuous multilead ST segment monitoring. *Crit Care Nurs Clin North Am* 1992; 4(2):313–323.

Brackett T, Condon N: Comparison of wedge turning frame and kinetic treatment table in the acute care of spinal cord injured patients. *Surg Neurol* 1984; 22:5356.

Champion H, Copes W, Sacco W: The major outcome study: Establishing national norms for Trauma Care. *J Trauma* 1990; 30(11):1356–1370.

Chisholm B: Stunned myocardium. *Focus Crit Care* 1990; 17(6):458–462.

Cruzzel J, Stotts N: Trial and error yields to knowledge. *Am J Nurs* 1990; 90(10):53–63.

Davidson J: Neuromuscular Blockade. *Focus Crit Care* 1991; 18(6):512–520.

Davis F, Youngstein K: *The injured brain.* New York: Biocom, Ltd., 1990.

Del Rossi A: Foreword. *Trauma Quart* 1990; 6(3): vii.

Dowe D, Curtas S, Meguid M: Trauma. In Blackburn GL (ed.) *Nutritional medicine: A case management approach.* Philadelphia, WB Saunders Co., 1989.

Earp J, Finlayson D: Relationship between urinary bladder and pulmonary artery temperatures: A preliminary study. *Heart Lung* 1991; 20(3):265–270.

Feroe D, Augustine S: Hypothermia in the PACU. *Crit Care Nurs Clin North Am* 1991; 3(1):135–144.

Fontaine D, McQuillan K: Positioning as a nursing therapy in trauma care. *Crit Care Nurs Clin North Am* 1989; 1(1):105–112.

Foreman M (ed): Gerontologic considerations. *Crit Care Nurs Quart* 1989; 12(1):189.

Gentilello L et al.: Effects of a rotating bed on the incidence of pulmonary complications in critically ill patients. *Crit Care Med* 1988; 16(8):783–786.

Gift A, Bolgiano S, Cunningham J: Sensations during chest tube removal. *Heart Lung* 1991; 20(2):131–137.

Goldberger D, Kruse L, Stender R: A survey of external fixator pin care techniques. *Clin Nurse Spec* 1987; 1(4):166–169.

Gregory J, Flancbaum L, Townsend C: Incidence and timing of hypothermia in trauma patients undergoing operations. *J Trauma* 1991; 31(6):795–800.

Grupp L, Perlanski E, Stewart R: Regulation of alcohol consumption by the renin-angiotensin system: A review of recent findings and a possible mechanism of action. *Neurosci Biobehav Rev* 1991; 15:265–275.

Halpern J: Administering methylprednisolone for acute spinal cord injuries. *JEN* 1991; 17(1):37–40.

Halvorsen L, Gunther R, Dubick M: Dose response characteristics of hypertonic saline dextran solutions. *J Trauma* 1991; 31(6):785–794.

Harris K, Booth F, Hassett J: Liver lacerations–a marker of severe but sometimes subtle intra-abdominal injuries in adults. *J Trauma* 1991; 31(7):894–901.

Henneman P, Marx J, Moore E: Diagnostic peritoneal lavage: Accuracy in predicting necessary laparotomy following blunt and penetrating trauma. *J Trauma* 1990; 30(11):1345–1355.

Helfman S et al.: Which drug prevents tachycardia and hypertension associated with tracheal intubation: Lidocaine, fentanyl, or esmolol? *Anesth Analg* 1991; 72(4):482–486.

Hind C: *Intensive care: A concise textbook.* London: Bailliere Tindall, 1987, p. 284.

Hogstel M: Emergency care. Pages 313–331 in *Nursing care of the older adult,* 2d ed, Hogstel M (ed). New York: Wiley, 1991.

Holtzclaw B: Shivering: A clinical nursing problem. *Nurs Clin North Am* 1990; 25(4):977–986.

Hunter J: Neuromuscular blocking drugs in intensive therapy. *Intens Ther Clin Monitor,* May 1989. Reprint.

Jackson M, Lynch P: In search of a rational approach. *Am J Nurs* 1990; 90(10):65–72.

Johansen BC et al (eds.): *Standards for critical care,* 3d ed. St. Louis: Mosby, 1988, pp. 449–492.

Kimura A, Otsuka T: Emergency center ultrasonography in the evaluation of hemoperitoneum: A prospective study. *J Trauma* 1991; 31(1):20–23.

Kirby D, Clifton G, Turner H: Early enteral nutrition after brain injury by percutaneous endoscopic gastrojejunostomy. *J Enteral Parenteral Nutr* 1991; 15(3):298–302.

Lee S: Intracranial pressure changes during positioning of patients with severe head injury. *Heart Lung* 1989; 18(4): 411–414.

Lookinland S: Hemodynamic and oxygen transport changes following endotracheal suctioning in trauma patients. *Nurs Res* 1991; 40(3):133–138.

Mackersie R, Karagianes T, Hoyt D: Prospective evaluation of epidural and intravenous administration of fentanyl for pain control and restoration of ventilatory function following multiple rib fractures. *J Trauma* 1991; 31(4):443–451.

May H: The critically injured patient. In *Emergency medicine.* New York: Wiley, 1984, p. 241.

McGuire R, Green B, Eismont F: Comparison of stability provided to the unstable spine by the kinetic therapy table and the Stryker frame. *Neurosurg* 1988; 22(5):842–844.

McSwain N, Belles A: Motorcycle helmets: Medical costs and the law. *J Trauma* 1990; 30(10):1189–1199.

Mirr M: Factors affecting decisions made by family members of patients with severe head injury. *Heart Lung* 1991; 20(3):228–235.

Mitchell P, Hodges L, Muwaswes M, Walleck C: *AANN's neuroscience nursing: Phenomena and practice.* Norwalk, CT: Appleton & Lange, 1988, pp. 446–447.

Muizelaar J et al.: Adverse effects of prolonged hyperventilation in patients with severe head injury: A randomized clinical trial. *J Neurosurg* 1991; 75:731–739.

Muizelaar J et al.: Pial arteriolar vessel diameter and CO_2 reactivity during prolonged hyperventilation in the rabbit. *J Neurosurg* 1988; 69:923–927.

Mukherji B, Sloviter H: A stable perfluorochemical blood substitute. *Transfusion* 1991; 31:324–326.

Norman E, Gadaleta D, Griffin C: An evaluation of three blood pressure methods in a stabilized acute trauma population. *Nurs Res* 1991; 40(2):86–89.

Reed L, Johnson T, Chen Y: Hypertonic saline alters plasma clotting times and platelet aggregation. *J Trauma* 1991; 31(1):8–14.

Rodriguez D, Clevenger F, Osler T. Obligatory negative nitrogen balance following spinal cord injury. *J Enteral Parenteral Nutr* 1991; 15(3):319–322.

Rodriguez J, Gibbons K, Bitzer L: Pneumonia: Incidence, risk factors, and outcome in injured patients. *J Trauma* 1991; 31(7):907–914.

Schmitz T: The semiprone position in ARDS: Five case-studies. *Crit Care Nurse* 1991; 11(5):22–33.

Shaver T et al.: Trauma case manager providers: Development and implementation as a nursing role in a community trauma center. *J Trauma* 1991; 31:10–36.

Songne E, Holmquist P: Comprehensive care by trauma nurse: Mission Hospital's ten year experience. *JEN* 1991; 17(2):73–79.

Stone K, Preusser B, Groch K: The effect of lung hyperinflation and endotracheal suctioning on cardiopulmonary hemodynamics. *Nurs Res* 1991; 40(2):76–80.

Sullivan J: Individual and family responses to acute spinal cord injury. *Crit Care Nurs Clin North Am* 1990; 2(1):407–414.

Trunkey D, Lewis F: *Current therapy of trauma.* Philadelphia: Decker, 1991.

Unkle D, Smejkal R, Snyder R: Blood antibodies and uncrossmatched type O blood. *Heart Lung* 1991; 20(3):284–286.

Vernale C, Packard S: Organ donation as gift exchange. *Image* 1990; 22(4):239–242.

Walleck C: Controversies in the management of the head-injured patient. *Crit Care Nurs Clin North Am* 1989; 1(1):67–74.

Walleck C: Neurologic considerations in the critical care phase. *Crit Care Nurs Clin North Am* 1990; 2(3):357–362.

Zador P: Alcohol-related relative risk of fatal driver injuries in relation to driver age and sex. *J Studies on Alcohol* 1991; 52(4):302–310.

Burns

American Burn Association: Specific optimal criteria for hospital resources for care of patients with burn injury. The Association, April 1976.

Brunner and Suddarth's textbook of medical-surgical nursing, 7th ed. Philadelphia: J.B. Lippincott, 1992. Chapter 52 (Management of patient with burn injury); pp. 1501–1539.

Davies J: *Physiological responses to burning injury.* London: New Academic Press, 1982, pp. 45–91, 108, 246, 396, 558–612.

Demling R: Fluid replacement in burned patients. *Surg Clin North Am* 1987; 67(2):15–70.

Dyer C, Roberts D: Thermal trauma. *Nurs Clin North Am* 1990; 25(1):85–117.

Hunt A, Eriksson E: Management of the burn wound. *Clinics of Plastic Surgery* 1986; 13(1):57–67.

Pruitt B: The diagnosis and treatment of infection in the burn patient. *Burns* 1984; 11:79–91.

Salisbury et al. (eds): *Manual of burn therapeutics: An interdisciplinary approach,* 1st ed. Boston/Toronto: Little, Brown, 1983, pp. 23–59.

Tompkins R, Burke J: Burn wound closure using permanent skin replacement materials. *World J Surg* 1992; 16(Jan-Feb):47–52.

Trofino R: *Nursing care of the burn-injured patient:* Philadelphia: Davis, 1991.

Pharmacology*

Designed for easy reference or review, this section offers vital information on drugs commonly used in critical care that are not specifically discussed in the text. Each drug table lists the *Common use, Mechanism of action, Dosage, Administration, Anticipated response, Side effects, Interactions,* and *Other pertinent information.* Specific nursing implications are italicized. Such nursing implications as "Obtain a thorough drug history to check for interaction" and "Teach patient about side effects of the drug" have not been listed in the tables. These implications apply in *every* situation where drugs are being administered and competent nursing care is being practiced. Since the nurse is held legally responsible for safe and effective drug administration, the reader should consult other sources as well as this reference section for pharmacologic management.

Certain drugs have been described as groups rather than individually due to their similarities other than dosages. This format eliminates unnecessary duplica-

tion and, more importantly, emphasizes the interrelationships of these drugs.

The authors and publisher have exerted every effort to ensure that drug selections and dosages set forth in this text are in accord with current recommendations and practice at the time of publication. (Note that pediatric doses are *not* included.) However, in view of ongoing research, changes in government regulations, and the constant flow of information relating to drug therapy and drug reactions, the reader is urged to check the package inserts of all drugs for any change in indications of dosage and for added warnings and precautions. This is particularly important when the recommended agent is a new and/or infrequently employed drug. Mention of a particular generic or brand name drug is not an endorsement, nor an implication that it is preferable to other named or unnamed agents.

The alphabetical index that follows lists the drugs' generic names, their trade names (in italics), and (when appropriate) group names. The appendix tables themselves are arranged alphabetically by generic name or group heading.

* Adapted and updated from Saxton D et al.: *The Addison-Wesley manual of nursing practice.* Menlo Park, CA: Addison-Wesley, 1983.

Index to Critical-Care Drugs

ACE (angiotensin-converting enzyme) inhibitors: captopril (Capoten), enalapril (Vasotec), lisinopril (Prinivil, Zestril)

Common use to lower high blood pressure or reduce afterload in congestive heart failure (CHF) unresponsive to conventional therapy.

Mechanism of action competitively inhibits angiotensin-converting enzyme (ACE) conversion of angiotensin I to angiotensin II, reducing vasoconstriction (arterial effect greater than venous, producing lowered systemic vascular resistance [SVR])

Dosage 1. *captopril: BP:* initially 25 mg three times daily, can be increased at intervals to 150 mg three times daily. Maximum dose: 450 mg/day; *CHF:* 6.25–25 mg initially, same dosage progression; usual dose: 50–100 mg three times daily. 2. *enalapril:* initially 2.5–5 mg daily, increased to 10–40 mg daily for hypertension or 5–20 mg daily for CHF; maximum dose: 40 mg/day. 3. *lisinopril:* 10 mg daily initially, increase slowly to 20–40 mg daily.

Administration oral

1. *Administer 1 hour before (preferred) or 2 hours after meals.* 2. *Monitor BP before giving.* 3. *Keep on bed rest and monitor BP for 3 hours after first dose.*

Anticipated response reduced blood pressure or reduced symptoms of congestive failure

1. *Most effective when given with diuretic. A beta-blocker may be added to combination.* 2. *At least two weeks required for full therapeutic effect.*

Side effects 1. *CNS:* headache, dizziness, fatigue. 2. *CV:* transient hypotension (especially in CHF), chest pain, tachycardia. **3.** *Dermatologic:* skin rash. **4.** *GI:* changes in taste, anorexia. **5.** *Hematologic:* eosinophilia and/or positive antinuclear antibody titers (accompanying skin rash). **6.** *Renal:* proteinuria. **7.** *Other:* cough.

1. *Measure urine protein (first voided specimen) before beginning therapy and every month for 9 months and periodically thereafter (especially in renal impairment or high dosage). Report positives.* **2.** *Obtain WBC counts with differential as monitored baseline, and then periodically.* **3.** *Use in CHF should be in combination with cardiac glycoside and diuretic.*

Interactions   **1.** With diuretics, other antihypertensives, and vasodilators, increased hypotension. **2.** Potassium supplements or potassium-sparing diuretics produce hyperkalemia. **3.** Prostaglandin inhibitors (nonsteroidal anti-inflammatory drugs [NSAIDs] and aspirin) reduce effectiveness of ACE inhibitors. **4.** Antacids decrease absorption of ACE inhibitors.

1. *Do not use with potassium supplements or potassium-sparing diuretics.* **2.** *Monitor blood pressure and dosage carefully when used with other drugs which lower BP.* **3.** *Space doses from antacids.*

Other   Use with caution in renal dysfunction *(reduce dosage)*, autoimmune disease (especially SLE), actual/potential immune deficiency, coronary or cerebrovascular disease, volume or sodium depletion.

Adenosine (Adenocard)

Common use   to restore normal sinus rhythm in paroxysmal supraventricular tachycardia (PSVT), including Wolff-Parkinson-White syndrome.
Mechanism of action   naturally occurring nucleoside which directly slows conduction through the AV node, interrupts reentry pathways, and restores normal sinus rhythm.

Dosage   **1.** (IV) 6 mg intravenous push (IVP); if SVT not converted in 1–2 minutes, 12 mg as second and third dose if required.
Administration   intravenous

1. *Give undiluted IVP over 1–2 seconds directly into vein. If given into IV line, use most proximal port and follow with 50 ml NS flush to ensure that the dose reaches the circulation. Store at room temperature.* **2.** *Monitor ECG continuously. Do not give repeat dose if high-degree AV block develops. Transient arrhythmias at time of conversion do not require intervention (PVCs, PACs, sinus bradycardia or tachycardia, skipped beats, or varying degrees of AV block).*

Anticipated response   restoration of normal sinus rhythm.

Use with caution in asthma (bronchoconstriction). Do not use in second- or third-degree AV block, sick sinus syndrome (without functioning artificial pacemaker), atrial flutter/fibrillation, or ventricular tachycardia.

Side effects   **1.** *CNS:* headache or lightheadedness (2%), dizziness, numbness, tingling or heaviness in arms. **2.** *CV:* palpitations, chest pressure or pain (7%), hypotension (<1%). **3.** *Dermatologic:* facial flushing, sweating. **4.** *GI:* nausea (3%), metallic taste. **5.** Hypersensitivity. **6.** *Ophthalmic:* blurred vision. **7.** *Respiratory:* dyspnea, hyperventilation, tight throat.

1. *Monitor BP before and after dose.* **2.** *Use anxiety-lowering techniques as needed due to critical nature of patient condition.* **3.** *Warn patient that transient sensations may occur, such as flushing, headache, shortness of breath, or pressure in the chest.*

Interactions   **1.** Atropine does not block adenosine's effect. **2.** Adenosine may not be effective when caffeine and theophylline are used because they competitively antagonize adenosine's effect. **3.** Dipyridamole potentiates adenosine's effect, requiring reduction of adenosine dose. **4.** Carbamazepine increases degree of AV block, may produce higher degrees of block.

Monitor closely for effect when caffeine, theophylline, or dipyridamole are being used. Monitor closely for AV block when carbamazepine is also taken.

Adrenal Corticosteroids (inhalation): beclomethasone (Beclovent, Vanceril), dexamethasone (Decadron Respihaler)

Common use   treatment of bronchial asthma that does not respond to nonsteroidal medications.
Mechanism of action   mechanism of local action is not clear; it may involve the systemic anti-inflammatory and immunosuppressant actions of these drugs.

Dosage   **1.** *beclomethasone:* (inhalation aerosol) 2 metered sprays 3 or 4 times a day, increased if necessary up to a total daily dose of 20 metered sprays. **2.** *dexamethasone:* (inhalation aerosol) 3 metered sprays 3 or 4 times a day, increased if necessary up to a total daily dose of 12 metered sprays.
Administration   inhalation.

1. *When transferring patients from systemic to inhalation adrenal corticosteroids, the systemic drug should be continued at full dose for at least 1 week after beginning inhalation therapy, and decreased very gradually after that. Monitor patient for signs of adrenal insufficiency.* **2.** *Give corticosteroid aerosol after bronchodilator aerosol, if ordered together.*

Anticipated response   improved pulmonary function.

1. *These drugs are unsuitable for acute asthmatic episodes.* **2.** *Significant improvement may not be evident for 1–4 weeks after the start of therapy.*

Side effects **1.** *GI:* irritation, dry mouth and nose, oral candidiasis. **2.** *Dermatologic:* skin rash (allergy). **3.** *Respiratory:* paradoxical bronchospasm, hoarseness.

1. *Rinse patient's mouth after each dose to prevent throat irritation and candidiasis.* **2.** *At high doses or in sensitive individuals, systemic adrenocorticosteroid effects are possible with these aerosols. See Adrenal corticosteroids, systemic, for a complete discussion.*

Interactions **1.** Inhalation aerosol forms of bronchodilators contain fluorocarbon propellants, as do adrenal corticosteroid aerosols. The use of both drugs close together can cause fluorocarbon toxicity. **2.** These aerosols may increase or decrease the effects of oral anticoagulants. **3.** Dexamethasone may increase the risk of GI side effects when used with nonsteroidal anti-inflammatory agents or alcohol. **4.** Dexamethasone may increase potassium loss when administered concurrently with any potassium-depleting diuretic. **5.** Dexamethasone may increase blood glucose and therefore antagonize the effects of antidiabetic drugs.

1. *Allow at least 15 minutes to elapse between bronchodilator and adrenal corticosteroid aerosols.* **2.** *Monitor potassium levels in the patient receiving potassium-depleting diuretics and these drugs.*

Adrenal Corticosteroids (systemic): betamethasone, corticotropin, cortisone, dexamethasone, hydrocortisone, methylprednisolone, prednisolone, prednisone, triamcinolone (There are many brand names for each drug.)

Common use in adrenal insufficiency, as anti-inflammatory or immunosuppressant agents in a wide variety of disorders, and in hypercalcemia, to reduce serum calcium level.

Mechanism of action exact mechanisms are unknown; these drugs interfere with inflammatory processes and suppress cell-mediated immune reactions, increase sodium and water retention and potassium excretion through actions on the renal distal tubules, decrease calcium absorption and increase calcium excretion, decrease bone formation and increase bone resorption, stimulate protein catabolism, mobilize fatty acids, and induce gluconeogenesis.

Dosage **1.** *betamethasone:* (oral) 0.5–9 mg daily in single or divided doses; (IM, IV) up to 12 mg daily. **2.** *corticotropin:* (IM) 40–80 USP units daily; (IV diagnostic aid) 10–25 USP units in 500 cc D$_5$W run over 8 hours. **3.** *cortisone:* (oral) 25–300 mg/day in single or divided doses; (IM) 20–300 mg/day. **4.** *dexamethasone:* (oral) 0.5–9 mg daily in single or divided doses; (IM) 8–16 mg of the acetate suspension, or 0.5–9 mg of the phosphate; (IV) 0.5–9 mg of the phosphate daily. **5.** *hydrocortisone:* (oral) 20–240 mg daily in single or divided doses; (IM) 15–240 mg of the suspension daily; (IM, IV, SC) 100–500 mg of the phosphate or sodium succinate, repeated every 2–6 hours; (rectal) 90–100 mg retention enema. **6.** *methylprednisolone:* (oral) 4–48 mg daily as single or divided doses; (IM) 40–120 mg of the acetate suspension at 1–4 week intervals; (IM, IV) 10–40 mg of the sodium succinate; (rectal) 40 mg 3–7 times a week. **7.** *prednisolone:* (oral) 5–60 mg daily as single or divided doses; (IM) 4–60 mg daily of the acetate or sodium phosphate; (IV) 4–60 mg daily of the sodium phosphate. **8.** *prednisone:* (oral) 5–60 mg daily in single or divided doses. **9.** *triamcinolone:* (oral) 4–48 mg daily in single or divided doses; (IM) 40–80 mg weekly.

Administration oral, intramuscular, intravenous, rectal.

1. *Administer IM injections deep into gluteal muscle to avoid local tissue atrophy. Rotate sites if repeated doses are necessary.* **2.** *IV forms have numerous incompatibilities; double check before giving in same IV line.* **3.** *Rapid IV injection can cause life-threatening cardiac dysrhythmias. Keep resuscitation equipment and medications on hand.*

Anticipated response See Common use, Mechanism of action, and Side effects. Adrenal corticosteroids are used for a wide variety of disorders.

Corticotropin should not be used in emergencies or when an immediate effect is needed.

Side effects **1.** *GI:* nausea, peptic ulceration, pancreatitis. **2.** *CV:* hypertension, edema, hypercholesterolemia. **3.** *Metabolic:* poor wound healing, increased blood glucose, abnormal fatty deposits, adrenal suppression. **4.** *Musculoskeletal:* muscle weakness, osteoporosis, growth suppression. **5.** *CNS:* depression, euphoria, insomnia, confusion, disorientation. **6.** *Ophthalmic:* increased intraocular pressure, cataracts, blurred vision. **7.** *Dermatologic:* hirsutism, acne, subcutaneous tissue atrophy. **8.** *Other:* increased susceptibility to infection; carcinogenic with long-term use.

1. *Administer oral doses with food to decrease GI irritation. The administration of antacids has not been shown to prevent severe GI problems in adrenal corticosteroid therapy.* **2.** *For prolonged use, a full 48-hr dose every other morning is preferred, to reduce side effects and secondary insufficiency. Give daily dose before 9 A.M. to coincide with diurnal effect of endogenous hormone.* **3.** *Adrenal recovery may occur within a week after very-short-term therapy; recovery may take a year or more after long-term administration, and some patients never fully recover their adrenal function. Adrenal function monitoring may be needed to assess patient's continued ability to respond to stress.* **4.** *A low-calorie, low-carbohydrate, low-fat, high-protein, or sodium-restricted diet may be necessary during long-term* *therapy. Potassium and/or calcium supplementation also may be needed.*

Interactions **1.** With alcohol, aspirin, or nonsteroidal anti-inflammatory drugs, increased risk of GI ulceration and hemorrhage. **2.** Phenobarbital, phenytoin, and rifampin increase glucocorticoid metabolism, reducing steroid effect. **3.** May increase or decrease the effects of oral anticoagulants. **4.** These drugs may antagonize the effects of antidiabetic drugs. **5.** Estrogen-containing medications may increase both the therapeutic and the toxic effects of adrenal corticosteroids. **6.** Adrenal corticosteroids increase the potential for digitalis toxicity. **7.** These drugs antagonize the diuretic effects of diuretics and enhance the hypokalemia of potassium-depleting diuretics. **8.** With other immunosuppressive agents, increased risk of infection and lymphomas. **9.** These drugs may antagonize the effects of potassium supplements. **10.** The administration of live virus vaccines may result in viral infection rather than immunization. With other immunizations, possible decreased or absent antibody response and increased risk of neurologic complications.

Many of the potential drug interactions involving the adrenal corticosteroids have serious consequences. Multiple drug therapy must be monitored very closely, and the benefits and risks of these combinations weighed carefully.

Albuterol (Proventil, Ventolin)

Common use relief of bronchospasm in patients with reversible obstructive airway disease, such as asthma.
Mechanism of action sympathomimetic agent, beta-adrenergic agonist, bronchodilator; directly relaxes bronchial smooth muscle.

Dosage (inhalation) 1 or 2 inhalations repeated every 4–6 hours; (oral) 2–8 mg 3 or 4 times a day.
Administration inhalation, oral.

1. Advise patient to take amount prescribed—excessive dosage may result in paradoxical bronchospasm. 2. Store away from heat and light. 3. Do not puncture or burn container. 4. Avoid contact with eyes. 5. Advise patient to notify physician if he or she becomes nonresponsive to usual dose or if condition worsens. 6. Use lower doses with the elderly.

Anticipated response relief of bronchospasm and wheezing.

Onset of action within 5–15 minutes by inhalation, within 30 minutes orally. Maximum effect within 60–90 minutes, and duration of action 3–6 hours after inhalation; orally, 2–3 hours to maximum effect, and 6 hours or more duration.

Side effects **1.** *CV:* tachycardia, hypertension, palpitations, angina, dysrhythmias, headache, chest pain. **2.** *CNS:*
tremor, nervousness, dizziness, insomnia. **3.** *GI:* heartburn, nausea, vomiting, unusual taste. **4.** *Respiratory:* paradoxical bronchospasm, drying or irritation of oropharynx. **5.** *GU:* difficult urination.

1. Monitor blood pressure and apical pulse. 2. Rinse mouth with water after each inhaled dose to relieve dry mouth.

Interactions **1.** Beta-blockers inhibit drug's effect. **2.** Additive effect when given with other sympathomimetic drugs. **3.** With monoamine oxidase inhibitors or tricyclic antidepressants, excessive and potentially dangerous hemodynamic responses. **4.** With digitalis glycosides, increased risk of dysrhythmias.

1. Beta-blockers generally should not be administered to people with obstructive lung disease. 2. Avoid concurrent use of albuterol and MAO inhibitors or tricyclic antidepressants. 3. Monitor the digitalized patient closely.

Other **1.** Patients who are hypersensitive to other sympathomimetics, or to fluorocarbon propellants, may be hypersensitive to albuterol. **2.** Use with caution in patients with cardiovascular disorders, diabetes mellitus, hyperthyroidism, or enlarged prostate. **3.** Used experimentally to delay preterm labor.

Aminocaproic Acid (Amicar)

Common use to control excessive bleeding.
Mechanism of action antihemorrhagic; inhibits plasminogen activator substances and inhibits fibrinolysin activity.

Dosage oral or IV, initially, 4–5 g over 1 hour followed by 1–1.5 g/hour until bleeding is controlled (up to 30 g within 24 hours).
Administration oral and intravenous.

1. Do not administer unless there is laboratory documentation of hyperfibrinolysis. 2. Never administer IV form undiluted. 3. Dilute solution for IV use with sterile water for injection, 5% dextrose and water, normal saline, or Ringer's solution. 4. To avoid thrombophlebitis, use care inserting IV needle, fixing its position, and maintaining the site.

Anticipated response control of bleeding.

1. Keep careful intake and output records to determine fluid loss. 2. Monitor coagulation studies carefully.

Side effects **1.** *CNS:* headache, tinnitus, dizziness, fatigue. **2.** *GI:* nausea, vomiting, cramps, diarrhea. **3.** *CV:* slow or irregular heartbeat, hypotension. **4.** *GU:* difficult or painful urination, oliguria.

1. Monitor vital signs and ECG continuously, and report hypotension or significant arrhythmias. Change in pulse rate

usually indicates too-rapid IV administration; slow the rate. **2.** *Urinary problems may indicate renal failure.*
Interactions no significant interactions noted.

Other Use with caution in cardiac, hepatic, or renal disease or in patients predisposed to thrombosis.

Aminophylline (Phyllocontin, Somophyllin, Truphylline)

Common use treatment of bronchial asthma, bronchospasm, COPD.
Mechanism of action bronchodilator; relaxes bronchial smooth muscle.

Dosage maintenance dosages (initial loading doses are higher):

Equivalent of Anhydrous Theophylline

	ORAL/RECTAL	IV
Smoker	4 mg/kg every 6 hours	0.7 mg/kg/hour
Nonsmoker	3 mg/kg every 8 hours	0.43 mg/kg/hour
Elderly	2 mg/kg every 8 hours	0.26 mg/kg/hour
CHF, liver failure	2 mg/kg every 12 hours	0.2 mg/kg/hour

Administration oral, intravenous, rectal.

1. *Before administering loading dose, ascertain if patient has recently been on theophylline therapy.* **2.** *Rectal absorption is erratic; rectal administration is not recommended.* **3.** *Do not use if solution is crystallized.* **4.** *Oral form is absorbed best on an empty stomach but can be given with meals if GI irritation develops.* **5.** *Give IV form at a rate no faster than 25 mg per minute. Monitor for chest pain, hypotension, cardiac arrhythmias; if noted, slow IV rate.* **6.** *Space doses over 24 hours.* **7.** *Dose must be individualized, due to narrow therapeutic range and wide patient variation.* **8.** *When changing from IV to oral dosing, the first oral dose should be given 4–6 hours after the IV infusion is completed. When using an extended-release oral form, the initial dose should be given at the time the IV infusion is discontinued.* **9.** *Enteric-coated or extended-release dosage forms should never be crushed or broken. If the patient cannot tolerate the whole pill, obtain an order for liquid aminophylline.*

Anticipated response **1.** *Increased ease of respiration.* **2.** Decreased rate of respiration.

Observe patient for improved ventilation: improved color, decreased pulse and respiratory rates, decreased use of accessory muscles for respiration, decreased anxiety.

Side effects **1.** *CNS:* anxiety, insomnia, headache, seizures. **2.** *CV:* palpitations, hypotension, dysrhythmias, tachycardia, hypotension, precordial pain. **3.** *GI:* bitter aftertaste, nausea, vomiting, anorexia, dyspepsia, feeling of gastric fullness, epigastric pain, bleeding. **4.** *GU:* diuresis.

1. *Monitor blood pressure and pulse and respiratory rates while patient is on therapy.* **2.** *GI side effects may diminish if taken with food.* **3.** *IV form should be diluted, and infused slowly to avoid severe hypotension.*

Interactions **1.** *When used with ephedrine or other sympathomimetics, excessive CNS stimulation may occur.* **2.** Mutual antagonism in effects on bronchial smooth muscle exists between aminophylline and beta-blocking drugs. **3.** Smoking tobacco or marijuana may increase aminophylline metabolism, necessitating dosage increases. **4.** Cimetidine, allopurinol, propranolol, or erythromycin may decrease aminophylline clearance, resulting in possible toxicity. **5.** Aminophylline increases lithium excretion, requiring lithium dosage adjustment. **6.** When given with caffeine, increased CNS side effects result.

Instruct patient not to use over-the-counter preparations without consulting a physician.

Other **1.** Aminophylline therapy may exacerbate cardiac disease or peptic ulcer; use with caution. **2.** Hepatic or renal disease, severe hypoxemia, or prolonged fever may decrease aminophylline clearance and result in toxic plasma concentrations. **3.** Monitoring of serum levels is highly recommended, due to wide variation in therapeutic dose and relatively narrow therapeutic serum level range. **4.** Monitor for tachycardia or dysrhythmias, anorexia, nausea, headache, or insomnia as signs of toxicity. If noted, draw serum levels before next dose, report, and hold dose if the level is greater than 20 mcg/ml.

Amiodarone (Cordarone)

Common use prevention and treatment of refractory ventricular dysrhythmias.
Mechanism of action antidysrhythmic; prolongs refractory period, slows AV conduction, suppresses automaticity in the Purkinje network.

Dosage (oral) 800–1,600 mg/day initially, in divided doses if necessary, until satisfactory patient response or side effects occur; decrease gradually over 1 month to a maintenance dose of 200–400 mg/day.
Administration oral.

Because of its delayed onset of action and complicated dosing, amiodarone is not recommended as a first-line antidysrhythmic drug.

Anticipated response control of dysrhythmia.

Side effects **1.** *Respiratory:* cough, dyspnea, SOB; potentially fatal pulmonary fibrosis. **2.** *CV:* tachycardia, bradycardia, other dysrhythmias. **3.** *Neurologic:* peripheral neuropathy, tremors, ataxia. **4.** *Ophthalmic:* microdeposits on cornea, blurred vision, dry eyes, photophobia. **5.** *Dermatologic:* photosensitivity, blue-gray coloration of skin, rash. **6.** *Metabolic:* hypothyroidism, hyperthyroidism. **7.** *GI:* anorexia, nausea, constipation. **8.** *CNS:* malaise, dizziness (without hypotension). **9.** *GU:* impotence, decreased libido.

1. Side effects may not be evident until therapy has continued for several days or weeks, and they may persist for several months after amiodarone withdrawal. 2. The elderly may experience more ataxia than younger adults. 3. Monitor for pulmonary toxicity: progressive dyspnea, fatigue, cough, chest pain, fever. Auscultate chest regularly; employ x-ray, pulmonary function studies, or bronchoscopy as needed if pulmonary toxicity is evident. 4. Protect skin from excess sunlight during therapy, and for several months afterwards. 5. Ophthalmoscopic exam is recommended prior to therapy and as a follow-up to ophthalmic signs and symptoms. 6. Monitor for and report signs of thyroid dysfunction: increased BP and HR, weight change, increased skin temperature, exopthalmos, increased GI motility, and urinary frequency. Thyroid function tests should be monitored as baseline and every 3–6 months, especially in elderly.

Interactions **1.** With other antidysrhythmic drugs, including beta-blockers and calcium channel blockers, possible additive cardiac effects and increased tachydysrhythmias. **2.** Amiodarone potentiates coumarin anticoagulants, and this effect can persist for weeks or months after amiodarone is discontinued. **3.** Amiodarone increases serum levels of the following drugs and may cause toxicity: digoxin, coumadin, quinidine, phenytoin, and procainamide. **4.** Potassium-depleting diuretics may increase risk of hypokalemia-related dysrhythmias.

1. Use with extreme caution with other antidysrhythmic drugs. 2. Decrease anticoagulant dose by one-third to one-half and monitor prothrombin time closely when amiodarone is given with anticoagulants. 3. When amiodarone is given with digoxin, quinidine, phenytoin, and procainamide, decrease the dose by 33–50%, and carefully monitor cardiac function and drug toxicity.

Other Do not use if severe bradycardia is present, unless controlled by a pacemaker.

Benzodiazepines: alprazolam (Xanax), chlordiazepoxide (Librium), clorazepate (Tranxene), diazepam (Valium), flurazepam (Dalmane), halazepam (Paxipam), lorazepam (Ativan), midazolam (Versed), oxazepam (Serax), prazepam (Centrax), temazepam (Restoril), triazolam (Halcion)

Common use treatment of anxiety, insomnia, and alcohol withdrawal; skeletal muscle relaxant; anticonvulsant; anesthesia adjunct.

Mechanism of action specific mechanisms of action are not completely established; appear to potentiate inhibitory neurotransmitter at specific benzodiazepine receptors in all levels of CNS, producing various levels of CNS depression.

Dosage **1.** *alprazolam:* (oral) 0.25–0.5 mg 3 times a day, increased gradually as needed. **2.** *chlordiazepoxide:* (oral) 5–25 mg 3 or 4 times a day; (IM, IV) 50–100 mg initially, followed by 25–50 mg 3 times a day if needed. **3.** *clorazepate:* 15–60 mg/day, divided. **4.** *diazepam:* (oral) 2–10 mg 3 or 4 times a day; (IM, IV) 2–10 mg, repeated in 3 or 4 hours as needed. **5.** *flurazepam;* (oral) 15–30 mg at bedtime. **6.** *halazepam:* 20–40 mg 3 or 4 times a day. **7.** *lorazepam:* (oral) 2–6 mg/day, divided with largest dose at bedtime; (IM) 50 mcg/kg; (IV) 44 mcg/kg or a total of 2 mg, whichever is less. **8.** *midazolam:* (IM) 70–80 mcg/kg 30–60 min. before surgery; (IV) 75–200 mcg/kg, administered slowly; (IV anesthesia adjunct) 150–600 mcg/kg **9.** *oxazepam:* (oral) 10–30 mg 3 or 4 times a day. **10.** *prazepam:* 20–60 mg/day, divided or at bedtime. **11.** *temazepam:* (oral) 15–30 mg at bedtime. **12.** *triazolam:* (oral) 0.125–0.5 mg at bedtime.

Administration oral, intramuscular, intravenous.

1. Begin with lower doses in elderly, debilitated, or very young patients or in those with impaired renal or hepatic function. 2. Parenteral administration, especially rapid IV administration, may cause apnea, hypotension, bradycardia, or cardiac arrest. Keep emergency equipment and medications on hand. 3. In general, avoid the IM route because of possible erratic absorption. 4. For IM chlordiazepoxide, prepare solution with the manufacturer's diluent only. 5. An IV solution of diazepam may precipitate; give as IV bolus only, do not dilute.

Anticipated response relief of anxiety; shortened time to fall asleep; prevention of most physical manifestations of alcohol withdrawal; relief of muscle spasm and pain; suppression of seizure activity; facilitated anesthesia.

Physical dependence will develop with regular use. Depending on the specific benzodiazepine, withdrawal symptoms may occur 2–20 days after abrupt discontinuance of the drug; therefore, gradual dosage reduction is necessary.

Side effects **1.** *CNS:* drowsiness, dizziness, confusion, paradoxical excitement, mental depression. **2.** *Ophthalmic:* blurred vision. **3.** *Musculoskeletal:* weakness, ataxia, clumsiness. **4.** *GI:* nausea, hiccups, constipation, dry mouth. **5.** *CV:* hypotension, dizziness. **6.** *Overdose:* confusion, drowsiness, shakiness, slurred speech, bradycardia, dyspnea, severe weakness.

Elderly and debilitated patients are more sensitive to the CNS effects of these drugs; use with caution.

Interactions **1.** *Increased CNS depression when used with other CNS depressants.* **2.** Possible additive hypotension with antihypertensives, diuretics, or other medications that lower blood pressure. **3.** Cimetidine, disulfiram, oral contraceptives, ketoconazole, metoprolol, propoxyphene, propranolol, and valproic acid may increase plasma level of benzodiazepines, thereby increasing their effects. **4.** With the anticonvulsants primidone, valproic acid, or carbamazepine, possible increased seizure activity or other change in seizure pattern. **5.** Possible digoxin toxicity may occur due to increased serum digoxin levels; monitor serum levels.

Use cautiously with interacting drugs, monitor carefully, and adjust doses as needed.

Other **1.** Avoid use during pregnancy; several benzodiazepines have been implicated in congenital malformations. **2.** These drugs may exacerbate mental depression, myasthenia gravis, narrow-angle glaucoma, or respiratory distress. **3.** Use with caution in history of drug abuse, suicidal tendencies, hepatic or renal dysfunction (lorazepam not recommended), open angle glaucoma, elderly patients, or limited respiratory reserve.

Beta-Adrenergic Blocking Agents: acebutolol (Sectral), atenolol (Tenormin), betaxolol (Kerlone), carteolol (Cartrol), esmolol (Brevibloc), labetolol (Normodyne, Trandate), metoprolol (Lopressor), nadolol (Corgard), penbutolol (Levatol), pindolol (Visken), propranolol (Inderal), timolol (Blocadren)

Common use[1] control of angina, dysrhythmias, hypertension, migraines, essential tremor; postmyocardial infarction cardiac preservation.

[1]Not all uses for all members of family; propranolol has widest range of approved uses.

Mechanism of action selectively block beta receptors in sympathetic nervous system without causing general inhibition of adrenergic activity.

Dosage **1.** *acebutolol:* 200–400 mg twice a day. **2.** *atenolol:* (oral) initially, 50 mg once a day, increased as needed to 100 mg once a day; (IV in acute MI) 5 mg, repeated in 10 min. **3.** *betaxolol:* 10 mg once a day, increased as needed to 20 mg daily. **4.** *carteolol:* 2.5 mg once a day, increased as needed to 10 mg. **5.** *esmolol:* (IV) 500 mcg/kg over 1 min, followed by 50 mcg/kg/min for 4 min; repeat loading dose, followed by 100 mcg/kg/min for 4 min; repeat titration, increasing infusion by 50 mcg/kg/min increments until end point (or 300 mcg/kg/min) reached; maintenance infusion: 25–50 mcg/kg/min. **6.** *labetolol:* (oral) 100–400 mg twice a day; (IV) 20-mg bolus over 2 minutes, followed by 40–80 mg every 10 minutes, titrated to BP response; or 2 mg/min up to a total dose of 50–300 mg. **7.** *metoprolol:* (oral) 100–450 mg once daily or divided into 2 doses; (IV) 5 mg every 2 minutes for 3 doses, then change to oral. **8.** *nadolol:* 40–320 mg daily. **9.** *penbutolol:* 20–40 mg once a day. **10.** *pindolol:* 10–60 mg daily, divided into 2–4 doses. **11.** *propranolol:* (oral) 30–640 mg divided into 3 or 4 doses; extended-release tablets, 80, 120, or 160 mg daily; (IV) 1–3 mg bolus, administered at 1 mg/min, repeated in 2 minutes and again in 4 hours as needed. **12.** *timolol:* 20–60 mg/day, divided into 2 doses.

Atenolol, betaxolol, and nadolol have longer half-lives: give only once a day.

Administration *oral; atenolol, betaxolol, esmolol, labetolol, metoprolol, and propranolol may also be given intravenously. Older people may be sensitive to the effects of beta-blocker drugs; adjust doses carefully.*

Anticipated response **1.** Slowed heart rate. **2.** Decreased blood pressure. **3.** Less frequent dysrhythmias. **4.** Decrease in rate of postmyocardial reinfarction and possibly mortality.

1. *Patients should be advised not to discontinue drug abruptly, because rebound angina or even myocardial infarction can occur; withdraw drug over at least 3 days, preferably 1–2 weeks.* **2.** *Some practitioners recommend gradual beta-blocker withdrawal 48 hours prior to surgery.* **3.** *Labetolol may cause pronounced hypotensive effects, because it blocks both alpha and beta receptors. Monitor closely.* **4.** *Give before meals, or be consistent in relation to food intake.* **5.** *Check heart rate (and BP during dosage adjustment) before administration; in stable patients, note cardiac response to exercise.*

Side effects **1.** *CNS:* weakness, fatigue, drowsiness, depression, insomnia, nightmares, confusion. **2.** *Respiratory:* bronchospasm. **3.** *GI:* nausea, dry mouth, diarrhea. **4.** *Metabolic:* hypoglycemia. **5.** *CV:* bradycardia, congestive heart failure, AV blocks, peripheral ischemia, fluid retention (high doses). **6.** *GU:* change in sexual response.

1. *Beta-blockers generally are contraindicated in patients with severe COPD or CHF, higher than first-degree heart block, or* *sinus bradycardia.* **2.** *Atenolol, betaxolol, and metoprolol are most "cardioselective" and are least likely to cause blood sugar or respiratory problems.* **3.** *Side effects are not dose related and increase with age and renal impairment.* **4.** *Use with caution in patients with a history of CHF, asthma, diabetes, or renal or hepatic impairment.*

Interactions **1.** With other antihypertensive drugs, including diuretics and phenothiazines, increased hypotension. **2.** Possible excessive bradycardia or heart block when given with digitalis. **3.** Mutual inhibition of effects when given with aminophylline. **4.** May potentiate antidiabetic drugs; dosage adjustment may be necessary. **5.** Antidysrhythmics may produce additive or antagonistic effects. **6.** Anticholinergics (antimuscarinics and tricyclic antidepressants) in large doses antagonize beta-blocker cardiac effect by reestablishing balance of sympathetic and parasympathetic action. **7.** Cimetidine, chlorpromazine, and oral contraceptives inhibit hepatic metabolism, increasing beta-blocker bioavailability. **8.** Epinephrine and other adrenergics may cause hypertension. **9.** Indomethacin and salicylates inhibit antihypertensive effect, possibly through prostaglandin inhibition. **10.** MAO inhibitors are contraindicated within 2 weeks.

Diabetics need to monitor blood sugar more closely due to hypoglycemia and masking of usual signs of low blood sugar, except sweating, hunger, and inability to concentrate.

Calcium Channel Blocking Agents: diltiazem (Cardizem), nicardipine (Cardene), nifedipine (Adalat, Procardia), nimodipine (Nimotop), verapamil (Calan, Isoptin)

Common use control of angina and hypertension; (verapamil) treatment of supraventricular tachycardia; (nimodipine) treatment of spasm due to subarachnoid hemorrhage.
Mechanism of action inhibit flow of calcium ions into cardiac and vascular smooth muscle cells, resulting in decreased muscle tone; also decreases AV conduction and prolongs refractory period

Dosage **1.** *diltiazem:* (oral) 30 mg 3–4 times a day, increased gradually as needed up to 360 mg daily. **2.** *nicardipine:* (oral) 20 mg 3 times a day, increased gradually 40 mg 3 times a day. **3.** *nifedipine:* (oral) 10 mg 3 times a day, increased gradually as needed up to 180 mg daily. **4.** *nimodipine:* (oral) 60 mg every 4 hours for 21 days. **5.** *verapamil:* (oral) 80 mg 3–4 times a day, increased gradually as needed up to 480 mg daily; (IV) initially, 5–10 mg over 2 minutes, with a 10-mg dose 30 minutes later if needed.
Administration oral (verapamil) IV.

1. *Advise patient not to discontinue these drugs abruptly.* **2.** *In elderly patients, administer IV dose over at least 3 minutes.* **3.** *Monitor ECG continuously during IV administration. Observe for PR prolongation or bradycardia.* **4.** *Give undiluted, IVP over 2 minutes.*

Anticipated response decrease in frequency of anginal episodes or dysrhythmias; improved coronary artery perfusion and decreased coronary artery spasm; peripheral vasodilatation and decreased blood pressure; depressed SA and AV nodal conduction (diltiazem and verapamil).

1. *Observe patient for reduction of anginal pain.* **2.** *Monitor blood pressure, especially during initial dose titration.* **3.** *Emphasize the benefits of weight loss, proper diet, exercise, and smoking cessation in control of angina and hypertension.*

Side effects **1.** *CNS:* dizziness, light-headedness, syncope, headache, nervousness. **2.** *CV:* hypotension, flushing, peripheral edema, palpitations, tachycardia, bradycardia. **3.** *GI:* nausea, constipation. **4.** *Musculoskeletal:* weakness. **5.** *Respiratory:* dyspnea, cough, nasal congestion. **6.** *Metabolic:* hypoglycemia. **7.** *Dermatologic:* urticaria, pruritis.

1. *Monitor BP, especially during initial therapy or when the dose is changed. Instruct patient to change position slowly to avoid orthostatic hypotension.* **2.** *Observe for peripheral edema.* **3.** *Monitor frequency, duration, and severity of anginal attacks.* **4.** *Have vasopressors available during initial therapy in case of severe hypotension.*

Interactions **1.** With beta-adrenergic blockers, possible dangerously prolonged AV conduction or congestive failure (especially in LV dysfunction). **2.** With other drugs that lower BP, additive hypotensive effect. **3.** With rifampin, decreased bioavailability of verapamil; monitor closely. **4.** With digitalis, increased serum digitalis level, resulting in possible toxicity. **5.** Verapamil both decreases lithium levels and increases neurotoxicity; use with caution. **6.** Calcium channel blockers, increase carbamazepine and theophylline levels, resulting in possible toxicity; reduce dose and monitor closely.

1. *Monitor serum digitalis levels if both drugs are given concurrently, and closely monitor cardiac status. Reduction of digitalis dose may be necessary.* **2.** *Monitor for signs of congestive heart failure if used with beta-adrenergic blocking agents.*

Calcium Chloride

Common use treatment of hypocalcemia and hyperkalemia; an adjunct drug in cardiac resuscitation.
Mechanism of action electrolyte replenisher; plays important role in impulse transmission, muscle contraction, and blood clotting.

Dosage 200–1,000 mg administered at no greater than 100 mg/min. Repeat in 1–3 days as needed for depletion; for hyperkalemic emergency, give 1–10 ml of 10% solution, titrated to ECG changes.
Administration intravenous.

1. Warm solution to body temperature before administering. 2. Infuse at a rate no greater than 100 mg/min.

Anticipated response correction of electrolyte imbalance.

Side effects 1. *GI:* bitter chalky taste, nausea. 2. *CV:* flushing, warmth. 3. *Neurologic:* tingling sensations. 4. *Overdose or intolerance:* bradycardia, cardiac arrest, hypotension, diarrhea, vomiting, mental depression, high urine output. 5. *Other:* sweating, burning sensation at injection site, necrosis at injection site.

1. Infuse slowly to decrease incidence of side effects. 2. Use a small-gauge needle and a large vein to minimize local irritation, and infuse slowly after confirming vein patency. 3. A serum calcium greater than 10.5 mg/100 ml is considered hypercalcemic. Initial treatment is conservative—withhold calcium. In serious hypercalcemia, employ hydration, loop diuretics, chelating agents, calcitonin, and corticosteroids as needed.

Interactions 1. Calcitonin will antagonize the effects of calcium chloride in hypercalcemia. 2. With vitamin D, other calcium-containing medications, or thiazide diuretics, possible hypercalcemia. 3. Calcium chloride may cause serious dysrhythmias in digitalized patients. 4. Calcium chloride antagonizes the effect of calcium channel blockers; it is used as antidote in overdose.

When calcium chloride is given to digitalized patients, carefully monitor cardiac function; avoid use if possible.

Other 1. Do not use in digitalis toxicity or ventricular fibrillation. 2. Use with caution if renal function is impaired, because of the danger of hypercalcemia.

Cromolyn Sodium (Intal)

Common use prophylactic treatment of asthma or exercise-induced bronchospasm.
Mechanism of action mast cell stabilizer; inhibits bronchoconstriction by preventing release of substances that mediate allergic response.

Dosage 20 mg (in capsule or solution) 4 times daily, or less than 1 hour before exercise.
Administration inhalation.

1. If a bronchodilator inhaler is also prescribed, use it 20–30 minutes prior to cromolyn. 2. Protect capsules from moisture,

and store at room temperature. 3. Teach patient correct use of inhaler: exhale before placing mouthpiece between lips, then inhale deeply with even breath. Hold breath and exhale. Repeat until powder is gone. 4. Rinse mouth after each dose to prevent throat irritation. 5. Full benefit of the drug may not be evident for 3–4 weeks.

Anticipated response reduction in frequency of asthmatic attacks.

Not effective in relieving acute attack. Cromolyn is not a bronchodilator or anti-inflammatory drug.

Side effects 1. *CNS:* dizziness, headache. 2. *Respiratory:* bronchospasm, cough, stuffy nose, throat irritation. 3. *Dermatologic:* skin rash, itching, swelling of lips or eyes. 4. *GI:* nausea, dry mouth. 5. *GU:* frequent or difficult urination.

Interactions none reported.

Other The inhalation-capsule form contains lactose. Patients who are lactose-intolerant may not tolerate this form.

Diazoxide (Hyperstat)

Common use lowers blood pressure in hypertensive crisis.
Mechanism of action antihypertensive; vasodilates venous and arterial vessels by directly relaxing vascular smooth muscle

Dosage 1–3 mg/kg, up to 150 mg, repeated as needed in 5–15 minutes.
Administration intravenous.

1. Administer IV bolus over 30 seconds, with patient lying down. Maintain patient in supine position for 15–30 minutes after administration. 2. Patient should be maintained on oral medication after blood pressure is under control.

Anticipated response rapid fall in blood pressure.

Monitor vital signs before each dose and every 5 min for 30 min after each dose, then hourly. Peak effect in 2–5 minutes, duration of action 2–12 hours.

Side effects 1. *CNS:* dizziness, light-headedness, flushing, drowsiness, confusion. 2. *CV:* sodium and water retention, tachycardia, hypotension. 3. *Metabolic:* hyperglycemia, hyperuricemia. 4. *GI:* nausea, vomiting, constipation, anorexia.

1. Weigh patient daily. 2. Instruct patient to rise slowly to avoid orthostatic hypotension. 3. Check blood sugar regularly; diabetics may require insulin coverage. 4. Keep norepinephrine on hand, and notify physician to treat severe hypotension. 5. Often administered with a diuretic (given IV 30–60 minutes prior to diazoxide) to potentiate antihypertensive effect and to prevent congestive heart failure from salt and water retention.

Interactions   **1.** May increase the effect of oral anticoagulants. **2.** Hypotension will be potentiated if given with other drugs that lower blood pressure. **3.** Thiazide or loop diuretics may increase the hyperglycemic, hyperuricemic, and antihypertensive effects of this drug. **4.** Antagonizes effects of antidiabetic drugs.

Other   Use with extreme caution in patients with poor cardiac reserve; coronary, renal, or cerebral insufficiency.

Digitalis Glycosides: digitoxin (Crystodigin), digoxin (Lanoxin, Lanoxicaps)

Common use   treatment of congestive heart failure, atrial fibrillation, and atrial flutter.

Mechanism of action   cardiotonic, antidysrhythmic; increases strength and force of cardiac contraction, causing increased cardiac output; decreases heart rate and lengthens atrioventricular and sinoatrial conduction time.

Dosage   **1.** *digitoxin:* (oral) loading: 0.6 mg, followed by 0.4 mg in 4–6 hours, followed by 0.2 mg at 4–6 hour intervals for total of 1.2–1.6 mg; maintenance: 0.05–0.3 mg every day. **2.** *digoxin:* (oral[1]) loading: 10–15 mcg/kg (8–12 mg/kg) over 24 hours, usually 0.75–1.25 mg; 50% in first dose, then 25% fractions at 6–8 hour intervals; maintenance: 0.125–0.5 mg daily; (IV) loading: 8–12 mcg/kg over 24 hours; 50% in first dose, then 25% fractions at 4–8 hour intervals, usually 0.5–1 mg; maintenance: 0.125–0.35 mg daily.

Administration   oral, intravenous.

1. Higher doses may be needed initially as loading doses. 2. Do not substitute digoxin for digitoxin or vice versa; these drugs cannot be interchanged without dosage revisions. 3. Do not change brands of either digoxin or digitoxin without consulting physician; differences in bioavailability can result in different therapeutic effects. 4. IM routes are usually avoided because of pain of injection and erratic rate of absorption. If absolutely necessary, administer deep IM and massage the site well afterwards.

Anticipated response   slowed heart rate, decreased edema, increased urine output, resolution of CHF symptoms, control of dysrhythmias.

1. Give digoxin IV push over 5 minutes. 2. Digoxin is safer than digitoxin in presence of liver disease. 3. Digitoxin is safer than digoxin in presence of renal disease. 4. Instruct patient about importance of weight control, regular exercise, and low-salt diet in controlling heart disease. 5. Note: Digitalized patients are

more sensitive than others to electrical countershock, and they are more likely to respond with ventricular dysrhythmias. If electrical intervention is necessary, begin with minimal energy levels and increase carefully. 6. Elderly or debilitated patients, those with impaired renal function, or those using electronic pacemakers may develop digitalis toxicity at lower doses than other patients. Monitor carefully.

Side effects   **1.** *GI:* anorexia, nausea, vomiting. **2.** *CV:* unusually slow pulse, dysrhythmias. **3.** *CNS:* lethargy, confusion. **4.** *Other:* gynecomastia, thrombocytopenia. **5.** Signs of toxicity include anorexia, nausea and vomiting, diarrhea, drowsiness, lethargy, fatigue, headache, confusion, personality changes, blurred vision, blue/green vision, photophobia, and dysrhythmias.

1. Take apical-radial pulse for 1 minute before administering drug; do not give if patient's pulse is too low (minimum safe pulse rate varies: know the patient's usual pulse range and check with prescriber for guidelines). 2. Low serum potassium and high serum calcium levels predispose patient to digitalis toxicity. Monitor serum potassium, renal function, ECG if toxicity suspected. First ECG signs of toxicity are ST sagging, PR prolongation, and possible bigeminal rhythm. 3. Therapeutic serum digitalis levels vary greatly from person to person, and digitalis toxicity is better diagnosed on the basis of signs and symptoms than on blood levels. 4. Toxicity: if no impairment of cardiac output is present, drug is withheld until serum level is therapeutic. If CO is impaired or dysrhythmias are potentially progressive, treatment may include bed rest, potassium, antidysrhythmics, or digoxin-immune Fab (digoxin-specific antigen-binding fragments that bind digoxin for excretion, given IV in equimolar quantities).

Interactions   *1. Quinidine and calcium channel blockers may increase effect of digitalis, possibly resulting in digitalis toxicity. 2.* Cholestyramine, antacids, or bran may decrease oral digitalis absorption. *3. Digitoxin only:* Rifampin (and possibly barbiturates) increase hepatic metabolism of digitoxin, resulting in decreased serum digitalis levels. **4.** Adrenocorticosteroids and potassium-depleting diuretics increase the possibility of digitalis toxicity because of their tendency to cause hypokalemia. **5.** Parenteral calcium salts, parenteral magnesium sulfate, other antidysrhythmic drugs, or sympathomimetics may increase the risk of cardiac dysrhythmias.

1. Adjust doses of digitalis or other drugs as needed. 2. Allow at least 2 hours to elapse from time of digitalis dose before administering antacids, cholestyramine, or bran. 3. Monitor serum potassium levels.

Disopyramide (Norpace)

Common use   suppression or prevention of recurrent ventricular dysrhythmias, such as premature ventricular contractions or ventricular tachycardia.

---

[1]Oral dosage stated for tablets and elixir (liquid-filled capsules in parentheses).

Mechanism of action antidysrhythmic agent; depresses myocardial responsiveness; normalizes regional cardiac electrical impulse conduction.

Dosage **1.** 150 mg every 6 hours, or 300 mg extended-release capsules every 12 hours; average daily doses range from 400–1,600 mg in divided doses. **2.** A 300-mg loading dose may be given for rapid control of dysrhythmias.
Administration oral.

1. Small patients and patients with moderate renal or hepatic insufficiency, cardiomyopathy, or possible cardiac decompensation usually require reduced doses. 2. Hypokalemia should be corrected before therapy is begun. 3. Monitor vital signs for potential hypotension and bradycardia during initial therapy; alert physician if significant (approximately 25%) widening of QRS complex or first-degree AV block is observed on ECG. 4. Contraindications: cardiogenic shock and second- or third-degree AV block.

Anticipated response maintenance of normal sinus rhythm; reduced frequency or duration of recurrent ventricular dysrhythmias.

Onset of effects takes 30 minutes to 3 hours.

Side effects **1.** *GU:* urinary hesitancy, frequency, or urgency, impotence. **2.** *CV:* hypotension, heart failure, conduction disturbances, dizziness. **3.** *GI:* constipation, dry mouth, hepatotoxicity. **4.** *CNS:* blurred vision, headache, confusion. **5.** *Other:* rash, hypoglycemia.

1. Observe for possible urinary retention, particularly among older males. 2. Caution patient to rise slowly from sitting or recumbent position to avoid orthostatic hypotension. 3. Patients with glaucoma may react with increased intraocular pressure; instruct them to report immediately any visual changes or eye pain. 4. Observe for signs of hepatotoxicity—for example, jaundice. 5. Caution patient against driving or operating machinery if dizziness or blurred vision occurs.

Interactions **1.** May produce profound heart failure or conduction delays (or block) when given with other antidysrhythmic drugs. **2.** Phenytoin, rifampin, and other hepatic enzyme inducers reduce disopyramide plasma levels. **3.** With oral anticoagulants, possible erratic anticoagulant effect.

1. Give cautiously with similar antidysrhythmic drugs. Do not administer within 48 hours before or 24 hours after verapamil. 2. Do not use with alcohol. 3. Use caution in giving oral anticoagulants with disopyramide.

Other worsening of heart failure may occur in patients with compromised ventricular function.

Epoetin Alfa (Epogen, Procrit)

Common use to treat anemia associated with deficiency of erythropoietin (in chronic renal failure [CRF]) or anemia related to AZT therapy.
Mechanism of action stimulates erythropoiesis in bone marrow, increasing circulating RBC count, hemoglobin, and hematocrit (Hct).

Dosage 50–100 U/kg 3 times weekly, dosage reduced when Hct reaches target range (30–33% in CRF, 36–40% with AZT); maintenance: individualized. Median dose: dialysis, 75 U/kg 3 times weekly; nondialysis, 75–150 U/kg weekly.
Administration subcutaneous, intravenous

Do not shake (shaking renders glycoprotein biologically inactive). Withdraw one dose per vial; do not reenter vial. Discard unused portion.

Anticipated response increase in hemoglobin and hematocrit levels.

Side effects **1.** *CNS:* headache, fatigue, dizziness, seizures. **2.** *CV:* hypertension, tachycardia, edema, chest pain. **3.** *Respiratory:* shortness of breath. **4.** *Musculoskeletal:* arthralgia. **5.** *GI:* nausea, diarrhea, vomiting. **6.** *GU:* resumption of menses (CRF).

1. Hct is monitored twice weekly during dosage adjustment and during dosage reduction; then regularly with stable Hct. CBC, BUN and creatinine, electrolytes, and serum chemistry (SMA-12) are monitored regularly. 2. Obtain baseline BP and monitor BP regularly during initiation of therapy and dosage adjustment; monitor BP periodically during therapy. 3. Dosage may be reduced during excessive rise of Hct (exceeding 36%) or rapid rise of Hct (more than 4 points in 2 weeks) to prevent exacerbation of hypertension or seizures. 4. Patients on hemodialysis may require increased heparin to prevent clotting in the artificial kidney or of the vascular access. 5. If no response to therapy, iron stores, transferrin saturation (> 20%), and serum ferritin (> 100 ng/ml) are evaluated. All patients eventually require supplemental iron.

Interactions none noted.

Heparin

Common use treatment and prevention of peripheral venous and arterial thrombi and pulmonary embolism; treatment of disseminated intravascular coagulation; to maintain patency of indwelling venous access devices.
Mechanism of action anticoagulant; prevents formation of fibrin and thrombin.

Dosage (SC) 10,000–20,000 units initially, then 8,000–10,000 units every 8 hours; (low-dose SC) 5,000 units 2 hours preoperatively, then every 8–12 hours postoperatively until ambulatory; (IV) 10,000 units initially, then 5,000–10,000 units every 4–6 hours; (continuous IV infusion) 20,000–40,000 units in 1,000-ml sodium chloride solution, infused over 24 hours titrated to coagulation values; (IV patency) 10–100 units after use or every 8–12 hours.

Administration　intravenous, subcutaneous.

1. Obtain report of partial thromboplastin time before administering (one-half hour before administration time); partial thromboplastin time values are usually maintained at 1½–2 times the control value. 2. When administration is SC, inject above iliac crest or in lower abdomen deep into fat; do not aspirate prior to injection; do not massage area. 3. Avoid IM route because of irregular absorption of drug, increased incidence of hematoma, and pain. 4. IV pump is recommended for continuous IV infusion. 5. After taking blood samples from patient, apply continuous pressure for 3–5 minutes. 6. Intermittent IV infusion may be given diluted and piggybacked into main IV line, or IV push (at max. rate of 1,000 U/min). 7. Do not use solution if discolored or if precipitate is present. 8. Heparin is strongly acidic and incompatible with many IV medications. Use separate infusion sites, or flush tubing carefully before and after each dose. 9. For heparin lock flush, use NS flush after medication and before heparin to avoid drug mixing.

Anticipated response　anticoagulation and prevention of embolism formation.

Have protamine sulfate available as antidote for frank bleeding; because heparin is short-acting, treatment of overdose is conservative unless frank bleeding occurs.

Side effects　1. *Hematologic:* hemorrhage, prolonged clotting time, thrombocytopenia (incidence higher with beef (15%) than with pork (5%). 2. *Dermatologic:* urticaria (allergy). 3. *CV:* vasospastic hypersensitivity, with pain and cyanosis of limbs (not reversed by protamine sulfate). 4. *Other:* with long-term therapy, possible hair loss or osteoporosis.

1. Check patient's urine and feces for overt signs of bleeding; watch for easy bruising, unexplained nosebleeds, prolonged menses, dizziness, severe headache. 2. People over 60, especially women, are more susceptible to hemorrhage during heparin therapy.

Interactions　1. *Aspirin, ibuprofen, indomethacin, phenylbutazone, and other antiplatelet drugs may increase risk of hemorrhage.* 2. With steroids and nonsteroidal anti-inflammatory agents, increased risk of GI hemorrhage because of these drugs' potential to cause GI ulceration.

Warn patient not to take OTC preparations that contain aspirin or ibuprofen.

Other　Contraindicated in bleeding disorders (except disseminated intravascular coagulation) and in severe uncontrolled hypertension or thrombocytopenia.

Histamine H_2 Antagonists: cimetidine (Tagamet), famotidine (Pepcid), nizatidine (Axid), ranitidine (Zantac)

Common use　treatment and prevention of gastric or duodenal ulcer and hypersecretory states.

Mechanism of action　histamine H_2 receptor antagonist; inhibits gastric acid secretion.

Dosage　1. *cimetidine:* (oral) 300 mg 4 times a day with meals and at bedtime, 400 mg 2 times daily; 400–800 mg at bedtime. (IM, IV) 300 mg every 6–8 hours. 2. *famotidine:* (oral) 40 mg at bedtime, 20–40 mg 2 times a day; (IV) 20 mg every 12 hours. 3. *nizatidine:* (oral) 150–300 mg at bedtime, or 150 mg twice a day. 4. *ranitidine:* (oral) 150 mg 2 times daily; 150–300 mg at bedtime; (IM, IV) 50 mg every 6–8 hours.

Administration　oral, intramuscular, intravenous.

1. Cigarette smoking reduces drug effectiveness. 2. Give with or after meals and at bedtime. 3. For IV, piggyback administration is preferred; use 50–100 ml of dextrose or saline; infuse over 15–20 minutes. 4. When administering IV push, dilute in 20 ml and inject over a 2-minute period (5 minutes for ranitidine). 5. Do not use for minor digestive complaints.

Anticipated response　relief of pain, healing of ulcers, prevention of recurrence.

In most cases, limit dosage to period of 8 weeks (pathologic hypersecretory states may need indefinite course of therapy).

Side effects　1. *GI:* transient diarrhea. 2. *GU:* rare gynecomastia. 3. *Hematologic:* rare blood dyscrasias. 4. *CNS:* headache, dizziness, confusion. 5. *CV:* hypotension or cardiac rate or rhythm changes may occur after too-rapid IV injection.

1. Side effects tend to be more common with cimetidine than with the second-generation (other) agents. 2. Assess pain relief. 3. Older patients are more susceptible to CNS side effects, especially with IV doses.

Interactions　1. Cimetidine may potentiate oral anticoagulants. 2. Antacids may decrease cimetidine absorption. 3. Cimetidine may increase blood levels of diazepam, lidocaine, phenytoin, propranolol, theophylline, triamtpere, and tricyclic antidepressants, possibly resulting in toxicity. 4. Cimetidine may decrease the absorption of ferrous salts, ketoconazole, and tetracyclines.

1. Monitor patient for adjustment of anticoagulant drug dosage with cimetidine. 2. Separate from antacid dose by at least 1 hour. 3. Monitor interacting drugs closely for toxic effects, and adjust doses as needed.

Phenytoin (Dilantin)

Common use   management of grand mal and psychomotor seizures, and status epilepticus; treatment of dysrhythmias.

Mechanism of action   anticonvulsant, exact mechanism unknown; believed to alter the movement of sodium ions across cell membranes, thereby stabilizing neuronal membranes and inhibiting seizure activity.

Dosage   (oral) 100 mg 3 times a day, increased as needed to 600 mg daily; (IV) (in status epilepticus) 150–200 mg, followed by 100–150 mg after 30 minutes if needed; (as antidysrhythmic) 50–100 mg every 10–15 minutes as needed and tolerated to a maximum of 1 gram.

Administration   oral, intravenous.

1. IV phenytoin should be administered at a rate no greater than 50 mg/min (anticonvulsant) and 25 mg/min (antidysrhythmic). Clear tubing with normal saline before and after each dose. 2. IV phenytoin precipitates easily in solution. If intermittent infusion, rather than bolus injections, is necessary, use normal saline solution, mix immediately before infusing for a concentration of 10 mg/ml, infuse within 4 hours, and use an in-line filter. 3. Avoid extravasation of phenytoin, as it is very caustic to tissues; avoid IM administration due to pain and poor absorption. 4. When discontinuing an anticonvulsant, gradual dosage reduction is necessary. 6. Oral absorption differs greatly among different brands of phenytoin. The prescribing physician should be informed of any brand change.

Anticipated response   decreased frequency of seizures, control of status epilepticus, or decreased dysrhythmias.

Side effects   **1.** *GI:* constipation, nausea, gingival hyperplasia, rare toxic hepatitis. **2.** *CNS:* drowsiness, fatigue, insomnia, dizziness, headache, diplopia. **3.** *Hematologic:* rare agranulocytosis, thrombocytopenia. **4.** *Musculoskeletal:* muscle twitching, bone fractures, or slowed growth. **5.** *Dermatologic:* lymphadenopathy; rare: excessive growth of body and facial hair. **6.** *Toxicity:* continuous rolling or back-and-forth movements of eyes, blurred vision, confusion, behavioral changes, hallucinations, slurred speech, ataxia, increased frequency of convulsions.

1. Administer oral forms with food or milk to decrease GI side effects. 2. Until drug's sedative effects are known, instruct patient to be careful in tasks requiring alertness. 3. Teach proper mouth and dental care, including regular teeth cleaning by a professional.

Interactions   **1.** Phenytoin increases the rate of metabolism of many other drugs, including adrenocorticoids, oral contraceptives and other estrogens, cyclosporine, dicumarol, digitoxin, disopyramide, tetracyclines, haloperidol, methadone, dopamine, furosemide, sulfonylureas, quinidine, and levodopa, and may decrease the therapeutic effects of these drugs. **2.** Salicylates, allopurinol, chloramphenicol, cimetidine, diazepam, disulfiram, ethanol (acute), INH, miconazole, phenylbutazone, succinimides, sulfonamides, trimethoprim, ibuprofen, and imipramine may increase the effects of phenytoin, resulting in toxicity. **3.** Antacids, barbiturates, antineoplastics, carbamazepine, calcium salts, diazoxide, ethanol (chronic), folic acid, theophylline, nitrofurantoin, pyridoxine, and valproic acid may decrease the serum level and effect of phenytoin. **4.** Monitor closely for increased lithium toxicity. **5.** Barbiturates have variable effects on phenytoin metabolism. **6.** Phenytoin decreases analgesia of meperidine and increases toxicity; avoid use if possible. **7.** Phenytoin inhibits metabolism of primidone, possibly producing toxicity; monitor closely if used together. **8.** Adjust phenytoin dose when tricyclic antidepressants are used; seizures may be precipitated otherwise. **9.** Chronic alcohol use may decrease phenytoin effects, while high-dose acute use may increase serum phenytoin.

1. Separate the doses of antacids and phenytoin by at least 2 hours. 2. If administered with lithium, closely monitor for lithium toxicity. 3. Carefully monitor phenytoin blood levels when phenobarbital or another barbiturate is part of the regimen.

Other   **1.** Teach good oral hygiene (daily brushing, flossing, and gum massage; an electric toothbrush works well) to reduce gum problems. **2.** Hydantoins administered before delivery increase the risk of life-threatening hemorrhage in the neonate.

Isoetharine (Bronkosol, Bronkometer)

Common use   treatment of chronic bronchitis, asthma, and emphysema.

Mechanism of action   sympathomimetic bronchodilator; relaxes bronchial smooth muscle.

Dosage   **1.** mesylate: 1 inhalation, repeated after 1–2 minutes, every 4 hours. **2.** hydrochloride salt: *hand nebulizer*—3–7 inhalations of 1% solution every 4 hours; *IPPB or oxygen aerosolization*—0.5–4 ml of 0.125–0.25% solution every 4 hours.

Administration   inhalation.

1. Avoid contact with eyes. 2. Instruct patient to use inhaler correctly (Exhale; deeply inhale on mouthpiece while squeezing bulb of inhaler; hold breath for several seconds; exhale slowly into the air.) 3. When drug is administered with oxygen, adjust flow of oxygen to 4–6 L/min for 15–20 minutes. Do not administer if solution is discolored or contains a precipitate.

Anticipated response   relief of bronchospasm, increased vital capacity, and decreased airway resistance.

1. Observe patient's respirations for rate and depth. 2. Vital capacity monitoring may be ordered to confirm effectiveness of drug. **3.** *Continued use of isoetharine may decrease its effectiveness, necessitating a switch to another drug.*

Side effects **1.** *CNS:* insomnia, tremor, headache, anxiety, dizziness. **2.** *CV:* palpitation, tachycardia, chest pain. **3.** *GI:* nausea. **4.** *Other:* sulfite preservative used in some brands can cause allergic reactions and worsen bronchospasm.

Elderly patients are more sensitive than younger adults to sympathomimetic effects.

Interactions **1.** Beta-blocking drugs will antagonize bronchodilating effect of this drug. **2.** With other adrenergic drugs, increased adrenergic effects and possible increase in uncomfortable side effects and/or toxicity. **3.** Inhalation-aerosol forms of adrenocorticoids contain fluorocarbon propellants, as does isoetharine, and the use of both drugs close together can cause fluorocarbon toxicity. **4.** May antagonize antihypertensive medications. **5.** With digitalis, increased risk of dysrhythmias.

1. *Allow at least 15 minutes to elapse between isoetharine and adrenocorticoid aerosols.* **2.** *Monitor cardiac status when isoetharine is used in digitalized patient.*

Ketorolac (Toradol)

Common use relieve moderate to severe short-term pain
Mechanism of action decreases stimulation of pain receptors by prostaglandins.

Dosage loading dose: 30–60 mg, followed by half of loading dose (15–30 mg) every 6 hours. Maximum dose: 150 mg/first day, then 120 mg/day.
Administration intramuscular; intravenous not yet approved.

1. *Apply pressure over injection site for 15–30 seconds after injection.* **2.** *Drug may be safely used with opiate analgesics.*

Anticipated response relief of pain and/or reduced need for narcotic analgesics.

1. *Effects are prolonged in the elderly; use lower doses (30 mg loading, followed by 15 mg every 6 hours).*

Side effects **1.** *CNS:* drowsiness, dizziness, headache, sweating. **2.** *GI:* nausea, dyspepsia, GI pain, diarrhea (> 1%); (< 1%): constipation, flatulence, peptic ulcer, GI bleeding. **3.** *CV:* edema. **4.** *GU:* increased urinary frequency. **5.** *Hematologic:* prolonged bleeding time. **6.** *Other:* myalgia, injection site pain (2%).

1. *Use with caution in active or recurrent GI lesions or bleeding disorders.* **2.** *Monitor for GI bleeding closely in patients with previous history, long-term use (not recommended), and elderly patients.*

Interactions **1.** Small risk of bleeding complications with oral anticoagulants. **2.** Increased NSAID blood level. **3.** Increased GI side effects with aspirin.

Monitor for GI side effects if used with aspirin; monitor for bleeding with oral anticoagulants.

Other Monitor renal function in renal insufficiency (lower doses), elderly patients, and all long-term use. Also monitor CBC in long-term use.

Loop Diuretics: bumetanide (Bumex), ethacrynic acid (Edecrin), furosemide (Lasix)

Common use treatment of congestive heart failure, essential hypertension, and edema, including acute pulmonary edema.
Mechanism of action inhibits reabsorption of electrolytes (Na^+, Cl^-, and K^+) and thereby increases excretion of water in renal tubules.

Dosage **1.** *bumetanide:* (oral) 0.5–2 mg daily; (IV, IM) 0.5–1 mg, repeated every 2–3 hours as needed. **2.** *ethacrynic acid:* (oral) 50–200 mg daily; (IV) 50 mg, repeated in 2–6 hours as needed. **3.** *furosemide:* (oral) 20–80 mg daily; (IV) 20–40 mg, repeated or increased at 2-hour intervals as needed.
Administration oral, intravenous, intramuscular.

1. *When administering IV, dilute with 5% dextrose or sodium chloride, or give undiluted.* **2.** *If solution is hazy (due to diluents with a pH below 5), discard.* **3.** *Discard reconstituted drug after 24 hours.* **4.** *IV solution is physically incompatible with whole blood or whole-blood derivatives, as well as a number of acidic drugs; check compatibility.* **5.** *Do not add drug to IV solution; inject through Y-tube or 3-way stopcock.* **6.** *Avoid IM or SC administration, because these routes will cause local irritation.* **7.** *Give oral doses in the morning; if divided, do not give dose later than 4 P.M.; do not give with food.*

Anticipated response diuresis.

1. *Onset of action after IV administration is within minutes; after oral administration, 30–60 minutes. Keep bedpan or urinal available, or Foley tubing patent.* **2.** *Explain to patient importance of low-sodium diet.* **3.** *Check patient's weight; keep accurate intake and output records, and monitor electrolyte levels.* **4.** *These drugs generally are prescribed for people who don't respond to thiazides, or for rapid mobilization of extreme edema.*

Side effects **1.** *CNS:* tinnitus, deafness (associated with rapid IVP or renal impairment; may not be reversible), headache, confusion, drowsiness, muscle cramps, lethargy. **2.** *GI:* abdominal cramps, dry mouth, thirst, diarrhea, nausea. **3.** *CV:* orthostatic hypotension, dizziness, circulatory collapse. **4.** *Metabolic:* hypokalemia, hyponatremia, hyperglycemia, hyperuricemia, hypocalcemia.

1. *Encourage intake of foods and fluids high in potassium.* **2.** *Potassium salts or potassium-sparing diuretic may be prescribed in lieu of dietary potassium supplementation.* **3.** *Check patient for signs of electrolyte depletion.* **4.** *Elderly patients are more sensitive than younger adults to hypotensive and electrolyte effects, and at greater risk of circulatory collapse.* **5.** *Monitor the patient's hearing during therapy, using audiometric testing if necessary.*

Interactions **1.** When taken with other nephrotoxic or ototoxic drugs, increased potential for toxicity. **2.** May potentiate antihypertensives and muscle relaxants. **3.** May cause cardiac dysrhythmias with digitalis. **4.** With corticosteroids, increased potassium loss. **5.** With lithium, increased serum lithium levels. **6.** With alcohol, barbiturates, or narcotics, possible increased orthostatic hypotension. **7.** Antagonizes antigout drugs. **8.** May increase or decrease the effects of anticoagulants or thrombolytic agents. **9.** May antagonize hypoglycemic medications. **10.** For furosemide only (in addition to above): with neuromuscular blocking agents, enhanced neuromuscular blockade.

Other **1.** Contraindicated in cases of anuria or severe renal disease. **2.** Furosemide usually is the first choice over ethacrynic acid, because it is easier to give IV and because it has a lower risk of ototoxicity. **3.** Diuretics do not prevent toxemia of pregnancy, and there is no evidence that they are useful in the treatment of toxemia. Contraindicated during pregnancy. **4.** These drugs may exacerbate lupus erythematosus.

Mannitol (Osmitrol)

Common use treatment of acute renal failure and cerebral edema; reduction of intraocular and intracranial pressure; in overdose, promotion of urinary excretion of toxic substances and prevention of renal damage.
Mechanism of action osmotic diuretic; increases osmotic pressure of glomerular filtrate, thereby decreasing renal tubular reabsorption of water; elevates blood plasma osmolality.

Dosage usual dose is 50–200 g as a 5–25% solution; adjust rate of administration to maintain urine flow of at least 30–50 ml/hour.
Administration intravenous.

1. *Begin with a test dose if inadequate renal function is suspected.* **2.** *Dissolve all crystals by warming ampules in hot water; cool to body temperature before administering.* **3.** *Use IV filter when administering a 15% or greater solution of mannitol.*

Anticipated response diuresis; decreased intraocular and intracranial pressure.

1. *Monitor urine output and specific gravity hourly throughout course of therapy.* **2.** *Monitor electrolytes.*

Side effects **1.** *GI:* thirst, nausea, vomiting, dry mouth. **2.** *CNS:* headache, dizziness, blurred vision. **3.** *Metabolic:* fluid and electrolyte imbalance. **4.** *CV:* circulatory overload with congestive heart failure, pulmonary edema, tachycardia, hypotension.

1. *Observe patient for signs of electrolyte imbalance.* **2.** *Monitor intake and output.* **3.** *Weigh patient daily.* **4.** *Monitor vital signs frequently.* **5.** *Monitor renal function.*

Interactions **1.** Mannitol increases lithium excretion; monitor for decreased therapeutic response. **2.** Mannitol solution may cause pseudoagglutination of blood during transfusion.

If blood and mannitol must be administered together, add at least 20 mEq of sodium chloride to each liter of mannitol solution.

Other Do not use mannitol if acute tubular necrosis, severe pulmonary congestion, or intracranial bleeding are present.

Metaproterenol Sulfate (Alupent)

Common use symptomatic treatment of bronchial asthma, bronchitis, emphysema.
Mechanism of action sympathomimetic bronchodilator; enhances beta-adrenergic receptor activity, resulting in bronchodilation, decreased airway resistance, and relief of bronchospasm.

Dosage acute episodes: **1.** *(inhalation aerosol) 2–3 inhalations no more often than every 3–4 hours. (Do not exceed 12 inhalations in 24 hours.)* **2.** (inhalation, solution, via hand nebulizer) 5–15 inhalations no more often than every 4 hours. **3.** (inhalation, solution, via IPPB) 0.2–0.3 ml no more often than every 4 hours. **4.** (oral) 20 mg 3–4 times a day.
Administration oral, via inhalation.

1. *Teach patient how to administer inhalation dose. (Exhale through nose; shake container; deeply inhale on mouthpiece; hold breath for several seconds; exhale slowly. Repeat in 2 minutes.)* **2.** *Store drug in light-resistant container.*

Anticipated response increased vital capacity.

Observe patient carefully for response to drug. If no response is apparent, or if respiratory distress worsens, discontinue drug immediately and contact physician.

Side effects **1.** *CNS:* nervousness, restlessness, dizziness, weakness, headache, drowsiness. **2.** *CV:* tachycardia, hypertension, angina, dysrhythmia. **3.** *GI:* nausea, vomiting. **4.** *Other:* sulfite preservative used in some brands can cause allergic reactions and worsen bronchospasm.

1. *Explain the importance of not overusing this drug.* **2.** *Elderly patients are more sensitive than younger adults to sympathomimetic effects.*

Interactions **1.** With beta-blocker drugs, mutual antagonism of effects. **2.** With other sympathomimetic drugs, possible increased effects (or side effects) of metaproterenol. **3.** Inhalation aerosol forms of adrenocorticoids contain fluorocarbon propellants, as does metaproterenol, and the use of both drugs close together can cause fluorocarbon toxicity. **4.** May antagonize the effects of antihypertensive or antianginal drugs. **5.** With digitalis, may increase the risk of dysrhythmias.

1. *Allow at least 15 minutes to elapse between metaproterenol and adrenocorticoid aerosols.* **2.** *Monitor cardiac status when metaproterenol is used in digitalized patients.*

Other Use with caution in individuals with hypertension, coronary disease, diabetes, or thyroid disease.

Metaraminol (Aramine)

Common use prevention and treatment of acute hypotension resulting from hemorrhage, shock, surgery, drug reactions, etc.

Mechanism of action sympathomimetic vasopressor; stimulates alpha-adrenergic receptors, increasing systolic and diastolic blood pressures.

Dosage (IM, SC) 2–10 mg; (IV bolus) 0.5–5 mg, followed by IV infusion; (IV infusion) 15–100 mg in 500 ml sodium chloride or D_5W, adjusting rate to BP response.

Administration Intravenous, intramuscular, subcutaneous.

1. *IV route is preferred; use large veins.* **2.** *Administer IV infusion with an infusion-control device.* **3.** *Too-rapid administration may cause pulmonary edema, dysrhythmias, and cardiac arrest.* **4.** *Correct blood volume depletion immediately or concurrently.* **5.** *Discard solution after 24 hours.* **6.** *Physically incompatible with barbiturates, penicillins, and phenytoin—administer via separate IV line, or flush tubing carefully.*

Anticipated response increased blood pressure and improved circulation.

Withdraw drug gradually to avoid recurrent hypotension.

Side effects **1.** *CV:* dysrhythmias; sloughing of tissue at injection site (in extravasation); hypotension with prolonged

use. **2.** *Overdose:* convulsions, severe hypertension, severe dysrhythmias. **3.** *Other:* sulfite preservative used in some brands can cause allergic reactions.

1. *In case of extravasation, infiltrate site with phentolamine.* **2.** *IV phentolamine can be used to counteract excessive hypertension.*

Interactions **1.** Alpha-adrenergic blockers such as phentolamine and prazosin will decrease the pressor effect of metaraminol. **2.** With a hydrocarbon inhalation anesthetic such as cyclopropane or halothane, increased risk of severe ventricular dysrhythmias. **3.** With beta-blockers, possible mutual inhibition, or hypertension, bradycardia, and heart block. **4.** With oxytoxics, increased risk of persistent hypertension. **5.** With MAO inhibitors, possible hypertensive crisis and intracranial hemorrhage. **6.** With guanethidine, possible enhanced pressor effect and hypertension. **7.** With tricyclic antidepressants, possible need for higher dose of metaraminol.

1. *Decrease metaraminol dose in patients who are receiving hydrocarbon anesthetics, and closely monitor cardiac function.* **2.** *Do not use with MAO inhibitors.*

Morphine Sulfate

Common use treatment of moderate to severe pain; as preoperative medication; to reduce preload in acute pulmonary edema secondary to left ventricular failure.

Mechanism of action narcotic analgesic; exact mechanism of action is unknown; alters perception of and emotional response to pain by occupying endorphin receptor sites in CNS that alter the release of afferent neurotransmitters.

Dosage (oral) 10–30 mg every 3–4 hours. (oral, extended release) 30 mg every 12 hours. (IM, SC) 5–20 mg every 3–4 hours. (IV bolus) 2.5–15 mg, diluted in 4–5 ml of water for injection. (IV infusion) 1–10 mg/hour initially, titrated up to 20–150 mg/hour. (rectal) 10–20 mg every 3–4 hours.

Administration oral, subcutaneous, intramuscular, intravenous, rectal.

1. *For analgesic effect, administer before pain peaks; inform patient that he or she may request medication.* **2.** *In chronic pain, around-the-clock dosing is more effective than p.r.n. administration.* **3.** *This drug is a controlled substance, Schedule II.* **4.** *Rapid IV injection can cause anaphylaxis, circulatory collapse, or cardiac arrest. Inject IV morphine slowly over a period of several minutes.* **5.** *Administer extended-release tablets whole, never crushed.* **6.** *Dosages are highly individualized, depending on the severity of pain, patient response, and degree of tolerance. Dosages listed above are initial ranges only.* **7.** *Use infusion controllers for titrated infusions; also use patient-controlled analgesia (PCA) pumps.*

Anticipated response relief of pain; vasodilatation

1. Use nondrug measures to increase patient's comfort: proper positioning, environmental temperature, and so on. 2. Physical dependence will develop with regular use. Taper dosage when drug is discontinued, to avoid withdrawal symptoms.

Side effects 1. *CNS:* dizziness, euphoria, mood changes, dysphoria, depressed cough reflex, sedation. 2. *CV:* bradycardia, orthostatic hypotension. 3. *GI:* nausea, vomiting, dry mouth, constipation, biliary spasm. 4. *GU:* urinary retention, urgency, impotence. 5. *Respiratory:* decreased respiratory rate and depth. 6. *Other:* tolerance, visual disturbances, miosis.

1. Observe patient for onset of side effects; report respiratory rate of less than 12/minute before parenteral administration. 2. Keep narcotic antagonist and resuscitative equipment on hand when administering drug. 3. Warn patient not to undertake tasks requiring alertness until drug's sedative effect has been assessed. 4. Begin a bowel regimen (usually, a stimulant laxative) at the time of initiation of around-the-clock dosing. 5. Elderly patients may be more sensitive to respiratory depressant effects. 6. Tolerance develops much more rapidly with parenteral dosage forms than with other forms. 7. If hypotension, dizziness, or nausea make the patient particularly uncomfortable, keep the patient recumbent during periods of the drug's peak effect.

Interactions 1. With other CNS depressants, increased CNS depression. 2. Additive hypotension when used with other drugs that decrease blood pressure. 3. With anticholinergics or other constipating drugs, increased risk of severe constipation, impaction, or paralytic ileus.

Other Use with caution in head injury or increased intracranial pressure, COPD, arrhythmias, shock, liver or kidney disease, Addison's disease, prostatic hypertrophy, pregnancy, acute abdomen, drug abuse history or emotional instability, severe inflammatory bowel disease, or the elderly.

Naloxone (Narcan)

Common use antidote for narcotic-induced respiratory depression.

Mechanism of action narcotic antagonist; exact mechanism of action is unknown; believed to work by competitive inhibition of narcotics at tissue receptor sites.

Dosage 0.1–0.2 mg, repeated every 2–3 minutes as needed; may be repeated at 1–2 hour intervals. (continuous IV) 0.4 mg/hr initially, titrated to patient response.

Administration intravenous, subcutaneous, intramuscular.

1. IV route is preferred for better dose titration. Initial IV bolus may be followed by repeat boluses, IV infusion, or IM injection.

2. Because narcotic duration of action may exceed that of naloxone, respiratory depression may recur; observe respiratory pattern before and after administration.

Anticipated response reversal of narcotic effects.

1. Will precipitate withdrawal symptoms in narcotic-dependent patients. 2. Prepare for agitation and combativeness as naloxone takes effect. 3. Naloxone will reverse analgesia as well as respiratory effects; if applicable, reinstitute pain control as soon as possible. 4. Use other resuscitative measures as needed.

Side effects 1. *GI:* nausea and vomiting (rare). 2. *CV:* tachycardia, hypertension. 3. *CNS:* nervousness, restlessness. *Nausea and vomiting only with high doses.*

Nitrates: erythrityl tetranitrate (Cardilate); isosorbide dinitrate (Isordil, Sorbitrate); nitroglycerin—oral (Nitro-Bid, Nitrospan), parenteral (Nitrostat IV, Tridil), transmucosal (Nitrogard), sublingual (Nitrostat), transdermal (Nitro-Bid, Nitrodisc, Nitro-Dur, Transderm-Nitro); pentaerythritol tetranitrate (Peritrate)

Common use treatment and prevention of angina pectoris.

Mechanism of action generalized peripheral vasodilatation results in decreased peripheral resistance and increased venous pooling, thus decreasing cardiac workload.

Dosage 1. *erythrityl tetranitrate:* (oral, sublingual) 5–10 mg 3–4 times a day. 2. *isosorbide dinitrate:* (oral) 5–10 mg every 6 hours; (chewable form) 5 mg every 2–3 hours; (extended-release) 40 mg every 8–12 hours; (sublingual or buccal) 2.5–5 mg every 2–3 hours. 3. *nitroglycerin:* (oral extended-release) 2.5–9 mg every 8–12 hours; (transmucosal extended-release) 1 mg every 3–5 hours; (sublingual) 150–600 mcg, repeated at 5-minute intervals as needed for angina relief; (ointment) 15–30 mg (2.5–5 cm) every 8 hours; (transdermal system) 1 dosage system every 24 hours; (intravenous) initially 5 mcg/min, increased at 3–5-minute intervals until desired effect is achieved or rate reaches 20 mcg/min. 4. *pentaerythritol tetranitrate:* (oral) 10–20 mg 4 times a day; (oral extended-release) 30–80 mg 2 times a day.

Administration oral, sublingual, transmucosal, transdermal, intravenous, topical.

1. Ointment: spread evenly over area skin at least 2 by 3 inches (6 by 6 inches recommended). Do not use fingers to apply ointment. Do not rub in ointment. Cover ointment with plastic wrap, taped or secured. If patient is able, teach patient to measure dosage and have patient do all measuring to ensure greater consistency in dosage. **2.** *Transdermal ointment or patches are best applied to skin that is not hairy and that is free of scars or lesions. Avoid the distal extremities and thick adipose tissue.* **3.** *Transdermal patches should never be trimmed in an attempt to modify dosage.* **4.** *Although newer forms of sublingual nitroglycerin have improved stability, the sublingual form generally should be replaced every 6 months to ensure continued effectiveness.* **5.** *Many people cannot digest extended-release dosage forms. A partially dissolved tablet or capsule may be found in the patient's stool. The patient's response to nitrate therapy should be determined through the use of regular dosage forms before an extended-release form is tried.* **6.** *Give oral forms on empty stomach, 1 hour before (preferred) or 2 hours after meals.* **7.** *IV nitroglycerin should be administered with an infusion monitoring device.* **8.** *Standard IV infusion sets are made of polyvinyl chloride (PVC) plastic and unpredictably absorb up to 80% of nitroglycerin from solution. Use glass bottles and non-PVC plastic for tubing and connections. Be aware that non-PVC plastic may be incompatible with consistent operation of the infusion monitoring device.* **9.** *Do not use filters.*

Anticipated response   decreased frequency (or, with nitroglycerin sublingual, prompt relief) of anginal pain.

1. *Long-acting forms will not provide relief during acute attack.* **2.** *Tolerance may develop with prolonged use. Discontinuing nitrate therapy briefly and then restarting may restore its effectiveness.*

Side effects   **1.** *CV:* orthostatic hypotension, headache, flushing, tachycardia, dizziness. **2.** *GI:* nausea. **3.** *Dermatologic:* skin irritation.

1. *Treat occasional headache with acetaminophen.* **2.** *Frequent headaches warrant decrease in level or frequency of dose, or change to nonnitrate antianginal medication.* **3.** *Advise patient to rise slowly to avoid orthostatic hypotension.* **4.** *Rotate transdermal sites to avoid skin irritation.* **5.** *Nurses or others administering topical nitroglycerin should avoid contact with the ointment or patch surface, and wash hands thoroughly after preparing the dose, to avoid transdermal absorption of the drug.* **6.** *During IV administration, monitor BP and HR constantly. Also monitor PCWP, if possible. A drop in PCWP precedes arterial hypotension; if PCWP falls, reduce or discontinue drug temporarily. Reduce dose gradually to prevent rebound symptoms or sudden changes in pressures.*

Interactions   **1.** With alcohol and other drugs that lower blood pressure, possible aggravated hypotension. **2.** Aspirin increases serum nitrate concentrations; use acetaminophen.

Other   **1.** Use cautiously with hepatic or renal disease and glaucoma. **2.** Use cautiously with recent MI; hypotension and tachycardia may aggravate ischemia.

Norepinephrine (Levophed)

Common use   treatment of severe hypotension, as in shock, cardiac arrest, and drug reactions.
Mechanism of action   Stimulates alpha- and beta$_1$ adrenergic receptors; vasoconstrictor, raises blood pressure, improves myocardial contractility and rate.

Dosage   adults: initially, 8–12 mcg/min; then adjust flow rate to maintain low-normal blood pressure; maintenance dose is usually about 2–4 mcg/min.
Administration   intravenous infusion.

1. *If possible, give into a large vein to avoid accidental extravasation.* **2.** *Mix with IV fluids that contain dextrose—for example, D_5W or D_5NS. (Dextrose protects against loss of the drug's potency in solution.)* **3.** *Individual response to this drug varies greatly, so titrate infusion rate to BP. Maintain systolic blood pressure (SBP) at 80–100 mm Hg (or 30–40 mm Hg below norm if previously hypertensive). Check peripheral pulses and urinary output at least hourly.* **4.** *Reduce infusion gradually when discontinuing drug.*

Anticipated response   increase in blood pressure; improved tissue perfusion.

1. *Blood flow to all areas except heart and brain may be reduced. Renal vasoconstriction occurs. Monitor accordingly.* **2.** *Treat underlying cause of shock as soon as possible.*

Side effects   **1.** *CV:* hypertension, angina, bradycardia, other dysrhythmias. **2.** *CNS:* headache, dizziness, restlessness. **3.** *Dermatologic:* skin necrosis (from severe vasoconstriction) if drug extravasates. **4.** *Other:* sulfite preservative used in preparing norepinephrine injection can cause allergic reactions.

1. *Monitor blood pressure, pulse, and ECG continuously during therapy.* **2.** *Monitor intake and output.* **3.** *In case of extravasation, inject solution of saline and phentolamine locally to try to prevent skin necrosis and sloughing.*

Interactions   **1.** *Hydrocarbon anesthetics such as halothane and cyclopropane sensitize the heart to the action of norepinephrine and may result in severe ventricular dysrhythmias.* **2.** With beta-blocker drugs, mutual inhibition, or hypertension, excessive bradycardia, and possible heart block. **3.** Alpha-adrenergic blockers eliminate pressor effects of norepinephrine; 5–10 mg of phentolamine may be added to each liter of norepinephrine infusion to prevent tissue sloughing without pressor loss. **4.** With oxytocin or tricyclic antidepressants, methyldopa, and possibly MAO inhibitors, possible prolonged and severe hypertension.

Avoid use with interacting drugs. If norepinephrine is essential in these patients, begin with a reduced dosage.

Other   Norepinephrine crosses the placenta and can cause fetal hypoxia.

Pancuronium Bromide (Pavulon)

Common use to facilitate mechanical ventilation; to aid in intubation; as adjunct to anesthesia.

Mechanism of action neuromuscular blocking agent; blocks nerve impulse transmission at myoneural junction, resulting in skeletal muscle paralysis.

Dosage 0.04–0.1 mg/kg; then increments of 0.01 mg/kg.
Administration intravenous.

1. Do not administer unless under direct supervision of physician experienced in the use of this drug. 2. Do not store in plastic containers. 3. Store in refrigerator. 4. Ventilatory assistance must be available. 5. Patient needs to be sedated during administration.

Anticipated response rapidly induced skeletal-muscle paralysis.

1. Monitor vital signs closely. 2. Anticholinesterase agents usually are used for reversal of paralysis. Observe patient closely after administration of antagonist for possible return of muscle relaxation.

Side effects 1. *CV:* tachycardia. 2. *Dermatologic:* transient rash. 3. *GI:* salivation. 4. *Neurologic:* prolonged neuromuscular blockade. 5. *Respiratory:* depression, apnea. 6. *Overdose:* deep respiratory depression, cardiovascular collapse.

Interactions 1. Possible intensified neuromuscular blockade when given with beta-blockers, procainamide, quinidine, aminoglycoside or polymixin antibiotics, inhalation anesthetics, high-dose lidocaine, phenothiazines, oral contraceptives, parenteral magnesium sulfate, or massive blood transfusions. 2. Additive respiratory depression with opiates or other drugs that depress respiration. 3. Diazepam reduces duration of neuromuscular blockade. 4. Possible increased cardiac dysrhythmias or cardiac arrest with digitalis and quinidine. 5. Hypokalemia may potentiate pancuronium effects.

1. When drugs that may enhance neuromuscular blockade are given concurrently or sequentially, the primary risk is incomplete reversal of neuromuscular blockade postoperatively. Monitor patient carefully. 2. Check serum potassium prior to administration. Use caution if potassium-depleting drugs, such as thiazide diuretics, loop diuretics, or corticosteroids, are administered.

Other Hyperthermia may intensify and prolong pancuronium's effect.

Procainamide (Pronestyl)

Common use treatment of premature ventricular contractions, ventricular tachycardia, paroxysmal atrial tachycardia, and atrial fibrillation.

Mechanism of action antidysrhythmic; depresses automaticity of heart muscle fibers; slows rate of atrioventricular conduction; increases refractory period.

Dosage 1. *(oral) Atrial: Loading dose: 1.25 g followed by 750 mg in 1 hour if no ECG change occurs; then 0.5–1 g every 2 hours until normal sinus rhythm is restored or toxic effects appear. Maintenance: either 0.5–1 g every 6 hours, or 50 mg/kg SR divided. (Sustained release [SR]) every 6–8 hours. Ventricular: loading: 1 g followed by 6 mg/kg every 3 hours; same for maintenance.* 2. *(IM)* 500–1,000 mg every 4–8 hours. 3. *(IV)* 100–500 mg, diluted and infused at 20–50 mg/min, then 1–6 mg/min as maintenance.
Administration oral, intramuscular, intravenous.

1. Patient should be placed on cardiac monitor during parenteral therapy. 2. Observe for indications of heart block or prolonged Q-T interval. 3. Constantly observe patient receiving drug as IV drip; discontinue IV when dysrhythmia is terminated, BP falls more than 15 mm Hg, or the ECG shows greater than 50% widening of QRS or PR prolongation. 4. Patient should be in supine position when drug is administered IV. 5. IV rate should not exceed 25 mg/min (some sources say 50 mg/min with great caution).

Anticipated response control of irregular cardiac activity.

Instruct patient to take this drug exactly as prescribed.

Side effects 1. *CNS:* confusion, depression, hallucinations, dizziness. 2. *CV:* hypotension (especially with IV form). 3. *GI:* nausea, vomiting, anorexia, diarrhea. 4. *Musculoskeletal:* systemic lupus erythematosis (SLE). 5. *Hematologic:* agranulocytosis, leukopenia, thrombocytopenia.

1. Elderly patients are more sensitive to the drug's hypotensive effects. 2. Patients on long-term therapy should have antinuclear antibody (ANA) titers measured at regular intervals or when SLE symptoms appear. Discontinue drug for rising titers or clinical signs of lupus. 3. Routinely monitor CBCs and cardiac function during long-term therapy. 4. Give tablets on empty stomach; if they cause gastric distress, they can be given with food. Administration in relation with food should be consistent.

Interactions 1. With other antidysrhythmics, possible additive or antagonistic effects. 2. With antihypertensives, additive hypotension. 3. Procainamide may inhibit the effects of antimyasthenic drugs on skeletal muscle. 4. May enhance the effects of neuromuscular blocking drugs. 5. With anticholinergics, additive effect. 6. Cimetidine and ranitidine increase serum levels of procainamide (NAPA, N–acetyl procainamide) with potential toxicity, especially in elderly; monitor closely and adjust dosage.

Other Use with caution in patients with congestive heart failure, renal disease, hepatic dysfunction, MI, hypotension, or SLE.

Quinidine: quinidine gluconate (Quinaglute), quinidine polygalacturonate (Cardioquin), quinidine sulfate (Cin-Quin)

Common use treatment of atrial dysrhythmias or premature ventricular contractions.
Mechanism of action antidysrhythmic agent; increases cardiac refractory period; slows A-V conduction; depresses automaticity.

Dosage **1.** *sulfate:* (oral) 200–600 mg every 2–3 hours initially, followed by 200–300 mg 3–4 times a day. **2.** *gluconate:* (IV) 16 mg/min. (1 ml/min. of 16 mg/ml dilution [800 mg in 40 ml D5W]) until arrhythmia terminated or adverse effects (see below); usually 300 mg; max. 750 mg. (IM) initially 600 mg, then 400 mg up to 12 times a day. (oral) 300–600 mg every 8–12 hours (SR). **3.** *polygalacturonate:* (oral) 275–825 mg every 3–4 hours initially, then gradually increase dose as needed.
Administration oral, intravenous, intramuscular.

1. Do not use discolored solutions. 2. Check apical rate and blood pressure before administration. 3. Utilize continuous ECG and BP monitoring during IV administration; discontinue IV and report immediately the following effects: QRS widening greater than 25% from baseline, disappearance of P waves, restoration of sinus rhythm, fall in HR to less than 120 beats per minute, or sudden onset or increase in ventricular ectopy. 4. IM administration not recommended due to muscle damage.

Anticipated response control of dysrhythmia.

Monitor ECG when initiating therapy.

Side effects **1.** *Hematologic:* blood dyscrasias. **2.** *CNS:* restlessness, vertigo, confusion. **3.** *CV:* hypotension, tachycardia, pallor. **4.** *GI:* nausea, vomiting, diarrhea, hypersalivation. **5.** *Other:* signs of toxicity include nausea, vomiting, tinnitus, dizziness, headache, fever, tremor, visual changes, widening QRS interval, ventricular ectopic beats, AV block.

1. Administer drug with food, to lessen GI irritation. 2. Notify physician if you suspect toxicity. Check blood levels of quinidine (normal levels are 2–6 mcg/ml).

Interactions **1.** With anticoagulants, possible increased anticoagulant effect. **2.** With digitalis, possible increased serum digitalis, resulting in toxicity. **3.** With urinary alkalizers such as sodium bicarbonate, other antacids, carbonic anhydrase inhibitors, thiazide diuretics, or large amounts of citrus fruit juices, increased serum quinidine and possible toxicity. **4.** With other antidysrhythmics, additive cardiac effects and possible hypotension. **5.** Quinidine antagonizes cholinergics; use with great caution, if at all. **6.** Cimetidine prolongs quinidine half-life. **7.** Quinidine may potentiate the effects of neuromuscular blocking agents. **8.** Potassium-containing medications may enhance quinidine effects, while hypokalemia tends to decrease quinidine effect. **9.** Phenytoin, rifampin, and phenobarbital decrease serum quinidine levels.

1. Use caution when giving quinidine with anticoagulants. 2. Monitor patient closely if quinidine must be given with cardiac glycosides; decrease digoxin dose as needed. 3. Adjust drug doses as needed when quinidine is given with other interacting drugs.

Other Do not give quinidine for digitalis-induced dysrhythmias; ectopic rhythms due to escape mechanisms; second- or third-degree heart block in the absence of a ventricular pacemaker, or intraventricular conduction defects.

Sodium Polystyrene Sulfonate (Kayexalate)

Common use treatment of hyperkalemia.
Mechanism of action antihyperkalemic; sodium in the resin is partially replaced by potassium and excreted.

Dosage **1.** (oral) 15 g up to 4 times daily diluted in water or sorbitol. **2.** (rectal) 25–100 g as needed.
Administration oral, rectal.

1. Chill solution for oral administration. 2. For rectal administration, prepare medication at room temperature. 3. Administer cleansing enema before and after Kayexalate enema; explain procedure to patient, and advise that minimum retention time is 30–60 minutes. Post-Kayexalate enema should be non-sodium and be administered via Y-tubing for continuous drainage. 4. A mild laxative given concurrently will help prevent constipation. Sorbitol acts as laxative and improves palatability when mixed with drug.

Anticipated response reduction of excessively high serum potassium level when resin is eliminated through bowel movement.

1. Not useful in emergency treatment because of slow action. 2. Monitor patient for signs and symptoms of electrolyte depletion. 3. Monitor serum potassium levels daily, and run periodic ECGs.

Side effects **1.** *GI:* anorexia, nausea, vomiting, constipation, fecal impaction. **2.** *Metabolic:* hypokalemia, sodium retention, and other electrolyte disturbances. **3.** *CNS:* confusion, irritability.

Sorbitol may be given with both forms to combat constipation.

Interactions **1.** With antacids and laxatives, possible reduction in sodium/potassium exchange and possible systemic alkalosis. **2.** Other drugs that affect potassium levels, such as intravenous sodium bicarbonate and insulin, should be used with caution.

Do not use this drug with antacids or laxatives that contain calcium or magnesium.

Terbutaline (Brethine, Bricanyl)

Common use management of bronchial asthma, bronchitis, emphysema.
Mechanism of action stimulates beta-adrenergic receptors, relaxes bronchial smooth muscle.

Dosage (oral) 2.5–5 mg 3 times a day, with a maximum of 15 mg daily; (SC) 0.25 mg repeated once after 15–30 minutes if necessary; (inhalation) 2 inhalations 60 seconds apart every 4–6 hours.
Administration oral, subcutaneous, inhalation.

1. *Space 3 daily doses 6 hours apart.* **2.** *Administer subcutaneously in deltoid region.* **3.** *Check heart rate and blood pressure before parenteral dose.*

Anticipated response decreased airway resistance; relief of bronchospasm.

Side effects **1.** *CNS:* tremors, dizziness, nervousness, drowsiness, anxiety, headache. **2.** *CV:* tachycardia, palpitations. **3.** *GI:* nausea, vomiting.

1. *Careful observation is essential when administered to patients with elevated blood pressure, dysrhythmias, or hyperthyroidism.* **2.** *Elderly patients are more sensitive than younger adults to sympathomimetic effects.*

Interactions **1.** Beta-blockers may antagonize this drug's bronchodilatory effect. **2.** With other sympathomimetic drugs, potentiation of effects and increased side effects. **3.** Inhalation aerosol forms of adrenocorticoids and terbutaline contain fluorocarbon propellants; concurrent use can lead to fluorocarbon toxicity. **4.** With hydrocarbon inhalation anesthetics such as halothane or cyclopropane, increased risk of severe ventricular dysrhythmias. **5.** Tricyclic antidepressants and MAO inhibitors potentiate terbutaline.

1. *Separate corticosteroid and terbutaline aerosols by at least 15 minutes.* **2.** *Monitor cardiac function as needed when terbutaline is given with interacting drugs.*

Other Use with caution in patients with a history of dysrhythmias, high blood pressure, convulsions, diabetes, or hyperthyroidism.

Thrombolytic Agents: streptokinase (Streptase), urokinase (Abbokinase), alteplase (Activase), anistreplase (Eminase)

Common use dissolution of coronary artery thrombi, acute pulmonary emboli, and deep venous thromboses, and clearance of intravenous catheter obstruction.
Mechanism of action activate plasmin, which in turn breaks down fibrin clots.

Dosage **1.** *streptokinase:* (coronary artery thrombi) intracoronary infusion of 20,000 IU bolus followed by infusion of 2,000 IU/min for 1 hour; (other) IV loading dose of 250,000 IU over 30 minutes, then maintenance dose of 100,000 IU/hour for up to 24–72 hours. (catheter obstruction) 100,000–250,000 IV, administered slowly. **2.** *urokinase:* (coronary artery thrombi) 6,000 IU/min, up to a usual total dose of 500,000 IU; (other) 4,400 IU/kg over 10 minutes, then 4,400 IU/kg/hour; (catheter obstruction) fill catheter with a solution of 5,000 IU/ml urokinase. **3.** *alteplase:* various protocols exist for cardiac use: for example, (1) 100 mg divided over 3 hours; 60% of dose in 1st hour, then 20%/hr over next 2 hours; (2) 60 mg over 1st hour (of which 6–10 mg is given as bolus over first 2 minutes), followed by 20 mg/hour in second and third hours. Maximum dose: less than 150 mg total. ([3] if patient weighs less than 65 kg): 1.25 mg/kg over 3 hours, (as above); (pulmonary embolism): 100 mg over 2 hours. **4.** *anistreplase:* (coronary) 30 units IVP over 2–5 minutes.
Administration intravenous.

1. *For best results after coronary artery thrombus, thrombolytics should be administered within 6 hours of myocardial infarct.* **2.** *These drugs are not used for superficial thrombophlebitis.* **3.** *Reconstitute immediately before use. Do not shake.* **4.** *Streptokinase: Reconstitute each vial in 5 ml NS; further dilute in 50 ml NS (1.5 million U in 100 ml)—up to 500 ml for continuous infusion (dilute in 45-ml increments).* **5.** *Urokinase: Reconstitute 250,000 U in 5.2 ml sterile water for injection without shaking (5,000 U in 1 ml for IV catheters). May be further diluted in up to 195 ml NS or D_5W.* **6.** *Alteplase: Using 18-gauge needle, reconstitute with sterile water (without preservatives, correct volume supplied with medication to provide concentration of 1 mg/ml. May be given IVP, or (preferred) diluted in saline or D_5W to 0.5 mg/ml for infusion. After total dose, flush line with 30 ml NS or D_5W over 30 minutes. Do not mix with any other drug. Discard after 8 hours.* **7.** *Anistreplase: Reconstitute with 5 ml sterile water for injection: give IVP over 4–5 minutes. Discard within 30 minutes of dilution.*

Anticipated response   dissolution of thrombi and emboli, with improved circulation to previously occluded vascular beds.

1. Monitor coagulation panels. 2. Action is almost immediate and persists up to 12 hours after infusion is discontinued. 3. The patient usually is kept on bedrest during therapy.

Side effects   1. *Hematologic:* bleeding. **2.** *Metabolic:* fever. **3.** *Other (except alteplase):* allergic reactions, including anaphylaxis, in sensitive patients; streptokinase is antigenic and induces antibody formation, and resistance to subsequent streptokinase therapy may persist for 3–6 months.

1. Keep antifibrinolysin aminocaproic acid (Amicar) on hand to reverse severe bleeding (with Streptokinase). 2. Blood should be available for transfusion in case of severe bleeding. 3. Check for blood in urine and stools, as well as at any traumatized areas, including IV sites. 4. The risk of hemorrhage is greater with these drugs than with heparin or the oral anticoagulants. 5. Elderly patients may have an increased risk of cerebral hemorrhage when these drugs are administered. 6. Monitor for allergic reaction (except for alteplase): rash, itching, flushing, nausea, musculoskeletal pain, difficulty breathing; and monitor vital signs including temperature (do not use aspirin for elevations). 7. Keep epinephrine 1:1000 units on hand in case of anaphylaxis. 8. For cardiac use, monitor for dysrhythmias (sign of reperfusion or ventricular ischemia), and decreased chest pain and ST segment normalization (signs of reperfusion).

Interactions   1. With other anticoagulants, possible uncontrolled, excessive bleeding. **2.** With other drugs that alter platelet function (aspirin, indomethacin, and so on), increased risk of bleeding.

1. Do not give with other anticoagulants. 2. Do not give with other drugs that alter platelet function (including OTC drugs containing aspirin).

Other   Absolute contraindications include active internal bleeding, known allergy, intracranial neoplasm, recent CVA, or trauma. Relative contraindications include major surgery within 10 days, recent GI bleed, uncontrolled hypertension, any condition with bleeding potential that would be difficult to manage, or pregnancy.

Warfarin (Coumadin, Panwarfin)

Common use   treatment of pulmonary emboli; prevention or treatment of venous thrombosis and atrial fibrillation with embolization.
Mechanism of action   interferes with activity of vitamin K, which in turn interferes with the formation of active procoagulation factors.

Dosage   2–10 mg daily (maintenance dose).

Administration   oral.

1. Prothrombin times are done daily at the start of therapy and then weekly; prothrombin times should not exceed 2½ times normal. (Best to maintain patient at 1½–2 times normal.) 2. Administer drug at same time daily. 3. Elderly and debilitated patients are extrasensitive to this drug's effects.

Anticipated response   decreased blood clotting, as evidenced by laboratory tests; prevention of thrombus formation and/or uneventful resolution of existing clots.

1. Inform patient of importance of complying with medication regimen and laboratory tests. 2. Onset of action may take up to 3 days.

Side effects   1. *GI:* cramps, nausea, vomiting, diarrhea. **2.** *Hematologic:* hemorrhage, leukopenia. **3.** *Other:* unusual hair loss.

1. Watch for signs of bleeding. 2. Instruct patient to shave with electric razor. 3. Instruct patient to carry card identifying ongoing anticoagulant therapy. 4. Avoid IM injections and repeated blood drawing. 5. Anticoagulant effect may increase during prolonged fever or diarrhea. Monitor patient closely for altered response to anticoagulants.

Interactions   Because warfarin is highly but weakly protein bound, there is potential for numerous drug interactions. In addition, any drugs that can affect platelets or vitamin K or that are ulcerogenic contribute to risk of bleeding. Therefore, prothrombin time should *always* be checked when anything is added to or subtracted from the regimen of the patient on warfarin.

Encourage patient to avoid self-medication and alcohol.

Other   1. Contraindicated during pregnancy; congenital malformations have been documented. **2.** Warfarin therapy is contraindicated when any of the following conditions exist: cerebral or aortic aneurysm, suspected cerebrovascular hemorrhage, any active bleeding, recent neurosurgery or ophthalmic surgery, known blood dyscrasias, uncontrolled hypertension. **3.** Use with caution in renal or hepatic function impairment, visceral carcinomas, severe diabetes, recent childbirth, or vitamin C or K deficiencies.

REFERENCES

Benson D, with Conte R: *Nursing Meds—91–92,* 2d ed. Norwalk, CT: Appleton & Lange, 1991.

Conte J, Barriere S: *Manual of antibiotics and infectious diseases,* 6th ed. Philadelphia: Lea & Febiger, 1986.

Drugdex, (Vol. 62–63), Micromedex, 1989–1990.

Gahart B: *Intravenous medications: A handbook for nurses and other allied health personnel,* 7th ed. St. Louis: Mosby, 1991.

Govoni L, Hayes J: *Drugs and nursing implications,* 6th ed. Norwalk, CT: Appleton & Lange, 1988.

Fraulini K: *After anesthesia: A guide for PACU, ICU, and medical-surgical nurses.* Norwalk, CT: Appleton & Lange, 1987.

Knoben J, Anderson P (eds): *Handbook of clinical drug data,* 6th ed. Hamilton, IL: Drug Intelligence Publications, 1988.

Koda-Kimble M, Katcher B, Young L: *Applied therapeutics for clinical pharmacists,* 3d ed. San Francisco: Applied Therapeutics, 1986.

McEvoy G et al. (eds): *Drug information 1991.* Bethesda: American Hospital Formulary Service, 1991.

Olin B et al. (eds): *Drug facts and comparisons.* St. Louis: Lippincott, 1991.

Rayburn W, Zuspan F. (eds): *Drug therapy in obstetrics and gynecology.* Norwalk, CT: Appleton & Lange, 1988.

Sanford J: *Guide to anti-microbial therapy.* Bethesda: Antimicrobial Therapy, Inc., 1989.

Trissel L: *Handbook on injectable drugs.* Bethesda: American Hospital Formulary Service, 1991; & Supplement.

Wicklund S, Devroye M (eds): *Nurses' drug alert.* Milburn, NJ: M.J. Powers, 1989–91.

Index

plantation, 571
Liver lobule, 549f, 549
Living wills, 43
Lobectomy, 237
LOC (level of consciousness)
    as acid-base imbalance sign or symptom,
        477–478
    in diabetes insipidus planning and car-
        ing, 506
    in diabetic ketoacidosis planning and
        caring, 492
    in intracranial surgery planning and car-
        ing, 134
    multiple organ systems failure hemato-
        logic effects and, 608
    in neuro-checks, 68–69, 71t, 135
    terms describing, 71t
Lomotil, 527
Loop of Henle, 413
Lorazepam, 108
Lower GI hemorrhage, 540–541
Lower motor neurons, 81
LPH (left posterior hemiblock), 313
LP (lumbar puncture), 82–83, 114
Lumbar puncture, 82–83, 114
Lund and Browder chart, 644, 646f
Lung markings, 174
Lungs. See also Pulmonary assessment; spe-
        cific pulmonary disorders
    acid-base imbalances and, 477
    anatomy of, 150–152, 152f, 153f, 154f
    biopsy, 178
    capacities of, 162f, 163
    collapse of, 175–176
    expansion of, 212
    multiple organ systems failure pulmo-
        nary effects and, 600
    scans, 176–177
    volumes of, 161f, 161
LVEDP (left ventricular end-diastolic pres-
        sure), 276–277
Lymphocytes, 511, 514f, 514–515, 519
Lymphokines, 512

Macrophages, 511f, 512, 513t, 523
Magnesium, 472
Magnesium imbalances, 472–473, 473t
Magnetic resonance imaging. See MRI
Major burns, 644
Major histocompatibility complex (MHC),
        515
Major trauma, 613
Mallory-Weiss syndrome, 540
Malnutrition. See also Nutrition
    immune system and, 518
    infection and, 574
    injury and, 574
    nursing diagnosis for, 574
    planning and caring for
        enteral feeding, 575t, 575–577
        nutritional supplementation, 574–575
        total parenteral nutrition, 577–578,
            579t, 580–584
    starvation physiology and, 573–574
Malpractice, 45

Mannitol, 99, 132, 398, 595
MAP (mean arterial pressure)
    autoregulation and, 92
    coronary perfusion pressure and, 91–92
    description of, 249
    elevation of, 144
    increased intracranial pressure and, 144
    regulation of, 252
    systematic vascular resistance and, 250,
        275
    vasodilators and, 143
Mask CPAP, 227
Mast cells, 511f, 511–512
MAST (military anti-shock trouser),
        621–622
Maximum inspiratory force (MIF), 163, 223
MDF (myocardial depressant factor), 589,
        599
Mean arterial pressure. See MAP
Mechanical valves, 396t, 396
Mechanical ventilation
    in acute asthma planning and caring,
        200
    complications, 227–230
    discontinuation of, 230–232
    evaluation of, 233
    expiratory maneuvers and, 226–227
    hemodynamic pressure in, 227, 228f
    procedure for, 223
    use of, 223
    ventilating modes in, 223–226, 226f
    ventilators for, 223, 225f
    weaning from, 232t, 233
Mechanism of injury
    in abdominal trauma, 638–639
    in chest trauma, 634–635
    definition of, 616
    in head injury, 626
    in spinal cord injury, 631
Mediastinal shift, 193
Medical diagnosis, 9–10
Medically questionable order, 46
Medulla, 62, 410, 413f
Medulla oblongata, 54f, 56
Melanin, 643
Melena, 541
Memory, 53, 56, 76, 626
Meningeal arteries, 59
Meninges, 57–58, 58f
Mental status examination, 77
Mentation, 76–78, 78t, 79t
Mentoring, 22–23
Metabolic acid, 474
Metabolic acidosis, 475t, 475, 482, 583
Metabolic alkalosis, 476t, 476, 482
Metabolic disorders, 484–485. See also spe-
        cific types
Metabolism
    calcium, 417
    definition of, 485
    multiple organ systems failure and,
        600–601
    on electrocardiogram, 305
    phosphorus, 417
Methimazole, 499

Methylprednisolone, 99, 451
MHC (major histocompatibility complex),
        515
MI (acute myocardial infarction)
    assessment of, 340–342, f342
    bedmaking and, 356
    diagnostic procedures for, 341–348, 356
    electrocardiogram and, 344f, 344–346,
        345f, 346f
    end-stage renal disease and, 433
    evaluation of, 356–357
    gerontology and, 340
    location and evolution of, 346–348
    nursing care plan for, 347–355
    nursing diagnosis for, 357
    planning and caring for, 356
    radionuclide studies in, 348, 356
    risk conditions for, 340
    serum enzymes and, 348
    signs and symptoms of, 340–341
Midazolam, 381
Midbrain, 54f, 56
Middle cerebral artery, 58–59, 60f
Middle fossa, 57f, 57
Midposition fixed pupils, 71, 72f
MIF (maximum inspiratory force), 163, 223
Military anti-shock trouser (MAST),
        621–622
Mineral abnormalities, 583
Minor burns, 644
Minor trauma, 612–613
Mitral area, 256f, 256
Mixed acid-base balance disorders, 477t,
        477, 479–480, 482–483
Mixed venous blood gases, 173f, 173t, 598
Mixed venous oxygen saturation, 171,
        172–173, 173f
M-mode (motion-mode) echocardiography,
        269
Moderate burns, 644
Monoclonal antibodies, 451–452, 529, 530f,
        608
Monocytes, 511f, 512
Monokines, 512
Morphine, 100, 625
MOSF (multiple organ systems failure)
    circulatory effects of, 599–600
    detection of, early, 598
    ethical issues in, 609
    gerontology and, 599
    hematologic effects of, 601–609, 604f,
        605f
    metabolic effects of, 600–601
    nursing diagnosis for, 600
    oxygen used in, 598–599
    pathophysiology, 598–599
    prevention of, 598
    prognosis, 609
    pulmonary effects of, 600
    renal effects of, 609
    shock therapy and, 608
    in trauma planning and caring, 624
Mothers Against Drunk Driving, 613
Motion-mode (M-mode) echocardiography,
        269

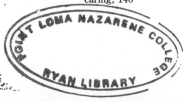